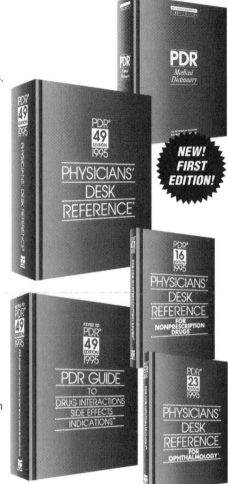

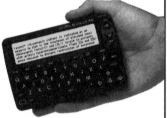
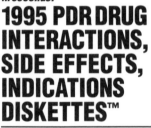

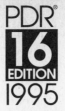

PDR 16 EDITION 1995

PHYSICIANS' DESK REFERENCE

FOR NONPRESCRIPTION DRUGS®

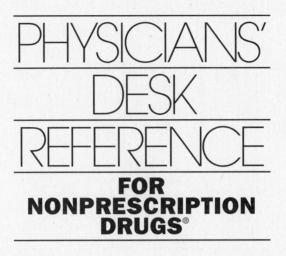

Medical Consultant
Ronald Arky, MD, Charles S. Davidson Professor of Medicine and Master, Francis Weld Peabody Society, Harvard Medical School

President and Chief Operating Officer, Drug Information Services Group: William J. Gole

Senior Vice President and General Manager: Thomas F. Rice
Product Manager: Stephen B. Greenberg
Associate Product Manager: Cy S. Caine
Sales Manager: James R. Pantaleo
Senior Account Manager: Michael S. Sarajian
Account Managers
Dikran N. Barsamian
Donald V. Bruccoleri
Lawrence C. Keary
Jeffrey M. Keller
P. Anthony Pinsonault
Anthony Sorce
Commercial Sales Manager: Robin B. Bartlett
Direct Marketing Manager: Robert W. Chapman
Vice President of Production: Steven R. Andreazza

Manager, Professional Data: Mukesh Mehta, RPh
Manager, Database Administration: Lynne Handler
Contracts and Special Services Director: Marjorie A. Duffy
Director of Production: Carrie Williams
Production Managers: Kimberly Hiller-Vivas, Tara L. Walsh
Format Editor: Gregory J. Westley
Index Editor: Jeffrey Schaefer
Art Associate: Joan K. Akerlind
Director of Corporate Communications: Gregory J. Thomas
Digital Photography: Shawn W. Cahill
Digital Prepress Processing: Joanne M. Pearson, Kevin J. Leckner
Editor, Special Projects: David W. Sifton

Officers of Medical Economics: President and Chief Executive Officer: Norman R. Snesil; Executive Vice President and Chief Financial Officer: J. Crispin Ashworth; Senior Vice President of Corporate Operations Group: John R. Ware; Senior Vice President of Corporate Business Development: Raymond M. Zoeller; Vice President of Information Services and Chief Information Officer: Edward J. Zecchini

ISBN: 1-56363-089-3

FOREWORD

Welcome to the sixteenth edition of *Physicians' Desk Reference For Nonprescription Drugs*. This companion volume to the main edition of *PDR* provides detailed information on nearly 700 over-the-counter remedies, as well as a number of home diagnostic tests and other medical aids for consumers.

This edition offers you an important new feature: an in-depth analysis of the changing role of over-the-counter drugs. The growing self-care movement among consumers, increasing cost pressures throughout the health care system, and the expanding number of Rx-to-OTC conversions have all conspired to make nonprescription drugs an ever more significant factor in the health care equation. This up-to-the-minute analysis, which can be found in Section 5, spells out the changes and examines their impact on medical therapy.

As the role of over-the-counter drugs continues to expand, we feel certain that you'll find *PDR For Nonprescription Drugs* to be an increasingly important part of your working reference library. In conjunction with *Physicians' Desk Reference* and *PDR* for *Ophthalmology*, it supplies you with America's most authoritative, comprehensive, and reliable database of product-specific drug information. In turn, this core database is fully indexed in the 1,500 page *PDR Guide to Drug Interactions • Side Effects • Indications™*. An invaluable addition to the *PDR* library of drug references, the *PDR Guide* permits fast, easy identification of an adverse reaction's probable source — and the approved alternatives for the problem medication.

Data from these printed references is also available in a variety of electronic formats:

- *Pocket PDR™* — A handheld personal database of key sections from the prescription-drug listings in PDR.

- *PDR Library* on *CD-ROM™* — Complete prescribing information from all PDR volumes — with the full contents of *The Merck Manual* and *Stedman's Medical Dictionary* as optional enhancements — all on one convenient disc for use on PC networks and individual PC's.

- *PDR Drug Interactions/Side Effects/Indications Diskettes™* — A powerful screening program for patient regimens of up to 20 drugs.

- *PDR Tape Services* — A preformatted text file suitable for integration in large mainframe-based information systems.

In the current cost-conscious health care environment, you should also be aware of the newest volume in the PDR family of references. Entitled *PDR Generics™*, this exhaustive pharmaceutical compendium includes generic monographs covering virtually all prescription drugs--plus brand/generic unit cost comparisons, average generic prices by package size for all therapeutically equivalent products, and average wholesale prices of all available supplies. Drugs in this volume are indexed by brand and generic name, therapeutic category, and indication. Off-label indications are included.

Also new and noteworthy is the *PDR® Medical Dictionary*, an authoritative reference that combines a complete medical lexicon with *PDR's* unparalleled database of brand and generic drug names.

For more information on any of these important references, please call, toll-free, 1-800-232-7379 or fax 201-573-4956.

PDR For Nonprescription Drugs is published annually by Medical Economics in cooperation with participating manufacturers. The function of the publisher is the compilation, organization, and distribution of product information obtained from manufacturers. Each product description has been prepared by the manufacturer, and edited and approved by the manufacturer's medical department, medical director, and/or medical consultant. During compilation of this information, the publisher has emphasized the necessity of describing products comprehensively, in order to provide all the facts necessary for sound and intelligent decision making. The descriptions seen here include all information made available by the manufacturer.

In organizing and presenting this material in *Physicians' Desk Reference For Nonprescription Drugs*, the publisher does not warrant or guarantee any of the products described, or perform any independent analysis in connection with any of the product information contained herein. *Physicians' Desk Reference For Nonprescription Drugs* does not assume, and expressly disclaims, any obligation to obtain and include any information other than that provided to it by the manufacturer. It should be understood that by making this material available the publisher is not advocating the use of any product described herein, nor is the publisher responsible for misuse of a product due to typographical error. Additional information on any product may be obtained from the manufacturer.

MEDICAL ECONOMICS

CONTENTS

MEDICAL ECONOMICS

SECTION 1

MANUFACTURERS' INDEX

Listed in this index are all manufacturers that have supplied information in this edition. Each company's entry includes the address, phone, and fax number of its headquarters and regional offices, as well as contacts for inquiries, orders, and emergency information. A list of the company's major over-the-counter products is also included.

The ◆ symbol marks drugs shown in the Product Identification Guide. If a company has two page numbers, the first refers to its photographs in the "Product Identification Guide," the second to its prescribing information.

**B. F. ASCHER & 503, 602
COMPANY, INC.**
15501 West 109th Street
Lenexa, KS 66219
Mailing Address:
P.O. Box 717
Shawnee Mission, KS 66201-0717
Address Inquiries to:
Joan F. Bowen: (913) 888-1880

OTC Products Available:
◆ Ayr Saline Nasal Drops
◆ Ayr Saline Nasal Mist
◆ Cough-X Lozenges
◆ Itch-X Gel
◆ Itch-X Spray
◆ Mobigesic Tablets
◆ Mobisyl Analgesic Creme
◆ Pen●Kera Creme
◆ Pretty Feet and Hands Sloughing Cream

ASTRA USA, INC. 503, 603
50 Otis Street
Westboro, MA 01581-4500
Address Inquiries to:
Professional Information Department:
(508) 366-1100
FAX (508) 366-7406
For Medical Emergencies Contact:
Medical Information Services
(800) 225-6333

OTC Products Available:
◆ Xylocaine Ointment 2.5%

AYERST LABORATORIES
Division of American Home Products
Corporation
685 Third Avenue
New York, NY 10017-4071

For information for Ayerst's consumer products, see product listings under Whitehall Laboratories.
Please turn to WHITEHALL LABORATORIES

**BAKER CUMMINS 503, 604
DERMATOLOGICALS, INC.**
8800 NW 36th Street
Miami, FL 33178
Address Inquiries to:
(305) 770-5202
FAX: (305) 770-5400
For Medical Emergencies Contact:
Medical Department: (305) 590-2254
(800) 842-6704
FAX: (305) 770-5400

OTC Products Available:
Acno Cleanser
Acno Lotion
Acticort Lotion 100
◆ Aquaderm Cream
◆ Aquaderm Lotion
◆ Aquaderm Sunscreen/Moisturizer SPF 15
Baker's Biopsy Punch (sizes 2, 3, 3.5, 4,
    5 and 6 mm)
Baker's DTM
P&S HC Gel
P&S HC Liquid
◆ P&S Liquid
P&S Plus Tar Gel
◆ P&S Shampoo
Panscol Medicated Lotion
Panscol Medicated Ointment
Phacid Shampoo
Ultra Derm Bath Oil
Ultra Derm Lotion
◆ Ultra Derm Moisturizer
◆ Ultra Mide 25 Extra Strength Moisturizer
Ultra Mide 25 Lotion
◆ X-Seb Shampoo

◆ X-Seb Plus Antidandruff Conditioning
    Shampoo
◆ X-Seb T Pearl Shampoo
◆ X-Seb T Plus Conditioning Shampoo

**BAUSCH & LOMB 503, 606
INCORPORATED**
Personal Products Division
1400 North Goodman Street
P.O. Box 450
Rochester, NY 14692-0450
OTC Products Available:
◆ Curel Lotion and Cream

**BAYER CORPORATION
CONSUMER CARE DIVISION**
(See MILES INC., CONSUMER CARE
DIVISION)

BEACH PHARMACEUTICALS. 607
Division of Beach Products, Inc.
Executive Office:
5220 South Manhattan Avenue
Tampa, FL 33611
(813) 839-6565
Manufacturing and Distribution:
Main Street at Perimeter Road
Conestee, SC 29605
Toll Free: (800) 845-8210
Address Inquiries to:
Victor De Oreo, R Ph, V.P., Sales:
(803) 277-7282
Richard Stephen Jenkins, Exec. V.P.:
(813) 839-6565

OTC Products Available:
Beelith Tablets

(◆) Shown in Product Identification Guide

BEIERSDORF INC. 503, 607
360 Dr. Martin Luther King Dr.
Norwalk, CT 06856-5529
Address Inquiries to:
Medical Division:
(203) 853-8008
FAX: (203) 854-8180

OTC Products Available:
◆ Aquaphor Healing Ointment
◆ Aquaphor Healing Ointment, Original
  Formula
Basis Facial Cleanser (Normal to Dry Skin)
Basis Intensive Hydrating Oil
Basis Multi Protective Balm
Basis Over Night Recovery Creme
Basis Soap-Combination Skin
Basis Soap-Extra Dry Skin
Basis Soap-Normal to Dry Skin
Basis Soap-Sensitive Skin
◆ Eucerin Cleansing Bar
◆ Eucerin Original Moisturizing Creme
◆ Eucerin Facial Moisturizing Lotion SPF 25
◆ Eucerin Original Moisturizing Lotion
◆ Eucerin Plus Alphahydroxy Moisturizing
  Lotion
◆ Eucerin Plus Alphahydroxy Moisturizing
  Creme
Nivea Bath Silk Bath Oil
Nivea Bath Silk Bath & Shower Gel
  (Extra-Dry Skin)
Nivea Bath Silk Bath & Shower Gel
  (Normal-to-Dry Skin)
Nivea Moisturizing Creme
Nivea Moisturizing Lotion (Extra Enriched)
Nivea Moisturizing Lotion (Original
  Formula)
Nivea Moisturizing Oil
Nivea Skin Oil
Nivea Sun After Sun Lotion
Nivea Sun SPF 15
Nivea Visage Facial Nourishing Creme
Nivea Visage Facial Nourishing Lotion

BLAINE COMPANY, INC. 608
1465 Jamike Lane
Erlanger, KY 41018
Address Inquiries to:
Mr. Alex M. Blaine: (606) 283-9437
FAX: (606) 283-9460

OTC Products Available:
Mag-Ox 400
Uro-Mag

BLAIREX LABORATORIES, INC. ... 609
4810 Tecumseh Lane
P.O. Box 15190
Evansville, IN 47716-0190
Address Inquiries to:
Bruce Faulkenberg, R.Ph.:
(800) 252-4739
FAX: (812) 474-6764
For Medical Emergency Contact:
Bruce Faulkenberg, R.Ph.:
(800) 252-4739
FAX: (812) 474-6764

OTC Products Available:
Broncho Saline
Nasal Moist

BLOCK DRUG COMPANY, INC. 609
257 Cornelison Avenue
Jersey City, NJ 07302
Address Inquiries to:
Steve Gattanella: (201) 434-3000
For Medical Emergencies Contact:
James Gingold: (201) 434-3000

OTC Products Available:
Arthritis Strength BC Powder

BC Cold Powder Multi-Symptom Formula
  (Cold-Sinus-Allergy)
BC Cold Powder Non-Drowsy Formula
  (Cold-Sinus)
BC Powder
Balmex Ointment
Maximum Strength Nytol Caplets
Nytol QuickCaps Caplets
Promise Sensitive Toothpaste
Cool Gel Sensodyne
Fresh Mint Sensodyne Toothpaste
Original Formula Sensodyne-SC
  Toothpaste
Sensodyne with Baking Soda
Tegrin Dandruff Shampoo
Tegrin Skin Cream & Tegrin Medicated
  Soap

BOCK PHARMACAL 504, 612
COMPANY
P.O. Box 419056
St. Louis, MO 63141-9056
Address Inquiries to:
(314) 579-0770

OTC Products Available:
◆ Emetrol

BOIRON, THE WORLD 504, 612
LEADER IN HOMEOPATHY
Headquarters and East Coast Branch
6 Campus Blvd., Building A
Newtown Square, PA 19073
Address Inquiries to:
John Durkin Demonceaux
East Coast Manager
(800) 258-8823
For Medical Emergencies Contact:
Mark Land
Technical Services Department:
(800) 258-8823
West Coast Branch
98C West Cochran Street
Simi Valley, CA 93065
(805) 582-9091
Address Inquiries to:
Ambroise Demonceaux
West Coast Manager

OTC Products Available:
Arnica & Calendula Gel
Chestal, the homeopathic cough syrup
  remedy
Coldcalm, the homeopathic cold remedy
Cyclease, the homeopathic cramp
  remedy
Hayfever, the homeopathic pollen-allergy
  remedy
Homeodent Anise and Lemon toothpaste
Natural Phases, the homeopathic PMS
  remedy
Nervousness, the homeopathic stress
  remedy
◆ Oscillococcinum
Quiétude the homeopathic insomnia
  remedy
Sinusitis, the homeopathic sinus remedy
Sportenine, the homeopathic sports
  remedy
Yeastaway, the homeopathic yeast
  remedy

BRISTOL-MYERS 504, 613
PRODUCTS
A Bristol-Myers Squibb Company
345 Park Avenue
New York, NY 10154
Address Inquiries to:
Bristol-Myers Products Division
Consumer Affairs Department
1350 Liberty Avenue
Hillside, NJ 07207
In Emergencies Call: (800) 468-7746

OTC Products Available:
Alpha Keri Moisture Rich Body Oil
Alpha Keri Moisture Rich Cleansing Bar
Alpha Keri Moisturizing Spray Mist
Alpha Keri Shower & Bath Gelee
Ammens Medicated Powder
Backache Caplets
BAN Antiperspirant Deodorant Cream
BAN Basic Non-Aerosol Antiperspirant
  Spray
BAN Roll-On Antiperspirant Deodorant
BAN Solid Antiperspirant Deodorant
◆ Bufferin Analgesic Tablets and Caplets
◆ Arthritis Strength Bufferin Analgesic
  Caplets
◆ Extra Strength Bufferin Analgesic Tablets
◆ Comtrex Multi-Symptom Cold Reliever
  Tablets/Caplets/Liqui-Gels/Liquid
◆ Allergy-Sinus Comtrex Multi-Symptom
  Allergy-Sinus Formula Tablets
Comtrex Multi-Symptomn Day/Night
  Caplet-Tablet
◆ Comtrex Multi-Symptom Non-Drowsy
  Caplets
◆ Comtrex Multi-Symptom Non-Drowsy
  Liqui-gels
Aspirin Free Excedrin Analgesic Caplets
Aspirin Free Excedrin Dual Caplets
◆ Excedrin Extra-Strength Analgesic Tablets
  & Caplets
◆ Excedrin P.M. Analgesic/Sleeping Aid
  Tablets, Caplets, Liquigels
Sinus Excedrin Analgesic, Decongestant
  Tablets & Caplets
◆ 4-Way Fast Acting Nasal Spray (regular &
  mentholated)
◆ 4-Way Long Lasting Nasal Spray
Fisherman's Friend Lozenges
Fostex 10% Benzoyl Peroxide Bar
Fostex 10% Benzoyl Peroxide (Vanish) Gel
Fostex 10% Benzoyl Peroxide Wash
Fostex Medicated Cleansing Bar
Fostex Medicated Cleansing Cream
KeriCort-10 Cream
Keri Facial Soap
◆ Keri Lotion - Original Formula
◆ Keri Lotion - Silky Smooth
◆ Keri Lotion - Sensitive Skin
Minit-Rub Analgesic Ointment
Mum Antiperspirant Cream Deodorant
Chewable NODOZ Tablets
No Doz Maximum Strength Caplets
Backache Caplets from Nuprin Analgesic
◆ Nuprin Ibuprofen/Analgesic Tablets &
  Caplets
Pazo Hemorrhoid Ointment &
  Suppositories
PreSun Active 15 and 30 Clear Gel
  Sunscreens
PreSun for Kids Lotion
PreSun 23 and PreSun For Kids, Spray
  Mist Sunscreens
PreSun 15 Moisturizing Sunscreen with
  Keri
PreSun 25 Moisturizing Sunscreen with
  Keri Moisturizer
PreSun 15 and 29 Sensitive Skin
  Sunscreens
PreSun 46 Moisturizing Sunscreen
◆ Theragran Antioxidant
Theragran Liquid
Theragran Stress Formula
◆ Theragran Tablets
◆ Theragran-M Tablets with Beta Carotene
◆ Therapeutic Mineral Ice, Pain Relieving
  Gel
Therapeutic Mineral Ice Exercise Formula,
  Pain Relieving Gel

W.K. BUCKLEY INC.......... 505, 624
P.O. Box 5022
Westport, CT 06880

(◆) Shown in Product Identification Guide

Address Inquiries to:
Customer Service Office:
(203) 454-5966
FAX: (203) 454-8625
For Medical Emergencies Contact:
Customer Service Office
(203) 454-5966
FAX: (203) 454-8625

OTC Products Available:
◆ Buckley's Mixture

BURROUGHS WELLCOME CO.
(See WARNER WELLCOME)

CAMPBELL LABORATORIES ..... 624 INC.
Address Inquiries to:
Richard C. Zahn, President
P.O. Box 812, FDR Station
New York, NY 10150-0812
(212) 688-7684

OTC Products Available:
Herpecin-L Cold Sore Lip Balm

CARE-TECH LABORATORIES...... 624
3224 South Kingshighway Boulevard
St. Louis, MO 63139
Address Inquiries to:
Sherry L. Brereton: (314) 772-4610
FAX: (314) 772-4613
For Medical Emergencies Contact:
Customer Service: (800) 325-9681
FAX: (314) 772-4613

OTC Products Available:
Barri-Care Antimicrobial Barrier Ointment
CC-500 Antibacterial Skin Cleanser for Dialysis Patient Care
Care Creme Antimicrobial Cream
Clinical Care Dermal Wound Cleanser
Concept Antimicrobial Skin Cleanser
Formula Magic Antibacterial Powder
Just Lotion - Highly Absorbent Aloe Vera Glycerine Based Skin Lotion
Loving Lather II Antibacterial Skin Cleanser
Loving Lotion Antibacterial Skin & Body Lotion
Orchid Fresh II Perineal/Ostomy Cleanser
Satin Antimicrobial Skin Cleanser for Diabetic/Cancer Patient Care
Skin Magic - Antimicrobial Body Rub & Emollient
Soft Skin Non-greasy Bath Oil with Rich Emollients for Severely Damaged Dermal Tissue
Swirlsoft Whirlpool Emollient for Dry Skin Conditions
Tech 2000 Antimicrobial Oral Rinse (No Alcohol, No Sodium)
Techni-Care Surgical Scrub and Wound Cleanser
Velvet Fresh Non-irritating Cornstarch Baby Powder

J. R. CARLSON .... 626 LABORATORIES, INC.
15 College Drive
Arlington Heights, IL 60004-1985
Address inquiries to:
David Lin　　　　　　　　(708) 255-1600
　　　　　　　FAX (708) 255-1605
For Medical Emergency Contact:
Customer Service　　　　(708) 255-1600
　　　　　　　FAX (708) 255-1605
OTC Products Available
ACES Antioxidant Soft Gels
E-Gems Soft Gels

CARTILAGE .... 505, 626 TECHNOLOGIES, INC
200 Clearbrook Road
Elmsford, NY 10523
Phone: (914) 592-7111
Fax: (914) 592-7166
OTC Products Available:
◆ Cartilade Shark Cartilage Capsules, Powder, and Caplets

CHESEBROUGH-POND'S USA .... 626 CO.
33 Benedict Place
Greenwich, CT 06830
Address Inquiries to:
Consumer Affairs: (800) 243-5804
For Medical Emergencies Contact:
(800) 243-5804

OTC Products Available:
Dermasil Dry Skin Concentrated Treatment
Dermasil Dry Skin Treatment Cream
Dermasil Dry Skin Treatment Lotion
Vaseline Intensive Care Lotion Extra Strength
Vaseline Petroleum Jelly Cream
Vaseline Pure Petroleum Jelly Skin Protectant

CHURCH & DWIGHT CO., INC. 627
469 North Harrison Street
Princeton, NJ 08543
Address Inquiries to:
Cathy Marino (609) 683-7015
For Medical Emergencies Contact:
HIS (800) 228-5635
Extension 7

OTC Products Available:
Arm & Hammer Pure Baking Soda

CIBA CONSUMER .... 505, 627 PHARMACEUTICALS
Division of CIBA-GEIGY Corporation
581 Main Street
Woodbridge, NJ 07095
Address Inquiries to:
Nancy Casper:
(908) 602-6000
FAX: (908) 602-6612
For Medical Emergencies Contact:
(908) 277-5000

OTC Products Available:
◆ Acutrim 16 Hour Steady Control Appetite Suppressant
◆ Acutrim Late Day Strength Appetite Suppressant
◆ Acutrim Maximum Strength Appetite Suppressant
Allerest Children's Chewable Tablets
Allerest Eye Drops
Allerest Headache Strength Tablets
Allerest Maximum Strength Tablets
Allerest No Drowsiness Tablets
Allerest Sinus Pain Formula
Allerest 12 Hour Caplets
Allerest 12 Hour Nasal Spray
◆ Americaine Hemorrhoidal Ointment
◆ Americaine Topical Anesthetic First Aid Ointment
◆ Americaine Topical Anesthetic Spray
◆ Arthritis Pain Ascriptin
◆ Maximum Strength Ascriptin
◆ Regular Strength Ascriptin Tablets
Bacid Capsules
◆ Caldecort Anti-Itch Hydrocortisone Cream
◆ Caldecort Anti-Itch Hydrocortisone Spray
◆ Caldecort Light Cream
◆ Caldesene Medicated Ointment
◆ Caldesene Medicated Powder

◆ Cruex Antifungal Cream
◆ Cruex Antifungal Powder
◆ Cruex Antifungal Spray Powder
◆ Desenex Antifungal Cream
◆ Desenex Antifungal Ointment
◆ Desenex Antifungal Powder
◆ Desenex Antifungal Spray Liquid
◆ Desenex Antifungal Spray Powder
Desenex Foot & Sneaker Deodorant Powder Plus
◆ Desenex Foot & Sneaker Deodorant Spray
Desenex Soap
◆ Prescription Strength Desenex Cream
◆ Prescription Strength Desenex Spray Powder and Spray Liquid
◆ Doan's Extra-Strength Analgesic
◆ Extra Strength Doan's P.M.
◆ Doan's Regular Strength Analgesic
◆ Dulcolax Suppositories
◆ Dulcolax Tablets
◆ Efidac/24
◆ Eucalyptamint Arthritis Pain Reliever (External Analgesic)
◆ Eucalyptamint Muscle Pain Relief Formula
◆ Fiberall Chewable Tablets, Lemon Creme Flavor
◆ Fiberall Fiber Wafers - Fruit & Nut
◆ Fiberall Fiber Wafers - Oatmeal Raisin
◆ Fiberall Powder, Natural Flavor
◆ Fiberall Powder, Orange Flavor
◆ Isoclor Timesule Capsules
◆ Kondremul
◆ Maalox Antacid Caplets
◆ Maalox Anti-Diarrheal Caplets
◆ Maalox Anti-Diarrheal Oral Solution
◆ Maalox Anti-Gas Tablets, Regular Strength
◆ Maalox Anti-Gas Tablets, Extra Strength
◆ Maalox Daily Fiber Therapy
Maalox Heartburn Relief Suspension
Maalox Heartburn Relief Tablets
◆ Maalox Magnesia and Alumina Oral Suspension
◆ Maalox Plus Tablets
◆ Extra Strength Maalox Antacid Plus Antigas Liquid and Tablets
◆ Myoflex External Analgesic Creme
◆ Nōstril 1/4% Mild Nasal Decongestant
◆ Nōstril 1/2% Regular Nasal Decongestant
Nōstrilla Long Acting Nasal Decongestant
◆ Nupercainal Hemorrhoidal and Anesthetic Ointment
◆ Nupercainal Hydrocortisone 1% Cream
◆ Nupercainal Pain Relief Cream
◆ Nupercainal Suppositories
◆ Otrivin Nasal Drops
◆ Otrivin Pediatric Nasal Drops
◆ Perdiem Fiber
◆ Perdiem
◆ Privine Nasal Solution and Drops
Privine Nasal Spray
Sinarest Tablets
Sinarest Extra Strength Tablets
Sinarest No Drowsiness Tablets
Sinarest 12 Hour Nasal Spray
◆ Slow Fe Tablets
◆ Slow Fe with Folic Acid
◆ Sunkist Children's Chewable Multivitamins - Complete
◆ Sunkist Children's Chewable Multivitamins - Plus Extra C
◆ Sunkist Children's Chewable Multivitamins - Plus Iron
◆ Sunkist Children's Chewable Multivitamins - Regular
◆ Sunkist Vitamin C - Chewable
◆ Sunkist Vitamin C - Easy to Swallow
◆ Ting Antifungal Cream
◆ Ting Antifungal Powder
◆ Ting Antifungal Spray Liquid
◆ Ting Antifungal Spray Powder
Vitron-C Tablets

(◆) Shown in Product Identification Guide

COLUMBIA **508, 650**
LABORATORIES, INC.
2665 South Bayshore Drive
Miami, FL 33133
Address Inquiries to:
Professional Services Department
For Medical Emergencies Contact:
(305) 964-6666

OTC Products Available:
◆ Diasorb Liquid
◆ Diasorb Tablets
◆ Legatrin PM
    Vaporizer in a Bottle Nasal Decongestant

DEL PHARMACEUTICALS, .. **508, 651**
INC.
A Subsidiary of Del Laboratories, Inc.
163 East Bethpage Road
Plainview, NY 11803
Address Inquiries to:
Peter Liman, V.P. Marketing:
(516) 293-7070
FAX: (516) 293-9018
For Medical Emergencies Contact:
Allen Williams
(516) 293-7070, Ext. 3275

OTC Products Available:
◆ ArthriCare Odor Free Rub
◆ ArthriCare Triple Medicated Rub
    Auro-Dri Ear Water-Drying Aid
    Auro Ear Wax Removal Aid
    Boil-Ease Pain Relieving Ointment
    Dermarest DriCort Anti-Itch Creme
    Dermarest Plus Gel
    Detane Desensitizing Lubricant
    Diaper Guard Skin Rash Ointment
    Exocaine Analgesic Rubs
    Off-Ezy Corn Remover
    Off-Ezy Wart Remover
    Baby Orajel Nighttime Formula
◆ Baby Orajel Teething Pain Medicine
◆ Baby Orajel Tooth & Gum Cleanser
    Orajel Denture Pain Medicine
◆ Orajel Maximum Strength Toothache
        Medication
◆ Orajel Mouth-Aid for Canker and Cold
        Sores
◆ Orajel Perioseptic Oxygenating Liquid
◆ Pronto Lice Killing Shampoo &
        Conditioner in One Kit
◆ Pronto Lice Killing Spray
    Propa pH Acne Medications
    Skin Shield Liquid Bandage
    Stye Ophthalmic Ointment
◆ Tanac Medicated Gel
◆ Tanac No Sting Liquid
    TripTone for Motion Sickness

EFFCON **508, 654**
LABORATORIES, INC.
P.O. Box 7509
Marietta, GA 30065-1509
Address Inquiries to:
Leigh Ann Buice: (800) 722-2428
FAX: (404) 499-0058
For Medical Emergency Contact:
Ed R. Burklow: (800) 722-2428
FAX: (404) 499-0058

OTC Products Available:
◆ Pin-X Pinworm Treatment

FISONS CORPORATION **654**
PRESCRIPTION PRODUCTS
755 Jefferson Road
Rochester, NY 14623
Mailing Address:
P.O. Box 1766
Rochester, NY 14603
Address Inquiries to:
Professional Services Department

P.O. Box 1766
Rochester, NY 14603
(716) 475-9000

OTC Products Available:
Delsym Extended-Release Suspension

FLEMING & COMPANY **654**
1600 Fenpark Dr.
Fenton, MO 63026
Address Inquiries to:
John J. Roth, M.D.: (314) 343-8200
For Medical Emergencies Contact:
John R. Roth, M.D.: (314) 343-8200

OTC Products Available:
Chlor-3 Condiment
Impregon Concentrate
Magonate Tablets and Liquid
Marblen Suspension Peach/Apricot
Marblen Tablets
Nephrox Suspension
Nicotinex Elixir
Ocean Nasal Mist
Purge Concentrate

FLEMMING **655**
PHARMACEUTICALS, INC.
Eleven Greenway Plaza, Suite 1115
Houston, TX 77046
Address inquiries to:
Consumer Affairs Department
                    (713) 621-1985
                FAX (713) 621-6726
For Medical Emergency Contact:
Dr. Miguel L. Gallegos
                    (713) 621-1985
                FAX (713) 621-6726
Branch Office:
1310 Ranch Road 620 South, Suite A-8
Austin, TX 78734
                    (512) 263-3585
                FAX (512) 263-3588
OTC Products Available
Capsin Topical Analgesic Lotion 0.025%
    and 0.075%.

GEBAUER COMPANY **508, 656**
9410 St. Catherine Avenue
Cleveland, OH 44104
Address Inquiries to:
(800) 321-9348
FAX: (216) 271-5335
For Medical Emergencies Contact:
(800) 321-9348
FAX: (216) 271-5335

OTC Products Available:
Dr. Caldwell Senna Laxative
◆ Salivart Saliva Substitute

GLENBROOK LABORATORIES
(See MILES INC)

A. C. GRACE COMPANY **656**
1100 Quitman Rd., P.O. Box 570
Big Sandy, TX 75755
Address Inquiries To:
Roy Erickson   (903) 636-4368
                    FAX (903) 636-4051
For Medical Emergencies Contact:
Roy Erickson   (903) 636-4368
                    FAX (903) 636-4051

OTC Products Available:
Unique E Vitamin E Capsules

HOGIL **508, 656**
PHARMACEUTICAL CORP.
One Byram Brook Place
Armonk, NY 10504

Address Inquiries To:
Tanya Castagna
(914) 273-9666
Fax (914) 273-9743
For Medical Emergencies Contact:
Dr. Gilbert Spector
(914) 273-9666
Fax (914) 273-9743

OTC Products Available:
◆ A-200 Lice Control Spray
    A-200 Lice Treatment Kit
◆ A-200 Lice Killing Shampoo
◆ InnoGel Plus
    Innomed Lice Treatment Kit
    Psor-A-Set Liquid, Shampoo, & Soap

IMMUNOSTICS, INC. **508, 657**
3505 Sunset Avenue
Ocean, NJ 07712

OTC Products Available:
◆ Hema-Screen
    Immuno HCG Detector

INTER-CAL CORPORATION **658**
533 Madison Avenue
Prescott, AZ 86301
Address Inquiries to:
Nancy J. Chandler: (520) 445-8063

OTC Products Available:
Ester-C Mineral Ascorbates Powder

JAMOL LABORATORIES INC.. ...... **658**
13 Ackerman Avenue
Emerson, NJ 07630

OTC Products Available:
Ponaris Nasal Mucosal Emollient

JOHNSON & JOHNSON **508, 658**
CONSUMER PRODUCTS,
INC.
Grandview Road
Skillman, NJ 08558
Address Inquiries: to:
Customer Information Services:
(800) 526-3967
For Medical Emergency Contact:
Customer Information Services:
(800) 526-3967

OTC Products Available:
    Clean & Clear Deep Action Cream
        Cleanser
    Clean & Clear Foaming Facial Cleanser
    Clean & Clear Invisible Blemish Treatment
        Maximum Strength and Sensitive Skin
    Clean & Clear Oil Controlling Astringent
        Regular and Sensitive Skin
    Clean & Clear Skin Balancing Moisturizer
        Regular and Sensitive Skin
◆ K-Y Jelly Personal Lubricant
◆ K-Y Plus Vaginal Contraceptive and
        Personal Lubricant
    Purpose Dual Treatment
        Mositurizer-Fragrance Free, SPF15
    Purpose Gentle Cleansing Bar
    Purpose Gentle Cleansing Wash

JOHNSON & JOHNSON • **508, 659**
MERCK CONSUMER
PHARMACEUTICALS CO.
Camp Hill Road
Fort Washington, PA 19034
Address Inquiries to:
Consumer Affairs Department:
(215) 233-7000
For Medical Emergencies Contact:
(215) 233-7000

OTC Products Available:
◆ ALternaGEL Liquid
◆ Dialose Tablets
◆ Dialose Plus Tablets

(◆) Shown in Product Identification Guide

- ◆ Mylanta Gas Relief Tablets
- ◆ Maximum Strength Mylanta Gas Relief Tablets
- ◆ Mylanta Gelcaps Antacid
- ◆ Mylanta Liquid
- ◆ Mylanta Natural Fiber Supplement
- ◆ Mylanta Soothing Lozenges
- ◆ Mylanta Tablets
- ◆ Mylanta Double Strength Liquid
- ◆ Mylanta Double Strength Tablets
- ◆ Infants' Mylicon Drops
- ◆ The Stuart Formula Tablets

KONSYL PHARMACEUTICALS, ... 663 INC.

4200 South Hulen
Ft. Worth, TX 76109
Address Inquiries: to:
Bill Steiber: (817) 763-8011 Ext. 23
FAX: (817) 731-9389

OTC Products Available:
Konsyl Fiber Tablets
Konsyl Powder Sugar Free Unflavored
Konsyl-D Powder Unflavored
Konsyl-Orange Ultra Fine Powder

LAVOPTIK COMPANY, INC........ 665

661 Western Avenue North
St. Paul, MN 55103
Address Inquiries to:
661 Western Avenue North
St. Paul, MN 55103-1694
(612) 489-1351
For Medical Emergencies Contact:
B. C. Brainard: (612) 489-1351
FAX: (612) 489-0760

OTC Products Available:
Lavoptik Eye Cup
Lavoptik Eye Wash

LEDERLE CONSUMER ...... 509, 665 HEALTH

Division of American Cyanamid Co.
One Cyanamid Plaza
Wayne, NJ 07470
Address Inquiries to:
Consumer Affairs Department
(8:30 AM - 4:30 PM Eastern time):
(800)-282-8805
For Medical Emergencies Contact:
Consumer Affairs Department
(8:30 AM - 4:30 PM Eastern time):
(800)-282-8805
For After Hours Emergencies Contact:
(914) 732-5000
Distribution Centers:
ATLANTA
Contact EASTERN (Philadelphia)
Distribution Center

CHICAGO
Bulk Address:
1100 East Business Center Drive
Mt. Prospect, IL 60056
Mail Address:
P.O. Box 7614
Mt. Prospect, IL 60056-7614
(800) 533-3753
(708) 827-8871
DALLAS
Bulk Address:
7611 Carpenter Freeway
Dallas, TX 75247
Mail Address:
P.O. Box 655731
Dallas, TX 75265
(800) 533-3753
(214) 631-2130
WESTERN
Bulk Address:
16218 Arthur Street

Cerritos, CA 90701
Mail Address:
P.O. Box 6042
Artesia, CA 90702-6042
(800) 533-3753
(310) 802-1128
EASTERN (Philadelphia)
Bulk and Mail Address:
202 Precision Drive
P.O. Box 993
Horsham, PA 19044
(800) 533-3753
(215) 672-5400

OTC Products Available:
- ◆ Caltrate 600
- ◆ Caltrate PLUS
- ◆ Caltrate 600 + D
- ◆ Centrum
- ◆ Centrum, Jr. (Children's Chewable) + Extra C
- ◆ Centrum, Jr. (Children's Chewable) + Extra Calcium
- ◆ Centrum, Jr. (Children's Chewable) + Iron
- ◆ Centrum Liquid
- ◆ Centrum Silver
- ◆ Centrum Singles Beta Carotene
- ◆ Centrum Singles Calcium
- ◆ Centrum Singles Vitamin C
- ◆ Centrum Singles Vitamin E
- ◆ Ferro-Sequels
- ◆ FiberCon Caplets
- Gevrabon Liquid
- ◆ Protegra Antioxidant Vitamin & Mineral Supplement
- ◆ Stresstabs
- ◆ Stresstabs + Iron
- ◆ Stresstabs + Zinc
- ◆ Zincon Dandruff Shampoo

LEVER BROTHERS.......... 511, 672

390 Park Avenue
New York, NY 10022
Address Inquiries to:
(212) 688-6000

OTC Products Available:
- ◆ Dove Bar
- ◆ Liquid Dove Beauty Wash
- ◆ Lever 2000
- ◆ Liquid Lever 2000
- ◆ Unscented Lever 2000

3M PERSONAL HEALTH .... 511, 672 CARE

Bldg. 515-3N-02
St. Paul, MN 55144-1000
Address Inquiries to:
Customer Service   (800) 537-2191
Product Orders or Returns:
(800) 832-2189
For Medical Emergencies Contact:
(612) 733-2882 (answered 24 hrs.)

OTC Products Available:
- ◆ Titralac Antacid Regular
- ◆ Titralac Antacid Extra Strength
- ◆ Titralac Plus Liquid
- ◆ Titralac Plus Tablets

MARLYN NUTRACEUTICALS...... 673

14851 North Scottsdale Road
Scottsdale, AZ 85254 USA
(800) 462-7596
(602) 991-0200

Address Inquiries to:
Kelly Easton: (602) 991-0200
FAX: (602) 991-0551

OTC Products Available:
4-Hair
4-Nails
Hep-Forte Capsules
Marlyn Formula 50 Capsules
Marlyn PMS
Osteo Fem
Pro-Skin-E (Face Capsule)
Wobenzym N

McNEIL CONSUMER .... 511, 673 PRODUCTS CO.

Division of McNeil-PPC, Inc.
Camp Hill Road
Fort Washington, PA 19034
(215) 233-7000
Address Inquiries to:
Consumer Affairs Department
Fort Washington, PA 19034
Manufacturing Divisions:
Fort Washington, PA 19034

Southwest Manufacturing Plant
4001 N. I-35
Round Rock, TX 78664

Road 183 KM 19.8
Barrios Montones
Las Piedras, Puerto Rico 00771

OTC Products Available:
- ◆ Arthritis Foundation Aspirin Free Caplets
- ◆ Arthritis Foundation Ibuprofen Tablets
- ◆ Arthritis Foundation NightTime Caplets
- ◆ Arthritis Foundation Safety Coated Aspirin Tablets
- ◆ Imodium A-D Caplets and Liquid
- ◆ Lactaid Caplets
- ◆ Lactaid Drops
- ◆ PediaCare Cold Allergy Chewable Tablets
- ◆ PediaCare Cough-Cold Chewable Tablets and Liquid
- ◆ PediaCare Infants' Decongestant Drops
- ◆ PediaCare Night Rest Cough-Cold Liquid
- ◆ Sine-Aid IB Ibuprofen Strength Caplets
- ◆ Sine-Aid Maximum Strength Sinus Headache Gelcaps, Caplets and Tablets
- ◆ Children's TYLENOL acetaminophen Chewable Tablets, Elixir, Suspension Liquid
- ◆ Children's TYLENOL Cold Multi Symptom Chewable Tablets and Liquid
- ◆ Children's TYLENOL Cold Plus Cough Multi Symptom Tablets and Liquid
- ◆ Infant's TYLENOL acetaminophen Drops and Suspension Drops
- ◆ TYLENOL Extended Relief Caplets
- ◆ TYLENOL, Extra Strength, acetaminophen Adult Liquid Pain Reliever
- ◆ TYLENOL, Extra Strength, acetaminophen Gelcaps, Caplets, Tablets, Geltabs
- ◆ TYLENOL, Extra Strength, Heacache Plus Pain Reliever with Antacid Caplets
- ◆ TYLENOL, Junior Strength, acetaminophen Coated Caplets, and Chewable Tablets
- ◆ TYLENOL Maximum Strength Allergy Sinus Medication Gelcaps and Caplets
- ◆ TYLENOL Maximum Strength Allergy Sinus NightTime Medication Caplets
- ◆ TYLENOL Maximum Strength Flu Gelcaps
- ◆ TYLENOL Maximum Strength Flu NightTime Gelcaps
- ◆ TYLENOL Maximum Strength Flu NightTime Hot Medication Packets
- ◆ TYLENOL, Maximum Strength, Sinus Medication Geltabs, Gelcaps, Caplets and Tablets
- ◆ TYLENOL Multi-Symptom Cold Medication Caplets and Tablets
- ◆ TYLENOL Multi-Symptom Cold Medication No Drowsiness Formula Caplets and Gelcaps

(◆) Shown in Product Identification Guide

McNEIL CONSUMER PRODUCTS CO.
—cont.
- ◆ TYLENOL Cold Multi-Symptom Hot Medication Liquid Packets
- ◆ TYLENOL Multi-Symptom Cough Medication
- ◆ TYLENOL Multi-Symptom Cough Medication with Decongestant
- ◆ TYLENOL, Regular Strength, acetaminophen Caplets and Tablets
- ◆ TYLENOL PM Extra Strength Pain Reliever/Sleep Aid Gelcaps, Caplets, Geltabs
- ◆ TYLENOL Severe Allergy Medication Caplets

MEAD JOHNSON 700
NUTRITIONALS
Mead Johnson & Company
A Bristol-Myers Squibb Company
2400 W. Lloyd Expressway
Evansville, IN 47721
(812) 429-5000
Address Inquiries to:
Scientific Information Section
Medical Department

OTC Products Available:
Enfamil Human Milk Fortifier
Enfamil Infant Formula
Enfamil With Iron Infant Formula
Enfamil Infant Formula Nursette
Enfamil Next Step Toddler Formula
Enfamil Premature Formula
Enfamil Premature Formula With Iron
Fer-In-Sol Iron Supplement Drops, Syrup, Capsules
Infalyle Oral Electrolyte Maintenance Solution made with Rice Syrup Solids
Lactofree Milk-Based, Lactose-Free Formula For Baby's 1st Year and Beyond
Lofenalac Iron Fortified Low Phenylalanine Diet Powder
Metabolic Modules, Special
  HIST 1
  HIST 2
  HOM 1
  HOM 2
  LYS 1
  LYS 2
  MSUD 1
  MSUD 2
  OS 1
  OS 2
  PKU 1
  PKU 2
  PKU 3
  Protein-Free Diet Powder (Product 80056)
  TYR 1
  TYR 2
  UCD 1
  UCD 2
Moducal Dietary Carbohydrate Powder
MSUD Diet Powder
Nutramigen Hypoallergenic Protein Hydrolysate Formula
Phenyl-Free Phenylalanine-Free Diet Powder
Poly-Vi-Sol Vitamins, Chewable Tablets and Drops (without Iron)
Poly-Vi-Sol Vitamins, Peter Rabbit Shaped Chewable Tablets (without Iron)
Poly-Vi-Sol Vitamins with Iron, Peter Rabbit Shaped Chewable Tablets
Poly-Vi-Sol Vitamins with Iron, Drops
Portagen Iron Fortified Powder with Medium Chain Triglycerides
Pregestimil Iron Fortified Protein Hydrolysate Formula with Medium Chain Triglycerides
Product 3200AB Low PHE/TYR Diet Powder

Product 3200K Low Methionine Diet Powder
Product 3232A Mono and Disaccharide-Free Diet Powder
ProSobee Soy Formula
ProSobee Soy Formula Nursette
Tempra 1 Acetaminophen Infant Drops
Tempra 2 Acetaminophen Toddlers Syrup
Tempra 3 Chewable Tablets, Regular or Double-Strength
Tri-Vi-Sol Vitamin Drops
Tri-Vi-Sol Vitamin Drops with Iron

MILES INC. 514, 701
CONSUMER HEALTHCARE PRODUCTS
1127 Myrtle Street
Elkhart, IN 46514
Address Inquiries to:
Consumer Affairs:
(800) 800-4793
For Medical Emergency Contact:
Miles Inc.:
(800) 800-4793

OTC Products Available:
- ◆ Alka-Mints Chewable Antacid
- ◆ Alka-Seltzer Effervescent Antacid and Pain Reliever
- ◆ Alka-Seltzer Extra Strength Effervescent Antacid and Pain Reliever
- ◆ Alka-Seltzer Gold Effervescent Antacid
- ◆ Alka-Seltzer Lemon Lime Effervescent Antacid and Pain Reliever
- ◆ Alka-Seltzer Plus Cold Medicine
- ◆ Alka-Seltzer Plus Cold Medicine Liqui-Gels
- ◆ Alka-Seltzer Plus Cold & Cough Medicine
- ◆ Alka-Seltzer Plus Cold & Cough Medicine Liqui-Gels
- ◆ Alka-Seltzer Plus Night-Time Cold Medicine
- ◆ Alka-Seltzer Plus Night-Time Cold Medicine Liqui-Gels
- ◆ Alka Seltzer Plus Sinus Medicine
- ◆ Bactine Antiseptic/Anesthetic First Aid Liquid
- ◆ Bactine First Aid Antibiotic Plus Anesthetic Ointment
- ◆ Bactine Hydrocortisone Anti-Itch Cream
- ◆ Bayer Children's Chewable Aspirin
- ◆ Genuine Bayer Aspirin Tablets & Caplets
- ◆ Extra Strength Bayer Arthritis Pain Regimen Formula
- ◆ Extra Strength Bayer Aspirin Caplets & Tablets
- ◆ Extended-Release Bayer 8-Hour Aspirin
- ◆ Extra Strength Bayer Plus Aspirin Caplets
- ◆ Extra Strength Bayer PM Aspirin
- ◆ Aspirin Regimen Bayer Adult Low Strength 81 mg Tablets
- ◆ Aspirin Regimen Bayer Regular Strength 325 mg Caplets
- ◆ Bayer Select Backache Pain Relief Formula
- ◆ Bayer Select Headache Pain Relief Formula
- ◆ Bayer Select Ibuprofen Pain Relief Formula
- ◆ Bayer Select Menstrual Multi-Symptom Formula
- ◆ Bayer Select Night Time Pain Relief Formula
- ◆ Bayer Select Sinus Pain Relief Formula
- ◆ Bronkaid Mist
- ◆ Bronkaid Mist Suspension
- ◆ Bronkaid Caplets
- ◆ Bugs Bunny Complete Children's Chewable Vitamins + Minerals with Iron and Calcium (Sugar Free)
- ◆ Bugs Bunny With Extra C Children's Chewable Vitamins (Sugar Free)
- ◆ Bugs Bunny Plus Iron Children's Chewable Vitamins (Sugar Free)
- ◆ Campho-Phenique Antiseptic Gel

- ◆ Campho-Phenique Cold Sore Gel
- ◆ Campho-Phenique Liquid
- ◆ Campho-Phenique Maximum Strength First Aid Antibiotic Plus Pain Reliever Ointment
- ◆ Dairy Ease Caplets and Tablets
- ◆ Dairy Ease Drops
- Dairy Ease Real Milk
- ◆ Domeboro Astringent Solution Effervescent Tablets
- ◆ Domeboro Astringent Solution Powder Packets
- ◆ Fergon Iron Supplement Tablets
- ◆ Flintstones Children's Chewable Vitamins
- ◆ Flintstones Children's Chewable Vitamins Plus Extra C
- ◆ Flintstones Children's Chewable Vitamins Plus Iron
- ◆ Flintstones Complete With Calcium, Iron & Minerals Children's Chewable Vitamins
- ◆ Flintstones Plus Calcium Children's Chewable Vitamins
- Haley's M-O, Regular & Flavored
- ◆ Maximum Strength Multi-Symptom Formula Midol
- Night Time Formula Midol PM
- ◆ PMS Multi-Symptom Formula Midol
- ◆ Teen Multi-Symptom Formula Midol
- ◆ Miles Nervine Nighttime Sleep-Aid
- ◆ Mycelex OTC Cream Antifungal
- ◆ Mycelex OTC Solution Antifungal
- ◆ Mycelex-7 Vaginal Cream Antifungal
- ◆ Mycelex-7 Vaginal Antifungal Cream with 7 Disposable Applicators
- ◆ Mycelex-7 Vaginal Inserts Antifungal
- ◆ Mycelex-7 Combination-Pack Vaginal Inserts & External Vulvar Cream
- NTZ Long Acting Nasal Spray & Drops 0.05%
- ◆ NāSal Moisturizer AF Nasal Drops
- ◆ NāSal Moisturizer AF Nasal Spray
- ◆ Neo-Synephrine Maximum Strength 12 Hour Nasal Spray
- ◆ Neo-Synephrine Maximum Strength 12 Hour Extra Moisturizing Nasal Spray
- ◆ Neo-Synephrine Maximum Strength 12 Hour Nasal Spray Pump
- ◆ Neo-Synephrine Nasal Drops, Pediatric, Mild, Regular & Extra Strength
- ◆ Neo-Synephrine Nasal Sprays, Pediatric, Mild, Regular & Extra Strength
- ◆ One-A-Day Essential Vitamins with Beta Carotene
- ◆ One-A-Day Extras Antioxidant
- ◆ One-A-Day Extras Garlic
- ◆ One-A-Day Extras Vitamin C
- ◆ One-A-Day Extras Vitamin E
- ◆ One-A-Day Maximum
- ◆ One-A-Day Men's
- ◆ One-A-Day Women's
- ◆ One-A-Day 55 Plus
- ◆ Phillips' Gelcaps
- ◆ Phillips' Milk of Magnesia Liquid
- ◆ Stri-Dex Antibacterial Cleansing Bar
- ◆ Stri-Dex Antibacterial Face Wash
- ◆ Stri-Dex Clear Gel
- ◆ Stri-Dex Maximum Strength Pads
- ◆ Stri-Dex Regular Strength Pads
- ◆ Stri-Dex Sensitive Skin Pads
- ◆ Stri-Dex Dual Textured Maximum Strength Pads
- ◆ Stri-Dex Super Scrub Pads—Oil Fighting Formula
- ◆ Vanquish Analgesic Caplets

MILES INC., DIAGNOSTICS 731
DIVISION
511 Benedict Avenue
Tarrytown, NY 10591
OTC Products Available:
Glucometer Elite
Glucometer Encore

(◆) Shown in Product Identification Guide

MURO PHARMACEUTICAL, ... 733
INC.
890 East Street
Tewksbury, MA 01876-1496
Address Inquiries to:
Professional Service Dept.:
(800) 225-0974
(508) 851-5981

OTC Products Available:
Bromfed Syrup
Guaifed Syrup
Guaitab Tablets
Salinex Nasal Mist and Drops

NATURE'S BOUNTY, ... 518, 734
INC.
90 Orville Drive
Bohemia, NY 11716
Address Inquiries to:
Professional Service Department:
(516) 567-9500
(800) 645-5412
FAX: (516) 563-1623

OTC Products Available:
ABC to Z
Acidophilus
Antioxidant 4000
B-Complex +C (Long Acting) Tablets
B-6 50 mg., 100 mg., 200 mg.
B-12 1000 mcg. Tablets
B-12 and B-12 Sublingual Tablets
B-50 Tablets
B-100 Tablets-Ultra B Complex
Beta-Carotene Capsules
Bounty Bears (Children's Chewables)
C-500 mg., C-1000 mg., C-1500 mg. &
  Time Release Formulas
Calcium Magnesium-Chelated Tablets
E-Oil 25,000 I.U.
◆ Ener-B Vitamin B_{12} Nasal Gel Dietary
  Supplement
EnerVite (High Performance Nutrition)
Ferrous Sulfate Tablets
Garlic Oil 15 gr. & 77 gr.
KLB6 Capsules
L-Lysine 500 mg. Tablets & 1000 mg.
  Tablets
Lecithin 1200 mg. Capsules
M-KYA (For Leg Cramps)
Niacin 50 mg., 100 mg., & 250 mg.
Oat Bran 850 mg.
Odor Free Garlic
Oystercal-500 & Oystercal 500 + D
Shark Cartilage
Ultra Vita-Time Tablets
Vitamin A 10,000 I.U. & 25,000 I.U.
Vitamin E (Natural d-alpha tocopheryl)
Water Pill (Natural Diuretic)
Zinc 10 mg., 25 mg., 50 mg. Tablets

NICHE PHARMACEUTICALS, ... 735
INC.
200 N. Oak Street
P.O. Box 449
Roanoke, TX 76262
Address Inquiries to:
Steve F. Brandon: (817) 491-2770
FAX: (817) 491-3533
For Medical Emergencies Contact:
Gerald L. Beckloff, M.D.:
(817) 491-2770
FAX: (817) 491-3533

OTC Products Available:
MagTab SR Caplets

OHM LABORATORIES, ... 518, 735
INC.
Mailing:
P.O. Box 279
Franklin Park, NJ 08823

Locations:
1385 Livingston Ave
North Brunswick, NJ 08902
(908) 297-3030
464-C Black Horse Lane
South Brunswick, NJ 08852
(908) 297-3835
Address Inquiries to:
Arun Heble: (908) 297-3030
For Medical Emergencies Contact:
(908) 297-3030

OTC Products Available:
Bisacodyl Tablets 5 mg.
◆ Cramp End Tablets
Docusate Potassium with Casanthranol
  Capsules and Caplets
◆ Ibuprohm (Ibuprofen) Caplets, 200 mg
◆ Ibuprohm (Ibuprofen) Tablets, 200 mg
◆ Loperamide Hydrochloride Caplets, 2 mg
Ohmni-Scon Chewable Tablets, Extra
  Strength
Pseudoephedrine Hydrochloride Tablets
  30mg and 60mg
Senna Tablets
Tribuffered Aspirin
Trisudrine Tablets

ORTHO PHARMACEUTICAL .. 518, 736
CORPORATION
ADVANCED CARE
PRODUCTS
Route 202 South
Raritan, NJ 08869

OTC Products Available:
◆ Conceptrol Contraceptive Gel Single
  Use Applicators
◆ Conceptrol Contraceptive Inserts
◆ Delfen Contraceptive Foam
◆ Gynol II Extra Strength Contraceptive Jelly
◆ Gynol II Original Formula Contraceptive
  Jelly
◆ Ortho-Gynol Contraceptive Jelly

P & S LABORATORIES 741
210 West 131st Street
Los Angeles, CA 90061

(See STANDARD HOMEOPATHIC
COMPANY)

PARKE-DAVIS
(See WARNER WELLCOME)

THE PARTHENON COMPANY, ... 741
INC.
3311 West 2400 South
Salt Lake City, UT 84119
Address Inquiries to:
(801) 972-5184
FAX: (801) 972-4734
For Medical Emergency Contact:
Nick G. Mihalopoulos: (801) 972-5184

OTC Products Available:
Devrom Chewable Tablets

PFIZER CONSUMER 519, 741
HEALTH CARE DIVISION
Division of Pfizer Inc.
100 Jefferson Road
Parsippany, NJ 07054
Address Inquiries to:
Research and Development Dept.:
(201) 887-2100

OTC Products Available:
BenGay External Analgesic Products
Bonine Tablets
◆ Daily Care from DESITIN
◆ Desitin Cornstarch Baby Powder

◆ Desitin Ointment
Rheaban Maximum Strength Fast Acting
  Caplets
Rid Lice Control Spray
Rid Lice Killing Shampoo
Maximum Strength Unisom Sleepgels
Unisom Nighttime Sleep Aid
Unisom With Pain Relief-Nighttime Sleep
  Aid and Pain Reliever
◆ Visine Maximum Strength Allergy Relief
◆ Visine L.R. Eye Drops
◆ Visine Moisturizing Eye Drops
◆ Visine Original Eye Drops
Wart-Off Wart Remover

PHARMAVITE 519, 748
CORPORATION
15451 San Fernando Mission Blvd.
Mission Hills, CA 91345
Address Inquiries to:
PHARMAVITE
ATTN: Customer Service
P.O. Box 9606
Mission Hills, CA 91346-9606
1 (800) 423-2405
1 (800) 276-2878 Mon-Fri, 7:00-4:00
Pacific Time (For Consumer Use Only)

OTC Products Available:
Nature Made Vitamins
◆ Nature Made Antioxidant Formula
◆ Nature Made Essential Balance
  Multivitamin
Nutra E Skin Care Products
Private Label Vitamins
Sunny Maid Brand Vitamins

PLOUGH, INC
(See SCHERING-PLOUGH HEALTHCARE
PRODUCTS)

POLYMEDICA 748
PHARMACEUTICALS (USA),
INC.
Subsidiary of PolyMedica Industries, Inc.
11 State Street
Woburn, MA 01801
Address Inquiries to:
Dr. Arthur Siciliano: (617) 933-2020
FAX: (617) 933-7992
For Medical Emergencies Contact:
Dr. Arthur Siciliano: (617) 933-2020
FAX: (617) 933-7992

OTC Products Available:
Alconephrin Nasal Decongestant
Azo-Standard
Neopap Pediatric Suppositories

PREMIER, INC.................. 749
Greenwich Office Park One
Greenwich, CT 06831
Address Inquiries to:
Robert Albus: (203) 622-1211
FAX: (203) 622-0773
For Medical Emergency Contact:
Sergio Nacht, Ph.D.: (415) 366-2626
FAX: (415) 368-4470
Branch Office:
3696 Haven Avenue
Redwood City, CA 94063
(415) 366-2626
FAX: (415) 368-4470

OTC Products Available:
Every Step Foot Deodorant
Exact Vanishing and Tinted Creams

PROCTER & GAMBLE............ 749
P.O. Box 5516
Cincinnati, OH 45201
Address Inquiries to:
Charles Lambert (800) 358-8707

(◆) Shown in Product Identification Guide

PROCTER & GAMBLE—*cont.*

For Medical Emergencies:
Call Collect: (513) 558-2085

OTC Products Available:
Aleve
Children's Vicks Chloraseptic Sore Throat
Lozenges
Children's Vicks Chloraseptic Sore Throat
Spray
Children's Vicks DayQuil Allergy Relief
Children's Vicks NyQuil Cold/Cough Relief
Crest Sensitivity Protection Toothpaste
Extra Strength Vicks Cough Drops
Head & Shoulders Intensive Treatment
Dandruff Shampoo
Head & Shoulders Intensive Treatment
Dandruff Shampoo 2-in-1 plus
Conditioner
Maximum Strength Pepto-Bismol Liquid
Metamucil Effervescent Sugar Free,
Lemon-Lime Flavor
Metamucil Effervescent Sugar Free,
Orange Flavor
Metamucil Original Texture
Metamucil Powder, Orange Flavor
Metamucil Powder, Regular Flavor
Metamucil Smooth Texture Powder,
Orange Flavor
Metamucil Smooth Texture Powder,
Regular Flavor
Metamucil Smooth Texture Powder, Sugar
Free, Orange Flavor
Metamucil Smooth Texture, Citrus Flavor
Metamucil Smooth Texture, Sugar Free,
Citrus Flavor
Metamucil Wafers, Apple Crisp &
Cinnamon Spice Flavors
Oil of Olay Daily UV Protectant SPF 15
Beauty Fluid-Original and Fragrance
Free (Olay Co. Inc.)
Pediatric Vicks 44d Dry Hacking Cough &
Head Congestion
Pediatric Vicks 44e Chest Cough & Chest
Congestion
Pediatric Vicks 44m Cough & Cold Relief
Pepto Diarrhea Control
Pepto-Bismol Liquid, Tablets & Caplets
Percogesic Analgesic Tablets
Vicks 44 Dry Hacking Cough
Vicks 44 LiquiCaps Cough, Cold & Flu
Relief
Vicks 44 LiquiCaps Non-Drowsy Cough &
Cold Relief
Vicks 44D Dry Hacking Cough & Head
Congestion
Vicks 44E Chest Cough & Chest
Congestion
Vicks 44M Cough, Cold & Flu Relief
Vicks Chloraseptic Cough & Throat Drops
Vicks Chloraseptic Sore Throat Lozenges
Vicks Chloraseptic Sore Throat Spray, and
Gargle and Mouth Rinse
Vicks Cough Drops
Vicks DayQuil Allergy Relief 12-Hour
Extended Release Tablets
Vicks DayQuil Allergy Relief 4-Hour Tablets
Vicks DayQuil LiquiCaps Multi-Symptom
Cold/Flu Relief
Vicks DayQuil Multi-Symptom Cold/Flu
Relief–(Liquid)
Vicks DayQuil SINUS Pressure &
CONGESTION Relief
Vicks DayQuil SINUS Pressure & PAIN
Relief with IBUPROFEN
Vicks Nyquil Hot Therapy
Vicks NyQuil LiquiCaps Multi-Symptom
Cold/Flu Relief
Vicks NyQuil Multi-Symptom Cold/Flu
Relief - (Original & Cherry Flavor)
Vicks Sinex 12-Hour Nasal Decongestant
Spray and Ultra Fine Mist
Vicks Sinex Nasal Spray and Ultra Fine
Mist
Vicks Vapor Inhaler

Vicks VapoRub Cream
Vicks VapoRub Ointment
Vicks VapoSteam

QUINTEX 766
PHARMACEUTICALS, LTD.
1 Executive Drive
Fort Lee, NJ 07024
Tel.: (201) 947-8700
Fax: (201) 947-8779
Address Inquires To:
Customer Service
For Medical Emergencies Contact:
Professional Services

OTC Products Available:
Alcomed Tablets and Liquid
Analox 500 Caplets
Cap-Z Pure Lotion
Co-Complex DM Caplets
Congestrol D Tablets
Expressin 400 Caplets
Inspire Nasal Spray
Isohist 2.0 Tablets
Ivy Soothe Derma Spray
Nauquel Liquid
Nauzet 50 Tablets
PediaPressin Drops
Restyn 76 Caplets
Sinutrol 500 Caplets
Suppressin DM Caplets and Liquid
Suppressin DM Plus Liquid
Uro-Dyne 97.5 Tablets

REED & CARNRICK 519, 767
Division of Block Drug Company, Inc.
257 Cornelison Avenue
Jersey City, NJ 07302
Address Inquiries to:
Consumer & R&C Professional Affairs:
(201) 434-4000 X1821
FAX: (201) 434-3032
For Medical Emergencies Contact:
Reed & Carnrick Medical Dept.:
(800) 568-6133 X1993

OTC Products Available:
Dura Screen
◆ Phazyme Drops
Phazyme Tablets
Phazyme-95 Tablets
Phazyme-125 Chewable Tablets
Phazyme-125 Softgels Maximum Strength
ProctoFoam-NS (Non-Steroid)
Proxigel
R&C Lice Treatment Kit
R&C Shampoo
R&C Spray
Trichotine Liquid Vaginal Douche
Trichotine Powder Vaginal Douche

REQUA, INC. 768
Box 4008
1 Seneca Place
Greenwich, CT 06830
Address Inquiries to:
J. Geils: (203) 869-2445
(800) 321-1085
FAX: (203) 661-5630

OTC Products Available:
CharcoAid
CharcoAid 2000
Charcoal Tablets

RICHARDSON-VICKS, INC.
(See PROCTER & GAMBLE)

ROBERTS 519, 768
PHARMACEUTICAL
CORPORATION
4 Industrial Way West
Eatontown, NJ 07724

Address Inquiries to:
Customer Service Department:
(908) 389-1182
FAX: (908) 389-1014
(800) 828-2088
For Medical Emergencies Contact:
Medical Services Department:
(800) 992-9306

OTC Products Available:
Baciguent Topical Cream
Cheracol Cough Syrup
◆ Cheracol-D Cough Formula
Cheracol Nasal Spray Pump
◆ Cheracol Plus Head Cold/Cough Formula
Cheracol Sinus
Cheracol Sore Throat Spray
Cheracol Throat Discs
Citrocarbonate Antacid
Clocream Skin Protectant Cream
Clomycin Antibiotic Ointment
◆ Colace
Diostate D Tablets
◆ Haltran Tablets
Lipomul Oral Liquid
Myciguent Topical Cream
Orexin Tablets
◆ Peri-Colace
Probec-T Tablets
Procort Cream with Aloe
Procort Maximum Strength Cream
◆ Pyrroxate Caplets
Saluron
Salutensin
◆ Sigtab Tablets
◆ Sigtab-M Tablets
Squibb Cod Liver Oil
Squibb Glycerin Suppositories
Squibb Mineral Oil
Super D Perles
Zymacap Capsules

A. H. ROBINS 520, 773
CONSUMER PRODUCTS
American Home Products Corporation
Five Giralda Farms
Madison, N.J. 07940-0871
Address Inquiries to:
Consumer Affairs
Professional Samples:
(800) 343-0856
Other Information (800) 762-4672

OTC Products Available:
Allbee with C Caplets
Allbee C-800 Plus Iron Tablets
Allbee C-800 Tablets
Anacin Caplets
Anacin Tablets
Maximum Strength Anacin Tablets
Aspirin Free Anacin Caplets
Aspirin Free Anacin Gel Caplets
Aspirin Free Anacin Tablets
Aspirin Free Anacin P.M. Caplets
Chap Stick Lip Balm
Chap Stick Medicated Lip Balm
Chap Stick Sunblock 15 Lip Balm
Chap Stick Petroleum Jelly Plus
Chap Stick Petroleum Jelly Plus with
Sunblock 15
Dimacol Caplets
Dimetane Elixir
Dimetane Extentabs 8 mg
Dimetane Extentabs 12 mg
Dimetapp Allergy LiquiGels
Dimetapp Allergy Tablets
Dimetapp Decongestant LiquiGels
Dimetapp Decongestant Pediatric Drops
◆ Dimetapp Elixir
◆ Dimetapp Extentabs
Dimetapp Liqui-Gels

(◆) Shown in Product Identification Guide

Dimetapp Tablets
Dimetapp Cold & Allergy Chewable
Tablets
Dimetapp Cold & Flu Caplets
Dimetapp DM Elixir
Dimetapp Sinus Caplets
Robitussin
Robitussin Cold & Cough Liqui-Gels
Robitussin Cold, Cough & Flu Liqui-Gels
Robitussin Cough Calmers
Robitussin Cough Drops
Robitussin Liquid Center Cough Drops
Robitussin Maximum Strength Cough
Suppressant
Robitussin Maximum Strength Cough &
Cold
Robitussin Night Relief
Robitussin Pediatric Cough & Cold
Formula
Robitussin Pediatric Cough Suppressant
Robitussin Pediatric Night Relief
◆ Robitussin Severe Congestion Liqui-Gels
Robitussin Sugar-Free Cough Drops
Robitussin-CF
◆ Robitussin-DM
Robitussin-PE
Z-BEC Tablets

ROSS PRODUCTS 520, 780
DIVISION
Abbott Laboratories
Columbus, OH 43215-1724
Address Inquiries to:
Medical Director: (614) 624-7677

OTC Products Available:
Clear Eyes ACR Astringent/Lubricant
Redness Reliever Eye Drops
Clear Eyes Lubricant Eye Redness
Reliever Eye Drops
Ear Drops by Murine—(See Murine Ear
Wax Removal System/Murine Ear
Drops)
Murine Ear Drops
Murine Ear Wax Removal System
Murine Lubricant Eye Drops
Murine Plus Lubricant Redness Reliever
Eye Drops
◆ Pedialyte Oral Electrolyte Maintenance
Solution
◆ PediaSure and PediaSure with Fiber
Rehydralyte Oral Electrolyte Rehydration
Solution
Ross Pediatric Nutritional Products
Alimentum Protein Hydrolysate Formula
With Iron
Isomil Soy Formula With Iron
Isomil DF Soy Formula For Diarrhea
Isomil SF Sucrose-Free Soy Formula
With Iron
◆ PediaSure Complete Liquid Nutrition
◆ PediaSure With Fiber Complete Liquid
Nutrition
RCF Ross Carbohydrate Free Low-Iron
Soy Formula Base
Similac Low-Iron Infant Formula
Similac NeoCare Premature Infant
Formula with Iron
Similac PM 60/40 Low-Iron Infant
Formula
Similac Special Care With Iron 24
Premature Infant Formula Similac
Toddler's Best Milk-Based Nutritional
Beverage
Similac With Iron Infant Formula
◆ Similac Toddler's Best Milk-Based
Nutritional Beverage
Selsun Blue Dandruff Shampoo
Selsun Blue Dandruff Shampoo
Medicated Treatment Formula
Selsun Blue Extra Conditioning Formula
Dandruff Shampoo
Selsun Gold for Women Dandruff
Shampoo

Tronolane Anesthetic Cream for
Hemorrhoids
Tronolane Hemorrhoidal Suppositories

SANDOZ 520, 785
PHARMACEUTICALS
CORPORATION/
CONSUMER DIVISION
59 Route 10
East Hanover NJ 07936
Address Medical Inquiries to:
Medical Department
Sandoz Pharmaceuticals Corporation
East Hanover, NJ 07936
(201) 503-7500
Other Inquiries to:
(201) 503-7500
FAX: (201) 503-8265

OTC Products Available:
Acid Mantle Creme
◆ BiCozene Creme
Cama Arthritis Pain Reliever
◆ Dorcol Children's Cough Syrup
◆ Ex-Lax Chocolated Laxative Tablets
Extra Gentle Ex-Lax Laxative Pills
◆ Maximum Relief Formula Ex-Lax Laxative
Pills
◆ Regular Strength Ex-Lax Laxative Pills
◆ Ex-Lax Gentle Nature Laxative Pills
◆ Gas-X Chewable Tablets
Extra Strength Gas-X Chewable Tablets
◆ Tavist-1 12 Hour Relief Tablets
◆ Tavist-D 12 Hour Relief Tablets
◆ TheraFlu Flu and Cold Medicine
◆ TheraFlu Flu, Cold and Cough Medicine
◆ TheraFlu Maximum Strength Nighttime
Flu, Cold & Cough Medicine
◆ TheraFlu Maximum Strength Non-Drowsy
Formula Flu, Cold & Cough Medicine
◆ Thera Flu Maximum Strength, Non-Drowsy
Formula Flu, Cold and Cough Caplets
Triaminic Allergy Tablets
◆ Triaminic AM Cough and Decongestant
Formula
◆ Triaminic AM Decongestant Formula
◆ Triaminic Cold Tablets
◆ Triaminic Expectorant
◆ Triaminic Nite Light
◆ Triaminic Sore Throat Formula
◆ Triaminic Syrup
◆ Triaminic-12 Tablets
◆ Triaminic-DM Syrup
◆ Triaminicin Tablets
◆ Triaminicol Multi-Symptom Cold Tablets
◆ Triaminicol Multi-Symptom Relief
Ursinus Inlay-Tabs

SANOFI WINTHROP 794
PHARMACEUTICALS
Main Office
90 Park Avenue
New York, NY 10016
(212) 907-2000
Address Medical Inquiries to:
Product Information Services:
(800) 446-6267

OTC Products Available:
Drisdol
Zephiran Chloride Aqueous Solution
Zephiran Chloride Concentrate Solution
Zephiran Chloride Spray
Zephiran Chloride Tinted Tincture

SCANDINAVIAN NATURAL 797
HEALTH & BEAUTY PRODUCTS,
INC.
13 North Seventh Street
Perkasie, PA 18944
Address Inquires To:
Catherine Peklak:
(215) 453-2505

OTC Products Available:
Nasaline Preservative-Free Nasal Saline
Salix SST Lozenges Saliva Stimulant

SCHERING CORPORATION
(See SCHERING-PLOUGH HEALTHCARE
PRODUCTS)

SCHERING-PLOUGH 522, 797
HEALTHCARE PRODUCTS
110 Allen Road
Liberty Corner, NJ 07938
Address Product Requests to:
Public Relations: (908) 604-1836
For Medical Emergencies Contact:
Clinical Department:
(901) 320-2998

OTC Products Available:
◆ A and D Medicated Diaper Rash Ointment
◆ A and D Ointment
Afrin Cherry Scented Nasal Spray 0.05%
◆ Afrin Extra Moisturizing Nasal Spray
Afrin Menthol Nasal Spray, 0.05%
◆ Afrin Nasal Spray 0.05% and Nasal Spray
Pump
Afrin Nose Drops 0.05%
Afrin Saline Mist
Afrin Sinus
◆ Aftate for Athlete's Foot
◆ Aftate for Jock Itch
Aspergum
◆ Chlor-Trimeton Allergy Decongestant
Tablets
Chlor-Trimeton Allergy-Sinus Headache
Caplets
◆ Chlor-Trimeton Allergy Tablets
◆ Chooz Antacid Gum
◆ Complex 15 Therapeutic Moisturizing
Face Cream
◆ Complex 15 Therapeutic Moisturizing
Lotion
◆ Coricidin 'D' Decongestant Tablets
◆ Coricidin Tablets
◆ Correctol Extra Gentle Stool Softener
◆ Correctol Laxative Tablets & Caplets
Cushion Grip Denture Adhesive
◆ Di-Gel Antacid/Anti-Gas
◆ Drixoral Cold and Allergy Sustained-Action
Tablets
◆ Drixoral Cold and Flu Extended-Release
Tablets
◆ Drixoral Cough Liquid Caps
◆ Drixoral Cough + Congestion Liquid Caps
◆ Drixoral Cough + Sore Throat Liquid Caps
◆ Drixoral Non-Drowsy Formula
Extended-Release Tablets
◆ Drixoral Allergy/Sinus Extended Release
Tablets
◆ DuoFilm Liquid Wart Remover
◆ DuoFilm Patch Wart Remover
◆ DuoPlant Gel Plantar Wart Remover
◆ Duration 12 Hour Nasal Spray
Duration 12 Hour Nasal Spray Pump
◆ Feen-A-Mint Gum
Feen-A-Mint Laxative Pills
Gyne-Lotrimin Vaginal Cream
Gyne-Lotrimin Vaginal Cream with 7
Disposable Applicators
Gyne-Lotrimin Vaginal Cream in Prefilled
Applicators
Gyne-Lotrimin Vaginal Inserts
Gyne-Lotrimin Combination Pack
◆ Gyne-Moistrin Vaginal Moisturizing Gel
◆ Lotrimin AF Antifungal Cream, Lotion and
Solution
◆ Lotrimin AF Antifungal Spray Liquid, Spray
Powder, Powder and Jock Itch Spray
Powder
Muskol Insect Repellent Aerosol Liquid
Muskol Insect Repellent Lotion
Muskol Insect Repellent Pump Spray
◆ Shade Gel SPF 30 Sunblock
◆ Shade Lotion SPF 45 Sunblock

(◆) Shown in Product Identification Guide

SCHERING-PLOUGH HEALTHCARE PRODUCTS—cont.

- ◆ Shade UVAGUARD SPF 15 Suncreen Lotion
- ◆ St. Joseph Adult Chewable Aspirin (81 mg.)
  St. Joseph Aspirin-Free Fever Reducer for Children Chewable Tablets
  St. Joseph Cold Tablets for Children
  St. Joseph Cough Suppressant for Children
- ◆ Tinactin Aerosol Liquid 1%
- ◆ Tinactin Aerosol Powder 1%
- ◆ Tinactin Antifungal Cream, Solution & Powder 1%
  Tinactin Deodorant Powder Aerosol 1%
- ◆ Tinactin Jock Itch Cream 1%
- ◆ Tinactin Jock Itch Spray Powder 1%

SCOT-TUSSIN PHARMACAL ...... 810 CO., INC.

50 Clemence Street
Cranston, RI 02920-0217 (USA)
Mailing Address: P.O. Box 8217
Cranston, RI 02920-0217
Address Inquiries to:
(401) 942-8555
(401) 942-8556
(800) 638-SCOT (7268)
FAX: (401) 942-5690
For Medical Emergency Contact:
Dr. S. G. Scotti:
(800) 638-SCOT (7268)
FAX: (401) 942-5690

OTC Products Available:
Chlorpheniramine Maleate Sugar-Free Febrol SF and DF
Hayfebrol Allergy Relief Formula SF & DF
Romilar DM Cough & Cold Formula
Romilar DM Pediatric Sugar-Free
Romilar Infant Decongestant Sugar-Free
Scot-Tussin Allergy Relief Formula Sugar-Free and Dye-Free
Scot-Tussin DM Cough Chasers Lozenges Sugar-Free & Dye-Free
Scot-Tussin DM Sugar-Free
Scot-Tussin Expectorant Sugar-Free, Dye-Free, Alcohol-Free
Scot-Tussin Original Syrup (with sugar)
Scot-Tussin Sugar-Free Original
Vitalize Sugar-Free, Alcohol-Free, Dye-Free

SMART .... 524, 810 PHARMACEUTICALS, INC.

214 E. 16th Street
Vancouver, WA 98663

OTC Products Available:
- ◆ Healthprin Aspirin

SMITHKLINE BEECHAM .... 424, 810 CONSUMER HEALTHCARE, L.P.

Unit of SmithKline Beecham, Inc.
P.O. Box 1467
Pittsburgh, PA 15230
Address Consumer Inquiries to:
1-(800) 245-1040
Address Healthcare Professional Inquiries to:
1-(800) 378-4055
Address Healthcare Professional Sample Requests to:
1-(800) BEECHAM

OTC Products Available:
- ◆ CĒPASTAT Cherry Flavor Sore Throat Lozenges
- ◆ CĒPASTAT Extra Strength Sore Throat Lozenges

- ◆ CITRUCEL Orange Flavor
- ◆ CITRUCEL Sugar Free Orange Flavor
  Contac Continuous Action Nasal Decongestant/Antihistamine 12 Hour Capsules
- ◆ Contac Day Allergy/Sinus Caplets
- ◆ Contac Day & Night Cold/Flu Caplets
  Contac Day & Night Cold/Flu Night Caplets
- ◆ Contac Maximum Strength Continuous Action Decongestant/Antihistamine 12 Hour Caplets
- ◆ Contac Night Allergy/Sinus Caplets
- ◆ Contac Severe Cold and Flu Formula Caplets
- ◆ Contac Severe Cold & Flu Non-Drowsy
- ◆ Debrox Drops
- ◆ Ecotrin Enteric Coated Aspirin Maximum Strength Tablets and Caplets
- ◆ Ecotrin Enteric Coated Aspirin Regular Strength and Adult Low Strength Tablets
- ◆ Feosol Capsules
- ◆ Feosol Elixir
- ◆ Feosol Tablets
- ◆ Gaviscon Antacid Tablets
- ◆ Gaviscon-2 Antacid Tablets
- ◆ Gaviscon Extra Strength Relief Formula Antacid Tablets
- ◆ Gaviscon Extra Strength Relief Formula Liquid Antacid
- ◆ Gaviscon Liquid Antacid
- ◆ Gly-Oxide Liquid
  Massengill Disposable Douches
  Massengill Feminine Cleansing Wash
  Massengill Fragrance-Free and Baby Powder Scent Soft Cloth Towelettes
  Massengill Liquid Concentrate
- ◆ Massengill Medicated Disposable Douche
  Massengill Medicated Liquid Concentrate
  Massengill Medicated Soft Cloth Towelette
  Massengill Powder
  N'ICE Medicated Sugarless Sore Throat and Cough Lozenges
- ◆ Novahistine DMX
- ◆ Novahistine Elixir
- ◆ Panodol Tablets and Caplets
- ◆ Children's Panodol Chewable Tablets, Liquid, Infant's Drops
  Simron Capsules
  Simron Plus Capsules
- ◆ Sine-Off No Drowsiness Formula Caplets
- ◆ Sine-Off Sinus Medicine
  Singlet Tablets
- ◆ Sucrets Children's Cherry Flavored Sore Throat Lozenges
- ◆ Sucrets Maximum Strength Wintergreen and Sucrets Wild Cherry (Regular Strength) Sore Throat Lozenges
- ◆ Sucrets 4-Hour Cough Suppressant
- ◆ Teldrin 12 Hour Antihistamine/Nasal Decongestant Allergy Relief Capsules
- ◆ Tums Antacid Tablets
- ◆ Tums Anti-gas/Antacid Formula Tablets, Assorted Fruit
- ◆ Tums E-X Antacid Tablets
  Tums 500 Calcium Supplement
- ◆ Tums ULTRA Antacid Tablets

SMITHKLINE CONSUMER PRODUCTS

(See SMITHKLINE BEECHAM CONSUMER HEALTHCARE, L.P.)

E. R. SQUIBB & SONS, INC.

A Bristol-Myers Squibb Company
P.O. Box 4000
Princeton, NJ 08543-4000

Theragran line is now being distributed by BRISTOL-MYERS PRODUCTS.

STANDARD HOMEOPATHIC ...... 828 COMPANY

210 West 131st Street
Box 61067
Los Angeles, CA 90061
Address Inquiries to:
Jay Borneman:
(800) 624-9659
OTC Products Available:
Hyland's Arnicaid Tablets
Hyland's Bed Wetting Tablets
Hyland's Calms Forté Tablets
Hyland's ClearAc
Hyland's Colic Tablets
Hyland's Cough Syrup with Honey
Hyland's C-Plus Cold Tablets
Hyland's Diarrex Tablets
Hyland's EnurAid Tablets
Hyland's Teething Tablets
Hyland's Vitamin C for Children

STELLAR PHARMACAL .... 830 CORPORATION

1990 N.W. 44th Street
Pompano Beach, FL 33064-8712
Address Inquiries to:
Scott L. Davidson: (305) 972-6060
Customer Service & Order Department:
(800) 845-7827

OTC Products Available:
Star-Otic Ear Solution

STERLING HEALTH

(See MILES INC)

THOMPSON MEDICAL ...... 526, 830 COMPANY, INC.

222 Lakeview Avenue
West Palm Beach, FL 33401
Address Inquiries to:
Consumer Services

OTC Products Available:
Aqua-Ban Maximum Strength Tablets
Arthritis Hot
- ◆ Aspercreme Creme, Lotion Analgesic Rub
  Breathe Free
- ◆ Capzasin-P
  Control Caplets
- ◆ Cortizone for Kids
- ◆ Cortizone-5 Creme and Ointment
- ◆ Cortizone-10 Creme and Ointment
- ◆ Cortizone-10 External Anal Itch Relief
- ◆ Cortizone-10 Scalp Itch Formula
  Dexatrim Maximum Strength Caffeine-Free Caplets
- ◆ Dexatrim Maximum Strength Extended Duration Time Tablets
- ◆ Dexatrim Maximum Strength Plus Vitamin C/Caffeine-free Caplets
  Dexatrim Plus Vitamins Caplets
  Diar Aid Tablets
  Encare Vaginal Contraceptive Suppositories
  End Lice
- ◆ Hemorid For Women Cleanser
- ◆ Hemorid For Women Creme
- ◆ Hemorid For Women Suppositories
  Ibuprin
- ◆ NP-27 Cream, Solution & Spray Powder
- ◆ Sleepinal Night-time Sleep Aid Capsules and Softgels
  Sportscreme External Analgesic Rub Cream & Lotion
- ◆ Tempo Soft Antacid
  Tribiotic Plus

(◆) Shown in Product Identification Guide

TRANSDERMAL **835**
TECHNOLOGIES, INC.
P.O. Box 14804
North Palm Beach, FL 33408-0804

OTC Products Available:
Topical Analgesic Ointment

TRITON CONSUMER **835**
PRODUCTS, INC.
561 West Golf Road
Arlington Heights, IL 60005
Address Inquiries to:
Karen Shrader: (800) 942-2009
For Medical Emergencies Contact:
(800) 942-2009

OTC Products Available:
MG 217 Medicated Tar Shampoo
MG 217 Medicated Tar-Free Shampoo
MG 217 Psoriasis Ointment and Lotion
ProTech First-Aid Stik
Retro G Medicated Cold Sore Gel
Skeeter Stik Insect Bite Medication

UAS LABORATORIES **835**
5610 Rowland Road #110
Minnetonka, MN 55343

OTC Products Available:
DDS-Acidophilus

THE UPJOHN COMPANY **526, 836**
7000 Portage Road
Kalamazoo, MI 49001
For Medical and Pharmaceutical
Information, Including Emergencies:
(616) 329-8244
(616) 323-6615
Pharmaceutical Sales Areas
and Distribution Centers:
Atlanta (Chamblee)
GA 30341-2626 2626
(404) 451-4822
Boston (Wellesley)
MA 02181
(617) 431-7970
Buffalo (Amherst)
NY 14221
(716) 632-5942
Chicago (Oak Brook Terrace)
IL 60181
(708) 663-9300
Cincinnati, OH 45202
(513) 723-1010
Dallas (Irving)
TX 75062
(214) 256-0022
Denver, CO 80216
(303) 399-3113
Hartford (Enfield) CT 06082
(203) 741-3421
Honolulu, HI 96818
(808) 422-2777
Kalamazoo, MI 49001
(616) 384-9060
Kansas City (Overland Park) KS 66210
(913) 469-8863
Memphis, TN 38119
(901) 685-8192
New York (Uniondale) NY 11553
(914) 769-5400
Orlando, FL 32809
(407) 859-4591
Philadelphia (Berwyn) PA 19312
(215) 993-0100
Pittsburgh (Bridgeville) PA 15017
(412) 391-0411
Portland, OR 97232
(503) 232-2133
St. Louis, MO 63141
(816) 361-2287
San Francisco (Foster City)
CA 94404
(415) 377-0203

Shreveport, LA 71129
(318) 688-3700
Simi Valley, CA 93065
(805) 582-0072
Washington, DC 20011
(703) 849-1300

OTC Products Available:
◆ Cortaid Cream with Aloe
◆ Cortaid Lotion
◆ Cortaid Ointment with Aloe
◆ Cortaid Spray
◆ Maximum Strength Cortaid Cream
◆ Maximum Strength Cortaid Ointment
◆ Maximum Strength Cortaid Spray
◆ Doxidan Liqui-Gels
◆ Dramamine Chewable Tablets
◆ Children's Dramamine Liquid
◆ Dramamine Tablets
◆ Dramamine II Tablets
◆ Kaopectate Concentrated Anti-Diarrheal,
   Peppermint Flavor
◆ Kaopectate Concentrated Anti-Diarrheal,
   Regular Flavor
◆ Kaopectate Children's Liquid
◆ Kaopectate Maximum Strength Caplets
   Kaopectate 1-D
◆ Motrin IB Caplets, Tablets, and Geltabs
◆ Motrin IB Sinus
◆ Mycitracin Plus Pain Reliever
◆ Maximum Strength Mycitracin Triple
   Antibiotic First Aid Ointment
◆ Surfak Liqui-Gels

WAKUNAGA OF **527, 839**
AMERICA CO., LTD.
Subsidiary of Wakunaga Pharmaceutical
Co., Ltd.
23501 Madero
Mission Viejo, CA 92691
Address Inquiries to:
(800) 421-2998

OTC Products Available:
BeSure Caplets/Capsules
◆ Kyo-Dophilus
   Acidophilase Capsules: L. acidophilus,
      B. bifidum, amylase, protease, lipase
   Kyo-Dophilus Capsules: L. acidophilus,
      B. longum, B. bifidum
   Kyo-Dophilus Chewable Tablets: L.
      acidophilus
   Kyo-Green Powder: Barley & wheat grass,
      chlorella, kelp, brown rice
◆ Kyolic
   Kyo-Chrome Caplets: Aged garlic extract
      powder (500mg), niacin (20mg),
      chromium as picolinate (200mcg)
   Kyo-Chrome Capsules: Aged garlic
      extract powder (200mg), niacin
      (10mg), chromium as picolinate
      (100mcg)
   Kyolic Aged Garlic Extract, SGP (350mg)
   Kyolic Aged Garlic Extract Caplets: Aged
      garlic extract powder (600mg)
   Kyolic Aged Garlic Extract Flavor and
      Odor Modified Plain Liquid
   Kyolic Reserve Capsules: Aged garlic
      extract powder (600mg)
   Kyolic—Super Formula 100 Tablets &
      Caplets: Aged garlic extract powder
      (300mg), whey
   Kyolic—Super Formula 101 Garlic Plus:
      Tablets & Capsules: Aged garlic
      extract (270mg) whey, brewer's
      yeast, kelp, algin
   Kyolic—Super Formula 102 Tablets &
      Capsules: Aged garlic extract powder
      (350mg), amylase, protease,
      cellulase, lipase
   Kyolic—Super Formula 103 Capsules:
      Aged garlic extract powder (220mg),
      Ester C, astragalus, calcium
   Kyolic—Super Formula 104 Capsules:
      Aged garlic extract powder (300mg),
      lecithin

Kyolic—Super Formula 105 Capsules:
   Aged garlic extract powder (200mg),
   beta carotene, vitamin C, vitamin E,
   selenium, green tea
Kyolic—Super Formula 106 Capsules:
   Aged garlic extract powder (300mg),
   hawthorne berry, vitamin E, cayenne
   pepper
Ginkgo Biloba Plus Capsules: Ginkgo
   biloba extract, aged garlic extract
   (200mg), Siberian ginseng extract
Premium Kyolic-EPA Gel Caps: Aged
   garlic extract (120mg), fish oil
   (1000mg)

WALLACE **527, 840**
LABORATORIES
Half Acre Road
Cranbury, NJ 08512
Address Inquiries to:
Wallace Laboratories
Div. of Carter-Wallace, Inc.
P.O. Box 1001
Cranbury, NJ 08512
(609) 655-6000
For Medical Emergencies:
(800) 526-3840

OTC Products Available:
◆ Maltsupex Liquid, Powder & Tablets
◆ Ryna Liquid
◆ Ryna-C Liquid
◆ Ryna-CX Liquid

WARNER-LAMBERT **528, 842**
COMPANY
Consumer Health Products Group
201 Tabor Road
Morris Plains, NJ 07950
(See also Warner Wellcome)
Address Inquiries to:
Consumer Affairs

For Consumer Product Information Call:
1-(800) 524-2854
1-(800) 223-0182

OTC Products Available:
◆ Celestial Seasonings Soothers Throat
   Drops
◆ Halls Mentho-Lyptus Cough Suppressant
   Tablets
◆ Maximum Strength Halls Plus Cough
   Suppressant Tablets
◆ Halls Sugar Free Cough Suppressant
   Tablets
◆ Halls Vitamin C Drops
◆ Rolaids Tablets
◆ Rolaids (Calcium Rich/Sodium Free)
   Tablets

WARNER WELLCOME **528, 844**
Consumer HealthCare Products
Warner-Lambert Company
201 Tabor Road
Morris Plains, NJ 07950
(See also Warner-Lambert)
(201) 540-2000
For Product Information call:
1-(800) 524-2624
1-(800) 562-0266
1-(800) 773-1554
1-(800) 547-8374

OTC Products Available:
◆ Actifed Allergy Daytime/Nighttime Caplets
◆ Actifed Plus Caplets
◆ Actifed Plus Tablets
◆ Actifed Sinus Daytime/Nighttime Tablets
   and Caplets
   Actifed Syrup
◆ Actifed Tablets
   Agoral Liquid
◆ Anusol Hemorrhoidal Suppositories

(◆) Shown in Product Identification Guide

WARNER WELLCOME—*cont.*
- ◆ Anusol Ointment
- ◆ Anusol HC-1 Anti-Itch Hydrocortisone Ointment
- ◆ Benadryl Allergy Decongestant Liquid Medication
- ◆ Benadryl Allergy Decongestant Tablets
- ◆ Benadryl Allergy Liquid Medication
- ◆ Benadryl Allergy Kapseals
- ◆ Benadryl Allergy Tablets
- ◆ Benadryl Allergy Sinus Headache Formula Caplets
- ◆ Benadryl Dye-Free Allergy Liqui-gel Softgels
- ◆ Benadryl Dye-Free Allergy Liquid Medication
- ◆ Benadryl Itch Relief Cream, Children's Formula and Maximum Strength 2%
- ◆ Benadryl Itch Relief Spray, Children's Formula and Maximum Strength 2%
- ◆ Benadryl Itch Relief Stick Maximum Strength 2%
- ◆ Benadryl Itch Stopping Gel, Children's Formula and Maximum Strength 2%
- ◆ Benylin Adult Formula Cough Suppressant
- ◆ Benylin Expectorant
- ◆ Benylin Multisymptom
- ◆ Benylin Pediatric Cough Suppressant
- ◆ Borofax Skin Protectant Ointment
- ◆ Caladryl Clear Lotion
- ◆ Caladryl Cream For Kids
- ◆ Caladryl Lotion
- Corn Husker's Lotion
- ◆ e.p.t. Early Pregnancy Test
- Efferdent Antibacterial Denture Cleanser
- Empirin Aspirin Tablets
- ◆ Gelusil Liquid & Tablets
- Lavacol Rubbing Alcohol
- Listerex Acne Medication Lotion
- ◆ Listerine Antiseptic
- ◆ Cool Mint Listerine
- ◆ FreshBurst Listerine
- ◆ Listermint Alcohol-Free Mouthwash
- ◆ Lubriderm Bath and Shower Oil
- ◆ Lubriderm Care Lotion
- ◆ Lubriderm Moisture Recovery Alpha Hydroxy Formula Cream and Lotion
- ◆ Lubriderm Moisture Recovery GelCreme
- ◆ Lubriderm Seriously Sensitive Lotion
- Myadec Tablets
- ◆ Neosporin Ointment
- ◆ Neosporin Plus Maximum Strength Cream
- ◆ Neosporin Plus Maximum Strength Ointment
- ◆ Nix Creme Rinse
- ◆ Polysporin Ointment
- ◆ Polysporin Powder
- Proxacol-Hydrogen Peroxide Solution
- ◆ Replens Vaginal Moisturizer
- ◆ Sinutab Non-Drying Liquid Caps
- ◆ Sinutab Sinus Allergy Medication, Maximum Strength Tablets and Caplets
- ◆ Sinutab Sinus Medication, Maximum Strength Without Drowsiness Formula, Tablets & Caplets
- Sinutab Sinus Medication, Regular Strength Without Drowsiness Formula
- ◆ Sudafed Children's Liquid
- ◆ Sudafed Cold and Cough Liquidcaps
- ◆ Sudafed Cough Syrup
- ◆ Sudafed Plus Liquid
- ◆ Sudafed Plus Tablets
- ◆ Sudafed Severe Cold Formula Caplets
- ◆ Sudafed Severe Cold Formula Tablets
- ◆ Sudafed Sinus Caplets
- ◆ Sudafed Sinus Tablets
- ◆ Sudafed Tablets, 30 mg
- ◆ Sudafed Tablets, 60 mg
- ◆ Sudafed 12 Hour Caplets
- ◆ Tucks Clear Hemorrhoidal Gel
- ◆ Tucks Premoistened Hemorrhoidal/Vaginal Pads
- Tucks Take-Alongs

WELLNESS INTERNATIONAL ..... 865 NETWORK, LTD.
1501 Luna Road, Bldg. 102
Carrollton, TX 75006
Address Inquiries to:
Director, Product Development
(214) 245-1097
FAX (214) 389-3060

OTC Products Available:
Bio-Complex 5000 Gentle Foaming Cleanser
Bio-Complex 5000 Revitalizing Conditioner
Bio-Complex 5000 Revitalizing Shampoo
BioLean
BioLean Accelerator
BioLean LipoTrim
BioLean Meal
Food for Thought
Inches Away
StePHan Bio-Nutritional Daytime Hydrating Creme
StePHan Bio-Nutritional Eye-Firming Concentrate
StePHan Bio-Nutritional Nightime Moisture Creme
StePHan Bio-Nutritional Refreshing Moisture Gel
StePHan Bio-Nutritional Ultra Hydrating Fluid
StePHan Clarity
StePHan Elasticity
StePHan Elixir
StePHan Essential
StePHan Feminine
StePHan Flexibility
StePHan Lovpil
StePHan Masculine
StePHan Protector
StePHan Relief
StePHan Tranquility
Winrgy

WHITEHALL .... 531, 870 LABORATORIES INC.
American Home Products Corporation
Five Giralda Farms
Madison, NJ 07940-0871
Address Inquiries to:
Consumer Affairs
Professional Samples:
(800) 343-0856
Other Information:
(800) 322-3129

OTC Products Available:
- ◆ Advil Cold and Sinus Caplets and Tablets (formerly CoAdvil)
- ◆ Advil Ibuprofen Tablets and Caplets
- Anacin Caplets and Tablets (See A.H. Robins Consumer)
- Maximum Strength Anacin (See A.H. Robins Consumer)
- Aspirin Free Anacin, Maximum Strength (See A.H. Robins Consumer)
- Baby Anbesol
- Grape Baby Anbesol
- Anbesol Gel - Regular Strength
- Anbesol Gel - Maximum Strength
- Anbesol Liquid - Regular Strength
- Anbesol Liquid - Maximum Strength
- Arthritis Pain Formula, Maximum Strength Analgesic Caplets
- Bronitin Mist
- ◆ Clearblue Easy
- ◆ Clearplan Easy
- Compound W Gel
- Compound W Liquid
- Denorex Medicated Shampoo and Conditioner

Denorex Medicated Shampoo, Extra Strength
Denorex Medicated Shampoo, Extra Strength With Conditioners
Denorex Medicated Shampoo, Mountain Fresh Herbal Scent
Dermoplast Anesthetic Pain Relief Lotion
Dermoplast Anesthetic Pain Relief Spray
Dristan Cold Multi-Symptom Tablets
Dristan Maximum Strength Cold Multi-Symptom Gel Caplets
Dristan Maximum Strength Cold Non-Drowsiness Caplets
Dristan Maximum Strength Cold Non-Drowsiness Gel Caplets
Dristan Nasal Spray
Dristan 12-hour Nasal Spray
Dristan Sinus Caplets
Freezone Corn Remover
Heet Liniment
Kerodex Cream 51 (for dry or oily work)
Kerodex Cream 71 (for wet work)
Momentum Backache Formula
Outgro Solution
Oxipor VHC Psoriasis Lotion
Posture 600 mg
Posture-D 600 mg
Preparation H Cleansing Tissues
- ◆ Preparation H Hemorrhoidal Cream
- ◆ Preparation H Hemorrhoidal Ointment
- ◆ Preparation H Hemorrhoidal Suppositories
- ◆ Preparation H Hydrocortisone 1% Cream
- ◆ Primatene Dual Action Formula
- ◆ Primatene Mist
- ◆ Primatene Tablets
- Riopan Suspension
- Riopan Plus Suspension
- Riopan Plus D.S. Suspension
- ◆ Semicid Vaginal Contraceptive Inserts
- Sleep-eze 3 Tablets
- Today Vaginal Contraceptive Sponge

J.B. WILLIAMS .... 532, 875 COMPANY, INC.
65 Harristown Rd
Glen Rock, NJ 07452
Address Inquires To:
Consumer Affairs
1-800-254-8656
201-251-8100
Fax: 201-251-8097
OTC Products Available:
- ◆ Cēpacol Anesthetic Lozenges
- ◆ Cēpacol/Cēpacol Mint Mouthwash/Gargle
- ◆ Cēpacol Dry Throat Lozenges, Cherry Flavor
- ◆ Cēpacol Dry Throat Lozenges, Honey-Lemon Flavor
- ◆ Cēpacol Dry Throat Lozenges, Menthol-Eucalyptus Flavor
- ◆ Cēpacol Dry Throat Lozenges, Original Flavor

WINTHROP CONSUMER PRODUCTS
(See MILES INC)

WYETH-AYERST .... 532, 876 LABORATORIES
Division of American Home Products Corporation
P.O. Box 8299
Philadelphia, PA 19101
Address Inquiries to:
Professional Service: (610) 688-4400
For EMERGENCY Medical Information,
Day or night call: (610) 688-4400
For Medical/Pharmacy inquiries on marketed products call:
(800) 934-5556
8:30 AM to 4:30 PM (Eastern Standard Time)

(◆) Shown in Product Identification Guide

WYETH-AYERST LABORATORIES—*cont.*

WYETH-AYERST DISTRIBUTION CENTERS

(Do not use freight addresses for mailing orders.)

Atlanta, GA—P.O. Box 1773
Paoli, PA 19301-1773
(800) 666-7248
Freight Address:
100 Union Court
Kennesaw, GA 30144
Mail DEA order forms to:
P.O. Box 4365
Atlanta, GA 30302
Chicago, IL—P.O. Box 1773
Paoli, PA 19301-1773
(800) 666-7248
Freight Address:
745 N. Gary Avenue
Carol Stream, IL 60188
Mail DEA order forms to:
P.O. Box 140
Wheaton, IL 60189-0140
Dallas, TX—P.O. Box 1773
Paoli, PA 19301-1773
(800) 666-7248
Freight Address:
11240 Petal Street
Dallas, TX 75238
Mail DEA order forms to:
P.O. Box 650231
Dallas, TX 75265-0231
Hawaii—P.O. Box 1773
Paoli, PA 19301-1773
(800) 666-7248

Mail DEA order forms to:
96-1185 Waihona Street, Unit C1
Pearl City, HI 96782
Los Angeles, CA—P.O. Box 1773
Paoli, PA 19301-1773
(800) 666-7248

Freight Address:
6530 Altura Blvd.
Buena Park, CA 90622
Mail DEA order forms to: P.O. Box 5000
Buena Park, CA 90622-5000
Philadelphia, PA—P.O. Box 1773
Paoli, PA 19301-1773
(800) 666-7248

Freight Address:
31 Morehall Road
Frazer, PA 19355
Mail DEA order forms to:
P.O. Box 61
Paoli, PA 19301
Seattle, WA—P.O. Box 1773
Paoli, PA 19301-1773
(800) 666-7248

Freight Address:
19255 80th Ave. South
Kent, WA 98032
Mail DEA order forms to:
P.O. Box 5609
Kent, WA 98064-5609

OTC Products Available:
- ◆ Aludrox Oral Suspension
- ◆ Amphojel Suspension (Mint Flavor)
- ◆ Amphojel Suspension without Flavor
- ◆ Amphojel Tablets

- ◆ Basaljel Capsules
- ◆ Basaljel Suspension
- ◆ Basaljel Tablets
- ◆ Bonamil
- ◆ Cerose DM
- ◆ Collyrium for Fresh Eyes
- ◆ Collyrium Fresh
- ◆ Donnagel Liquid and Donnagel Chewable Tablets
- ◆ Nursoy, Soy Protein Isolate Formula for Infants, Concentrated Liquid, Ready-to-Feed, and Powder
- ◆ SMA Iron Fortified Infant Formula, Concentrated, Ready-to-Feed and Powder
- ◆ SMA Lo-Iron Infant Formula, Concentrated, Ready-to-Feed, and Powder
- ◆ Stuart Prenatal Tablets
- ◆ Wyanoids Relief Factor Hemorrhoidal Suppositories

ZILA 533, 882
PHARMACEUTICALS, INC.
5227 North 7th Street
Phoenix, AZ 85014-2817
Address Inquiries to:
Ed Pomerantz,
Vice President, Marketing:
(602) 266-6700

OTC Products Available:
DermaFlex Topical Anesthetic Gel
PeriGel Toothpaste
- ◆ Zilactin Medicated Gel
- ◆ Zilactin-B Medicated Gel with Benzocaine
- ◆ Zilactin-L Liquid

(◆) Shown in Product Identification Guide

MEDICAL ECONOMICS

SECTION 2

PRODUCT NAME INDEX

This index includes all entries in the "Product Information" section. Products are listed alphabetically by brand name.

If two page numbers appear, the first refers to the product's photograph, the second to its prescribing information.

- **Bold page numbers** indicate full prescribing information.

- *Italic page numbers* signify partial information.

Italic Page Number Indicates Brief Listing

Italic Page Number Indicates Brief Listing

Italic Page Number Indicates Brief Listing

Italic Page Number Indicates Brief Listing

Italic Page Number Indicates Brief Listing

Italic Page Number Indicates Brief Listing

Italic Page Number Indicates Brief Listing

Italic Page Number Indicates Brief Listing

Italic Page Number Indicates Brief Listing

Italic Page Number Indicates Brief Listing

SECTION 3

PRODUCT CATEGORY INDEX

This index cross-references each brand by prescribing category. All entries in the "Product Information" section are included. In each category, all fully described products are listed first, followed by those with only partial descriptions.

If two page numbers appear, the first refers to the product's photograph, the second to its prescribing information.

• **Bold page numbers** indicate full prescribing information.

• *Italic page numbers* signify partial information.

The categories employed in this index were established by the OTC Review process of the United States Food and Drug Administration. Classification of products within these categories has been determined in cooperation with the products' manufacturers or, when necessary, by the publisher alone.

A

ACNE PRODUCTS
(see
DERMATOLOGICALS, ACNE PREPARATIONS)

ALLERGY RELIEF PRODUCTS
(see COLD & COUGH PREPARATIONS; NASAL
SPRAYS; OPHTHALMIC PREPARATIONS)

ANALGESICS
ACETAMINOPHEN & COMBINATIONS
Actifed Plus Caplets
(WARNER WELLCOME) **528, 845**
Actifed Plus Tablets
(WARNER WELLCOME) **528, 845**
Arthritis Foundation Aspirin Free
Caplets (McNeil Consumer) .. **511, 673**
Arthritis Foundation NightTime
Caplets (McNeil Consumer) .. **511, 674**
Bayer Select Headache Pain
Relief Formula
(Miles Consumer) **515, 716**
Bayer Select Menstrual
Multi-Symptom Formula
(Miles Consumer) **516, 716**
Bayer Select Night Time Pain
Relief Formula
(Miles Consumer) **516, 716**
Aspirin Free Excedrin Analgesic
Caplets
(Bristol-Myers Products) **504, 618**
Excedrin Extra-Strength Analgesic
Tablets & Caplets
(Bristol-Myers Products) **505, 619**
Excedrin P.M. Analgesic/Sleeping
Aid Tablets, Caplets, Liquigels
(Bristol-Myers Products) **504, 620**
Maximum Strength
Multi-Symptom Formula Midol
(Miles Consumer) **517, 722**

PMS Multi-Symptom Formula
Midol (Miles Consumer) **517, 723**
Teen Multi-Symptom Formula
Midol (Miles Consumer) **517, 722**
Panodol Tablets and Caplets
(SmithKline Beecham
Consumer) **525, 824**
Children's Panadol Chewable
Tablets, Liquid, infant's Drops
(SmithKline Beecham
Consumer) **525, 824**
Percogesic Analgesic Tablets
(Procter & Gamble) **754**
Children's TYLENOL
acetaminophen Chewable
Tablets, Elixir, Suspension
Liquid
(McNeil Consumer) **512, 679**
Infant's TYLENOL acetaminophen
Drops and Suspension Drops
(McNeil Consumer) **512, 679**
TYLENOL Extended Relief Caplets
(McNeil Consumer) **513, 684**
TYLENOL, Extra Strength,
acetaminophen Adult Liquid
Pain Reliever (McNeil
Consumer) **513, 684**
TYLENOL, Extra Strength,
acetaminophen Gelcaps,
Caplets, Tablets, Geltabs
(McNeil Consumer) **513, 687**
TYLENOL, Extra Strength,
Heacache Plus Pain Reliever
with Antacid Caplets
(McNeil Consumer) **514, 685**
TYLENOL, Junior Strength,
acetaminophen Coated
Caplets, and Chewable
Tablets
(McNeil Consumer) **512, 688**
TYLENOL Maximum Strength Flu
Gelcaps
(McNeil Consumer) **513, 692**

TYLENOL Maximum Strength Flu
NightTime Gelcaps
(McNeil Consumer) **513, 694**
TYLENOL Maximum Strength Flu
NightTime Hot Medication
Packets (McNeil Consumer) .. **513, 693**
TYLENOL, Regular Strength,
acetaminophen Caplets and
Tablets (McNeil Consumer).... **513, 699**
TYLENOL PM Extra Strength Pain
Reliever/Sleep Aid Gelcaps,
Caplets, Geltabs
(McNeil Consumer) **514, 686**
Unisom With Pain Relief-Nighttime
Sleep Aid and Pain Reliever
(Pfizer Consumer) **745**
Vanquish Analgesic Caplets
(Miles Consumer) **518, 731**
ACETAMINOPHEN WITH ANTACIDS
TYLENOL, Extra Strength,
Heacache Plus Pain Reliever
with Antacid Caplets
(McNeil Consumer) **514, 685**
ASPIRIN
Arthritis Foundation Safety
Coated Aspirin Tablets
(McNeil Consumer) **511, 675**
Bayer Children's Chewable
Aspirin (Miles Consumer) **515, 711**
Genuine Bayer Aspirin Tablets &
Caplets (Miles Consumer)...... **515, 713**
Extra Strength Bayer Arthritis Pain
Regimen Formula
(Miles Consumer) **515, 711**
Extra Strength Bayer Aspirin
Caplets & Tablets
(Miles Consumer) **515, 712**
Extended-Release Bayer 8-Hour
Aspirin (Miles Consumer) **515, 712**
Extra Strength Bayer PM Aspirin
(Miles Consumer) **515, 713**

Italic Page Number **Indicates Brief Listing**

Italic Page Number **Indicates Brief Listing**

Italic Page Number **Indicates Brief Listing**

Italic Page Number **Indicates Brief Listing**

Italic Page Number **Indicates Brief Listing**

Italic Page Number **Indicates Brief Listing**

Italic Page Number **Indicates Brief Listing**

Italic Page Number **Indicates Brief Listing**

Italic Page Number **Indicates Brief Listing**

Italic Page Number **Indicates Brief Listing**

Italic Page Number **Indicates Brief Listing**

Italic Page Number **Indicates Brief Listing**

Italic Page Number **Indicates Brief Listing**

Italic Page Number **Indicates Brief Listing**

Italic Page Number **Indicates Brief Listing**

Italic Page Number **Indicates Brief Listing**

Italic Page Number **Indicates Brief Listing**

SECTION 4

ACTIVE INGREDIENTS INDEX

This index cross-references each brand by its generic ingredients. All entries in the "Product Information" section are included. Under each generic heading, all fully described products are listed first, followed by those with only partial descriptions.

If two page numbers appear, the first refers to the product's photograph, the second to its prescribing information.

- **Bold page numbers** indicate full prescribing information.

- *Italic page numbers* signify partial information.

Classification of products under these headings has been determined in cooperation with the products' manufacturers or, if necessary, by the publisher alone.

Italic Page Number **Indicates Brief Listing**

Italic Page Number **Indicates Brief Listing**

Italic Page Number **Indicates Brief Listing**

Italic Page Number **Indicates Brief Listing**

Italic Page Number **Indicates Brief Listing**

Italic Page Number **Indicates Brief Listing**

Italic Page Number **Indicates Brief Listing**

Italic Page Number **Indicates Brief Listing**

Italic Page Number **Indicates Brief Listing**

Italic Page Number **Indicates Brief Listing**

Italic Page Number **Indicates Brief Listing**

Italic Page Number **Indicates Brief Listing**

Italic Page Number **Indicates Brief Listing**

Italic Page Number **Indicates Brief Listing**

Italic Page Number **Indicates Brief Listing**

Italic Page Number **Indicates Brief Listing**

Italic Page Number **Indicates Brief Listing**

NONPRESCRIPTION DRUGS: THEIR IMPACT AND USE

Each year, Americans spend over $13 billion on non-prescription drugs, an amount that increases by 8 percent to 10 percent annually. This growth is fueled in part by two important trends: the self-care movement and an increase in the number of OTC (over-the-counter) products, mainly through Rx-to-OTC switches and product line extensions. It's important for physicians and pharmacists to be aware of these trends, and to understand how and why patients use OTCs. Because consumers turn to you as a drug expert, you play a critical role in providing counseling on the safe and effective use of medications. The information and guidance you provide can help lead to positive outcomes and help prevent costly and potentially harmful drug misuse by your patients.

This chapter is designed to help you more thoroughly understand the nonprescription drug market and the drugs themselves.

The first section, "The Changing OTC Market," discusses the growth of the OTC marketplace and factors contributing to this increase, including:

■ the growing self-care movement among consumers;
■ the increasing availability of new products and categories of products, mainly due to Rx-to-OTC switches;
■ the cost effectiveness of OTCs in the face of rising health care costs.

The second part, "Consumer Perceptions and OTC Use," focuses on how consumers perceive and use OTCs, the effect of demographics on OTC utilization, and sales volumes by product category.

Section three, "Establishing Safety and Effectiveness," provides an overview of the approval process for OTC and switched products, as well as labeling, packaging, and marketing regulations.

"Patient Counseling: A Critical Role for Physicians and Pharmacists" outlines the growing need for patient counseling on OTC use, and explains how you can help fill this critical information gap. The effect of OTCs on physicians' and pharmacists' practices is also covered.

Finally, "The Future of OTCs" examines trends and issues that are likely to affect the nonprescription drug industry into the next century, as well as likely sources of future drugs and the kinds of new drugs that may soon become available over-the-counter.

Chapter 1: The Changing OTC Market

Most medications used in the United States today are nonprescription, or over-the-counter (OTC), drugs. In fact, six of every ten medications bought in the U.S. are nonprescription. Studies show that the rate of OTC use is steadily increasing, fueling market growth of eight percent to ten percent each year.

There are a number of factors propelling this growth, including a growing number of new products and classes of products, heightened interest among consumers in their own care, and a national health care agenda geared toward controlling costs. Indeed, the relatively low cost of OTCs contributes greatly to their success. For despite the wide use of nonprescription drugs (accounting for 30 percent of all drug expenditures), total spending for OTC medications takes less than two cents of the U.S. health care dollar. Over-the-counter drugs are thus one of the most cost-effective segments of health care.

These forces, combined with the overall safety and efficacy of the drugs, mean that OTC drugs will likely only increase in importance to consumers and manufacturers. U.S. and global sales figures support this.

Worldwide, OTC sales reached $32.5 billion in 1993. In the U.S. in 1993, nonprescription drugs were a $13.3 billion industry. Nonprescription drugs represent a growing market as well. Sales in the U.S. increased 40 percent between 1986 and 1991. In both 1992 and 1993, worldwide OTC sales increased by over $1 billion.

What Is an OTC?

Under current law, there are only two classes of drugs available on the market: OTC's—those safe for consumers to use on the basis of their labeling alone—and Rx—those that cannot be used safely without a physician's prescription.

To be marketed in the U.S., an OTC must be effective for its intended use and provide a margin of safety when used as directed.

Differences between OTC and Rx Drugs

Generally, OTC drugs pose minimum risk and possess a higher safety profile than Rx drugs, which are typically more toxic and defined as safe in the context of specific benefit-risk ratios. Another important distinction between the two classes of drugs is that OTCs are used to treat complaints or illnesses for which users recognize their own symptoms and level of relief; conditions treated by Rx drugs are usually more difficult to self-assess.

Nonprescription drugs differ from prescription drugs in other ways as well:

■ Labeling for an OTC, unlike an Rx, must, by law, provide all the information a consumer needs for safe and effective use.

■ OTC drugs are advertised directly to consumers, whereas Rx medications have traditionally been marketed to health professionals. This distinction is blurring, however, as drug companies make use of "institutional" advertising to alert consumers about prescription products with the recommendation to "ask your doctor." Common examples are advertisements for such Rx products as Rogaine and Seldane. These ads are strictly regulated and restricted in what they can tell consumers.

■ OTCs are far more numerous than Rx drugs. There are about 300,000 OTC drugs (including different package sizes, dose strengths, and forms) currently on the market. Prescription drugs, on the other hand, number about 65,000.

A Brief History of the Two-Class System

The Federal Food, Drug, and Cosmetic Act (passed in 1938) is the primary law governing drugs sold in the U.S. The act prohibits the sale of drugs that are contaminated, misbranded, or otherwise dangerous to health; establishes minimum standards of strength, quality, and purity; and sets up specifications for labeling. According to this law, a drug is suitable for nonprescription use if it is not habit-forming and can be used safely by laymen without professional supervision.

The 1938 legislation, however, left it to drug manufacturers to make the distinction, and it wasn't until 1951 that federal law set up specific standards for determining whether or not a drug should be sold on a prescription-only basis. The 1951 Durham-Humphrey amendments established a consumer's right to self-treatment with safe and effective OTCs. It also stated that if a drug is safe and effective, and if labeling can be written so that a consumer may use it without professional supervision, it must be available over-the-counter.

Prescription drugs, on the other hand, were defined by the 1951 amendment as:

■ certain habit-forming drugs (listed by name in the act);
■ drugs not safe for use except under a physician's supervision because of toxicity or other potential harmful effects, the method of use, or other measures necessary to use;
■ drugs limited to prescription use under a new drug application.

Today, the Food and Drug Administration (FDA) through its various divisions, review boards, and committees devoted to OTCs, reviews data required to establish safety, effectiveness, and proper labeling for OTCs and approves proposed manufacturer labeling. (The approval process and safety and efficacy of OTCs are discussed in more detail later.)

Self-Care, Self-Medication

The self-care movement is one of the prime movers behind the rise of OTCs. Americans want more control over their own health, and studies show that they are more involved in their own care, a trend that is leading to better lifestyle choices and a growing awareness of preventive measures. Not surprisingly, today's consumer is also better informed about health issues than previous generations.

According to a survey published in the pharmacy news publication *Drug Topics,* nearly all consumers say they practice self-medication at some time; and over three-quarters do so frequently (see figure 1).

Figure 1
Frequency with which Americans Practice Self-Care

Frequency	% of Consumer
Frequently	76%
Occasionally	17%
Rarely	4%
Never	1%
No Response	2%

Source: Gannon, K., "Exclusive Consumer OTC Survey: Who's Buying What" *Drug Topics,* January 8, 1990.

And that trend is growing: A quarter of those polled said they self-medicate more now than in the past (see figure 2).

Figure 2
The Trend toward Self-Care

Increase in Self-Care	% of Consumers
Substantial Increase	13%
Increase	13%
No Change	66%
Decrease	5%
No Response	3%

Source: Gannon, K., "Exclusive Consumer OTC Survey: Who's Buying What" *Drug Topics,* January 8, 1990.

Over-the-counter medications play an important role in this self-care movement. A survey of over 1,500 Americans conducted by the Heller Research Group examined how consumers handle common health complaints. It revealed that the average person suffers six common health problems in any given two-week period, and over one-third (38 percent) of these are treated with an OTC (see figure 3).

Figure 3
Treatment of Common Health Complaints with OTCs

Treatment	1983	1992
Treated with an OTC	35%	38%
Not treated	37%	30%
Treated with home remedy	14%	16%
Treated with previous Rx	11%	13%
Sought professional help	9%	17%

Source: Heller Research Group. "Self-Medication in the 90s: Practices and Perceptions." New York, 1992

Nonprescription drugs are therefore the most common alternative used by consumers to treat everyday ailments. The trend toward self-care may also be accelerated as the average age of the population increases. Certainly, the "aging of America" and a concomitant increase in chronic health problems will have an impact on OTC use. The elderly, in particular, rely on cost-effective treatment options as their incomes shrink and their health complaints proliferate with age.

The Heller study also showed that consumers are achieving healthier lifestyles. It said, for example, that Americans are changing the way they eat by adopting diets that are lower in fat and cholesterol. Consumers are also smoking less, exercising more and taking more vitamins and other dietary supplements.

Cost-Effectiveness of OTCs

One of the main benefits of over-the-counter drugs is their relatively low cost, a factor that has contributed greatly to their success and growing popularity in the marketplace. This relative low cost has also generated significant savings within the health care system. It's estimated, for example, that OTCs saved the nation $10.5 billion in health care costs in 1987 alone. This figure includes savings on prescription drugs, doctor visits, lost work time, insurance costs, and travel. Today, OTCs are estimated to save $20 billion each year. These numbers take on even greater significance when they are considered in the context of rising health care costs.

In 1991, total health care expenditures topped $750 billion or 13 percent of all national spending on goods and services (GNP) for that year. By 1993, health care costs reached an astounding $903 billion. Of that amount, however, over-the-counter drugs accounted for a tiny portion—$13 billion, or less than two cents of each U.S. health care dollar. And while other health care costs have risen dramatically year after year, OTC prices have increased by 4 percent or less each year since 1986 (excluding 1989, when prices jumped 5 percent).

The low cost of OTCs makes them very attractive to consumers, who are concerned with both costs and health. In fact, a typical OTC costs the consumer

Figure 4

The OTC Market in 1993, by Product Category

Category	Dollar Sales (in thousands)	% Change over previous year
Internal analgesics	$2,722,443	6.2
Cold/sinus/cough drops	2,080,191	13.4
Vitamins	1,668,896	17.3
Miscellaneous remedies	830,479	3.7
Antacids	824,555	4.8
Laxatives	739,763	6.0
Cold/allergy/sinus powder	492,497	9.4
Cough syrup	462,140	10.3
Nasal spray	348,805	4.9
External analgesic rubs	193,905	4.0
Miscellaneous remedy tablets	192,509	16.9
Miscellaneous health treatments	184,630	0.1
Miscellaneous health tablets	150,394	(0.1)

Source: Information Resources Inc., Chicago, 1994

less than $4, compared with $24 for an average prescription drug. In addition, consumers spend only about $47 a year on OTCs. According to a Nielsen Marketing Research study done in 1993, it costs only 11 cents to treat a headache with one dose of an OTC, 12 cents to relieve an upset stomach, and 20 cents per dose to fight symptoms of a cold or cough. These economical alternatives give consumers a wide range of choice as they seek to control their own health and health-care decisions.

Increasing Number of OTCs

Increased use of OTCs by health- and cost-conscious consumers is not the only factor driving the OTC market. The number and variety of OTCs are also swelling.

Today, there are about 300,000 different OTC products being marketed in the United States. The array changes constantly in response to shifting demographics, outbreaks of flu and other communicable conditions, and consumer trends and perceptions.

Even though the market is subject to rapid change, the latest research gives some indication of how it is carved up (see figure 4). Internal analgesics lead the field in OTC sales, accounting for $2.7 billion in sales in 1993. Other high-volume product categories are cold/sinus/cough drops ($2.0 billion), vitamins ($1.7 billion), antacids ($825.5 million),

and laxatives ($739.7 million). Those product categories showing the greatest increase over the previous year include vitamins (17 percent), cold/sinus/cough drops (13 percent), and cough syrup (10 percent).

One important sales trend gaining momentum—and providing consumers with even more OTC alternatives—is the private label. These are OTC products sold under a store name and generally offered at competitive prices. In 1991, private labels accounted for 10 percent of total drugstore Health and Beauty Care sales, and in some categories of products, up to 13 percent of sales.

Impact of Rx-to-OTC Switching

Another important trend in the growing OTC market is the fairly new practice of switching prescription drugs to OTC status. This process makes entire new categories of treatments available to consumers without a prescription.

Although many new drugs have been introduced since World War II, virtually all have been marketed as prescription drugs. Then, about a decade ago, the FDA adopted a policy of switching drugs from prescription to OTC status. This policy has had a tremendous impact on the OTC market, with 52 ingredients or dosages switched to OTC status and over 25 more pending. Today, more than 450 OTC products use ingredients and dosages available by prescription-only 15 years ago. And more than 70 petitions from manufacturers to switch ingredients are expected in the next five years.

Important recent switches include topical hydrocortisone, antihistamines, and analgesics, including ibuprofen and naproxen. Figure 5 shows other products that are likely candidates for a future OTC switch.

Figure 5
CANDIDATES FOR FUTURE OTC SWITCH

Category: Cold, Allergy, Sinus, and Asthma

Active Ingredient	Description	Product Examples	Manufacturers
Albuterol	Bronchodilator	Proventil Ventolin	Schering-Plough Glaxo
Cromolyn sodium	Anti-allergy	Intal Nasalcrom	Fisons Fisons
Loratadine	Non-sedating antihistamine	Claritin	Schering-Plough
Theophylline	Bronchodilator	Theo-Dur	Key

Category: Analgesics

Active Ingredient	Description	Product Examples	Manufacturers
Diflunisal	NSAID	Dolobid	J&J-Merck
Indomethacin	NSAID	Indocin	J&J-Merck
Piroxicam	NSAID	Feldene	Pfizer
Sulindac	NSAID	Clinoril	J&J-Merck

Category: Gastrointestinal Drugs

Active Ingredient	Description	Product Examples	Manufacturers
Cimetidine	Anti-ulcer	Tagamet	SmithKline Beecham
Famotidine	Anti-ulcer	Pepcid	J&J-Merck
Nizatidine	Anti-ulcer	Axid	Whitehall Labs
Ranitidine (HCl)	Anti-ulcer	Zantac	Glaxo, Sandoz
Sucralfate	Anti-ulcer	Carafate	MMD

Category: Antifungals and Antiinfectives

Active Ingredient	Description	Product Examples	Manufacturers
Econazole	Antifungal	Spectazole	Ortho
Ketoconazole	Antifungal	Nizoral	Janssen
Methenamine mandelate	Urinary tract infection	Mandelamine	Parke-Davis
Nystatin	Anti-fungal	Mycostatin	BMS

Category: Other

Active Ingredient	Description	Product Examples	Manufacturers
Carisoprodol	Muscle relaxant	Soma	Wallace Laboratories
Cyclobenzaprine HCl	Muscle relaxant	Flexeril	J&J-Merck
Cholestyramine	Cholesterol-lowering	Cholybar	Parke-Davis
Nicotine polacrilex	Smoking -cessation	Nicorette	MMD
Sulfacetamide sodium	Ocular anti-infective	Bleph-10 Sulamyd	Allergan Schering-Plough
Minoxidil	Hair loss treatment	Rogaine	Upjohn

Source: FIND/SVP Inc. "The Market for Rx-to-OTC Switches." September, 1993.

Effect of Switching on Costs and Care

The range of health problems that can be treated with OTCs has grown dramatically in the last ten years, and switches have played an important role in this growth. Consumers are very aware of these newly available switched products. They perceive them as strong, cost-effective medications. According to the Heller survey, close to 60 percent of consumers say they believe switches make it possible for them to save money, and almost two-thirds (64 percent) say they favor the process of Rx to OTC switching. Consumers also said that they buy more switches, by a margin of two to one, when they are available.

The effect of switches on health care costs has also been tremendous. For example, the net annual savings from the switch of cough-cold medicines to OTC status is estimated at about three-quarters of a billion dollars. Another example is the 1979 switch of 1/2 percent hydrocortisone that saved American consumers more than $1 billion in the first three years after the change.

The Line Extension Strategy

Line extensions are another important strategy that drug makers are using to bring new products to the shelves of the nation's 750,000 OTC outlets, pharmacies, supermarkets, convenience stores, and mass merchandisers. This is the practice of extending an established brand name to an entire line of nonprescription products. Thus, an extra-strength or non-drowsy formulation may be marketed under a pre-existing product name. The success of this practice is based on the trust that consumers develop for specific brand names leading them to purchase other products with the same brand name.

The FDA, however, has expressed concern about whether this proliferation of products confuses consumers. The Nonprescription Drug Manufacturers Association (NDMA), a Washington, DC-based trade association representing OTC makers, claims that line extensions are useful to consumers, since they offer new solutions and more choices for common complaints. It cites, for example, the use of clear labeling and explanatory advertising to prevent confusion about line extensions and other new products, and also points to a growing number of published guides to medications and self-care, such as *PDR for Nonprescription Drugs.*

Chapter 2: Consumer Perceptions and OTC Use

Studies that have explored the ways consumers use and perceive nonprescription medicines shed light on the following issues:

■ Americans' use of OTCs in comparison to other nationalities;

■ OTCs as serious medicine;

■ Safety and correctness of nonprescription drug use;

■ Effect of age, sex, and economic status on self-medication habits;

■ Product choice and availability;

■ Impact of the rise of managed care and the national movement toward health care reform.

Important and far-reaching trends in these areas may be changing the way nonprescription—and prescription—drugs are used. In addition, the role that physicians and pharmacists play in the use of OTCs is paramount, and is discussed in a separate section.

Use Highest in the U.S.

Americans use more OTCs than people in other countries, according to a study comparing 14 national surveys on self-medication (see figure 1). The review ascribes this usage to the fact that the U.S. is the only country lacking a national health care program. It concludes: "Many U.S. citizens must pay for both doctor visits and prescription medicines; others [U.S. citizens] must pay a percentage of these costs. As a result, for common conditions, many Americans consider self-treatment with over-the-counter medicines a cost-saving alternative to doctor visits and prescription drugs."

Figure 1
Use of OTCs for Common Health Complaints: A Worldwide Comparison

Country	Percent of Consumers Using OTCs
United States	33%
Australia	28%
Germany	28%
Spain	24%
United Kingdom	24%
Sweden	24%
Switzerland	22%
Mexico	21%
Italy	20%
Japan	16%

Source: World Federation of Proprietary Medicine Manufacturers. "Health Care, Self-Care and Self-Medication" 1991

Other consumer surveys bear out the importance of cost. In a national Gallup poll, nearly half of those surveyed cited low cost as the greatest advantage to using an OTC. Other important features are convenience (cited by 29 percent) and the fact that OTCs eliminate the need for a doctor's visit (23 percent).

Conditions for which OTCs are used are similar throughout the world. In all countries surveyed, the common cold is the most frequently reported ailment for which OTCs are used, followed by headache, digestive problems, and body aches and pains.

Satisfied Customers

OTCs can treat or cure about 400 different common health complaints. The average consumer reports suffering from about six of these every two weeks, ranging from headaches, which are treatable with an OTC according to more than three-quarters of consumers (76 percent), to dry skin and sinus problems (56 percent and 54 percent respectively) (see figure 2). By category, respiratory and feminine complaints are most likely to be treated with a nonprescription medication (see figure 3).

Figure 2
Top Ten Problems Most Likely to be Treated with OTCs

Complaint	Percent Who Would Treat with OTCs
Headache	76%
Athlete's foot	69%
Lip problems	68%
Common cold	63%
Chronic dandruff	59%
Pre-menstrual	58%
Menstrual	57%
Upset Stomach	57%
Painful/dry skin	56%
Sinus problems	54%

Source: Heller Research Group. "Self-Medication in the 90s: Practices and Perceptions." New York, 1992

Figure 3
Major Categories for which OTCs are used

Condition	Percent Treated with OTCs
Respiratory	50%
Feminine	50%
Pain	46%
Digestive	44%
Eye/ear/mouth	41%
Skin	33%
General well being	8%

Source: Heller Research Group. "Self Medication in the 90s: Practices and perceptions." New York, 1992

American consumers also say that OTCs are effective treatment for these conditions. Americans are, in fact, more satisfied with OTCs than consumers in other countries (see figure 4). Of all 14 countries surveyed, the U.S. had the highest level of satisfaction with nonprescription drugs.

Figure 4
Percentage of Consumers, by Country, who are Satisfied with OTCs.

Country	%
United States	92%
Mexico	90%
United Kingdom	83%
Canada	80%
Australia	75%

Source: World Federation of Proprietary Medicine Manufacturers. "Health Care, Self-Care and Self-Medication" 1991

In a survey conducted in the U.S., 94 percent of those surveyed said they would retake OTCs they've used previously, and more than nine out of ten reported that they were satisfied with the products they had used. Indeed, nearly three-quarters of Americans say they believe OTCs are as effective as prescription medications.

Finally, studies have also probed the reasons consumers stop taking an OTC. Ninety percent of those surveyed said they discontinued use because the problem went away. Only 3 percent said they used a medicine that did not work.

The Safe Use of OTCs

No drug is completely safe, and consumers have shown that they appreciate the potential risk of taking any medication. In one survey, 94 percent of American consumers said that care must be used when taking medications, even those that are not prescription drugs. Ninety-five percent disagreed with the statement that "it is safe to take as many OTCs as you wish."

Over-medication with nonprescription drugs is rare among consumers. According to the Heller study, seven out of ten respondents prefer to fight symptoms without taking medications at all, and nine out of ten said they know all medications should only be used when absolutely necessary. In the same survey, 85 percent said it is nonetheless important to have nonprescription medications available to help relieve minor medical problems.

Americans rate second only to residents of the UK when it comes to reading the label before using an OTC, according to national surveys. Ninety-six percent of U.S. consumers said they read OTC labels, compared with 97 percent in the U.K. Many U.S. studies have confirmed this fact, reporting percentages ranging from 88 percent to 93 percent.

National surveys also show that:

■ Americans generally take less than the maximum recommended daily dose when using OTC analgesics. (For colds, menstruation, and headache, the average number of tablets taken ranges from four to six; for arthritis, rheumatism, and backache, the average number taken each day of use is five);
■ Nearly all OTCs are used for considerably less time than the standard ten-day limit-of-use warning;
■ Consumer knowledge about OTCs is more accurate than consumer knowledge of many other areas, including banking, nutrition, and insurance. In comparative studies, consumers show a solid understanding, with scores of 75 percent or higher, for over half of the drug questions;
■ Consumers read labels more carefully now than in the past.

Demographics of OTC Use

The way consumers approach self-medication with a nonprescription drug is affected by age, sex, and economic status, among other factors.

For example, the level of OTC use remains fairly constant with age, although younger consumers tend to use OTCs for acute conditions, whereas the elderly turn to them more often for chronic conditions.

The level of usage and conditions for which OTCs are used do differ with gender. Women not only buy more OTCs than men, they also use them more and use them to treat different types of conditions. Women take OTCs for anxiety, indigestion and stom-

Figure 5
Recent Additions to the OTC Market

Ingredient	Category	Products
Clemastine fumarate	Antihistamine	Tavist-1
Clemastine fumarate with phenylpropanolamine HCl	Antihistamine/decongestant	Tavist -D
Clotrimazole	Anticandidal	Gyne-Lotrimin, Mycelex-7
Hydrocortisone acetate	Antipruritic	Anusol, Caldecort
Miconazole nitrate	Anticandidal	Monistat 7
Naphazoline HCl with pheniramine maleate	Antihistamine/decongestant eye drop	Opcon A
Naproxen	Internal analgesic/antipyretic	Aleve
Permethrin	Pediculicide	Nix

Source: Nonprescription Drug Manufacturers Association, 1994

ach complaints, headaches, fatigue, sleep problems, arthritis, lip and skin conditions, and weight control. Among men, OTCs are used predominantly for aches and pains, cuts, and colds.

Economic status also affects how OTCs are used. Americans covered by Medicaid, for example, are less likely to take an OTC. They are more likely to seek a physician's care or use a prescription medication that is already in the home.

Increasing Product Choices

New categories and forms of OTCs in the market also affect consumer's self-medication choices. New drugs and whole new categories of products provide consumers with a growing number of effective alternatives for self-care. These new entities also increase the importance of physicians and pharmacists as OTC counselors.

Most of today's new nonprescription drugs contain ingredients that have recently been switched to OTC status. (Examples of these new OTCs are listed in figure 5.) And as noted above, consumer acceptance of switches is exceptionally high. For example, two feminine antifungal ingredients—clotrimazole and miconazole nitrate—became available over-the-counter in 1991. These products, which provide women with an entirely new class of over-the-counter remedies for treating vaginal infections, accounted for about 90 percent of Health and Beauty Care new-

item sales volume in drugstores and other outlets in the year they appeared on the market.

The high use of switched products by consumers is also strongly demonstrated by a survey of top-selling OTCs. In 1992, 14 of the 15 best-selling OTCs introduced since 1975 were either switched brands or switch-related products, as shown in figure 6.

Figure 6
Consumer Preference for Switched Products

In 1992, 14 of the 15 best selling OTCs introduced since 1975 were either switched brands or switch-related products.

Product	1992 Sales (in millions)
Advil	$320
Monistat 7	114
Benadryl	92
Sudafed	92
Motrin IB*	87
Imodium AD	85
Dimetapp	77
Nuprin	67
Afrin	62
Gyne-Lotrimin	53
Oxy-line	52
Drixoral	49
Chlor-Trimeton	44
Actifed	44
Comtrex**	35

*Switch-related
**New proprietary product
Source: Sudler & Hennessy, New York, 1992

Effects of Health Care Reform and Managed Care

Two trends that have affected every segment of health care delivery are health care reform and managed care. Since these trends are still evolving, their impact on the OTC market cannot yet be determined, but some outcomes can reasonably be projected.

Managed care probably has less of a direct effect on the use of OTCs than on other segments of health care since most third-party health care plans do not include coverage for nonprescription drugs. By contrast, prescription drugs are often closely managed by the use of drug formularies through financial incentives to members to use less expensive products, mail order pharmacies, and generics; and through drug utilization review. Nonetheless, because of the cost-effectiveness of OTCs, it is likely that their use will increase as health care costs rise and efforts to contain costs are exerted by payers and national reform programs. Self-medication will most likely be recognized as part of the solution to the problems of rising costs and limited access.

Managed care may also increase OTC use in another indirect way. Managed care typically uses capitated plans in which physicians and pharmacists are paid a flat rate per member by the managed care administrator, regardless of the amount of care provided. Plan members may also be given financial incentives to use fewer plan services. As a result, both providers and plan members often have an incentive to contain costs and use fewer of the medical services and products covered by the plan. Self-medication may therefore become more accepted and encouraged under this type of managed care reimbursement system.

By contrast, traditional fee-for-service health insurance plans provide reimbursement based on utilization rates. Under this system, self-care is, in effect, a form of competition for physicians and pharmacists since it decreases office visits and prescription drug use.

In addition, although most consumers are not reimbursed by health insurance companies for OTCs, nonprescription drugs nonetheless generally end up costing less than a prescription since the copay and/or deductible on an Rx drug usually exceeds the average price of an OTC.

Finally, health care reform, in an effort to make health care affordable and accessible, may also encourage the process of switching Rx products to over-the-counter status. In fact, experts predict that this trend may put a high number of new OTC products on the market in the near future.

Chapter 3: Establishing Safety and Effectiveness

Every over-the-counter medication marketed in the U.S. must meet rigorous safety and efficacy standards set by the Food and Drug Administration (FDA). Manufacturers are required by law to follow strict labeling, packaging, and advertising regulations. In addition, the industry has created voluntary standards and specific guidelines for many aspects of product safety and effective use. The high safety profile and effectiveness that consumers count on in OTC medicines are thus the result of a collaborative effort between the government and the pharmaceutical industry.

History of Government Regulation

The first U.S. drug law—the Food and Drugs Act of 1906—required only that drug products meet standards of purity and strength. Under this law, fraudulent labeling was the only basis for removing a product from the market and even in these cases, the burden of proof rested with the government.

In 1938, the more comprehensive Federal Food, Drug, and Cosmetic Act was passed. The legislation followed closely on the heels of a tragedy in which 107 people, mostly children, were poisoned by "elixir sulfanilamide," which contained ethylene glycol, a colorless syrupy alcohol used as an antifreeze in heating and cooling systems. The new law required drug companies to demonstrate the safety of all new products—before they were marketed. This was to be accomplished by making the drug meet the preapproval requirements of a new drug application (NDA). (Pre-existing drugs were grandfathered in under the new law.) The legislation also eliminated the need for the government to show intent to defraud in cases of mislabeling; provided tolerances for necessary poisonous substances; authorized factory inspections; and added court injunctions to existing seizure and prosecution provisions for violators.

It wasn't until 1951 that certain drugs were required to be labeled as prescription only. The Durham-Humphrey Amendments were added to federal law to provide for those medications that are unsafe to take without a physician's supervision. The amendments state that if a drug is safe and effective and can be labeled for use without professional supervision, it must be available over-the-counter.

OTC Drug Review

Providing evidence of safety prior to marketing was therefore required as early as 1938. However, it wasn't until 1962 that proof of efficacy was required as well. In that year, another amendment to the 1938 law required manufacturers to prove the effectiveness of a drug before it is marketed. Shortly thereafter, the FDA contracted for a review of all drugs, including OTCs that had been grandfathered in by the 1938 law. After 512 OTCs were evaluated, 75 percent were found to lack evidence of effectiveness. As a result, the FDA broadened its review to include all OTC products.

The FDA Division of OTC Evaluation chose to review the 700 or so active ingredients found in OTCs, rather than each of the 300,000 products on the market. This effort, which is still in progress, consists of classifying nonprescription drugs into 81 treatment categories (antacids, internal analgesics, etc.), and evaluating all the active ingredients in those categories in order to establish dosage and labeling regulations for each of them.

In the case of multiple indications or dosages, the ingredients are covered in more than one category. Diphenhydramine HCl, for example, has indications as a sleep aid, antitussive, antiemetic, and antihistamine, and is thus discussed in each of those categories.

The first phase of OTC review, which took place from 1972 to 1981, also established panels of outside experts to evaluate the OTC ingredients. Their review placed OTC products into one of three categories:

■ Category I: generally recognized as safe and effective for the therapeutic indication claimed;
■ Category II: not generally recognized as safe and effective, or having unacceptable indications;
■ Category III: insufficient data to permit final classification.

OTC Monographs and Nonmonographs

During the second phase of OTC review, which continues today, the FDA reviews the panels' findings and publishes in the Federal Register tentative monographs establishing dosage and labeling requirements. After considering objections and comments, a final monograph is published in the *Code of Federal Regulations*. Of the 81 product monographs to be published, 18 have been completed to date. Products that contain ingredients without a final monograph are marketed on a provisional basis and are subject to the requirements of a final monograph.

All OTC monographs consist of Subpart A, which includes regulations common to all OTCs, general warning labeling requirements, and a list of permissible inactive ingredients for the category. Subpart B identifies active ingredients that may be used within the category and acceptable combinations with other active ingredients. Subpart C contains indications, warnings and precautions, directions for use, dosages, dose frequency, and any specialized labeling requirements. Subpart D includes testing procedures, if any are required for the category, such as acid-neutralizing tests for antacids.

Once a monograph is final, any manufacturer may market a product without preapproval, provided the product meets the monograph's standards. Products that use new drug delivery systems or formulations, such as timed-release products, however, require a new drug application and separate approval.

In some cases, "nonmonographs" have been published following this stringent review process. A nonmonograph indicates that an ingredient or category of products fails to demonstrate safety and/or efficacy. The OTC review has resulted in nonmonographs—concomitant removal of products from the market—in a number of product categories:

■ anticholinergics;
■ aphrodisiacs;
■ camphorated oil;
■ daytime sedatives;
■ hair loss prevention products;
■ halogenated salicylanilides;
■ oral insect repellants;
■ stomach acidifiers;
■ sweet spirits of nitre;
■ topical hormones;
■ zirconium aerosols.

OTC Switching Procedures

The process of switching a prescription drug to nonprescription status also establishes its safety and efficacy as an OTC. (See figure 1 for a list of all 52 ingredients that have been switched to date.)

There are a number of mechanisms used to switch an Rx product.

■ The FDA advisory panels for OTC drug review may recommend that a drug be switched. This type of review is responsible for about 40 of the switches to date, including hydrocortisone, diphenhydramine, nystatin, and oxymetazoline.

■ A full NDA can be submitted for a current Rx drug in a new dosage or formulation. Since the FDA requires costly new studies for switches to be approved under a full NDA, it also grants the sponsor exclusive marketing rights for a period of years following approval. This mechanism, which deals with products rather than ingredients, is behind the approval of a number of new OTC products, including ibuprofen, loperamide, permethrin, micozole, and clotrimazole. Full NDAs will probably be preferred by manufacturers for future switches, since it gives them marketing exclusivity and thus an edge over their competition.

■ A supplemental NDA may be filed by a holder of an approved original or abbreviated application for a closely related product.

■ An abbreviated NDA may be submitted for products that are identical to an existing Rx product. This is used mainly for near duplicates of an Rx drug.

■ The FDA can determine that an Rx is unnecessary for an existing drug. Requests for this type of switch can come from a company, or any interested party. However, there have been no switches resulting from this mechanism since 1971.

Drugs are switched to over-the-counter status on a case-by-case basis. General criteria that act as informal guidelines for the process include an acceptable margin of safety, lack of toxicity, adequate labeling, treatment of recognizable symptoms, a simple treatment regimen, and the potential savings that a switch might yield to consumers and to the health care system.

To ensure that OTCs receive the same level of regulatory priority as Rx drugs, the FDA restructured the Division of OTC Drug Evaluation to form the Office of OTC Drug Evaluation in 1991. This new office provides a forum for reviewing a drug's status. A committee of outside experts was established at the same time to advise the FDA on nonprescription drugs.

Industry Self Regulation

Federal regulation is just one aspect of OTC safety and effectiveness. Since 1934, member companies of the Nonprescription Drug Manufacturers Association (NDMA) have established voluntary guidelines covering a variety of marketing issues, including packaging, labeling, distribution, and advertising. Today, there are twelve voluntary guidelines used extensively by the industry. The most recently implemented are guidelines to improve readability of labels. Other areas of voluntary regulation include:

■ advertising codes;
■ package sizes of certain OTCs;
■ "label flags" for those products with significant changes;
■ complaint protocols;
■ money-back guarantees;
■ safety closures for products that may be harmful to children;
■ standardization of children's aspirin products;
■ disclosure of the quantities of active ingredients;
■ disclosure of inactive ingredients;
■ bulk mail sampling;
■ expiration dates;
■ product identification of solid dosage OTC products.

Labeling and Packaging: Issues and Regulations

Labeling for nonprescription drugs must either include all the required elements indicated in an OTC monograph or receive preapproval through an NDA. Labels are required by law to provide detailed information on ingredients, product use, dosages, dose frequencies, possible reactions, contraindications, and other warnings, if applicable (see figure 2).

Despite these regulations, some labeling issues, such as label clarity, continue to cause concern. Studies show that about 90 percent of consumers read OTC labels (96 percent in the case of children's medicine labels). Nonetheless, about 10 percent of consumers say that OTC labels are too difficult to understand. Although many OTC labels are written on a ninth-grade level, the average consumer reads at only the eighth grade level, and 20 percent of

Figure 1

Ingredients Switched from Rx Status to OTC

Ingredient	Adult Dosage	Product Category	Product Examples and Manufacturer
Acidulated phosphate fluoride rinse*	0.02% fluoride in aqueous solution (topical)	Dental rinse	
Brompheniramine maleate	4 mg/4-6 h (oral)	Antihistamine	Dimetane (A.H. Robins)
Chlorphedianol HCl	25 mg/6-8 h (oral)	Antitussive	
Chlorpheniramine maleate	4 mg/4-6 h (oral)	Antihistamine	Allerest (Pharmacraft), Chlor-Trimeton (Schering), Contac (Menley & James), Sudafed Plus (Burroughs Wellcome)
Chlorpheniramine maleate (NDA)	12 mg/12 h (oral timed-release)	Antihistamine	Triaminic 12 (Dorsey)
Clemastine fumarate (NDA)	1.34 mg/12 h	Antihistamine	Tavist-1 (Sandoz)
Clemastine fumarate phenylpropanolamine HCl (NDA)	1.34 mg/12 h	Antihistamine with decongestant	Tavist D (Sandoz)
Clotrimazole (NDA)	1% lotion/cream 2x/day	Antifungal	Lotrimin AF (Schering)
Clotrimazole (NDA)	1% cream; 100 mg inserts	Anticandidal	Gyne-Lotrimin (Schering), Mycelex-7 (Miles)
Dexbrompheniramine maleate	2 mg/4-6 h (oral)	Antihistamine	
Dexbrompheniramine maleate (NDA)	3 mg/6-8 h (oral)	Antihistamine	Drixoral Plus (Schering)
Dexbrompheniramine maleate (NDA)	6 mg/12 h (oral timed-release)	Antihistamine	Drixoral (Schering)
Diphenhydramine HCl (NDA)	25 mg/4 hr (oral)	Antitussive	Benylin (Parke-Davis)
Diphenhydramine HCl	50 mg/single dose only (oral)	Sleep Aid	Sominex 2 (Beecham), Sleep-eze 3 (Whitehall)
Diphenhydramine HCl	25-50 mg/4-6 h (oral)	Antiemetic	
Diphenhydramine HCl	25-50 mg/4-6 h (oral)	Antihistamine	Benadryl 25 (Parke-Davis)
Diphenhydramine monocitrate	76 mg/single dose only (oral)	Sleep Aid	
Doxylamine succinate (NDA)	25 mg/single dose only (oral)	Sleep Aid	Unisom (Pfizer)
Doxylamine succinate	7.5-12.5 mg/4-6 h (oral)	Antihistamine	Nyquil (Vicks)
Dyclonine HCl*	0.05-0.1% in rinse, mouthwash, gargle, or spray 3-4x/day; 1-3 mg as lozenge	Oral Anesthetic	Sucrets Maximum Strength Lozenges (Beecham)
Ephedrine sulfate	0.1-1.25% (topical)	Anorectal/Vaso-constrictor	
Epinephrine HCl	0.005 to 0.01% (topical)	Anorectal/Vaso-constrictor	
Haloprogin	1.0% (topical)	Antifungal	
Hydrocortisone*	0.25-0.50% (topical)	Antipruritic	Cortaid (Upjohn), Lanacort (Combe)
Hydrocortisone*	above 0.50-1.0% (topical)	Antipruritic	
Hydrocortisone acetate*	0.25-0.50% (topical)	Antipruritic	Bactine (Miles), Caldecort (Pharmacraft)
Hydrocortisone acetate*	above 0.50-1.0% (topical)	Antipruritic	
Ibuprofen (NDA)	200 mg/4-6 h (oral)	Internal analgesic	Advil (Whitehall), Nuprin (Bristol-Myers)
Liposperse cholecystokinetic (hydrogenated soybean oil and lecithin)	12.4g powder dissolved in 2-3 oz. water 20 minutes before gall bladder x-ray		

Figure 1

Ingredients Switched from Rx Status to OTC, continued

Ingredient	Adult Dosage	Product Category	Product Examples and Manufacturer
Loperamide (NDA)	4 mg, then 2 mg; max. 8 mg/day (oral)	Antidiarrheal	Imodium A-D (Johnson & Johnson)
Miconazole nitrate	2.0% (topical)	Antifungal	Micatin (Ortho)
Miconazole nitrate (NDA)	2.0% cream; 100 mg inserts	Anticandidal	Monistat 7 (Ortho)
Naphazoline HCl with pheniramine maleate	0.027% naphazoline HCl/ 0.315% pheniramine maleate	Antihistamine/ decon-gestant, eye drop	Opcon A (Bausch &Lomb)
Naproxen (NDA)	200 mg/8-12 h (oral)	Internal analgesic; antipyretic	Aleve (Proctor & Gamble)
Oxymetazoline HCl*	0.05% aqueous solution (topical)	Nasal decongestant	Afrin (Schering), Duration (Plough), Dristan Long Lasting (Whitehall), Neo-Synephrine 12 Hour (Winthrop)
Oxymetazoline HCl (NDA)	0.025% solution/drops (topical)	Ocular vasoconstrictor	Ocuclear (Schering)
Permethrin (NDA)	1% cream rinse	Pediculicide	Nix (Burroughs-Wellcome)
Phenylephrine HCl*	0.5 mg in aqueous solution (topical)	Anorectal vasoconstrictor	
Phenylpropanolamine HCl (NDA)	75 mg/12 h (oral timed-release)	Nasal decongestant	Triaminic 12 (Dorsey)
Povidone iodine (NDA)	10% sponge (new dosage form)	Antimicrobial	E-Z Scrub 241 (Deseret)
Pseudophedrine HCl*	60 mg/4 or 4-6 h (oral); 240 mg max./24 h	Nasal decongestant	Sudafed (Burroughs Wellcome), Neo-Synephrinol (Winthrop)
Pseudophedrine HCl (NDA)	120 mg/12 h (oral timed-release)	Nasal decongestant	Actifed (Burroughs Wellcome)
Pseudophedrine sulfate*	60 mg/4 or 4-6 h (oral)	Nasal decongestant	Afrinol (Schering), Chlor-Trimeton (Schering)
Pseudophedrine sulfate (NDA)	120 mg/12 h (oral timed-release)	Nasal decongestant	Afrinol Repetabs (Schering)
Pyrantel pamoate	11 mg/kilo body weight; max. dose 1g (oral)	Anthelmintic	Antiminth (Pfizer)
Sodium fluoride rinse*	0.05% aqueous solution (topical)	Dental rinse	Fluorigard (Colgate-Palmolive)
Stannous fluoride gel*	0.4% aqueous solution (topical)	Dental rinse	
Stannous fluoride rinse*	0.1% aqueous solution (topical)	Dental Rinse	Stan Care (Block)
Tioconazole (NDA)	1% cream	Antifungal	TZ-3 (Pfizer)
Triprolidine HCl*	2.5 mg/4-6 h	Antihistamine	Actifed Capsules (Burroughs Wellcome), Actidil Syrup and Capsules (Burroughs Wellcome)
Triprolidine HCl (NDA)	5 mg/12 h	Antihistamine	Actifed 12 Hour Capsules (Burroughs Wellcome)
Xylometazoline HCl*	0.01% aqueous solution (topical)	Nasal decongestant	Orrivin (CIBA)

* FDA approval for OTC marketing is on an interim basis pending adoption of a final monograph

(NDA) Denotes switched under a new drug application

Source: Nonprescription Drug Manufacturers Association, "Ingredients & Dosages Transferred from Rx to OTC Status as a Consequence of the U.S. Food and Drug Administration's Review of Nonprescription Drug Products." Washington, DC, 1994

What's on the Label

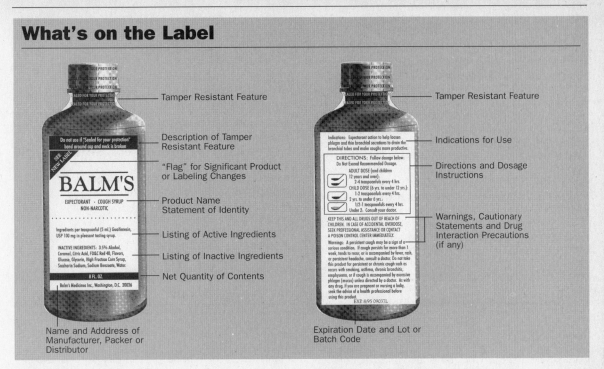

Tamper Resistant Feature

Description of Tamper Resistant Feature

"Flag" for Significant Product or Labeling Changes

Product Name Statement of Identity

Listing of Active Ingredients

Listing of Inactive Ingredients

Net Quantity of Contents

Name and Adddress of Manufacturer, Packer or Distributor

Tamper Resistant Feature

Indications for Use

Directions and Dosage Instructions

Warnings, Cautionary Statements and Drug Interaction Precautions (if any)

Expiration Date and Lot or Batch Code

Americans are functionally illiterate. Label readability can also be affected by such factors as poor vision and inadequate lighting in retail settings, particularly for the elderly.

The OTC industry has actively sought ways to help resolve readability issues. In 1990, the NDMA established a special task force to recommend label improvements. The resulting voluntary guidelines established specific requirements for layout, design, typography, and printing, to assist manufacturers in making labels as legible as possible.

Perhaps even more critical is product tampering. The first main incidence of OTC tampering occurred in Chicago in 1982, and led to swift enactment of tamper-resistant packaging regulations by the FDA. Federal laws also beefed up jail terms and fines for product tampering.

The OTC industry also responded vigorously to the Chicago poisonings and to subsequent tampering cases. In addition to designing tamper-resistant packaging at a cost of approximately $1 billion, individual companies offered large cash rewards for information, and the industry set up tampering hotlines for consumers and launched a massive public education campaign. The results have been positive, and OTC tampering has decreased significantly since 1982. In addition, consumers approve of the methods used to deter tampering. A national survey of 1,500 consumers indicated that tamper-resistant containers and consumer education were the best possible solutions to the tampering problem.

Marketing and Advertising OTCs

United States law allows OTC makers to advertise their products directly to consumers under the authority of the Federal Trade Commission (FTC). Reviews by this body are conducted for all OTC ads on a case-by-case basis after the ads are used, and are subject to the same truth in advertising guidelines as any other product.

An international study recently assessed the impact of advertising on OTC use. It indicated that use of nonprescription medicines is no greater in those countries that allow consumer advertising than in those that don't. Sweden and Switzerland, which restrict OTC advertising, for example, have the same level of OTC use as countries with consumer ads. The study concluded that advertising OTCs directly to consumers does not lead to overuse or misuse.

Some states have also proposed laws that would place new requirements on OTC makers. The pharmacy news magazine, *Drug Topics*, reported in 1994 that 68 such proposals had been made in the previous 18 months. These include a bill in New York requiring special label warnings for the elderly and a bill in Texas calling for bittering agents in topical OTCs. As a whole, the industry has criticized what it calls the evolution of 50 "mini-FDAs" that it believes individual state legislation would bring. According to industry leaders, present federal laws and regulation work effectively to protect consumers against unsafe, ineffective, or mislabeled medicines. They argue that state regulations are not only an unnecessary replication of FDA efforts, but would also mean chaos for the interstate commerce in OTCs.

Chapter 4: Patient Counseling:
A Critical Role for Physicians and Pharmacists

The Consumer's Self-Medication Bill of Rights, drafted by the Nonprescription Drug Manufacturers Association, states: "Next to safe and effective products, information is the most important commodity in self-care/self-medication." And as OTC use increases and the number of available products grows, consumers will require more information than ever to choose the right products and use them effectively and safely. For most consumers, that information comes from their health care providers. Physicians and pharmacists are in an ideal and unique position to provide patients with informed and up-to-date OTC advice. Through effective patient counseling on OTC use, physicians and phamacists can help improve medical outcomes and prevent costly incidents of drug misuse.

A Growing Need For Information

For most consumers, information on nonprescription drugs comes from product labels and advertising, but these can be confusing or incomplete. Consumers thus rely on the one-to-one relationship they possess with their doctors and pharmacists for additional information.

New products, line extensions, and OTC switches are just some of the factors that may overwhelm even the most well-informed patient. In 1993, for example, 97 percent of all pharmacists surveyed across the nation said that line extensions for adult cough/cold/flu preparations led to significant confusion among their customers. Switches for children's cough/cold preparations caused even more problems.

Such confusion, multiplied by the number of products on the market, can foster potential medical misadventures, including:

■ use of an inappropriate medication;
■ use of an inappropriate dosage;
■ use of an OTC that is contraindicated;
■ drug-drug interactions;
■ inappropriate duration of OTC use;
■ side effects.

In addition, although all consumers need counseling on OTCs, many have special needs. Groups requiring special attention include:

■ patients with comprehension problems (20 percent of consumers are illiterate and nearly 10 percent say they are sometimes confused by OTC labels);
■ blind and other visually impaired patients;
■ deaf and other hearing-impaired patients;
■ the elderly;
■ children;
■ patients with comprehension deficits;
■ pregnant or nursing patients.

For these patients, self-medicating safely may pose difficulties, and counseling from a physician or pharmacist is particularly important.

All consumers, however, have occasional questions about nonprescription medications. These range from requests for product recommendations to questions about cost. (Figure 1 lists the most commonly asked questions.) According to one national survey, almost two-thirds (65 percent) of consumers ask their physician for OTC advice and over half (54 percent) consult their pharmacist. (The total exceed 100 percent, since many consumers consult both physicians and pharmacists.) Consumers place a high value on the advice they receive. The same study revealed that 58 percent of patients are extremely satisfied with their doctor's advice, and 61 percent give the same high grade to pharmacists.

Figure 1
Commonly Asked Questions About OTCs

Question	Percent of Pharmacists receiving the question
Recommendations for the best OTC product for a specific ailment	94%
Side effects	54%
Dosage/duration of therapy	37%
Information on medical conditions	36%
Cost of OTC	35%

Source: Cardinale, V. "Pharmacists as OTC Counselors," *Drug Topics* (suppl.), 1994

OTCs and Physicians

Nearly all (97 percent) physicians recommend OTCs to their patients, according to a recent survey by the international business consulting firm Kline & Co. They do so, in fact, for 27 percent of all their patients. As the professionals that consumers count on most, physicians and pharmacists play an important role in how OTCs are used. In turn, physician and pharmacy practices are also affected by the wide availability and effectiveness of these medications.

Americans take about one-tenth of their health problems to physicians. For the remainder of injuries and illness, they resort to no treatment or self-treatment; and 70 percent say they self-medicate regularly. For physicians, OTCs have a direct impact on the number of patients they see and the reasons for those office visits.

One study found that MD visits for the common cold dropped by 110,000 a year between 1976 and 1989. The study attributed the decrease to the high number of switched drugs available for treating cold symptoms. The number of visits for other ailments, including serious respiratory conditions, did not decrease in the same period. Another survey revealed that over half (54 percent) of Americans believe that new, switched OTCs saved them trips to the doctor.

Self-medication and seeking out a health care professional are not mutually exclusive. In fact, both approaches are increasing in frequency. Apparently, as their awareness grows, consumers place more reliance on physicians, as well as OTCs. For physicians, OTCs may often serve to screen out those patients with minor, self-treatable conditions, and free up valuable practice time for conditions that do require professional attention.

Some over-the-counter products actually encourage consumers to seek medical care. The greater availability of self-diagnostic and self-monitoring products, for example, serve to increase office visits by alerting patients to the need for a doctor's attention.

Finally, the impact of OTCs on physicians' practices in the future may be even greater under managed care programs. Capitated reimbursement systems, in which providers are reimbursed per enrollee, encourage practitioners to contain costs, reduce unnecessary services, and write fewer and less costly prescriptions. Under managed care, therefore, self-medication may be seen as an important component of cost-containment.

OTCs and Pharmacists

Year after year in national Gallup polls, consumers vote pharmacists the most trusted professional. It's not surprising that 98 percent of pharmacists say their customers generally or always follow their advice on OTCs and purchase the products they recommend.

Pharmacists are also the most accessible health care provider for consumers, and many prefer buying

Figure 2

Product Categories Causing Confusion Among Consumers

Product Category	% of pharmacists asked for recommendation	Average number of recommenations per month
Adult cough/cold	100	29
Adult cold	100	28
Allergy relief	100	23
Sinus remedies	99	2
Ibuprofens	99	20
Antacids	99	12
Antidiarrheals	99	1
Children's cough	98	21
Acetaminophens	98	19
Throat lozenges	98	13
Stool softeners/laxatives	98	10
Children's cold	96	21
Athlete's foot	95	8
Jock itch	95	6
Canker/cold sore	94	8
Bulk laxatives	92	8
Hemorrhoidal	92	6
Aspirins	91	13
Vaginal antifungals	91	7
Flu	90	15
Topical anesthetics	90	9
Pediculicides	87	8
Ear drops	87	6
Wart removers	87	6
Toothache/teething	85	7
Pregnancy test kits	83	6
Suntan/sunscreen	81	8
Asthma	81	6
Infant oral rehydration	81	5
Blood glucose monitors	79	5
Irritant/stimulant laxatives	77	6
Acne	74	5
Diet aids/weight loss	58	8
Saline laxatives	50	5
Antiplaque/gingivitis	47	3
Ovulation test kits	44	3
Fluoride dental rinses	38	3

Source: Gannon, K. "I Recommend . . . What R.Ph.'s suggest in OTCs," *Drug Topics*, August 16, 1993

their OTCs in a pharmacy because a pharmacist is on hand to provide counseling. There are, for instance, over three-quarters of a million OTC outlets, and only about 10 percent of these are pharmacies. Yet, about 45 percent of all the nation's OTCs are bought in drugstores. Consumers clearly go out of their way to purchase OTCs in a pharmacy.

Consumers often rely on their pharmacist to provide counseling on an OTC until they can make an appointment with a physician, and nearly all pharmacists report that patients occasionally or frequently come to them for OTC advice as an alternative to consulting their physician. In fact, patient counseling by pharmacists is a growing practice. In one recent study, pharmacists were shown to have made an average of 450 more OTC recommendations than they had in the previous year. In 1992, the number of OTC consultations per pharmacist reached 3,888—or almost 672 million per year nationwide—and the level is still rising. In 1993, over half (53 percent) of all pharmacists polled said that they were providing more OTC counseling and that three-quarters of the time, the customer initiated the exchange. In addition, consumers ask pharmacists for help with every category of OTC product. Figure 2 ranks the percentage of pharmacists who were asked to make a product recommendation in that category. It also shows the average number of recommendations made per month.

OTCs are a crucial element in pharmacy practice. About 30 percent of pharmacy revenues come from OTC sales, and for chain drugstores the number is even higher. In addition, pharmacy owners who report expanding OTC sales cite pharmacist counseling as the number one reason for the increase.

With the rise of interest in pharmaceutical care, in which pharmacists are part of a health care team that plans, implements, and monitors patient care, some pharmacists today receive reimbursement for the time they spend counseling a patient. And many pharmacy plans provide financial incentives to pharmacists who encourage use of less expensive Rx or OTC medications. All of these factors may work to encourage OTC counseling by pharmacists in the near future, and may certainly change the way they dispense medications.

Figure 3

What Physicians Want to Know About OTCs

Physicians indicate that they often need more information about an OTC before making a recommendation to their patients. These categories were ranked as most important.

Type of Information	% of Physicians
Side effects, contraindications, symptoms and treatment of overdose	89
Clinical data from an independent source	77
Dosing, directions for use, how supplied	73
Direct comparison to similar products	50
Patient acceptance, compliance	41
Unique physical characteristics	41
Consumer pricing information	37
Reputation of company marketing the product	30
Unique packaging features	19
Clinical data from manufacturer	15
Differences in consumer and professional labeling	9
Type of consumer promotion and support	7
Market share data	2

Source: Griffie, K.G. "How Healthcare Providers Influence Drug Use," Kline & Co., Fairfield, NJ 1993

Counseling Obstacles

Despite the increase in OTC use, and in patient counseling, studies show that consumers do not always receive the help they need from their health care providers. Physicians, constrained by time and the amount of other information that must be exchanged during a phone consultation or office visit, may neglect to discuss the OTCs their patients use.

Pharmacists also face busy schedules, and studies show that they cite time constraints as the main barrier to OTC counseling. Other obstacles for pharmacists include lack of reimbursement for counseling services, a need for more education on OTCs, and the absence of a physical area that provides privacy. Pharmacists report that insufficient staff and lack of management support are further disincentives for counseling.

Poor communication skills on the part of physicians and pharmacists may also impede effective patient counseling. The following elements of good communication can enhance the counseling process:

■ Listen to patients, ask them for details and clarification, and repeat their answers to confirm your understanding.

■ Assess the knowledge level of your patient. This process can often uncover special problems, such as a reading disability.

■ Use nontechnical terms with patients, and ask them to repeat the instructions you've given them.

■ Provide clearly-written instructions whenever possible. Oral instructions are often quickly forgotten.

■ Stay up-to-date on OTC products, and use current reference books, journals, product information from manufacturers, and other necessary sources, for the most recent and complete information. (Physicians and pharmacists both indicate that they would like to know more about the OTC products they recommend for their patients. Figure 3, for example, shows the percentage of doctors who seek more information on particular OTC topics.)

Finally, one useful aspect of patient counseling is often underused by pharmacists and physicians alike. This is the practice of recommending a companion OTC when a prescription is written or dispensed. Despite the benefits that companion OTCs can provide a patient, half of all pharmacists say they never recommend them. Many nonprescription drugs, however, can help control side effects and improve the efficacy of Rx drugs. Companion OTC recommendations also provide a useful service to patients, help build loyalty, encourage communication, and, for pharmacies, boost OTC sales. (Figure 4 shows which categories of OTC drugs can be helpful with which categories of Rx drugs.)

Figure 4
OTC Companions

OTCs are often overlooked for the relief they can bring from Rx drug side effects, or the added effectiveness they can bring to prescription drugs. Some examples are:

OTC Category	Prescription Drug Category
Antacids	Gastrointestinal drugs
Antacids	Anti-inflammatory drugs
Antacids	Glucocorticoids
Diabetes testing products and supplies	Antidiabetics
Anti-infective agents	Antifungals
Laxatives and vitamins	Cholesterol-lowering drugs
Antacids and analgesics	Rx analgesics
Analgesics	Cardiovascular drugs

Chapter 5: The Future of OTCs

By 2010, OTC sales are expected to reach $28 billion, more than double today's volume. Sales and use will be driven by the development of new technologies and treatments and by ongoing changes in society and how we view and use health care.

New Treatments and New Technologies

Powerful new products, will be the driving force behind the growing popularity of OTCs and self-medication. These products will come from a number of sources. Switches, for example, have already added 52 ingredients to the market, and as many as 70 new applications are expected in the next five years. If approved, these will provide consumers with:

■ new combinations of existing ingredients, for example, hydrocortisone and an antifungal;
■ new formulations, for example, stronger dosages or time-released versions of existing drugs;
■ new ingredients, such as the NSAID, diflunisal, and the asthma medication, aminophylline;
■ entirely new classes of OTC medications, e.g., antivirals (acyclovir).

Many proposed switches are already in process and may be granted over-the-counter status in the near future. These include medications for treating sleep disorders, obesity, smoking, anxiety, arthritis, diabetes, ulcers, asthma, and cardiovascular conditions. Other medications pending approval are dermatological, ophthalmological, genitourinal, and cholesterol-lowering agents. The availability of these strong medications will give consumers an even greater degree of control over their own care, and at a low price. By the year 2000, in fact, it's estimated that switches will have saved the U.S. $34 billion in health care costs.

Another vital source of future medications is biotechnology. Since the first successful genetic engineering experiment took place in California in 1973, this method of drug development is being adopted in every biological research institution in the nation. In fact, the number of applications for approval of biotechnology drugs actually outstripped the number of applications for traditional drugs in the early 1990s. Although most of these genetically engineered medicines are designed to treat serious conditions that require a physician's care, refinements such as the development of peptides that can be taken orally will undoubtedly lead to new OTC drugs in the future. Promising leads for tomorrow's biotechnology drugs include breakthroughs in immunomodulators, anticancer drugs, antivirals, anti-inflammatories, hormones, tissue repair treatments, and antithrombotics.

Along with new ingredients and treatments, new ways to deliver medications are also the subject of intense research. Some of these innovative delivery systems, such as transdermal patches and aerosols, are already being used in prescription medications. Studies are also underway on specially coated molecules that are either more rapidly absorbed or designed to stay in the body longer. Molecular sponges and tiny pumps inserted under the skin may also be used some day, and researchers are experimenting with piggy-backing molecules on existing drugs, to produce products that are less toxic or more effective.

Certainly, other countries must also be counted as a potential source for future OTCs. Today, there are about 35 OTCs that are marketed only outside the U.S. Subject to FDA approval, however, they could eventually become available to American consumers.

Future Trends in the OTC Market

A number of societal trends will also shape the OTC market of tomorrow.

■ As the 58 million members of the baby boomer generation reach old age, their reliance on OTC treatments, especially for chronic conditions such as arthritis and diabetes, will undoubtedly grow significantly.
■ We can expect a continued emphasis on wellness and self-care with a heightened interest in prevention and in medications that enhance quality of life. Currently available and newly developed diagnostic and monitoring products will also play a large role in self-care.
■ The "information revolution" will lead to better-informed patients and more self-treatment and self-diagnosis.

Figure 1
A Surge in Biotech Drugs

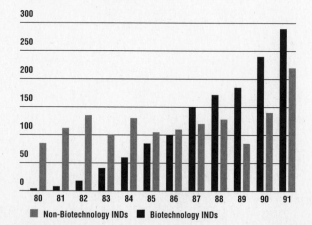

Non-Biotechnology INDs ■ Biotechnology INDs

■ The number of new nonprescription products, as well as their increasing strength and sophistication, will require greater understanding and increased education among consumers and continued reliance on health care providers for expertise and advice.

■ The OTC market could also be affected by a push from pharmacies and other groups to establish a third class of drugs that would be available only through pharmacies. Manufacturers strongly oppose the proposal as anticonsumer, anticompetitive, unnecessary, and a threat to the industry. The FDA has rejected the idea several times over the past two decades but in many other countries there are already three or more classes of drugs.

■ With or without health care reform legislation, the trend toward managed care, with its emphasis on cost containment, is already having an impact on OTC use. In this cost-conscious environment, we can expect to see an increasing emphasis on the approval and use of OTC products and self-treatment in general.

Conclusion

Whatever the source of future OTCs, one thing is certain: tomorrow's consumers will have a wide array of new nonprescription drug products from which to choose. They will play an increasingly important role in the self-treatment of your patients. Keeping abreast of these new therapeutic alternatives will become an ever more critical part of cost-effective patient care and counseling.

Sources

Chapter One

Heller Research Group. Self-medication in the '90s: Practices and perceptions. New York, 1992.

Nielsen North America, 1991.

Nonprescription Drug Manufacturers Association, 1993.

Gannon, K. Exclusive consumer OTC survey: Who's buying what. *Drug Topics,* Jan. 8, 1990.

Find/SVP Inc. The market for Rx-to-OTC switches. September, 1993.

Sudler & Hennessy. Switches vs. non-switches: Results and insights. New York, 1992.

Temin, P. Realized benefits from switching drugs. *J. Law Econ.* (25)2, 1992.

Information Resources, Inc. Chicago, 1994.

U.S. Bureau of Statistics, 1993.

Kline & Co. Economic benefit of self-medication. Fairfield, New Jersey, 1993.

Kline & Co. Fairfield, New Jersey, 1991.

Chapter Two

World Federation of Proprietary Medicine Manufacturers. Health Care, Self-Care and Self Medication, 1991.

Market Research Corporation of America. Health care remedies usage study. February, 1990.

Consumer Federation of America. September, 1990.

Gallup Organization. *American Health,* March, 1989.

Gallup Organization. *American Health,* 1991.

Heller Research Group. Self-Medication in the '90s: Practices and perceptions. New York, 1992.

Holt G.A., Beck D., Williams M.M. Interview analysis regarding health status, health needs and health care utilization of ambulatory elderly. 40th Annual Conference of the National Council of Aging, Washington, DC, April, 1990.

Shanas E., Maddox G. Aging, health, and the organization of health resources. In: Binstock R., Shanas E., eds. *Handbook of Aging and the Social Sciences.* Van Nostrand Reinhold, New York, 1985.

Princeton Survey Research Associates. *Prevention,* 1992.

Gannon K. The Rx-to-OTC switch race: Drugstores setting the pace. *Drug Topics,* November 22, 1993.

Sudler & Hennessy. New York, 1992.

Rosendahl I. The private label story. *Drug Topics* June 13, 1994.

Chapter Three

Gannon K. Shelf busters: Analyzing nonprescription drug trends. *Drug Topics* January 25, 1993.

Nonprescription Drug Manufacturers Association. Ingredients & dosages transferred from Rx to OTC status as a consequence of the U.S. Food and Drug Administration's Review of Nonprescription Drug Products. Washington DC, 1994.

Nonprescription Drug Manufacturers Association. *Voluntary Codes and Guidelines of the OTC Medicines Industry.* Washington DC.

Nonprescription Drug Manufacturers Association. *Self-Medication's Role in U.S. Health Care.* Washington DC.

Cardinale V. Self-medication: Trend to be reckoned with, not wrecked. *Drug Topics* April 5, 1993.

Gannon K. NDMA's Cope upholds consumer's 'rights' on OTCs. Drug Topics June 13, 1994.

Mercill A.W. Regulation of nonprescription drug products in the United States. Presented at the World Federation of Proprietary Medicine Manufacturers, March 6, 1990.

Princeton Survey Research Associates, 1992.

Code of Federal Regulations. April 1, 1994.

Heller Research Group. Self-medication in the '90s: Practices and perceptions. New York, 1992.

Farley D. Benefit vs. risk: How FDA approves new drugs. *The FDA Consumer.* 1989.

Walden J.T. Impact of tampering on the OTC industry. *The Nielsen Researcher.* Fall, 1986.

Epstein D. More counseling called for in medicating the illiterate. *Drug Topics* November, 1988.

Chapter Four

Gannon K. What R.Ph.s suggest in OTCs. *Drug Topics,* August 16, 1993.

IMS America. National Disease and Therapeutic Index, 1990.

Temin, P. Realized benefits from switching drugs. *J. Law Econ.* (25)2, 1992.

Gannon K. Pharmacists step up level of counseling on OTCs. *Drug Topics,* September 20, 1993.

Cardinale V. Pharmacists as OTC Counselors, *Drug Topics* (suppl.). 1994.

Gannon K. What do patient want to know about OTCs? *Drug Topics,* August 21, 1989

Epstein D. More counseling called for in medicating the illiterate. *Drug Topics,* November, 1988.

Schering Laboratories. *What's Right with Pharmacy.* The Schering Report VII, Kenilworth, New Jersey.

Griffie K.G. *How Healthcare Providers Influence Drug Use.* Kline & Co., Fairfield, New Jersey, 1993.

Chapter Five

Nonprescription Drug Manufacturers Association. The U.S. system of drug distribution. Washington, DC, 1994.

Kline & Co., Fairfield, New Jersey, 1993.

Nonprescription Drug Manufacturers Association. Self-Medication's Role in U.S. Health Care. Washington, DC, 1993.

Eckian A.G. *The Frontiers of Rx-to-OTC Switch.* Presented at the Research and Scientific Development Conference, Nonprescription Drug Manufacturers Association, December 12, 1986.

Nonprescription Drug Manufacturers Association. Rx-to-OTC switch: The right trend for the '90s. Washington DC, 1993.

Ringel M. Changing disease patterns, shifting demographics: Effects on laboratory practices. *Clin. Lab. Mgt. Rev.* September/October, 1994.

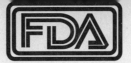

U.S. FOOD AND DRUG ADMINISTRATION

Professional and Consumer Information Numbers

Medical Product Reporting Programs

MedWatch (24 hour service) 800-332-1088
Reporting of problems with drugs, devices, biologics (except vaccines), medical foods, dietary supplements.

Vaccine Adverse Event Reporting (24 hour service)..............................800-822-7967
Reporting of vaccine-related problems.

Mandatory Medical Device Reporting...301-427-7500
Reporting required from User facilities regarding device-related deaths and serious injuries.

Veterinary Adverse Drug Reaction Program 301-594-0749
Reporting of adverse drug events in animals.

Medical Advertising Information (24 hour service).................................800-238-7332
Inquiries from health professionals regarding product promotion.

Information for Health Professionals

Center for Drugs Executive Secretariat 301-594-1012
Information on human drugs including hormones.

Center for Biologics Executive Secretariat 301-594-1800
Information on biological products including vaccines and blood.

Center for Devices and Radiological Health 301-443-4190
Automated request for information on medical devices and radiation-emitting products.

Office of Orphan Products Development 301-443-4718
Information on products for rare diseases.

Office of Health Affairs Medicine Staff 301-443-5470
Information for health professionals on FDA activities.

General Information

General Consumer Inquiries 301-443-3170
Consumer information on regulated products/issues.

Freedom of Information 301-443-6310
Request for publicly available FDA documents.

Office of Public Affairs...301-443-1130
Interviews/press inquiries on FDA activities.

Breast Implant Inquiries (24 hour service) 800-332-3541
Prerecorded message/request information.

Seafood Hotline (24 hour service)..800-332-4010
Prerecorded message/request information (English/Spanish).

All numbers accessible 8:00 a.m. to 4:30 p.m. eastern time, except where otherwise noted.

MEDICAL ECONOMICS

STATE BOARDS OF PHARMACY

Questions on local regulations governing prescription and over-the-counter drugs, controlled substances, and pharmacy licensure can often be answered by your local state board of pharmacy. For your convenience, a contact name, address, and phone number for each state board is listed in the directory that follows.

ALABAMA

Jerry Moore, R.Ph.
Executive Secretary
1 Perimeter Park S.,
Suite 425 S
Birmingham, AL 35243
Tel.: 205-967-0130
Fax: 205-967-1009

ALASKA

Clay Kent
Licensing Examiner
Dept. of Commerce and
Economic
Development
Division of Occupational
Licensing
P.O. Box 110806
Juneau, AK 99811-0806
Tel.: 907-465-2589
Fax: 907-465-2974

ARIZONA

L. A. Lloyd, R.Ph.
Executive Director
5060 N. 19th Ave.,
Suite 101
Phoenix, AZ 85015
Tel.: 602-255-5125
Fax: 602-255-5740

ARKANSAS

Lester Hosto P.D.
Executive Director
101 E. Capitol Ave.,
Suite 218
Little Rock, AR 72201
Tel.: 501-682-0190
Fax: 501-682-0195

CALIFORNIA

Patricia Harris
Executive Officer
400 "R" St., Suite 4070
Sacramento, CA 95814
Tel.: 916-445-5014
Fax: 916-327-6308

COLORADO

D. L. Simmons
Program Administrator
1560 Broadway,
Suite 1310
Denver, CO 80202-5146
Tel.: 303-894-7750
Fax: 303-894-7764

CONNECTICUT

Margaret Soracchi, R.Ph.
Board Administrator
State Office Bldg.,
Room G-3A
165 Capitol Ave.
Hartford, CT 06106
Tel.: 203-566-3290
Fax: 203-566-7630

DELAWARE

Bonnie Wallner, R.Ph.
Executive Secretary
P.O. Box 637
Dover, DE 19903
Tel.: 302-739-4798
Fax: 302-739-3071

DISTRICT OF COLUMBIA

Barbara Hagans
Contact Representative
614 "H" St. NW,
Room 923
Washington, DC 20001
Tel.: 202-727-7832
Fax: 202-727-7662

FLORIDA

John D. Taylor, R.Ph.
Exective Director
Health Care
Administration
Board of Pharmacy
1940 N. Monroe St.
Northwood Center
Tallahassee, FL 32399-
0775
Tel.: 904-488-7546
Fax: 904-922-7865

GEORGIA

Gregg W. Schuder
Executive Director
166 Pryor St. SW
Atlanta, GA 30303
Tel.: 404-656-3912
Fax: 404-651-9532

HAWAII

Charlene Tamanaha
Exective Officer
P.O. Box 3469
Honolulu, HI 96801
Tel.:808-586-2698

IDAHO

R. K. Markuson, R.Ph.
Director
P.O. Box 83720
Boise, ID 83720-0067
Tel.: 208-334-2356
Fax: 208-334-3536

ILLINOIS

Ed Duffy, R.Ph.
Exective Administrator
Drug Compliance
Illinois Dept. of
Professional Regulation
100 W. Randolph,
Suite 9-300
Chicago, IL 60601
Tel.: 312-814-4573
Fax: 312-814-3145

INDIANA

Frances L. Kelly
Director
402 W. Washington St.,
Room 041
Indianapolis, IN 46204
Tel.: 317-233-4403
Fax: 317-233-4236

IOWA

Lloyd K. Jessen, R.Ph.,
J.D.
1209 East Court Ave.
Executive Hills West
Des Moines, IA 50319
Tel.: 515-281-5944
Fax: 515-281-4609

KANSAS

Tom Hitchcock
Exective Secretary
900 Jackson St., Room 513
Topeka, KS 66612-1231
Tel.: 913-296-4056
Fax: 913-296-8420

KENTUCKY

Ralph E. Bouvette,
R.Ph., Ph.D., J.D.
Exective Director
1228 U.S. Hwy. 127 S.
Frankfort, KY 40601
Tel.: 502-564-3833
Fax: 502-564-2032

LOUISIANA

Howard B. Bolton, R.Ph.
Executive Director
5615 Corporate Blvd.,
8th Floor
Baton Rouge, LA 70808
Tel.: 504-925-6496
Fax: 504-925-6499

MAINE

Susan Greenlaw
Board Clerk
Dept. of Professional
and Financial
Regulations
Board of Commissioners
of the Profession of
Pharmacy
State House Station #35
Augusta, ME 04333
Tel.: 207-582-8723
Fax: 207-624-8637

MARYLAND

Tamara Banks
Administrative Officer
4201 Patterson Ave.
Baltimore, MD 21215
Tel.: 410-764-4755
Fax: 410-358-6207

MASSACHUSETTS

Charles R. Young, R.Ph.
Acting Exective Director
100 Cambridge St.,
Room 1514
Boston, MA 02202
Tel.: 617-727-9955
Fax: 617-727-2197

MICHIGAN

Patrick Gaven, R.Ph.
Chairman
611 W. Ottawa St.
P.O. Box 30018
Lansing, MI 48909
Tel.: 517-373-9102
Fax: 517-373-2179

MINNESOTA

David E. Holmstrom,
R.Ph., J.D.
Executive Director
2700 University Ave. W.,
Rm. 107
St. Paul, MN 55114-1079
Tel.: 612-642-0541
Fax: 612-643-3530

MISSISSIPPI

William L. Stevens
Eective Director
2310 Highway 80 W.
C & F Plaza, Suite D
Jackson, MS 39204
Tel.: 601-354-6750
Fax: 601-354-6071

MISSOURI

Kevin E. Kinkade, R.Ph.
Exective Director
P.O. Box 625
Jefferson City, MO 65102
Tel.: 314-751-0091
Fax: 314-526-3464

MONTANA

Warren R. Amole, Jr.,
R.Ph.
Exective Director
111 N. Last Chance Gulch
Helena, MT 59620-0513
Tel.: 406-444-1698
Fax: 406-444-1667

NEBRASKA

Katherine A. Brown
Executive Secretary
Board of Examiners in
Pharmacy
P.O. Box 95007
301 Centennial Mall S.
Lincoln, NE 68509
Tel.: 402-471-2115
Fax: 402-471-0383

NEVADA

Keith W. MacDonald,
R.Ph.
Executive Secretary
1201 Terminal Way,
Suite 212
Reno, NV 89502-3257
Tel.: 702-322-0691
Fax: 702-322-0895

NEW HAMPSHIRE

Paul G. Boisseau, R.Ph.
Executive Director
57 Regional Dr.
Concord, NH 03301
Tel.: 603-271-2350
Fax: 603-271-2856

NEW JERSEY

H. Lee Gladstein, R.Ph.
Exective Director
124 Halsey St., 6th Fl.
P.O. Box 45013
Newark, NJ 07102
Tel.: 201-504-6450
Fax: 201-648-3355

NEW MEXICO

Richard W. Thompson
Executive Director
1650 University Blvd. NE
Suite 400-B
Albuquerque, NM 87102
Tel.: 505-841-9102
Fax: 505-841-9113

NEW YORK

Lawrence H. Mokhiber,
R.Ph.
Executive Secretary
Cultural Education Center
Room 3035
Albany, NY 12230
Tel.: 518-474-3848
Fax: 518-473-6995

NORTH CAROLINA

David R. Work, R.Ph.
Exective Director
P.O. Box 459
Carrboro, NC 27510-0459
Tel.: 919-942-4454
Fax: 919-967-5757

NORTH DAKOTA

William J. Grosz, Sc.D.,
R.Ph.
Executive Director
P.O. Box 1354
Bismarck, ND 58502
Tel.: 701-258-1535
Fax: 701-258-9312

OHIO

Franklin Z. Wickham,
R.Ph.
Exective Director
77 S. High St., 17th Floor
Columbus, OH 43266
Tel.: 614-466-4143
Fax: 614-752-4836

OKLAHOMA

Bryan Potter, R.Ph.
Executive Secretary
4545 N. Lincoln Blvd.,
Suite 112
Oklahoma City, OK 73105
Tel.: 405-521-3815
Fax: 405-521-3758

OREGON

Ruth Vandever, R.Ph.
Exective Director
State Office Bldg.,
Suite 425
800 NE Oregon St., #9
Portland, OR 97232
Tel.: 503-731-4032
Fax: 503-731-4067

PENNSYLVANIA

Richard Marshman,
R.Ph.
Exective Secretary
P.O. Box 2649
Harrisburg, PA 17105
Tel.: 717-783-7157
Fax: 717-783-4853

PUERTO RICO

Arnalo LaLuc
President
Call Box 10200
Santurce, PR 00908
Tel.: 809-725-8161
       Ext. 2245
Fax: 809-725-7903

RHODE ISLAND

Mario Casinelli, Jr.,
R.Ph.
Chairman of the Board
Department of Health
Division of Drug Control
Three Capitol Hill,
Room 304
Providence, RI 02908
Tel.: 401-277-2837
Fax: 401-277-2499

SOUTH CAROLINA

Joseph L. Mullinax, R.Ph.
Administator
S.C.L.L.R./Board of
Pharmacy
1026 Sumter St.,
Room 209
P.O. Box 11927
Columbia, SC 29211
Tel.: 803-734-1010
Fax: 803-734-1552

SOUTH DAKOTA

Galen Jordre, R.Ph.
Secretary
P.O. Box 518
Pierre, SD 57501-0518
Tel.: 605-224-2338
Fax: 605-224-1280

TENNESSEE

J. Floyd Ferrell, Jr., R.Ph.
Director
500 James Robertson
Pkwy.
Nashville, TN 37243
Tel.: 615-741-2718
Fax: 615-741-6470

TEXAS

Fred S. Brinkley, Jr., R.Ph.
Exective Director
8505 Cross Park Dr.,
Suite 110
Austin, TX 78754
Tel.: 512-832-0661
Fax: 512-832-0855

UTAH

David E. Robinson
Director
Utah Dept. of Commerce
Division of Occupational
and Professional Licensing
160 E. 300 S.
P.O. Box 45805
Salt Lake City, UT
84145-0805
Tel.: 801-530-6628
Fax: 801-530-6511

VERMONT

Carla Preston
Staff Assistant
109 State St.
Montpelier, VT 05609
Tel.: 802-828-2875
Fax: 802-828-2496

VIRGINIA

Scotti W. Milley, R.Ph.
Exective Director
6606 W. Broad St.
Richmond, VA 23230
Tel.: 804-662-9911
Fax: 804-662-9313

WASHINGTON

Donald H. Williams,
R.Ph.
Executive Director
P.O. Box 47863
Olympia, WA 98504
Tel.: 206-753-6834
Fax: 206-586-4359

WEST VIRGINIA

Sam Kapourales, R.Ph.
President
236 Capitol St.
Charleston, WV 25301
Tel.: 304-558-0558
Fax: 304-558-0572

WISCONSIN

Pat Schenck
Program Assistant
Wisconsin Dept. of
Registration and
Licensing
P.O. Box 8935
1400 E. Washington Ave.
Madison, WI 53708
Tel.: 608-266-2811
Fax: 608-267-0644

WYOMING

Marilynn H. Mitchell,
R.Ph.
Exective Director
1720 S. Poplar St.,
Suite 5
Casper, WY 82601
Tel.: 307-234-0294
Fax: 307-234-7226

PRODUCT IDENTIFICATION GUIDE

To aid in quick identification, this section provides full-color, actual-size photographs of tablets and capsules. A variety of other dosage forms and packages are shown at less than actual size. In all, the section contains a total of more than 1,000 photos.

Products in this section are arranged alphabetically by manufacturer. In some instances, not all dosage forms and sizes are pictured. Letters or numbers representing the manufacturer's identification code are followed by an asterisk.

For more information on any of the products in this section, please turn to the "Product Information" section, or check directly with the manufacturer. For easy reference, the page number of each product's text entry appears with its photographs.

While every effort has been made to guarantee faithful reproduction of the photos in this section, changes in size, color, and design are always a possibility. Be sure to confirm a product's identity with the manufacturer or your pharmacist.

Manufacturer's Index

ASCHER & CO., INC.

B.F. Ascher & Co., Inc.
P. 602

Available in 50 mL Saline Nasal Drops
and 50 mL Nasal Mist
Ayr®

B.F. Ascher & Co., Inc.
P. 602

Cough Suppressant and
Sore Throat Relief Lozenges
COUGH-X®

B.F. Ascher & Co., Inc.
P. 602

Available in: 35.4 g (1.25 oz) tube gel
and New 2 Fl. oz (59.1 mL) spray.
ITCH-X®

B.F. Ascher & Co., Inc.
P. 602

Analgesic Tablets
Available in: 18's, 50's & 100's
Mobigesic®

B.F. Ascher & Co., Inc.
P. 603

Analgesic Creme
Available in 1.25 oz., 3.5 oz.
and 8 oz. size
Mobisyl®

B.F. Ascher & Co., Inc.
P. 603

Therapeutic Creme for
Chronic Dry Skin
Available in: 8 fl.oz. bottle
PEN·KERA®

B.F. Ascher & Co., Inc.
P. 603

3 fl.oz.
Removes Rough Skin
Pretty Feet and Hands®

ASTRA

Astra USA, Inc.
P. 603

2.5% Ointment
Available in 35 gram Tube
Xylocaine®
(lidocaine)

BAKER CUMMINS

Baker Cummins Dermatologicals, Inc.
P. 604

Lotion, Cream and
Sunscreen Moisturiser (SPF 15)
Aquaderm®

Baker Cummins Dermatologicals, Inc.
P. 604

Liquid and Shampoo
P & S®

Baker Cummins Dermatologicals, Inc.
P. 605

Moisturizer
**Ultra Derm®/
Ultra Mide 25®**

Baker Cummins Dermatologicals, Inc.
P. 605

Shampoo
X-Seb®/X-Seb® Plus

Baker Cummins Dermatologicals, Inc.
P. 606

Shampoo
**X-Seb T® Pearl/
X-Seb T® Plus**

BAUSCH & LOMB

Bausch & Lomb
P. 606

Dry Skin Care Lotion and Creme
Fragrance Free (Shown) and
Original formulas
Curél®

BEIERSDORF

Beiersdorf Inc.
P. 607

Healing Ointments For Dry Skin,
Minor Cuts and Burns
Aquaphor®

Beiersdorf Inc.
P. 607

Cleansing Bar
Eucerin®

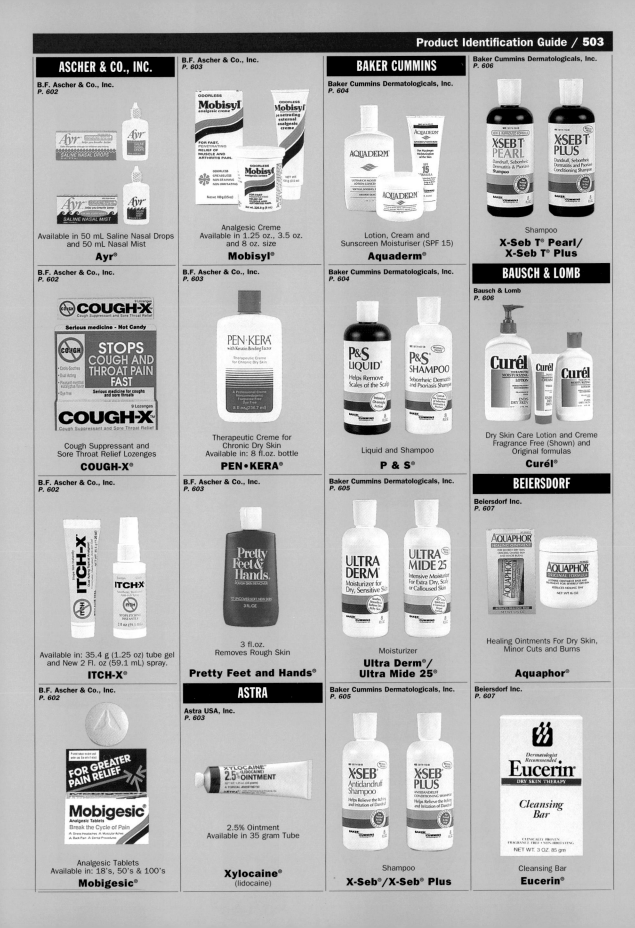

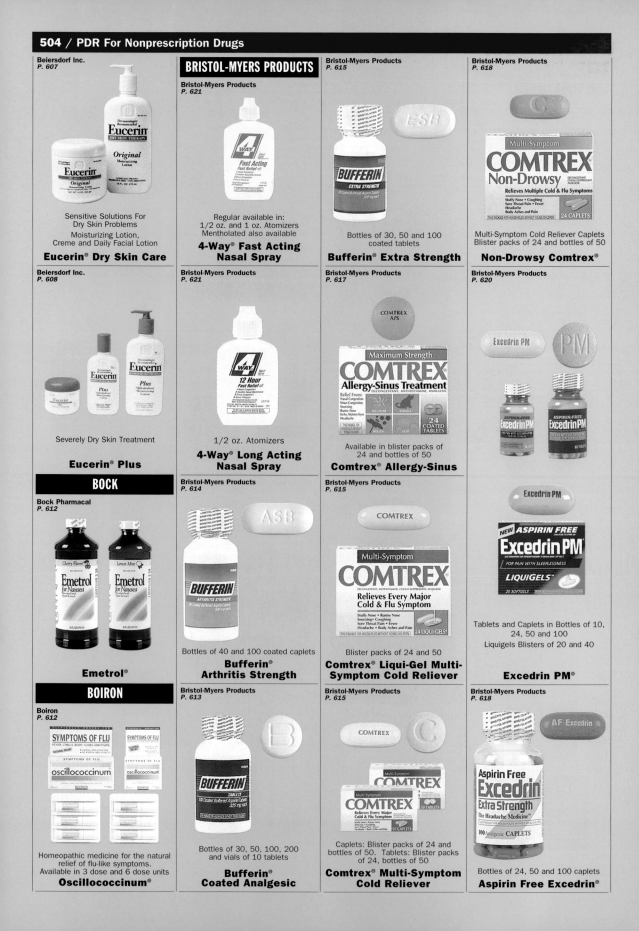

Beiersdorf Inc.
P. 607

Sensitive Solutions For
Dry Skin Problems
Moisturizing Lotion,
Creme and Daily Facial Lotion
Eucerin® Dry Skin Care

Beiersdorf Inc.
P. 608

Severely Dry Skin Treatment

Eucerin® Plus

BOCK

Bock Pharmacal
P. 612

Emetrol®

BOIRON

Boiron
P. 612

Homeopathic medicine for the natural
relief of flu-like symptoms.
Available in 3 dose and 6 dose units
Oscillococcinum®

BRISTOL-MYERS PRODUCTS

Bristol-Myers Products
P. 621

Regular available in:
1/2 oz. and 1 oz. Atomizers
Mentholated also available
**4-Way® Fast Acting
Nasal Spray**

Bristol-Myers Products
P. 621

1/2 oz. Atomizers
**4-Way® Long Acting
Nasal Spray**

Bristol-Myers Products
P. 614

Bottles of 40 and 100 coated caplets
**Bufferin®
Arthritis Strength**

Bristol-Myers Products
P. 613

Bottles of 30, 50, 100, 200
and vials of 10 tablets
**Bufferin®
Coated Analgesic**

Bristol-Myers Products
P. 615

Bottles of 30, 50 and 100
coated tablets
Bufferin® Extra Strength

Bristol-Myers Products
P. 617

Available in blister packs of
24 and bottles of 50
Comtrex® Allergy-Sinus

Bristol-Myers Products
P. 615

Blister packs of 24 and 50
**Comtrex® Liqui-Gel Multi-
Symptom Cold Reliever**

Bristol-Myers Products
P. 615

Caplets: Blister packs of 24 and
bottles of 50. Tablets: Blister packs
of 24, bottles of 50
**Comtrex® Multi-Symptom
Cold Reliever**

Bristol-Myers Products
P. 618

Multi-Symptom Cold Reliever Caplets
Blister packs of 24 and bottles of 50
Non-Drowsy Comtrex®

Bristol-Myers Products
P. 620

Tablets and Caplets in Bottles of 10,
24, 50 and 100
Liquigels Blisters of 20 and 40
Excedrin PM®

Bristol-Myers Products
P. 618

Bottles of 24, 50 and 100 caplets
Aspirin Free Excedrin®

Bristol-Myers Products
P. 619

Bottles of 12, 24, 50, 100, 175
and 275, metal tins of 12
and vials of 10 tablets
Extra Strength Excedrin®

Bristol-Myers Products
P. 622

For Dry Skin Care
6.5, 11 and 15 oz. 20 oz. size
for Original Formula
Silky Smooth and Fragrance Free
Keri® Lotion

Bristol-Myers Products
P. 622

Bottles of 24, 50, 100, 150
and vials of 10 tablets
Nuprin®

Bristol-Myers Products
P. 623

Complete Formula with Beta Carotene
High Potency Multivitamin Formula
Theragran®

Bristol-Myers Products
P. 623

Complete Formula with Antioxidants
High Potency Multivitamin
Formula with Minerals
Theragran-M®

Bristol-Myers Products
P. 623

Theragran® Antioxidant

Bristol-Myers Products
P. 623

Available in: 3.5 oz., 8 oz.
and 16 oz. Pain Relieving Gel
Therapeutic Mineral Ice®

W.K. BUCKLEY, INC.

W.K. Buckley, Inc.
P. 624

8 Fl. oz. and 4 Fl. oz.
Buckley's® Mixture

CARTILAGE

Cartilage Technologies, Inc.
P. 626

Available in Capsules and Caplets of
42's, 90's, 180's, 360's and Powder
200 g, 400 g, 500 g,
and 1400 g
Cartilade®

CIBA CONSUMER

Ciba Consumer
P. 628

Appetite Suppressants
Caffeine Free/Works all Day
Acutrim®

Ciba Consumer
P. 629

Ointment 3/4 oz. and Spray 2 oz.
Also available in
Hemorrhoidal Ointment 1 oz.
Americaine®

Ciba Consumer
P. 629

Bottles of 60, 100, 160,
225 & 500 Tablets
**Regular Strength
Ascriptin®**

Ciba Consumer
P. 630

Bottles of 36, 50 & 85 Caplets
**Maximum Strength
Ascriptin®**

Ciba Consumer
P. 631

Bottles of 60, 100,
225 & 500 Caplets
**Arthritis Pain
Ascriptin®**

Ciba Consumer
P. 631

Caldecort and Caldecort Light® Cream
1.5 oz. Spray
Caldecort®

Ciba Consumer
P. 632

Medicated Powder and Ointment
Also available in 2 oz. and 4 oz. powder
Caldesene®

Ciba Consumer
P. 632

Antifungal Spray and Squeeze
Powder & Cream
Relieves Itching, Chafing, Rash
Cures Jock Itch

Cruex®

Ciba Consumer
P. 633

Backache Analgesic
Relieves Backache
Regular/Extra Strength/Nighttime

Doan's® & Doan's® P.M.

Ciba Consumer
P. 636

Powder and Wafers

Fiberall®

Ciba Consumer
P. 643

Ciba Consumer
P. 632

Spray Powder, Cream,
Ointment & Spray Liquid
Cures Athlete's Foot

Desenex®

Ciba Consumer
P. 634

Tablets & Suppositories

Dulcolax® Laxative

Ciba Consumer
P. 637

Plain (Mineral Oil)
Lubricant Laxative

Kondremul®

Lemon Creme, Assorted &
Cherry Creme Flavors in
Bottles of 50 & 100 Tablets
Rollpacks of 3 in assorted Lemon and
Creme Flavors Only

**Maalox® Antacid
Plus Anti-Gas**

Ciba Consumer
P. 633

Spray Powder, Cream
& Liquid Spray
Cures Athlete's Foot

**Prescription Strength
Desenex®**

Ciba Consumer
P. 635

Nasal Decongestant

Efidac/24®

Ciba Consumer
P. 638

Blister Packs of 24's and Bottles of
50's Antacid Caplets

Maalox® Antacid Caplets

Ciba Consumer
P. 638

Mint Creme Tablets and Assorted
Flavors in 38's, 75's

**Extra Strength Maalox®
Antacid Plus Anti-Gas**

Ciba Consumer
P. 633

Foot & Sneaker Deodorant
Soothes, Cools, Comforts
and Absorbs Moisture

Desenex®

Ciba Consumer
P. 635

Alpine Breeze, Powder Fresh
and Arthritis Pain External Analgesics

Eucalyptamint®

Ciba Consumer
P. 642

Mint & Cherry Creme
Available in 12 & 26 oz.

Maalox® Antacid

Ciba Consumer
P. 638

Mint Creme, Cherry Creme and Lemon
Creme All available in 12 & 26 oz.

**Extra Strength Maalox®
Plus Anti-Gas**

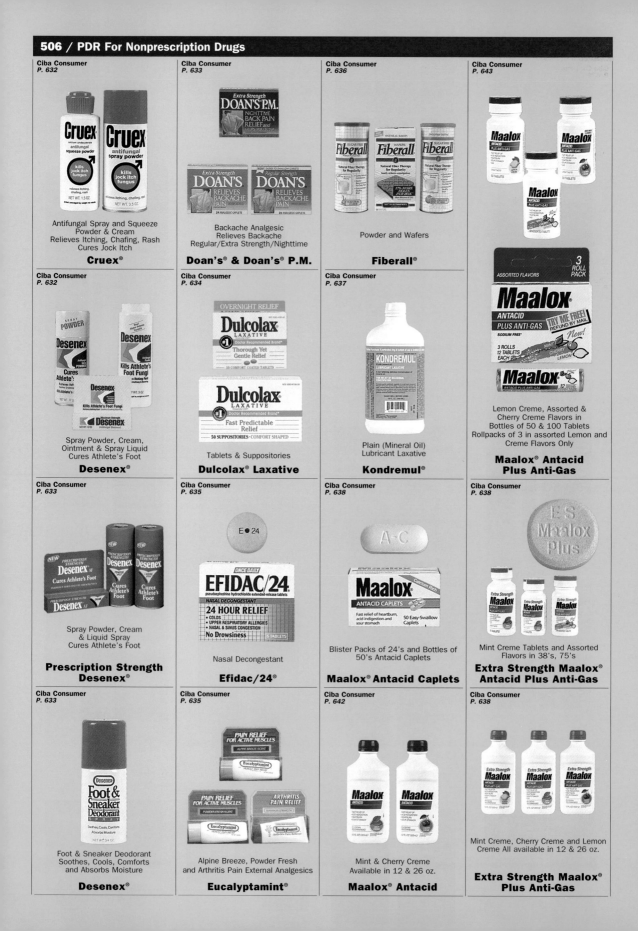

Ciba Consumer
P. 639

Available in 2 oz. and 4 oz. liquid
(cherry flavored) w/dosage cup
6 and 12 Caplets

Maalox® Anti-Diarrheal

Ciba Consumer
P. 640

Peppermint and Lemon Flavor
Regular Strength 12's & 48's
Extra Strength 10's

Maalox® Anti-Gas

Ciba Consumer
P. 641

Orange and Citrus Flavors
Bulk-Producing Psyllium Fiber
Regular & Sugar Free

**Maalox® Daily
Fiber Therapy**

Ciba Consumer
P. 643

External Analgesic Cream
Available in 2 oz. and 4 oz. tubes,
8 oz. and 16 oz. jars

Myoflex®

Ciba Consumer
P. 644

Children's & Regular
Metered Pump Spray
Also available in Nostrilla®
12 Hour Metered Pump Spray

Nóstril®

Ciba Consumer
P. 645

For fast, soothing relief of anal itch.

Nupercainal®

Ciba Consumer
P. 645

1 1/2 oz. Pain Relief Cream
Prompt, temporary relief of painful
sunburn, minor burns, scrapes, scratches,
and nonpoisonous insect bites.

Nupercainal®

Ciba Consumer
P. 644

Hemmorhoidal & Anesthetic
Available in: Ointment 2 oz. & 1 oz.
Suppositories: boxes of 12 & 24

Nupercainal®

Ciba Consumer
P. 645

Nasal Decongestant Drops
Pediatric Drops and Nasal Spray

Otrivin®

Ciba Consumer
P. 646

100% Natural Vegetable Laxative
250 gm and 6-6gm packets

Perdiem®

Ciba Consumer
P. 646

100% Natural
Daily Fiber Source
available in 250 gm only

Perdiem® Fiber

Ciba Consumer
P. 647

Fast
relief
of
stuffy
nose

**Privine®
nasal drops**
naphazoline HCl, USP
Nasal Decongestant

.83 fl oz (25ml)

Also available in Nasal Spray

Privine®

Ciba Consumer
P. 648

Slow Release Iron and Slow Release
Iron & Folic Acid

Slow Fe®

Ciba Consumer
P. 649

Children's Multivitamins
Regular + Extra C + Iron Complete

Sunkist®

Ciba Consumer
P. 649

250 & 500 mg Chewable Tablets;
500 mg Easy to Swallow Caplets;
60 mg Chewable Tablets (11 Tablet Roll)

**Sunkist® Vitamin C
Citrus Complex**

Ciba Consumer
P. 650

Cream, Powder, Spray Liquid & Powder
For Athlete's Foot & Jock Itch

Ting®

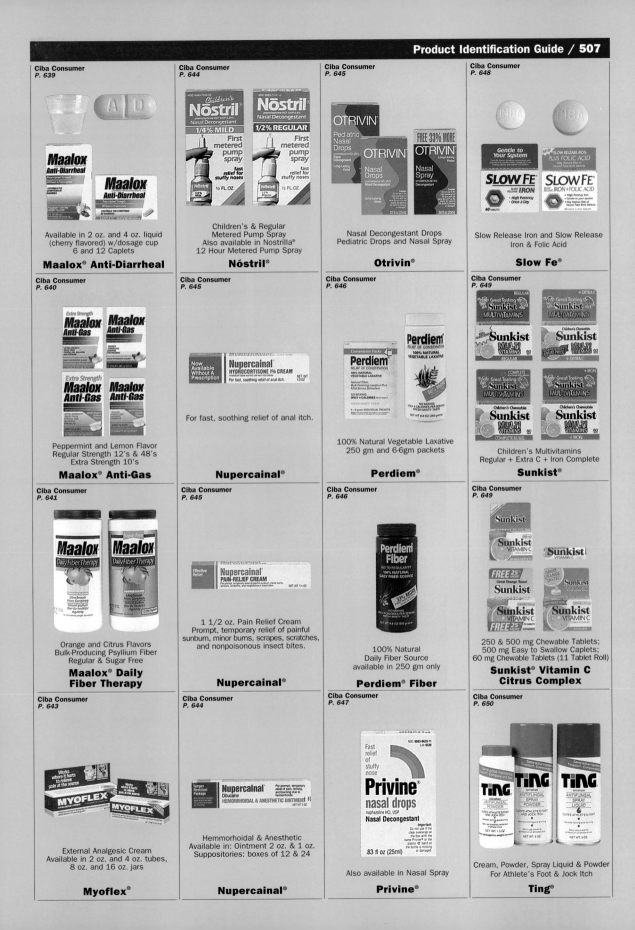

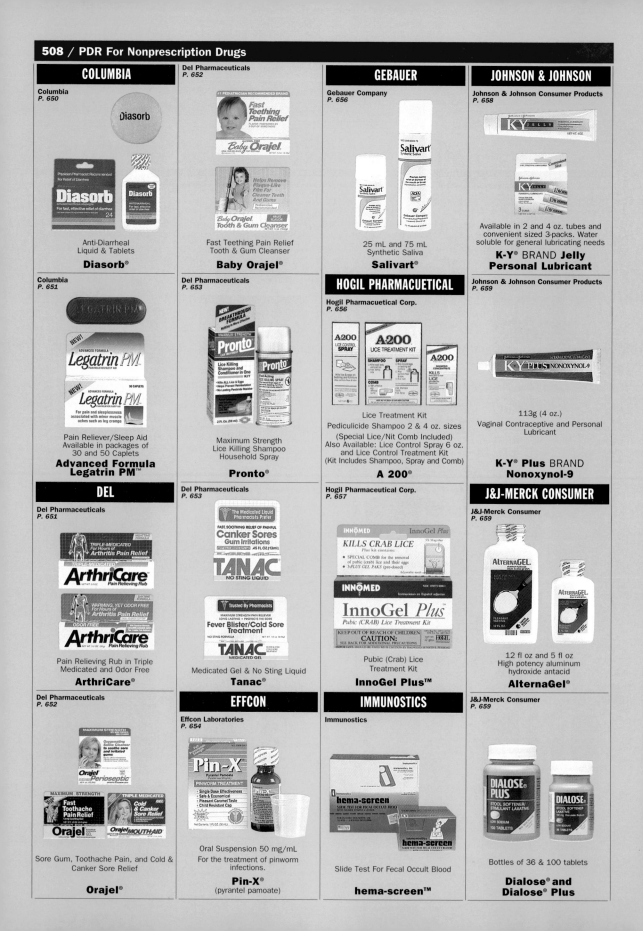

COLUMBIA

Columbia
P. 650

Anti-Diarrheal
Liquid & Tablets

Diasorb®

Columbia
P. 651

Pain Reliever/Sleep Aid
Available in packages of
30 and 50 Caplets

**Advanced Formula
Legatrin PM™**

DEL

Del Pharmaceuticals
P. 651

Pain Relieving Rub in Triple
Medicated and Odor Free

ArthriCare®

Del Pharmaceuticals
P. 652

Sore Gum, Toothache Pain, and Cold &
Canker Sore Relief

Orajel®

Del Pharmaceuticals
P. 652

Fast Teething Pain Relief
Tooth & Gum Cleanser

Baby Orajel®

Del Pharmaceuticals
P. 653

Maximum Strength
Lice Killing Shampoo
Household Spray

Pronto®

Del Pharmaceuticals
P. 653

Medicated Gel & No Sting Liquid

Tanac®

EFFCON

Effcon Laboratories
P. 654

Oral Suspension 50 mg/mL
For the treatment of pinworm
infections.

Pin-X®
(pyrantel pamoate)

GEBAUER

Gebauer Company
P. 656

25 mL and 75 mL
Synthetic Saliva

Salivart®

HOGIL PHARMACUETICAL

Hogil Pharmacuetical Corp.
P. 656

Lice Treatment Kit
Pediculicide Shampoo 2 & 4 oz. sizes
(Special Lice/Nit Comb Included)
Also Available: Lice Control Spray 6 oz.
and Lice Control Treatment Kit
(Kit Includes Shampoo, Spray and Comb)

A 200®

Hogil Pharmacuetical Corp.
P. 657

Pubic (Crab) Lice
Treatment Kit

InnoGel Plus™

IMMUNOSTICS

Immunostics

Slide Test For Fecal Occult Blood

hema-screen™

JOHNSON & JOHNSON

Johnson & Johnson Consumer Products
P. 658

Available in 2 and 4 oz. tubes and
convenient sized 3-packs. Water
soluble for general lubricating needs

**K-Y® BRAND Jelly
Personal Lubricant**

Johnson & Johnson Consumer Products
P. 659

113g (4 oz.)
Vaginal Contraceptive and Personal
Lubricant

**K-Y® Plus BRAND
Nonoxynol-9**

J&J-MERCK CONSUMER

J&J-Merck Consumer
P. 659

12 fl oz and 5 fl oz
High potency aluminum
hydroxide antacid

AlternaGEL®

J&J-Merck Consumer
P. 659

Bottles of 36 & 100 tablets

**Dialose® and
Dialose® Plus**

J&J-Merck Consumer
P. 662

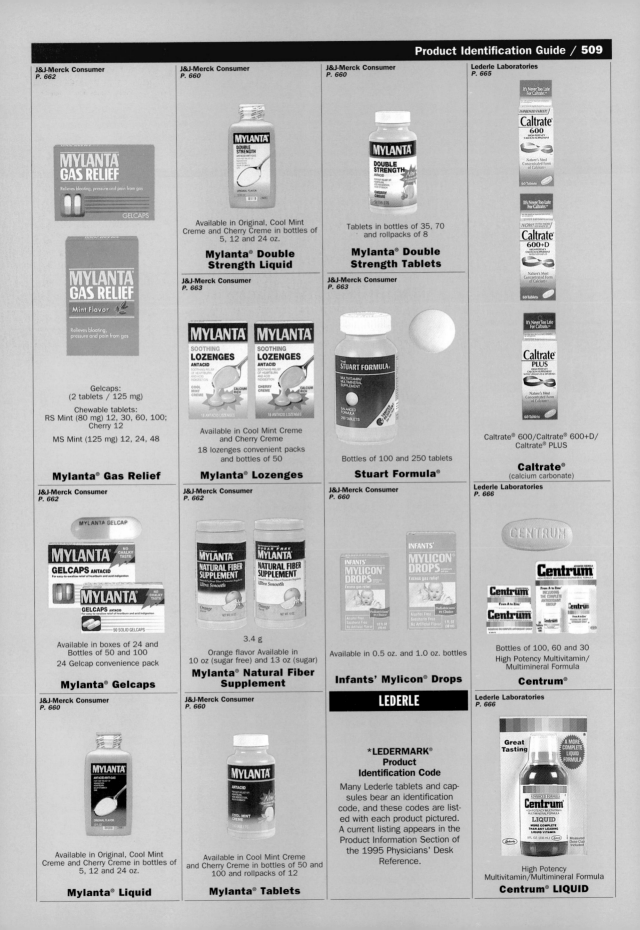

Gelcaps:
(2 tablets / 125 mg)
Chewable tablets:
RS Mint (80 mg) 12, 30, 60, 100;
Cherry 12

MS Mint (125 mg) 12, 24, 48

Mylanta® Gas Relief

J&J-Merck Consumer
P. 662

Available in boxes of 24 and
Bottles of 50 and 100
24 Gelcap convenience pack

Mylanta® Gelcaps

J&J-Merck Consumer
P. 660

Available in Original, Cool Mint
Creme and Cherry Creme in bottles of
5, 12 and 24 oz.

Mylanta® Liquid

J&J-Merck Consumer
P. 660

Available in Original, Cool Mint
Creme and Cherry Creme in bottles of
5, 12 and 24 oz.

**Mylanta® Double
Strength Liquid**

J&J-Merck Consumer
P. 663

Available in Cool Mint Creme
and Cherry Creme
18 lozenges convenient packs
and bottles of 50

Mylanta® Lozenges

J&J-Merck Consumer
P. 662

3.4 g
Orange flavor Available in
10 oz (sugar free) and 13 oz (sugar)

**Mylanta® Natural Fiber
Supplement**

J&J-Merck Consumer
P. 660

Available in Cool Mint Creme
and Cherry Creme in bottles of 50 and
100 and rollpacks of 12

Mylanta® Tablets

J&J-Merck Consumer
P. 660

Tablets in bottles of 35, 70
and rollpacks of 8

**Mylanta® Double
Strength Tablets**

J&J-Merck Consumer
P. 663

Bottles of 100 and 250 tablets

Stuart Formula®

J&J-Merck Consumer
P. 660

Available in 0.5 oz. and 1.0 oz. bottles

Infants' Mylicon® Drops

LEDERLE

***LEDERMARK®
Product
Identification Code**

Many Lederle tablets and capsules bear an identification
code, and these codes are listed with each product pictured.
A current listing appears in the
Product Information Section of
the 1995 Physicians' Desk
Reference.

Lederle Laboratories
P. 665

Caltrate® 600/Caltrate® 600+D/
Caltrate® PLUS

Caltrate®
(calcium carbonate)

Lederle Laboratories
P. 666

Bottles of 100, 60 and 30

High Potency Multivitamin/
Multimineral Formula

Centrum®

Lederle Laboratories
P. 666

High Potency
Multivitamin/Multimineral Formula

Centrum® LIQUID

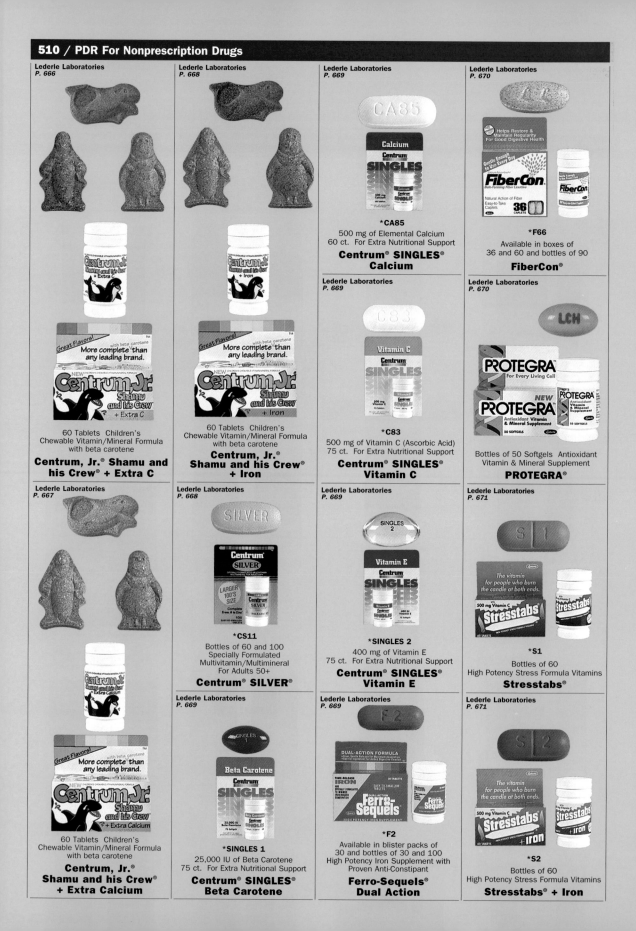

Lederle Laboratories
P. 666

60 Tablets Children's
Chewable Vitamin/Mineral Formula
with beta carotene

Centrum, Jr.® Shamu and his Crew® + Extra C

Lederle Laboratories
P. 667

60 Tablets Children's
Chewable Vitamin/Mineral Formula
with beta carotene

**Centrum, Jr.®
Shamu and his Crew®
+ Extra Calcium**

Lederle Laboratories
P. 668

60 Tablets Children's
Chewable Vitamin/Mineral Formula
with beta carotene

**Centrum, Jr.®
Shamu and his Crew®
+ Iron**

Lederle Laboratories
P. 668

*CS11
Bottles of 60 and 100
Specially Formulated
Multivitamin/Multimineral
For Adults 50+

Centrum® SILVER®

Lederle Laboratories
P. 669

*SINGLES 1
25,000 IU of Beta Carotene
75 ct. For Extra Nutritional Support

**Centrum® SINGLES®
Beta Carotene**

Lederle Laboratories
P. 669

*CA85
500 mg of Elemental Calcium
60 ct. For Extra Nutritional Support

**Centrum® SINGLES®
Calcium**

Lederle Laboratories
P. 669

*C83
500 mg of Vitamin C (Ascorbic Acid)
75 ct. For Extra Nutritional Support

**Centrum® SINGLES®
Vitamin C**

Lederle Laboratories
P. 669

*SINGLES 2
400 mg of Vitamin E
75 ct. For Extra Nutritional Support

**Centrum® SINGLES®
Vitamin E**

Lederle Laboratories
P. 669

*F2
Available in blister packs of
30 and bottles of 30 and 100
High Potency Iron Supplement with
Proven Anti-Constipant

**Ferro-Sequels®
Dual Action**

Lederle Laboratories
P. 670

*F66
Available in boxes of
36 and 60 and bottles of 90

FiberCon®

Lederle Laboratories
P. 670

Bottles of 50 Softgels Antioxidant
Vitamin & Mineral Supplement

PROTEGRA®

Lederle Laboratories
P. 671

*S1
Bottles of 60
High Potency Stress Formula Vitamins

Stresstabs®

Lederle Laboratories
P. 671

*S2
Bottles of 60
High Potency Stress Formula Vitamins

Stresstabs® + Iron

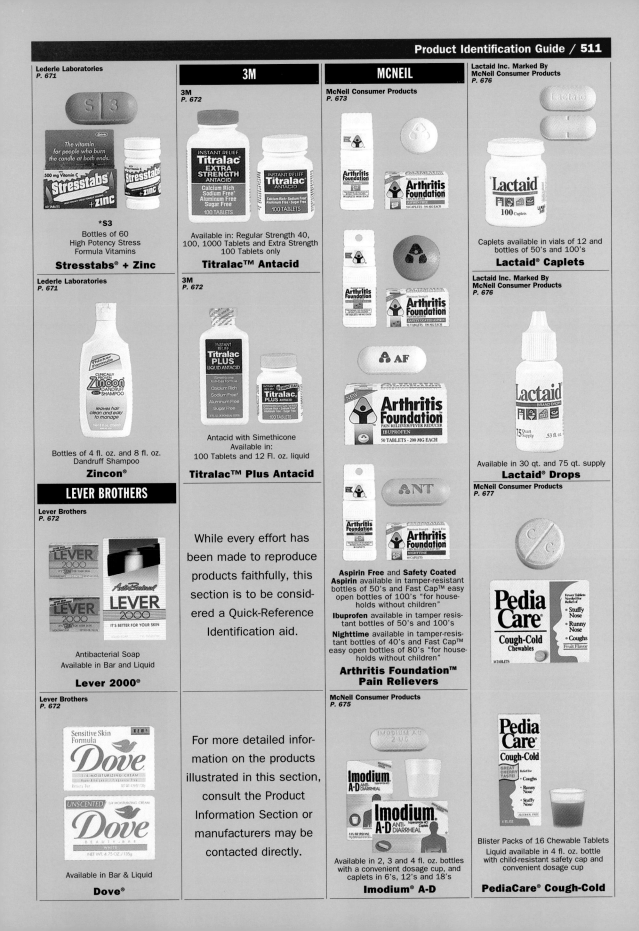

Lederle Laboratories
P. 671

*S3
Bottles of 60
High Potency Stress
Formula Vitamins

Stresstabs® + Zinc

Lederle Laboratories
P. 671

Bottles of 4 fl. oz. and 8 fl. oz.
Dandruff Shampoo

Zincon®

LEVER BROTHERS

Lever Brothers
P. 672

Antibacterial Soap
Available in Bar and Liquid

Lever 2000®

Lever Brothers
P. 672

Available in Bar & Liquid

Dove®

3M

3M
P. 672

Available in: Regular Strength 40,
100, 1000 Tablets and Extra Strength
100 Tablets only

Titralac™ Antacid

3M
P. 672

Antacid with Simethicone
Available in:
100 Tablets and 12 Fl. oz. liquid

Titralac™ Plus Antacid

While every effort has been made to reproduce products faithfully, this section is to be considered a Quick-Reference Identification aid.

For more detailed information on the products illustrated in this section, consult the Product Information Section or manufacturers may be contacted directly.

MCNEIL

McNeil Consumer Products
P. 673

Aspirin Free and **Safety Coated Aspirin** available in tamper-resistant bottles of 50's and Fast Cap™ easy open bottles of 100's "for households without children"
Ibuprofen available in tamper resistant bottles of 50's and 100's
Nighttime available in tamper-resistant bottles of 40's and Fast Cap™ easy open bottles of 80's "for households without children"

Arthritis Foundation™ Pain Relievers

McNeil Consumer Products
P. 675

Available in 2, 3 and 4 fl. oz. bottles with a convenient dosage cup, and caplets in 6's, 12's and 18's

Imodium® A·D

Lactaid Inc. Marked By McNeil Consumer Products
P. 676

Caplets available in vials of 12 and bottles of 50's and 100's

Lactaid® Caplets

Lactaid Inc. Marked By McNeil Consumer Products
P. 676

Available in 30 qt. and 75 qt. supply

Lactaid® Drops

McNeil Consumer Products
P. 677

Blister Packs of 16 Chewable Tablets
Liquid available in 4 fl. oz. bottle with child-resistant safety cap and convenient dosage cup

PediaCare® Cough-Cold

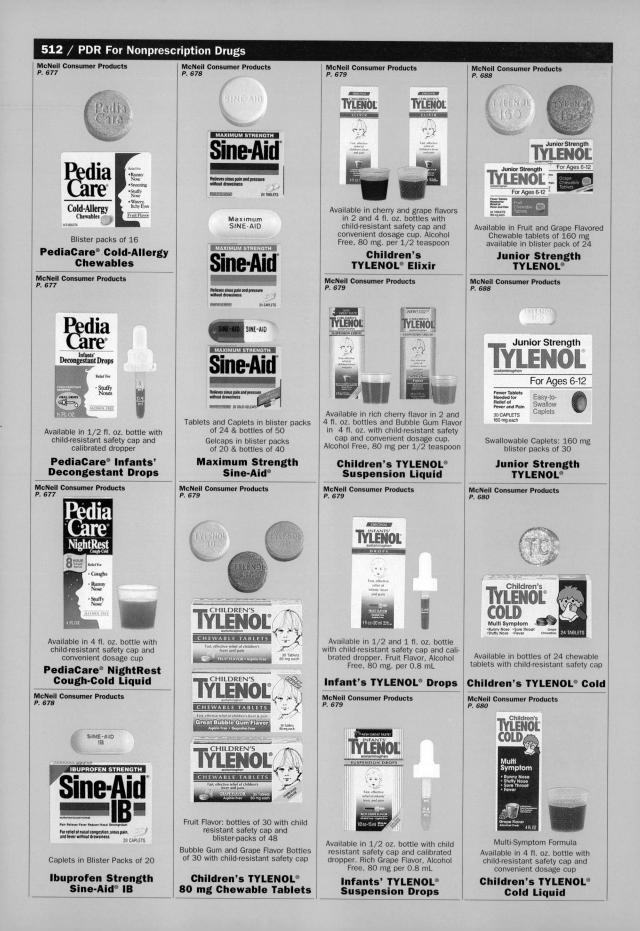

McNeil Consumer Products
P. 677

Blister packs of 16

PediaCare® Cold-Allergy Chewables

McNeil Consumer Products
P. 677

Available in 1/2 fl. oz. bottle with child-resistant safety cap and calibrated dropper

PediaCare® Infants' Decongestant Drops

McNeil Consumer Products
P. 677

Available in 4 fl. oz. bottle with child-resistant safety cap and convenient dosage cup

PediaCare® NightRest Cough-Cold Liquid

McNeil Consumer Products
P. 678

Caplets in Blister Packs of 20

Ibuprofen Strength Sine-Aid® IB

McNeil Consumer Products
P. 678

Tablets and Caplets in blister packs of 24 & bottles of 50

Gelcaps in blister packs of 20 & bottles of 40

Maximum Strength Sine-Aid®

McNeil Consumer Products
P. 679

Fruit Flavor: bottles of 30 with child resistant safety cap and blister-packs of 48

Bubble Gum and Grape Flavor Bottles of 30 with child-resistant safety cap

Children's TYLENOL® 80 mg Chewable Tablets

McNeil Consumer Products
P. 679

Available in cherry and grape flavors in 2 and 4 fl. oz. bottles with child-resistant safety cap and convenient dosage cup. Alcohol Free, 80 mg. per 1/2 teaspoon

Children's TYLENOL® Elixir

McNeil Consumer Products
P. 679

Available in rich cherry flavor in 2 and 4 fl. oz. bottles and Bubble Gum Flavor in 4 fl. oz. with child-resistant safety cap and convenient dosage cup. Alcohol Free, 80 mg per 1/2 teaspoon

Children's TYLENOL® Suspension Liquid

McNeil Consumer Products
P. 679

Available in 1/2 and 1 fl. oz. bottle with child-resistant safety cap and calibrated dropper. Fruit Flavor, Alcohol Free, 80 mg. per 0.8 mL

Infant's TYLENOL® Drops

McNeil Consumer Products
P. 679

Available in 1/2 oz. bottle with child resistant safety cap and calibrated dropper. Rich Grape Flavor, Alcohol Free, 80 mg per 0.8 mL

Infants' TYLENOL® Suspension Drops

McNeil Consumer Products
P. 688

Available in Fruit and Grape Flavored Chewable tablets of 160 mg available in blister pack of 24

Junior Strength TYLENOL®

McNeil Consumer Products
P. 688

Swallowable Caplets: 160 mg blister packs of 30

Junior Strength TYLENOL®

McNeil Consumer Products
P. 680

Available in bottles of 24 chewable tablets with child-resistant safety cap

Children's TYLENOL® Cold

McNeil Consumer Products
P. 680

Multi-Symptom Formula
Available in 4 fl. oz. bottle with child-resistant safety cap and convenient dosage cup

Children's TYLENOL® Cold Liquid

McNeil Consumer Products
P. 681

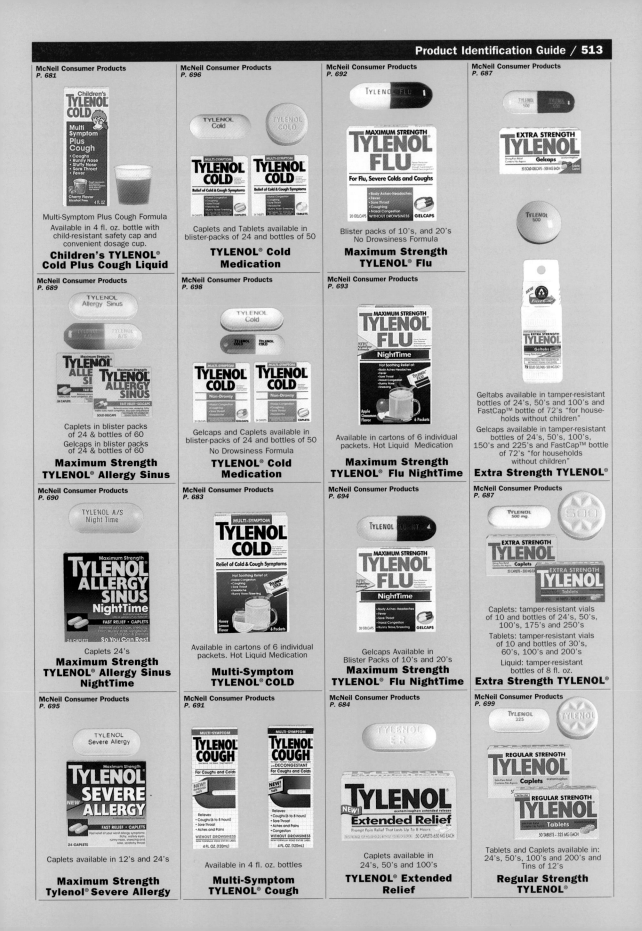

Multi-Symptom Plus Cough Formula
Available in 4 fl. oz. bottle with
child-resistant safety cap and
convenient dosage cup.
**Children's TYLENOL®
Cold Plus Cough Liquid**

McNeil Consumer Products
P. 696

Caplets and Tablets available in
blister-packs of 24 and bottles of 50
**TYLENOL® Cold
Medication**

McNeil Consumer Products
P. 692

Blister packs of 10's, and 20's
No Drowsiness Formula
**Maximum Strength
TYLENOL® Flu**

McNeil Consumer Products
P. 687

Geltabs available in tamper-resistant
bottles of 24's, 50's and 100's and
FastCap™ bottle of 72's "for households without children"

Gelcaps available in tamper-resistant
bottles of 24's, 50's, 100's,
150's and 225's and FastCap™ bottle
of 72's "for households
without children"
Extra Strength TYLENOL®

McNeil Consumer Products
P. 689

Caplets in blister packs
of 24 & bottles of 60
Gelcaps in blister packs
of 24 & bottles of 60
**Maximum Strength
TYLENOL® Allergy Sinus**

McNeil Consumer Products
P. 698

Gelcaps and Caplets available in
blister-packs of 24 and bottles of 50
No Drowsiness Formula
**TYLENOL® Cold
Medication**

McNeil Consumer Products
P. 693

Available in cartons of 6 individual
packets. Hot Liquid Medication
**Maximum Strength
TYLENOL® Flu NightTime**

McNeil Consumer Products
P. 690

Caplets 24's
**Maximum Strength
TYLENOL® Allergy Sinus
NightTime**

McNeil Consumer Products
P. 683

Available in cartons of 6 individual
packets. Hot Liquid Medication
**Multi-Symptom
TYLENOL® COLD**

McNeil Consumer Products
P. 694

Gelcaps Available in
Blister Packs of 10's and 20's
**Maximum Strength
TYLENOL® Flu NightTime**

McNeil Consumer Products
P. 687

Caplets: tamper-resistant vials
of 10 and bottles of 24's, 50's,
100's, 175's and 250's

Tablets: tamper-resistant vials
of 10 and bottles of 30's,
60's, 100's and 200's

Liquid: tamper-resistant
bottles of 8 fl. oz.
Extra Strength TYLENOL®

McNeil Consumer Products
P. 695

Caplets available in 12's and 24's
**Maximum Strength
Tylenol® Severe Allergy**

McNeil Consumer Products
P. 691

Available in 4 fl. oz. bottles
**Multi-Symptom
TYLENOL® Cough**

McNeil Consumer Products
P. 684

Caplets available in
24's, 50's and 100's
**TYLENOL® Extended
Relief**

McNeil Consumer Products
P. 699

Tablets and Caplets available in:
24's, 50's, 100's and 200's and
Tins of 12's
**Regular Strength
TYLENOL®**

McNeil Consumer Products
P. 685

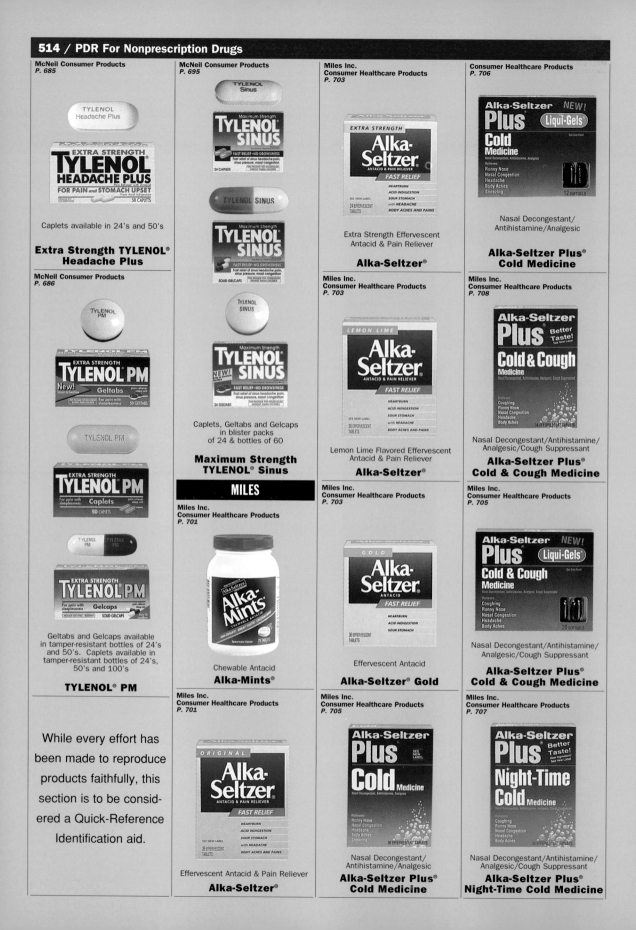

Caplets available in 24's and 50's

**Extra Strength TYLENOL®
Headache Plus**

McNeil Consumer Products
P. 686

Geltabs and Gelcaps available
in tamper-resistant bottles of 24's
and 50's. Caplets available in
tamper-resistant bottles of 24's,
50's and 100's

TYLENOL® PM

While every effort has
been made to reproduce
products faithfully, this
section is to be consid-
ered a Quick-Reference
Identification aid.

McNeil Consumer Products
P. 695

Caplets, Geltabs and Gelcaps
in blister packs
of 24 & bottles of 60

**Maximum Strength
TYLENOL® Sinus**

MILES

Miles Inc.
Consumer Healthcare Products
P. 701

Chewable Antacid
Alka-Mints®

Miles Inc.
Consumer Healthcare Products
P. 701

Effervescent Antacid & Pain Reliever
Alka-Seltzer®

Miles Inc.
Consumer Healthcare Products
P. 703

Extra Strength Effervescent
Antacid & Pain Reliever

Alka-Seltzer®

Miles Inc.
Consumer Healthcare Products
P. 703

Lemon Lime Flavored Effervescent
Antacid & Pain Reliever

Alka-Seltzer®

Miles Inc.
Consumer Healthcare Products
P. 703

Effervescent Antacid

Alka-Seltzer® Gold

Miles Inc.
Consumer Healthcare Products
P. 705

Nasal Decongestant/
Antihistamine/Analgesic

**Alka-Seltzer Plus®
Cold Medicine**

Consumer Healthcare Products
P. 706

Nasal Decongestant/
Antihistamine/Analgesic

**Alka-Seltzer Plus®
Cold Medicine**

Miles Inc.
Consumer Healthcare Products
P. 708

Nasal Decongestant/Antihistamine/
Analgesic/Cough Suppressant

**Alka-Seltzer Plus®
Cold & Cough Medicine**

Miles Inc.
Consumer Healthcare Products
P. 705

Nasal Decongestant/Antihistamine/
Analgesic/Cough Suppressant

**Alka-Seltzer Plus®
Cold & Cough Medicine**

Miles Inc.
Consumer Healthcare Products
P. 707

Nasal Decongestant/Antihistamine/
Analgesic/Cough Suppressant

**Alka-Seltzer Plus®
Night-Time Cold Medicine**

Miles Inc.
Consumer Healthcare Products
P. 707

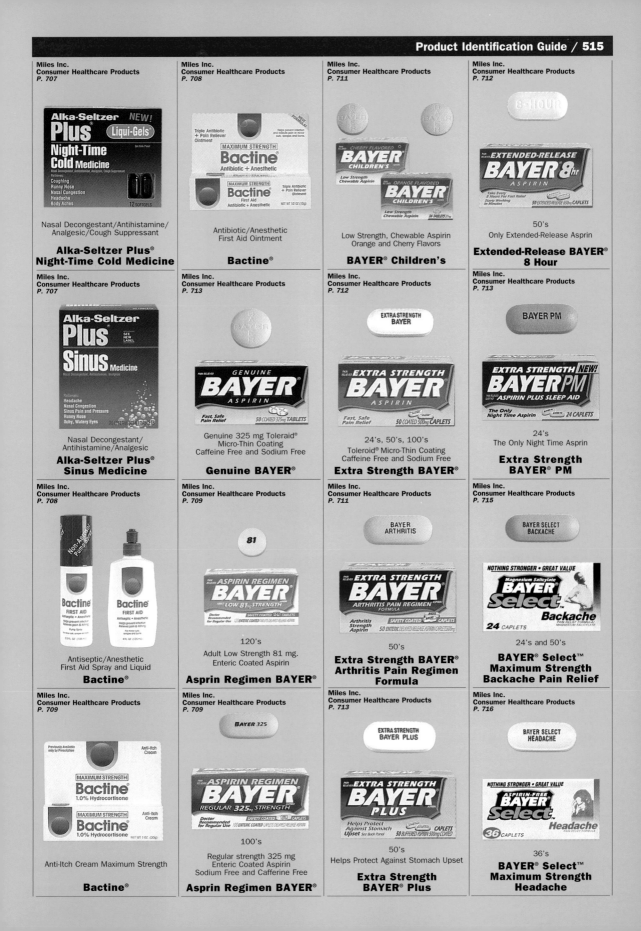

Nasal Decongestant/Antihistamine/
Analgesic/Cough Suppressant

**Alka-Seltzer Plus®
Night-Time Cold Medicine**

Miles Inc.
Consumer Healthcare Products
P. 707

Nasal Decongestant/
Antihistamine/Analgesic

**Alka-Seltzer Plus®
Sinus Medicine**

Miles Inc.
Consumer Healthcare Products
P. 708

Antiseptic/Anesthetic
First Aid Spray and Liquid

Bactine®

Miles Inc.
Consumer Healthcare Products
P. 709

Anti-Itch Cream Maximum Strength

Bactine®

Miles Inc.
Consumer Healthcare Products
P. 708

Antibiotic/Anesthetic
First Aid Ointment

Bactine®

Miles Inc.
Consumer Healthcare Products
P. 713

Genuine 325 mg Toleraid®
Micro-Thin Coating
Caffeine Free and Sodium Free

Genuine BAYER®

Miles Inc.
Consumer Healthcare Products
P. 709

120's
Adult Low Strength 81 mg.
Enteric Coated Aspirin

Asprin Regimen BAYER®

Miles Inc.
Consumer Healthcare Products
P. 709

100's
Regular strength 325 mg
Enteric Coated Aspirin
Sodium Free and Cafferine Free

Asprin Regimen BAYER®

Miles Inc.
Consumer Healthcare Products
P. 711

Low Strength, Chewable Aspirin
Orange and Cherry Flavors

BAYER® Children's

Miles Inc.
Consumer Healthcare Products
P. 712

24's, 50's, 100's
Toleroid® Micro-Thin Coating
Caffeine Free and Sodium Free

Extra Strength BAYER®

Miles Inc.
Consumer Healthcare Products
P. 711

50's

**Extra Strength BAYER®
Arthritis Pain Regimen
Formula**

Miles Inc.
Consumer Healthcare Products
P. 713

50's
Helps Protect Against Stomach Upset

**Extra Strength
BAYER® Plus**

Miles Inc.
Consumer Healthcare Products
P. 712

50's
Only Extended-Release Asprin

**Extended-Release BAYER®
8 Hour**

Miles Inc.
Consumer Healthcare Products
P. 713

24's
The Only Night Time Aspirin

**Extra Strength
BAYER® PM**

Miles Inc.
Consumer Healthcare Products
P. 715

24's and 50's

**BAYER® Select™
Maximum Strength
Backache Pain Relief**

Miles Inc.
Consumer Healthcare Products
P. 716

36's

**BAYER® Select™
Maximum Strength
Headache**

Miles Inc.
Consumer Healthcare Products
P. 715

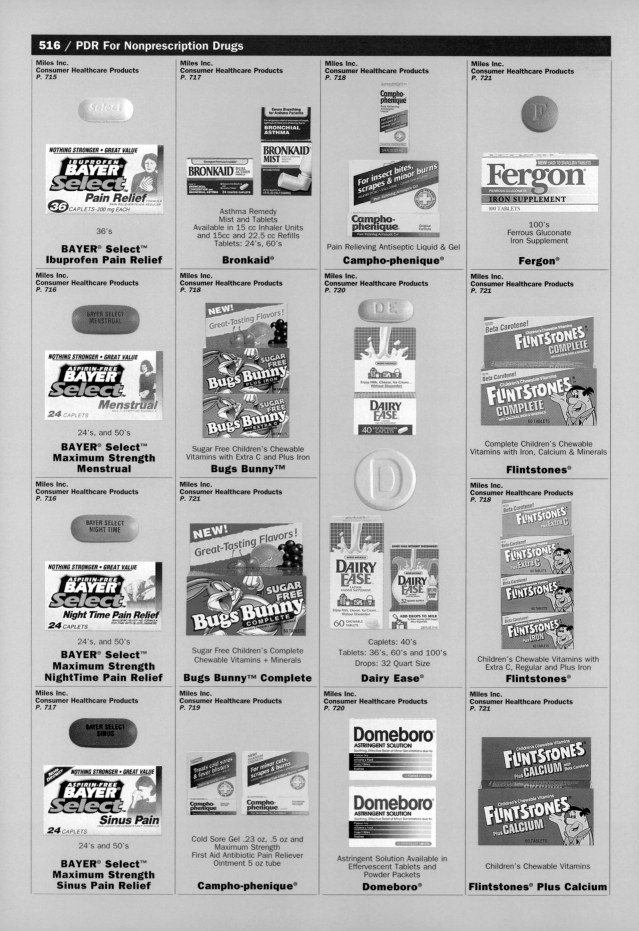

36's

**BAYER® Select™
Ibuprofen Pain Relief**

Miles Inc.
Consumer Healthcare Products
P. 716

24's, and 50's

**BAYER® Select™
Maximum Strength
Menstrual**

Miles Inc.
Consumer Healthcare Products
P. 716

24's, and 50's

**BAYER® Select™
Maximum Strength
NightTime Pain Relief**

Miles Inc.
Consumer Healthcare Products
P. 717

24's and 50's

**BAYER® Select™
Maximum Strength
Sinus Pain Relief**

Miles Inc.
Consumer Healthcare Products
P. 717

Asthma Remedy
Mist and Tablets
Available in 15 cc Inhaler Units
and 15cc and 22.5 cc Refills
Tablets: 24's, 60's

Bronkaid®

Miles Inc.
Consumer Healthcare Products
P. 718

Sugar Free Children's Chewable
Vitamins with Extra C and Plus Iron

Bugs Bunny™

Miles Inc.
Consumer Healthcare Products
P. 721

Sugar Free Children's Complete
Chewable Vitamins + Minerals

Bugs Bunny™ Complete

Miles Inc.
Consumer Healthcare Products
P. 719

Cold Sore Gel .23 oz, .5 oz and
Maximum Strength
First Aid Antibiotic Pain Reliever
Ointment 5 oz tube

Campho-phenique®

Miles Inc.
Consumer Healthcare Products
P. 718

Pain Relieving Antiseptic Liquid & Gel

Campho-phenique®

Miles Inc.
Consumer Healthcare Products
P. 720

Caplets: 40's
Tablets: 36's, 60's and 100's
Drops: 32 Quart Size

Dairy Ease®

Miles Inc.
Consumer Healthcare Products
P. 720

Astringent Solution Available in
Effervescent Tablets and
Powder Packets

Domeboro®

Miles Inc.
Consumer Healthcare Products
P. 721

100's
Ferrous Gluconate
Iron Supplement

Fergon®

Miles Inc.
Consumer Healthcare Products
P. 721

Complete Children's Chewable
Vitamins with Iron, Calcium & Minerals

Flintstones®

Miles Inc.
Consumer Healthcare Products
P. 718

Children's Chewable Vitamins with
Extra C, Regular and Plus Iron

Flintstones®

Miles Inc.
Consumer Healthcare Products
P. 721

Children's Chewable Vitamins

Flintstones® Plus Calcium

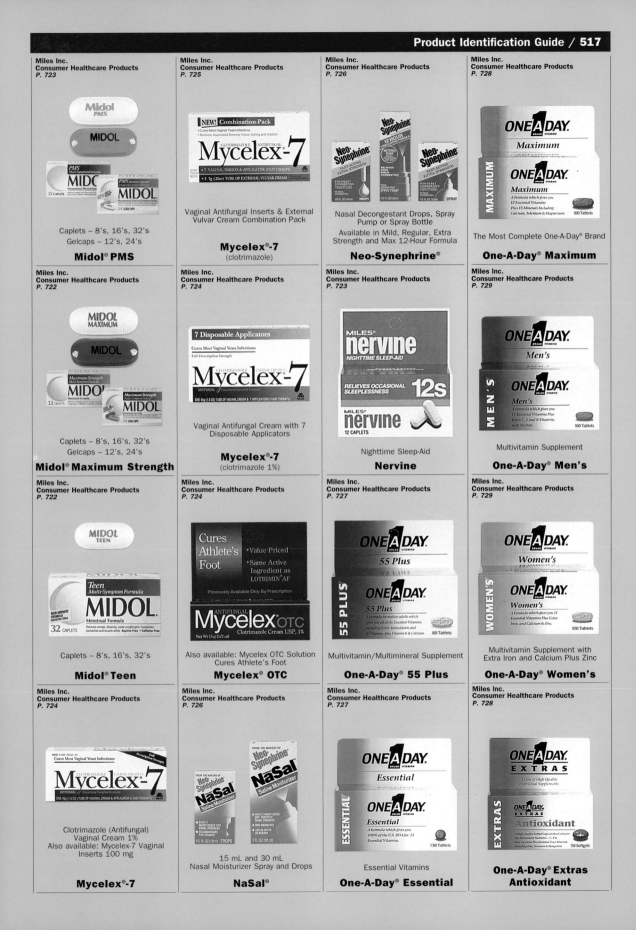

Miles Inc.
Consumer Healthcare Products
P. 723

Caplets – 8's, 16's, 32's
Gelcaps – 12's, 24's

Midol® PMS

Miles Inc.
Consumer Healthcare Products
P. 722

Caplets – 8's, 16's, 32's
Gelcaps – 12's, 24's

Midol® Maximum Strength

Miles Inc.
Consumer Healthcare Products
P. 722

Caplets – 8's, 16's, 32's

Midol® Teen

Miles Inc.
Consumer Healthcare Products
P. 724

Clotrimazole (Antifungal)
Vaginal Cream 1%
Also available: Mycelex-7 Vaginal
Inserts 100 mg

Mycelex®-7

Miles Inc.
Consumer Healthcare Products
P. 725

NEW! Combination-Pack

Vaginal Antifungal Inserts & External
Vulvar Cream Combination Pack

Mycelex®-7
(clotrimazole)

Miles Inc.
Consumer Healthcare Products
P. 724

7 Disposable Applicators

Vaginal Antifungal Cream with 7
Disposable Applicators

Mycelex®-7
(clotrimazole 1%)

Miles Inc.
Consumer Healthcare Products
P. 724

Cures Athlete's Foot
• Value Priced
• Same Active Ingredient as LOTRIMIN®AF
Previously Available Only By Prescription

Also available: Mycelex OTC Solution
Cures Athlete's Foot

Mycelex® OTC

Miles Inc.
Consumer Healthcare Products
P. 726

From the makers of Neo-Synephrine
NaSal

15 mL and 30 mL
Nasal Moisturizer Spray and Drops

NaSal®

Miles Inc.
Consumer Healthcare Products
P. 726

Nasal Decongestant Drops, Spray
Pump or Spray Bottle
Available in Mild, Regular, Extra
Strength and Max 12-Hour Formula

Neo-Synephrine®

Miles Inc.
Consumer Healthcare Products
P. 723

Nighttime Sleep-Aid

Nervine

Miles Inc.
Consumer Healthcare Products
P. 727

Multivitamin/Multimineral Supplement

One-A-Day® 55 Plus

Miles Inc.
Consumer Healthcare Products
P. 727

Essential Vitamins

One-A-Day® Essential

Miles Inc.
Consumer Healthcare Products
P. 728

The Most Complete One-A-Day® Brand

One-A-Day® Maximum

Miles Inc.
Consumer Healthcare Products
P. 729

Multivitamin Supplement

One-A-Day® Men's

Miles Inc.
Consumer Healthcare Products
P. 729

Multivitamin Supplement with
Extra Iron and Calcium Plus Zinc

One-A-Day® Women's

Miles Inc.
Consumer Healthcare Products
P. 728

**One-A-Day® Extras
Antioxidant**

Miles Inc.
Consumer Healthcare Products
P. 728

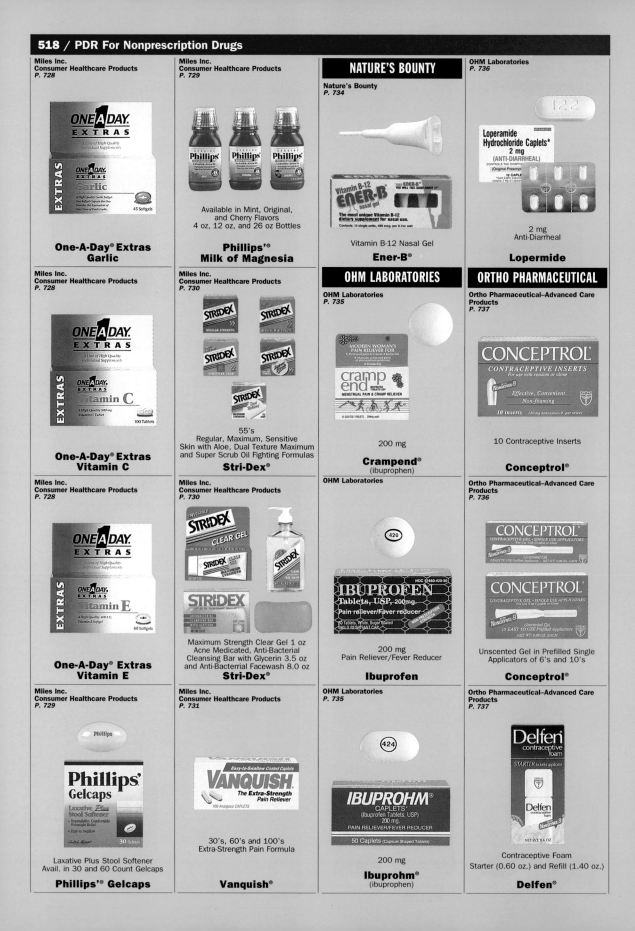

**One-A-Day® Extras
Garlic**

Miles Inc.
Consumer Healthcare Products
P. 728

**One-A-Day® Extras
Vitamin C**

Miles Inc.
Consumer Healthcare Products
P. 728

**One-A-Day® Extras
Vitamin E**

Miles Inc.
Consumer Healthcare Products
P. 729

Laxative Plus Stool Softener
Avail. in 30 and 60 Count Gelcaps

Phillips'® Gelcaps

Miles Inc.
Consumer Healthcare Products
P. 729

Available in Mint, Original,
and Cherry Flavors
4 oz, 12 oz, and 26 oz Bottles

**Phillips'®
Milk of Magnesia**

Miles Inc.
Consumer Healthcare Products
P. 730

55's
Regular, Maximum, Sensitive
Skin with Aloe, Dual Texture Maximum
and Super Scrub Oil Fighting Formulas

Stri-Dex®

Miles Inc.
Consumer Healthcare Products
P. 730

Maximum Strength Clear Gel 1 oz
Acne Medicated, Anti-Bacterial
Cleansing Bar with Glycerin 3.5 oz
and Anti-Bacterial Facewash 8.0 oz

Stri-Dex®

Miles Inc.
Consumer Healthcare Products
P. 731

30's, 60's and 100's
Extra-Strength Pain Formula

Vanquish®

NATURE'S BOUNTY

Nature's Bounty
P. 734

Vitamin B-12 Nasal Gel

Ener-B®

OHM LABORATORIES

OHM Laboratories
P. 735

200 mg

Crampend®
(ibuprofen)

OHM Laboratories

200 mg
Pain Reliever/Fever Reducer

Ibuprofen

OHM Laboratories
P. 735

200 mg

Ibuprohm®
(ibuprophen)

OHM Laboratories
P. 736

2 mg
Anti-Diarrheal

Lopermide

ORTHO PHARMACEUTICAL

Ortho Pharmaceutical–Advanced Care
Products
P. 737

10 Contraceptive Inserts

Conceptrol®

Ortho Pharmaceutical–Advanced Care
Products
P. 736

Unscented Gel in Prefilled Single
Applicators of 6's and 10's

Conceptrol®

Ortho Pharmaceutical–Advanced Care
Products
P. 737

Contraceptive Foam
Starter (0.60 oz.) and Refill (1.40 oz.)

Delfen®

Ortho Pharmaceutical–Advanced Care Products
P. 738

2.5 and 3.8 oz.
Original Formula

Gynol II®

Ortho Pharmaceutical–Advanced Care Products
P. 739

Extra Strength
2.85 oz. Tube with Applicator

Gynol II®

Ortho Pharmaceutical–Advanced Care Products
P. 740

Contraceptive Jelly
3.8 oz. Tube

Ortho-Gynol®

PFIZER

Pfizer Consumer Health Care
P. 742

Diaper Rash Prevention Ointment

**Daily Care™
from DESITIN®**

Pfizer Consumer Health Care
P. 742

Diaper Rash Ointment

DESITIN®

Pfizer Consumer Health Care
P. 742

**DESITIN® Cornstarch
Baby Powder**

Pfizer Consumer Health Care
P. 746

Original, Long Lasting,
Allergy Relief and Moisturizing

Visine®

PHARMAVITE

Pharmavite
P. 748

Vitamins C, E and Beta Carotene
Package of 60 Softgels

**Nature Made®
Antioxidant Formula**

Pharmavite
P. 748

Complete High Potency
Multivitamin Multimineral
Bottles of 100 + 30

**Nature Made®
Essential Balance®**

REED & CARNRICK

Reed & Carnrick
P. 767

Available in 1 oz. and 1/2 oz. bottles
A liquid antiflatulent suitable for
relieving infant gas symptoms and for
those who prefer liquid dosage forms.

Phazyme® Drops

ROBERTS

Roberts Pharmaceutical Corp.
P. 769

2 oz., 4 oz., 6 oz. Cough Formula
Also available Cheracol Plus
Head Cold/Cough Formula 4 oz., 6 oz.

Cheracol D®

Roberts Pharmaceutical Corp.
P. 770

Stool softener – 50mg/100mg
100 mg available:
Two tone color 30, 60, 100, 250, 1000
50 mg available: 30, 60, 250
Available in Liquid and Syrup

Colace®

Roberts Pharmaceutical Corp.
P. 771

Bottles of 30: 200 mg Tablets

Haltran®

Roberts Pharmaceutical Corp.
P. 771

Bottles of 30, 60, 250, 1000
Laxative and Stool Softener
Available in Syrup

Peri-Colace®

Roberts Pharmaceutical Corp.
P. 772

Nasal Decongestant/
Antihistamine/Analgesic
Bottles of 24 and 500 Caplets

Pyrroxate®

Roberts Pharmaceutical Corp.
P. 772

Bottles of 100 Tablets
High Potency Vitamin Supplement
Also Available in Sigtab

Sigtab®-M

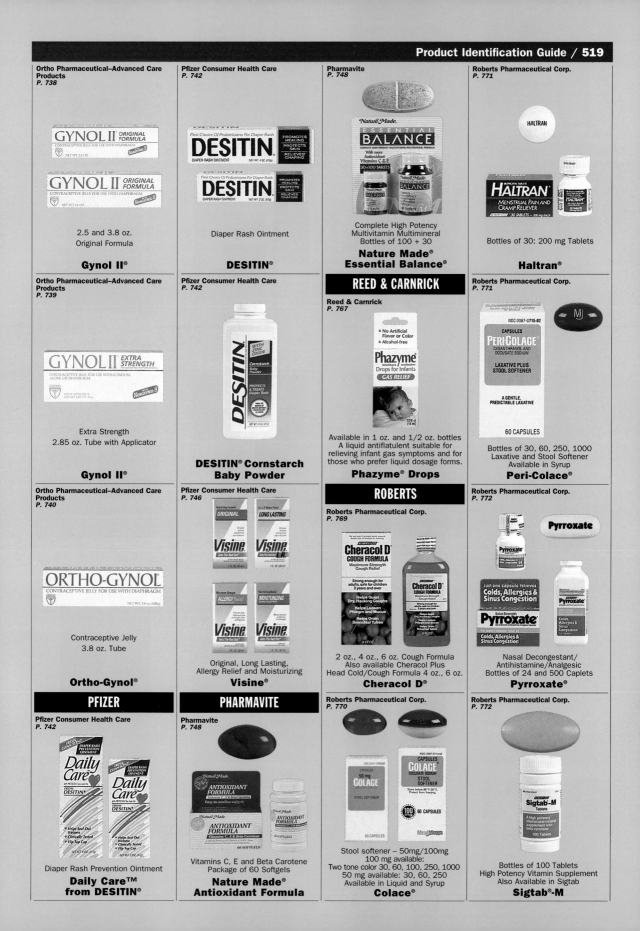

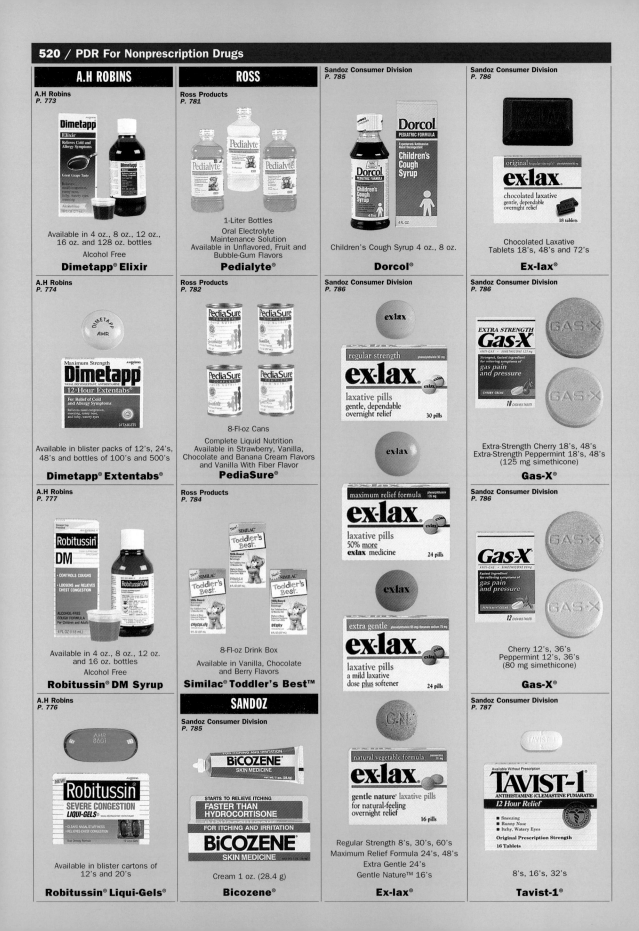

A.H ROBINS

A.H Robins
P. 773

Available in 4 oz., 8 oz., 12 oz.,
16 oz. and 128 oz. bottles

Alcohol Free

Dimetapp® Elixir

A.H Robins
P. 774

Available in blister packs of 12's, 24's,
48's and bottles of 100's and 500's

Dimetapp® Extentabs®

A.H Robins
P. 777

Available in 4 oz., 8 oz., 12 oz.
and 16 oz. bottles

Alcohol Free

Robitussin® DM Syrup

A.H Robins
P. 776

Available in blister cartons of
12's and 20's

Robitussin® Liqui-Gels®

ROSS

Ross Products
P. 781

1-Liter Bottles
Oral Electrolyte
Maintenance Solution
Available in Unflavored, Fruit and
Bubble-Gum Flavors

Pedialyte®

Ross Products
P. 782

8-Fl-oz Cans

Complete Liquid Nutrition
Available in Strawberry, Vanilla,
Chocolate and Banana Cream Flavors
and Vanilla With Fiber Flavor

PediaSure®

Ross Products
P. 784

8-Fl-oz Drink Box

Available in Vanilla, Chocolate
and Berry Flavors

Similac® Toddler's Best™

SANDOZ

Sandoz Consumer Division
P. 785

FOR ITCHING AND IRRITATION

STARTS TO RELIEVE ITCHING
**FASTER THAN
HYDROCORTISONE**

FOR ITCHING AND IRRITATION

**BiCOZENE®
SKIN MEDICINE**

Cream 1 oz. (28.4 g)

Bicozene®

Sandoz Consumer Division
P. 785

Children's Cough Syrup 4 oz., 8 oz.

Dorcol®

Sandoz Consumer Division
P. 786

Regular Strength 8's, 30's, 60's
Maximum Relief Formula 24's, 48's
Extra Gentle 24's
Gentle Nature™ 16's

Ex-lax®

Sandoz Consumer Division
P. 786

Chocolated Laxative
Tablets 18's, 48's and 72's

Ex-lax®

Sandoz Consumer Division
P. 786

Extra-Strength Cherry 18's, 48's
Extra-Strength Peppermint 18's, 48's
(125 mg simethicone)

Gas-X®

Sandoz Consumer Division
P. 786

Cherry 12's, 36's
Peppermint 12's, 36's
(80 mg simethicone)

Gas-X®

Sandoz Consumer Division
P. 787

8's, 16's, 32's

Tavist-1®

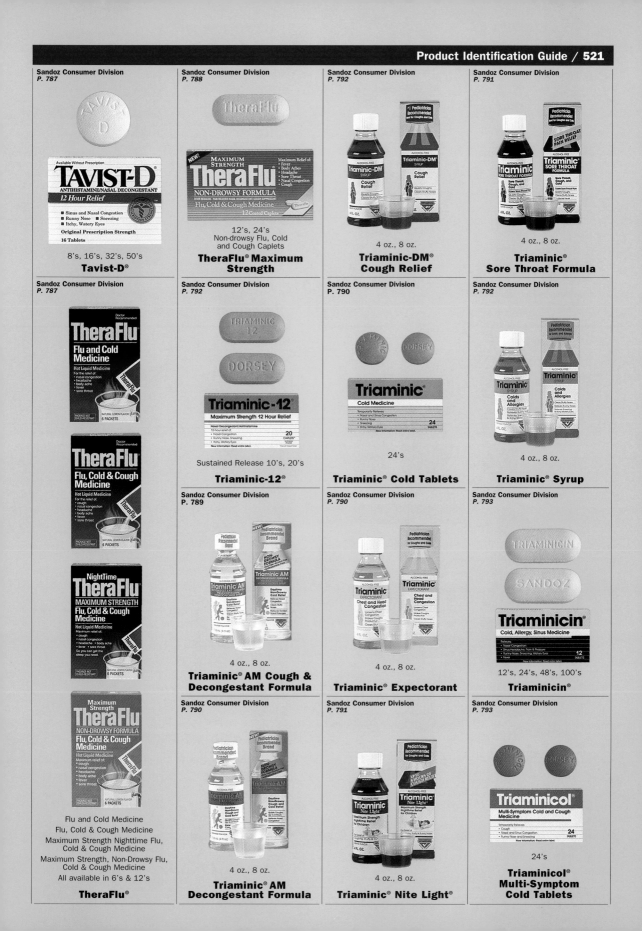

Sandoz Consumer Division
P. 787

Available Without Prescription
TAVIST-D®
ANTIHISTAMINE/NASAL DECONGESTANT
12 Hour Relief
■ Sinus and Nasal Congestion
■ Runny Nose ■ Sneezing
■ Itchy, Watery Eyes
Original Prescription Strength
16 Tablets

8's, 16's, 32's, 50's
Tavist-D®

Sandoz Consumer Division
P. 788

NEW!
MAXIMUM STRENGTH
TheraFlu®
NON-DROWSY FORMULA
FEVER REDUCER·PAIN RELIEVER·NASAL DECONGESTANT·COUGH SUPPRESSANT
Flu, Cold & Cough Medicine
12 Coated Caplets
Maximum Relief of:
► Fever
► Body Aches
► Headache
► Sore Throat
► Nasal Congestion
► Cough

12's, 24's
Non-drowsy Flu, Cold
and Cough Caplets
**TheraFlu® Maximum
Strength**

Sandoz Consumer Division
P. 792

4 oz., 8 oz.
**Triaminic-DM®
Cough Relief**

Sandoz Consumer Division
P. 791

4 oz., 8 oz.
**Triaminic®
Sore Throat Formula**

Sandoz Consumer Division
P. 787

TheraFlu
Flu and Cold Medicine
Hot Liquid Medicine
For the relief of:
• nasal congestion
• headache
• body ache
• fever
• sore throat
NATURAL LEMON FLAVOR
6 PACKETS

TheraFlu
Flu, Cold & Cough Medicine
Hot Liquid Medicine
For the relief of:
• cough
• nasal congestion
• headache
• body ache
• fever
• sore throat
NATURAL LEMON FLAVOR
6 PACKETS

NightTime
TheraFlu
MAXIMUM STRENGTH
Flu, Cold & Cough Medicine
Hot Liquid Medicine
Maximum relief of:
• cough
• nasal congestion
• headache • body ache
• fever • sore throat
So you can get the
sleep you need.
NATURAL LEMON FLAVOR
6 PACKETS

Maximum Strength
TheraFlu
NON-DROWSY FORMULA
Flu, Cold & Cough Medicine
Hot Liquid Medicine
Maximum relief of:
• cough
• nasal congestion
• headache
• body ache
• fever
• sore throat
NATURAL LEMON FLAVOR
6 PACKETS

Flu and Cold Medicine
Flu, Cold & Cough Medicine
Maximum Strength Nighttime Flu,
Cold & Cough Medicine
Maximum Strength, Non-Drowsy Flu,
Cold & Cough Medicine
All available in 6's & 12's
TheraFlu®

Sandoz Consumer Division
P. 792

TRIAMINIC 12
DORSEY
Triaminic-12®
Maximum Strength 12 Hour Relief
Nasal Decongestant/Antihistamine
12-hour relief of:
• Nasal Congestion
• Runny Nose, Sneezing
• Itchy, Watery Eyes
New information: Read entire label.
20 CAPLETS

Sustained Release 10's, 20's
Triaminic-12®

Sandoz Consumer Division
P. 789

4 oz., 8 oz.
**Triaminic® AM Cough &
Decongestant Formula**

Sandoz Consumer Division
P. 790

4 oz., 8 oz.
**Triaminic® AM
Decongestant Formula**

Sandoz Consumer Division
P. 790

TRIAMINIC
DORSEY
Triaminic®
Cold Medicine
Temporarily Relieves:
• Nasal and Sinus Congestion
• Sneezing
• Itchy, Watery Eyes
New information: Read entire label.
24 TABLETS

24's
Triaminic® Cold Tablets

Sandoz Consumer Division
P. 790

4 oz., 8 oz.
Triaminic® Expectorant

Sandoz Consumer Division
P. 791

4 oz., 8 oz.
Triaminic® Nite Light®

Sandoz Consumer Division
P. 792

4 oz., 8 oz.
Triaminic® Syrup

Sandoz Consumer Division
P. 793

TRIAMINICIN
SANDOZ
Triaminicin®
Cold, Allergy, Sinus Medicine
Relieves:
• Nasal Congestion
• Sinus Headache, Pain & Pressure
• Runny Nose, Sneezing, Watery Eyes
• Fever
New information: Read entire label.
12 TABLETS

12's, 24's, 48's, 100's
Triaminicin®

Sandoz Consumer Division
P. 793

TRIAMINIC
DORSEY
Triaminicol®
Multi-Symptom Cold and Cough
Medicine
Temporarily Relieves:
• Cough
• Nasal and Sinus Congestion
• Runny Nose and Sneezing
New information: Read entire label.
24 TABLETS

24's
**Triaminicol®
Multi-Symptom
Cold Tablets**

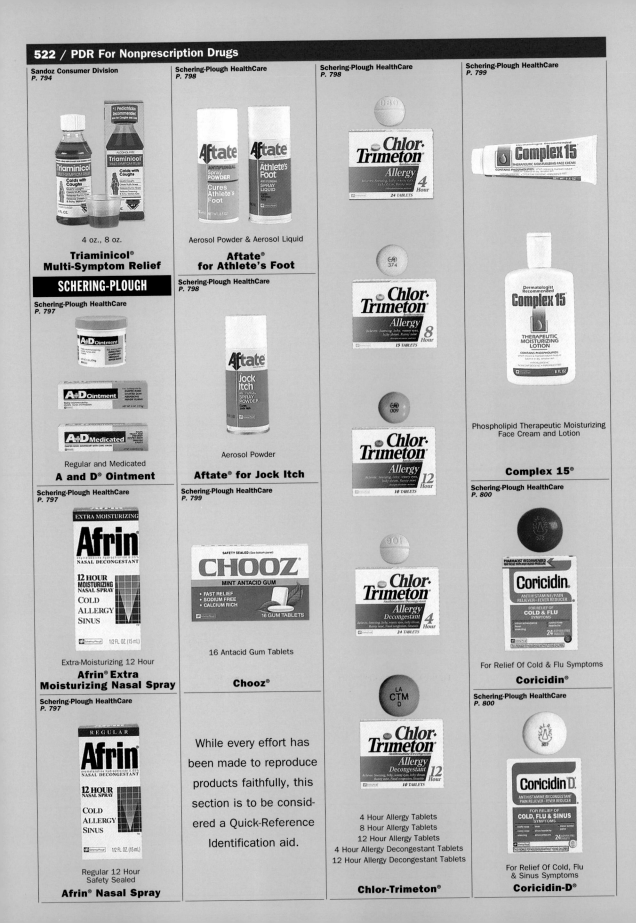

Sandoz Consumer Division
P. 794

4 oz., 8 oz.
Triaminicol®
Multi-Symptom Relief

SCHERING-PLOUGH

Schering-Plough HealthCare
P. 797

Regular and Medicated
A and D® Ointment

Schering-Plough HealthCare
P. 797

Extra-Moisturizing 12 Hour
Afrin® Extra Moisturizing Nasal Spray

Schering-Plough HealthCare
P. 797

Regular 12 Hour
Safety Sealed
Afrin® Nasal Spray

Schering-Plough HealthCare
P. 798

Aerosol Powder & Aerosol Liquid
Aftate®
for Athlete's Foot

Schering-Plough HealthCare
P. 798

Aerosol Powder
Aftate® for Jock Itch

Schering-Plough HealthCare
P. 799

16 Antacid Gum Tablets
Chooz®

While every effort has been made to reproduce products faithfully, this section is to be considered a Quick-Reference Identification aid.

Schering-Plough HealthCare
P. 798

4 Hour Allergy Tablets
8 Hour Allergy Tablets
12 Hour Allergy Tablets
4 Hour Allergy Decongestant Tablets
12 Hour Allergy Decongestant Tablets

Chlor-Trimeton®

Schering-Plough HealthCare
P. 799

Phospholipid Therapeutic Moisturizing Face Cream and Lotion

Complex 15®

Schering-Plough HealthCare
P. 800

For Relief Of Cold & Flu Symptoms

Coricidin®

Schering-Plough HealthCare
P. 800

For Relief Of Cold, Flu & Sinus Symptoms

Coricidin-D®

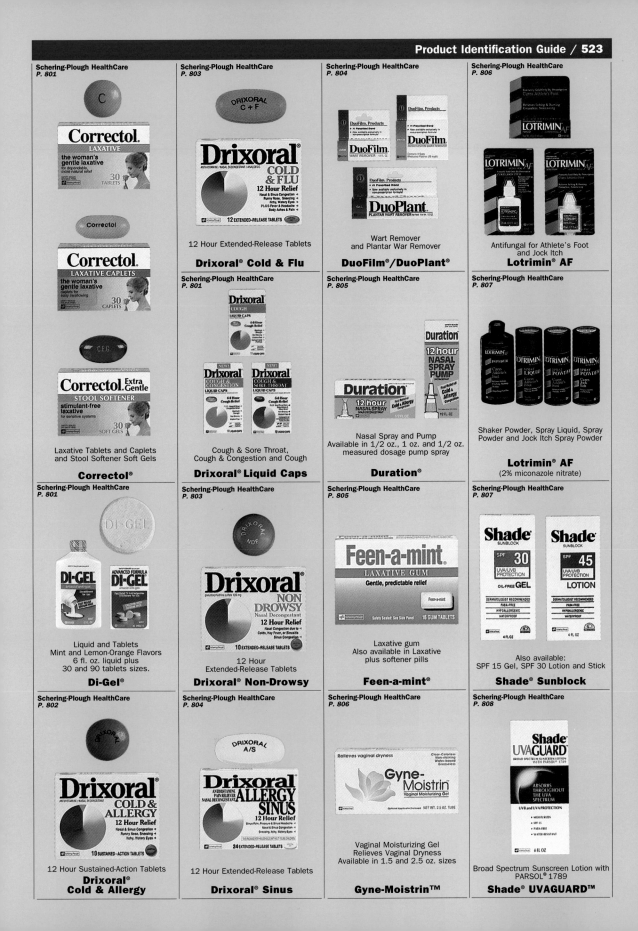

Schering-Plough HealthCare
P. 801

the woman's gentle laxative
for dependable, once natural relief
30 TABLETS

LAXATIVE CAPLETS
the woman's gentle laxative
caplets for easy swallowing
30 CAPLETS

Correctol Extra Gentle
STOOL SOFTENER
stimulant-free laxative
for sensitive systems
30 SOFT GELS

Laxative Tablets and Caplets
and Stool Softener Soft Gels
Correctol®

Schering-Plough HealthCare
P. 801

DI-GEL
ADVANCED FORMULA DI-GEL

Liquid and Tablets
Mint and Lemon-Orange Flavors
6 fl. oz. liquid plus
30 and 90 tablets sizes.
Di-Gel®

Schering-Plough HealthCare
P. 802

Drixoral®
COLD & ALLERGY
12 Hour Relief
10 SUSTAINED-ACTION TABLETS

12 Hour Sustained-Action Tablets
**Drixoral®
Cold & Allergy**

Schering-Plough HealthCare
P. 803

DRIXORAL C + F

Drixoral®
COLD & FLU
12 Hour Relief
12 EXTENDED-RELEASE TABLETS

12 Hour Extended-Release Tablets
Drixoral® Cold & Flu

Schering-Plough HealthCare
P. 801

Drixoral COUGH LIQUID CAPS

NEW! Drixoral COUGH & CONGESTION LIQUID CAPS

NEW! Drixoral COUGH & SORE THROAT CAPS

Cough & Sore Throat,
Cough & Congestion and Cough
Drixoral® Liquid Caps

Schering-Plough HealthCare
P. 803

DRIXORAL NDF

Drixoral®
NON DROWSY
Nasal Decongestant
12 Hour Relief
10 EXTENDED-RELEASE TABLETS

12 Hour
Extended-Release Tablets
Drixoral® Non-Drowsy

Schering-Plough HealthCare
P. 804

DUOFILM A/S

DuoFilm. Products
DuoFilm.
WART REMOVER

DuoFilm. Products
DuoFilm.
PATCH SYSTEM WART REMOVER

DuoFilm. Products
DuoPlant.
PLANTAR WART REMOVER

Wart Remover
and Plantar War Remover
DuoFilm®/DuoPlant®

Schering-Plough HealthCare
P. 805

Duration
12 hour
NASAL SPRAY PUMP

Duration
12 hour
NASAL SPRAY

Nasal Spray and Pump
Available in 1/2 oz., 1 oz. and 1/2 oz.
measured dosage pump spray
Duration®

Schering-Plough HealthCare
P. 805

Feen-a-mint.
LAXATIVE GUM
Gentle, predictable relief
16 GUM TABLETS

Laxative gum
Also available in Laxative
plus softener pills
Feen-a-mint®

Schering-Plough HealthCare
P. 806

DRIXORAL A/S

Relieves vaginal dryness
Gyne-Moistrin
Vaginal Moisturizing Gel
Clear-Colorless
Non-staining
Water-based
Greaseless
Optional Applicator Enclosed   NET WT. 2.5 OZ. TUBE

Vaginal Moisturizing Gel
Relieves Vaginal Dryness
Available in 1.5 and 2.5 oz. sizes
Gyne-Moistrin™

Schering-Plough HealthCare
P. 806

LOTRIMIN AF

LOTRIMIN AF   LOTRIMIN AF

Antifungal for Athlete's Foot
and Jock Itch
Lotrimin® AF

Schering-Plough HealthCare
P. 807

LOTRIMIN AF POWDER   LOTRIMIN AF SPRAY LIQUID   LOTRIMIN AF SPRAY POWDER   LOTRIMIN AF SPRAY POWDER

Shaker Powder, Spray Liquid, Spray
Powder and Jock Itch Spray Powder
Lotrimin® AF
(2% miconazole nitrate)

Schering-Plough HealthCare
P. 807

Shade
SUNBLOCK
SPF 30
UVA/UVB PROTECTION
OIL-FREE GEL
DERMATOLOGIST RECOMMENDED
PABA-FREE
HYPOALLERGENIC
WATERPROOF
4 FL OZ

Shade
SUNBLOCK
SPF 45
UVA/UVB PROTECTION
LOTION
DERMATOLOGIST RECOMMENDED
PABA-FREE
HYPOALLERGENIC
WATERPROOF
4 FL OZ

Also available:
SPF 15 Gel, SPF 30 Lotion and Stick
Shade® Sunblock

Schering-Plough HealthCare
P. 808

Shade
UVAGUARD
BROAD SPECTRUM SUNSCREEN LOTION
WITH PARSOL 1789
ABSORBS THROUGHOUT THE UVA SPECTRUM
UVB and UVA PROTECTION
• MOISTURIZES
• SPF 15
• PABA-FREE
• WATER-RESISTANT
4 FL OZ

Broad Spectrum Sunscreen Lotion with
PARSOL® 1789
Shade® UVAGUARD™

Schering-Plough HealthCare
P. 804

DRIXORAL A/S

Drixoral®
ALLERGY SINUS
12 Hour Relief
24 EXTENDED-RELEASE TABLETS

12 Hour Extended-Release Tablets
Drixoral® Sinus

Schering-Plough HealthCare
P. 808

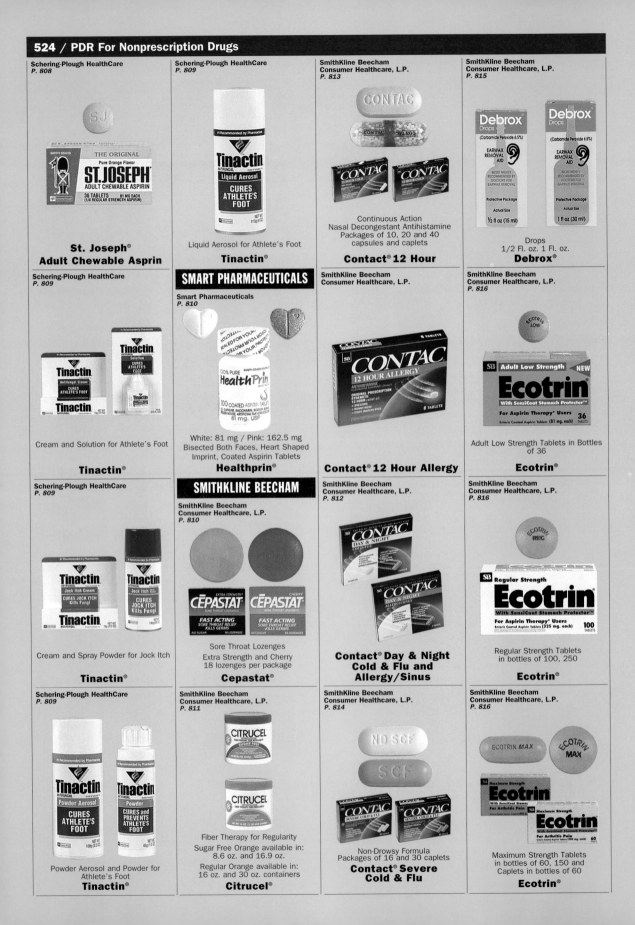

St. Joseph®
Adult Chewable Asprin

Schering-Plough HealthCare
P. 809

Cream and Solution for Athlete's Foot

Tinactin®

Schering-Plough HealthCare
P. 809

Cream and Spray Powder for Jock Itch

Tinactin®

Schering-Plough HealthCare
P. 809

Powder Aerosol and Powder for
Athlete's Foot

Tinactin®

Schering-Plough HealthCare
P. 809

Liquid Aerosol for Athlete's Foot

Tinactin®

SMART PHARMACEUTICALS

Smart Pharmaceuticals
P. 810

White: 81 mg / Pink: 162.5 mg
Bisected Both Faces, Heart Shaped
Imprint, Coated Aspirin Tablets

Healthprin®

SMITHKLINE BEECHAM

SmithKline Beecham
Consumer Healthcare, L.P.
P. 810

Sore Throat Lozenges
Extra Strength and Cherry
18 lozenges per package

Cepastat®

SmithKline Beecham
Consumer Healthcare, L.P.
P. 811

Fiber Therapy for Regularity
Sugar Free Orange available in:
8.6 oz. and 16.9 oz.
Regular Orange available in:
16 oz. and 30 oz. containers

Citrucel®

SmithKline Beecham
Consumer Healthcare, L.P.
P. 813

Continuous Action
Nasal Decongestant Antihistamine
Packages of 10, 20 and 40
capsules and caplets

Contact® 12 Hour

SmithKline Beecham
Consumer Healthcare, L.P.

Contact® 12 Hour Allergy

SmithKline Beecham
Consumer Healthcare, L.P.
P. 812

**Contact® Day & Night
Cold & Flu and
Allergy/Sinus**

SmithKline Beecham
Consumer Healthcare, L.P.
P. 814

Non-Drowsy Formula
Packages of 16 and 30 caplets

**Contact® Severe
Cold & Flu**

SmithKline Beecham
Consumer Healthcare, L.P.
P. 815

Drops
1/2 Fl. oz. 1 Fl. oz.

Debrox®

SmithKline Beecham
Consumer Healthcare, L.P.
P. 816

Adult Low Strength Tablets in Bottles
of 36

Ecotrin®

SmithKline Beecham
Consumer Healthcare, L.P.
P. 816

Regular Strength Tablets
in bottles of 100, 250

Ecotrin®

SmithKline Beecham
Consumer Healthcare, L.P.
P. 816

Maximum Strength Tablets
in bottles of 60, 150 and
Caplets in bottles of 60

Ecotrin®

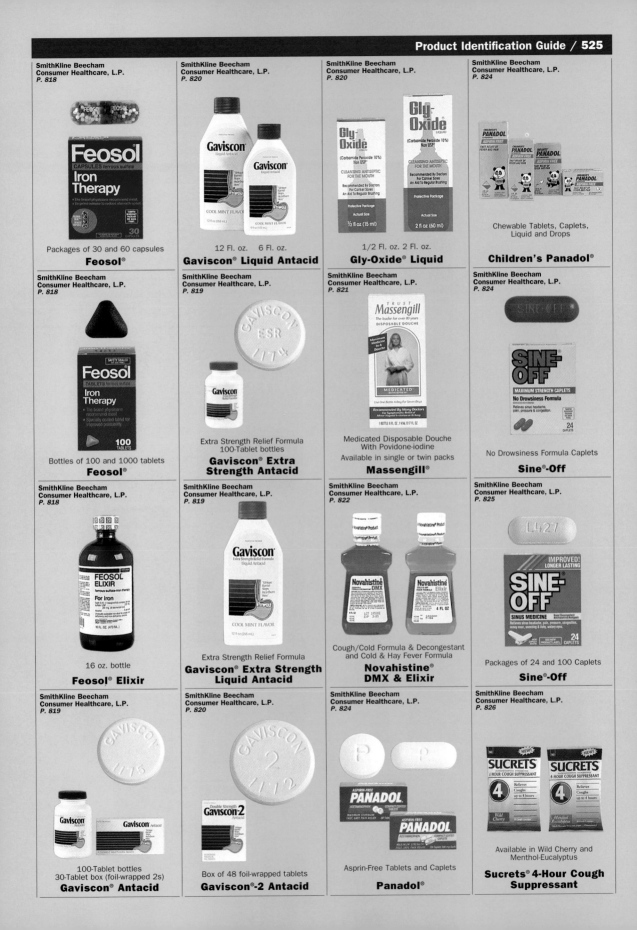

SmithKline Beecham
Consumer Healthcare, L.P.
P. 818

Packages of 30 and 60 capsules
Feosol®

SmithKline Beecham
Consumer Healthcare, L.P.
P. 818

Bottles of 100 and 1000 tablets
Feosol®

SmithKline Beecham
Consumer Healthcare, L.P.
P. 818

16 oz. bottle
Feosol® Elixir

SmithKline Beecham
Consumer Healthcare, L.P.
P. 819

100-Tablet bottles
30-Tablet box (foil-wrapped 2s)
Gaviscon® Antacid

SmithKline Beecham
Consumer Healthcare, L.P.
P. 820

12 Fl. oz.   6 Fl. oz.
Gaviscon® Liquid Antacid

SmithKline Beecham
Consumer Healthcare, L.P.
P. 819

Extra Strength Relief Formula
100-Tablet bottles
**Gaviscon® Extra
Strength Antacid**

SmithKline Beecham
Consumer Healthcare, L.P.
P. 819

Extra Strength Relief Formula
**Gaviscon® Extra Strength
Liquid Antacid**

SmithKline Beecham
Consumer Healthcare, L.P.
P. 820

Box of 48 foil-wrapped tablets
Gaviscon®-2 Antacid

SmithKline Beecham
Consumer Healthcare, L.P.
P. 820

1/2 Fl. oz. 2 Fl. oz.
Gly-Oxide® Liquid

SmithKline Beecham
Consumer Healthcare, L.P.
P. 821

Medicated Disposable Douche
With Povidone-iodine
Available in single or twin packs
Massengill®

SmithKline Beecham
Consumer Healthcare, L.P.
P. 822

Cough/Cold Formula & Decongestant
and Cold & Hay Fever Formula
**Novahistine®
DMX & Elixir**

SmithKline Beecham
Consumer Healthcare, L.P.
P. 824

Asprin-Free Tablets and Caplets
Panadol®

SmithKline Beecham
Consumer Healthcare, L.P.
P. 824

Chewable Tablets, Caplets,
Liquid and Drops
Children's Panadol®

SmithKline Beecham
Consumer Healthcare, L.P.
P. 824

No Drowsiness Formula Caplets
Sine®-Off

SmithKline Beecham
Consumer Healthcare, L.P.
P. 825

Packages of 24 and 100 Caplets
Sine®-Off

SmithKline Beecham
Consumer Healthcare, L.P.
P. 826

Available in Wild Cherry and
Menthol-Eucalyptus
**Sucrets® 4-Hour Cough
Suppressant**

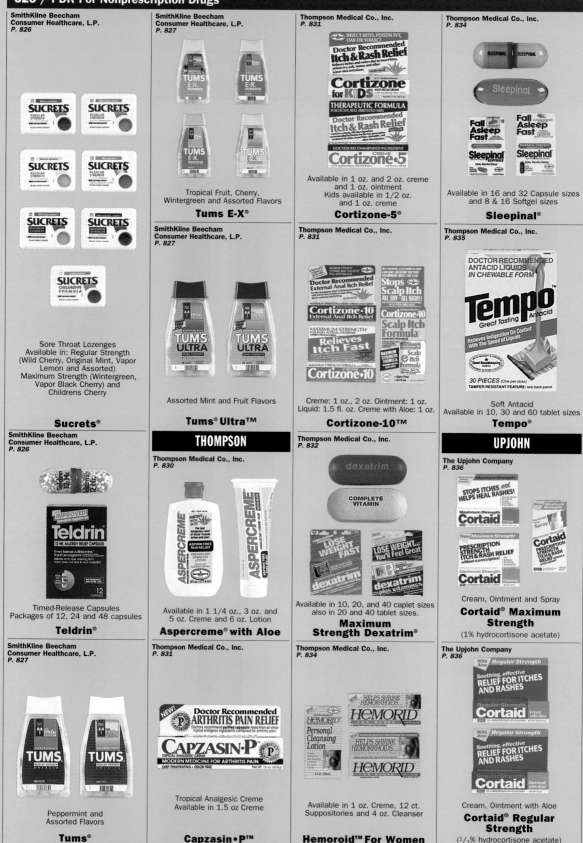

SmithKline Beecham Consumer Healthcare, L.P.
P. 826

Sore Throat Lozenges
Available in: Regular Strength
(Wild Cherry, Original Mint, Vapor Lemon and Assorted)
Maximum Strength (Wintergreen, Vapor Black Cherry) and Childrens Cherry

Sucrets®

SmithKline Beecham Consumer Healthcare, L.P.
P. 826

Timed-Release Capsules
Packages of 12, 24 and 48 capsules

Teldrin®

SmithKline Beecham Consumer Healthcare, L.P.
P. 827

Peppermint and Assorted Flavors

Tums®

SmithKline Beecham Consumer Healthcare, L.P.
P. 827

Tropical Fruit, Cherry, Wintergreen and Assorted Flavors

Tums E-X®

SmithKline Beecham Consumer Healthcare, L.P.
P. 827

Assorted Mint and Fruit Flavors

Tums® Ultra™

THOMPSON

Thompson Medical Co., Inc.
P. 830

Available in 1 1/4 oz., 3 oz. and 5 oz. Creme and 6 oz. Lotion

Aspercreme® with Aloe

Thompson Medical Co., Inc.
P. 831

Tropical Analgesic Creme
Available in 1.5 oz Creme

Capzasin•P™

Thompson Medical Co., Inc.
P. 831

Available in 1 oz. and 2 oz. creme and 1 oz. ointment
Kids available in 1/2 oz. and 1 oz. creme

Cortizone-5®

Thompson Medical Co., Inc.
P. 831

Creme: 1 oz., 2 oz. Ointment: 1 oz.
Liquid: 1.5 fl. oz. Creme with Aloe: 1 oz.

Cortizone-10™

Thompson Medical Co., Inc.
P. 832

Available in 10, 20, and 40 caplet sizes
also in 20 and 40 tablet sizes.

Maximum Strength Dexatrim®

Thompson Medical Co., Inc.
P. 834

Available in 1 oz. Creme, 12 ct.
Suppositories and 4 oz. Cleanser

Hemoroid™ For Women

Thompson Medical Co., Inc.
P. 834

Available in 16 and 32 Capsule sizes
and 8 & 16 Softgel sizes

Sleepinal®

Thompson Medical Co., Inc.
P. 835

Soft Antacid
Available in 10, 30 and 60 tablet sizes

Tempo®

UPJOHN

The Upjohn Company
P. 836

Cream, Ointment and Spray

Cortaid® Maximum Strength

(1% hydrocortisone acetate)

The Upjohn Company
P. 836

Cream, Ointment with Aloe

Cortaid® Regular Strength

($^1/_2$% hydrocortisone acetate)

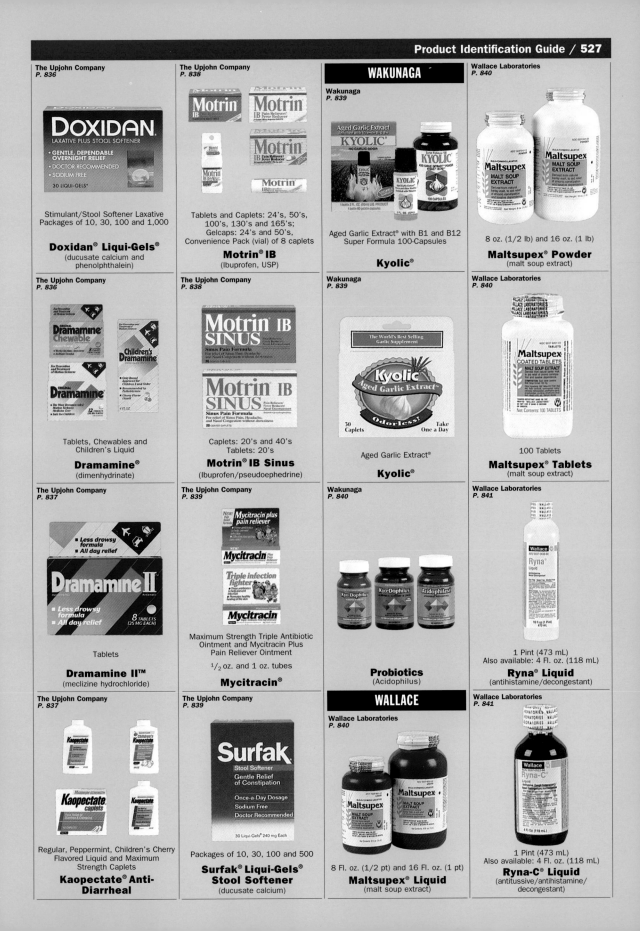

The Upjohn Company
P. 836

Stimulant/Stool Softener Laxative
Packages of 10, 30, 100 and 1,000

Doxidan® Liqui-Gels®
(ducusate calcium and
phenolphthalein)

The Upjohn Company
P. 836

Tablets, Chewables and
Children's Liquid

Dramamine®
(dimenhydrinate)

The Upjohn Company
P. 837

Tablets

Dramamine II™
(meclizine hydrochloride)

The Upjohn Company
P. 837

Regular, Peppermint, Children's Cherry
Flavored Liquid and Maximum
Strength Caplets

**Kaopectate® Anti-
Diarrheal**

The Upjohn Company
P. 838

Tablets and Caplets: 24's, 50's,
100's, 130's and 165's;
Gelcaps: 24's and 50's,
Convenience Pack (vial) of 8 caplets

Motrin® IB
(Ibuprofen, USP)

The Upjohn Company
P. 838

Caplets: 20's and 40's
Tablets: 20's

Motrin® IB Sinus
(Ibuprofen/pseudoephedrine)

The Upjohn Company
P. 839

Maximum Strength Triple Antibiotic
Ointment and Mycitracin Plus
Pain Reliever Ointment
$^1/_2$ oz. and 1 oz. tubes

Mycitracin®

The Upjohn Company
P. 839

Packages of 10, 30, 100 and 500

**Surfak® Liqui-Gels®
Stool Softener**
(ducusate calcium)

WAKUNAGA

Wakunaga
P. 839

Aged Garlic Extract® with B1 and B12
Super Formula 100-Capsules

Kyolic®

Wakunaga
P. 839

Aged Garlic Extract®

Kyolic®

Wakunaga
P. 840

Probiotics
(Acidophilus)

WALLACE

Wallace Laboratories
P. 840

8 Fl. oz. (1/2 pt) and 16 Fl. oz. (1 pt)

Maltsupex® Liquid
(malt soup extract)

Wallace Laboratories
P. 840

8 oz. (1/2 lb) and 16 oz. (1 lb)

Maltsupex® Powder
(malt soup extract)

Wallace Laboratories
P. 840

100 Tablets

Maltsupex® Tablets
(malt soup extract)

Wallace Laboratories
P. 841

1 Pint (473 mL)
Also available: 4 Fl. oz. (118 mL)

Ryna® Liquid
(antihistamine/decongestant)

Wallace Laboratories
P. 841

1 Pint (473 mL)
Also available: 4 Fl. oz. (118 mL)

Ryna-C® Liquid
(antitussive/antihistamine/
decongestant)

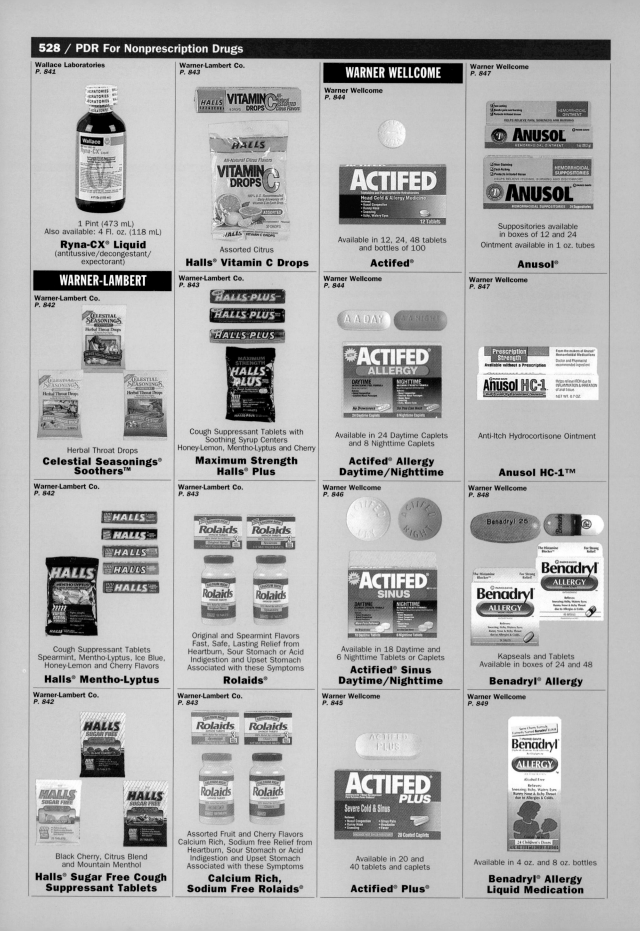

Wallace Laboratories
P. 841

1 Pint (473 mL)
Also available: 4 Fl. oz. (118 mL)

Ryna-CX® Liquid
(antitussive/decongestant/
expectorant)

WARNER-LAMBERT

Warner-Lambert Co.
P. 842

Herbal Throat Drops

**Celestial Seasonings®
Soothers™**

Warner-Lambert Co.
P. 842

Cough Suppressant Tablets
Spearmint, Mentho-Lyptus, Ice Blue,
Honey-Lemon and Cherry Flavors

Halls® Mentho-Lyptus

Warner-Lambert Co.
P. 842

Black Cherry, Citrus Blend
and Mountain Menthol

**Halls® Sugar Free Cough
Suppressant Tablets**

Warner-Lambert Co.
P. 843

Assorted Citrus

Halls® Vitamin C Drops

Warner-Lambert Co.
P. 843

Cough Suppressant Tablets with
Soothing Syrup Centers
Honey-Lemon, Mentho-Lyptus and Cherry

**Maximum Strength
Halls® Plus**

Warner-Lambert Co.
P. 843

Original and Spearmint Flavors
Fast, Safe, Lasting Relief from
Heartburn, Sour Stomach or Acid
Indigestion and Upset Stomach
Associated with these Symptoms

Rolaids®

Warner-Lambert Co.
P. 843

Assorted Fruit and Cherry Flavors
Calcium Rich, Sodium free Relief from
Heartburn, Sour Stomach or Acid
Indigestion and Upset Stomach
Associated with these Symptoms

**Calcium Rich,
Sodium Free Rolaids®**

WARNER WELLCOME

Warner Wellcome
P. 844

Available in 12, 24, 48 tablets
and bottles of 100

Actifed®

Warner Wellcome
P. 844

Available in 24 Daytime Caplets
and 8 Nighttime Caplets

**Actifed® Allergy
Daytime/Nighttime**

Warner Wellcome
P. 846

Available in 18 Daytime and
6 Nighttime Tablets or Caplets

**Actifed® Sinus
Daytime/Nighttime**

Warner Wellcome
P. 845

Available in 20 and
40 tablets and caplets

Actifed® Plus®

Warner Wellcome
P. 847

Suppositories available
in boxes of 12 and 24
Ointment available in 1 oz. tubes

Anusol®

Warner Wellcome
P. 847

Anti-Itch Hydrocortisone Ointment

Anusol HC-1™

Warner Wellcome
P. 848

Kapseals and Tablets
Available in boxes of 24 and 48

Benadryl® Allergy

Warner Wellcome
P. 849

Available in 4 oz. and 8 oz. bottles

**Benadryl® Allergy
Liquid Medication**

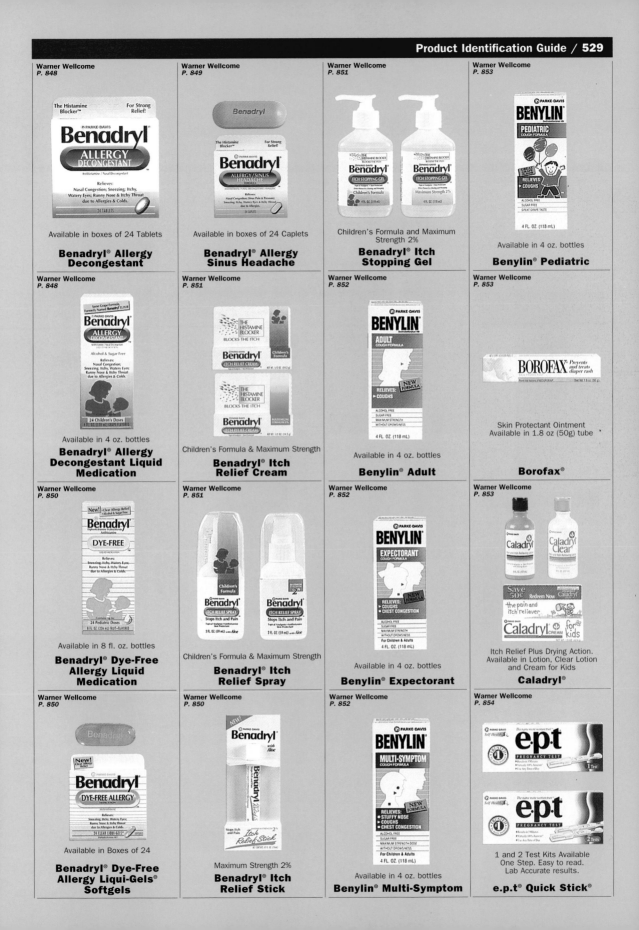

Warner Wellcome
P. 848

Available in boxes of 24 Tablets

**Benadryl® Allergy
Decongestant**

Warner Wellcome
P. 848

Available in 4 oz. bottles

**Benadryl® Allergy
Decongestant Liquid
Medication**

Warner Wellcome
P. 850

Available in 8 fl. oz. bottles

**Benadryl® Dye-Free
Allergy Liquid
Medication**

Warner Wellcome
P. 850

Available in Boxes of 24

**Benadryl® Dye-Free
Allergy Liqui-Gels®
Softgels**

Warner Wellcome
P. 849

Available in boxes of 24 Caplets

**Benadryl® Allergy
Sinus Headache**

Warner Wellcome
P. 851

Children's Formula & Maximum Strength

**Benadryl® Itch
Relief Cream**

Warner Wellcome
P. 851

Children's Formula & Maximum Strength

**Benadryl® Itch
Relief Spray**

Warner Wellcome
P. 850

Maximum Strength 2%

**Benadryl® Itch
Relief Stick**

Warner Wellcome
P. 851

Children's Formula and Maximum
Strength 2%

**Benadryl® Itch
Stopping Gel**

Warner Wellcome
P. 852

Available in 4 oz. bottles

Benylin® Adult

Warner Wellcome
P. 852

Available in 4 oz. bottles

Benylin® Expectorant

Warner Wellcome
P. 852

Available in 4 oz. bottles

Benylin® Multi-Symptom

Warner Wellcome
P. 853

Available in 4 oz. bottles

Benylin® Pediatric

Warner Wellcome
P. 853

Skin Protectant Ointment
Available in 1.8 oz (50g) tube

Borofax®

Warner Wellcome
P. 853

Itch Relief Plus Drying Action.
Available in Lotion, Clear Lotion
and Cream for Kids

Caladryl®

Warner Wellcome
P. 854

1 and 2 Test Kits Available
One Step. Easy to read.
Lab Accurate results.

e.p.t® Quick Stick®

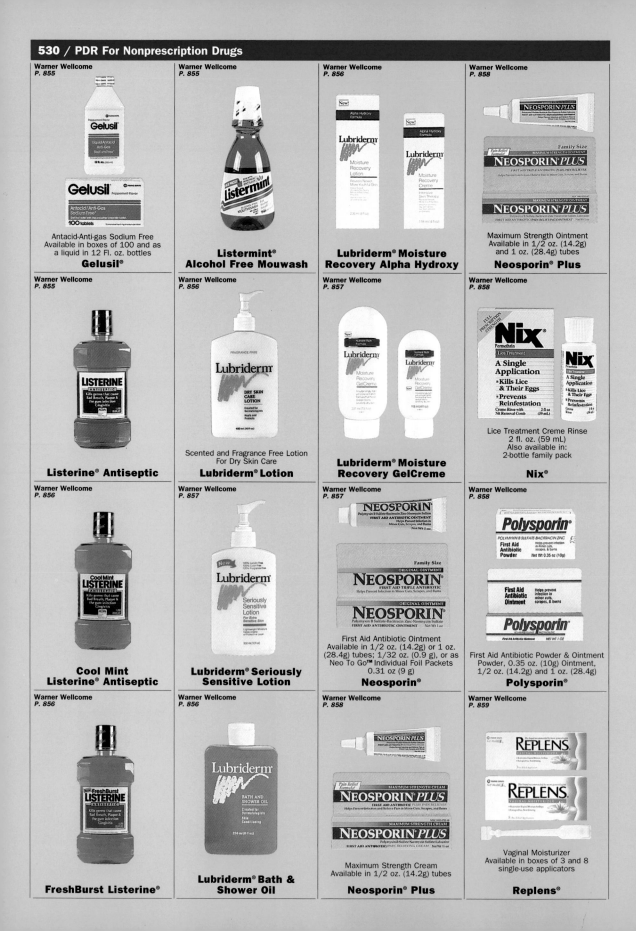

Warner Wellcome
P. 855

Antacid-Anti-gas Sodium Free
Available in boxes of 100 and as
a liquid in 12 Fl. oz. bottles
Gelusil®

Warner Wellcome
P. 855

**Listermint®
Alcohol Free Mouwash**

Warner Wellcome
P. 856

**Lubriderm® Moisture
Recovery Alpha Hydroxy**

Warner Wellcome
P. 858

Maximum Strength Ointment
Available in 1/2 oz. (14.2g)
and 1 oz. (28.4g) tubes
Neosporin® Plus

Warner Wellcome
P. 855

Listerine® Antiseptic

Warner Wellcome
P. 856

Scented and Fragrance Free Lotion
For Dry Skin Care
Lubriderm® Lotion

Warner Wellcome
P. 857

**Lubriderm® Moisture
Recovery GelCreme**

Warner Wellcome
P. 858

Lice Treatment Creme Rinse
2 fl. oz. (59 mL)
Also available in:
2-bottle family pack
Nix®

Warner Wellcome
P. 856

**Cool Mint
Listerine® Antiseptic**

Warner Wellcome
P. 857

**Lubriderm® Seriously
Sensitive Lotion**

Warner Wellcome
P. 857

First Aid Antibiotic Ointment
Available in 1/2 oz. (14.2g) or 1 oz.
(28.4g) tubes; 1/32 oz. (0.9 g), or as
Neo To Go™ Individual Foil Packets
0.31 oz (9 g)
Neosporin®

Warner Wellcome
P. 858

First Aid Antibiotic Powder & Ointment
Powder, 0.35 oz. (10g) Ointment,
1/2 oz. (14.2g) and 1 oz. (28.4g)
Polysporin®

Warner Wellcome
P. 856

FreshBurst Listerine®

Warner Wellcome
P. 856

**Lubriderm® Bath &
Shower Oil**

Warner Wellcome
P. 858

Maximum Strength Cream
Available in 1/2 oz. (14.2g) tubes
Neosporin® Plus

Warner Wellcome
P. 859

Vaginal Moisturizer
Available in boxes of 3 and 8
single-use applicators
Replens®

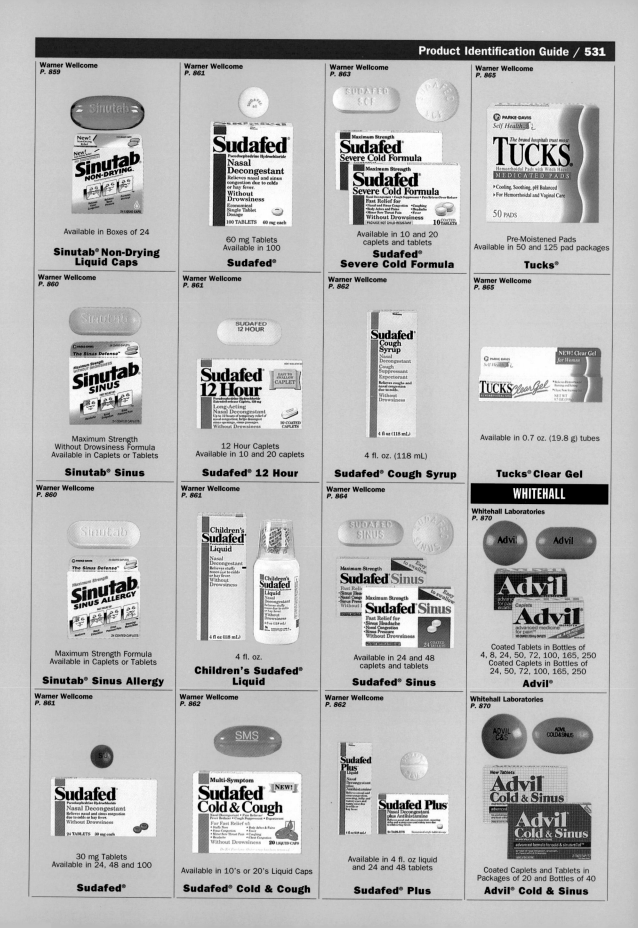

Warner Wellcome
P. 859

Available in Boxes of 24

**Sinutab® Non-Drying
Liquid Caps**

Warner Wellcome
P. 860

Maximum Strength
Without Drowsiness Formula
Available in Caplets or Tablets

Sinutab® Sinus

Warner Wellcome
P. 860

Maximum Strength Formula
Available in Caplets or Tablets

Sinutab® Sinus Allergy

Warner Wellcome
P. 861

30 mg Tablets
Available in 24, 48 and 100

Sudafed®

Warner Wellcome
P. 861

60 mg Tablets
Available in 100

Sudafed®

Warner Wellcome
P. 861

12 Hour Caplets
Available in 10 and 20 caplets

Sudafed® 12 Hour

Warner Wellcome
P. 861

4 fl. oz.

**Children's Sudafed®
Liquid**

Warner Wellcome
P. 862

Available in 10's or 20's Liquid Caps

Sudafed® Cold & Cough

Warner Wellcome
P. 863

Available in 10 and 20
caplets and tablets

**Sudafed®
Severe Cold Formula**

Warner Wellcome
P. 862

4 fl. oz. (118 mL)

Sudafed® Cough Syrup

Warner Wellcome
P. 864

Available in 24 and 48
caplets and tablets

Sudafed® Sinus

Warner Wellcome
P. 862

Available in 4 fl. oz liquid
and 24 and 48 tablets

Sudafed® Plus

Warner Wellcome
P. 865

Pre-Moistened Pads
Available in 50 and 125 pad packages

Tucks®

Warner Wellcome
P. 865

Available in 0.7 oz. (19.8 g) tubes

Tucks® Clear Gel

WHITEHALL

Whitehall Laboratories
P. 870

Coated Tablets in Bottles of
4, 8, 24, 50, 72, 100, 165, 250
Coated Caplets in Bottles of
24, 50, 72, 100, 165, 250

Advil®

Whitehall Laboratories
P. 870

Coated Caplets and Tablets in
Packages of 20 and Bottles of 40

Advil® Cold & Sinus

Whitehall Laboratories
P. 871

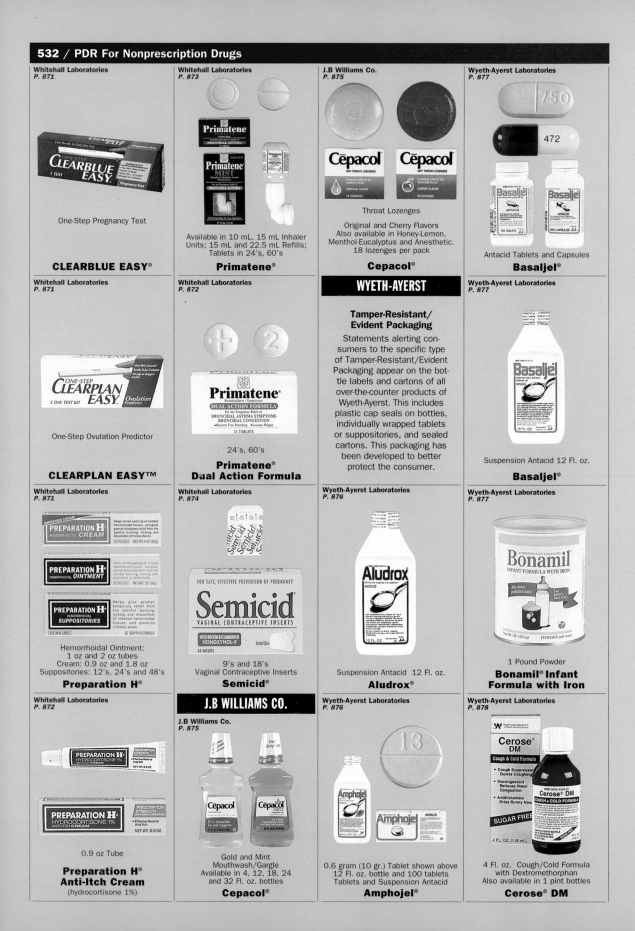

One-Step Pregnancy Test

CLEARBLUE EASY®

Whitehall Laboratories
P. 871

One-Step Ovulation Predictor

CLEARPLAN EASY™

Whitehall Laboratories
P. 871

Hemorrhoidal Ointment:
1 oz and 2 oz tubes
Cream: 0.9 oz and 1.8 oz
Suppositories: 12's, 24's and 48's

Preparation H®

Whitehall Laboratories
P. 872

0.9 oz Tube

**Preparation H®
Anti-Itch Cream**
(hydrocortisone 1%)

Whitehall Laboratories
P. 873

Available in 10 mL, 15 mL Inhaler
Units; 15 mL and 22.5 mL Refills;
Tablets in 24's, 60's

Primatene®

Whitehall Laboratories
P. 872

24's, 60's

**Primatene®
Dual Action Formula**

Whitehall Laboratories
P. 874

9's and 18's
Vaginal Contraceptive Inserts

Semicid®

J.B WILLIAMS CO.

J.B Williams Co.
P. 875

Gold and Mint
Mouthwash/Gargle
Available in 4, 12, 18, 24
and 32 Fl. oz. bottles

Cepacol®

J.B Williams Co.
P. 875

Throat Lozenges

Original and Cherry Flavors
Also available in Honey-Lemon,
Menthol-Eucalyptus and Anesthetic.
18 lozenges per pack

Cepacol®

WYETH-AYERST

**Tamper-Resistant/
Evident Packaging**

Statements alerting con-
sumers to the specific type
of Tamper-Resistant/Evident
Packaging appear on the bottle labels and cartons of all
over-the-counter products of
Wyeth-Ayerst. This includes
plastic cap seals on bottles,
individually wrapped tablets
or suppositories, and sealed
cartons. This packaging has
been developed to better
protect the consumer.

Wyeth-Ayerst Laboratories
P. 876

Suspension Antacid 12 Fl. oz.

Aludrox®

Wyeth-Ayerst Laboratories
P. 876

0.6 gram (10 gr.) Tablet shown above
12 Fl. oz. bottle and 100 tablets
Tablets and Suspension Antacid

Amphojel®

Wyeth-Ayerst Laboratories
P. 877

Antacid Tablets and Capsules

Basaljel®

Wyeth-Ayerst Laboratories
P. 877

Suspension Antacid 12 Fl. oz.

Basaljel®

Wyeth-Ayerst Laboratories
P. 877

1 Pound Powder

**Bonamil® Infant
Formula with Iron**

Wyeth-Ayerst Laboratories
P. 878

4 Fl. oz. Cough/Cold Formula
with Dextromethorphan
Also available in 1 pint bottles

Cerose® DM

Wyeth-Ayerst Laboratories
P. 879

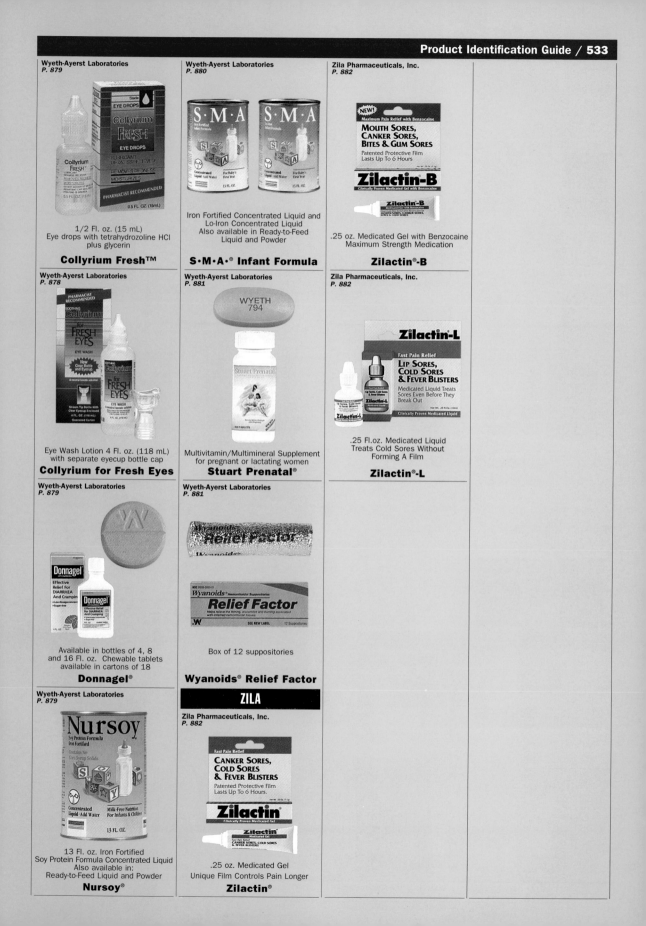

1/2 Fl. oz. (15 mL)
Eye drops with tetrahydrozoline HCl
plus glycerin

Collyrium Fresh™

Wyeth-Ayerst Laboratories
P. 878

Eye Wash Lotion 4 Fl. oz. (118 mL)
with separate eyecup bottle cap

Collyrium for Fresh Eyes

Wyeth-Ayerst Laboratories
P. 879

Available in bottles of 4, 8
and 16 Fl. oz. Chewable tablets
available in cartons of 18

Donnagel®

Wyeth-Ayerst Laboratories
P. 879

13 Fl. oz. Iron Fortified
Soy Protein Formula Concentrated Liquid
Also available in:
Ready-to-Feed Liquid and Powder

Nursoy®

Wyeth-Ayerst Laboratories
P. 880

Iron Fortified Concentrated Liquid and
Lo-Iron Concentrated Liquid
Also available in Ready-to-Feed
Liquid and Powder

S•M•A•® Infant Formula

Wyeth-Ayerst Laboratories
P. 881

WYETH
794

Multivitamin/Multimineral Supplement
for pregnant or lactating women

Stuart Prenatal®

Wyeth-Ayerst Laboratories
P. 881

Box of 12 suppositories

Wyanoids® Relief Factor

ZILA

Zila Pharmaceuticals, Inc.
P. 882

.25 oz. Medicated Gel
Unique Film Controls Pain Longer

Zilactin®

Zila Pharmaceuticals, Inc.
P. 882

NEW!
Maximum Pain Relief with Benzocaine
MOUTH SORES,
CANKER SORES,
BITES & GUM SORES
Patented Protective Film
Lasts Up To 6 Hours
Zilactin-B

.25 oz. Medicated Gel with Benzocaine
Maximum Strength Medication

Zilactin®-B

Zila Pharmaceuticals, Inc.
P. 882

Zilactin®-L
Fast Pain Relief
LIP SORES,
COLD SORES
& FEVER BLISTERS
Medicated Liquid Treats
Sores Even Before They
Break Out

.25 Fl.oz. Medicated Liquid
Treats Cold Sores Without
Forming A Film

Zilactin®-L

MEDICAL ECONOMICS

PRODUCT INFORMATION

This section provides information on medications, testing kits, and other medical products designed for home use by consumers. It is made possible through the courtesy of the manufacturers whose products appear on the following pages. The information concerning each product has been prepared, edited, and approved by the medical department, medical director, and/or medical counsel of each manufacturer.

The product descriptions in this section comply with labeling regulations. They are designed to provide all information necessary for informed use, including, when applicable, active ingredients, indications, actions, warnings, cautions, drug interactions, symptoms and treatment of oral overdosage, dosage and directions for use, professional labeling, and how supplied. In some cases, additional information has been supplied to complement the standard labeling.

In compiling this section, the publisher has emphasized the necessity of describing products comprehensively. The descriptions seen here include all information made available by the manufacturer. The publisher does not warrant or guarantee any product described here, and does not perform any independent analysis of the information provided. Inclusion of a product in this book does not represent an endorsement, and the publisher does not necessarily advocate the use of any product listed.

B.F. Ascher & Company, Inc.

15501 WEST 109th STREET
LENEXA, KS 66219
Mailing address:
P.O. BOX 717
SHAWNEE MISSION, KS
66201-0717

AYR® Saline Nasal Mist and Drops
[ār]

AYR Mist or Drops restores vital moisture to provide prompt relief for dry, crusted and inflamed nasal membranes due to chronic sinusitis, colds, low humidity, overuse of nasal decongestant drops and sprays, allergies, minor nose bleeds and other minor nasal irritations. AYR provides a soothing way to thin thick secretions and aid their removal from the nose and sinuses. AYR can be used as often as needed without the side effects associated with overuse of decongestant nose drops and sprays.

SAFE AND GENTLE ENOUGH FOR CHILDREN AND INFANTS

AYR Drops are particularly convenient for easy application with infants and children. AYR is formulated to prevent stinging, burning and irritation of delicate nasal tissue, even that of babies.

Directions For Use: SPRAY—Squeeze twice in each nostril as often as needed. Hold bottle upright. To spray, give the bottle short, firm squeezes. Take care not to aspirate nasal contents back into bottle. DROPS—Two to four drops in each nostril every two hours as needed, or as directed by your physician.

AYR is a specially formulated, buffered, isotonic saline solution containing sodium chloride 0.65% adjusted to the proper tonicity and pH with monobasic potassium phosphate/sodium hydroxide buffer to prevent nasal irritation. AYR also contains the non-irritating antibacterial and antifungal preservatives thimerosal and benzalkonium chloride and is formulated with deionized water.

How Supplied: AYR Mist in 50 ml spray bottles, AYR Drops in 50 ml dropper bottles.

Shown in Product Identification Guide, page 503

COUGH-X®

Active Ingredients: Each lozenge contains dextromethorphan hydrobromide 5 mg and benzocaine 2 mg. Also contains: Corn syrup, eucalyptus oil, menthol, propylene glycol and sucrose.

Indications: Temporarily suppresses cough due to minor throat and bronchial irritants. Also, for the temporary relief of occasional minor irritation and sore throat.

Warnings: A persistent cough may be a sign of a serious condition. If cough persists for more than 1 week, tends to recur or if sore throat is severe, persists for more than 2 days or if cough and/or sore throat is accompanied or followed by fever, persistent headache, rash, swelling, nausea or vomiting, consult a physician. Do not take this product for persistent or chronic cough such as occurs with smoking, asthma, emphysema or if cough is accompanied by excessive phlegm (mucus) unless directed by a physician. Do not exceed recommended dosage. Do not use this product if you have a history of allergy to local anesthetics such as procaine, butacaine, benzocaine or other "caine" anesthetics. As with any drug, if you are pregnant or nursing a baby, seek the advice of a health professional before using this product. KEEP THIS AND ALL DRUGS OUT OF REACH OF CHILDREN. In case of accidental overdose, seek professional assistance or contact a Poison Control Center immediately.

Drug Interaction Precaution: Do not use this product if you are now taking a prescription monoamine oxidase inhibitor (MAOI) (certain drugs for depression, psychiatric or emotional conditions, or Parkinson's disease), or for 2 weeks after stopping the MAOI drug. If you are uncertain whether your prescription drug contains an MAOI, consult a health professional before taking this product.

Directions: Allow lozenge to dissolve slowly in the mouth. Adults and children 6 years of age and older: One lozenge every 2 hours as needed not to exceed 12 lozenges in 24 hours or as directed by a physician. Children 2 to 6 years of age: One lozenge every 4 hours not to exceed 6 lozenges in 24 hours or as directed by a physician. Children under 2 years of age: Consult a physician.

How Supplied: Available in pleasant-tasting menthol eucalyptus flavor. 9 individually-wrapped lozenges come packaged in a carton.
Shown in Product Identification Guide, page 503

ITCH-X® Gel & Spray
Dual-acting, itch-relieving gel and spray with aloe vera

Active Ingredients: Benzyl alcohol 10% and pramoxine HCl 1%.

Inactive Ingredients: Gel: aloe vera gel, carbomer 934, diaolidinyl urea, FD&C blue #1, methylparaben, propylene glycol, propylparaben, SD alcohol 40, styrene/acrylate copolymer, triethanolamine, and water.
Spray: Aloe vera gel, SD alcohol 40 and water.

Indications: For the temporary relief of pain and itching associated with minor skin irritations, allergic itches, rashes, hives, minor burns, insect bites, poison ivy, poison oak, and poison sumac.

Warnings: For external use only. Avoid contact with the eyes. Do not apply to open wounds or damaged skin. If condition worsens, or if symptoms persist for more than 7 days or clear up and occur again within a few days, discontinue use of this product and consult a physician. KEEP THIS AND ALL DRUGS OUT OF THE REACH OF CHILDREN. In case of accidental ingestion, seek professional assistance or contact a Poison Control Center immediately.
Additional Warning for Spray: Flammable, keep away from fire or flame.

Directions: Adults and children 2 years of age and older: Apply to affected area not more than 3 to 4 times daily. Children under 2 years of age: consult a physician.

How Supplied: Gel: 35.4g (1.25 oz) tube
Spray: 59.1 mL (2 fl oz) pump spray bottle.
Shown in Product Identification Guide, page 503

MOBIGESIC® Tablets
[mō′bĭ-jē′zĭk]
Pain reliever–Fever reducer

Indications: For the temporary relief of minor aches and pains associated with headache, muscular aches, backache, toothache, colds, premenstrual and menstrual cramps and for the minor pain from arthritis, and to reduce fever.

Directions: Adults and children 12 years of age and older: Oral dosage is 1 or 2 tablets every 4 hours while symptoms persist, not to exceed 10 tablets in 24 hours. Drink a full glass of water with each dose. Children 6 to under 12 years of age: Oral dosage is 1 tablet every 4 hours while symptoms persist, not to exceed 5 tablets in 24 hours. Drink water with each dose. Children under 6 years of age: Consult a physician.

Warnings: Do not take this product for pain for more than 10 days (5 days for children 6 to under 12 years of age) or for fever for more than 3 days unless directed by a physician. If pain or fever persists or gets worse, if new symptoms occur, or if redness or swelling is present, consult a physician because these could be signs of a serious condition. Children and teenagers who have or are recovering from chicken pox, flu symptoms or flu should NOT use this product. If nausea, vomiting or fever occur, consult a physician because these sysmptoms could be an early sigm of Reye syndrome, a rare but serious illness. If ringing in the ears or a loss of hearing occurs, consult a physician before taking any more of this product. Do not take this product if you have stomach problems (such as hearburn, upset stomach or stomach pain) that persist or recur, or if you have ulcers or bleeding problems, unless directed by a physician.

Drug Interaction Precaution: Do not take this product if you are taking a prescription drug for anticoagulation (thinning of the blood), diabetes, gout or arthritis unless directed by a physician. Do not take this product if you are allergic to salicylates (including aspirin) unless directed by a physician. May cause excitability especially in children. Do not take this product, unless directed by a physician, if you have a breathing problem such as emphysema or chronic bronchitis, or if you have glaucoma or difficulty in urination due to enlargement of the prostate gland. May cause drowsiness; alcohol, sedatives and tranquilizers may increase the drowsiness effect. Avoid alcoholic beverages while taking this product. Do not take this product if you are taking sedatives or tranquilizers, without first consulting your physician. Use caution when driving a motor vehicle or operating machinery. KEEP THIS AND ALL DRUGS OUT OF THE REACH OF CHILDREN. In case of accidental overdose, seek professional assistance or contact a Poison Control Center immediately. As with any drug, if you are pregnant or nursing a baby, seek the advice of a health professional before using this product.

Active Ingredients: Each tablet contains magnesium salicylate 325 mg and phenyltoloxamine citrate 30 mg. Also contains: Micro crystalline cellulose, magnesium stearate and colloidal silicon dioxide.

How Supplied: Packages of 18's; bottles of 50's and 100's.
Shown in Production Identifiction Guide, page 503

MOBISYL® Analgesic Creme
[mō'bĭ-sĭl]
Penetrates to the site of pain to bring relief.

Active Ingredient: Trolamine salicylate 10%. Also Contains: Glycerin, methylparaben, mineral oil, polysorbate 60, propylparaben, sorbitan stearate, sorbitol, stearic acid, and water.

Description: MOBISYL is a greaseless, odorless, penetrating, non-burning, non-irritating analgesic creme.

Indications: For adults and children, 12 years of age and older, MOBISYL is indicated for the temporary relief of minor aches and pains of muscles and joints, such as simple backache, lumbago, arthritis, neuralgia, strains, bruises and sprains.

Actions: MOBISYL penetrates fast into sore, tender joints and muscles where pain originates. It works to reduce inflammation. Helps soothe stiff joints and muscles and gets you going again.

Warnings: For external use only. Avoid contact with the eyes. Discontinue use if condition worsens or if symptoms persist for more than 7 days, and consult a physician. Do not use on children under 12 years of age except under the advice and supervision of a physician. In case of accidental ingestion, seek professional assistance or contact a Poison Control Center immediately. Close cap tightly.

KEEP THIS AND ALL DRUGS OUT OF THE REACH OF CHILDREN. Store at room temperature.

Dosage and Administration: Place a liberal amount of MOBISYL Creme in your palm and massage into the area of pain and soreness three or four times a day, especially before retiring. MOBISYL may be worn under clothing or bandages.

How Supplied: MOBISYL is available in 35.4g (1.25 oz) tubes, 100g (3.5 oz) tubes, 226.8g (8 oz) jars.
Shown in Product Identification Guide, page 503

PEN•KERA® Creme with Keratin Binding Factor
A Therapeutic Moisturizing Creme for Chronic Dry Skin

Ingredients: Water, octyl palmitate, glycerin, mineral oil, polysorbate 60, sorbitan stearate, polyamino sugar condensate, urea, wheat germ glycerides, carbomer 940, triethanolamine, DMDMH, iodo propynyl butyl carbamate, diazolidinyl urea, and dehydroacetic acid.

Indications: PEN•KERA Therapeutic Creme for Chronic Dry Skin contains Keratin Binding Factor, a polyamino sugar condensate and urea, which is synthesized to match the same biological components as those found in skin. The Keratin Binding Factor in PEN•KERA Creme replaces the missing elements of dehydrated skin which absorb and retain moisture. The Keratin Binding Factor actually simulates the natural moisturizing mechanism of the skin, relieving itching, flaking, sensitive, dry skin symptoms.
PEN•KERA is fragrance-free, dye-free, paraben-free, lanolin-free, non-comedogenic and non-greasy for smooth, fast absorption.

Dosage and Administration: Apply in a thin layer. Because it penetrates quickly and is non-greasy, PEN•KERA may be used under make-up or sun screens. Regular use will reduce the frequency of application and quantity required to achieve moisturized skin.

Precautions: FOR EXTERNAL USE ONLY

How Supplied: PEN•KERA Therapeutic Creme is available in 8 oz. bottles.
Shown in Product Identification Guide, page 503

PRETTY FEET & HANDS®

For rough, dry skin and calluses, hand lotions or moisturizers aren't always enough. But Pretty Feet & Hands does what a moisturizer doesn't.
It rolls off that rough, dry skin from feet, elbows, knees and hands. Uncovers soft, new skin underneath.

Directions for use: Shake before using. Use a generous amount of Pretty Feet & Hands and rub thoroughly into rough skin until it rolls off. Contains no abrasives or alcohol.

Contains: Water, paraffin, magnesium aluminum silicate palmitic acid, stearic acid, trolamine, methylparaben, propylparaben, fragrance.
Shown in Product Identification Guide, page 503

EDUCATIONAL MATERIAL

The following Patient Information Materials are available to physicians, pharmacists and consumers:
"How to Administer Nose Drops to an Infant" in English and Spanish
"Chronic Sinusitis" – Tips for alleviating sinus problems
"Dry, Irritated Nasal Passages"
"Decongestant Rebound" – Overuse of topical nasal decongestants
"Tension Headache: Break the Cycle of Stress-tension Headache"
"Chronic Dry Skin" – You don't have to live with it.
"Coping with Arthritis"
"Sports Injuries" – Types of injuries and how to avoid them.
"Urinary Tract Infection" – What it is and coping with it.
"IBS" – What it is and what you can do about it.
Write: Patient Information, B. F. Ascher & Co., Inc., P.O. Box 717, Shawnee Mission, KS 66201-0717

Astra USA, Inc.
50 OTIS ST.
WESTBORO, MA 01581-4500

XYLOCAINE® (lidocaine) 2.5%
[zī'lo-caine]
OINTMENT

For temporary relief of pain and itching due to minor burns, sunburn, minor cuts, abrasions, insect bites and minor skin irritations.

Composition: Lidocaine 2.5% in a water miscible ointment vehicle consisting of polyethylene glycols and propylene glycol.

Action and Uses: A topical anesthetic ointment for fast, temporary relief of pain and itching due to minor burns, sunburn, minor cuts, abrasions, insect bites and minor skin irritations. The ointment can be easily removed with water.

Administration and Dosage: Xylocaine 2.5% Ointment should be applied liberally over the affected areas. Use enough to provide temporary relief and reapply Xylocaine 2.5% Ointment as needed for continued relief.

Continued on next page

Astra—Cont.

Important Warning: *Use only as directed by a physician in persistent, severe or extensive skin disorders. In case of accidental ingestion seek professional assistance or contact a poison control center immediately.* **KEEP OUT OF THE REACH OF CHILDREN.**

Caution: *Do not use in the eyes. Not for prolonged use. If the condition for which this preparation is used persists, or if a rash or irritation develops, discontinue use and consult a physician.*

How Supplied: 1.25 ounce tubes containing 2.5% lidocaine base in water soluble carbowaxes.
Shown in Product Identification Guide, page 503

Ayerst Laboratories
**Division of American Home
Products Corporation
685 THIRD AVE.
NEW YORK, NY 10017-4071**

For information for Ayerst's consumer products, see product listings under Whitehall Laboratories.
Please turn to Whitehall Laboratories, page 870.

Baker Cummins Dermatologicals, Inc.
**8800 NW 36TH ST.
MIAMI, FL 33178**

AQUADERM® LOTION

Description: Special concentrated formula for maximum moisturization. Developed and tested by dermatologists, this unique combination of natural concentrates restores moisture to the skin. Aquaderm creates younger-looking, younger-feeling skin. Non-greasy. Hypoallergenic. Noncomedogenic (will not cause acne).

Directions: Apply to hands and body morning or night or both.

Ingredients: Water, Caprylic/Capric Triglyceride, Methyl Gluceth-10, Glyceryl Stearate, Dimethicone, Petrolatum, Mineral Oil, PPG-20 Methyl Glucose Ether Distearate, Squalane, PEG-50 Stearate, Stearic Acid, Sodium Hyaluronate, Lecithin, Sodium Polyglutamate, Magnesium Aluminum Silicate, Carbomer 934, Dichlorobenzyl Alcohol, Cetyl Alcohol, BHT, Diazolidinyl Urea, Xanthan Gum, Menthol, Tetrasodium EDTA, Sodiuim Hydroxide.

How Supplied: 7.5 oz. Bottle (NDC 58174-201-75)
Shown in Product Identification Guide, page 503

AQUADERM® Sunscreen/ Moisturizer SPF 15

Description: Aquaderm® Sunscreen/ Moisturizer developed by leading dermatologists to deliver maximum moisturization. Regular daily use of Aquaderm's dual action moisturizer and sunscreen protects and preserves your youthful appearance. This specially developed formula contains sunscreens (SPF 15) that shield your skin from UVA and UVB rays, to protect it from wrinkles and reduce skin damage and possible skin cancer. Aquaderm® Sunscreen/Moisturizer is safe and effective, hypo-allergenic, non-comedogenic, Parabens-free, and will not leave an artificial-feeling film. Aquaderm® Sunscreen/Moisturizer is especially suited for patients undergoing Retin-A® therapy, who require maximum moisturization and sun protection.

Directions: Apply as needed. Compatible for daily use under make-up.

Active Ingredients: Octyl Methoxycinnamate, 7.5%, Oxybenzone, 6%, in a moisturizing cream base.

Warnings: FOR EXTERNAL USE ONLY. Avoid contact with eyes. If irritation develops, discontinue use. Keep this and all drugs out of the reach of children. In case of accidental ingestion, seek professional assistance or contact a Poison Control Center immediately.
Retin-A® is a registered trademark of Johnson & Johnson

How Supplied: 3.5 oz. tube (58174-205-35)
Shown in Product Identification Guide, page 503

AQUADERM® Cream
CLINICALLY PROVEN FOR ALL SKIN TYPES, FRAGRANCE FREE.

Description: Special concentrated facial formula for maximum moisturization. Developed and tested by dermatologists, this unique combination of natural concentrates restores moisture to facial skin. Aquaderm creates younger-looking, younger-feeling skin. Non-greasy. Hypoallergenic. Noncomedogenic (will not cause acne).

Directions: Apply to face or other dry areas morning or night or both.

Ingredients: Water, Caprylic/Capric Triglyceride, Methyl Gluceth-10, Glyceryl Stearate, Mineral Oil, Squalane, PPG-20 Methyl Glucose Ether Distearate, Dimethicone, Stearic Acid, PEG-50 Stearate, Sodium Hyaluronate, Lecithin, Sodium Polyglutamate, Magnesium Aluminum Silicate, Carbomer 934, Dichlorobenzyl Alcohol, Cetyl Alcohol, BHT, Diazolidinyl Urea, Xanthan Gum, Menthol, Sodium Hydroxide, Tetrasodium EDTA.

How Supplied: 4 oz. Jar (NDC 58174-202-04)
Shown in Product Identification Guide, page 503

P&S Liquid®

Description: P&S Liquid® used regularly, helps loosen and remove scales on the scalp.

Directions: Apply liberally to scalp each night before retiring. Massage gently to loosen scales. Leave on overnight and shampoo the next morning. Use daily as needed.

Ingredients: Mineral Oil • Water • Fragrance • Glycerin • Phenol • Sodium Chloride • D&C Yellow #11 • D&C Red #17 • D&C Green #6.

Caution: Do not apply to large portions of body surfaces. Discontinue use if excessive skin irritation develops. Avoid contact with eyes or mucous membranes. Keep out of the reach of children. In case of accidental ingestion, seek professional assistance or contact a Poison Control Center immediately.
FOR EXTERNAL USE ONLY. SHAKE WELL BEFORE USING

How Supplied: 8 fl. oz. Bottle (58174-401-08); 4 fl. oz. Bottle (58174-401-04)
Shown in Product Identification Guide, page 503

P&S® PLUS Tar Gel

Description: **PAS® PLUS** helps stop the itching, irritation, and skin flaking associated with seborrheic dermatitis and psoriasis. Non-Staining formula.

Indications: For relief of skin and scalp itching, irritation and flaking associated with seborrheic dermatitis and psoriasis.

Active Ingredient: 8% Coal Tar Solution (equivalent to 1.6% Crude Coal Tar).

Directions: Apply to affected areas one to four times daily or as directed by a physician.

Warnings: FOR EXTERNAL USE ONLY. Avoid contact with the eyes. If contact occurs, rinse eyes thoroughly with water. If condition worsens or does not improve after regular use of this product as directed, consult a physician. Use caution in exposing skin to sunlight after applying this product. It may increase your tendency to sunburn for up to 24 hours after application. Do not use for prolonged periods without consulting a physician. Do not use this product in or around the rectum or in the genital area or groin except on the advice of a physician. Do not use this product with other forms of psoriasis therapy such as ultraviolet radiation or prescription drugs unless directed to do so by a physician. If condition covers a large area of the body, consult your physician before using this product.

Caution: Keep this and all drugs out of reach of children. In case of accidental ingestion, seek professional assistance or contact a Poison Control Center immediately.

How Supplied: 3.5 oz. tube (NDC 58174-409-35)

P&S® Shampoo

Description: P&S® Shampoo relieves the itching, irritation and skin flaking associated with seborrheic dermatitis of the scalp. It also relieves the itching, redness, and scaling associated with psoriasis of the scalp. P&S® Shampoo may be used alone as well as following treatment with P&S® Liquid. Its rich conditioning formula improves hair's manageability and helps prevent tangles.

Indications: For relief of the symptoms of seborrheic dermatitis and psoriasis.

Active Ingredient: 2% Salicylic Acid.

Directions: For best results use at least twice a week or as directed by a physician. Wet hair, apply to scalp and massage vigorously. Rinse and repeat.

Warnings: FOR EXTERNAL USE ONLY. Avoid contact with eyes. If contact occurs, rinse eyes thoroughly with water. If condition worsens or does not improve after regular use of this product as directed, consult a physician. If condition covers a large area of the body, consult your physician before using this product. Do not use on children under 2 years of age except as directed by a physician.

Caution: Keep this and all drugs out of reach of children. In case of accidental ingestion, seek professional assistance or contact a Poison Control Center immediately.

How Supplied: 8 fl. oz. Bottle (NDC 58174-407-08); 4 fl. oz. Bottle (NDC 58174-407-04)
Shown in Product Identification Guide, page 503

ULTRA DERM® Moisturizer

Description: ULTRA DERM® LOTION combines lubricants and moisturizers in a formula that soothes, smooths and softens dry, itchy skin.

Directions: Apply as often as needed or as directed by a physician. Smooths readily into the skin.

Ingredients: Water • Propylene Glycol • Mineral Oil • Lanolin Oil • Petrolatum • Glycerin • Glyceryl Stearate • PEG-50 Stearate • Propylene Glycol Stearate SE • Cetyl Alcohol • Sorbitan Laurate • Potassium Sorbate • Phosphoric Acid • Tetrasodium EDTA • Fragrance.

Warnings: FOR EXTERNAL USE ONLY. Avoid contact with the eyes; if contact occurs, rinse eyes thoroughly with water.

Caution: Keep out of the reach of children. In case of accidental ingestion, seek

professional assistance or contact a Poison Control Center immediately.

How Supplied: 8 fl. oz. Bottle (NDC 58174-101-08)
Shown in Product Identification Guide, page 503

ULTRA MIDE 25® LOTION

Description: ULTRA MIDE 25® LOTION, contains ingredients to soften and moisturize areas of very dry, rough or calloused skin. This unique keratolytic formula (U.S. Patent #4,672,078) contains a stabilized form of urea (25%) to help prevent the stinging and irritation often associated with moisturizers containing urea. ULTRA MIDE 25® Lotion contains no parabens.

Directions: Apply 4 times daily, or as directed by a physician. Each application should be rubbed in completely.

Ingredients: Water • Urea • Mineral Oil • Glycerin • Propylene Glycol • PEG-50 Stearate • Butyrolactone • Hydrogenated Lanolin • Sorbitan Laurate • Glyceryl Stearate • Magnesium Aluminum Silicate • Propylene Glycol Stearate SE • Cetyl Alcohol • Fragrance • Diazolidinyl Urea • Tetrasodium EDTA.

FOR EXTERNAL USE ONLY
Keep out of reach of children. Discontinue use if irritation occurs. Caution should be taken when used near the eyes. In case of accidental ingestion, seek professional assistance or contact a Poison Control Center immediately.

How Supplied: 8 fl. oz. Bottle (NDC 58174-402-08)
Shown in Product Identification Guide, page 503

ULTRA MIDE 25® Extra Strength Moisturizer

Ingredients: Water, Urea, Mineral Oil, Glycerin, Propylene Glycol, PEG-50 Stearate, Butyrolactone, Hydrogenated Lanolin, Sorbitan Laurate, Glyceryl Stearate, Magnesium Aluminum Silicate, Propylene Glycol Stearate SE, Cetyl Alcohol, Fragrance, Diazolidinyl Urea, Tetrasodium EDTA.

Indications: Intensive moisturizer for extra dry, scaly or calloused skin. Contains ingredients to soften and moisturize areas of very dry, rough, cracked or calloused skin. This unique keratolytic patented formula contains a stabilized form of urea (25%) to help prevent the stinging and irritation often associated with moisturizers containing urea. ULTRA MIDE 25® Lotion contains no parabens.

Warnings: FOR EXTERNAL USE ONLY. Keep out of reach of children. Discontinue use if irritation occurs. Caution should be taken when used near the eyes. In case of accidental ingestion, seek professional assistance or contact a Poison Control Center immediately.

Directions for Use: Apply four times daily, or as directed by a physician. Each application should be rubbed in completely.

How Supplied: 8 fl. oz. bottle (58174-420-08)

X–SEB® Shampoo

Description: X-SEB® Antidandruff Shampoo provides relief of the itching and scalp flaking associated with dandruff. This unique formulation is gentle enough for daily use leaving hair healthy looking and manageable.

Indications: For relief of the symptoms of dandruff.

Active Ingredient: 1% Pyrithione Zinc

Directions: For best results, use X-SEB® Antidandruff Shampoo at least twice a week or as directed by a physician. Wet hair, apply to scalp and massage vigorously. Rinse and repeat.

Warnings: FOR EXTERNAL USE ONLY. Avoid contact with the eyes. If contact occurs, rinse eyes thoroughly with water. If condition worsens or does not improve after regular use of this product as directed, consult a physician. Do not use on children under 2 years of age except as directed by a physician.

Caution: Keep this and all drugs out of the reach of children. In case of accidental ingestion, seek professional assistance or contact a Poison Control Center immediately.

How Supplied: 8 fl. oz. Bottle (NDC 58174-106-08); 4 fl. oz. Bottle (NDC 58174-106-04)
Shown in Product Identification Guide, page 503

X-SEB® PLUS Antidandruff Conditioning Shampoo

Description: X-SEB® PLUS Antidandruff Conditioning Shampoo provides relief of the itching and scalp flaking associated with dandruff. Ideal for dry, brittle hair. This unique formulation is gentle enough for daily use giving hair extra body, a healthy look and ease of manageability.

Indications: For relief of the symptoms of dandruff.

Active Ingredient: 1% Pyrithione Zinc

Directions: For best results, use X-SEB® PLUS Antidandruff Conditioning Shampoo at least twice a week or as directed by a physician. Wet hair, apply to scalp and massage vigorously. Rinse and repeat.

Warnings: FOR EXTERNAL USE ONLY. Avoid contact with the eyes. If contact occurs, rinse eyes thoroughly with water. If condition worsens or does not improve after regular use of this

Continued on next page

Baker Cummins Derm.—Cont.

product as directed, consult a physician. Do not use on children under 2 years of age except as directed by a physician.

Caution: Keep this and all drugs out of the reach of children. In case of accidental ingestion, seek professional assistance or contact a Poison Control Center immediately.

How Supplied: 8 oz. Bottle (NDC 58174-116-08); 4 oz Bottle (NDC 58174-116-04)

Shown in Product Identification Guide, page 503

X–SEB T® Pearl Shampoo

Description: X-SEB T® Pearl Shampoo helps stop the itching, irritation, redness and scalp flaking and scaling associated with dandruff, seborrheic dermatitis and psoriasis. This formulation is designed to be a mild, gentle cleansing base leaving hair healthy looking and manageable. X-SEB T® Pearl Shampoo will not discolor or damage hair that has been color treated or permed.

Indications: For relief of the symptoms of dandruff, seborrheic dermatitis and psoriasis.

Active Ingredient: 10% Coal Tar Solution (equivalent to 2% Crude Coal Tar).

Directions: For best results, use X-SEB T® Pearl Shampoo at least twice a week or as directed by physician. Wet hair, apply to scalp and massage vigorously. Rinse and repeat.

Warnings: FOR EXTERNAL USE ONLY. Avoid contact with the eyes. If contact occurs, rinse eyes thoroughly with water. If condition worsens or does not improve after regular use of this product as directed, consult a physician. Use caution in exposing skin to sunlight after applying this product. It may increase your tendency to sunburn for up to 24 hours after application. Do not use for prolonged periods without consulting a physician. Do not use this product with other forms of psoriasis therapy such as ultraviolet radiation or prescription drugs unless directed to do so by a physician. If condition covers a large area of the body, consult your physician before using this product. Do not use on children under 2 years of age except as directed by a physician.

Caution: Keep this and all drugs out of the reach of children. In case of accidental ingestion, seek professional assistance or contact a Poison Control Center immediately.

How Supplied: 8 fl. oz. Bottle (NDC 58174-104-08); 4 fl. oz. Bottle (NDC 58174-104-04)

Shown in Product Identification Guide, page 503

X-SEB T® PLUS
Conditioning Shampoo

Description: X-SEB T® PLUS Conditioning Shampoo relieves the itching, irritation and skin flaking associated with dandruff, seborrheic dermatitis and psoriasis. This formulation is designed to effectively treat scaly conditions in a mild, gentle cleansing base leaving hair healthy looking and manageable. X-SEB T® PLUS Conditioning Shampoo will not discolor or damage hair that has been color treated or permed.

Indications: For relief of the symptoms of dandruff, seborrheic dermatitis and psoriasis.

Active Ingredient: 10% Coal Tar Solution (equivalent to 2% Crude Coal Tar)

Directions: For best results, use X-SEB T® PLUS Conditioning Shampoo at least twice a week or as directed by a physician. Wet hair, apply to scalp and massage vigorously. Rinse and repeat.

Warnings: FOR EXTERNAL USE ONLY. Avoid contact with the eyes. If contact occurs, rinse eyes thoroughly with water. If condition worsens or does not improve after regular use of this product as directed, consult a physician. Use caution in exposing skin to sunlight after applying this product: it may increase your tendency to sunburn for up to 24 hours after application. Do not use for prolonged periods without consulting a physician. Do not use this product with other forms of psoriasis therapy such as ultraviolet radiation or prescription drugs unless directed to do so by a physician. If condition covers a large area of the body, consult your physician before using this product. Do not use on children under 2 years of age except as directed by a physician.

Caution: Keep this and all drugs out of the reach of children. In case of accidental ingestion, seek professional assistance or contact a Poison Control Center immediately.

How Supplied: 8 fl. oz. Bottle (NDC 58174-115-08); 4 fl. oz. Bottle (NDC 58174-115-04)

Shown in Product Identification Guide, page 503

UNKNOWN DRUG?
Consult the
Product Identification Guide
(Gray Pages)
for full-color photos of
leading over-the-counter
medications

Bausch & Lomb Incorporated
Personal Products Division
ROCHESTER, NY 14692-0450

CURÉL® Therapeutic Moisturizing Lotion and Cream

Indications: For control of dry skin symptoms, Curél delivers extra effective moisturization that with regular use, ends dry skin for most people.

Actions: Curél's unique cationic emulsion base enables it to be faster absorbing and more substantive to dry skin, all without a greasy after-feel. Curél is rich in humectant and occlusive ingredients, which help skin retain natural moisture and help heal dry skin problems like chapping, soreness, cracking, and erythema. Clinical skin hydration studies have shown that Curél moisturizes better than other leading therapeutic lotions, giving extra effective moisturization for softer, healthier skin. Dermatologist tested and recommended, Curél contains no mineral oil or lanolin and all ingredients are non-comedogenic. Available in lightly fragranced Original Formula and Fragrance Free.

Contents: Original Formula: Deionized Water, Glycerin, Quaternium-5, Petrolatum, Isopropyl Palmitate, 1-Hexadecanol, Dimethicone, Sodium Chloride, Fragrance, Methyl Paraben, Propyl Paraben.

Fragrance Free: Deionized Water, Glycerin, Quaternium-5, Petrolatum, Isopropyl Palmitate, 1-Hexadecanol, Dimethicone, Sodium Chloride, Methyl Paraben, Propyl Paraben.

Directions for Use: Apply as often as needed. Especially effective when applied after bathing while skin is still damp. For external use only.

How Supplied: Original Formula:
Cream— 2.5 oz. tube;
Lotion— 6 oz. and 10 oz. fliptop bottles
13 oz. pump bottle

Fragrance Free:
Cream— 2.5 oz. tube;
Lotion— 6 oz. fliptop bottle
13 oz. pump bottle
For Toll-Free Product Information: Call 1-800-572-2931

Shown in Product Identification Guide, page 503

Bayer Corporation
Consumer Care Division
See
Miles Inc.
Consumer Care Division

Beach Pharmaceuticals
Division of Beach Products, Inc.
5220 SOUTH MANHATTAN AVE. TAMPA, FL 33611

BEELITH Tablets
MAGNESIUM SUPPLEMENT WITH PYRIDOXINE HCl
Each tablet supplies 362 mg (30 mEq) of magnesium and 25 mg of pyridoxine HCL.

Description: Each tablet contains magnesium oxide 600 mg and pyridoxine hydrochloride (Vitamin B_6) 25 mg equivalent to B_6 20 mg. *Also, microcrystalline cellulose, sodium starch glycolate, D&C Yellow #10, FD&C Yellow #6 (Sunset Yellow), titanium dioxide, and other ingredients.* Each tablet yields 362 mg of magnesium and supplies 90% of the Adult U.S. Recommended Daily Allowance (RDA) for magnesium and 1000% of the Adult RDA for vitamin B_6.

Indications: As a dietary supplement for patients with magnesium and/or vitamin B_6 deficiencies resulting from malnutrition, alcoholism, magnesium depleting drugs and inadequate nutritional intake or absorption.

Dosage: One tablet daily or as directed by a physician.

Drug Interaction Precautions: Do not take this product if you are presently taking a prescription drug without consulting your physician or other health professional.

Warnings: If you have kidney disease, take only under the supervision of a physician. Excessive dosage may cause laxation. **KEEP OUT OF THE REACH OF CHILDREN.**

How Supplied: Golden yellow, film coated tablet with the name **BEACH** and the number **1132** printed on each tablet. Packaged in bottles of 100 (NDC 0486-1132-01) tablets.

Beiersdorf Inc.
360 Dr. Martin Luther King Dr. NORWALK, CT 06856-5529

AQUAPHOR®— OTC
Original Formula Ointment
NDC Numbers— 10356-020-01
10356-020-02

Composition: Petrolatum, mineral oil, mineral wax and wool wax alcohol.

Actions and Uses: Aquaphor is a stable, neutral, odorless, anhydrous ointment base. Miscible with water or aqueous solutions, Aquaphor will absorb several times its own weight, forming smooth, creamy water-in-oil emulsions. In its pure form, Aquaphor is recommended for use as a topical preparation to help heal severely dry skin. Aquaphor contains no preservatives, fragrances or known irritants.

Administration and Dosages: Use Aquaphor alone or in compounding virtually any ointment using aqueous solutions, or in combination with other oil-based substances and all common topical medications. Apply Aquaphor liberally to affected area.

Precautions: For external use only. Avoid contact with eyes. Not to be applied over third degree burns, deep or puncture wounds, infections or lacerations. If condition worsens or does not improve within 7 days, patient should consult a doctor.

How Supplied: 16 oz. jar—List No. 45585
5 lb. jar—List. No. 45586
Shown in Product Identification Guide, page 503

AQUAPHOR OTC
Healing Ointment
NDC Number—10356-021-01

Composition: Petrolatum, Mineral Oil, Mineral Wax, Wool Wax Alcohol, Panthenol, Bisabolol, Glycerin.

Actions and Uses: Aquaphor Healing Ointment is specially formulated for faster healing of severely dry skin, cracked skin and minor burns. It is recommended for patients suffering from severe skin chapping and from skin disorders that result in severely dry skin. This formula is also indicated as a follow-up skin treatment for patients undergoing radiation therapy or other drying/burning medical therapies. It is preservative-free, fragrance-free and hypoallergenic.[1]

Administration and Dosage: Use Aquaphor Healing Ointment whenever a mild healing agent is needed. Apply liberally to affected areas two to three times a day. In the case of minor wounds, clean area prior to application.

Precautions: For external use only. Avoid contact with the eyes. Not to be applied over third degree burns, deep or puncture wounds, infections or lacerations. If condition worsens or does not improve within seven days, patient should consult a physician.

How Supplied: 1.75 oz. tube
1. Data on file, BDF Inc
Shown in Product Identification Guide, page 503

EUCERIN® BAR OTC
[ū 'sir-in]
Cleansing Bar

Indications: Use with warm water to cleanse skin.

Active Ingredient: Eucerite®

Contains: Disodium Lauryl Sulfosuccinate, Sodium Cocoyl Isethionate, Cetearyl Alcohol, Corn Starch, Glyceryl Stearate, Paraffin, Water, Titanium Dioxide, Octyldodecanol, Cyclopentadecanolide, Lanolin Alcohol, Bisabolol.

Actions and Uses: Eucerin® Cleansing Bar has been specially formulated for use on sensitive skin. The formulation contains Eucerite®, a special blend of ingredients that closely resemble the natural oils of the skin, thus providing excellent moisturizing properties. This formulation is fragrance-free and non-comedogenic. Additionally, the pH value of Eucerin Cleansing Bar is neutral so as not to affect the skin's normal acid mantle.

Directions: Use during shower, bath, or regular cleansing.

How Supplied: 3 ounce bar.
List number 3852
Shown in Product Identification Guide, page 503

EUCERIN® Creme OTC
[ū 'sir-in]
Original Moisturizing Creme
NDC Numbers—10356-090-01
10356-090-05
10356-090-04
10356-090-07

Indications: Use daily to help relieve dry and very dry skin.

Composition: Triple Purified Water, Petrolatum, Mineral Oil, Ceresin, Lanolin Alcohol, Methylchloroisothiazolinone, Methylisothiazolinone.

Actions and Uses: A gentle, non-comedogenic, fragrance-free water-in-oil emulsion. Eucerin can be used as a treatment for dry skin associated with eczema, psoriasis, chapped or chafed skin, sunburn, windburn and itching associated with dryness.[1]

Administration and Dosages: Apply freely to affected areas of the skin as often as necessary.

Precautions: For external use only. Discontinue use if signs of irritation occur.

How Supplied: 16 oz. jar—List Number 0090
8 oz. jar—List Number 3774
4 oz. jar—List Number 3797
2 oz. tube—List Number 3868
1. Data on File.
Shown in Product Identification Guide, page 504

EUCERIN® OTC
FACIAL MOISTURIZING LOTION SPF 25
NDC Number—10356-972-01

Indications: Use daily to help relieve dry skin and provide broad spectrum sun protection.

Composition:
Active Ingredients: Octyl Methoxycinnamate, Octyl Salicylate, Titanium Dioxide.

Continued on next page

Beiersdorf—Cont.

Other Ingredients: Water, Octyldodecyl Neopentanoate, Dioctyl Malate, Glycerin, Petrolatum, Zinc Oxide, Cetearyl Alcohol, DEA-Cetyl Phosphate, PEG-40 Castor Oil, Glyceryl Stearate, Sodium Hyaluronate, Lactic Acid, Lanolin Alcohol, Sodium Cetearyl Sulfate, Xanthan Gum, Methicone, Dimethicone, EDTA, Sodium Hydroxide, Methylchloroisothiazolinone, Methylisothiazolinone.

Actions and Uses: Eucerin Facial Moisturizing Lotion SPF 25 is fragrance-free and non-comedogenic, with a unique sun screen (titanium dioxide) to protect skin from UVA and UVB light. It is specially formulated for dry, sensitive skin or for those undergoing therapies which irritate delicate facial skin. This light, oil-in-water formula is non-greasy and is easily absorbed into the skin.

Administration and Dosage: Apply Eucerin Facial Moisturizing Lotion SPF 25 twice a day (especially in the morning), to nourish and moisture skin and protect it from harmful UVA and UVB rays.

Precautions: For external use only. Avoid contact with eyes. Keep out of the reach of children. Discontinue use if signs of irritation occur.

How Supplied: 4-oz. bottle.—List No. 03972
Shown in Product Identification Guide, page 504

EUCERIN® Lotion OTC
[*ū'sir-in*]
Original Moisturizing Lotion
NDC Numbers—10356-793-01
　　　　　　　10356-793-04

Indications: Use daily to help relieve dry skin.

Composition: Water, Mineral Oil, Isopropyl Myristate, PEG-40 Sorbitan Peroleate, Glyceryl Lanoleate, Sorbitol, Propylene Glycol, Cetyl Palmitate, Magnesium Sulfate, Aluminum Stearate, Lanolin Alcohol, BHT, Methylchloroisothiazolinone, Methylisothiazolinone.

Actions and Uses: Eucerin Lotion is a non-comedogenic, fragrance-free, unique water-in-oil formulation that will help to alleviate and soothe dry skin, and provide long-lasting moisturization.

Administration and Dosage: Use daily on dry skin.

Precautions: For external use only. Discontinue use if signs of irritation occur.

How Supplied: 8 fluid oz. plastic bottle—List Number 3793
16 fluid oz. plastic bottle—List number 3794
Shown in Product Identification Guide, page 504

EUCERIN PLUS CREME OTC
Moisturizing Alphahydroxy Creme
NDC 10356-036-01

Indications: Use daily to help relieve severely dry, flaky skin.

Composition: Water, Mineral Oil, Urea, Magnesium Stearate, Ceresin, Polyglyceryl-3 Diisostearate, Sodium Lactate, Isopropyl Palmitate, Benzyl Alcohol, Panthenol, Bisabolol, Lanolin Alcohol, Magnesium Sulfate.

Caution: For external use only. Avoid contact with eyes and areas where skin is inflamed or cracked. Discontinue use if signs of irritation occur. Keep out of reach of children.

Action and Uses: Eucerin Plus Creme is a unique alpha-hydroxy acid moisturizing creme (2.5% sodium lactate, 10% urea) that is clinically proven to relieve severely dry, flaky skin conditions[1]. Unlike other alpha-hydroxy acid mositurizers, Eucerin Plus Creme has low irritation potential, is fragrance-free and non-comedogenic.

Administration and Dosage: Use daily on severely dry, scaly skin.

Precautions: Avoid contact with eyes or areas where skin is inflamed or cracked. Discontinue use if signs of irritation occur. For external use only. Keep out of reach of children.

How Supplied: 4 oz. jar—List No. 03611
1. Data on file.
Shown in Product Identification Guide, page 504

EUCERIN PLUS LOTION OTC
Alphahydroxy Moisturizing Lotion
NDC 10356-967-01

Indications: Use daily to help relieve severely dry, flaky skin.

Composition: Water, Mineral Oil, PEG-7 Hydrogenated Castor Oil, Isohexadecane, Sodium Lactate 5%, Urea 5%, Glycerin, Isopropyl Palmitate, Panthenol, Ozokerite, Magnesium Sulfate, Lanolin Alcohol, Bisabolol, Methylchloroisothiazolinone, Methylisothiazolinone.

Action and Uses: Eucerin Plus Lotion in a unique alpha-hydroxy acid moisturizing lotion (5% Sodium Lactate, 5% Urea) that is clinically proven to relieve severely dry, flaky skin conditions.[1] Unlike other alpha-hydroxy acid moisturizing lotions, Eucerin Plus has low irritation potential, is fragrance free and non-comedogenic.

Administration and Dosage: Use daily on severely dry, flaky skin.

Precautions: Avoid contact with eyes or areas where skin is inflamed or cracked. Discontinue use if signs of irritation occur. For external use only. Keep out of reach of children.

How Supplied: 6 oz bottle—List No. 03967
1. Data on File.
Shown in Product Identification Guide, page 504

Blaine Company, Inc.
1465 JAMIKE LANE
ERLANGER, KY 41018

MAG-OX 400

Description: Each tablet contains Magnesium Oxide 400 mg. U.S.P. (Heavy), or 241.3 mg. Elemental Magnesium (19.86 mEq.)

Indications and Usage: Hypomagnesemia, magnesium deficiencies and/or magnesium depletion during therapy with diuretics and/or digitalis, aminoglycosides, amphotericin B, cyclosporin, chemotherapy, and during pregnancy, PMS, menopause, diabetes, hyperoxaluria, malnutrition, weight/strength training, restricted diet, or alcoholism.

Warnings: Do not use this product except under the advice and supervision of a physician if you have a kidney disease. May have laxative effect.

Dosage: Adult dose 1 or 2 tablets daily with meals or as directed by a physician.

Professional Labeling: Serum magnesium levels do not accurately represent total body, tissue, or bone magnesium levels.

How Supplied: Bottles of 100, 1000, and hospital unit dose (U.D. 100s)

URO-MAG

Description: Each capsule contains Magnesium Oxide 140 mg. U.S.P. (Heavy), or 84.5 mg. Elemental Magnesium (6.93 mEq.)

Indications and Usage: Hypomagnesemia, magnesium deficiencies and/or magnesium depletion during therapy with diuretics and/or digitalis, aminoglycosides, amphotericin B, cyclosporin, chemotherapy, and during pregnancy, PMS, menopause, diabetes, hyperoxaluria, malnutrition, weight/strength training, restricted diet, or alcoholism.

Warnings: Do not use this product except under the advice and supervision of a physician if you have a kidney disease. May have laxative effect.

Dosage: Adult dose 3–4 capsules daily with meals or as directed by a physician.

Professional Labeling: Serum magnesium levels do not accurately represent total body, tissue, or bone magnesium levels.

How Supplied: Bottles of 100 and 1000.

EDUCATIONAL MATERIAL

Cardiovascular system charts, female reproductive system charts, samples, and literature available to physicians upon request.

Blairex Laboratories, Inc.
4810 TECUMSEH LANE
P.O BOX 15190
EVANSVILLE, IN 47716-0190

BRONCHO SALINE®
0.9% Sodium Chloride Aerosol
for the dilution of bronchodilator
inhalation solutions. Sterile
normal saline for diluting
bronchodilator solutions
for oral inhalation.

Description: Broncho Saline® is for patients using bronchodilator solutions for oral inhalation that require dilution with sterile normal saline solution. Broncho Saline is a sterile liquid solution consisting of 0.9% sodium chloride for oral inhalation with a pH of 4.5 to 7.5. Not to be used for injection.

How Supplied: Broncho Saline® comes in 90cc (mL) and 240cc (mL) Pressurized Containers.
Store between 15–25°C (59–77°F). Keep out of reach of children. See WARNINGS.

NASAL MOIST®
Sodium Chloride 0.65%

Description: Isotonic saline solution buffered with sodium bicarbonate. Preserved with Benzyl alcohol.

Actions and Uses: Use for dry nasal membranes caused by chronic sinusitis, allergy, asthma, dry air, oxygen therapy. May be used as often as needed.

Directions: Squeeze twice into each nostril as needed.

How Supplied: 45 mL (1.5 oz.) plastic squeeze bottle.

UNKNOWN DRUG?
Consult the
Product Identification Guide
(Gray Pages)
for full-color photos of
leading over-the-counter
medications

Block Drug Company, Inc.
257 CORNELISON AVENUE
JERSEY CITY, NJ 07302

BALMEX® OINTMENT
for diaper rash

Description: Balmex® contains Zinc Oxide (11.3%) in a unique formulation including Peruvian Balsam suitable for topical application for the treatment and prevention of diaper rash.

Indications and Uses: Balmex helps treat and prevent diaper rash in four ways: 1. Soothes irritation. 2. Provides protection. 3. Promotes healing. 4. Reduces inflammation.
The zinc oxide based formulation provides a protective barrier on the skin against the natural causes of irritation. Balmex spreads on smooth and wipes off the baby easily, without causing irritation to the affected area. Balmex tactile properties promote compliance amongst mothers, and clinical studies have demonstrated that Balmex is effective in treating diaper rash.

Directions: At the first sign of diaper rash or redness apply Balmex three or more times daily as needed. To help prevent diaper rash, apply Balmex liberally as often as necessary, with each diaper change, especially at bedtime or anytime when exposure to wet diapers may be prolonged.

Warnings: Avoid contact with the eyes. For external use only. If condition worsens or does not improve within 7 days, contact a physician. Keep out of reach of children.

Active Ingredient: Zinc Oxide.

Inactive Ingredients: Balsam (Specially Purified Balsam Peru), Beeswax, Benzoic Acid, Bismuth Subnitrate, Mineral Oil, Purified Water, Silicone, Synthetic White Wax, and other ingredients.

How Supplied: 2 oz. (57 g.) and 4 oz. (113 g.) tubes and 16 oz. (454 g.) jars.

BC® POWDER
ARTHRITIS STRENGTH BC® POWDER
BC® COLD POWDER

Description: BC® POWDER: Active Ingredients: Each powder contains Aspirin 650 mg, Salicylamide 195 mg and Caffeine 32 mg. ARTHRITIS STRENGTH BC® POWDER: Active Ingredients: Each powder contains Aspirin 742 mg, Salicylamide 222 mg and Caffeine 36 mg. BC® COLD POWDER MULTI-SYMPTOM FORMULA (COLD-SINUS ALLERGY)
BC® COLD POWDER NON-DROWSY FORMULA (COLD-SINUS)
BC Cold Powder Multi-Symptom Formula (Cold-Sinus-Allergy) Active Ingredients: Aspirin 650 mg, Phenylpropanolamine Hydrochloride 25 mg, and Chlor-

pheniramine Maleate 4 mg per powder. BC Cold Powder Non-Drowsy Formula (Cold-Sinus) Active Ingredients: Aspirin 650 mg and Phenylpropanolamine Hydrochloride 25 mg per powder.

Indications: BC Powder is for relief of simple headache; for temporary relief of minor arthritic pain, neuralgia, neuritis and sciatica; for relief of muscular aches, discomfort and fever of colds; and for relief of normal menstrual pain and pain of tooth extraction.
Arthritis Strength BC Powder is specially formulated to fight occasional minor pain and inflammation of arthritis. Like original formula BC, Arthritis Strength BC provides fast temporary relief of minor arthritis pain and inflammation, neuralgia, neuritis and sciatica; relief of muscular aches, discomfort and fever of colds; and pain of tooth extraction.
BC Cold Powder Multi-Symptom (Cold-Sinus-Allergy) is for relief of cold symptoms such as body aches, fever, nasal congestion, sneezing, running nose, and watery itchy eyes. BC Cold Powder Non-Drowsy Formula (Cold-Sinus) is for relief of such symptoms as body aches, fever, and nasal congestions.

BC® Powder, Arthritis Strength BC® Powder:

Warnings: BC Powder and Arthritis Strength BC® Powder: Children and teenagers should not use this medicine for chicken pox or flu symptoms before a doctor is consulted about Reye Syndrome, a rare but serious illness reported to be associated with aspirin. Do not take this product if you are allergic to aspirin. If pain persists for more than 10 days or redness is present, discontinue use of this product and consult a physician immediately. Keep this and all medication out of children's reach. As with any drug, if you are pregnant or nursing a baby, consult your physician before using this product. IT IS ESPECIALLY IMPORTANT NOT TO USE ASPIRIN DURING THE LAST 3 MONTHS OF PREGNANCY UNLESS SPECIFICALLY DIRECTED TO DO SO BY A DOCTOR BECAUSE IT MAY CAUSE PROBLEMS IN THE UNBORN CHILD OR COMPLICATIONS DURING DELIVERY.

BC Cold Powder Line:

Warnings: Children and teenagers should not use BC for chicken pox or flu symptoms before a doctor is consulted about Reye Syndrome, a rare but serious illness reported to be associated with aspirin. Keep BC and all medicines out of children's reach. In case of accidental overdose, contact a physician immediately.
As with any drug, if you are pregnant or nursing a baby seek the advice of a health professional before using BC.
IT IS ESPECIALLY IMPORTANT NOT TO USE ASPIRIN DURING THE LAST 3 MONTHS OF PREGNANCY UNLESS SPECIFICALLY DIRECTED

Continued on next page

Block Drug—Cont.

TO DO SO BY A DOCTOR BECAUSE IT MAY CAUSE PROBLEMS IN THE UNBORN CHILD OR COMPLICATIONS DURING DELIVERY.
Nervousness, dizziness or sleeplessness may occur if recommended dosage is exceeded. If symptoms do not improve within 7 days, or are accompanied by fever that lasts more than 3 days, or if new symptoms occur, consult a physician before continuing use. Do not take BC if you are sensitive to aspirin, or have heart disease, high blood pressure, thyroid disease, diabetes, asthma, glaucoma, emphysema, chronic pulmonary disease, shortness of breath, difficulty in breathing or difficulty in urination due to enlargement of the prostate gland, or if you are presently taking a prescription antihypertensive or antidepressant drug containing a monoamine oxidase inhibitor unless directed by a doctor. BC Cold Powder Multi-Symptom with antihistamine may cause drowsiness. Avoid alcoholic beverages while taking this product. Use caution when driving a motor vehicle or operating machinery.

Overdosage: In case of accidental overdosage, contact a physician or poison control center immediately.

Dosage and Administration: BC® Powder, Arthritis Strength BC® Powder, BC® Cold Powder Line:
Place one powder on tongue and follow with liquid. If you prefer, stir powder into glass of water or other liquid. May be used every three to four hours, up to 4 powders each 24 hours. For children under 12, consult a physician.

How Supplied: BC Powder: Available in tamper resistant overwrapped envelopes of 2 or 6 powders, as well as tamper resistant boxes of 24 and 50 powders.
Arthritis Strength BC Powder: Available in tamper resistant over wrapped envelopes of 6 powders, and tamper resistant overwrapped boxes of 24 and 50 powders.
BC Cold Powder Line:
Available in tamper-resistant overwrapped envelopes of 6 powders, as well as tamper-resistant boxes of 24 powders.

Maximum Strength NYTOL® Caplets

Active Ingredient: Doxylamine succinate, 25 mg per caplet.

Indications: Helps to reduce difficulty in falling asleep.

Warnings: DO NOT TAKE THIS PRODUCT IF YOU HAVE ASTHMA, GLAUCOMA, OR ENLARGEMENT OF THE PROSTATE GLAND EXCEPT UNDER THE ADVICE AND SUPERVISION OF A PHYSICIAN. If sleeplessness persists continuously for more than two weeks, consult your physician. Insomnia may be a symptom of serious underlying medical illness. Do not take this product if presently taking any other drug, without consulting your physician or pharmacist. Take this product with caution if alcohol is being consumed. As with any drug, if you are pregnant or nursing a baby, seek the advice of a health professional before using this product. For adults only. Do not give to children under 12 years of age.
Keep this and all drugs out of the reach of children. In case of accidental overdose, seek professional assistance or contact a Poison Control Center immediately.

Caution: This product contains an antihistamine and will cause drowsiness. It should be used only at bedtime.

Dosage and Administration: Adults and children 12 years of age and over, take 1 Maximum Strength NYTOL caplet 30 minutes before going to bed. Take once daily or as directed by a physician.

How Supplied: Available in packages of 8 and 16 caplets.

NYTOL® QUICKCAPS™ CAPLETS

Active Ingredient: Diphenhydramine Hydrochloride, 25 mg per caplet.

Indications: For relief of occasional sleeplessness. Diphenhydramine Hydrochloride is an antihistamine with anticholinergic and sedative effects which induces drowsiness and helps in falling asleep.

Warnings: Do not give children under 12 years of age. If sleeplessness persists continuously for more than 2 weeks, consult your doctor. Insomnia may be a symptom of serious underlying medical illness. Do not take this product, unless directed by a doctor, if you have a breathing problem such as emphysema or chronic bronchitis, or if you have glaucoma or difficulty in urination due to enlargement of the prostate gland. Avoid alcoholic beverages while taking this product. Do not take this product if you are taking tranquilizers or sedatives, without first consulting your doctor. In case of accidental overdose seek professional assistance or contact a poison control center immediately. As with any drug, if your are pregnant or nursing a baby, seek the advice of a health professional before using this product. Keep this and all drugs out of the reach of children.

Drug Interaction: Alcohol and other drugs which cause CNS depression will heighten the depressant effect of this product. Monoamine oxidase (MAO) inhibitors will prolong and intensify the anticholinergic effects of antihistamines.

Symptoms and Treatment of Oral Overdosage: In adults overdose may cause CNS depression resulting in hypnosis and coma. In children CNS hyperexcitability may follow sedation; the stimulant phase may bring tremor, delirium and convulsions. Gastrointestinal reactions may include dry mouth, appetite loss, nausea and vomiting. Respiratory distress and cardiovascular complications (hypotension) may be evident. Treatment includes inducing emesis, and controlling symptoms.

Dosage and Administration: Adults and children 12 years of age and over, take 2 NYTOL with DPH at bedtime if needed, or as directed by a physician.

How Supplied: Available in tamper resistant packages of 16, 32, and 72 caplets NYTOL with DPH.

PROMISE® SENSITIVE TOOTHPASTE
For Sensitive Teeth and Cavity Prevention

Active Ingredients: Potassium Nitrate and Sodium Monofluorophosphate in a pleasantly mint-flavored dentifrice.

Promise contains Potassium Nitrate for relief of dentinal hypersensitivity resulting from the exposure of tooth dentin due to periodontal surgery, cervical (gumline) erosion, abrasion or recession which causes pain on contact with hot, cold, or tactile stimuli. Promise also contains Sodium Monofluorophosphate for cavity prevention.

Indications: Promise builds increasing protection against painful sensitivity of the teeth to cold, heat, acids, sweets or contact and aids in the prevention of dental cavities.

Actions: Promise significantly reduces tooth hypersensitivity, with response to therapy evident after two weeks of use. Controlled double-blind clinical studies provide substantial evidence of the safety and effectiveness of Promise. The current theory on mechanism of action is that the potassium nitrate in Promise has an effect on neural transmission, interrupting the signal which would result in the sensation of pain. Sodium Monofluorophosphate protects the tooth surfaces to prevent cavities.

Warning: Sensitive teeth may indicate a serious problem that may need prompt care by a dentist. See your dentist if the problem persists or worsens. Do not use this product longer than 4 weeks unless recommended by a dentist or physician. **Keep this and all drugs out of the reach of children.**

Directions: Adults and children 12 years of age and older:
Apply at least a 1-inch strip of the product onto a soft bristle toothbrush. Brush teeth thoroughly for at least 1 minute twice a day (morning and evening) or as recommended by a dentist or doctor. Make sure to brush all sensitive areas of the teeth. Children under 12 years of age: Consult a dentist or physician.

How Supplied: Promise Sensitive is supplied in 1.6 oz. (46 g), 3.0 oz. (85 g) and 4.5 oz. (128 g) tubes.

ORIGINAL FORMULA SENSODYNE® –SC
Toothpaste for Sensitive Teeth

Description: Each tube contains strontium chloride hexahydrate (10%) in a pleasantly flavored cleansing/polishing desensitizing dentifrice.

Actions/Indications: Tooth hypersensitivity is a condition in which individuals experience pain from exposure to hot, cold stimuli, from chewing fibrous foods, or from tactile stimuli (e.g. toothbrushing.) Hypersensitivity may also be caused by a reaction to sweet or acidic foods (OSMOTIC) stimuli. · Hypersensitivity usually occurs when the protective enamel covering on teeth wears away (which happens most often at the gum line) or if gum tissue recedes and exposes the dentin underneath.
Running through the dentin are microscopic small "tubules" which, according to many authorities, carry the pain impulses to the nerve of the tooth.
Sensodyne–SC provides a unique ingredient—strontium chloride—which is believed to be deposited in the tubules where it blocks the pain. The longer Sensodyne–SC is used, the more of a barrier it helps build against pain.
The effect of Sensodyne–SC may not be manifested immediately and may require a few weeks or longer of use for relief to be obtained. A number of clinical studies in the U.S. and other countries have provided substantial evidence of the performance attributes of Sensodyne–SC. Complete relief of hypersensitivity has been reported in approximately 65% of users and measurable relief or reduction in hypersensitivity in approximately 90%. The Original Formula has been commercially available for over 30 years. The ADA Council on Dental Therapeutics has given Sensodyne–SC the Seal of Acceptance as an effective desensitizing dentifrice in otherwise normal teeth.

Contraindications: Subjects with severe dental erosion should brush properly and lightly with any dentifrice to avoid further removal of tooth structure.

Dosage and Administration: Adults and children 12 years of age and older: Apply at least a 1-inch strip of the product onto a soft bristle toothbrush. Brush teeth thoroughly for at least 1 minute twice a day (morning and evening) or as recommended by a dentist or physician. Make sure to brush all sensitive areas of the teeth. Children under 12 years of age: consult a dentist or physician.

Warnings: Sensitive teeth may indicate a serious problem that may need prompt care by a dentist. See your dentist if the problem persists or worsens. Do not use this product longer than 4 weeks unless recommended by a dentist or doctor.
Keep this and all drugs out of the reach of children.

How Supplied: SENSODYNE–SC Toothpaste is supplied in 2.1 oz. (60 g), 4.0 oz. (113 g), and 6.0 oz. (170 g).

FRESH MINT SENSODYNE® COOL GEL SENSODYNE® SENSODYNE® WITH BAKING SODA
Toothpaste for Sensitive Teeth and Cavity Prevention
Desensitizing Dentrifice

Active Ingredients: 5% Potassium Nitrate and Sodium Monofluorophosphate (Fresh Mint) or Sodium Fluoride (Cool Gel and Baking Soda) in a pleasantly mint-flavored dentifrice.
Fresh Mint Sensodyne, Cool Gel Sensodyne and Sensodyne with Baking Soda contain Potassium Nitrate for relief of dentinal hypersensitivity resulting from the exposure of tooth dentin due to periodontal surgery, cervical (gum line) erosion, abrasion or recession which causes pain on contact with hot, cold, or tactile stimuli and fluoride for cavity prevention. Fresh Mint Sensodyne has been given the Seal of Acceptance by the ADA Council on Dental Therapeutics as an effective desensitizing dentifrice for otherwise normal teeth.

Actions: Fresh Mint Sensodyne, Cool Gel Sensodyne and Sensodyne with Baking Soda significantly reduce tooth hypersensitivity, with response to therapy evident after two weeks of use. Controlled double-blind clinical studies provide substantial evidence of the safety and effectiveness of potassium nitrate. The current theory on mechanism of action is that potassium nitrate has an effect on neural transmission, interrupting the signal which would result in the sensation of pain. Fluorides are anticariogenic, forming fluoroapatite in the outer surface of the dental enamel which is resistant to acids and caries.

Warnings: Sensitive teeth may indicate a serious problem that may need prompt care by a dentist. See your dentist if the problem persists or worsens. Do not use this product longer than 4 weeks unless recommended by a dentist or physician. Keep this and all drugs out of the reach of children.

Dosage and Administration: Adults and children 12 years of age and older: Apply at least a 1-inch strip of the product onto a soft bristle toothbrush. Brush teeth thoroughly for at least 1 minute twice a day (morning and evening) or as recommended by a dentist or doctor. Make sure to brush all sensitive areas of the teeth. Children under 12 years of age: consult a dentist or physician.

How Supplied: Fresh Mint Sensodyne is supplied in 2.1 (60 g), 4.0 (113 g) and 6.0 oz. (170 g) tubes and in 4.0 oz. pumps. Cool Gel and Sensodyne with Baking Soda are available in 2.1 (60 g), 4.0 (113 g) and 6.0 oz. (170 g) tubes.

TEGRIN® DANDRUFF SHAMPOO TEGRIN® FOR PSORIASIS SKIN CREAM AND MEDICATED SOAP

Description: Tegrin® Dandruff Shampoo contains 7% coal tar solution equivalent to 1.1% coal tar, in a pleasantly scented, high-foaming, cleansing shampoo base with emollients, conditioners and other formula components.
Tegrin® for Psoriasis Skin Cream and Medicated Soap each contain 5% coal tar solution, equivalent to 0.8% coal tar. The Cream also contains alcohol (4.9% and 4.7%, respectively).

Actions/Indications: Coal Tar is obtained in the destructive distillation of bituminous coal and is a highly effective agent for controlling the flaking and itching of the scalp associated with dandruff, seborrheic dermatitis and psoriasis. The action of coal tar is believed to be keratolytic, antiseptic, antipruritic and astringent. The coal tar solution used in Tegrin Dandruff Shampoo is prepared in such a way as to reduce the pitch and other irritant components found in crude coal tar without reduction in therapeutic potency.
Coal tar solution has been used clincially for many years as a remedy for dandruff and for scaling associated with scalp disorders such as seborrhea and psoriasis. Its mechanism of action has not been fully established, but it is believed to retard the rate of turnover of epidermal cells with regular use. A number of clinical studies have demonstrated the performance attributes of Tegrin Dandruff Shampoo against dandruff and seborrheic dermatitis. In addition to relieving the above symptoms, Tegrin shampoo, used regularly, maintains scalp and hair cleanliness and leaves the hair lustrous and manageable.

Warnings: *All Tegrin® products:* For external use only. Avoid contact with eyes. If contact occurs, rinse eyes thoroughly with water. If condition worsens or does not improve after regular use of this product as directed, consult a doctor. Use caution in exposing skin to sunlight after applying this product. It may increase tendency to sunburn for up to 24 hours after application. Do not use for prolonged periods without consulting a doctor. Do not use this product with other forms of psoriasis therapy, such as ultraviolet radiation or prescription drugs, unless directed by a doctor. Keep out of reach of children. In case of accidental ingestion, seek professional assistance or contact a Poison Control Center immediately.
Tegrin® for Psoriasis Skin Cream and Medicated Soap: If the condition covers a large area of the body, consult a doctor before using this product. (See other Warnings above).

Directions: Shake Tegrin Dandruff Shampoo well. Wet hair thoroughly. Rub Tegrin liberally into hair and scalp.

Continued on next page

Block Drug—Cont.

Rinse thoroughly. Briskly massage a second application of the shampoo into a rich lather. Rinse thoroughly. For best results use at least twice a week or as directed by a doctor.

Apply Tegrin for Psoriasis cream to affected areas one to four times daily or as directed by a doctor. Use Tegrin Soap on affected areas in place of your regular soap.

How Supplied: Tegrin Dandruff Shampoo is supplied in 7 fl. oz. (207 ml) plastic bottles.

Tegrin Cream 2 oz. (57 g) and 4.4 oz. (124 g) tubes, Tegrin Soap 4.5 oz. (127 g) bars.

Bock Pharmacal Company
P.O. BOX 419056
ST. LOUIS, MO 63141-9056

EMETROL®
(Phosphorated Carbohydrate Solution)
For the relief of nausea associated with upset stomach

Description: EMETROL is an oral solution containing balanced amounts of dextrose (glucose) and levulose (fructose) and phosphoric acid with controlled hydrogen ion concentration. Available in original lemon-mint or cherry flavor.

Ingredients: Each 5 mL teaspoonful contains dextrose (glucose), 1.87 g; levulose (fructose), 1.87 g; phosphoric acid, 21.5 mg; and the following inactive ingredients: glycerin, methylparaben, purified water; D&C yellow No. 10 and natural lemon-mint flavor in lemon-mint Emetrol; FD&C red No. 40 and artificial cherry flavor in cherry Emetrol.

Action: EMETROL quickly relieves nausea by local action on the wall of the hyperactive G.I. tract. There is no delay in therapeutic action such as that associated with systemic drugs.

Indications: For the relief of nausea due to upset stomach from intestinal flu, stomach flu, and food or drink indiscretions. For other conditions, take only as directed by your physician.

Advantages:
1. **Fast Action**—works quickly through local action relaxing hyperactive muscles of the G.I. tract.
2. **Effectiveness**—clinically proven to stop nausea.
3. **Safety**—all natural active ingredients won't mask symptoms of organic pathology. No salicylates makes Emetrol safe for children and teens with flu or fever. No known drug interactions.
4. **Convenience**—no ℞ required.
5. **Patient Acceptance**—pleasant tasting lemon-mint or cherry flavor.

Usual Adult Dose: One or two tablespoons. Repeat every 15 minutes until distress subsides.

Usual Children's Dose: One or two teaspoons. Repeat dose every 15 minutes until distress subsides.

Important: For maximum effectiveness never dilute EMETROL or drink fluids of any kind immediately before or after taking a dose.

Caution: Not to be taken for more than one hour (5 doses) without consulting a physician. If upset stomach continues or recurs frequently, consult a physician promptly as it may be a sign of a serious condition.

WARNING: KEEP THIS AND ALL MEDICATIONS OUT OF THE REACH OF CHILDREN. As with any drug, if you are pregnant or nursing a baby, seek the advice of a health professional before using this product.

This product contains fructose and should not be taken by persons with hereditary fructose intolerance (HFI).

> **This product contains sugar and should not be taken by diabetics except under the advice and supervision of a physician.**

In case of accidental overdose, contact a poison control center, emergency medical facility, or physician immediately for advice.

How Supplied: Each 5 mL teaspoonful of EMETROL contains dextrose (glucose), 1.87 g; levulose (fructose), 1.87 g; and phosphoric acid, 21.5 mg in a yellow, lemon-mint or red, cherry-flavored syrup.

Yellow, Lemon-Mint
NDC 0563-2113-04—Bottle of 4 fluid ounces (118 mL)
NDC 0563-2113-08—Bottle of 8 fluid ounces (236 mL)
NDC 0563-2113-16—Bottle of 1 pint (473 mL)

Red, Cherry
NDC 0563-2114-04—Bottle of 4 fluid ounces (118 mL)
NDC 0563-2114-08—Bottle of 8 fluid ounces (236 mL)
NDC 0563-2114-16—Bottle of 1 pint (473 mL)

Store at room temperature.

NOTICE: Each bottle is protected by a printed band around the cap. Do not use if band is damaged or missing.

Shown in Product Identification Guide, page 504

> **IF YOU SUSPECT AN INTERACTION...**
> The 1,400-page
> *PDR Guide to Drug Interactions* •
> *Side Effects* • *Indications*
> can help.
> Use the order form
> in the front of this book.

Boiron, The World Leader In Homeopathy
6 CAMPUS BLVD.
BUILDING A
NEWTOWN SQUARE, PA 19073

OSCILLOCOCCINUM®
[ah-sill 'o-cox-see 'num ']

Active Ingredient: Anas Barbariae Hepatis et Cordis Extractum HPUS 200C

Indications: For the relief of flu-like symptoms such as fever, chills, body aches and pains.

Actions: Like most Homeopathic medicine, Oscillococcinum® acts gently by stimulating the patient's natural defense mechanisms.

Warnings: If symptoms persist for more than three days or worsen, consult your physician. Keep all medication out of reach of children. As with any drug if you are pregnant or nursing a baby, seek professional advice before using this product.

Dosage and Administration: (Adults and Children over 2 years)
At the onset of symptoms, place the entire contents of one tube in your mouth and allow to dissolve under your tongue. Repeat every 6 hours as necessary. For maximum results, Oscillococcinum® should be taken early, at the onset of symptoms, and at least 15 minutes before or 1 hour after meals.

How Supplied: boxes of 3 unit doses or 6 unit doses of 0.04 oz. (1 gram) each (NDC #0220-9280-32 and NDC #0220-9288-33) Tamper-resistant package.
Manufactured by Boiron, France.
Distributor: Boiron, Newtown Square, PA

Shown in Product Identification Guide, page 504

> **EDUCATIONAL MATERIAL**

Boiron Product Catalogue
General description of the most popular Boiron products.
***Oscillococcinum* ® Brochure**
Brochure on Oscillococcinum® describing clinical research on the product and its general use.
"What Is Homeopathy?"
Booklet free to physicians and pharmacists.
"An Introduction to Homeopathy for the Practicing Pharmacist"
A free continuing education booklet for pharmacists.

Bristol-Myers Products
(A Bristol-Myers Squibb Company)
345 PARK AVENUE
NEW YORK, NY 10154

ALPHA KERI®
Moisture Rich Body Oil

Composition: Contains mineral oil, Hydroloc™ brand of Westwood's PEG-4 dilaurate, lanolin oil, fragrance, benzophenone-3, D&C green 6.

Indications: ALPHA KERI is a water-dispersible oil for the care of dry skin. ALPHA KERI effectively deposits a thin, uniform, emulsified film of oil over the skin. This film lubricates and softens the skin. ALPHA KERI Moisture Rich Body Oil is an all-over skin moisturizer. Only Alpha Keri contains Hydroloc™—the unique emulsifier that provides a more uniform distribution of the therapeutic oils to moisturize dry skin. ALPHA KERI is valuable as an aid for dry skin and mild skin irritations.

Directions for Use: ALPHA KERI *should always be used with water, either added to water or rubbed on to wet skin.* Because of its inherent cleansing properties it is not necessary to use soap when ALPHA KERI is being used.
For external use only.
Label directions should be followed for use in shower, bath and cleansing.

Precaution: The patient should be warned to guard against slipping in tub or shower.

How Supplied: 4 fl. oz., 8 fl. oz., 12 fl. oz., and 16 fl. oz., plastic bottles. Also available in non-aerosol pump spray, 3.5 oz.

BACKACHE CAPLETS

Composition: Each caplet contains Magnesium Salicylate Tetrahydrate 580 mg (equivalent to 467 mg of anhydrous Magnesium Salicylate)
Other Ingredients: Carnauba Wax, Hydrogenated Vegetable Oil, Hydroxypropyl Methylcellulose, Magnesium Stearate, Microcrystalline Cellulose, Polyethylene Glycol, Polysorbate 80, Titanium Dioxide

Indications: For the temporary relief of minor aches and pains associated with backache and muscular aches (e.g., sprains and strains).

Directions: Adults: 2 caplets with water every 6 hours while symptoms persist, not to exceed 8 caplets in 24 hours or as directed by a doctor. Children under 12: Consult a doctor.

Warnings: Children and teenagers should not use this medicine for chicken pox or flu symptoms before a doctor is consulted about Reye syndrome, a rate but serious illness. **KEEP THIS AND ALL OTHER MEDICATIONS OUT OF THE REACH OF CHILDREN. IN CASE OF ACCIDENTAL OVERDOSE, SEEK PROFESSIONAL ASSISTANCE OR CONTACT A POISON CONTROL CENTER IMMEDIATELY.** As with any drug, if you are pregnant or nursing a baby, seek the advice of a health professional before using this product. Do not take this product for more than 10 days unless directed by a doctor. If pain persists or gets worse, if new symptoms occur, or if redness or swelling is present, consult a doctor because these could be signs of a serious condition. Do not take this product if you are allergic to salicylates (including aspirin), have asthma, have stomach problems (such as heartburn, upset stomach or stomach pain) that persists or recur, or if you have ulcers or bleeding problems, unless directed by a doctor. If ringing in the ears or loss of hearing occurs, consult a doctor before taking any more of this product.

Drug Interaction Precaution: Do not take this product if you are taking a prescription drug for anticoagulation (thinning of blood), diabetes, gout or arthritis unless directed by a doctor.

How Supplied: BACKACHE is a white caplet with the logo "N-BACK" debossed on one side.
NDC 19810–0579–1   Blister cards of 24's
NDC 19810–0579–2   Bottles of 50's
The bottles of 50's are packaged in child resistant closures; the blister cards of 24's are recommended for households without young children and are packaged without a child resistant closure. Store at room temperature.

BUFFERIN®
[bŭf′fĕr-ĭn]
Analgesic

Composition:
Active Ingredient: Each coated tablet or caplet contains Aspirin 325 mg in a formulation buffered with Calcium Carbonate, Magnesium Oxide and Magnesium Carbonate.
Other Ingredients: Benzoic Acid, Citric Acid, Corn Starch, FD&C Blue No. 1, Hydroxypropyl Methylcellulose, Magnesium Stearate, Mineral Oil, Polysorbate 20, Povidone, Propylene Glycol, Simethicone Emulsion, Sodium Phosphate, Sorbitan Monolaurate, Titanium Dioxide. May also contain: Carnauba Wax, Zinc Stearate.

Indications: For fast temporary relief of headaches, minor arthritis pain and inflammation, muscle aches, pain and fever of colds, menstrual pain and toothaches.

Directions: Adults: 2 tablets or caplets with water every 4 hours as needed, not to exceed 12 tablets or caplets a day. Children under 12: Consult a doctor.

Warnings: Children and teenagers should not use this medicine for chicken pox or flu symptoms before a doctor is consulted about Reye syndrome, a rare but serious illness reported to be associated with aspirin. KEEP THIS AND ALL OTHER MEDICATIONS OUT OF THE REACH OF CHILDREN. IN CASE OF ACCIDENTAL OVERDOSE, SEEK PROFESSIONAL ASSISTANCE OR CONTACT A POISON CONTROL CENTER IMMEDIATELY. As with any drug, if you are pregnant or nursing a baby, seek the advice of a health professional before using this product. **IT IS ESPECIALLY IMPORTANT NOT TO USE ASPIRIN DURING THE LAST 3 MONTHS OF PREGNANCY UNLESS SPECIFICALLY DIRECTED TO DO SO BY A DOCTOR BECAUSE IT MAY CAUSE PROBLEMS IN THE UNBORN CHILD OR COMPLICATIONS DURING DELIVERY.** Do not take this product for pain for more than 10 days or for fever for more than 3 days unless directed by a doctor. If pain or fever persists or gets worse, if new symptoms occur, or if redness or swelling is present, consult a doctor because these could be signs of a serious condition. Do not take this product if you are allergic to aspirin, have asthma, have stomach problems (such as heartburn, upset stomach or stomach pain) that persist or recur, or if you have ulcers or bleeding problems, unless directed by a doctor. If ringing in the ears or loss of hearing occurs, consult a doctor before taking or giving any more of this product.

Drug Interaction Precaution: Do not take this product if you are taking a prescription drug for anticoagulation (thinning of blood), diabetes, gout or arthritis unless directed by a doctor.

How Supplied: BUFFERIN is supplied as:
Coated circular white tablet with letter "B" debossed on one surface.
NDC 19810-0093-3 Bottle of 30's
NDC 19810-0093-4 Bottle of 50's
NDC 19810-0073-5 Bottle of 100's
NDC 19810-0073-6 Bottle of 200's
NDC 19810-0073-0 Vials of 10
Coated scored white caplet with letter "B" debossed on each side of scoring.
NDC 19810-0072-7 Bottle of 30's
NDC 19810-0072-8 Bottle of 50's
NDC 19810-0072-3 Bottle of 100's
All consumer sizes have child resistant closures except 100's for tablets and 50's for caplets which are sizes recommended for households without young children. Store at room temperature.
Also described in *PDR* for prescription drugs.

Professional Labeling

1. BUFFERIN® FOR RECURRENT TRANSIENT ISCHEMIC ATTACKS

Indication: For reducing the risk of recurrent transient ischemic attacks (TIA's) or stroke in men who have had transient ischemia of the brain due to fibrin platelet emboli. There is inadequate evidence that aspirin or buffered aspirin is effective in reducing TIA's in women at the recommended dosage. There is no evidence that aspirin or buff-

Continued on next page

Bristol-Myers—Cont.

ered aspirin is of benefit in the treatment of completed strokes in men or women.

Clinical Trials: The indication is supported by the results of a Canadian study (1) in which 585 patients with threatened stroke were followed in a randomized clinical trial for an average of 26 months to determine whether aspirin or sulfinpyrazone, singly or in combination, was superior to placebo in preventing transient ischemic attacks, stroke, or death. The study showed that, although sulfinpyrazone had no statistically significant effect, aspirin reduced the risk of continuing transient ischemic attacks, stroke, or death by 19 percent and reduced the risk of stroke or death by 31 percent. Another aspirin study carried out in the United States with 178 patients, showed a statistically significant number of "favorable outcomes," including reduced transient ischemic attacks, stroke, and death (2).

Precautions: Patients presenting with signs and symptoms of TIA's should have a complete medical and neurologic evaluation. Consideration should be given to other disorders that resemble TIA's. Attention should be given to risk factors: it is important to evaluate and treat, if appropriate, other diseases associated with TIA's and stroke, such as hypertension and diabetes.

Concurrent administration of absorbable antacids at therapeutic doses may increase the clearance of salicylates in some individuals. The concurrent administration of nonabsorbable antacids may alter the rate of absorption of aspirin, thereby resulting in a decreased acetylsalicylic acid/salicylate ratio in plasma. The clinical significance of these decreases in available aspirin is unknown. Aspirin at dosages of 1,000 milligrams per day has been associated with small increases in blood pressure, blood urea nitrogen, and serum uric acid levels. It is recommended that patients placed on long-term aspirin treatment be seen at regular intervals to assess changes in these measurements.

Adverse Reactions: At dosages of 1,000 milligrams or higher of aspirin per day, gastrointestinal side effects include stomach pain, heartburn, nausea and/or vomiting, as well as increased rates of gross gastrointestinal bleeding.

Dosage and Administration: Adult oral dosage for men is 1,300 milligrams a day, in divided doses of 650 milligrams twice a day or 325 milligrams four times a day.

References:
(1) The Canadian Cooperative Study Group. "A Randomized Trial of Aspirin and Sulfinpyrazone in Threatened Stroke," *New England Journal of Medicine,* 299:53–59, 1978.
(2) Fields, W.S., et al., "Controlled Trial of Aspirin in Cerebral Ischemia," *Stroke* 8:301–316, 1977.

2. BUFFERIN® FOR MYOCARDIAL INFARCTION

Indication: Aspirin is indicated to reduce the risk of death and/or nonfatal myocardial infarction in patients with a previous infarction or unstable angina pectoris.

Clinical Trials: The indication is supported by the results of six, large, randomized multicenter, placebo-controlled studies[1–7] involving 10,816, predominantly male, post-myocardial infarction (MI) patients and one randomized placebo-controlled study of 1,266 men with unstable angina. Therapy with aspirin was begun at intervals after the onset of acute MI varying from less than 3 days to more than 5 years and continued for periods of from less than one year to four years. In the unstable angina study, treatment was started within 1 month after the onset of unstable angina and continued for 12 weeks and complicating conditions such as congestive heart failure were not included in the study.

Aspirin therapy in MI patients was associated with about a 20 percent reduction in the risk of subsequent death and/or nonfatal reinfarction, a median absolute decrease of 3 percent from the 12 to 22 percent event rates in the placebo groups. In the aspirin-treated unstable angina patients the reduction in risk was about 50 percent, a reduction in the event rate of 5% from the 10% rate in the placebo group over the 12 weeks of the study.

Daily dosage of aspirin in the post-myocardial infarction studies was 300 mg. in one study and 900 and 1500 mg. in five studies. A dose of 325 mg. was used in the study of unstable angina.

Adverse Reactions: Gastrointestinal Reactions: Doses of 1000 mg. per day of aspirin caused gastrointestinal symptoms and bleeding that in some cases were clinically significant. In the largest post-infarction study (The Aspirin Myocardial Infarction Study (AMIS) with 4,500 people), the percentage incidences of gastrointestinal symptoms for the aspirin (1000 mg. of a standard, solid-tablet formulation) and placebo-treated subjects, respectively, were: stomach pain (14.5%; 4.4%); heartburn (11.9%; 4.8%); nausea and/or vomiting (7.6%; 2.1%); hospitalization for gastrointestinal disorder (4.8%; 3.5%). In the AMIS and other trials, aspirin treated patients had increased rates of gross gastrointestinal bleeding. Symptoms and signs of gastrointestinal irritation were not significantly increased in subjects treated for unstable angina with buffered aspirin in solution.

Cardiovascular and Biochemical:
In the AMIS trial, the dosage of 1000 mg. per day of aspirin was associated with small increases in systolic blood pressure (BP) (average 1.5 to 2.1 mm) and diastolic BP (0.5 to 0.6 mm), depending upon whether maximal or last available readings were used. Blood urea nitrogen and uric acid levels were also increased, but by less than 1.0 mg%.

Subjects with marked hypertension or renal insufficiency had been excluded from the trial so that the clinical importance of these observations for such subjects or for any subjects treated over more prolonged periods is not known. It is recommended that patients placed on long-term aspirin treatment, even at doses of 300 mg. per day, be seen at regular intervals to assess changes in these measurements.

Administration and Dosage: Although most of the studies used dosages exceeding 300 mg., two trials used only 300 mg. and pharmacologic data indicate that this dose inhibits platelet function fully. Therefore, 300 mg. or a conventional 325 mg. aspirin dose is a reasonable, routine dose that would minimize gastrointestinal adverse reactions.

References: 1. Elwood P.C., et al., "A Randomized Controlled Trial of Acetylsalicylic Acid in the Secondary Prevention of Mortality from Myocardial Infarction," *British Medical Journal,* 1:436–440, 1974. 2. The Coronary Drug Project Research Group, "Aspirin in Coronary Heart Disease," *Journal of Chronic Disease,* 29:625–642, 1976. 3. Breddin K, et al., "Secondary Prevention of Myocardial Infarction; Comparison of Acetylsalicylic Acid Phenprocoumon and Placebo," *Thromb. Haemost.,* 41:225–236, 1979. 4. Aspirin Myocardial Infarction Study Research Group, "A Randomized, Controlled Trial of Aspirin in Persons Recovered from Myocardial Infarction," *Journal American Medical Association,* 243:661–669, 1980. 5. Elwood P.C., and Sweetnam, P.M., "Aspirin and Secondary Mortality after Myocardial Infarction," *Lancet,* pp. 1313–1315, December 22–29, 1979. 6. The Persantine-Aspirin Reinfarction Study Research Group. "Persantine and Aspirin in Coronary Heart Disease," *Circulation* 62;449–460, 1980. 7. Lewis H.D., et al., "Protective Effects of Aspirin Against Acute Myocardial Infarction and Death in Men with Unstable Angina, Results of a Veterans Administration Cooperative Study," *New England Journal of Medicine,* 309;396–403, 1983.

Shown in Product Identification Guide, page 504

Arthritis Strength BUFFERIN®
[bŭf´fĕr-ĭn]
Analgesic

Composition:
Active Ingredient: Aspirin (500 mg) in a formulation buffered with Calcium Carbonate, Magnesium Oxide and Magnesium Carbonate.
Other Ingredients: Benzoic Acid, Citric Acid, Corn Starch, FD&C Blue No. 1, Hydroxypropyl Methylcellulose, Magnesium Stearate, Mineral Oil, Polysorbate 20, Povidone, Propylene Glycol, Simethicone Emulsion, Sodium Phosphate, Sorbitan Monolaurate, Titanium Dioxide.

May also contain: Carnauba Wax, Zinc Stearate.

Indications: For fast temporary relief of the minor aches and pains, stiffness, swelling and inflammation of arthritis.

Directions: Adults: 2 caplets with water every 6 hours as needed, not to exceed 8 caplets a day. Children under 12: Consult a doctor.

Warnings: Children and teenagers should not use this medicine for chicken pox or flu symptoms before a doctor is consulted about Reye syndrome, a rare but serious illness reported to be associated with aspirin. KEEP THIS AND ALL OTHER MEDICATIONS OUT OF THE REACH OF CHILDREN. IN CASE OF ACCIDENTAL OVERDOSE, SEEK PROFESSIONAL ASSISTANCE OR CONTACT A POISON CONTROL CENTER IMMEDIATELY. As with any drug, if you are pregnant or nursing a baby, seek the advice of a health professional before using this product.

IT IS ESPECIALLY IMPORTANT NOT TO USE ASPIRIN DURING THE LAST 3 MONTHS OF PREGNANCY UNLESS SPECIFICALLY DIRECTED TO DO SO BY A DOCTOR BECAUSE IT MAY CAUSE PROBLEMS IN THE UNBORN CHILD OR COMPLICATIONS DURING DELIVERY. Do not take this product for pain for more than 10 days or for fever for more than 3 days unless directed by a doctor. If pain or fever persists or gets worse, if new symptoms occur, or if redness or swelling is present, consult a doctor because these could be signs of a serious condition. Do not take this product if you are allergic to aspirin, have asthma, have stomach problems (such as heartburn, upset stomach or stomach pain) that persist or recur, or if you have ulcers or bleeding problems, unless directed by a doctor. If ringing in the ears or loss of hearing occurs, consult a doctor before taking any more of this product.

Drug Interaction Precaution: Do not take this product if you are taking a prescription drug for anticoagulation (thinning of blood), diabetes, gout or arthritis unless directed by a doctor.

How Supplied: Arthritis Strength BUFFERIN® is supplied as:
Plain white coated caplet "ASB" debossed on one side.
NDC 19810-0051-1 Bottle of 40's
NDC 19810-0051-2 Bottle of 100's
The 40 caplet size does not have a child resistant closure and is recommended for households without young children.
Store at room temperature.
Shown in Product Identification Guide, page 504

Extra Strength BUFFERIN®
[bŭf'fĕr-ĭn]
Analgesic

Composition:
Active Ingredient: Aspirin (500 mg) in a formulation buffered with Calcium Carbonate, Magnesium Oxide and Magnesium Carbonate.
Other Ingredients: Benzoic Acid, Citric Acid, Corn Starch, FD&C Blue No. 1, Hydroxypropyl Methylcellulose, Magnesium Stearate, Mineral Oil, Polysorbate 20, Povidone, Propylene Glycol, Simethicone Emulsion, Sodium Phosphate, Sorbitan Monolaurate, Titanium Dioxide. May also contain: Carnauba Wax, Zinc Stearate.

Indications: For fast temporary relief of headaches, minor arthritis pain and inflammation, muscle aches, pain and fever of colds, menstrual pain and toothaches.

Directions: Adults: 2 tablets with water every 6 hours as needed, not to exceed 8 tablets a day. Children under 12: Consult a doctor.

Warnings: Children and teenagers should not use this medicine for chicken pox or flu symptoms before a doctor is consulted about Reye syndrome, a rare but serious illness reported to be associated with aspirin. KEEP THIS AND ALL OTHER MEDICATIONS OUT OF THE REACH OF CHILDREN. IN CASE OF ACCIDENTAL OVERDOSE, SEEK PROFESSIONAL ASSISTANCE OR CONTACT A POISON CONTROL CENTER IMMEDIATELY. As with any drug, if your are pregnant or nursing a baby, seek the advice of a health professional before using this product. IT IS ESPECIALLY IMPORTANT NOT TO USE ASPIRIN DURING THE LAST 3 MONTHS OF PREGNANCY UNLESS SPECIFICALLY DIRECTED TO DO SO BY A DOCTOR BECAUSE IT MAY CAUSE PROBLEMS IN THE UNBORN CHILD OR COMPLICATIONS DURING DELIVERY. Do not take this product for more than 10 days or for fever for more than 3 days unless directed by a doctor. If pain or fever persists or gets worse, if new symptoms occur, or if redness or swelling is present, consult a doctor because these could be signs of a serious condition. Do not take this product if you are allergic to aspirin, have asthma, have stomach problems (such as heartburn, upset stomach or stomach pain) that persist or recur, or if you have ulcers or bleeding problems, unless directed by a doctor. If ringing in the ears or loss of hearing occurs, consult a doctor before taking any more of this product.

Drug Interaction Precaution: Do not take this product if you are taking a prescription drug for anticoagulation (thinning of blood), diabetes, gout or arthritis unless directed by a doctor.

How Supplied: Extra Strength BUFFERIN® is supplied as:

White elongated coated tablet with "ESB" debossed on one side.
NDC 19810-0074-1 Bottle of 30's
NDC 19810-0074-4 Bottle of 50's
NDC 19810-0074-3 Bottle of 100's
All sizes have child resistant closures except 50's which is recommended for households without young children.
Store at room temperature.
Shown in Product Identification Guide, page 504

COMTREX® Maximum Strength
[cŏm'trĕx]
Multi-Symptom Cold Reliever

Composition: Each tablet, caplet, liqui-gel and fluidounce (30 ml.) contains:
[See table at bottom of next page.]

Indications: COMTREX® provides temporary relief of these major cold and flu symptoms: nasal and sinus congestion, runny nose, sneezing, coughing, minor sore throat pain, headache, fever, body aches and pain.

Directions:
Tablets or Caplets: Adults: 2 tablets or caplets every 6 hours while symptoms persist, not to exceed 8 tablets or caplets in 24 hours, or as directed by a doctor. Children under 12: Consult a doctor.
Liqui-Gel: Adults: 2 liqui-gels every 6 hours while symptoms persist, not to exceed 8 liqui-gels in 24 hours, or as directed by a doctor. Children under 12: Consult a doctor.
Liquid: Adults: One fluidounce (30 ml) in medicine cup provided or 2 tablespoons every 6 hours while symptoms persist, not to exceed 4 doses in 24 hours. Children under 12: Consult a doctor.

Warnings: KEEP THIS AND ALL OTHER MEDICATIONS OUT OF THE REACH OF CHILDREN. IN CASE OF ACCIDENTAL OVERDOSE, SEEK PROFESSIONAL ASSISTANCE OR CONTACT A POISON CONTROL CENTER IMMEDIATELY. PROMPT MEDICAL ATTENTION IS CRITICAL FOR ADULTS AS WELL AS FOR CHILDREN EVEN IF YOU DO NOT NOTICE ANY SIGNS OR SYMPTOMS. As with any drug, if you are pregnant or nursing a baby, seek the advice of a health professional before using this product. Do not give this product to children under 12 years of age or use for more than 7 days (or for fever for more than 3 days), unless directed by a doctor. If symptoms do not improve or are accompanied by a fever that lasts for more than 3 days, if new symptoms occur, or if redness or swelling is present, consult a doctor. Do not exceed recommended dosage because at higher doses nervousness, dizziness or sleeplessness may occur. A persistent cough may be a sign of a serious condition. If cough persists for more than 7 days, tends to recur, or is accompanied by rash, persistent headache, fever that lasts for more than 3 days, or if new symptoms occur, consult a doctor.

Continued on next page

Bristol-Myers—Cont.

Do not take this product for persistent or chronic cough such as occurs with smoking, asthma or emphysema, or if cough is accompanied by excessive phlegm (mucus/sputum) unless directed by a doctor. If sore throat is severe, persists for more than 2 days, is accompanied or followed by a fever, headache, rash, nausea or vomiting, consult a doctor promptly. Do not take this product unless directed by a doctor, if you have a breathing problem such as emphysema or chronic bronchitis or if you have heart disease, high blood pressure, thyroid disease, diabetes, glaucoma, or difficulty in urination due to enlargement of the prostate gland. May cause marked drowsiness; alcohol, sedatives, and tranquilizers may increase the drowsiness effect. Avoid alcoholic beverages, while taking this product. Do not take this product if you are taking sedatives or tranquilizers without first consulting your doctor. Use caution when driving a motor vehicle or operating machinery. May cause excitability, especially in children.

Drug Interaction Precaution: Do not use this product if you are now taking a prescription monoamine oxidase inhibitor (MAOI) (certain drugs for depression, psychiatric or emotional conditions, or Parkinson's disease), or for 2 weeks after stopping the MAOI drug. If you are uncertain whether your prescription drug contains an MAOI, consult a health professional before taking this product.

Overdose:
MUCOMYST (acetylcysteine) As An Antidote For Acetaminophen Overdose)

Acetaminophen is rapidly absorbed from the upper gastrointestinal tract with peak plasma levels occurring between 30 and 60 minutes after therapeutic doses and usually within 4 hours following an overdose. The parent compound, which is nontoxic, is extensively metabolized in the liver to form principally the sulfate and glucuronide conjugates which are also nontoxic and are rapidly excreted in the urine. A small fraction of an ingested dose is metabolized in the liver by the cytochrome P-450 mixed function oxidase enzyme system to form a reactive, potentially toxic, intermediate metabolite which preferentially conjugates with hepatic glutathione to form the nontoxic cysteine and mercapturic acid derivatives which are then excreted by the kidney. Therapeutic doses of acetaminophen do not saturate the glucuronide and sulfate conjugation pathways and do not result in the formation of sufficient reactive metabolite to deplete glutathione stores. However, following ingestion of a large overdose (150 mg/kg or greater) the glucuronide and sulfate conjugation pathways are saturated resulting in a larger fraction of the drug being metabolized via the P-450 pathway. The increased formation of reactive metabolite may deplete the hepatic stores of glutathione with subsequent binding of the metabolite to protein molecules within the hepatocyte resulting in cellular necrosis. Acetylcysteine has been shown to reduce the extent of liver injury following acetaminophen overdose. Early symptoms following a potentially hepatotoxic overdose may include: nausea, vomiting, diaphoresis and general malaise. Clinical and laboratory evidence of hepatic toxicity may not be apparent until 48 to 72 hours postingestion. In adults and adolescents, regardless of the quantity of acetaminophen reported to have been ingested, administer MUCOMYST® acetylcysteine immediately. MUCOMYST acetylcysteine therapy should be initiated and continued for a full course of therapy. Its effectiveness depends on early administration, with benefit seen principally in patients treated within 16 hours of the overdose. If acetaminophen plasma assay capability is not available, and the estimated acetaminophen ingestion exceeds 150 mg/kg, MUCOMYST acetylcysteine therapy should be initiated and continued for a full course of therapy.

For full prescribing information, refer to the MUCOMYST package insert. Do not await the results of assays for acetaminophen level before initiating treatment with MUCOMYST acetylcysteine. The following additional procedures are recommended: The stomach should be emptied promptly by lavage or by induction of emesis with syrup of ipecac. A serum acetaminophen assay should be obtained as early as possible, but no sooner than four hours following ingestion. Liver function studies should be obtained initially and repeated at 24-hour intervals.

For additional emergency information call your regional poison center or toll-free (1-800-525-6115) to the Rocky Mountain Poison Center for assistance in diagnosis and for directions in the use of MUCOMYST acetylcysteine as an antidote.

How Supplied:
COMTREX® is supplied as:
Yellow tablet with letter "C" debossed on one surface.

	COMTREX Per Tablet or Caplet	COMTREX Liquid-Gel per Liqui-Gel	COMTREX Liquid Per Fl. Ounce
Acetaminophen:	500 mg.	500 mg.	1000 mg.
Pseudoephedrine HCl:	30 mg.	—	60 mg.
Phenylpropanolamine HCl:	—	12.5 mg.	—
Chlorpheniramine Maleate:	2 mg.	2 mg.	4 mg.
Dextromethorphan HBr:	15 mg.	15 mg.	30 mg.

Tablet/Caplet
Benzoic Acid
Carnauba Wax
Corn Starch
D&C Yellow No. 10 Lake
FD&C Red No. 40 Lake
Hydroxypropyl Methylcellulose
Magnesium Stearate

Methylparaben

Mineral Oil
Polysorbate 20
Povidone
Propylene Glycol
Propylparaben
Simethicone Emulsion
Sorbitan Monolaurate
Stearic Acid
Titanium Dioxide
May also contain:
Crospovidone
Hydroxypropyl cellulose
Silicon Dioxide

Liqui-Gels
D&C Yellow No. 10
FD&C Red No. 40
Gelatin
Glycerin
Polyethylene Glycol
Povidone
Propylene Glycol

Silicon Dioxide

Sorbitol
Titanium Dioxide
Water

Liquid
Alcohol (10% by volume)
Benzoic acid
D&C Yellow No. 10
FD&C Blue No. 1
FD&C Red No. 40
Flavors
Glycerin
Polyethylene Glycol
Povidone
Saccharin Sodium
Sodium Citrate
Sucrose
Water

NDC 19810-0092-1 Blister packages of 24's
NDC 19810-0092-2 Bottles of 50's
Coated yellow caplet with "Comtrex" printed in red on one side.
NDC 19810-0055-1 Blister packages of 24's
NDC 19810-0055-2 Bottles of 50's
Yellow Liqui-Gel with "Comtrex" printed in red on one side.
NDC 19810-0431-1 Blister packages of 24's
NDC 19810-0431-2 Blister packages of 50's
Clear Red Cherry Flavored liquid:
NDC 19810-0527-1 6 oz. plastic bottles.
All sizes packaged in child resistant closures except for 24's for tablets, caplets and liqui-gels which are sizes recommended for households without young children. Store caplets, tablets and liquid at room temperature.
Store liqui-gels below 86° F. (30° C.). Keep from freezing.

Shown in Product Identification Guide, page 504

ALLERGY–SINUS COMTREX
Maximum Strength
[cŏm 'trĕx]
Multi-Symptom Allergy/Sinus Formula

Composition:
Active Ingredients: Each coated tablet contains 500 mg acetaminophen, 30 mg pseudoephedrine HCl, 2 mg chlorpheniramine maleate.
Other Ingredients: Benzoic acid, carnauba wax, corn starch, D&C yellow No. 10 lake, FD&C blue No. 1 lake, FD&C Red No. 40 lake, hydroxypropyl methylcellulose, mineral oil, polysorbate 20, povidone, propylene glycol, simethicone emulsion, sodium citrate, sorbitan monolaurate, stearic acid, titanium dioxide. May also contain: crospovidone, D&C yellow No. 10, erythorbic acid, FD&C blue No. 1, magnesium stearate, methylparaben, microcrystalline cellulose, polysorbate 80, propylparaben, silicon dioxide, wood cellulose.

Indications:
ALLERGY-SINUS COMTREX provides temporary relief of these upper respiratory allergy, hay fever, and sinusitis symptoms: sneezing, itchy watery eyes, runny nose, headache, nasal and sinus pressure and congestion.

Directions: Adults: 2 tablets every 6 hours while symptoms persist, not to exceed 8 tablets in 24 hours, or as directed by a doctor. Children under 12 years of age: Consult a doctor.

Warnings: KEEP THIS AND ALL OTHER MEDICATIONS OUT OF THE REACH OF CHILDREN. IN CASE OF ACCIDENTAL OVERDOSE, SEEK PROFESSIONAL ASSISTANCE OR CONTACT A POISON CONTROL CENTER IMMEDIATELY. PROMPT MEDICAL ATTENTION IS CRITICAL FOR ADULTS AS WELL AS FOR CHILDREN EVEN IF YOU DO NOT NOTICE ANY SIGNS OR SYMPTOMS. As with any drug, if you are pregnant or nursing a baby, seek the advice of a health professional before using this product. Do not take this product for more than 7 days unless directed by a doctor. If symptoms do not improve or are accompanied by a fever that lasts for more than 3 days, or if new symptoms occur, consult a doctor. Do not exceed recommended dosage because at higher doses nervousness, dizziness or sleeplessness may occur. May cause excitability especially in children. Do not take this product unless directed by a doctor if you have a breathing problem such as emphysema, or chronic bronchitis, or if you have heart disease, high blood pressure, thyroid disease, diabetes, shortness of breath, or difficulty in urination due to enlargement of the prostate gland. May cause drowsiness; alcohol, sedatives and tranquilizers may increase the drowsiness effect. Avoid alcoholic beverages, while taking this product. Do not take this product if you are taking sedatives or tranquilizers without first consulting your doctor. Use caution when driving a motor vehicle or operating machinery.

Drug Interaction Precaution: Do not use this product if you are now taking a prescription monoamine oxidase inhibitor (MAOI) (certain drugs for depression, psychiatric or emotional conditions, or Parkinson's disease), or for 2 weeks after stopping the MAOI drug. If you are uncertain whether your prescription drug contains an MAOI, consult a health professional before taking this product.

Overdose:
MUCOMYST (acetylcysteine) As An Antidote For Acetaminophen Overdose)
Acetaminophen is rapidly absorbed from the upper gastrointestinal tract with peak plasma levels occurring between 30 and 60 minutes after therapeutic doses and usually within 4 hours following an overdose. The parent compound, which is nontoxic, is extensively metabolized in the liver to form principally the sulfate and glucuronide conjugates which are also nontoxic and are rapidly excreted in the urine. A small fraction of an ingested dose is metabolized in the liver by the cytochrome P-450 mixed function oxidase enzyme system to form a reactive, potentially toxic, intermediate metabolite which preferentially conjugates with hepatic glutathione to form the nontoxic cysteine and mercapturic acid derivatives which are then excreted by the kidney. Therapeutic doses of acetaminophen do not saturate the glucuronide and sulfate conjugation pathways and do not result in the formation of sufficient reactive metabolite to deplete glutathione stores. However, following ingestion of a large overdose (150 mg/kg or greater) the glucuronide and sulfate conjugation pathways are saturated resulting in a larger fraction of the drug being metabolized via the P-450 pathway. The increased formation of reactive metabolite may deplete the hepatic stores of glutathione with subsequent binding of the metabolite to protein molecules within the hepatocyte resulting in cellular necrosis. Acetylcysteine has been shown to reduce the extent of liver injury following acetaminophen overdose. Early symptoms following a potentially hepatotoxic overdose may include: nausea, vomiting, diaphoresis and general malaise. Clinical and laboratory evidence of hepatic toxicity may not be apparent until 48 to 72 hours postingestion. In adults and adolescents, regardless of the quantity of acetaminophen reported to have been ingested, administer MUCOMYST® acetylcysteine immediately. MUCOMYST acetylcysteine therapy should be initiated and continued for a full course of therapy. Its effectiveness depends on early administration, with benefit seen principally in patients treated within 16 hours of the overdose. If acetaminophen plasma assay capability is not available, and the estimated acetaminophen ingestion exceeds 150 mg/kg, MUCOMYST acetylcysteine therapy should be initiated and continued for a full course of therapy.
For full prescribing information, refer to the MUCOMYST package insert. Do not await the results of assays for acetaminophen level before initiating treatment with MUCOMYST acetylcysteine. The following additional procedures are recommended: The stomach should be emptied promptly by lavage or by induction of emesis with syrup of ipecac. A serum acetaminophen assay should be obtained as early as possible, but no sooner than four hours following ingestion. Liver function studies should be obtained initially and repeated at 24-hour intervals.
For additional emergency information call your regional poison center or toll-free (1-800-525-6115) to the Rocky Mountain Poison Center for assistance in diagnosis and for directions in the use of MUCOMYST acetylcysteine as an antidote.

How Supplied: Allergy-Sinus COMTREX® is supplied as:
Coated green tablets with "Comtrex A/S" printed in black on one side.
NDC 19810-0774-1 Blister packages of 24's
NDC 19810-0774-2 Bottles of 50's
All sizes packaged in child resistant closures except 24's which are sizes recommended for households without young children.
Store at room temperature.

Shown in Product Identification Guide, page 504

Continued on next page

Bristol-Myers—Cont.

Non-Drowsy COMTREX®
Maximum Strength

Each caplet or liqui-gel contains:
[See table below.]

Other ingredients (Caplet): Benzoic Acid, Carnauba wax, Corn Starch, D&C Yellow No. 10 Lake, Hydroxypropyl Methylcellulose, Magnesium Stearate, Methylparaben, Povidone, Propylene Glycol, Propylparaben, Simethicone Emulsion, Stearic acid, Titanium Dioxide.
May also contain: Crospovidone, D&C Red #30 Lake, FD&C Red No. 40 lake, Hydroxy propylcellulose, Mineral oil, Polysorbate 20, Silicon Dioxide, Sorbitan Monolaurate

Other Ingredients (Liqui-gel): FD&C Yellow No. 6, Gelatin, Glycerin, Polyethylene Glycol, Povidone, Propylene Glycol, Silicon Dioxide, Sorbitol, Titanium Dioxide, Water

Indications: For temporary relief of major cold and flu symptoms without drowsiness, to relieve stuffy nose and sinus congestion, to quiet cough, to relieve headache, fever, minor sore throat pain and body aches and pain.

Warnings: KEEP THIS AND ALL OTHER MEDICATIONS OUT OF THE REACH OF CHILDREN. IN CASE OF ACCIDENTAL OVERDOSE, SEEK PROFESSIONAL ASSISTANCE OR CONTACT A POISON CONTROL CENTER IMMEDIATELY. PROMPT MEDICAL ATTENTION IS CRITICAL FOR ADULTS AS WELL AS FOR CHILDREN EVEN IF YOU DO NOT NOTICE ANY SIGNS OR SYMPTOMS. As with any drug, if you are pregnant or nursing a baby, seek the advice of a health professional before using this product. Do not give this product to children under 12 years of age or use for more than 7 days or for fever for more than 3 days unless directed by a doctor. If symptoms do not improve or are accompanied by fever that lasts for more than 3 days, if new symptoms occur or if redness or swelling is present, consult a doctor. Do not exceed recommended dosage because at higher doses nervousness, dizziness or sleeplessness may occur. A persistent cough may be a sign of a serious condition. If cough persists for more than 7 days, tends to recur or is accompanied by rash, persistent headache, fever that lasts for more than 3 days, or if new symptoms occur, consult a doctor. Do not take this product for persistent or chronic cough such as occurs with smoking, asthma or emphysema, or if cough is accompanied by excessive phlegm (mucus/sputum) unless directed by a doctor. If sore throat is severe, persists for more than 2 days, is accompanied or followed by a fever, headache, rash, nausea or vomiting, consult a doctor promptly. Do not take this product if you have heart disease, high blood pressure, thyroid disease, diabetes or difficulty in urination due to enlargement of the prostate gland unless directed by a doctor.

DRUG INTERACTION PRECAUTION: Do not use this product if you are now taking a prescription monoamine oxidase inhibitor (MAOI) (certain drugs for depression, psychiatric or emotional conditions, or Parkinson's disease), or for 2 weeks after stopping the MAOI drug. If you are uncertain whether your prescription drug contains an MAOI, consult a health professional before taking this product.

Directions: Adults: 2 caplets or liqui-gels every 6 hours while symptoms persist, not to exceed 8 caplets or liquigels in 24 hours, or as directed by doctor. **Children under 12:** Consult a doctor.

Overdose: MUCOMYST (acetylcysteine) As An Antidote For Acetaminophen Overdose)

Acetaminophen is rapidly absorbed from the upper gastrointestinal tract with peak plasma levels occurring between 30 and 60 minutes after therapeutic doses and usually within 4 hours following an overdose. The parent compound, which is nontoxic, is extensively metabolized in the liver to form principally the sulfate and glucuronide conjugates which are also nontoxic and are rapidly excreted in the urine. A small fraction of an ingested dose is metabolized in the liver by the cytochrome P-450 mixed function oxidase enzyme system to form a reactive, potentially toxic, intermediate metabolite which preferentially conjugates with hepatic glutathione to form the nontoxic cysteine and mercapturic acid derivatives which are then excreted by the kidney. Therapeutic doses of acetaminophen do not saturate the glucuronide and sulfate conjugation pathways and do not result in the formation of sufficient reactive metabolite to deplete glutathione stores. However, following ingestion of a large overdose (150 mg/kg or greater) the glucuronide and sulfate conjugation pathways are saturated resulting in a larger fraction of the drug being metabolized via the P-450 pathway. The increased formation of reactive metabolite may deplete the hepatic stores of glutathione with subsequent binding of the metabolite to protein molecules within the hepatocyte resulting in cellular necrosis. Acetylcysteine has been shown to reduce the extent of liver injury following acetaminophen overdose. Early symptoms following a potentially hepatotoxic overdose may include: nausea, vomiting, diaphoresis and general malaise. Clinical and laboratory evidence of hepatic toxicity may not be apparent until 48 to 72 hours postingestion. In adults and adolescents, regardless of the quantity of acetaminophen reported to have been ingested, administer MUCOMYST® acetylcysteine immediately. MUCOMYST acetylcysteine therapy should be initiated and continued for a full course of therapy. Its effectiveness depends on early administration, with benefit seen principally in patients treated within 16 hours of the overdose. If acetaminophen plasma assay capability is not available, and the estimated acetaminophen ingestion exceeds 150 mg/kg, MUCOMYST acetylcysteine therapy should be initiated and continued for a full course of therapy.

For full prescribing information, refer to the MUCOMYST package insert. Do not await the results of assays for acetaminophen level before initiating treatment with MUCOMYST acetylcysteine. The following additional procedures are recommended: The stomach should be emptied promptly by lavage or by induction of emesis with syrup of ipecac. A serum acetaminophen assay should be obtained as early as possible, but no sooner than four hours following ingestion. Liver function studies should be obtained initially and repeated at 24-hour intervals.

For additional emergency information call your regional poison center or toll-free (1-800-525-6115) to the Rocky Mountain Poison Center for assistance in diagnosis and for directions in the use of MUCOMYST acetylcysteine as an antidote.

How Supplied: Non-Drowsy Comtrex® is supplied as:
Coated orange caplet with letter "C" debossed on one surface.
NDC 19810-0046-1 Blister packages of 24's
NDC 19810-0046-2 Bottles of 50's
Liquigel printed with "COMTREX"
NDC 19810-0008-1 Blister packages of 24's
NDC 19810-0008-2 Blister packages of 50's
The 24 size does not have a child resistant closure and is recommended for households without young children.
Store at room temperature.

Shown in Product Identification Guide, page 504

Aspirin Free EXCEDRIN®

Composition: Each caplet contains Acetaminophen 500 mg. and Caffeine 65 mg. Other Ingredients: Benzoic Acid, Carnauba Wax, Corn Starch, Croscarmellose Sodium, D&C Red No. 27 Lake, D&C Yellow No. 10 Lake, FD&C Blue No. 1 Lake, Hydroxypropyl Methylcellulose, Magnesium Stearate, Methylparaben, Microcrystalline Cellulose, Propylparaben, Saccharin Sodium, Simethicone

Active:	Comtrex Non-Drowsy per caplet	Comtrex Non-Drowsy per liqui-gel
Acetaminophen	500 mg	500 mg
Pseudoephedrine HCL	30 mg	—
Dextromethorphan HBr	15 mg	15 mg
Phenylpropanolamine HCL	—	12.5 mg

Emulsion, Stearic Acid, Titanium Dioxide. May also contain: Erythorbic Acid, Mineral Oil, Polyethylene Glycol, Polysorbate 20, Polysorbate 80, Povidone, Propylene Glycol, Sorbitan Monolaurate.

Indications: For temporary relief of the pain of headache, sinusitis, colds, muscular aches, menstrual discomfort, toothaches and minor arthritis pain.

Directions: Adults: 2 caplets every 6 hours while symptoms persist, not to exceed 8 caplets in 24 hours, or as directed by a doctor. Children under 12 years of age: Consult a doctor.

Warnings: KEEP THIS AND ALL OTHER MEDICATIONS OUT OF THE REACH OF CHILDREN. IN CASE OF ACCIDENTAL OVERDOSE, SEEK PROFESSIONAL ASSISTANCE OR CONTACT A POISON CONTROL CENTER IMMEDIATELY. PROMPT MEDICAL ATTENTION IS CRITICAL FOR ADULTS AS WELL AS FOR CHILDREN EVEN IF YOU DO NOT NOTICE ANY SIGNS OR SYMPTOMS. As with any drug, if you are pregnant or nursing a baby, seek the advice of a health professional before using this product. Do not take this product for pain for more than 10 days or for fever for more than 3 days unless directed by a doctor. If pain or fever persists or gets worse, if new symptoms occur, or if redness or swelling is present, consult a doctor because these could be signs of a serious condition. Consult a dentist promptly for toothache.

Overdose:
MUCOMYST (acetylcysteine) As An Antidote For Acetaminophen Overdose)
Acetaminophen is rapidly absorbed from the upper gastrointestinal tract with peak plasma levels occurring between 30 and 60 minutes after therapeutic doses and usually within 4 hours following an overdose. The parent compound, which is nontoxic, is extensively metabolized in the liver to form principally the sulfate and glucuronide conjugates which are also nontoxic and are rapidly excreted in the urine. A small fraction of an ingested dose is metabolized in the liver by the cytochrome P-450 mixed function oxidase enzyme system to form a reactive, potentially toxic, intermediate metabolite which preferentially conjugates with hepatic glutathione to form the nontoxic cysteine and mercapturic acid derivatives which are then excreted by the kidney. Therapeutic doses of acetaminophen do not saturate the glucuronide and sulfate conjugation pathways and do not result in the formation of sufficient reactive metabolite to deplete glutathione stores. However, following ingestion of a large overdose (150 mg/kg or greater) the glucuronide and sulfate conjugation pathways are saturated resulting in a larger fraction of the drug being metabolized via the P-450 pathway. The increased formation of reactive metabolite may deplete the hepatic stores of glutathione with subsequent binding of the

metabolite to protein molecules within the hepatocyte resulting in cellular necrosis. Acetylcysteine has been shown to reduce the extent of liver injury following acetaminophen overdose. Early symptoms following a potentially hepatotoxic overdose may include: nausea, vomiting, diaphoresis and general malaise. Clinical and laboratory evidence of hepatic toxicity may not be apparent until 48 to 72 hours postingestion. In adults and adolescents, regardless of the quantity of acetaminophen reported to have been ingested, administer MUCOMYST® acetylcysteine immediately. MUCOMYST acetylcysteine therapy should be initiated and continued for a full course of therapy. Its effectiveness depends on early administration, with benefit seen principally in patients treated within 16 hours of the overdose. If acetaminophen plasma assay capability is not available, and the estimated acetaminophen ingestion exceeds 150 mg/kg, MUCOMYST acetylcysteine therapy should be initiated and continued for a full course of therapy.
For full prescribing information, refer to the MUCOMYST package insert. Do not await the results of assays for acetaminophen level before initiating treatment with MUCOMYST acetylcysteine. The following additional procedures are recommended: The stomach should be emptied promptly by lavage or by induction of emesis with syrup of ipecac. A serum acetaminophen assay should be obtained as early as possible, but no sooner than four hours following ingestion. Liver function studies should be obtained initially and repeated at 24-hour intervals.
For additional emergency information call your regional poison center or toll-free (1-800-525-6115) to the Rocky Mountain Poison Center for assistance in diagnosis and for directions in the use of MUCOMYST acetylcysteine as an antidote.

How Supplied: Aspirin Free EXCEDRIN® is supplied as: Coated red caplets with "AF Excedrin" printed in white on one side.
NDC 19810-0089-1 Bottles of 24's
NDC 19810-0089-2 Bottles of 50's
NDC 19810-0089-3 Bottles of 100's
All sizes packaged in child resistant closures except 100's which is recommended for households without young children. Store at room temperature.
Shown in Product Identification Guide, page 504

EXCEDRIN® Extra-Strength Analgesic
[ĕx "cĕd 'rĭn]

Composition:
Each tablet or caplet contains Acetaminophen 250 mg.: Aspirin 250 mg.; and Caffeine 65 mg.
Other Ingredients: (Tablets or Caplets) Benzoic Acid, FD&C Blue No. 1, Hydroxypropyl Methylcellulose, Microcrystal-

line Cellulose, Mineral Oil, Polysorbate 20, Povidone, Propylene Glycol, Saccharin Sodium, Simethicone Emulsion, Sorbitan Monolaurate, Stearic Acid, Titanium Dioxide. May Also Contain: Carnauba Wax, Hydroxypropylcellulose.

Indications: For temporary relief of the pain of headache, sinusitis, colds, muscular aches, menstrual discomfort, toothaches and minor arthritis pain.

Directions: Adults: 2 tablets or caplets with water every 6 hours while symptoms persist, not to exceed 8 tablets or caplets in 24 hours, or as directed by a doctor. Children under 12 years of age: Consult a doctor.

Warnings: Children and teenagers should not use this medicine for chickenpox or flu symptoms before a doctor is consulted about Reye syndrome, a rare but serious illness reported to be associated with aspirin. KEEP THIS AND ALL OTHER MEDICATIONS OUT OF THE REACH OF CHILDREN. IN CASE OF ACCIDENTAL OVERDOSE, SEEK PROFESSIONAL ASSISTANCE OR CONTACT A POISON CONTROL CENTER IMMEDIATELY. PROMPT MEDICAL ATTENTION IS CRITICAL FOR ADULTS AS WELL AS FOR CHILDREN EVEN IF YOU DO NOT NOTICE ANY SIGNS OR SYMPTOMS. As with any drug, if you are pregnant or nursing a baby, seek the advice of a health professional before using this product. IT IS ESPECIALLY IMPORTANT NOT TO USE ASPIRIN DURING THE LAST 3 MONTHS OF PREGNANCY UNLESS SPECIFICALLY DIRECTED TO DO SO BY A DOCTOR BECAUSE IT MAY CAUSE PROBLEMS IN THE UNBORN CHILD OR COMPLICATIONS DURING DELIVERY. Do not take this product for pain for more than 10 days or for fever for more than 3 days unless directed by a doctor. If pain or fever persists or gets worse, if new symptoms occur, or if redness or swelling is present, consult a doctor because these could be signs of a serious condition. Consult a dentist promptly for toothache. Do not take this product if you are allergic to aspirin, have asthma, have stomach problems (such as heartburn, upset stomach or stomach pain) that persist or recur, or if you have ulcers or bleeding problems, unless directed by a doctor. If ringing in the ears or loss of hearing occurs, consult a doctor before taking any more of this product.

Drug Interaction Precaution: Do not take this product if you are taking a prescription drug for anticoagulation (thinning of blood), diabetes, gout or arthritis unless directed by a doctor.

Overdose:
MUCOMYST (acetylcysteine As An Antidote For Acetaminophen Overdose)
Acetaminophen is rapidly absorbed from the upper gastrointestinal tract with peak plasma levels occurring between 30

Continued on next page

Bristol-Myers—Cont.

and 60 minutes after therapeutic doses and usually within 4 hours following an overdose. The parent compound, which is nontoxic, is extensively metabolized in the liver to form principally the sulfate and glucuronide conjugates which are also nontoxic and are rapidly excreted in the urine. A small fraction of an ingested dose is metabolized in the liver by the cytochrome P-450 mixed function oxidase enzyme system to form a reactive, potentially toxic, intermediate metabolite which preferentially conjugates with hepatic glutathione to form the nontoxic cysteine and mercapturic acid derivatives which are then excreted by the kidney. Therapeutic doses of acetaminophen do not saturate the glucuronide and sulfate conjugation pathways and do not result in the formation of sufficient reactive metabolite to deplete glutathione stores. However, following ingestion of a larger overdose (150 mg/kg or greater) the glucuronide and sulfate conjugation pathways are saturated resulting in a larger fraction of the drug being metabolized via the P-450 pathway. The increased formation of reactive metabolite may deplete the hepatic stores of glutathione with subsequent binding of the metabolite to protein molecules within the hepatocyte resulting in cellular necrosis. Acetylcysteine has been shown to reduce the extent of liver injury following acetaminophen overdose. Early symptoms following a potentially hepatotoxic overdose may include nausea, vomiting, diaphoresis and general malaise. Clinical and laboratory evidence of hepatic toxicity may not be apparent until 48 to 72 hours postingestion. In adults and adolescents, regardless of the quantity of acetaminophen reported to have been ingested, administer MUCOMYST® acetylcysteine immediately. MUCOMYST acetylcysteine therapy should be initiated and continued for a full course of therapy. Its effectiveness depends on early administration, with benefit seen principally in patients treated within 16 hours of the overdose.

If acetaminophen plasma assay capability is not available, and the estimated acetaminophen ingestion exceeds 150 mg/kg, MUCOMYST acetylcysteine therapy should be initiated and continued for a full course of therapy.

For full prescribing information, refer to the MUCOMYST package insert. Do not await the results of assays for acetaminophen level before initiating treatment with MUCOMYST acetylcysteine. The following additional procedures are recommended. The stomach should be emptied promptly by lavage or by induction of emesis with syrup of ipecac. A serum acetaminophen assay should be obtained as early as possible, but no sooner than four hours following ingestion. Liver function studies should be obtained initially and repeated at 24-hour intervals.

For additional emergency information call your regional poison center or toll-free (1-800-525-6115) to the Rocky Mountain Poison Center for assistance in diagnosis and for directions in the use of MUCOMYST acetylcysteine as an antidote.

How Supplied: Extra Strength EXCEDRIN® is supplied as:
White circular tablet with letter "E" debossed on one side.
NDC 19810-0700-2 Bottles of 12's
NDC 19810-0782-3 Bottles of 24's
NDC 19810-0782-4 Bottles of 50's
NDC 19810-0700-5 Bottles of 100's
NDC 19810-0061-9 Bottles of 175's
NDC 19810-0700-1 A metal tin of 12's
NDC 19810-0772-1 Vials of 10's
Coated white caplets with "Excedrin" printed in red on one side.
NDC 19810-0002-1 Bottles of 24's
NDC 19810-0002-2 Bottles of 50's
NDC 19810-0002-8 Bottles of 100's
NDC 19810-0091-1 Bottles of 175's
All sizes packaged in child resistant closures except 100's for tablets, 50's for caplets which are sizes recommended for households without young children.
Store at room temperature.

Shown in Product Identification Guide, page 505

EXCEDRIN P.M.®
[ĕx "cĕd 'rĭn]
Analgesic Sleeping Aid

Composition: Each tablet, and caplet [See table top left next page]

Indications: For temporary relief of occasional headaches and minor aches and pains with accompanying sleeplessness.

Directions:
Tablets or Caplets:
Adults, 2 tablets, caplets or liquigels at bedtime if needed or as directed by a doctor.

Warnings: KEEP THIS AND ALL OTHER MEDICATIONS OUT OF THE REACH OF CHILDREN. IN CASE OF ACCIDENTAL OVERDOSE, SEEK PROFESSIONAL ASSISTANCE OR CONTACT A POISON CONTROL CENTER IMMEDIATELY. PROMPT MEDICAL ATTENTION IS CRITICAL FOR ADULTS AS WELL AS FOR CHILDREN EVEN IF YOU DO NOT NOTICE ANY SIGNS OR SYMPTOMS. As with any drug, if you are pregnant or nursing a baby, seek the advice of a health professional before using this product. Do not give this product to children under 12 years of age or use for more than 10 days unless directed by a doctor. Consult a doctor if symptoms persist or get worse or if new ones occur, or if sleeplessness persists continuously for more than 2 weeks because these may be symptoms of serious underlying medical illnesses. Do not take this product if you have asthma, glaucoma, emphysema, chronic pulmonary disease, shortness of breath, difficulty in breathing, or difficulty in urination due to enlargement of the prostate gland unless directed by a doctor. Avoid alcoholic beverages while taking this product. Do not take this product if you are taking sedatives or tranquilizers, without first consulting your doctor.

Overdose:
MUCOMYST (acetylcysteine) As An Antidote For Acetaminophen Overdose)
Acetaminophen is rapidly absorbed from the upper gastrointestinal tract with peak plasma levels occurring between 30 and 60 minutes after therapeutic doses and usually within 4 hours following an overdose. The parent compound, which is nontoxic, is extensively metabolized in the liver to form principally the sulfate and glucuronide conjugates which are also nontoxic and are rapidly excreted in the urine. A small fraction of an ingested dose is metabolized in the liver by the cytochrome P-450 mixed function oxidase enzyme system to form a reactive, potentially toxic, intermediate metabolite which preferentially conjugates with hepatic glutathione to form the nontoxic cysteine and mercapturic acid derivatives which are then excreted by the kidney. Therapeutic doses of acetaminophen do not saturate the glucuronide and sulfate conjugation pathways and do not result in the formation of sufficient reactive metabolite to deplete glutathione stores. However, following ingestion of a large overdose (150 mg/kg or greater) the glucuronide and sulfate conjugation pathways are saturated resulting in a larger fraction of the drug being metabolized via the P-450 pathway. The increased formation of reactive metabolite may deplete the hepatic stores of glutathione with subsequent binding of the metabolite to protein molecules within the hepatocyte resulting in cellular necrosis. Acetylcysteine has been shown to reduce the extent of liver injury following acetaminophen overdose. Early symptoms following a potentially hepatotoxic overdose may include: nausea, vomiting, diaphoresis and general malaise. Clinical and laboratory evidence of hepatic toxicity may not be apparent until 48 to 72 hours postingestion. In adults and adolescents, regardless of the quantity of acetaminophen reported to have been ingested, administer MUCOMYST® acetylcysteine immediately. MUCOMYST acetylcysteine therapy should be initiated and continued for a full course of therapy. Its effectiveness depends on early administration, with benefit seen principally in patients treated within 16 hours of the overdose.

If acetaminophen plasma assay capability is not available, and the estimated acetaminophen ingestion exceeds 150 mg/kg, MUCOMYST acetylcysteine therapy should be initiated and continued for a full course of therapy.

For full prescribing information, refer to the MUCOMYST package insert. Do not await the results of assays for acetaminophen level before initiating treatment

EXCEDRIN® PM
Per Tablet or Caplet

Acetaminophen 500 mg.
Diphenhydramine Citrate: 38 mg.
Other Ingredients: —

Tablet or Caplet

Benzoic Acid
Carnauba Wax
Corn Starch
D&C Yellow No. 10 Aluminum Lake
FD&C Blue No. 1 Aluminum Lake
Hydroxypropyl Methylcellulose
Magnesium Stearate
Methyparaben,
    pregelatinized starch.
Propylparaben
Simethicone Emulsion
Stearic Acid
Titanium Dioxide

May also contain:
D & C Yellow No. 10
FD & C Blue No. 1
Polyethylene Glycol
Polysorbate 80
Propylene Glycol

EXCEDRIN PM
Per Liquigel

Acetaminophen 500 mg.
Diphenhydramine HCl 25 mg.
Other Ingredients:

D & C Red No. 33
FD & C Blue No. 1
FD & C Green No. 3
Gelatin
Glycerin
Polyethylene Glycol
Povidone
Propylene Glycol
Silicon Dioxide
Sorbitol
Titanium Dioxide
Water

with MUCOMYST acetylcysteine. The following additional procedures are recommended: The stomach should be emptied promptly by lavage or by induction of emesis with syrup of ipecac. A serum acetaminophen assay should be obtained as early as possible, but no sooner than four hours following ingestion. Liver function studies should be obtained initially and repeated at 24-hour intervals.

For additional emergency information call your regional poison center or toll-free (1-800-525-6115) to the Rocky Mountain Poison Center for assistance in diagnosis and for directions in the use of MUCOMYST acetylcysteine as an antidote.

How Supplied: EXCREDRIN P.M.® is supplied as:
Light blue circular coated tablets with "PM" debossed on one side.
NDC 19810-0763-6 Bottles of 10's
NDC 19810-0764-3 Bottles of 24's
NDC 19810-0763-4 Bottles of 50's
NDC 19810-0764-4 Bottles of 100's
Light blue coated caplet with "Excedrin P.M." imprinted on one side.
NDC 19810-0032-5 Bottles of 24's
NDC 19810-0032-3 Bottles of 50's
NDC 19810-0032-6 Bottles of 100's

Light blue liquigels:
NDC 19810-1023-1 20's
NDC 19810-1023-2 40's
All sizes packaged in child resistant closures except 50's tablets and caplets which are recommended for households without young children.
Store at room temperature
Shown in Product Identification Guide, page 504

4-WAY® Fast Acting Nasal Spray

Composition:
Phenylephrine hydrochloride 0.5%, naphazoline hydrochloride 0.05%, pyrilamine maleate 0.2%, in a buffered solution. Also Contains: Benzalkonium Chloride, Boric Acid, Sodium Borate, Water. Also available in a mentholated formula containing Phenylephrine hydrochloride 0.5%, naphazoline hydrochloride 0.05%, pyrilamine maleate 0.2%, in a buffered solution. Also Contains: Benzalkonium Chloride, Boric Acid, Camphor, Eucalyptol, Menthol, Poloxamer 188, Polysorbate 80, Sodium Borate, Water.

Indications: For prompt, temporary relief of nasal congestion due to the common cold, sinusitis, hay fever or other upper respiratory allergies.

Directions and Use Instructions:
Directions: Adults: Spray twice into each nostril not more often than every 6 hours. Do not give to children under 12 years of age unless directed by a doctor.
Use Instructions: For Metered Pump—Remove protective cap. Hold bottle with thumb at base and nozzle between first and second fingers. With head upright, insert metered pump spray nozzle into nostril. Depress pump all the way down, with a firm even stroke and sniff deeply. Repeat in other nostril. Do not tilt head backward while spraying. Wipe tip clean after each use. Note: This bottle is filled to correct level for proper pump action. Before using the first time, remove the protective cap from the tip and prime the metered pump by depressing pump firmly several times.
Use Instructions: For Atomizer—With head in a normal upright position, put atomizer tip into nostril. Squeeze bottle with firm, quick pressure while inhaling.

Warnings: KEEP THIS AND ALL OTHER MEDICATIONS OUT OF THE REACH OF CHILDREN. IN CASE OF ACCIDENTAL OVERDOSE OR INGESTION, SEEK PROFESSIONAL ASSISTANCE OR CONTACT A POISON CONTROL CENTER IMMEDIATELY. Do not exceed recommended dosage because burning, stinging, sneezing, or increase of nasal discharge may occur. The use of this container by more than one person may spread infection. Do not use this product for more than 3 days. If symptoms persist, consult a doctor. Adults and children who have heart disease, high blood pressure, thyroid disease, diabetes, or difficulty in urination due to enlargement of the prostate gland should not use this product unless directed by a doctor.

How Supplied:
Regular formula:
NDC 19810-0047-1 Atomizer of ½ fluid ounce.
NDC 19810-0047-2 Atomizer of 1 fluid ounce.
New Mentholated formula:
NDC 19810-0049-1 Atomizer of ½ fluid ounce.
Store at room temperature.
Shown in Product Identification Guide, page 504

4-WAY® Long Lasting Nasal Spray

Composition: Oxymetazoline Hydrochloride 0.05% in a buffered isotonic aqueous solution. Phenylmercuric Acetate 0.002% added as a preservative.
Also Contains: Benzalkonium Chloride, Glycine, Sorbitol, Water.

Indications: For prompt, temporary relief of nasal congestion due to the common cold, sinusitis, hay fever or other upper respiratory allergies.

Continued on next page

Bristol-Myers—Cont.

Directions and Use Instructions:

Directions: Adults and children 6 to under 12 years of age (with adult supervision): 2 or 3 sprays in each nostril not more often than every 10 to 12 hours. Do not exceed 2 applications in any 24-hour period. Children under 6 years of age: Consult a doctor.

Use Instructions:

With head in a normal, upright position, put atomizer tip into nostril. Squeeze bottle with firm, quick pressure while inhaling.

Warnings: KEEP THIS AND ALL OTHER MEDICATIONS OUT OF THE REACH OF CHILDREN. IN CASE OF ACCIDENTAL OVERDOSE OR INGESTION, SEEK PROFESSIONAL ASSISTANCE OR CONTACT A POISON CONTROL CENTER IMMEDIATELY. Do not exceed recommended dosage because burning, stinging, sneezing, or increase of nasal discharge may occur. The use of this container by more than one person may spread infection. Do not use this product for more than 3 days. If symptoms persist, consult a doctor. Adults and children who have heart disease, high blood pressure, thyroid disease, diabetes, or difficulty in urination due to enlargement of the prostate gland should not use this product unless directed by a doctor.

How Supplied: 4-WAY Long Lasting Nasal Spray is supplied as:

NDC 19810-0728-1 Atomizer of ½ fluid ounce.

Store at room temperature.

Shown in Product Identification Guide, page 504

KERI LOTION
Skin Lubricant—Moisturizer

Available in three formulations:
KERI Original

Composition: Water, mineral oil, propylene glycol, PEG-40 stearate, glyceryl stearate/PEG-100 stearate, PEG-4 dilaurate, laureth-4, lanolin oil, methyl paraben, carbomer , propylparaben, fragrance triethanolamine, dioctyl sodium sulfosuccinate, quaternium-15.

Direction for Use: Apply wherever skin feels dry, rough or irritated. For external use only.

KERI Silky Smooth recommended for daily use on dry skin.

Composition: Water, petrolatum, glycerin, dimethicone, steareth-2, cetyl alcohol, benzyl alcohol, laureth-23, magnesium aluminum silicate, carbomer, fragrance, sodium hydroxide, quaternium-15.

Directions for Use: Apply liberally after bathing, before bed or whenever skin feels dry. Use daily on hands, arms, legs, or anywhere skin feels dry for softer, smoother, healthier-looking skin. For external use only.

KERI Sensitive Skin

Composition: Water, petrolatum, glycerin, dimethicone, steareth-2, cetyl alcohol, benzyl alcohol, laureth-23, magnesium aluminum silicate, tocopheryl linoleate, carbomer, BHT, sodium hydroxide, disodium EDTA, quaternium-15.

Directions for Use: Apply liberally after bathing, before bed or whenever skin feels dry. Use daily on hands, arms, legs, or anywhere skin feels dry for softer, smoother, healthier-looking skin. For external use only.

How Supplied: KERI Lotion Original 6½ oz., 11 oz., 15 oz. and 20 oz. plastic bottles. KERI Silky Smooth 6½ oz., 11 oz. and 15 oz. plastic bottles. KERI Sensitive Skin 6½ oz., 11 oz. and 15 oz. plastic bottles.

Shown in Product Identification Guide, page 505

NO DOZ® Maximum Strength Caplets

Composition: Each caplet contains 200 mg. Caffeine. Other ingredients: Benzoic Acid, Corn Starch, FD&C Blue No. 1, Flavors, Hydroxypropyl Methylcellulose, Microcrystalline Cellulose, Propylene Glycol, Simethicone Emulsion, Stearic Acid, Sucrose, Titanium Dioxide. May also contain: Carnauba Wax, Mineral Oil, Polysorbate 20, Povidone, Sorbitan Monolaurate.

Indications: Helps restore mental alertness or wakefulness when experiencing fatigue or drowsiness.

Directions: Adults: one-half to one caplet not more often than every 3 to 4 hours.

Warnings: KEEP THIS AND ALL OTHER MEDICATIONS OUT OF THE REACH OF CHILDREN. IN CASE OF ACCIDENTAL OVERDOSE, SEEK PROFESSIONAL ASSISTANCE OR CONTACT A POISON CONTROL CENTER IMMEDIATELY. As with any drug, if you are pregnant or nursing a baby, seek the advice of a health professional before using this product. Do not give to children under 12 years of age. For occasional use only. Not intended for use as a substitute for sleep. If fatigue or drowsiness persists or continues to occur, consult a doctor. The recommended dose of this product contains about as much caffeine as a cup of coffee. Limit the use of caffeine-containing medications, foods, or beverages while taking this product because too much caffeine may cause nervousness, irritability, sleeplessness and, occasionally, rapid heart beat.

How Supplied: NO DOZ® Maximum Strength is supplied as: White coated caplets with "NO DOZ" debossed on one side. The opposite side is scored.
19810-0064-4 Bottles of 16's
19810-0064-5 Bottles of 36's
19810-0064-6 Bottles of 60's
Store at room temperature.

NUPRIN®
(ibuprofen)
Analgesic

Warning: ASPIRIN SENSITIVE PATIENTS. Do not take this product if you have had a severe allergic reaction to aspirin, e.g.—asthma, swelling, shock or hives, because even though this product contains no aspirin or salicylates, cross-reactions may occur in patients allergic to aspirin.

Composition: Each tablet or caplet contains ibuprofen USP, 200 mg. **Other Ingredients:** Carnauba wax, cornstarch, D&C Yellow No. 10, FD&C Yellow No. 6, hydroxypropyl methylcellulose, propylene glycol, silicon dioxide, stearic acid, titanium dioxide.

Indications: For the temporary relief of minor aches and pains associated with the common cold, headache, toothache, muscular aches, backache, for the minor pain of arthritis, for the pain of menstrual cramps and for reduction of fever.

Additional Warnings: The following warnings are stated on the Nuprin label: Do not take for pain for more than 10 days or for fever for more than 3 days unless directed by a doctor. If pain or fever persists or gets worse, if new symptoms occur, or if the painful area is red or swollen, consult a doctor. These could be signs of serious illness. If you are under a doctor's care for any serious condition, consult a doctor before taking this product. As with aspirin and acetaminophen, if you have any condition which requires you to take prescription drugs or if you have had any problems or serious side effects from taking any non-prescription pain reliever, do not take NUPRIN without first discussing it with your doctor. If you experience any symptoms which are unusual or seem unrelated to the condition for which you took ibuprofen, consult a doctor before taking any more of it. Although ibuprofen is indicated for the same conditions as aspirin and acetaminophen, it should not be taken with them except under a doctor's direction. Do not combine this product with any other ibuprofen-containing product. As with any drug, if you are pregnant or nursing a baby, seek the advice of a health professional before using this product. IT IS ESPECIALLY IMPORTANT NOT TO USE IBUPROFEN DURING THE LAST 3 MONTHS OF PREGNANCY UNLESS SPECIFICALLY DIRECTED TO DO SO BY A DOCTOR BECAUSE IT MAY CAUSE PROBLEMS IN THE UNBORN CHILD OR COMPLICATIONS DURING DELIVERY. Keep this and all drugs out of the reach of children. In case of accidental overdose, seek professional assistance or contact a poison control center immediately.

Caution: Store at room temperature. Avoid excessive heat 40°C (104°F).

Directions: Adults: Take 1 tablet or caplet every 4 to 6 hours while symptoms persist. If pain or fever does not respond to 1 tablet or caplet, 2 tablets or caplets may be used but do not exceed 6 tablets or caplets in 24 hours, unless directed by a doctor. The smallest effective dose should be used. Take with food or milk if occasional and mild heartburn, upset stomach, or stomach pain occurs with use. Consult a doctor if these symptoms are more than mild or if they persist. Children: Do not give this product to children under 12 except under the advice and supervision of a doctor.

How Supplied:
NUPRIN® is supplied as:
Golden yellow round tablets with "NU-PRIN" printed in black on one side.
NDC 19810-0767-2 Bottles of 24's
NDC 19810-0767-3 Bottles of 50's
NDC 19810-0767-4 Bottles of 100's
NDC 19810-0767-9 Vials of 10's
Golden yellow caplets with "NUPRIN" printed in black on one side.
NDC 19810-0796-1 Bottles of 24's
NDC 19810-0796-2 Bottles of 50's
NDC 19810-0796-3 Bottles of 10's
All sizes packaged in child resistant closures except 24's for tablets and 24's for caplets, which are sizes recommended for households without young children.
Store at room temperature. Avoid excessive heat 40°C. (104°F.).
Distributed by Bristol-Myers Company
Shown in Product Identification Guide, page 505

THERAGRAN® ANTIOXIDANT
Softgel
Multivitamin Complement

SOFTGEL CONTENTS: For Adults—Percentage of US Recommended Daily Allowance

Vitamins	Quantity	U.S. RDA
Vitamin A	5000 I.U.	100%
(as Beta Carotene)		
Vitamin C	250mg	417%
Vitamin E	200 I.U.	667%
Minerals		
Zinc	7.5mg	50%
Copper	1mg	50%
Manganese	1.5mg	*
Selenium	15mcg	*

* U.S. RDA not established

Ingredients: dl-alpha tocopheryl acetate, ascorbic acid, beeswax, beta carotene, copper oxide, dicalcium phosphate dihydrate, FD&C blue #1, FD&C red #40, gelatin, glycerine, lecithin, manganese sulfate, sodium selenate, titanium dioxide, vegetable oil (partially hydrogenated cottonseed and soybean oils), water, zinc oxide.

Warning: KEEP OUT OF THE REACH OF CHILDREN
Recommended Adult Intake: 1 Softgel daily.

How Supplied: Bottles of 50

Storage: Store below 86 F. (30 C.). Keep from freezing.
Shown in Product Identification Guide, page 505

THERAGRAN® TABLETS
(High Potency Multivitamin Formula)

FOR ADULTS—PERCENTAGE OF U.S. RECOMMENDED DAILY ALLOWANCE

Vitamins	Quantity	US RDA
Vitamin A	5000 IU	100%
(as Acetate and Beta Carotene)		
Vitamin B₁	3 mg	200%
Vitamin B₂	3.4 mg	200%
Vitamin B₆	3 mg	150%
Vitamin B₁₂	9 mcg	150%
Vitamin C	90 mg	150%
Vitamin D	400 I.U.	100%
Vitamin E	30 I.U.	100%
Niacin	20 mg	100%
Folic Acid	400 mcg	100%
Pantothenic Acid	10.0 mg	100%
Biotin	30 mcg	10%

Ingredients: Lactose, ascorbic acid, microcrystalline cellulose, gelatin, dl-alpha-tocopheryl acetate, niacinamide, starch, calcium pantothenate, sodium caseinate, hydroxypropyl methylcellulose, sucrose, povidone, pyridoxine hydrochloride, riboflavin, silicon dioxide, magnesium stearate, thiamine mononitrate, vitamin A acetate, polyethylene glycol, triacetin, stearic acid, titanium dioxide, annatto, beta carotene, FD&C Red 40, folic acid, biotin, ergocalciferol, cyanocobalamin.

Warning: Close tightly and keep out of reach of children.

Recommended Adult Intake—1 tablet daily.

How Supplied: Packs of 130; and Unimatic® cartons of 100.

Storage: Store at room temperature; avoid excessive heat.
Shown in Product Identification Guide, page 505

COMPLETE FORMULA THERAGRAN-M® TABLETS
(High Potency Multivitamin Formula with Minerals)

TABLET CONTENTS:
FOR ADULTS—PERCENTAGE OF U.S. RECOMMENDED DAILY ALLOWANCE

Vitamins	Quantity	US RDA
Vitamin A	5000 IU	100%
(20% as Beta Carotene)		
Vitamin B₁	3 mg	200%
(Thiamine)		
Vitamin B₂	3.4 mg	200%
(Riboflavin)		
Vitamin B₆	3 mg	150%
Vitamin B₁₂	9 mcg	150%
Vitamin C	90 mg	150%
Vitamin D	400 IU	100%
Vitamin E	30 IU	100%
Niacin	20 mg	100%
Folate	400 mcg	100%
Pantothenic Acid	10.0 mg	100%
Biotin	30 mcg	10%

Minerals		
Iron	27 mg	150%
Copper	2 mg	100%
Iodine	150 mcg	100%
Zinc	15 mg	100%
Magnesium	100 mg	25%
Calcium	40 mg	4%
Phosphorus	31 mg	3%
Chromium	15 mcg	*
Molybdenum	15 mcg	*
Selenium	10 mcg	*
Manganese	5 mg	*
ELECTROLYTES		
Chloride	7.5 mg	*
Potassium	7.5 mg	Less than 1%

*US RDA not established.

Ingredients: Magnesium oxide, dibasic calcium phosphate, lactose, ascorbic acid, ferrous fumarate, gelatin, dl-alpha tocopheryl, acetate, crospovidone, niacinamide, hydroxypropyl methylcellulose, zinc oxide, povidone, manganese sulfate, potassium starch, chloride, calcium pantothenate, cupric sulfate, pyridoxine hydrochloride, magnesium stearate, sucrose, silicon dioxide, riboflavin, thiamine mononitrate, stearic acid, polyethylene glycol, triacetin, Vitamin A acetate, FD&C Red 40, potassium citrate, beta carotene, titanium dioxide, folic acid, potassium iodide, FD&C Blue No. 2, chromic chloride, sodium molybdate, biotin, sodium selenate, ergocalciferol, cyanocobalamin

Warning: Close tightly and keep out of reach of children. Contains Iron, which can be harmful or fatal to children in large doses. In case of accidental overdose, seek professional assistance or contact a poison control center immediately.

Usage: For adults—1 tablet daily

How Supplied: Packs of 90, 130 and 240.

Storage: Store at room temperature; avoid excessive heat.
Shown in Product Identification Guide, page 505

THERAPEUTIC MINERAL ICE®

Composition:
Active Ingredient: Menthol 2%
Other Ingredients: Ammonium Hydroxide, Carbomer 934, Cupric Sulfate, FD&C Blue No. 1, Isopropyl Alcohol, Magnesium Sulfate, Sodium Hydroxide, Thymol, Water.

Indications: For the temporary relief of minor aches and pains of muscles and joints associated with arthritis, simple backache, strains, bruises, sprains and sports injuries. **USE ONLY AS DIRECTED. Read all warnings before use.**

Warnings: KEEP OUT OF THE REACH OF CHILDREN. For external use only. Not for internal use. Avoid contact with eyes and mucous membranes.

Continued on next page

Bristol-Myers—Cont.

Do not use with other ointments, creams, sprays, or liniments. **Do not use with Heating Pads or Heating Devices.** If condition worsens, or if symptoms persist for more than 7 days, or clear up and occur again within a few days, discontinue use of this product and consult your doctor. Do not apply to wounds or damaged skin. Do not bandage tightly. If you have sensitive skin, consult doctor before use. If skin irritation develops, discontinue use and consult your doctor. As with any drug, if you are pregnant or nursing a baby, seek the advice of a health professional before using this product. Keep cap tightly closed. Do not use, pour, spill or store near heat or open flame. **Note:** You can always use Mineral Ice as directed, but its use is never intended to replace your doctor's advice.

Directions: Adults and children 2 years of age and older: Clean skin of all other ointments, creams, sprays, or liniments. Apply to affected areas not more than 3 to 4 times daily. May be used with wet or dry bandages or with ice packs. No protective cover needed. Children under 2 years of age: Consult a doctor.

How Supplied:
NDC 19810-0034-4 3.5 oz.
NDC 19810-0034-2 8 oz.
NDC 19810-0034-3 16 oz.
Store at room temperature.
Shown in Product Identification Guide, page 505

W.K. Buckley, Inc.
P.O. BOX 5022
WESTPORT, CT 06881-5022

BUCKLEY'S MIXTURE

Each teaspoonful (5mL) contains 12.5 mg dextromethorphan hydrobromide in a sugar-free base. Also contains: ammonium carbonate, camphor, Canada balsam, carrageenan, glycerine, menthol, pine needle oil, sodium butylparaben and sodium propylparaben (as preservatives), sodium saccharin, tincture of calcium, water.

Indications: Temporarily relieves coughs due to minor throat and bronchial irritation as may occur with a cold.

Dosage and Administration: ADULT: One and a half teaspoonsful every four hours. CHILDREN: 6 to 12 years—Three quarters of a teaspoonful every four hours. Do not exceed recommended dosage or give to children under 6 years of age unless directed by a physician.

Warnings: A persistent cough may be a sign of a serious condition. If a cough persists for more than 1 week, tends to recur, or is accompanied by fever, rash, or persistent headache, consult a doctor. Do not take this product for persistent or chronic cough such as occurs with smoking, asthma, emphysema, or if a cough is accompanied by excessive phlegm (mu-

cus) unless directed by a doctor. As with any drug, if you are pregnant or nursing a baby, seek professional advice before using this product.

Drug Interaction Precaution: Do not take this product if you are presently taking a prescription monoamine oxidase inhibitor without first consulting your doctor.

Keep this and all drugs out of reach of children: In case of accidental overdose, seek professional assistance or contact a poison control center immediately. Store at controlled room temperature between 15°C and 30°C (59°F and 86°F).

How Supplied: Bottles of 4 fl oz and 8 fl oz.

Shown in Product Identification Guide, page 505

Campbell Laboratories Inc.
700 W. HILLSBORO BLVD.
(#2-107)
DEERFIELD BEACH, FL 33441

HERPECIN-L® Cold Sore Lip Balm
[*her "puh-sin-el "*]

PRODUCT OVERVIEW

Key Facts: HERPECIN-L Lip Balm is a convenient, easy-to-use treatment for perioral herpes simplex infections. Sunscreens provide an SPF of 15.

Major Uses: HERPECIN-L not only treats cold sores, sun and fever blisters, but with prophylactic use, its sunscreens also protect to help prevent them. Users report early use at the prodromal stages of an attack will often abort the lesions and prevent scabbing. Prescribe: Apply "early, often and liberally."

Safety Information: For topical use only. A rare sensitivity may occur.

PRESCRIBING INFORMATION
HERPECIN-L® Cold Sore Lip Balm

Composition: A soothing, emollient, lip balm incorporating the sunscreen, Padimate O, and allantoin, in a balanced, slightly acidic lipid base that includes petrolatum and titanium dioxide at a cosmetically acceptable level. (Does not contain any caines, antibiotics, phenol or camphor.) (NDC 38083-777-31)

Actions and Uses: HERPECIN-L relieves dryness and chapping by providing a lipid barrier to help restore normal moisture balance to the lips. Skin protectants help to soften the crusts and scabs of "cold sores." The sunscreen is effective in 2900-3200 AU range while titanium dioxide, though at low levels, helps to block, scatter and reflect the sun's rays. Applied as a lip balm, SPF is 15. Reapply often during sun exposure.

Administration: (1) *Recurrent "cold sores, sun and fever blisters":* Simply put, use **soon** and **often**. Frequent sufferers report that with *prophylactic* use

(BID/PRN), attacks are fewer and less severe. Most recurrent herpes labialis patients are aware of the prodromal symptoms: tingling, itching, burning. At this stage, or if the lesion has already developed, HERPECIN-L should be applied liberally as often as convenient —at least *every hour.* (2) *Outdoor protection:* Apply before and during sun exposure, after swimming and again at bedtime (h.s.). (3) *Dry, chapped lips:* Apply as needed.

Adverse Reactions: If sensitive to any of the ingredients, discontinue use.

Contraindications: None.

How Supplied: 2.8 gm. swivel tubes.

Samples Available: Yes. (Request on professional letterhead or Rx pad.)

Care-Tech Laboratories
Div. of Consolidated Chemical, Inc.
3224 SOUTH KINGSHIGHWAY BOULEVARD
ST. LOUIS, MO 63139

BARRI–CARE®

Composition: Active Ingredient: Chloroxylenol
Inactive Ingredients: Petrolatum, Water, Paraffin, Propylene Glycol, Milk Protein, Cod Liver Oil, Aloe Vera Gel, Fragrance, Potassium Hydroxide, Methyl Paraben, Propyl Paraben, Vitamin A & D_3, (E) dl Alpha-Tocopheryl Acetate, (E) dl-Alpha-Tocopherol, D&C Yellow #11 and D&C Red #17.

Actions and Uses: Barri-Care is an antimicrobial ointment formulated to provide a moisture proof barrier against urine, detergent irritants, feces and drainage from wounds or skin lesions. Proven antimicrobial action against E. coli, MRSA, S. aureus and Pseudomonas aeruginosa. Protects perineal area of the incontinent patient from painful skin rashes and relieves irritation around stoma sites. Utilize on Grades I–IV pressure ulcers to halt skin breakdown. Can be used also on minor burns. Will not melt under feverish conditions.

Precautions: External Use Only. Non-Toxic. Avoid eye contact.

Directions: Cleanse affected area with Satin thoroughly. Apply ointment topically to affected area. Reapply 2–3 times daily or as directed by physician.

How Supplied: 1 ounce tubes, 4 oz. tubes, 8 oz. jar. NDC #46706-206

CARE CREME®

Composition: Active Ingredient: Chloroxylenol
Inactive Ingredients: Water, Cetyl Alcohol, Lanolin Oil, Cod Liver Oil, Sodium Laureth Sulfate, Triethanolamine, Propylene Glycol, Petrolatum, Lanolin Alcohol, Methyl Gluceth 20 Distearate, Beeswax, Citric Acid, Methyl Paraben, Fra-

grance, Propyl Paraben, Vitamins A, D$_3$ and E-dl Alpha-Tocopherol.

Actions and Uses: Care Creme is an antimicrobial skin care creme specially formulated for use on severely dry skin such as Sjogren's Syndrome, atopic dermatitis, psoriasis, minor burns, urine or fecal exposure, scaling and inter-tissue ammonia related rash. Extremely effective on oncology radiation burns. Use at first sign of reddened skin or initial breakdown. Vitamin and oil enriched to promote skin integrity. Contains no metallic ions. Provides moisture and vitamin enriched wound treatment.

Precautions: Non-toxic, External Use Only. Avoid use around eye area.

Directions: Cleanse affected area with Satin and gently massage Care Creme into skin until completely absorbed or as directed by physician.

How Supplied: 1 ounce tubes, 4 oz. tubes, 9 oz. jar. NDC #46706-205

CLINICAL CARE® WOUND CLEANSER

Composition: Active Ingredient: Benzethonium Chloride
Inactive Ingredients: Water, Amphoteric 2, Aloe Vera Gel, DMDM Hydantoin, Citric Acid.

Actions and Uses: Clinical Care is an antimicrobial, emulsifying solution which aids in removing debris and particulate matter from open, dermal wounds. Clinical Care inhibits the growth of pathogenic organisms. Proven effective at eliminating S. aureus, P. aeruginosa, S. typhimurium, Aspergillus, E. coli, MRSA, S. pyogenes and K. pneumonia. Will not produce dermal irritation.

Precautions: External Use Only. Non-Toxic. No contra-indicators.

Directions: Spray affected area as necessary to debride. Use sterile gauze to gently remove debris and necrotic tissue at dermal surface.

How Supplied: 4 oz. spray, 12 oz. spray

CONCEPT®

Composition: Active Ingredient: Chloroxylenol
Inactive Ingredients: Water, Amphoteric 9, Polysorbate 20, PEG-150 Distearate, Cocamide DEA, Cocoyl Sarcosine, Fragrance, D&C Green #5.

Actions and Uses: Concept is a geriatric shampoo and body wash for patients whose skin is irritated by soaps and harsh detergents. Concept is non-eye irritating and reduces bacteria on the skin. Excellent for replenishing moisture in dry, flaky dermal tissues and eliminating body odors. Utilize on children over 6 months of age to address rashing or atopic dermatitis. Excellent for use on HIV and oncology patients.

Precautions: External Use Only. Non-Toxic.

Directions: Use in normal manner of bathing and shampooing. Rinse thoroughly.

How Supplied: 8 oz., Gallons

FORMULA MAGIC®

Composition: Active Ingredient: Benzethonium Chloride
Inactive Ingredients: Talc, Mineral Oil, Magnesium Carbonate, Fragrance, DMDM Hydantoin.

Actions and Uses: Formula Magic is primarily a geriatric care powder and nursing lubricant. Aids in preventing excoriation, friction chafing and eliminating odor. Antibacterial action proven effective at 99.9% inhibition where Formula Magic is applied. Excellent for use on diabetic patients, feet and under breasts to relieve redness and skin irritation.

Precautions: Non-irritating to skin, non-toxic, slightly irritating to eyes.

Directions: Apply liberally to body and rub gently into skin.

How Supplied: 4 oz. and 12 oz. NDC #46706-202

ORCHID FRESH II®
Perineal/Ostomy Cleanser

Composition: Active Ingredient: Benzethonium Chloride
Inactive Ingredients: Water, Amphoteric 2, DMDM Hydantoin, Fragrance, Citric Acid.

Actions and Uses: Orchid Fresh II is an amphoteric, topical antimicrobial cleansing solution which gently cleans and emulsifies feces and urine on the incontinent patient. Use also on stoma sites and ostomy bags to deodorize and eliminate odor. Outstanding antimicrobial action on Pseudomonas, E. coli, Staphylococcus aureus, MRSA, etc. Orchid Fresh II will aid in reducing skin breakdown.

Precautions: External Use Only, Non-Toxic—Non-Dermal Irritating

Directions: Spray topically and remove feces and urine with warm, moist washcloth. Spray directly on peristomal skin areas, clean gently and pat dry. Utilize Care Creme on reddened skin areas.

How Supplied: 4 oz., 8 oz., 16 oz. and Gallons NDC #46706-115

SATIN® ANTIMICROBIAL SKIN CLEANSER

Composition: Active Ingredient: Chloroxylenol
Inactive Ingredients: Water, Sodium Laureth Sulfate, Cocamidopropyl Betaine, PEG-8, Cocamide DEA, Glycol Stea-

rate, Lanolin Oil, Tetrasodium EDTA, D&C Yellow #10.

Actions and Uses: Satin has been specially formulated for use on sensitive or aging dermal tissue, atopic dermatitis and psoriasis. Effective in eliminating gram-positive and gram-negative pathogens such as E. coli, S. aureus, Pseudomonas, etc. Contains emollients to replenish natural oils and proteins. Satin also eliminates skin odor and dry, itchy skin.

Precautions: No contra-indicators. External use only. Non-Toxic.

Directions: Use during shower, bath or regular cleansing or as directed by physician.

How Supplied: 4 oz., 8 oz., 12 oz. 16 oz., 1 Gallon NDC #46706-101

TECHNI–CARE® SURGICAL SCRUB

Composition: Active Ingredient: Chloroxylenol 3%
Inactive Ingredients: Water, Sodium Lauryl Sulfate, Cocamide DEA, Propylene Glycol, Cocamidopropyl Betaine, Cocamidopropyl PG-Dimonium Chloride Phosphate, Citric Acid, Tetrasodium EDTA, Aloe Vera Gel, Hydrolyzed Animal Protein, D&C Yellow #10.

Actions and Uses: Techni-Care represents entirely new technology in a broad-spectrum, topical, antiseptic microbicide for skin degerming. 99.99% Bacterial reduction in 30 second contact usage. Techni-Care may be used for disinfection of wounds, for pre-op and post-op along with surgical scrub applications. Non-staining and non-irritating to dermal tissue. Techni-Care conditions dermal tissue and promotes more rapid rate of healing.

Precautions: Non-Toxic, Non-Irritating, External Use Only. Can be used safely around ears and eyes or as directed by a physician.

Directions: Apply, lather and rinse well. For pre-op, apply and let dry, no rinsing required.

How Supplied: 20 mL packets, 8 oz., 16 oz., 32 oz., Gallons and peel paks

---

UNKNOWN DRUG?
Consult the
Product Identification Guide
(Gray Pages)
for full-color photos of
leading over-the-counter
medications

J. R. Carlson Laboratories, Inc.
15 COLLEGE DR.
ARLINGTON HEIGHTS, IL 60004

ACES®
Vitamin, Antioxidants

Description: ACES provides four natural antioxidant nutrients.

Two Soft Gels Contain: % U.S. RDA

Beta-Carotene
(Pro-Vitamin A) 10,000 IU 200%
Vitamin C (Calcium
Ascorbate) 1,000 mg 1667%
Vitamin E (d-Alpha
Tocopherol) 400 IU 1333%
Selenium
(L-Selenomethionine) 100 mcg .... *

RDA: Recommended Daily Allowance -
Adults
*U.S. RDA not determined

The nutrients in ACES are: Beta-Carotene (Pro-vitamin A) derived from tiny sea plants or algae (D. salina) grown in the fresh ocean waters off southern Australia; Vitamin C provided as the gentle, buffered calcium ascorbate; Vitamin E 100% natural-source from soy, the most biologically active form; and Selenium, organically bound with the essential nutrient methionine to promote assimilation.

Suggested Use: For dietary supplementation, take two soft gels daily, preferably at mealtime.
CORN-Free, WHEAT-Free, MILK-Free, SUGAR-Free, YEAST-Free, PRESERVATIVE-Free, Soft Gel Contents: Nutrients listed above, soybean oil, vegetable stearin, lecithin, beeswax, Soft Gel Shell: Beef gelatin, glycerin, water, carob.

How Supplied: In bottles of 50, 90, 200, and 360.
Also available as ACES (R) plus ZINC.

E-GEMS®
Vitamins, Antioxidants

Description: 100% natural-source vitamin E (d-alpha tocopheryl acetate) soft gels. Available in 8 strengths: 30IU, 100IU, 200IU, 400IU, 600IU, 800IU, 1000IU, 1200IU.

How Supplied: Supplied in a variety of bottle sizes.

**Rx DRUG INFORMATION
AT THE TOUCH OF BUTTON**
Join the thousands of doctors
using the handheld, electronic
Pocket PDR.
Use the order form
in the front of this book.

Cartilage Technologies, Inc.
200 CLEARBROOK ROAD
ELMSFORD, NY 10523

CARTILADE® Shark Cartilage Powder, Capsules & Caplets

Available in: POWDER: 200g, 500g, 1400g; CAPSULES: 42's, 90's, 180's, 360's; CAPLETS: 42's, 90's, 180's, 360's

Indication: As a Dietary Supplement

Description: CARTILADE®, 100% pure Shark Cartilage, powder, capsules & caplets contain no sugar, salt, color, or preservatives, and is low in sodium, and fat and cholesterol free. The detectable preservative residue is controlled and kept within the limits allowed in food items as per guidance in 40 CFR 180.151. The active ingredient in CARTILADE® is Shark Cartilage, a natural dietary supplement, which is composed primarily of protein, calcium, phosphorus and a family of carbohydrates called mucopolysaccharides. CARTILADE® can be added to the diet as a natural supplment of calcium and phosphorus, and is free of adverse side effects.

Directions as a Dietary Supplement: POWDER: 4.4g, stirred in an 8oz glass of cool water, fruit juice or vegetable juice, and taken orally, preferably 15 minutes before breakfast.
CAPSULES/CAPLETS: Two (2) capsules/caplets, taken orally, preferably 15 minutes before each meal, three (3) times a day.

How Supplied:
POWDER: Packaged in high density, polyethylene (HDPE) bottles.
CAPSULES: Hard gel, two piece capsules, packaged in HDPE bottles. Each capsule contains 740mg of CARTILADE®.
CAPLETS: Packaged in HDPE bottles. Contains 740mg of CARTILADE®.

% US RDA:

	Powder 4.4g	Capsules 6 caps/day	Caplets 6 c.l/day
Protein	3	4	3
Calcium	90	90	90
Phosphorus	40	40	40
Magnesium	4	4	4
Zinc	2	2	2

Contraindications: If you are pregnant, nursing a baby, recovering from recent surgery or have a heart-circulatory condition, consult a health care professional before using this product.

Shown in Product Identification Guide, page 505

Chesebrough-Pond's USA Co.
33 BENEDICT PLACE
GREENWICH, CT 06830

DERMASIL™ DRY SKIN TREATMENT LOTION

Active Ingredient: dimethicone

Other Ingredients: water, petrolatum, glycerin, mineral oil, stearic acid, sunflower seed oil, glycol stearate, cetyl acetate, glyceryl stearate, TEA, lecithin, borage seed oil, cholesterol, ascorbyl, palmitate, carbomer, PEG-40 stearate, cetyl alcohol, acetylated lanolin alcohol, magnesium aluminum silicate, palmarosa oil, rose extract, sweet almond oil, sandalwood oil, vanilla, ethylene brassylate, stearamide amp, disodium EDTA, methylparaben, propylparaben, DMDM hydantoin.

Indications/Actions: Suitable for severe dry skin, and control of symptoms such as chapping, cracking, flaking, roughness, redness, soreness, and the itch associated with dry skin. This lotion contains four systems to control, and provide long-lasting relief from severe dry skin:
* Occlusives to block moisture loss from the skin's surface
* Humectant to bind water in the skins outermost layers
* Skin lipids to enhance the skin's natural ability to retain moisture
* EFA's an important component of the skin's moisture barrier
Hypoallergenic and fragrance free.

Directions: Apply as needed to areas of dry skin. Use in combination with Dermasil concentrated Treatment on patches of extreme dryness, such as fingertips and knuckles.

Warnings: Keep out of reach of children. For external use only. Avoid contact with eyes. If condition worsens or does not improve within seven days, consult a doctor or pharmacist. Not to be applied over deep or puncture wounds, infections or lacerations.

How Supplied: 8 oz. (236 ml.)
4 oz. (118 ml.)

DERMASIL™ DRY SKIN TREATMENT CREAM

Active Ingredient: Dimethicone

Other Ingredients: Water, petrolatum, myreth-3 myristate, glycerin, sunflower seed oil, cetearyl alcohol, TEA, lecithin, borage seed oil, cholesterol, stearic acid, carbomer, ceteareth-20, palmarosa oil, rose extract, sweet almond oil, sandalwood oil, vanilla, ethylene brassylate, methylparaben, propylparaben, DMDM hydantoin.

Indications/Actions: Suitable for severe dry skin, and control of symptoms such as chapping, cracking, flaking, roughness, soreness, and the itching associated with dry skin. This cream contains four systems to control, and provide long-lasting relief from severe dry skin:

- Occlusives to block moisture loss from the skin's surface
- Humectant to bind water in the skin's outermost layers
- Skin lipids to enhance the skin's natural ability to retain moisture
- EFA's an important compound of the skin's moisture barrier

Hypoallergenic and fragrance free.

Directions: Apply as needed to areas of dry skin. Use in combination with Dermasil Treatment on patches of extreme dryness, such as fingertips and knuckles.

Warning: Keep out of reach of children. For external use only. Avoid contact with eyes. If condition worsens or does not improve within seven days, consult a doctor or pharmacist. Not to be applied over deep or puncture wounds, infections and lacerations.

How Supplied: 4 oz. (113 g.)
2 oz. (56 g.)

DERMASIL™ DRY SKIN TREATMENT
Concentrated Treatment

Active Ingredients: Glycerin, dimethicone

Other Ingredients: Cyclomethicone, water, sunflower seed oil, petrolatum, oleth-10, soya sterol, borage seed oil, lecithin, tocopheryl acetate (Vitamin E acetate), retinyl palmitate (Vitamin A palmitate), cholecalciferol (Vitamin D$_3$), ascorbyl palmitate, stearic acid, TEA, carbomer, corn oil, disodium EDTA, methylparaben, DMDM hydantoin, iodopropynyl butylcarbamate.

Indications/Actions: Suitable for severe dry skin, and the control of symptoms such as chapping, cracking, flaking, roughness, redness, soreness, and the itching associated with dry skin. This concentrated treatment contains four systems to control and provide long-lasting relief from severe dry skin:

- Occlusives to block moisture loss from the skin's surface
- Humectant to bind water in the skin's outermost layers
- Skin lipids to enhance the skin's natural ability to retain moisture
- EFA's an important component of the skin's moisture barrier

Hypoallergenic and fragrance free.

Directions: Apply sparingly. Use in combination with Dermasil Lotion or Cream on patches of extreme dryness, such as fingertips and knuckles.

Warnings: Keep out of reach of children. For external use only. Avoid contact with eyes. If condition worsens or does not improve within seven days, consult a doctor or pharmacist. Not to be applied over deep or puncture wounds, infections or lacerations.

How Supplied: 1 oz. (28 g.)

VASELINE® INTENSIVE CARE®
Extra Strength LOTION

Active Ingredient: Dimethicone

How Supplied: 6 oz., 10 oz. and 15 oz.

VASELINE®
100% Pure Petroleum Jelly Skin Protectant

Composition: White Petrolatum U.S.P.

How Supplied: 1 oz. and 2.5 oz. plastic tubes. (NDC 0521-8120-01, -31). 1.75 oz., 3.75 oz., 7.5 oz., and 13 oz. plastic jars (NDC 0521-8120-24, -28, -29, -32).

VASELINE PETROLEUM JELLY CREAM
CREAMY FORMULA

Active Ingredient: Petrolatum

How Supplied: 4.75 oz (134 g)
4.5 oz (127 g)
2 oz (57 g)
.85 oz (24 g)

Church & Dwight Co., Inc.
**469 N. HARRISON STREET
PRINCETON, NJ 08540**

ARM & HAMMER®
Pure Baking Soda

Active Ingredient: Sodium Bicarbonate U.S.P.

Indications: For alleviation of acid indigestion, also known as heartburn or sour stomach. Not a remedy for other types of stomach complaints such as nausea, stomachache, abdominal cramps, gas pains, or stomach distention caused by overeating and/or overdrinking. In the latter case, one should not ingest solids, liquids or antacid but rather refrain from all physical activity and—if uncomfortable—call a physician.

Actions: ARM & HAMMER® Pure Baking Soda provides fast-acting, effective neutralization of stomach acids. Each level ½ teaspoon dose will neutralize 20.9 mEq of acid.

Warnings: Except under the advice and supervision of a physician: (1) do not administer to children under five years of age, (2) do not take more than eight level ½ teaspoons per person up to 60 years old or four level ½ teaspoons per person 60 years or older in a 24-hour period, (3) do not use this product if you are on a sodium restricted diet, (4) do not use the maximum dose for more than two weeks, (5) do not ingest food, liquid or any antacid when stomach is overly full to avoid possible injury to the stomach.

Dosage and Administration: Level ½ teaspoon in ½ glass (4 fl. oz.) of water every two hours up to maximum dosage or as directed by a physician. Accurately measure level ½ teaspoon. Each level ½ teaspoon contains 20.9 mEq (.476 gm) sodium.

How Supplied: Available in 8 oz., 16 oz., 32 oz., and 64 oz. boxes.

CIBA Consumer Pharmaceuticals
**Division of CIBA-GEIGY Corporation
MACK WOODBRIDGE II
581 MAIN STREET
WOODBRIDGE, NJ 07095**

ALLEREST® MAXIMUM STRENGTH TABLETS, NO DROWSINESS TABLETS, HEADACHE STRENGTH TABLETS, SINUS PAIN FORMULA TABLETS, CHILDREN'S CHEWABLE TABLETS AND 12 HOUR CAPLETS

Active Ingredients:
Maximum Strength Tablets —Chlorpheniramine maleate 2 mg, pseudoephedrine HCl 30 mg.
No Drowsiness Tablets —Acetaminophen 325 mg, pseudoephedrine HCl 30 mg.
Headache Strength Tablets —Acetaminophen 325 mg, chlorpheniramine maleate 2 mg, pseudoephedrine HCl 30 mg.
Sinus Pain Formula Tablets — Acetaminophen 500 mg, chlorpheniramine maleate 2 mg, pseudoephedrine HCl 30 mg.
Children's Chewable Tablets —Chlorpheniramine maleate 1 mg, phenylpropanolamine HCl 9.4 mg.
12 Hour Caplets —Chlorpheniramine maleate 12 mg, phenylpropanolamine HCl 75 mg.

Other Ingredients:
Maximum Strength Tablets —Blue 1 lake, dibasic calcium phosphate, magnesium stearate, microcrystalline cellulose, povidone, pregelatinized starch, sodium starch glycolate. *No Drowsiness and Headache Strength Tablets* —Magnesium stearate, microcrystalline cellulose, povidone, pregelatinized starch. *Sinus Pain Formula Tablets* —Magnesium stearate, microcrystalline cellulose, povidone, pregelatinized starch, sodium starch glycolate. *Children's Chewable Tablets* —Calcium stearate, citric acid, flavor, magnesium trisilicate, mannitol, saccharin sodium, sorbitol.

Continued on next page

The full prescribing information for each CIBA Consumer Pharmaceuticals product is contained herein and is that in effect as of December 15, 1994

CIBA Consumer—Cont.

12 Hour Caplets —Carnauba wax, colloidal silicon dioxide, lactose, methylcellulose, polyethylene glycol, povidone, Red 30, stearic acid, titanium dioxide, Yellow 6.

Indications: *Maximum Strength, Headache Strength, Sinus Pain Formula, Children's Chewable Tablets and 12 Hour Caplets* —Temporarily relieves nasal congestion, runny nose, sneezing, itching of the nose or throat, and itchy, watery eyes due to hay fever or other upper respiratory allergies; also *Headache Strength and Sinus Pain Formula Tablets* —For the temporary relief of minor aches, pains, and headache; also *12 Hour Caplets* —For temporary relief of nasal congestion due to the common cold, hay fever or other upper respiratory allergies, or associated with sinusitis.
No Drowsiness Tablets —Temporarily relieves nasal congestion due to hay fever, other upper respiratory allergies, or the common cold, or associated with sinusitis. For the temporary relief of minor aches, pains, and headache.

Warnings: *All Products* —Do not exceed recommended dosage because at higher doses, nervousness, dizziness, or sleeplessness may occur. Do not take this product if you have heart disease, high blood pressure, thyroid disease, diabetes, or difficulty in urination due to enlargement of the prostate gland, unless directed by a physician. As with any drug, if you are pregnant or nursing a baby, seek the advice of a health professional before using this product. **Keep this and all drugs out of the reach of children.** In case of accidental overdose, seek professional assistance or contact a Poison Control Center immediately. Prompt medical attention (for products containing acetaminophen) is critical for adults as well as children even if you do not notice any signs or symptoms. And, *All Products Except No Drowsiness Tablets* —Do not take this product if you have a breathing problem such as emphysema or chronic bronchitis, or if you have glaucoma, unless directed by a physician. May cause excitability, especially in children. May cause drowsiness; alcohol, sedatives, and tranquilizers may increase the drowsiness effect. Avoid alcoholic beverages while taking this product. Do not take this product if you are taking sedatives or tranquilizers, without first consulting your physician. Use caution when driving a motor vehicle or operating machinery.
Maximum Strength Tablets, Children's Chewable Tablets and 12 Hour Caplets —Do not take this product for more than 7 days. If symptoms do not improve or are accompanied by fever, consult a physician.
Headache Strength, Sinus Pain Formula, and No Drowsiness Tablets —Do not take this product for more than 10 days (for adults) or 5 days (for children). If symptoms do not improve or are accompanied

by fever that lasts more than 3 days, or if new symptoms occur, consult a physician.

Drug Interaction Precaution: *All Products* —Do not take this product if you are presently taking a prescription drug for high blood pressure or depression, without first consulting your physician; and *Children's Chewable Tablets* —Do not take this product if you are presently taking another medication containing phenylpropanolamine.

Directions: Dose as follows while symptoms persist, or as directed by a physician.
Maximum Strength, No Drowsiness and Headache Strength Tablets —Adults and children 12 years of age and over: 2 tablets every 4 to 6 hours, not to exceed 8 tablets in 24 hours. Children 6 to under 12 years of age: 1 tablet every 4 to 6 hours, not to exceed 4 tablets in 24 hours. Children under 6 years of age: Consult a physician.
Sinus Pain Formula Tablets —Adults and children 12 years of age and over: 2 tablets every 6 hours, not to exceed 8 tablets in 24 hours. Children under 12 years of age: Consult a physician.
Children's Chewable Tablets —Children 6 to under 12 years of age: 2 tablets every 4 to 6 hours, not to exceed 8 tablets in 24 hours. Children under 6 years of age: Consult a physician.
12 Hour Caplets —Adults and children 12 years of age and over: 1 caplet swallowed whole every 12 hours, not to exceed 2 caplets in 24 hours.

How Supplied:
Maximum Strength Tablets —Boxes of 24, 48, and 72.
No Drowsiness Tablets —Boxes of 20.
Headache Strength Tablets —Boxes of 24.
Sinus Pain Formula Tablets —Boxes of 20.
Children's Chewable Tablets —Boxes of 24.
12 Hour Caplets —Boxes of 10.
ALLEREST is a registered trademark of Ciba-Geigy Corporation

ACUTRIM® 16 HOUR* STEADY CONTROL APPETITE SUPPRESSANT TABLETS
Caffeine Free

ACUTRIM® MAXIMUM STRENGTH APPETITE SUPPRESSANT TABLETS
Caffeine Free

ACUTRIM LATE DAY® STRENGTH* APPETITE SUPPRESSANT TABLETS
Caffeine Free

Description: ACUTRIM® tablets are an aid to appetite control in conjunction with a sensible weight loss program. ACUTRIM® tablets deliver their maximum strength dosage of appetite suppressant at a precisely controlled rate.

This timed release is scientifically targeted to effectively distribute the appetite suppressant all day.*
ACUTRIM makes it easier to follow the kind of reduced calorie diet needed for best weight control results.
A diet plan developed by an expert dietician is included in the package for your personal use as a further aid.

Formula: Each ACUTRIM® tablet contains: Active Ingredient—phenylpropanolamine HCl 75 mg (appetite suppressant, time release).
Inactive Ingredients—ACUTRIM® 16 HOUR Steady Control: Cellulose Acetate, Hydroxypropyl Methylcellulose, Stearic Acid—ACUTRIM® MAXIMUM STRENGTH: Cellulose Acetate, D&C Yellow #10, FD&C Blue #1, FD&C Yellow #6, Hydroxypropyl Methylcellulose, Povidone, Propylene Glycol, Stearic Acid, Titanium Dioxide—ACUTRIM LATE DAY® Strength: Cellulose Acetate, FD&C Yellow #6, Hydroxypropyl Methylcellulose, Isopropyl Alcohol, Propylene Glycol, Riboflavin, Stearic Acid, Titanium Dioxide.

Directions: Adult oral dosage is **one tablet** at mid-morning with a full glass of water. SWALLOW EACH TABLET WHOLE; DO NOT DIVIDE, CRUSH, CHEW, OR DISSOLVE THE TABLET. Exceeding the recommended dose has not been shown to result in greater weight loss. This product's effectiveness is directly related to the degree to which you reduce your usual daily food intake. Attempts at weight reduction which involve the use of this product should be limited to periods not exceeding 3 months, because this should be enough time to establish new eating habits. Read and follow important Diet Plan enclosed.
WARNINGS: FOR ADULT USE ONLY. Do not take more than one tablet per day (24 hours). Exceeding the recommended dose may cause serious health problems. Do not give this product to children under 12 years of age. Persons between 12 and 18 are advised to consult their physician before using this product. If nervousness, dizziness, sleeplessness, palpitations or headache occurs, stop taking this medication and consult your physician. If you are being treated for high blood pressure, depression, or an eating disorder or have heart disease, diabetes, or thyroid disease, do not take this product except under the supervision of a physician. As with any drug, if you are pregnant or nursing a baby, seek the advice of a health professional before using this product.
DRUG INTERACTION PRECAUTION: If you are taking a cough/cold or allergy medication containing any form of phenylpropanolamine, or any type of nasal decongestant, do not take this product. Do not take this product if you are taking any prescription drug, except under the advice and supervision of a physician. Do not use this product if you are presently taking a prescription monoamine oxidase inhibitor (MAOI) for

depression or for two weeks after stopping use of a MAOI without first consulting a physician.

KEEP THIS AND ALL MEDICATION OUT OF THE REACH OF CHILDREN. In case of accidental overdose, seek professional assistance or contact a Poison Control Center immediately.

How Supplied: Tamper-evident blister packages of 20 and 40 tablets. Do not use if individual seals are broken.
DO NOT STORE ABOVE 30°C (86°F). PROTECT FROM MOISTURE.
*Peak strength and extent of duration relate solely to blood levels.
Shown in Product Identification Guide, page 505

AMERICAINE® HEMORRHOIDAL OINTMENT
[a-mer'i-kān]

Active Ingredient: Benzocaine 20%.

Other Ingredients: Benzethonium chloride, polyethylene glycol 300, polyethylene glycol 3350.

Indications: For the temporary relief of local pain, itching and soreness associated with hemorrhoids and anorectal inflammation.

Warnings: If condition worsens, or does not improve within 7 days, consult a physician. Do not exceed the recommended daily dosage unless directed by a physician. In case of bleeding, consult a physician promptly. Do not put this product into the rectum by using fingers or any mechanical device or applicator. Certain persons can develop allergic reactions to ingredients in this product. If the symptom being treated does not subside or if redness, irritation, swelling, pain, or other symptoms develop or increase, discontinue use and consult a physician. **Keep this and all drugs out of the reach of children.** In case of accidental ingestion, seek professional assistance or contact a Poison Control Center immediately.

Directions: *Adults:* When practical, cleanse the affected area with mild soap and warm water and rinse thoroughly. Gently dry by patting or blotting with toilet tissue or a soft cloth before application of this product. Apply externally to the affected area up to 6 times daily. *Children under 12 years of age:* Consult a physician.

How Supplied: *Hemorrhoidal Ointment* —1 oz. tube.
Store at 15°–30°C (59°–86°F).
AMERICAINE is a registered trademark of Ciba-Geigy Corporation.
Shown in Product Identification Guide, page 505

AMERICAINE® TOPICAL ANESTHETIC SPRAY AND FIRST AID OINTMENT
[a-mer'i-kān]

Active Ingredient: Benzocaine 20%.

Other Ingredients: *Spray* —isobutane (propellant), polyethylene glycol 300, propane (propellant). *Ointment* —Benzethonium chloride, polyethylene glycol 300, polyethylene glycol 3350.

Indications: For the temporary relief of pain and itching associated with minor cuts, scrapes, burns, sunburn, insect bites, or minor skin irritations.

Warnings: For external use only. Avoid contact with the eyes. If condition worsens, or if symptoms persist for more than 7 days or clear up and occur again within a few days, discontinue use of this product and consult a physician. **Keep this and all drugs out of the reach of children.** In case of accidental ingestion, seek professional assistance or contact a Poison Control Center immediately. *For Spray only* —Contents under pressure. Do not puncture or incinerate. Flammable mixture; do not use near fire or flame. Do not store at temperature above 120°F. Use only as directed. Intentional misuse by deliberately concentrating and inhaling the contents can be harmful or fatal.

Directions: Adults and children 2 years of age and older: Apply liberally to affected area not more than 3 to 4 times daily. Children under 2 years of age: Consult a physician.

How Supplied: *Topical Anesthetic Spray* —⅔ oz., 2 oz. and 4 oz. aerosol containers. *First Aid Ointment* —¾ oz. tube, which is a clear, fragrance-free gel formula that is nonstaining, easy to apply, and is easily removed with soap and water.
Store at 15°–30°C (59°–86°F).
AMERICAINE is a registered trademark of Ciba-Geigy Corporation.
Shown in Product Identification Guide, page 505

Regular Strength ASCRIPTIN®
[ă"skrĭp'tin]
Analgesic
Aspirin buffered with Maalox®for stomach comfort

Active Ingredients: Each tablet contains Aspirin (325 mg), buffered with Maalox® (Alumina-Magnesia) and Calcium Carbonate.

Inactive Ingredients: Hydroxypropyl Methylcellulose, Magnesium Stearate, Microcrystalline Cellulose, Starch, Talc, Titanium Dioxide, and other ingredients.

Description: Ascriptin is an excellent analgesic, antipyretic, and anti-inflammatory agent for general use, particularly where there is concern over aspirin-induced gastric distress. Coated tablets make swallowing easy.

Indications: As an analgesic for the temporary relief of minor pain in such conditions as headache, neuralgia, minor injuries, and dysmenorrhea. As an analgesic and antipyretic in adult colds. As an analgesic and anti-inflammatory agent for the minor aches and pains of arthritis and other rheumatic diseases. As an inhibitor of platelet aggregation, see MI's and TIA's indications.

Usual Adult Dose: Two tablets with water every 4 hours while symptoms persist; do not exceed 12 tablets in 24 hours, or as directed by a doctor. For children under twelve, consult a doctor.

WARNINGS: Children and teenagers should not use this medicine for chicken pox or flu symptoms before a doctor is consulted about Reye syndrome, a rare but serious illness reported to be associated with aspirin. Keep this and all medicines out of children's reach. If pain persists more than 10 days, redness or swelling is present, fever persists more than 3 days, or symptoms worsen, consult a doctor immediately. If you are under medical care or have a history of stomach, kidney, or bleeding disorders or asthma, consult a doctor before using. Do not use if allergic to aspirin. As with any drug, if you are pregnant or nursing a baby, consult a doctor before using. **IT IS ESPECIALLY IMPORTANT NOT TO USE ASPIRIN DURING THE LAST 3 MONTHS OF PREGNANCY UNLESS SPECIFICALLY DIRECTED TO DO SO BY A DOCTOR BECAUSE IT MAY CAUSE PROBLEMS IN THE UNBORN CHILD OR COMPLICATIONS DURING DELIVERY.** If ringing in the ears or loss of hearing occurs, consult a doctor before taking any more of this product. **In case of accidental overdose, contact a doctor immediately.**
Drug Interaction Precaution: Do not use if taking a prescription drug for anticoagulation (blood thinning), diabetes, gout or arthritis, or a tetracycline antibiotic unless directed by a doctor.

Professional Labeling
ASCRIPTIN FOR MYOCARDIAL INFARCTION

Indication: Aspirin is indicated to reduce the risk of death and/or non-fatal myocardial infarction in patients with a previous infarction or unstable angina pectoris.

Clinical Trials: The indication is supported by the results of six, large, randomized multicenter, placebo-controlled studies[1-7] involving 10,816, predominantly male, post-myocardial infarction (MI) patients and one randomized placebo-controlled study of 1,266 men with

Continued on next page

The full prescribing information for each CIBA Consumer Pharmaceuticals product is contained herein and is that in effect as of December 15, 1994

CIBA Consumer—Cont.

unstable angina. Therapy with aspirin was begun at intervals after the onset of acute MI varying from less than 3 days to more than 5 years and continued for periods of from less than one year to four years. In the unstable angina study, treatment was started within 1 month after the onset of unstable angina and continued for 12 weeks and patients with complicating conditions such as congestive heart failure were not included in the study.

Aspirin therapy in MI patients was associated with about a 20 percent reduction in the risk of subsequent death and/or nonfatal reinfarction, a median absolute decrease of 3 percent from the 12 to 22 percent event rates in the placebo groups. In the aspirin-treated unstable angina patients the reduction in risk was about 50 percent, a reduction in the event rate of 5% from the 10% rate in the placebo group over the 12 weeks of the study.

Daily dosage of aspirin in the post-myocardial infarction studies was 300 mg. in one study and 900 and 1500 mg. in five studies. A dose of 325 mg. was used in the study of unstable angina.

Adverse Reactions: Gastrointestinal Reactions:

Doses of 1000 mg. per day of aspirin caused gastrointestinal symptoms and bleeding that in some cases were clinically significant. In the largest post-infarction study (The Aspirin Myocardial Infarction Study (AMIS) with 4,500 people), the percentage incidences of gastrointestinal symptoms for the aspirin (1000 mg. of a standard, solid-tablet formulation) and placebo-treated subjects, respectively, were: stomach pain (14.5%; 4.4%); heartburn (11.9%; 4.8%); nausea and/or vomiting (7.6%; 2.1%); hospitalization for gastrointestinal disorder (4.8%; 3.5%). In the AMIS and other trials, aspirin treated patients had increased rates of gross gastrointestinal bleeding. Symptoms and signs of gastrointestinal irritation were not significantly increased in subjects treated for unstable angina with buffered aspirin in solution.

Cardiovascular and Biochemical:

In the AMIS trial, the dosage of 1000 mg. per day of aspirin was associated with small increases in systolic blood pressure (BP) (average 1.5 to 2.1 mm) and diastolic BP (0.5 to 0.6 mm), depending upon whether maximal or last available readings were used. Blood urea nitrogen and uric acid levels were also increased, but by less than 1.0 mg%.

Subjects with marked hypertension or renal insufficiency had been excluded from the trial so that the clinical importance of these observations for such subjects or for any subjects treated over more prolonged periods is not known. It is recommended that patients placed on long-term aspirin treatment, even at doses of 300 mg. per day, be seen at regular intervals to assess changes in these measurements.

Dosage and Administration: Although most of the studies used dosages exceeding 300 mg, two trials used only 300 mg, and pharmacologic data indicate that this dose inhibits platelet function fully. Therefore, 300 mg or a conventional 325-mg aspirin dose is a reasonable, routine dose that would minimize gastrointestinal adverse reactions. This use of aspirin applies to both solid, oral dosage forms (buffered and plain aspirin), and buffered aspirin in solution.

References: 1. Elwood P.C., et al., "A Randomized Controlled Trial of Acetylsalicylic Acid in the Secondary Prevention of Mortality from Myocardial Infarction," *British Medical Journal,* 1:436–440, 1974. 2. The Coronary Drug Project Research Group, "Aspirin in Coronary Heart Disease," *Journal of Chronic Disease,* 29:625–642, 1976. 3. Breddin K. et al., "Secondary Prevention of Myocardial Infarction; Comparison of Acetylsalicylic Acid Phenprocoumon and Placebo," *Thromb, Haemost.,* 41:225–236. 1979. 4. Aspirin Myocardial Infarction Study Research Group, "A Randomized. Controlled Trial of Aspirin in Persons Recovered from Myocardial Infarction." *Journal American Medical Association,* 243:661–669, 1980. 5. Elwood P.C., and Sweetnam, P.M., "Aspirin and Secondary Mortality after Myocardial Infartion," *Lancet,* pp. 1313–1315, December 22–29, 1979. 6. The Persantine-Aspirin Reinfarction Study Research Group "Persantine and Aspirin in Coronary Heart Disease," *Circulation* 62;449–460. 1980. 7. Lewis H.D., et al., "Protective Effects of Aspirin Against Acute Myocardial Infarction and Death in Men with Unstable Angina, Results of a Veterans Administration Cooperative Study." *New England Journal of Medicine,* 309;396–403, 1983.

ASCRIPTIN FOR RECURRENT TIA's IN MEN

Indications: For reducing the risk of recurrent transient ischemic attacks (TIA's) or stroke in men who have had transient ischemia of the brain due to fibrin platelet emboli. There is inadequate evidence that aspirin or buffered aspirin is effective in reducing TIA's in women at the recommended dosage. There is no evidence that aspirin or buffered aspirin is of benefit in the treatment of completed strokes in men or women.

Clinical Trials: The indication is supported by the results of a Canadian study (1) in which 585 patients with threatened stroke were followed in a randomized clinical trial for an average of 26 months to determine whether aspirin or sulfinpyrazone, singly or in combination was superior to placebo in preventing transient ischemic attacks, stroke, or death. The study showed that, although sulfinpyrazone had no statistically significant effect, aspirin reduced the risk of continuing transient ischemic attacks, stroke, or death by 19 percent and reduced the risk of stroke or death by 31 percent. Another aspirin study carried

out in the United States with 178 patients, showed a statistically significant number of "favorable outcomes" including reduced transient ischemic attacks, stroke, and death (2).

Precautions: (1) Patients presenting with signs and symptoms of TIA's should have a complete medical and neurologic evaluation. Consideration should be given to other disorders which resemble TIA's. **(2)** Attention should be given to risk factors; it is important to evaluate and treat, if appropriate, other diseases associated with TIA's and stroke such as hypertension and diabetes. **(3)** Concurrent administration of absorbable antacids at therapeutic doses may increase the clearance of salicylates in some individuals. The concurrent administration of nonabsorbable antacids may alter the rate of absorption of aspirin, thereby resulting in a decreased acetylsalicylic acid/salicylate ratio in plasma. The clinical significance on TIA's of these decreases in available aspirin is unknown.

Aspirin at dosages of 1,000 milligrams per day has been associated with small increases in blood pressure, blood urea nitrogen, and serum uric acid levels. It is recommended that patients placed on long-term aspirin treatment be seen at regular intervals to assess changes in these measurements.

Adverse Reactions: At dosages of 1,000 milligrams or higher of aspirin per day, gastrointestinal side effects include stomach pain, heartburn, nausea and/or vomiting, as well as increased rates of gross gastrointestinal bleeding.

Dosage: Adults dosage for men is 1300 mg a day, in divided doses of 650 mg twice a day or 325 mg four times a day.

References: (1) The Canadian Cooperative Study Group. "A Randomized Trial of Aspirin and Sulfinpyrazone in Threatened Stroke," *New England Journal of Medicine,* 299:53–59, 1978. (2) Fields, W.S., et al., "Controlled Trial of Aspirin in Cerebral Ischemia," *Stroke* 8:301–316, 1977.

How Supplied: Bottles of 60 tablets (0067-0145-60), 100 tablets (0067-0145-68), 160 (0067-0145-30) and 225 tablets (0067-0145-77).
Bottles of 500 tablets (0067-0145-74) without child-resistant closures (for arthritic patients).

Shown in Product Identification Guide, page 505

**Maximum Strength
ASCRIPTIN®
Analgesic
Aspirin Buffered with Maalox®
for Stomach Comfort**

Active Ingredients: Each coated caplet contains Aspirin (500 mg), buffered with Maalox®(Alumina-Magnesia) and Calcium Carbonate.

Inactive Ingredients: Hydroxypropyl Methylcellulose, Magnesium Stearate, Microcrystalline Cellulose, Starch, Talc, Titanium Dioxide, and other ingredients.

Description: Maximum Strength Ascriptin contains the maximum dose of aspirin for fast, effective pain relief, and is buffered with Maalox for stomach comfort. Coated caplets make swallowing easy.

Indications: Use Maximum Strength Ascriptin for temporary relief of minor pain in headache, neuralgia, minor injuries, dysmenorrhea, discomfort and fever of ordinary colds. Also provides relief from the minor aches and pains of arthritis and rheumatism.

Usual Adult Dose: Two caplets with water every 6 hours while symptoms persist, not to exceed 8 caplets in 24 hours, or as directed by a doctor. For children under 12, consult a doctor.

WARNINGS: Children and teenagers should not use this medicine for chicken pox or flu symptoms before a doctor is consulted about Reye syndrome, a rare but serious illness reported to be associated with aspirin. Keep this and all medicines out of children's reach. If pain persists more than 10 days, redness or swelling is present, fever persists more than 3 days, or symptoms worsen, consult a doctor immediately. If you are under medical care or have a history of stomach, kidney, or bleeding disorders or asthma, consult a doctor before using. Do not use if allergic to aspirin. As with any drug, if you are pregnant or nursing a baby, consult a doctor before using.

IT IS ESPECIALLY IMPORTANT NOT TO USE ASPIRIN DURING THE LAST 3 MONTHS OF PREGNANCY UNLESS SPECIFICALLY DIRECTED TO DO SO BY A DOCTOR BECAUSE IT MAY CAUSE PROBLEMS IN THE UNBORN CHILD OR COMPLICATIONS DURING DELIVERY. If ringing in the ears or loss of hearing occurs, consult a doctor before taking any more of this product. **In case of accidental overdose, contact a doctor immediately.** *Drug interaction precaution:* Do not use if taking a prescription drug for anticoagulation (blood thinning), diabetes, gout or arthritis, or a tetracycline antibiotic unless directed by a doctor.

Professional Labeling see detail under Regular Strength Ascriptin®

How Supplied: Bottles of 60 tablets (0067-0145-60), 100 tablets (0067-0145-68), 160 (0067-0145-30) and 225 tablets (0067-0145-77).
Bottles of 500 tablets (0067-0145-74) without child-resistant closures (for arthritic patients).
Shown in Product Identification Guide, page 505

ARTHRITIS PAIN ASCRIPTIN®
Analgesic
Aspirin buffered with extra Maalox® for extra stomach comfort

Active Ingredients: Each caplet contains Aspirin (325 mg), buffered with Maalox® (Alumina-Magnesia) and Calcium Carbonate.

Inactive Ingredients: Hydroxypropyl Methylcellulose, Magnesium Stearate, Microcrystalline Cellulose, Starch, Talc, Titanium Dioxide, and other ingredients.

Description: Arthritis Pain Ascriptin is a highly buffered analgesic, anti-inflammatory, and antipyretic agent which relieves the minor pain associated with rheumatoid arthritis, osteoarthritis, and other arthritic conditions. It is formulated with more Maalox® than Regular Strength Ascriptin to provide increased neutralization of gastric acid, thus reducing the likelihood of GI disturbance. Coated caplets make swallowing easy.

Indications: As an analgesic, anti-inflammatory, and antipyretic agent to relieve the minor pain associated with rheumatoid arthritis, osteoarthritis, and other arthritic conditions.

Usual Adult Dose: Two caplets with water, every 4 hours while symptoms persist, not to exceed 12 caplets in 24 hours, or as directed by the physician for arthritis therapy. For children under twelve, consult a doctor.

WARNINGS: Children and teenagers should not use this medicine for chicken pox or flu symptoms before a doctor is consulted about Reye syndrome, a rare but serious illness reported to be associated with aspirin. Keep this and all medicines out of children's reach. If pain persists more than 10 days, redness or swelling is present, fever persists more than 3 days, or symptoms worsen, consult a doctor immediately. If you are under medical care or have a history of stomach, kidney, or bleeding disorders or asthma, consult a doctor before using. Do not use if allergic to aspirin. As with any drug, if you are pregnant or nursing a baby, consult a doctor before using. **IT IS ESPECIALLY IMPORTANT NOT TO USE ASPIRIN DURING THE LAST 3 MONTHS OF PREGNANCY UNLESS SPECIFICALLY DIRECTED TO DO SO BY A DOCTOR BECAUSE IT MAY CAUSE PROBLEMS IN THE UNBORN CHILD OR COMPLICATIONS DURING DELIVERY.** If ringing in the ears or loss of hearing occurs, consult a doctor before taking any more of this product. **In case of accidental overdose, contact a doctor immediately.** *Drug Interaction Precaution:* Do not use if taking a prescription drug for anticoagulation (blood thinning), diabetes, gout or arthritis, or a tetracycline antibiotic unless directed by a doctor.

Professional Labeling see detail under Regular Strength Ascriptin®

How Supplied: Bottles of 60 tablets (0067-0145-60), 100 tablets (0067-0145-68), 160 (0067-0145-30) and 225 tablets (0067-0145-77).
Bottles of 500 tablets (0067-0145-74) without child-resistant closures (for arthritic patients).
Shown in Product Identification Guide, page 505

CALDECORT® ANTI-ITCH CREAM AND SPRAY;
CALDECORT LIGHT® CREAM
[kal 'de-kort]

Active Ingredient: *Cream* —Hydrocortisone acetate (equivalent to hydrocortisone 1%). *Light Cream* —Hydrocortisone acetate (equivalent to hydrocortisone ½%). *Spray* —Hydrocortisone 1%.

Other Ingredients: *Cream* —Isopropyl myristate, methylparaben, polysorbate 60, propylparaben, purified water, sorbitan monostearate, sorbitol solution, stearic acid. *Light Cream* —Aloe vera gel, isopropyl myristate, methylparaben, polysorbate 60, propylparaben, purified water, sorbitan monostearate, sorbitol solution, stearic acid. *Spray* —Isobutane (propellant), isopropyl myristate, SD alcohol 40-B 62.7% (w/w).

Indications: For the temporary relief of itching associated with minor skin irritations, inflammation, and rashes due to eczema, insect bites, poison ivy, poison oak, poison sumac, soaps, detergents, cosmetics, jewelry, seborrheic dermatitis, psoriasis, and for external feminine itching. Other uses of this product should be only under the advice and supervision of a doctor.

Warnings: For external use only. Avoid contact with the eyes. If condition worsens, or if symptoms persist for more than 7 days or clear up and occur again within a few days, stop use of this product and do not begin use of any other hydrocortisone product unless you have consulted a doctor. Do not use for the treatment of diaper rash. Consult a doctor. Do not use if you have a vaginal discharge. Consult a doctor. **Keep this and all drugs out of the reach of children.** In case of accidental ingestion, seek professional assistance or contact a Poison Control Center immediately. *For Spray only* —Avoid contact with the eyes or on other mucous membranes. Contents under pressure. Do not puncture or incinerate. Flammable mixture, do not use near fire or flame. Do not store at temperature above 120°F. Use only as directed. Intentional misuse by deliberately concentrat-

Continued on next page

The full prescribing information for each CIBA Consumer Pharmaceuticals product is contained herein and is that in effect as of December 15, 1994

CIBA Consumer—Cont.

ing and inhaling the contents can be harmful or fatal.

Directions: *Cream and Light Cream:* Adults and children 2 years of age and older: Apply to affected area not more than 3 or 4 times daily. Children under 2 years of age: Do not use, consult a doctor. *Spray:* Shake well, hold 4″ to 6″ from affected area. Apply to affected area not more than 3 to 4 times daily. Children under 2 years of age: Do not use, consult a doctor.

How Supplied: *Cream* —½ oz. and 1 oz. tubes. *Light Cream* —½ oz. tubes. *Spray* —1.5 oz. aerosol container. CALDECORT and CALDECORT LIGHT are registered trademarks of Ciba-Geigy Corporation.

Shown in Product Identification Guide, page 505

CALDESENE® MEDICATED POWDER AND OINTMENT
[*kal 'de-sēn*]

Active Ingredients: *Powder* —Calcium undecylenate 10%. *Ointment* —White petrolatum 53.9%; zinc oxide 15%.

Other Ingredients: *Powder* — Fragrance, talc. *Ointment* —Cod liver oil, fragrance, lanolin, methylparaben, propylparaben, talc.

Indications: Caldesene Medicated Powder is indicated to help relieve, treat and prevent diaper rash, prickly heat and chafing. Caldesene Ointment helps relieve, treat and prevent diaper rash, protects sensitive skin against wetness, and soothes chafed skin.

Actions: Only Caldesene Medicated Powder contains calcium undecylenate, an antimicrobial that inhibits growth of the organisms frequently associated with diaper rash. Also forms a protective coating to repel moisture, and helps treat and prevent chafing and prickly heat. Caldesene Ointment is specially formulated to soothe and treat diaper rash while protecting sensitive skin against wetness. Unlike other ointments containing zinc oxide, Caldesene Ointment has a mild fragrance and is easily removed from the diaper area with soap and water.

Warnings: For external use only. Avoid contact with eyes. If condition worsens or does not improve within 7 days, consult a physician. **Keep this and all drugs out of the reach of children.** In case of accidental ingestion, seek professional assistance or contact a Poison Control Center immediately.
Powder only: Keep powder away from child's face to avoid inhalation, which can cause breathing problems. Do not use on broken skin.
Ointment only: Do not apply over deep or puncture wounds, infections and lacerations.

Directions: Use on baby after every bath or diaper change as directed by a pediatrician. Cleanse and thoroughly dry baby's skin, then smooth on Caldesene. Powder only: Apply powder close to the body away from child's face. (Shake bottle—don't squeeze—to apply powder to your hand or directly into the diaper.)

How Supplied: *Medicated Powder* — 2 oz (57 g) and 4 oz (113 g) shaker containers. *Medicated Ointment* —1.25 oz (35 g). CALDESENE is a registered trademark of Ciba-Geigy Corporation.

Shown in Product Identification Guide, page 505

CRUEX® ANTIFUNGAL POWDER, SPRAY POWDER AND CREAM
[*kru 'ex*]

Active Ingredients: *Powder* —Undecylenate 10%, as calcium undecylenate. *Spray Powder* —Total undecylenate 19%, as undecylenic acid and zinc undecylenate. *Cream*—Total undecylenate 20%, as undecylenic acid and zinc undecylenate.

Other Ingredients: *Powder* —Colloidal silicon dioxide, fragrance, isopropyl myristate, talc. *Spray Powder* —Fragrance, isobutane (propellant), isopropyl myristate, menthol, talc, trolamine. *Cream* —Fragrance, glycol stearate SE, lanolin, methylparaben, PEG-8 laurate, PEG-6 stearate, propylparaben, sorbitol solution, stearic acid, trolamine, purified water, white petrolatum.

Indications: Cures jock itch. Relieves itching, chafing, and burning. Soothes irritation. Cruex powders also absorb perspiration.

Warnings: Do not use on children under 2 years of age unless directed by a doctor. For external use only. Avoid contact with the eyes. If irritation occurs, or if there is no improvement within 2 weeks, discontinue use and consult a doctor. **Keep this and all drugs out of the reach of children.** In case of accidental ingestion, seek professional assistance or contact a Poison Control Center immediately. *For Spray Powder only*—Avoid inhaling. Avoid contact with the eyes or other mucous membranes. Contents under pressure. Do not puncture or incinerate. Flammable mixture, do not use near fire or flame. Do not expose to heat or temperatures above 49°C (120°F.) Use only as directed. Intentional misuse by deliberately concentrating and inhaling the contents can be harmful or fatal.

Directions: Clean the affected area and dry thoroughly. Apply a thin layer of the product over affected area twice daily (morning and night) or as directed by a doctor. Supervise children in the use of this product. Use daily for 2 weeks. If condition persists longer, consult a doctor. This product is not effective on the scalp or nails.

How Supplied: *Powder* —1.5 oz (43 g) plastic squeeze bottle. *Spray Pow-*

der —1.8 oz (51 g), 3.5 oz (99 g) and 5.5 oz (156 g) aerosol containers. *Cream* —½ oz (14 g) tube.
CRUEX is a registered trademark of Ciba-Geigy Corporation.

Shown in Product Identification Guide, page 506

DESENEX® ANTIFUNGAL POWDER, SPRAY POWDER, CREAM, OINTMENT, AND SPRAY LIQUID
[*dess 'i-nex*]

Active Ingredients: *Cream, Ointment, Powder, and Spray Powder,* —Total undecylenate 25%, as undecylenic acid and zinc undecylenate. *Spray Liquid* —Tolnaftate 1%.

Other Ingredients: *Cream, Ointment* —Fragrance, glycol stearate SE, lanolin, methylparaben, PEG-8 laurate, PEG-6 stearate, propylparaben, purified water, sorbitol solution, stearic acid, trolamine, white petrolatum. *Powder* —Fragrance, talc. *Spray Powder* —Fragrance, isobutane (propellant), isopropyl myristate, menthol, talc, trolamine. *Spray Liquid* —BHT, fragrance, isobutane (propellant), polyethylene glycol 400, SD alcohol 40-B (41% w/w).

Indications: Proven clinically effective in the treatment of athlete's foot (tinea pedis). Relieves the painful itching, burning, cracking and discomfort associated with athlete's foot. Desenex Spray Liquid prevents the recurrence of athlete's foot with daily use.

Warnings: Do not use on children under 2 years of age unless directed by a doctor. For external use only. Avoid contact with the eyes. If irritation occurs, or if there is no improvement within 4 weeks, discontinue use and consult a doctor. **Keep this and all drugs out of the reach of children.** In case of accidental ingestion, seek professional assistance or contact a Poison Control Center immediately. *For Spray Powder* and *Spray Liquid*—Avoid inhaling. Avoid contact with the eyes or other mucous membranes. Contents under pressure. Do not puncture or incinerate. Flammable mixture, do not use near fire or flame. Do not expose to heat or temperatures above 49°C (120°F). Use only as directed. Intentional misuse by deliberately concentrating and inhaling the contents can be harmful or fatal.

Directions: Clean the affected area and dry thoroughly. Apply a thin layer of the product over affected area twice daily (morning and night) or as directed by a doctor. Supervise children in the use of this product. Pay special attention to the spaces between the toes. Wear well-fitting, ventilated shoes and change shoes and socks at least once daily. Use daily for 4 weeks. If condition persists longer, consult a doctor. This product is not effective on the scalp or nails. To prevent recurrence of athlete's foot, spray a thin layer of Desenex Spray Liquid to feet once or twice daily (morning and/or night) following the above directions.

How Supplied: *Cream* —½ oz (14 g) tube. *Ointment* —½ oz (14 g) and 1 oz (28 g) tubes. *Powder* —1.5 oz (43 g) and 3 oz (85 g) shaker containers. *Spray Powder* —2.7 oz (77 g) and 5.5 oz (156 g) aerosol containers. *Spray Liquid* —3 oz (85 g) aerosol container.
DESENEX is a registered trademark of Ciba-Geigy Corporation.

Shown in Product Identification Guide, page 506

DESENEX® FOOT & SNEAKER DEODORANT SPRAY
[*dess 'i-nex*]

Ingredients: Isobutane (propellant), SD alcohol 40-B, talc, aluminum chlorohydrex, silica, diisopropyl adipate, fragrance, menthol, tartaric acid.

Description: Foot & Sneaker Deodorant Spray cools and comforts feet, helping them feel clean and refreshed. Helps foster good foot hygiene with regular use. Specially formulated to absorb wetness, deodorize and relieve the discomfort of hot, perspiring, active feet. Sprays on like a liquid—dries quickly to a fine powder.

Directions: Shake well, hold 6 inches from area and spray onto soles of your feet and between your toes daily. Also, spray liberally over entire area of shoes or sneakers before wearing.

Warnings: Avoid spraying in eyes or other mucous membranes. Contents under pressure. Do not puncture or incinerate. Flammable mixture, do not use near fire or flame. Do not expose to heat or temperatures above 49°C (120°F). Use only as directed. Intentional misuse by deliberately concentrating and inhaling the contents can be harmful or fatal. **Keep out of reach of children.**

How Supplied: *Desenex Foot & Sneaker Deodorant Spray Powder* —3 oz (85 g) aerosol container. Also available, Desenex Foot & Sneaker Deodorant Powder Plus with an antifungal—2 oz (57 g) shaker container.
DESENEX is a registered trademark of Ciba-Geigy Corporation.

Shown in Product Identification Guide, page 506

PRESCRIPTION STRENGTH DESENEX® AF ANTIFUNGAL CREAM, PRESCRIPTION STRENGTH DESENEX® SPRAY POWDER AND SPRAY LIQUID

Active Ingredients: *Cream* —Clotrimazole 1%. *Spray Powder and Spray Liquid* —Miconazole Nitrate 2%.

Inactive Ingredients: *Cream* —Cetostearyl alcohol, cetyl esters wax, 2-octyldodecanol, polysorbate-60, sorbitan mon-ostearate, purified water and, as a preservative, benzyl alcohol (1%). *Spray Powder* —Aloe vera gel, aluminum starch octenylsuccinate, isopropyl myristate, propylene carbonate, SD alcohol 40-B (10% w/w), sorbitan monooleate, stearalkonium hectorite. *Spray Liquid* —Polyethylene glycol 300, polysorbate 20, SD alcohol 40-B (15% w/w).

Propellant: *Spray Powder* —Isobutane/propane. *Spray Liquid* —Dimethyl ether.

Indications: *Cream* —Cures athlete's foot (tinea pedis), jock itch (tinea cruris), and ringworm (tinea corporis). For effective relief of the itching cracking, burning, and discomfort which can accompany these conditions. *Spray Powder and Spray Liquid* —Proven clinically effective in the treatment of athlete's foot (tinea pedis) and ringworm (tinea corporis). Relieves the itching, scaling, burning, and discomfort that can accompany athlete's foot. Prescription Strength Desenex® Spray Powder is specially formulated to aid the drying of moist areas of the feet.

Warnings: Do not use on children under 2 years of age unless directed by a doctor. For external use only. Avoid contact with the eyes. If irritation occurs, or if there is no improvement within 4 weeks (for athlete's foot or ringworm) or within 2 weeks (for jock itch), discontinue use and consult a doctor. **Keep this and all drugs out of the reach of children.** In case of accidental ingestion, seek professional assistance or contact a Poison Control Center immediately. Use only as directed. *For Spray Powder and Spray Liquid* —Avoid inhaling. Avoid contact with the eyes or other mucous membranes. Contents under pressure. Do not puncture or incinerate. Flammable mixture, do not use near fire or flame. Do not expose to heat or temperatures above 49°C (120°F). Use only as directed. Intentional misuse by deliberately concentrating and inhaling the contents can be harmful or fatal.

Directions: Clean the affected area and dry thoroughly. Apply a thin layer of the product over affected area twice daily (morning and night) or as directed by a doctor. Supervise children in the use of this product. Pay special attention to the spaces between the toes. Wear well-fitting, ventilated shoes and change shoes and socks at least once daily. Use daily for 4 weeks. If condition persists longer, consult a doctor. This product is not effective on the scalp or nails.

How Supplied: *Cream* —15 g (½ oz). *Spray Powder* —85 g (3 oz). *Spray Liquid* —100 g (3.5 oz).
DESENEX is a registered trademark of Ciba-Geigy Corporation.

Shown in Product Identification Guide, page 506

EXTRA STRENGTH DOAN'S®
Analgesic Caplets

Indications: For temporary relief of minor backache pain.

Directions: Adults—Two caplets with water every 6 hours while symptoms persist, not to exceed 8 caplets during a 24-hour period or as directed by a doctor. Children under 12: consult a doctor.

Warnings: Children and teenagers should not use this medicine for chicken pox or flu symptoms before a doctor is consulted about Reye syndrome, a rare but serious illness. As with any drug, if you are pregnant or nursing a baby, seek the advice of a health professional before using this product. Do not take this product for pain for more than 10 days unless directed by a doctor. If pain or fever persists or gets worse, if new symptoms occur, or if redness or swelling is present, consult a doctor because these could be signs of a serious condition. Do not take this product if you are allergic to salicylates (including aspirin), have stomach problems (such as heartburn, upset stomach, or stomach pain) that persist or recur, or if you have ulcers or bleeding problems, unless directed by a doctor. If ringing in the ears or a loss of hearing occurs, consult a doctor before taking any more of this product.
KEEP THIS AND ALL MEDICINES OUT OF THE REACH OF CHILDREN. In case of accidental overdose, seek professional assistance or contact a Poison Control Center immediately.

Drug Interaction Precaution: Do not take this product if you are taking a prescription drug for anticoagulation (thinning of the blood), diabetes, gout, or arthritis unless directed by a doctor.

Active Ingredient: Each caplet contains Magnesium Salicylate Tetrahydrate 580 mg. (equivalent to 467.2 mg. of anhydrous Magnesium Salicylate).

Also Contains: Magnesium Stearate, Microcrystalline Cellulose, Opadry White, Polyethylene Glycol, Stearic Acid.

Shown in Product Identification Guide, page 506

**Extra Strength
DOAN'S® P.M.
Magnesium Salicylate/
Diphenhydramine
Analgesic/Sleep Aid Caplets**

Indications: For temporary relief of minor back pain accompanied by sleeplessness.

Continued on next page

The full prescribing information for each CIBA Consumer Pharmaceuticals product is contained herein and is that in effect as of December 15, 1994

CIBA Consumer—Cont.

Directions: Adults and children 12 years of age or older: Take 2 caplets with water at bedtime if needed, or as directed by a doctor.

Warnings: Children and teenagers should not use this medicine for chicken pox or flu symptoms before a doctor is consulted about Reye syndrome, a rare but serious illness. KEEP THIS AND ALL OTHER MEDICATIONS OUT OF THE REACH OF CHILDREN. IN CASE OF ACCIDENTAL OVERDOSE, SEEK PROFESSIONAL ASSISTANCE OR CONTACT A POISON CONTROL CENTER IMMEDIATELY. DO NOT GIVE THIS PRODUCT TO CHILDREN UNDER 12 YEARS OF AGE. As with any drug, if you are pregnant or nursing a baby, seek the advice of a health professional before using this product. Do not take this product for pain for more than 10 days unless directed by a doctor. If pain or fever persists or gets worse, if new symptoms occur, or if redness or swelling is present, consult a doctor because these could be signs of a serious condition. If sleeplessness persists continuously for more than 2 weeks, consult your doctor. Insomnia may be a symptom of serious underlying medical illness. Do not take this product, unless directed by a doctor, if you have a breathing problem such as emphysema or chronic bronchitis, or if you have glaucoma, difficulty in urination due to enlargement of the prostate gland, stomach problems (such as heartburn, upset stomach, or stomach pain) that persist or recur, ulcers or bleeding problems, or if you are allergic to aspirin or salicylates. If ringing in the ears or a loss of hearing occurs, consult a doctor before taking any more of this product. Avoid alcoholic beverages while taking this product. Do not take this product if you are taking sedatives or tranquilizers without first consulting your doctor.

Drug Interaction Precaution: Do not take this product if you are taking a prescription drug for anticoagulation (thinning of the blood), diabetes, gout, or arthritis unless directed by a doctor.

Active Ingredients: Each caplet contains Magnesium Salicylate Tetrahydrate 580mg. (equivalent to 467.2mg. of anhydrous Magnesium Salicylate) and Diphenhydramine HCl 25mg.

Also Contains: Carnauba Wax, Colloidal Silicon Dioxide, Croscarmellose Sodium, Microcrystalline Cellulose, Magnesium Stearate, Opadry Blue, Stearic Acid, Talc.

Shown in Product Identification Guide, page 506

REGULAR STRENGTH DOAN'S®
Analgesic Caplets

Indications: For temporary relief of minor backache pain.

Directions: Adults—Two caplets every 4 hours while symptoms persist, not to exceed 12 caplets during a 24-hour period or as directed by a doctor. Children under 12: consult a doctor.

Warning: Children and teenagers should not use this medicine for chicken pox or flu symptoms before a doctor is consulted about Reye syndrome, a rare but serious illness. As with any drug, if you are pregnant or nursing a baby, seek the advice of a health professional before using this product. Do not take this product for pain for more than 10 days unless directed by a doctor. If pain or fever persists or gets worse, if new symptoms occur, or if redness or swelling is present, consult a doctor because these could be signs of a serious condition. Do not take this product if you are allergic to salicylates (including aspirin), have stomach problems (such as heartburn, upset stomach, or stomach pain) that persist or recur, or if you have ulcers or bleeding problems, unless directed by a doctor. If ringing in the ears or a loss of hearing occurs, consult a doctor before taking any more of this product. KEEP THIS AND ALL MEDICINES OUT OF THE REACH OF CHILDREN. In case of accidental overdose, seek professional assistance or contact a Poison Control Center immediately.

Drug Interaction Precaution: Do not take this product if you are taking a prescription drug for anticoagulation (thinning of the blood), diabetes, gout, or arthritis unless directed by a doctor.

Active Ingredient: Each caplet contains Magnesium Salicylate Tetrahydrate 377 mg. (equivalent to 303.7 mg of anhydrous Magnesium Salicylate).

Also Contains: FD&C Yellow #6, Magnesium Stearate, Microcrystalline Cellulose, Opadry Light Green, Polyethylene Glycol, Stearic Acid.
Store at 15°–30°C (59°–86°F). PROTECT FROM MOISTURE.

Shown in Product Identification Guide, page 506

DULCOLAX®
[*dul'co-lax*]
brand of bisacodyl USP
Tablets of 5 mg
Suppositories of 10 mg
Laxative

Ingredients: Each enteric coated tablet contains: Active: Bisacodyl USP 5 mg. Also contains: Acacia, acetylated monoglyceride, carnauba wax, cellulose acetate phthalate, corn starch, D&C Red No. 30 aluminum lake, D&C Yellow No. 10 aluminum lake, dibutyl phthalate, docusate sodium, gelatin, glycerin, iron oxides, kaolin, lactose, magnesium stearate, methylparaben, pharmaceutical glaze, polyethylene glycol, povidone, propylparaben, sodium benzoate, sorbitan monooleate, sucrose, talc, titanium dioxide, white wax.

Each suppository contains: Active: Bisacodyl USP 10 mg. Also contains: Hydrogenated vegetable oil.
SODIUM CONTENT: Tablets and suppositories contain less than 0.2 mg per dosage unit and are thus dietetically sodium free.

Indications: For the relief of occasional constipation and irregularity. Physicians should refer to the "Professional Labeling" section for additional indications and information.

Directions:
Tablets
Adults and children 12 years of age and over: Take 2 or 3 tablets (usually 2) in a single dose once daily.
Children 6 to under 12 years of age: Take 1 tablet once daily.
Children under 6 years of age: Consult a physician.
Expect results in 8–12 hours if taken at bedtime or within 6 hours if taken before breakfast.
Suppositories
Adults and children 12 years of age and over: 1 suppository once daily. Remove foil wrapper. Lie on your side and, with pointed end first, push suppository high into the rectum so it will not slip out. Retain it for 15 to 20 minutes. If you feel the suppository must come out immediately, it was not inserted high enough and should be pushed higher.
Children 6 to under 12 years of age: ½ suppository once daily.
Children under 6 years of age: Consult a physician.
If the suppository seems soft, hold in foil wrapper under cold water for one or two minutes. In the presence of anal fissures or hemorrhoids, suppository may be coated at the tip with petroleum jelly before insertion.

Warnings: Do not use laxative products when abdominal pain, nausea, or vomiting are present unless directed by a physician. Restoration of normal bowel function by using this product may cause abdominal discomfort including cramps. Laxative products should not be used for a period longer than 1 week unless directed by a physician. Rectal bleeding or failure to have a bowel movement after use of a laxative may indicate a serious condition. If this occurs, discontinue use and consult your physician. As with any drug, if you are pregnant or nursing a baby, seek the advice of a health care professional before using this product. KEEP THIS AND ALL MEDICATION OUT OF THE REACH OF CHILDREN. In case of accidental overdose or ingestion, seek professional assistance or contact a poison control center immediately. For tablets: Do not chew or crush. Do not give to children under 6 years of age unless directed by a physician. Do not take this product within 1 hour after taking an antacid or milk.

How Supplied: Dulcolax, brand of bisacodyl: Yellow, enteric-coated tablets of 5

mg in boxes of 10, 25, 50 and 100; suppositories of 10 mg in boxes of 4, 8, 16 and 50.
NDC 0083-6200 (tablets)
NDC 0083-6100 (suppositories)

Note: Store Dulcolax suppositories and tablets at temperatures below 77°F (25°C). Avoid excessive humidity.

Also Available: Dulcolax® Bowel Prep Kit. Each kit contains:

1 Dulcolax suppository of 10 mg bisacodyl;
4 Dulcolax tablets of 5 mg bisacodyl;
Complete patient instructions.

PROFESSIONAL LABELING:

Description and Clinical Pharmacology: Dulcolax is a contact stimulant laxative, administered either orally or rectally, which acts directly on the colonic mucosa to produce normal peristalsis throughout the large intestine. The active ingredient in Dulcolax, bisacodyl, is a colorless, tasteless compound that is practically insoluble in water or alkaline solution. Its chemical name is: bis(p-acetoxyphenyl)-2-pyridylmethane. Bisacodyl is very poorly absorbed, if at all, in the small intestine following oral administration, nor in the large intestine following rectal administration. On contact with the mucosa or submucosal plexi of the large intestine, bisacodyl stimulates sensory nerve endings to produce parasympathetic reflexes resulting in increased peristaltic contractions of the colon. It has also been shown to promote fluid and ion accumulation in the colon, which increases the laxative effect. A bowel movement is usually produced approximately 6 hours after oral administration (8–12 hours if taken at bedtime), and approximately 15 minutes to 1 hour after rectal administration, providing satisfactory cleansing of the bowel which may, under certain circumstances, obviate the need for colonic irrigation.

Indications and Usage: For use as part of a bowel cleansing regimen in preparing the patient for surgery or for preparing the colon for x-ray endoscopic examination. Dulcolax will not replace the colonic irrigations usually given patients before intracolonic surgery, but is useful in the preliminary emptying of the colon prior to these procedures.
Also for use as a laxative in postoperative care (i.e., restoration of normal bowel hygiene), antepartum care, postpartum care, and in preparation for delivery.

Contraindications: Stimulant laxatives, such as Dulcolax, are contraindicated for patients with acute surgical abdomen, appendicitis, rectal bleeding, or intestinal obstruction.

Precautions: Long-term administration of Dulcolax is not recommended in the treatment of chronic constipation.

Dosage and Administration:
Preparation for x-ray endoscopy: For barium enemas, no food should be given following oral administration to prevent reaccumulation of material in the cecum, and a suppository should be administered one to two hours prior to examination.
Children under 6 years of age: Oral administration is not recommended due to the requirement to swallow tablets whole. For rectal administration, the suppository dosage is 5 mg (½ of 10 mg suppository) in a single daily dose.

Shown in Product Identification Guide, page 506

EFIDAC/24
Nasal decongestant

Indications: Provides temporary relief of nasal congestion due to the common cold, hay fever, or other upper respiratory allergies, and nasal congestion associated with sinusitis; reduces swelling of nasal passages; shrinks swollen membranes; relieves sinus pressure; and temporarily restores freer breathing through the nose.

Directions: Adults and children 12 years and over: Take just one tablet with fluid every 24 hours. DO NOT EXCEED ONE TABLET IN 24 HOURS. SWALLOW EACH TABLET WHOLE; DO NOT DIVIDE, CRUSH, CHEW, OR DISSOLVE THE TABLET. The tablet does not completely dissolve and may be seen in the stool (this is normal). Not for use in children under 12 years of age.

Warnings: DO NOT EXCEED RECOMMENDED DOSAGE because at higher doses nervousness, dizziness, or sleeplessness may occur. Do not take this product for more than 7 days. If symptoms do not improve or are accompanied by fever, consult a physician. Do not take this product if you have heart disease, high blood pressure, thyroid disease, diabetes, or difficulty in urination due to enlargement of the prostate gland, unless directed by a physician.
Rarely, tablets of this kind may cause bowel obstruction (blockage), usually in people with severe narrowing of the bowel (esophagus, stomach or intestine). If you have had obstruction or narrowing of the bowel, do not take this product without consulting your physician. Contact your physician if you experience persistent abdominal pain or vomiting. As with any drug, if you are pregnant or nursing a baby, seek the advice of a health professional before using this product.
KEEP THIS AND ALL DRUGS OUT OF THE REACH OF CHILDREN. In case of accidental overdose, seek professional assistance or contact a Poison Control Center immediately.

Drug Interaction Precaution: Do not use this product if you are now taking a prescription monoamine oxidase inhibitor (MAOI) (certain drugs for depression, psychiatric or emotional conditions, or Parkinson's disease), or for 2 weeks after stopping the MAOI drug. If you are uncertain whether your prescription drug contains an MAOI, consult a health professional before taking this product.

Store in a dry place between 4°–30°C (39°–86°F).
QUESTIONS? Please write Consumer Affairs at the address below.
Distributed by: Ciba Consumer Pharmaceuticals, 581 Main Street, Woodbridge, NJ 07095

Active Ingredient: Each Efidac 24 tablet contains 240 mg Pseudoephedrine Hydrochloride

Inactive Ingredients: Cellulose, cellulose acetate, FD&C Blue #1, hydroxypropl cellulose, hydroxypropl methylcellulose, magnesium stearate, polyethylene glycol, polysorbate 80, povidone, sodium chloride, and titanium dioxide.

Shown in Product Identification Guide, page 506

EUCALYPTAMINT®
Arthritis Pain Reliever
Maximum Strength
External Analgesic

Description: Maximum Strength topical analgesic that provides hours of effective relief.

Active Ingredient: Natural Menthol (16%)

Inactive Ingredients: Lanolin and Eucalyptus Oil

Indications: For the temporary relief of minor aches and pains of muscles and joints associated with arthritis.

Directions: Adults and children 2 years of age and older: Gently massage a conservative amount into affected area not more than 3 to 4 times daily.
Children under 2 years of age: Consult a physician.

Warning: FOR EXTERNAL USE ONLY. Avoid contact with eyes. Do not apply to wounds or damaged skin. Do not bandage tightly. Do not use with heating pads or heating devices. If condition worsens, or if symptoms persist for more than 7 days, discontinue use of this product and consult a physician. Keep this and all drugs out of the reach of children. In case of accidental ingestion, seek professional assistance or contact a Poison Control Center immediately. Store at room temperature 15°–30°C (59°–86°F). Do not freeze. It is normal for the consistency of Eucalyptamint to vary with temperature changes. If thickening does occur, warm the tube in the palms of your hands or run under warm water.

How Supplied: Eucalyptamint Ointment is supplied in a 2 oz. easy to squeeze tube.

Shown in Product Identification Guide, page 506

Continued on next page

The full prescribing information for each CIBA Consumer Pharmaceuticals product is contained herein and is that in effect as of December 15, 1994

CIBA Consumer—Cont.

EUCALYPTAMINT®
Muscle Pain Relief Formula
External Analgesic

Description: A uniquely scented gel creme formulation providing hours of effective pain relief for overworked muscles.

Active Ingredient: Menthol 8%

Other Ingredients: Carbomer 980, Eucalyptus Oil, Fragrance, Propylene Glycol, SD 3A Alcohol, Triethanolamine, TWEEN 80, Water.

Indications: For the temporary relief of minor aches and pains of muscles associated with simple backache, strains, sprains and sports injuries.

Directions: Adults and children 2 years of age and older. Shake tube with cap facing downward. Gently massage a conservative amount into affected area not more than 3 to 4 times daily. Children under 2 years of age: Consult a physician.

Warning: FOR EXTERNAL USE ONLY. Avoid contact with eyes. Do not apply to wounds or damaged skin. Do not bandage tightly. Do not use with heating pads or heating devices. If condition worsens, or if symptoms persist for more than 7 days, discontinue use of this product and consult a physician. Keep this and all drugs out of the reach of children. In case of accidental ingestion, seek professional assistance or contact a Poison Control Center immediately. Store at room temperature 15°–30°C (59°–86°F). DO NOT FREEZE.

How Supplied: Eucalyptamint Muscle Pain Relief Formula is supplied in 2.25 oz. bottles and is available in two scents: Alpine Breeze and Powder Fresh. *Eucalyptamint is a registered trademark of Ciba-Geigy.*

Shown in Product Identification Guide, page 506

FIBERALL® Chewable Tablets
[fi'ber-all]
Sodium Free, No chemical stimulants, less than 6 calories per tablet
Lemon Creme Flavor

Description: Fiberall Chewable Tablets are a bulk-forming, nonirritant laxative which contain less than 1.5 grams of sugar per tablet. The active ingredient is calcium polycarbophil, a bulk-forming man-made fiber with no chemical stimulant. The smooth gelatinous bulk formed by Fiber-all Chewable Tablets encourages peristaltic activity and a more normal elimination of the bowel contents.

Active Ingredient: Each tablet contains 1250 mg Calcium Polycarbophil (equivalent to 1000 mg polycarbophil)

Inactive Ingredients: Crospovidone, dextrose, flavors, magnesium stearate and yellow No. 10 aluminum lake.

Indications: Fiberall Chewable Tablets are indicated for the management of chronic constipation, temporary constipation caused by illness or pregnancy, irritable bowel syndrome, and for constipation related to duodenal ulcer or diverticulosis. Fiberall Chewable Tablets are also indicated for stool softening in patients with hemorrhoids or after anorectal surgery.

Actions: After the tablet is chewed it readily disperses and acts without irritants or stimulants. Polycarbophil absorbs water in the gastrointestinal tract to form a gelatinous bulk which encourages a more normal bowel movement.

Directions: Take this product (child or adult dose) with at least 8 ounces (a full glass) of water or other fluid. Taking this product without enough liquid may cause choking. See Warnings.

Dosage and Administration: *Adults and children 12 years and older:* chew and swallow 1 tablet, 1–4 times a day. *Children 6 to under 12 years:* one-half the usual adult dose or as recommended by a physician. *Children under 6:* consult a physician. **Drink a full glass (8 fl oz) of liquid with each dose.** Drinking additional liquid helps Fiberall work even more effectively. Continued use for 2 to 3 days may be desired for maximum laxative benefits.

Warnings: Taking this product without adequate fluid may cause it to swell and block your throat or esophagus and may cause choking. Do not take this product if you have difficulty in swallowing. If you experience chest pain, vomiting or difficulty in swallowing or breathing after taking this product, seek immediate medical attention.

Contraindications: Fecal impaction or intestinal obstruction. Any disease state in which consumption of extra calcium is contraindicated.

Drug Interactions: This product contains calcium, which may interact with some forms of TETRACYCLINE if taken concomitantly. The tetracycline product should be taken 1 hour before or 2–3 hours after taking a Fiberall Chewable Tablet.

How Supplied: Boxes containing 18 tablets.

FIBERALL® Fiber Wafers
[fi'ber-all]
Fruit & Nut, Oatmeal Raisin

Description: Fiberall Fiber Wafers are a bulk-forming, nonirritant laxative. The active ingredient is psyllium hydrophilic mucilloid, a dietary fiber extracted from the seed husk of blond psyllium seed *(Plantago ovata).* The smooth gelatinous bulk formed by Fiberall Wafers encourages peristaltic activity and a more normal elimination of the bowel contents.

One (1) Fiberall Fiber Wafer contains 3.4 g of psyllium hydrophilic mucilloid in a good-tasting wafer form, of which approximately 2.2 g is soluble fiber. One wafer is equivalent to one teaspoonful of Fiberall Powder.

Inactive Ingredients: Fruit & Nut Flavor: Baking powder, brown sugar, butter flavor, cinnamon, corn syrup, crisp rice, dried ground apricots, flour, glycerin, granulated sugar, granulated walnuts, lecithin, margarine, molasses, oats, salt, vegetable oil shortening (soybean and cottonseed oil), water and wheat bran. Fiberall Fruit & Nut Fiber Wafers contain approximately 79 calories and 110 mg of sodium per wafer.

Oatmeal Raisin Flavor: Baking powder, cinnamon, cinnamon flavor, cloves, corn syrup, flour, glycerin, granulated sugar, lecithin, molasses, oats, raisins, vegetable oil shortening (soybean and cottonseed oil), water and wheat bran. Fiberall Oatmeal Raisin Fiber Wafers contain approximately 78 calories and 30 mg of sodium per wafer.

Indications: Fiberall Fiber Wafers are indicated for the management of chronic constipation, temporary constipation caused by illness or pregnancy, irritable bowel syndrome, and for constipation related to duodenal ulcer or diverticulosis. Fiberall Wafers are also indicated for stool softening in patients with hemorrhoids or after anorectal surgery.

Actions: The homogenous high-fiber formula of Fiberall Fiber Wafers, eaten with 8 oz of a beverage of the patient's choice, acts without irritants or stimulants in the gastrointestinal tract.

Directions: Take this product (child or adult dose) with at least 8 ounces (a full glass) of water or other fluid. Taking this product without enough liquid may cause choking. See Warnings.

Dosage and Administration: The recommended dosage for adults is one to two Fiberall Fiber Wafers 1 to 3 times daily, with a full 8 oz glass of water or other liquid with each wafer. The recommended daily dose for children 6 to under 12 years old is one-half the usual adult dose (with liquid), or as recommended by a physician. For children under 6, consult a physician. Drinking additional liquid is recommended and helps Fiberall work even more effectively. Two to three days' usage may be required for optimal laxative benefits.

Warnings: Taking this product without adequate fluid may cause it to swell and block your throat or esophagus and may cause choking. Do not take this product if you have difficulty in swallowing. If you experience chest pain, vomiting or difficulty in swallowing or breathing after taking this product, seek immediate medical attention.

Contraindications: Fecal impaction or intestinal obstruction.

Precaution: As with any grain product, inhaled or ingested psyllium powder may cause an allergic reaction in individuals sensitive to it.

How Supplied: Boxes containing 14 wafers.

Shown in Product Identification Guide, page 506

FIBERALL® Powder, Orange or Natural Flavor
[fi'ber-all]

Description: Fiberall is a bulk-forming, nonirritant laxative which contains no sugar. The active ingredient is psyllium hydrophilic mucilloid, a dietary fiber extracted from the seed husk of blond psyllium seed *(Plantago ovata)*. The smooth gelatinous bulk formed by Fiberall encourages peristaltic activity and a more normal elimination of the bowel contents.

The recommended dose contains 3.4 g psyllium hydrophilic mucilloid, of which approximately 2.2 g is soluble fiber.

Active Ingredients: Psyllium hydrophilic mucilloid.

Inactive Ingredients: Natural Flavor: Citric acid, flavor, polysorbate 60 and wheat bran. Orange Flavor: Beta-carotene, citric acid, flavor, polysorbate 60, saccharin, wheat bran and yellow No. 6 lake. Each dose contains less than 10 mg of sodium, less than 60 mg of potassium, and provides less than 6 calories (10 calories for Orange).

Indications: Fiberall is indicated for the management of chronic constipation, temporary constipation caused by illness or pregnancy, irritable bowel syndrome, and for constipation related to duodenal ulcer or diverticulosis. Fiberall is also indicated for stool softening in patients with hemorrhoids or after anorectal surgery.

Actions: The homogenous, high-fiber formula of Fiberall is readily dispersed in liquids and acts without irritants or stimulants in the gastro-intestinal tract.

Directions: Take this product (child or adult dose) with at least 8 ounces (a full glass) of water or other fluid. Taking this product without enough liquid may cause choking. See Warnings.

Dosage and Administration:

Adults: Natural: Place one scoopful filled to the line (5 g) or one slightly rounded teaspoonful in a glass and add 8 oz. of cool water or other liquid. Stir to mix. Orange: Place one level scoopful (5.9 g) or one rounded teaspoonful in glass and add liquid as above. Take orally one to three times daily according to individual response.

Children 6 to under 12 years old: One-half the usual adult dose (with liquid) or as recommended by a physician. Drinking additional liquid is recommended and helps Fiberall work even more effectively. Two to three days' usage may be required for maximum laxative benefits.

New Users: Start by taking 1 dose each day. Gradually increase to 3 doses per day if needed or recommended by doctor. If minor gas or bloating occurs, reduce the amount taken until system adjusts.

Warnings: Taking this product without adequate fluid may cause it to swell and block your throat or esophagus and may cause choking. Do not take this product if you have difficulty in swallowing. If you experience chest pain, vomiting or difficulty in swallowing or breathing after taking this product, seek immediate medical attention.

Contraindications: Fecal impaction or intestinal obstruction.

Precaution: As with any grain product, inhaled or ingested psyllium powder may cause an allergic reaction in individuals sensitive to it.

How Supplied: Powder, in 10 or 15 oz containers.

Shown in Product Identification Guide, page 506

ISOCLOR® TIMESULE® Capsules
[is'ō-klōr]

Active Ingredients: Chlorpheniramine maleate 8 mg and phenylpropanolamine hydrochloride 75 mg.

Inactive Ingredients: Benzyl alcohol, butyl paraben, edetate calcium disodium, gelatin, methyl paraben, pharmaceutical glaze, propyl paraben, sodium lauryl sulfate, sodium propiomate, starch, sucrose and other ingredients.

Indications: For the temporary relief of nasal congestion due to the common cold, hay fever, or other upper respiratory allergies and associated with sinusitis. Helps decongest sinus openings, sinus passages and promotes nasal and/or sinus drainage; temporarily restores freer breathing through the nose. For the temporary relief of running nose, sneezing, itching of the nose or throat, and itchy and watery eyes as may occur in allergic rhinitis (such as hay fever).

Warnings: Do not give this product to children under 12 years except under the advice and supervision of a physician. Do not exceed the recommended dosage because at higher doses, nervousness, dizziness, or sleeplessness may occur. If symptoms do not improve within seven days or are accompanied by high fever, consult a physician before continuing use. Do not take this product if you have high blood pressure, heart disease, diabetes, thyroid disease, asthma, glaucoma or difficulty in urination due to enlargement of the prostate gland except under the advice and supervision of a physician. Do not take this product if you are taking another medication containing phenylpropanolamine. Avoid alcoholic beverages while taking this product. Avoid driving a motor vehicle or operating heavy machinery. This preparation may cause drowsiness; this preparation may cause excitability, especially in children. As with any drug, if you are pregnant or nursing a baby, seek the advice of a health professional before using this product.

Keep this and all drugs out of the reach of children. In case of accidental overdose, seek professional assistance or contact a Poison Control Center immediately.

Drug Interaction Precaution: Do not take this product if you are presently taking a prescription antihypertensive or antidepressant drug containing a monoamine oxidase inhibitor except under the advice and supervision of a physician.

Directions: Adults and children over 12 years of age: one capsule every 12 hours. Do not exceed two capsules in 24 hours.

How Supplied: Packaged on blister cards in cartons of 10's and 20's, and bottles of 100.
ISOCLOR® and TIMESULE® are registered trademarks of Ciba-Geigy Corporation.
Distributed by:
Ciba Consumer Pharmaceuticals

KONDREMUL®

Active Ingredient: Mineral Oil (55%).

Inactive Ingredients: Acacia, benzoic acid, carrageenan (Irish Moss), ethyl vanillin, glycerin, mapleine triple oil, purified water, vanillin.

Indications: For relief of occasional constipation. This product generally produces bowel movement in 6–8 hours.

Actions: Promotes gentle, predicatable regularity of normal bowel movement. Pleasant tasting and smooth acting, it passes through stomach and upper intestine without upset or dehydration.

Warning: Do not take with meals. Do not administer to children under 6 years of age, to pregnant women, to bedridden patients or to persons with difficulty swallowing. Do not use this product when abdominal pain, nausea or vomiting are present, unless directed by a physician. Laxative products should not be used for a period longer than 1 week unless directed by a physician. If you have noticed a sudden change in bowel habits that persist over a period of 2 weeks, consult a physician before using a laxative. Rectal bleeding or failure to have a bowel movement after use of a laxative may indicate a serious condition. Discontinue

Continued on next page

The full prescribing information for each CIBA Consumer Pharmaceuticals product is contained herein and is that in effect as of December 15, 1994

CIBA Consumer—Cont.

use and consult a physican. As with any drug, if you are pregnant or nursing a baby, seek the advice of a health care professional before using this product. KEEP THIS AND ALL DRUGS OUT OF THE REACH OF CHILDREN. In case of accidental overdose, seek professional assistance or contact a poison control center immediately.

Drug Interaction Precaution: Do not use this product if you are presently taking a stool softener laxative.

Directions: Shake well before using. Adults and children over 12 years of age: two to five tablespoonsful (30–75ml). Children 6 to under 12 years of age: two to five teaspoonsful (10–25ml). The dose may be taken as a single dose or in divided doses.
Children under 6 years of age: consult a physician.
Store at room temperature 15°–30°C (59°–86°F).
Distrubution by:
Ciba Consumer Pharmaceuticals
Woodbridge, NJ 07095
Shown in Product Identification Guide, page 506

MAALOX® Antacid Caplets
Antacid

Description: Maalox® antacid caplets provide fast, effective relief of acid indigestion, heartburn, and sour stomach. Because they are easy-to-swallow caplets, there is no chalky aftertaste.

Active Ingredients: Each caplet contains 1000 mg calcium carbonate.

Inactive Ingredients: Corn starch, croscarmellose, magnesium stearate and sodium lauryl sulfate. Contains not more than 0.4 mEq sodium per caplet. [See chart below]

Indications: For the relief of acid indigestion, heartburn, sour stomach and upset stomach associated with these symptoms.

Directions for Use: Take 1 caplet as needed or as directed by physician.

Minimum Recommended Dosage: Maalox Antacid Caplets Per caplet	
Acid neutralizing capacity	NLT 20.0 mEq/ caplet
Sodium content	NMT 5mg / caplet

CAPLETS SHOULD NOT BE CHEWED.

Patient Warnings: Do not take more than 8 caplets in a 24-hour period or use the maximum dosage for more than 2 weeks except under the advice and super-

vision of a physician. If you have a history of calcium stones or decreased renal function, consult a physician before use. Keep this and all drugs out of the reach of children.

Drug Interaction Precaution: Calcium antacid salts can decrease absorption of beta-adrenergic blockers and Dilantin. Thiazide diuretics can cause hypercalcemia by decreasing renal excretion of calcium antacids. The milk-alkali syndrome can occur with prolonged sodium bicarbonate use and/or homogenized milk containing Vitamin D.

Drug Interaction Precaution: Antacids may interact with certain prescription drugs. If you are presently taking a prescription drug, do not take this product without checking with your physician or other health professional.

Professional Labeling: Indicated for the symptomatic relief of hyperacidity associated with the diagnosis of peptic ulcer, gastritis, peptic esophagitis, gastric hyperacidity, and hiatal hernia.

How Supplied: Maalox Antacid Caplets are available in blister packs of 24 caplets (0067-0183-24) and plastic bottle of 50 caplets (0067-0183-50).

Storage: Store at room temperature. Protect from moisture.
Shown in Product Identification Guide, page 506

EXTRA STRENGTH MAALOX® ANTACID PLUS ANTI-GAS
Alumina, Magnesia and Simethicone Oral Suspension and Tablets, Antacid/Anti-Gas

Liquids	Tablets
☐ Lemon Creme	Mint Creme
Cherry Creme	Cherry
Mint Creme	Lemon Creme

☐ Physician-proven Maalox® formula for antacid effectiveness.
☐ Simethicone, at a recognized clinical dose, for antiflatulent action.

Description: Extra Strength Maalox® Antacid Plus Anti-Gas, a balanced combination of magnesium and aluminum hydroxides plus simethicone, is a non-constipating antacid/anti-gas product to provide symptomatic relief of hyperacidity plus alleviation of gas symptoms. Available in liquid form in Cherry Creme, Mint Creme or Lemon Creme flavors, and in tablet form in the Mint Creme, Cherry, and Lemon Creme flavors.

Composition: To provide symptomatic relief of hyperacidity plus alleviation of gas symptoms, each teaspoonful/tablet contains:

Active Ingredients	Extra Strength Maalox® Antacid Plus Per Tsp. (5 mL)	Extra Strength Maalox® Anti-Gas Per Tablet
Magnesium Hydroxide	450 mg	350 mg
Aluminum Hydroxide (equivalent to dried gel, USP)	500 mg	350 mg
Simethicone	40 mg	30 mg

Inactive Ingredients: FD&C Red No. 40, flavors, methylparaben, propylparaben, purified water, saccharin, sorbitol, and other ingredients. May also contain citric acid.
Extra Strength Maalox® Plus Tablets: Citric acid, confectioners' sugar, D&C Yellow No. 10, dextrose, FD&C Blue No. 1, flavors, glycerin, hydrogenated vegetable oil, magnesium stearate, mannitol, saccharin sodium, sorbitol, starch, talc.
Assorted flavor tablets: Confectioner's sugar, colors, dextrose, flavors, glycerin, magnesium stearate, mannitol, saccharin sodium, sorbitol, starch, talc. May also contain citric acid.

Directions for Use: Chew 1 to 3 tablets 4 times a day, 20 minutes to 1 hour after meals and at bedtime, or as directed by a physician.

Patient Warnings: Do not take more than 8 tablets in a 24-hour period or use the maximum dosage for more than 2 weeks or use if you have kidney disease except under the advice and supervision of a physician. Keep this and all drugs out of the reach of children.

Drug Interaction Precaution: Antacids may interact with certain prescription drugs. If you are presently taking a prescription drug, do not take this product without checking with your physician or other health professional. Do not take this product if you are presently taking a prescription antibiotic drug containing any form of tetracycline.
To aid in establishing proper dosage schedules, the following information is provided:

Minimum Recommended Dosage: Extra Strength Maalox® Antacid Plus Anti-Gas	Per 2 Tsp. (10 mL)	Per Tablet
Acid neutralizing capacity	58.1 mEq	18.6 mEq

Sodium content*	< 2 mg	< 1.7 mg
Sugar content	None	0.72 g
Lactose content	None	None

*Dietetically insignificant.

Professional Labeling

Indications: As an antacid for symptomatic relief of hyperacidity associated with the diagnosis of peptic ulcer, gastritis, peptic esophagitis, gastric hyperacidity, heartburn, or hiatal hernia. As an antiflatulent to alleviate the symptoms of gas, including postoperative gas pain.

Advantages: Among antacids, Extra Strength Maalox® Plus Suspension and Extra Strength Maalox® Plus Tablets are uniquely palatable—an important feature which encourages patients to follow your dosage directions. Extra Strength Maalox® Plus Suspension and Extra Strength Maalox® Plus Tablets have the time-proven, nonconstipating, sodium-free* Maalox® formula—useful for those patients suffering from the problems associated with hyperacidity. Additionally, Extra Strength Maalox® Plus Suspension and Extra Strength Maalox® Plus Tablets contain simethicone to alleviate discomfort associated with entrapped gas.

Warnings:
(i) Prolonged use of aluminum-containing antacids in patients with renal failure may result in or worsen dialysis osteomalacia. Elevated tissue aluminum levels contribute to the development of the dialysis encephalopathy and osteomalacia syndromes. Small amounts of aluminum are absorbed from the gastrointestinal tract and renal excretion of aluminum is impaired in renal failure. Aluminum is not well removed by dialysis because it is bound to albumin and transferrin, which do not cross dialysis membranes. As a result, aluminum is deposited in bone, and dialysis osteomalacia may develop when large amounts of aluminum are ingested orally by patients with impaired renal function.
(ii) Aluminum forms insoluble complexes with phosphate in the gastrointestinal tract, thus decreasing phosphate absorption. Prolonged use of aluminum-containing antacids by normophosphatemic patients may result in hypophosphatemia if phosphate intake is not adequate. In its more severe forms, hypophosphatemia can lead to anorexia, malaise, muscle weakness, and osteomalacia.

Extra Strength Maalox® Antacid Plus Anti-Gas Suspension

Directions for Use: Two to four teaspoonfuls, taken twenty minutes to one hour after meals and at bedtime, or as directed by a physician.

Patient Warnings: Do not take more than 12 teaspoonfuls in a 24-hour period or use the maximum dosage for more than 2 weeks or use if you have kidney disease except under the advice and supervision of a physician. Keep this and all drugs out of the reach of children.

Extra Strength Maalox® Antacid Plus Anti-Gas Tablets

Directions for Use: Chew one to three tablets twenty minutes to one hour after meals and at bedtime, or as directed by a physician.

Patient Warnings: Do not take more than 12 tablets in a 24-hour period or use the maximum dosage for more than two weeks or use if you have kidney disease except under the advice and supervision of a physician. Keep this and all drugs out of the reach of children.

Drug Interaction Precaution: Antacids may interact with certain prescription drugs. If you are presently taking a prescription drug, do not take this product without checking with your physician or other health professional. Do not take this product if you are presently taking a prescription antibiotic drug containing any form of tetracycline.

How Supplied:
Extra Strength Maalox® Plus Suspension
Available in Lemon Creme in the following sizes: 5 fl. oz. (148 mL) (0067-0333-62), 12 fl. oz. (355 mL) (0067-0333-71), and 26 fl. oz. (769 mL) (0067-0333-44).
Cherry Creme is available in plastic bottles of 5 fl. oz. (148 mL) (0067-0336-62, 12 fl. oz. (355 mL) (0067-0336-71), and 26 fl. oz. (769 mL) (0067-0336-44).
Mint Creme is available in plastic bottles of 5 fl. oz. (148 mL) (0067-0338-62), 12 fl. oz. (355 mL) (0067-0338-71) and 26 fl. oz. (769 mL) (0067-0338-44).
Extra Strength Maalox® Antacid Plus Anti-Gas Mint Creme Tablets are available in flip-top bottles of 38 tablets (0067-0345-38) and 75 tablets (0067-0345-75).

Shown in Product Identification Guide, page 506

MAALOX™ ANTI-DIARRHEAL
(Loperamide Hydrochloride)
Oral Solution

Description: Maalox™ Anti-Diarrheal relieves diarrhea for both adults and children 6 years of age and older, in many cases with just one dose. Maalox Anti-Diarrheal contains Loperamide Hydrochloride, previously available only in a leading prescription product. Loperamide Hydrochloride has been prescribed for millions of people, and has proven to be an exceptionally safe and effective anti-diarrheal medication.
Maalox Anti-Diarrheal is a non-chalky, cherry flavored, clear liquid.

Actions: Maalox Anti-Diarrheal contains Loperamide Hydrochloride which has been clinically proven to slow intestinal motility. It also affects water and electrolyte movement through the bowel.

Indications: Maalox Anti-Diarrheal controls the symptoms of diarrhea.

Active Ingredient: Loperamide Hydrochloride 1 mg per teaspoonful (5 ml).

Inactive Ingredients: Alcohol 5.25%, citric acid, flavors, glycerin, methylparaben and purified water. May contain sodium hydroxide to adjust pH.

Directions for use: A dose cup is provided to accurately measure doses as noted below. Drink plenty of clear fluids to help prevent dehydration, which may accompany diarrhea.
Adults and children 12 years of age and older —
Take 4 teaspoonfuls (1 dosage cup) after the first loose bowel movement and 2 teaspoonfuls after each subsequent loose bowel movement, but no more than 8 teaspoonfuls per day for no more than 2 days.
Children 9–11 years (60–95 lbs.) —
Take 2 teaspoonfuls (½ dosage cup) after the first loose bowel movement and 1 teaspoonful after each subsequent loose bowel movement. Do not exceed 6 teaspoonfuls per day.
Children 6–8 years (48–59 lbs.) —
Take 2 teaspoonfuls (½ dosage cup) after the first loose bowel movement and 1 teaspoonful after each subsequent loose bowel movement. Do not exceed 4 teaspoonfuls per day.
Children under 6 years (up to 47 lbs.) —
Consult a physician. Not intended for use in children under 6 years old.

Warnings: DO NOT USE FOR MORE THAN TWO DAYS UNLESS DIRECTED BY A PHYSICIAN. Do not use if diarrhea is accompanied by high fever (greater than 101°), or if blood is present in the stool, or if you have had a rash or other allergic reaction to Loperamide Hydrochloride. If you are taking antibiotics or have a history of liver disease, consult a physician before using this product. As with any drug, if you are pregnant or nursing a baby, seek the advice of a health professional before using this product. In case of accidental overdose, seek professional assistance or contact poison control center immediately.

Overdosage: Overdosage of loperamide HCl in man may result in constipation, CNS depression and nausea. A slurry of activated charcoal administered promptly after ingestion of loperamide hydrochloride can reduce the amount of drug which is absorbed. If vomiting occurs spontaneously upon ingestion, a slurry of 100 grams of activated charcoal should be administered orally as soon as fluids can be retained. If vomiting has not occurred, and CNS de-

Continued on next page

The full prescribing information for each CIBA Consumer Pharmaceuticals product is contained herein and is that in effect as of December 15, 1994

CIBA Consumer—Cont.

pression is evident, gastric lavage should be performed followed by administration to 100 grams of the activated charcoal slurry through the gastric tube. In the event of overdosage, patients should be monitored for signs of CNS depression for at least 24 hours. Children may be more sensitive to central nervous system effects than adults. If CNS depression is observed, naloxone may be administered. If responsive to naloxone, vital signs must be monitored carefully for recurrence of symptoms of drug overdose for at least 24 hours after the last dose of naloxone.

How Supplied: Cherry flavored liquid (2 fl oz and 4 fl oz) in tamper resistant bottles and child resistant safety caps and dosage cup.

Shown in Product Identification Guide, page 507

MAALOX™ ANTI-DIARRHEAL
Loperamide Hydrochloride
Caplets, 2mg

Description: Maalox™ Anti-Diarrheal relieves diarrhea for both adults and children 6 years of age and older, in many cases with just one dose. Maalox Anti-Diarrheal contains Loperamide Hydrochloride, previously available only in a leading prescription product. Loperamide Hydrochloride has been prescribed for millions of people, and has proven to be an exceptionally safe and effective anti-diarrheal medication.

Actions: Maalox Anti-Diarrheal contains loperamide hydrochloride which has been clinically proven to slow intestinal motility. It also affects water and electrolyte movement through the bowel.

Indications: Maalox Anti-Diarrheal controls the symptoms of diarrhea.

Active Ingredient: Loperamide Hydrochloride 2 mg per caplet.

Inactive Ingredients: Corn starch, lactose, magnesium stearate, microcrystalline cellulose, FD&C Blue #1 and D&C Yellow #10.

Directions for Use: Follow specific dosing information below, and drink plenty of clear fluids to help prevent dehydration, which may accompany diarrhea.
Adults and children 12 years of age and older—
Take 2 caplets after the first loose bowel movement and 1 caplet after each subsequent loose bowel movement, but no more than 4 caplets a day for no more than 2 days.
Children 9–11 years (60–95 lbs.)—Take 1 caplet after the first loose bowel movements and ½ caplet after each subsequent loose bowel movement, but no more than 3 caplets a day for no more than 2 days.

Children 6–8 years (48–59 lbs.)—Take 1 caplet after the first loose bowel movement and ½ caplet after each subsequent loose bowel movement, but no more than 2 caplets a day for no more than 2 days.
Children under 6 years (up to 47 lbs.)—Consult a physician. Not intended for use in children under 6 years old.

Warnings: DO NOT USE FOR MORE THAN TWO DAYS UNLESS DIRECTED BY A PHYSICIAN. Do not use if diarrhea is accompanied by high fever (greater than 101°), or if blood is present in the stool, or if you have had a rash or other allergic reaction to Loperamide Hydrochloride. If you are taking antibiotics or have a history of liver disease, consult a physician before using this product. As with any drug, if you are pregnant or nursing a baby, seek the advice of a health professional before using this product. Keep this and all drugs out of the reach of children. In case of accidental overdose, seek professional assistance or contact poison control center immediately.

Overdosage: Overdosage of loperamide HCl may result in constipation, CNS depression and nausea. A slurry of activated charcoal administered promptly after ingestion of loperamide hydrochloride can reduce the amount of drug which is absorbed. If vomiting occurs spontaneously upon ingestion, a slurry of 100 grams of activated charcoal should be administered orally as soon as fluids can be retained. If vomiting has not occurred, and CNS depression is evident, gastric lavage should be performed followed by administration to 100 grams of the activated charcoal slurry through the gastric tube. In the event of overdosage, patients should be monitored for signs of CNS depression for at least 24 hours. Children may be more sensitive to central nervous system effects than adults. If CNS depression is observed, naloxone may be administered. If responsive to naloxone, vital signs must be monitored carefully for recurrence of symptoms of drug overdose for at least 24 hours after the last dose of naloxone.

How Supplied: Cartons of 6 and 12 caplets.

Shown in Product Identification Guide, page 507

MAALOX™ ANTI-GAS
(Simethicone)
Tablets (Regular Strength)

Description: Maalox Anti-Gas relieves the painful symptoms of bloating, pressure, and fullness, commonly referred to as gas. It is formulated with the active ingredient that diffuses the excess gas in the stomach and digestive tract.

Active Ingredient: Simethicone (80 mg per tablet)

Inactive Ingredients: Corn starch, D&C Red No. 27, aluminum lake, flavor,

gelatin, mannitol, sucrose, and tribasic calcium phosphate.

Indications: For relief of painful symptoms of excess gas in the digestive tract. Such gas is frequently caused by excessive swallowing of air or by eating foods that disagree.
Maalox™ Anti-Gas acts in the stomach and intestines to change the surface tension of gas bubbles enabling them to coalesce: thus, the gas is freed and is eliminated more easily by belching or passing flatus.

Directions for Use: Chew 1 to 2 tablets thoroughly 4 times daily after meals and at bedtime or as directed by a physician. May also be taken as needed, up to 6 tablets daily.
If symptoms persist, contact your physician. **DO NOT EXCEED 6 TABLETS A DAY UNLESS DIRECTED BY A PHYSICIAN.**

Warnings: Keep this and all drugs out of the reach of children.

How Supplied: Cartons of 12 and 48 tablets.

Shown in Product Identification Guide, page 507

EXTRA STRENGTH MAALOX™ ANTI-GAS
(Simethicone) Tablets

Description: Maalox Anti-Gas relieves the painful symptoms of bloating, pressure, and fullness commonly referred to as gas. It is formulated with the active ingredient that diffuses the excess gas in the stomach and digestive tract.

Active Ingredient: Simethicone (150 mg per tablet)

Inactive Ingredients: Corn starch, D&C red No. 27, aluminum lake, flavor, gelatin, mannitol, sucrose and tribasic calcium phosphate.

Indications: For relief of painful symptoms of bloating, pressure, and fullness, commonly referred to as gas. Such gas is frequently caused by excessive swallowing of air or by eating foods that disagree.
Maalox™ Anti-Gas acts in the stomach and intestines to change the surface tension of gas bubbles enabling them to coalesce: thus, the gas is freed and is eliminated more easily by belching or passing flatus.

Directions for Use: Chew 1 tablet thoroughly. Use after meals or at bedtime, or as directed by a physician. May also be taken as needed, up to 3 tablets daily. If symptoms persist, contact your physician.

Warnings: Keep this and all drugs out of the reach of children.

How Supplied: Cartons of 10 tablets.
Shown in Product Identification Guide, page 507

Forms	Inactive Ingredients	Dosage	How Supplied	Per Dose Information
Maalox™ Daily Fiber Therapy Orange Flavor Powder	Citric Acid, D&C Yellow No. 10, FD&C Yellow No. 6, Flavoring, Sucrose	One rounded tablespoonful (12g) in 8 ounces of liquid up to 3 times per day	Canisters: 13 Ounce/30 Doses 20.3 Ounce/48 Doses Packettes: Cartons of Three Single Dose Packets	Calories: 35 Carbohydrates: 8g Fat: 100 mg
Maalox™ Daily Fiber Therapy Citrus Flavor Powder	Citric Acid, D&C Yellow No. 10, Flavoring, Sucrose	One rounded tablespoonful (12g) in 8 ounces of liquid up to 3 times per day	Canisters: 13 Ounce/30 Doses 20.3 Ounce/48 Doses	Calories: 35 Carbohydrates: 8g Fat: 100mg
Maalox™ Daily Fiber Therapy Orange Flavor Sugar Free Powder	Aspartame, Citric Acid, D&C Yellow No. 10, FD&C Yellow No. 6, Flavoring, Maltodextrin	One rounded teaspoonful (5.8g) in 8 ounces of liquid up to 3 times per day	Canisters: 10 Ounce/48 Doses Packettes: Cartons of Three Single Dose Packets	Calories: 9 Carbohydrates: 2g Fat: 100mg Phenylalanine: 21mg
Maalox™ Daily Fiber Therapy Citrus Flavor Sugar Free Powder	Aspartame, Citric Acid, D&C Yellow No. 10, Flavoring, Maltodextrin	One rounded teaspoonful (5.8g) in 8 ounces of liquid up to 3 times per day	Canisters: 10 Ounce/48 Dose	Calories: 9 Carboyhdrates: 2g Fat: 100mg Phenylalanine: 21mg

MAALOX™ DAILY FIBER THERAPY
(psyllium hydrophilic mucilloid)

Description: Maalox™ Daily Fiber Therapy is a bulk-producing, natural psyllium fiber encouraging normal elimination naturally, without chemical stimulants. It contains hydrophilic mucilloid fiber which is derived from the husk of the psyllium seed. It is a finely ground, ultra-smooth powder that mixes easily. It provides a daily source of soluble fiber that is effective in restoring and maintaining regularity.

Actions: Maalox Daily Fiber Therapy promotes natural elimination due to its bulking effect in the colon. The bulking effect is due to both the water-holding capacity of undigested fiber and the increased bacterial mass following partial fiber digestion. This results in enlargement of the lumen of the colon, thereby decreasing intraluminal pressure and speeding colonic transit in constipated patients.

Indications: Maalox Daily Fiber Therapy is indicated in the management of chronic constipation, in irritable bowel syndrome, as adjunctive therapy in constipation of diverticular disease, in the bowel management of patients with hemorrhoids, and for constipation during pregnancy, convalescence, and senility.

Contraindications: Intestinal obstruction, fecal impaction.
For Maalox™ Citrus and Orange flavored sugar free powders—Phenylketonurics: Contains 21 mg Phenylalanine per tablespoonful.

Warnings: TAKING THIS PRODUCT WITHOUT ADEQUATE FLUID MAY CAUSE IT TO SWELL AND BLOCK YOUR THROAT OR ESOPHAGUS AND MAY CAUSE CHOKING. DO NOT TAKE THIS PRODUCT IF YOU HAVE DIFFICULTY IN SWALLOWING. IF YOU EXPERIENCE CHEST PAIN, VOMITING, OR DIFFICULTY IN SWALLOWING OR BREATHING AFTER TAKING THIS PRODUCT, SEEK IMMEDIATE MEDICAL ATTENTION.
Patients are advised they should not use the product without consulting a doctor when abdominal pain, nausea, or vomiting are present, if they have noticed a sudden change in bowel habits that persists over a period of 2 weeks, or rectal bleeding, or if they have been diagnosed with esophageal narrowing or have difficulty in swallowing.
Patients are advised to consult a physician if constipation persists for longer than 1 week, as this may be a sign of serious medical condition.
Psyllium products may cause allergic reaction in people sensitive to inhaled or ingested psyllium. Keep this and all medications out of the reach of children.

Precaution: *Notice to Health Care Professionals:* To minimize the potential for allergic reaction, health care professionals who frequently dispense powdered psyllium products should avoid inhaling airborne dust while dispensing these products. *Handling and Dispensing:* To minimize generating airborne dust, spoon product from the canister into a glass according to label directions.

Dosage & Administration: MIX THIS PRODUCT (CHILD OR ADULT DOSE) WITH AT LEAST 8 OUNCES (A FULL GLASS) OF WATER OR OTHER FLUID. MIXING THIS PRODUCT WITHOUT ENOUGH LIQUID MAY CAUSE CHOKING. SEE WARNINGS. Recommended dosage is for sugar-free product 1 rounded teaspoonful or for sucrose product 1 rounded tablespoonful. The appropriate dose should be mixed with 8 ounces of water or your favorite cool beverage. Drinking another glass of liquid is helpful.
Children (6–12 years of age) should take ½ the adult dose with 8 ounces of liquid up to 3 times daily.

New Users: Start by taking 1 dose each day. Gradually increase to 3 doses per day if needed or recommended by your doctor. If minor gas or bloating occurs, reduce the amount you take until your system adjusts. Also useful in the treatment of disorders other than constipation, when recommended by a physician.

How Supplied: See chart on following page.
[See table above.]
Shown in Product Identification Guide, page 507

MAALOX® HEARTBURN RELIEF
Heartburn Relief™ Antacid Tablets

Description: Maalox® Heartburn Relief tablets are specially formulated to provide fast, effective relief of heartburn, acid indigestion, and sour stomach.

Active Ingredients: Each tablet contains aluminum hydroxide-magnesium

Continued on next page

The full prescribing information for each CIBA Consumer Pharmaceuticals product is contained herein and is that in effect as of December 15, 1994

CIBA Consumer—Cont.

carbonate codried gel 180 mg and magnesium carbonate 160 mg. It is formulated in a pleasant, cool mint flavor.

Inactive Ingredients: Compressible sugar, corn starch, D&C Yellow No. 10, FD&C Blue No. 2, flavors, magnesium alginate, magnesium stearate, potassium bicarbonate.

Minimum Recommended Dosage: Maalox Heartburn Relief Antacid Tablets Per 2 tablets	
Acid neutralizing Capacity	NLT 14.7 mEq
Sodium	NMT 6mg

Directions for Use: Chew 2–4 tablets thoroughly, after meals and at bedtime, or as directed by physician. For best results, follow with a half glass (4 fl. oz.) of water or other cool liquid.

Patient Warnings: Do not take more than 16 tablets in a 24-hour period or use the maximum dosage for more than 2 weeks or use if you have kidney disease except under the advice and supervision of a physician.

Drug Interaction Precaution: Antacids may interact with certain prescription drugs. If you are presently taking a prescription drug, do not take this product without checking with your physician or other health professional.

Professional Labeling:

Warnings: Prolonged use of aluminum-containing antacids in patients with renal failure may result in or worsen dialysis osteomalacia. Elevated tissue aluminum levels contribute to the development of the dialysis encephalopathy and osteomalacia syndromes. Small amounts of aluminum are absorbed from the gastrointestinal tract and renal excretion of aluminum is impaired in renal failure. Aluminum is not well removed by dialysis because it is bound to albumin and transferrin, which do not cross dialysis membranes. As a result, aluminum is deposited in bone and dialysis osteomalacia may develop when large amounts of aluminum are ingested orally by patients with impaired renal function. Aluminum forms insoluble complexes with phosphate in the gastrointestinal tract, thus decreasing phosphate absorption. Prolonged use of antacids containing aluminum by normophosphatemic patients may result in hypophosphatemia if phosphate intake is not adequate. In its more severe forms, hypophosphatemia can lead to anorexia, malaise, muscle weakness, and osteomalacia.

How Supplied: Maalox HRF antacid tablets are available in plastic bottles of 30 tablets (0067-0353-30), 60 tablets

(0067-0353-60) and blister packs of 12 tablets (0067-0353-12).

MAALOX® HEARTBURN RELIEF
Suspension (Antacid)

Description: Maalox® Heartburn Relief provides symptomatic relief of heartburn, acid indigestion and/or sour stomach.

Active Ingredients: Each 10 ml (2 teaspoonfuls) contains aluminum hydroxide-magnesium carbonate codried gel 280 mg and magnesium carbonate USP 350 mg. It is formulated in a pleasant, cool mint flavor to help provide a cooling and soothing sensation as it goes down the esophagus.

Inactive Ingredients: Calcium carbonate, calcium saccharin, FD&C Blue No. 1, FD&C Yellow No. 5 (tartrazine) as a color additive, flavors, magnesium alginate, methyl and propyl parabens, potassium bicarbonate, purified water, sorbitol and other ingredients.

Minimum Recommended Dosage: Maalox Heartburn Relief Suspension Per 2 tsp. (10 mL)	
Acid neutralizing capacity	NLT 17 mEq
Sodium content	NMT 5 mg

Directions for Use: Two to four teaspoonfuls 4 times a day, taken 20 min to 1 hour after meals and at bedtime, or as directed by a physician.

Patient Warnings: Do not take more than 16 teaspoonfuls in a 24-hour period or use the maximum dosage for more than 2 weeks or use if you have kidney disease except under the advice and supervision of a physician. Keep this and all drugs out of the reach of children.

Drug Interaction Precaution: Antacids may interact with certain prescription drugs. If you are presently taking a prescription drug, do not take this product without checking with your physician or other health professional.

Professional Labeling:

Warnings:
Prolonged use of aluminum-containing antacids in patients with renal failure may result in or worsen dialysis osteomalacia. Elevated tissue aluminum levels contribute to the development of the dialysis encephalopathy and osteomalacia syndromes. Small amounts of aluminum are absorbed from the gastrointestinal tract and renal excretion of aluminum is impaired in renal failure. Aluminum is not well removed by dialysis because it is bound to albumin and transferrin, which do not cross dialysis membranes. As a result, aluminum is deposited in bone,

and dialysis osteomalacia may develop when large amounts of aluminum are ingested orally by patients with impaired renal function.

Aluminum forms insoluble complexes with phosphate in the gastrointestinal tract, thus decreasing phosphate absorption. Prolonged use of antacids containing aluminum by normophosphatemic patients may result in hypophosphatemia if phosphate intake is not adequate. In its more severe forms, hypophosphatemia can lead to anorexia, malaise, muscle weakness, and osteomalacia.

How Supplied: Maalox® Heartburn Relief is available in a 10 fl oz plastic bottle (0067-0350-71).

MAALOX®
Magnesia and Alumina
Oral Suspension
Antacid

Liquids
Mint Flavored
Cherry Creme

Description: Maalox® is used for the relief of acid indigestion, heartburn, sour stomach and upset stomach associated with these symptoms.

Active Ingredients	Maalox Suspension 5 mL teaspoon
Magnesium Hydroxide	200 mg.
Aluminum Hydroxide (equivalent to dried gel, USP)	225 mg.

Inactive Ingredients: Flavors, methylparaben, propylparaben, saccharin, sorbitol, purified water and other ingredients. May also contain citric acid.

Minimum Recommended Dosage: Maalox Suspension Per 2 Tsp. (10 mL)	
Acid neutralizing capacity	NLT 26.6 mEq
Sodium content	NMT 2 mg

Professional Labeling

Indications: As an antacid for symptomatic relief of hyperacidity associated with the diagnosis of peptic ulcer, gastritis, peptic esophagitis, gastric hyperacidity, heartburn, or hiatal hernia.

Professional Labeling (cont'd)

Warnings: (i) Prolonged use of aluminum-containing antacids in patients with renal failure may result in or worsen dialysis osteomalacia. Elevated tissue aluminum levels contribute to the development of the dialysis encephalopathy and osteomalacia syndromes. Small amounts of aluminum are absorbed from the gastrointestinal tract and renal excretion of aluminum is impaired in renal failure. Aluminum is not well removed by dialysis because it is bound to albumin and transferrin, which do not cross dialysis membranes. As a result, aluminum is deposited in bone, and dialysis osteomalacia may develop when large amounts of aluminum are ingested orally by patients with impaired renal function. (ii) Aluminum forms insoluble complexes with phosphate in the gastrointestinal tract, thus decreasing phosphate absorption. Prolonged use of aluminum-containing antacids by normophosphatemic patients may result in hypophosphatemia if phosphate intake is not adequate. In its more severe forms, hypophosphatemia can lead to anorexia, malaise, muscle weakness, and osteomalacia.

Directions for Use. Two to four teaspoonfuls, four times a day, taken 20 minutes to 1 hour after meals and at bedtime, or as directed by a physician.

Patient Warnings: Do not take more than 16 teaspoonfuls in a 24-hour period or use the maximum dosage for more than 2 weeks or use if you have kidney disease except under the advice and supervision of a physician. Keep this and all drugs out of the reach of children.

Drug Interaction Precaution: Antacids may interact with certain prescription drugs. If you are presently taking a prescription drug, do not take this product without checking with your physician or other health professional.

How Supplied:
Maalox Mint Flavored Suspension is available in plastic bottles of 12 oz (0067-0330-71) and 26 oz (0067-0330-44).
Maalox Cherry Creme Flavored Suspension is available in plastic bottles of 12 oz (0067-0331-71) and 26 oz (0067-0331-44).

Shown in Product Identification Guide, page 506

MAALOX® Plus
Alumina, Magnesia and Simethicone Tablets,
Rhône-Poulenc Rorer
Antacid/Anti-Gas

Tablets
  Lemon Creme
  Cherry Creme, Mint Creme
☐ **Physician-proven Maalox® formula for antacid effectiveness.**
☐ **Simethicone, at a recognized clinical dose, for antiflatulent action.**
Description: Maalox® Plus, a balanced combination of magnesium and aluminum hydroxides plus simethicone, is a non-constipating antacid/anti-gas which comes in pleasant tasting flavors.
Composition: To provide symptomatic relief of hyperacidity plus alleviation of gas symptoms, each tablet contains:

Active Ingredients	Maalox® Plus Per Tablet
Magnesium Hydroxide	200 mg
Aluminum Hydroxide (equivalent to dried gel, USP)	200 mg
Simethicone	25 mg

Inactive Ingredients: Maalox® Plus Tablets: Citric acid, confectioners' sugar, D&C Red No. 30, D&C Yellow No. 10, dextrose, flavors, glycerin, magnesium stearate, mannitol, saccharin sodium, sorbitol, starch, talc.
To aid in establishing proper dosage schedules, the following information is provided:

Minimum Recommended Dosage:	Per Tablet
Acid neutralizing capacity	NLT 10.65 mEq
Sodium content*	NMT <1 mg
Sugar content	0.57 g
Lactose content	None

*Dietetically insignificant.

Directions for Use: Chew 1 to 4 tablets 4 times a day, 20 minutes to 1 hour after meals and at bedtime, or as directed by a physician.

Patient Warnings: Do not take more than 16 tablets in a 24-hour period or use the maximum dosage for more than 2 weeks or use if you have kidney disease except under the advice and supervision of a physician. Keep this and all drugs out of the reach of children.

Drug Interaction Precaution: Antacids may interact with certain prescription drugs. If you are presently taking a prescription drug, do not take this product without checking with your physician or other health professional. Do not take this product if you are presently taking a prescription antibiotic drug containing any form of tetracycline.

Professional Labeling

Indications: As an antacid for symptomatic relief of hyperacidity associated with the diagnosis of peptic ulcer, gastritis, peptic esophagitis, gastric hyperacidity, heartburn, or hiatal hernia. As an antiflatulent to alleviate the symptoms of gas, including postoperative gas pain.

Warnings: Prolonged use of aluminum-containing antacids in patients with renal failure may result in or worsen

dialysis osteomalacia. Elevated tissue aluminum levels contribute to the development of the dialysis encephalopathy and osteomalacia syndromes. Small amounts of aluminum are absorbed from the gastrointestinal tract and renal excretion of aluminum is impaired in renal failure. Aluminum is not well removed by dialysis because it is bound to albumin and transferrin, which do not cross dialysis membranes. As a result, aluminum is deposited in bone, and dialysis osteomalacia may develop when large amounts of aluminum are ingested orally by patients with impaired renal function. Aluminum forms insoluble complexes with phosphate in the gastrointestinal tract, thus decreasing phosphate absorption. Prolonged use of aluminum-containing antacids by normophosphatemic patients may result in hypophosphatemia if phosphate intake is not adequate. In its more severe forms, hypophosphatemia can lead to anorexia, malaise, muscle weakness, and osteomalacia.

Advantages: Maalox® Plus Tablets are uniquely palatable—an important feature which encourages patients to follow your dosage directions. Maalox® Plus Tablets have the time-proven, non-constipating, sodium-free* Maalox® formula—useful for those patients suffering from the problems associated with hyperacidity. Additionally, Maalox® Plus Tablets contain simethicone to alleviate discomfort associated with entrapped gas.

How Supplied: Maalox® Plus Lemon Creme Tablets are available in plastic bottles of 50 tablets (0067-0339-50) and 100 tablets (0067-0339-67), convenience packs of 12 tablets (0067-0339-19), tray of 12 rolls (0067-0339-23), and 3 roll packs of 36 tablets (0067-0339-33).
Maalox Plus Cherry Creme Tablets are available in plastic bottles of 50 tablets (0067-0341-50) and 100 tablets (0067-0341-68), tray of 12 rolls (0067-0341-23) and 3 roll packs of 36 tablets (0067-0341-33).

Shown in Product Identification Guide, page 506

MYOFLEX® EXTERNAL ANALGESIC CREME
[mī'ō-flex]

Description: Odorless, stainless and non-burning topical pain reliever.

Active Ingredient: Trolamine salicylate 10%.

Other Ingredients: Cetyl alcohol, disodium EDTA, fragrance, propylene glycol, purified water, sodium lauryl sulfate, stearyl alcohol, white wax.

Continued on next page

The full prescribing information for each CIBA Consumer Pharmaceuticals product is contained herein and is that in effect as of December 15, 1994

CIBA Consumer—Cont.

Indications: For the temporary relief of minor aches and pains of muscles and joints associated with simple backache, arthritis, strains and sprains.

Warning: FOR EXTERNAL USE ONLY. Do not apply to irritated skin or if excessive irritation develops. Avoid contact with eyes. If condition worsens, or if symptoms persist for more than 7 days or clear up and occur again within a few days, discontinue use of this product and consult a physician. Keep this and all other medication out of the reach of children. In case of accidental ingestion, seek professional assistance or contact a Poison Control Center immediately. As with any drug, if you are pregnant or nursing a baby, seek the advice of a health professional before using this product.

Directions: Use only as directed. **Adults and children 2 years of age and older:** Apply to affected area not more than three to four times daily. Affected areas may be wrapped loosely with two- or three-inch elastic bandage. **Children under 2 years of age:** Consult a physician.
Protect from freezing or excessive heat. Store at controlled room temperature 15°–30°C (59°–86°F).

How Supplied: Myoflex Creme is supplied in 2 oz. and 4 oz. easy-squeeze tubes, and 8 oz. and 16 oz. jars.
MYOFLEX is a registered trademark of Ciba-Geigy Corporation.
Shown in Product Identification Guide, page 507

NŌSTRIL® Nasal Decongestant
[nō'stril]
phenylephrine HCl, USP

Active Ingredient: phenylephrine HCl 0.25% (¼% Mild strength) or phenylephrine HCl 0.5% (½% Regular strength). Also contains benzalkonium chloride 0.004% as a preservative, boric acid, sodium borate, water.

Indications: For temporary relief of nasal congestion due to the common cold, hay fever, other upper respiratory allergies, or associated with sinusitis.

Actions: NŌSTRIL metered pump spray for nasal decongestion delivers measured, uniform doses. The medication constricts the smaller arterioles of the nasal passages, producing a gentle, predictable, decongestant effect. Nŏstril penetrates and shrinks swollen membranes, restoring freer breathing and unclogs sinus passages, bringing the effective medication in contact with inflamed, swollen tissues. It will not hurt tender membranes since it is formulated to match the pH of normal nasal secretions. The one-way pump helps prevent draw-back contamination of the medication.

Warnings: Do not exceed recommended dosage because burning, stinging, sneezing, or increased nasal discharge may occur. Do not use for more than 3 days. If symptoms persist, consult a physician. Use of the dispenser by more than one person may spread infection. Do not use this product if you have heart disease, high blood pressure, thyroid disease, diabetes or difficulty in urination due to enlargement of the prostate gland, unless directed by a physician. Keep this and all drugs out of reach of children.

Symptoms and Treatment of Oral Overdosage: In case of accidental ingestion, seek professional assistance or consult a poison control center immediately.

Dosage and Administration:
¼% Mild—Adults and children 6 to under 12 years of age (with adult supervision): 2 or 3 sprays in each nostril not more often than every 4 hours. Children under 6 years of age: consult a doctor.
½% Regular—Adults: 2 or 3 sprays in each nostril not more often than every 4 hours. Do not give to children under 12 years of age unless directed by a doctor. Remove protective cap. Hold bottle with thumb at base and nozzle between first and second fingers. With head upright, insert nozzle into nostril. Depress pump 2 or 3 times, all the way down, and sniff deeply. Repeat in other nostril. Before using the first time, prime pump by depressing it firmly several times.

How Supplied: Metered nasal pump spray in white plastic bottles of ½ fl. oz. (15 ml) packaged in tamper-resistant outer cartons.
0.25% (¼% Mild strength) for children 6 years and over and adults who prefer a milder decongestant.
0.5% (½% Regular strength) for adults and children 12 years or older.
Shown in Product Identification Guide, page 507

NŌSTRILLA® Long Acting
[nō-stril'a]
Nasal Decongestant
oxymetazoline HCl, USP

Active Ingredient: oxymetazoline HCl 0.05%. Also contains benzalkonium chloride 0.02% as a preservative, glycine, sorbitol solution, water. (Mercury preservatives are not used in this product.)

Indications: For temporary relief of nasal congestion due to the common cold, hay fever, other upper respiratory allergies, or associated with sinusitis.

Actions: NŌSTRILLA metered pump spray for nasal decongestion delivers measured, uniform doses. The medication constricts the smaller arterioles of the nasal passages, producing a prolonged (up to 12 hours), gentle, predictable, decongestant effect. Nŏstrilla penetrates and shrinks swollen membranes, restoring freer breathing and unclogs sinus passages, bringing the effective medication in contact with inflamed, swollen tissues. It will not hurt tender membranes since it is formulated to match the pH of normal nasal secretions. Use at bedtime restores freer nasal breathing through the night. The one-way pump helps prevent draw-back contamination of the medication.

Warnings: Do not exceed recommended dosage because burning, stinging, sneezing or increased nasal discharge may occur. Do not use for more than 3 days. If symptoms persist, consult a physician. Use of the dispenser by more than one person may spread infection. Do not use this product if you have heart disease, high blood pressure, thyroid disease, diabetes or difficulty in urination due to enlargement of the prostate gland unless directed by a doctor. Keep this and all drugs out of reach of children.

Symptoms and Treatment of Oral Overdosage: In case of accidental ingestion, seek professional assistance or contact a poison control center immediately.

Dosage and Administration: Adults and children 6 to under 12 years of age (with adult supervision): 2 or 3 sprays in each nostril not more often than every 10 to 12 hours. Do not exceed 2 applications in any 24-hour period. Children under 6 years of age: consult a doctor. Remove protective cap. Hold bottle with thumb at base and nozzle between first and second fingers. With head upright, insert nozzle into nostril. Depress pump 2 or 3 times, all the way down, and sniff deeply. Repeat in other nostril. Before using the first time, prime pump by depressing it firmly several times.

How Supplied: Metered nasal pump spray in white plastic bottles of ½ fl. oz. (15 ml) packaged in tamper-resistant outer cartons.

NUPERCAINAL®
Dibucaine
Hemorrhoidal and Anesthetic Ointment

Active Ingredient: 1% dibucaine USP. Also contains: acetone sodium bisulfite, lanolin, light mineral oil, purified water, and white petrolatum.

Indications: For prompt, temporary relief of pain, itching and burning due to hemorrhoids or other anorectal disorders. May also be used topically for temporary relief of pain and itching associated with sunburn, minor burns, cuts, scrapes, insect bites, or minor skin irritation.

Directions: Adults: When practical, cleanse the affected area with mild soap and water and rinse thoroughly. Gently dry by patting or blotting with toilet tissue or a soft cloth before application of this product. Puncture tube seal with cap or sharp object. Apply externally to the affected area up to 3 or 4 times daily.

Children 2–12: Do not use except under the advice and supervision of a physician. DO NOT USE IN INFANTS UNDER 2 YEARS OF AGE OR LESS THAN 35 LBS. WEIGHT.

Warnings: IF SWALLOWED, CONSULT A PHYSICIAN OR POISON CONTROL CENTER IMMEDIATELY. **Do not use in or near the eyes.** If condition worsens or does not improve within 7 days, consult a physician. Do not put this product into the rectum by using fingers or any mechanical device. Do not exceed recommended daily dosage unless directed by a physician. Certain persons can develop allergic reactions to ingredients in this product. If the symptom being treated does not subside or if redness, irritation, swelling, pain, bleeding or other symptoms develop or increase, discontinue use and consult a physician promptly. As with any drug, if you are pregnant or nursing a baby, seek the advice of a health care professional before using this product. KEEP THIS AND ALL MEDICATION OUT OF REACH OF CHILDREN.

How Supplied: Nupercainal Hemorrhoidal and Anesthetic Ointment is available in tubes of 1 and 2 ounces. See crimp of tube for lot number and expiration date. Store between 15°–30°C (59°–86°F).
NDC 0083-5812.
Distributed by: Ciba Consumer Pharmaceuticals, 581 Main Street, Woodbridge, NJ 07095
Made in Canada
Shown in Product Identification Guide, page 507

NUPERCAINAL
HYDROCORTISONE 1% CREAM
Anti-Itch Cream

Indications: For the temporary relief of external anal itching. May also be used for the temporary relief of itching associated with minor skin irritations and rashes due to eczema, insect bites, poison ivy, poison oak, poison sumac, soaps, detergents, cosmetics, jewelry, seborrheic dermatitis, or psoriarsis. Other uses of this product should be only under the advice and supervision of a physician.

Directions: Adults: When practical, cleanse the affected area with mild soap and warm water and rinse thoroughly. Gently dry by patting or blotting with toilet tissue or a soft cloth before application of this product. Apply to affected area not more than 3 to 4 times daily. Children under 12 years of age: Consult a physician.

Warnings: For external use only. Avoid contact with the eyes. If condition worsens, or if symptoms persist for more than 7 days or clear up and occur again within a few days, stop use of this product and do not begin use of any other hydrocortisone product unless you consulted a physician. Do not use for the

treatment of diaper rash; consult a physician. Do not exceed the recommended daily dosage unless directed by a physician. In case of bleeding, consult a physician promptly. Do not put this product into the rectum by using fingers or any mechanical device or applicator. KEEP THIS AND ALL MEDICATION OUT OF REACH OF CHILDREN. In case of accidental ingestion, seek professional assistance or contact a poison control center immediately.

Active Ingredient: 1% Hydrocortisone Acetate USP.

Inactive Ingredients: Cetostearyl Alcohol, Sodium Lauryl Sulfate, White Petrolatum, Propylene Glycol, Purified Water.

How Supplied: Nupercainal Hydrocortisone Cream is available in a 1 ounce tube. See crimp of tube for lot number and expiration date.
Store at room temperature 15–30°C (59°–86°F).
NDC 0083-5700-96
Distributed by: Ciba Consumer Pharmaceuticals, 581 Main Street, Woodbridge, NJ 07095
Made in Canada
Shown in Product Identification Guide, page 507

NUPERCAINAL®
Pain-Relief Cream

Active Ingredient: 0.5% dibucaine USP.

Inactive Ingredients: acetone sodium bisulfite, fragrance, glycerin, potassium hydroxide, purified water, stearic acid, and trolamine.

Indications: For prompt, temporary relief of pain and itching due to sunburn, minor burns, cuts, scrapes, scratches, and nonpoisonous insect bites.

Directions: Puncture tube seal with cap or sharp object. Apply to affected area, rub in gently. **Do not use in or near eyes.**

Caution: IF SWALLOWED, CONSULT A PHYSICIAN OR POISON CONTROL CENTER IMMEDIATELY. Not for prolonged use. Not more than ⅔ tube should be applied in 24 hours for adults or ⅙ tube to a child. If the symptom being treated does not subside or rash, irritation, swelling, pain, or other symptoms develop or increase, discontinue use and consult a physician.

How Supplied: Nupercainal Pain-Relief Cream is available in tubes of 1½ ounces. See crimp of tube for lot number and expiration date. Store between 15°–30°C (59°–86°F).
NDC 0083-5830-91.
Distributed by: Ciba Consumer Pharmaceuticals, 581 Main Street, Woodbridge, NJ 07095
Shown in Product Identification Guide, page 507

NUPERCAINAL®
Suppositories

Indications: Nupercainal Rectal Suppositories give temporary relief of itching, burning, and discomfort associated with hemorrhoids or other anorectal disorders.

Active Ingredients: 2.1 grams cocoa butter, NF and .25 gram zinc oxide.

Inactive Ingredients: acetone sodium bisulfite and bismuth subgallate.

Directions: ADULTS—When practical, cleanse the affected area. Tear one suppository at the "V" cut, peel foil downward and remove foil wrapper before inserting into the rectum. Gently insert the suppository rectally, rounded end first. Use one suppository up to 6 times daily or after each bowel movement. CHILDREN UNDER 12 YEARS OF AGE—Consult a physician.

WARNING: IF ACCIDENTALLY SWALLOWED, CONSULT A PHYSICIAN OR POISON CONTROL CENTER IMMEDIATELY.
If condition worsens or does not improve within 7 days, consult a physician. Do not exceed the recommended daily dosage unless directed by a physician. In case of bleeding consult a physician promptly. As with any drug, if you are pregnant or nursing a baby, seek the advice of a health professional before using this product.
Keep this and all medications out of reach of children.

How Supplied: Nupercainal Suppositories are available in tamper-evident packages of 12 and 24.
Do not store above 30°C (86°F).
NDC 0083-5841-25
C86-42 (Rev. 9/86)
Shown in Product Identification Guide, page 507

OTRIVIN®
xylometazoline hydrochloride USP
Nasal Spray and Nasal Drops 0.1%
Pediatric Nasal Drops 0.05%
Nasal Decongestant

One application provides rapid and long-lasting relief of nasal congestion for up to 10 hours.
Quickly clears stuffy noses due to common cold, sinusitis, hay fever.
Nasal congestion can make life miserable—you can't breathe, smell, taste, or sleep comfortably. That is why Otrivin is so helpful. It clears away that stuffy feeling.
Otrivin has been prescribed by doctors for many years. Here is how you use it:

Continued on next page

The full prescribing information for each CIBA Consumer Pharmaceuticals product is contained herein and is that in effect as of December 15, 1994

CIBA Consumer—Cont.

Nasal Spray 0.1%—for adults and children 12 years and older. Spray 2 or 3 times into each nostril every 8–10 hours. With head upright, squeeze sharply and firmly while inhaling (sniffing) through the nose. For adult use only.

Nasal Drops 0.1%—for adults and children 12 years and older. Put 2 or 3 drops into each nostril every 8 to 10 hours. Tilt head as far back as possible. Immediately bend head forward toward knees, hold for a few seconds, then return to upright position.

Do not give Nasal Spray 0.1% or Nasal Drops 0.1% to children under 12 years except under the advice and supervision of a physician.

Pediatric Nasal Drops 0.05%—for children 2 to 12 years of age. Put 2 or 3 drops into each nostril every 8 to 10 hours. Tilt head as far back as possible. Immediately bend head forward toward knees, hold a few seconds, then return to upright position.

Do not give this product to children under 2 years except under the advice and supervision of a physician.

Otrivin Nasal Spray/Nasal Drops contain 0.1% xylometazoline hydrochloride, USP. Also contains benzalkonium chloride, dibasic sodium phosphate, disodium edetate, monobasic sodium phosphate, purified water and sodium chloride. They are available in an unbreakable plastic spray package of 0.66 fl oz (20 ml) and in a plastic dropper bottle of 0.83 fl oz (25 ml).

Otrivin Pediatric Nasal Drops contain 0.05% xylometazoline hydrochloride, USP. Also contains benzalkonium chloride, dibasic sodium phosphate, disodium edetate, monobasic sodium phosphate, purified water and sodium chloride. It is available in a plastic dropper bottle of 0.83 fl oz (25 ml).

Warnings: Do not exceed recommended dosage, because symptoms such as burning, stinging, sneezing, or increase of nasal discharge may occur. Do not use this product for more than 3 days. If symptoms persist, consult a physician. The use of this dispenser by more than one person may cause infection.

Keep this and all medicines out of the reach of children. Overdosage in young children may cause marked sedation. In case of accidental ingestion, seek professional assistance or contact a Poison Control Center immediately.

Caution: Do not use if the clear overwrap with the name Otrivin® or the printed band on the bottle is missing or damaged.

Shown in Product Identification Guide, page 507

PERDIEM®
[pĕr "dē 'ŭm]

Indication: For relief of constipation. Perdiem®, with its 100% natural, gentle action provides comfortable relief from constipation. Perdiem® is a unique combination of bulk-forming fiber and natural stimulant. The vegetable mucilages of Perdiem® soften the stool and provide pain-free evacuation of the bowel with no chemical stimulants. Perdiem® is also effective as an aid to elimination for the hemorrhoid or fissure patient prior to and following surgery.

Composition: Perdiem® contains as its active ingredients, 82% psyllium (Plantago Hydrocolloid) a natural grain and 18% senna (Cassia Pod Concentrate), a natural vegetable derivative. Each rounded teaspoonful (6.0 g) contains approximately 3.25 g psyllium, 0.74 g senna, 1.8 mg of sodium, 35.5 mg of potassium, and only 4 calories. Perdiem® is "Dye-Free" and contains no artificial sweeteners.

Inactive Ingredients: Acacia, iron oxides, natural flavors, paraffin, sucrose, talc.

Directions for Use: TAKE THIS PRODUCT (CHILD OR ADULT DOSE) WITH AT LEAST 8 OUNCES (A FULL GLASS) OF COOL WATER OR OTHER FLUID. TAKING THIS PRODUCT WITHOUT ENOUGH LIQUID MAY CAUSE CHOKING. SEE WARNINGS.
Adults and Children 12 years and older: In the evening and/or before breakfast, 1 to 2 rounded teaspoonfuls of Perdiem (in full or partial doses) should be placed in the mouth and swallowed with at least 8 ounces of cool liquid. Perdiem should not be chewed.
Children 7 to 11 years: One (1) rounded teaspoon one to two times daily with at least 8 ounces of cool liquid.

For Severe Cases of Constipation: Perdiem may be taken more frequently, up to 2 rounded teaspoonfuls every 6 hours not to exceed 5 teaspoonfuls in a 24-hour period. Perdiem generally takes effect within 12 hours; in severe cases, 24 to 72 hours may be required for optimal relief.

Warnings: TAKING THIS PRODUCT WITHOUT ADEQUATE FLUID MAY CAUSE IT TO SWELL AND BLOCK YOUR THROAT OR ESOPHAGUS AND MAY CAUSE CHOKING. DO NOT TAKE THIS PRODUCT IF YOU HAVE DIFFICULTY IN SWALLOWING. IF YOU EXPERIENCE CHEST PAIN, VOMITING, OR DIFFICULTY IN SWALLOWING OR BREATHING AFTER TAKING THIS PRODUCT, SEEK IMMEDIATE MEDICAL ATTENTION.
Frequent or prolonged use without the direction of a doctor is not recommended. If use of this product for one week has produced no effect, discontinue use and consult a doctor.

If you have noticed a sudden change in bowel habits that persists over a two week period, consult a doctor before using any laxative product.
Do not use in patients with a history of psyllium allergy. Psyllium allergy is rare but can be severe. If an allergic reaction occurs, discontinue use and consult a doctor immediately.
Consult a physician before using any laxative or bulk fiber product in the presence of rectal bleeding or undiagnosed abdominal pain, nausea or vomiting.
Keep this and all drugs out of the reach of children. In case of accidental overdose, seek professional assistance or contact a poison control center immediately.
If you are pregnant or nursing a baby, seek the advice of a health professional before using this product and consider using Perdiem Fiber.

For Patients Habituated to Strong Purgatives: Two rounded teaspoonfuls of Perdiem® in the morning and evening may be required along with half the usual dose of the purgative being used. The purgative should be discontinued as soon as possible and the dosage of Perdiem® granules reduced when and if bowel tone shows lessened laxative dependence.

For Colostomy Patients: To ensure formed stools, give one to two rounded teaspoonfuls of Perdiem® in the evening.

For Clinical Regulation: For patients confined to bed, for those of inactive habits, and in the presence of cardiovascular disease where straining must be avoided, one rounded teaspoonful of Perdiem® taken once or twice daily will provide regular bowel habits.

How Supplied: Granules: 250-gram (8.8 oz) (0067-0690-70) plastic container, 6 single serving packets 6 gm (0067-0690-16) and 20 single serving packets 6 gm (0067-0690-17).
Shown in Product Identification Guide, page 507

PERDIEM® FIBER
[pĕr "dē 'ŭm]

Indications: Perdiem® Fiber provides gentle relief from simple, chronic, and spastic constipation. In addition, it relieves constipation associated with convalescence, pregnancy, and advanced age. Perdiem® Fiber is also indicated for use in special diets lacking in residue fiber to aid regularity and in the management of constipation associated with irritable bowel syndrome, diverticular disease, hemorrhoids, and anal fissures. Perdiem® Fiber is a 100% natural bulk-forming fiber that gently helps maintain regularity and prevents constipation. Perdiem® Fiber's unique form is easy to swallow and requires no mixing but must be followed by at least 8 ounces (a full glass) of water or other cool liquid. Perdiem® Fiber contains no chemical stimulants and may be used daily by those who may lack sufficient dietary fiber. When recommended by a doctor, Perdiem® Fiber is also useful for the treatment of bowel disorders other than constipation.

Composition: Perdiem® Fiber contains as its active ingredient 100% psyllium (Plantago Hydrocolloid), a natural grain with no chemical stimulants. Each rounded teaspoonful (6.0 g) contains approximately 4 g of psyllium, 1.8 mg of sodium, 36.1 mg of potassium, and only 4 calories. Perdiem® Fiber is "Dye-Free" and contains no artificial sweeteners.

Inactive Ingredients: Acacia, iron oxides, natural flavors, paraffin, sucrose, talc, titanium dioxide.

Directions for Use: TAKE THIS PRODUCT (CHILD OR ADULT DOSE) WITH AT LEAST 8 OUNCES (A FULL GLASS) OF COOL WATER OR OTHER FLUID. TAKING THIS PRODUCT WITHOUT ENOUGH LIQUID MAY CAUSE CHOKING. SEE WARNINGS.
Adults and children 12 years and older: In the evening and/or before breakfast, 1 to 2 rounded teaspoonfuls of Perdiem® Fiber (in full or partial doses) should be placed in the mouth and swallowed with at least 8 ounces of cool liquid. Perdiem® Fiber should not be chewed.
Children 7 to 11 years: One (1) rounded teaspoonful one to two times daily with at least 8 ounces of cool liquid.

For Severe Cases of Constipation: Perdiem® Fiber may be taken more frequently, up to 2 rounded teaspoonfuls every 6 hours not to exceed 5 teaspoonfuls in a 24-hour period. Perdiem® Fiber generally takes effect within 12 hours; in severe cases, 24 to 72 hours may be required to provide optimal relief.
During Pregnancy: Because of its natural ingredients and bulking action, Perdiem® Fiber is effective for expectant mothers—follow directions.

Warnings: TAKING THIS PRODUCT WITHOUT ADEQUATE FLUID MAY CAUSE IT TO SWELL AND BLOCK YOUR THROAT OR ESOPHAGUS AND MAY CAUSE CHOKING. DO NOT TAKE THIS PRODUCT IF YOU HAVE DIFFICULTY IN SWALLOWING. IF YOU EXPERIENCE CHEST PAIN, VOMITING, OR DIFFICULTY IN SWALLOWING OR BREATHING AFTER TAKING THIS PRODUCT, SEEK IMMEDIATE MEDICAL ATTENTION.
Frequent or prolonged use without the direction of a doctor is not recommended. If use of this product for one week has produced no effect, discontinue use and consult a doctor.
If you have noticed a sudden change in bowel habits that persists over a two week period, consult a doctor before using any laxative product.
Do not use in patients with a history of psyllium allergy. Psyllium allergy is rare but can be severe. If an allergic reaction occurs, discontinue use and consult a doctor immediately.
Consult a physician before using any laxative or bulk fiber product in the presence of rectal bleeding or undiagnosed abdominal pain, nausea or vomiting.
Keep this and all drugs out of the reach of children. In case of accidental overdose, seek professional assistance or contact a poison control center immediately.

After Rectal Surgery: The vegetable mucilages of Perdiem® Fiber soften the stool and provide pain-free evacuation of the bowel. Perdiem® Fiber is effective as an aid to elimination for the hemorrhoid or fissure patient prior to and following surgery.

For Clinical Regulation: For patients confined to bed—after an operation for example—and for those of inactive habits, 1 rounded teaspoonful of Perdiem® Fiber taken 1–2 times daily will ensure regular bowel habits.

How Supplied: Granules: 250-gram (8.8 oz) (0067-0795-70) plastic container, 6 single serving packets 6 gm (0067-0795-09) and 20 single serving packets 6 gm (0067-0795-10).

Shown in Product Identification Guide, page 507

PRIVINE®
naphazoline hydrochloride, USP
0.05% Nasal Solution
0.05% Nasal Spray
Nasal Decongestant

Privine is a nasal decongestant that comes in three forms: Nasal Drops (in a bottle with a dropper), Nasal Spray (in a plastic squeeze bottle) and Nasal Solution (in a 16 fl oz bottle). All are for prompt, and prolonged relief of nasal congestion due to common colds, sinusitis, hay fever, etc.
Privine is an effective nasal decongestant **when you use it in the recommended dosage.** If you use too much, too long, or too often, Privine may be harmful to your nasal mucous membranes and cause burning, stinging, sneezing or an increased runny nose.
Do not use Privine by mouth.
IF NASAL STUFFINESS PERSISTS AFTER 3 DAYS OF TREATMENT, DISCONTINUE USE AND CONSULT A DOCTOR.
Keep this and all medications out of the reach of children. Do not use Privine in children under 12 years of age, except with the advice and supervision of a doctor.

Caution: Do not use Privine if you have glaucoma.
OVERDOSAGE IN YOUNG CHILDREN MAY CAUSE MARKED SEDATION AND IF SEVERE, EMERGENCY TREATMENT MAY BE NECESSARY. IN CASE OF ACCIDENTAL INGESTION, SEEK PROFESSIONAL ASSISTANCE OR CONTACT A POISON CONTROL CENTER IMMEDIATELY.

How to use Nasal Drops.
Use only 1 to 2 drops in each nostril. Do not repeat this dosage more than every 6 hours. Squeeze rubber bulb to fill dropper with proper amount of medication. For best results, tilt head as far back as possible and put 1 to 2 drops of solution into your right nostril. Then lean head forward, inhaling and turning your head to the left. Refill dropper by squeezing bulb. Now tilt head as far back as possible and put 1 to 2 drops of solution into your left nostril. Then lean head forward, inhaling, and turning your head to the right.
The Privine dropper bottle is designed to make administration of the proper dosage easy. Privine will not cause sleeplessness, so you may use it before going to bed.

Important: After use, be sure to rinse the dropper with very hot water. This helps prevent contamination of the bottle with bacteria from nasal secretions. Use of the dispenser by more than one person may spread infection.

Note: Privine Nasal Solution may be used with glass, plastic, stainless steel and specially treated metals used in atomizers. Do not let the solution come in contact with reactive metals, especially aluminum. If solution becomes discolored, it should be discarded.
How to use Nasal Spray.
Spray 1 or 2 times in each nostril, not more often than every 6 hours. Avoid overdosage. Follow directions for use carefully. For best results do **not** shake the plastic squeeze bottle.
Remove cap. With head held upright, spray twice into each nostril. Squeeze the bottle sharply and firmly while sniffing through the nose.
Privine Nasal Drops contain 0.05% naphazoline HCl, USP. It also contains benzalkonium chloride, dibasic sodium phosphate, disodium edetate, monobasic sodium phosphate, purified water and sodium chloride.
Privine Nasal Solution contains 0.05% naphazoline hydrochloride, USP. It also contains benzalkonium chloride, disodium edetate dihydrate, hydrochloric acid, purified water, sodium chloride, and trolamine. It is available in bottles of 16 fl. oz. (473 ml).
Privine Nasal Spray contains 0.05% naphazoline hydrochloride USP. It also contains benzalkonium chloride, dibasic sodium phosphate, disodium edetate, monobasic sodium phosphate, purified water, and sodium chloride. It is available in plastic squeeze bottles of 0.66 fl oz (20 ml).

Caution: Do not use if the clear overwrap on the box with the name Privine®

Continued on next page

The full prescribing information for each CIBA Consumer Pharmaceuticals product is contained herein and is that in effect as of December 15, 1994

CIBA Consumer—Cont.

or the printed band on the bottle is missing or damaged.

Shown in Product Identification Guide, page 507

SINAREST® TABLETS, EXTRA STRENGTH TABLETS AND NO DROWSINESS TABLETS
[*sīn 'a-rest*]

Active Ingredients:
Tablets —Acetaminophen 325 mg, chlorpheniramine maleate 2 mg, pseudoephedrine HCl 30 mg.
Extra Strength Tablets —Acetaminophen 500 mg, chlorpheniramine maleate 2 mg, pseudoephedrine HCl 30 mg.
No Drowsiness Tablets —Acetaminophen 500 mg, pseudoephedrine HCl 30 mg.

Other Ingredients:
All Products —Magnesium stearate, microcrystalline cellulose, povidone, pregelatinized starch.
Extra Strength and No Drowsiness Tablets also contain—Sodium starch glycolate. *Tablets and Extra Strength Tablets* also contain—Yellow 6 lake, Yellow 10 lake.

Indications:
Tablets and Extra Strength Tablets —Temporarily relieves nasal congestion, runny nose, sneezing, itching of the nose and throat, and itchy, watery eyes due to hay fever or other upper respiratory allergies, or associated with sinusitis. For temporary relief of minor aches, pains, and headache.
No Drowsiness Tablets —Temporarily relieves nasal congestion due to hay fever or other upper respiratory allergies, or associated with sinusitis. For temporary relief of minor aches, pains, and headache.

Warnings: All Products:—Do not take this product for more than 10 days (for adults) or 5 days (for children). Do not exceed recommended dosage because at higher doses, nervousness, dizziness, or sleeplessness may occur. If symptoms do not improve or are accompanied by fever that lasts for more than 3 days, or if new symptoms occur, consult a physician. Do not take this product if you have heart disease, high blood pressure, thyroid disease, diabetes, or difficulty in urination due to enlargement of the prostate gland, unless directed by a physician. As with any drug, if you are pregnant or nursing a baby, seek the advice of a health professional before using this product. **Keep this and all drugs out of the reach of children.** In case of accidental overdose, seek professional assistance or contact a Poison Control Center immediately. Prompt medical attention is critical for adults as well as children even if you do not notice any signs or symptoms. Also, *Tablets and Extra Strength Tablets* —Do not take this product, unless directed by a physician, if you have a breathing problem such as emphysema or chronic bronchitis, or if you have glaucoma. May cause excitability, especially in children. May cause drowsiness; alcohol, sedatives, and tranquilizers may increase the drowsiness effect. Avoid alcoholic beverages while taking this product. Do not take this product if you are taking sedatives or tranquilizers, without first consulting your physician. Use caution when driving a motor vehicle or operating machinery.

Drug Interaction Precautions: *All Products* —Do not take this product if you are presently taking a prescription drug for high blood pressure or depression, without first consulting your physician.

Directions: Dose as follows while symptoms persist, or as directed by a physician.
Tablets and No Drowsiness Tablets —Adults and children 12 years of age and older: 2 tablets every 4 to 6 hours, not to exceed 8 tablets in 24 hours. Children 6 to under 12 years of age: 1 tablet every 4 to 6 hours, not to exceed 4 tablets in 24 hours. Children under 6 years of age: Consult a physician.
Extra Strength —Adults and children 12 years of age and older: 2 tablets every 6 hours, not to exceed 8 tablets in 24 hours. Children under 12 years of age: Consult a physician.

How Supplied:
Tablets —Boxes of 20, 40, and 80.
Extra Strength Tablets —Boxes of 24.
No Drowsiness Tablets —Boxes of 20.
SINAREST is a registered trademark of Ciba-Geigy Corporation

SLOW FE®
Slow Release Iron Tablets

Description: SLOW FE supplies ferrous sulfate for the treatment of iron deficiency and iron deficiency anemia with a significant reduction in the incidence of the common side effects of oral iron preparations. The wax matrix delivery system of SLOW FE is designed to maximize the release of ferrous sulfate in the duodenum and the jejunum where it is best tolerated and absorbed. SLOW FE has been clinically shown to be associated with a lower incidence of constipation, diarrhea and abdominal discomfort when compared to regular iron tablets and the leading capsule.

Formula: Each tablet contains 160 mg. dried ferrous sulfate USP, equivalent to 50 mg. elemental iron. Also contains cetostearyl alcohol, colloidal silicon dioxide, hydroxypropyl methylcellulose, shellac, lactose, magnesium stearate, polyethylene glycol.

Dosage: ADULTS—one or two tablets daily or as recommended by a physician. A maximum of four tablets daily may be taken. CHILDREN—one tablet daily. Tablets must be swallowed whole.

Warning: Close tightly and keep out of reach of children. Contains iron, which can be harmful or fatal to children in large doses. In case of accidental overdose, seek professional assistance or contact a Poison Control Center immediately. The treatment of any anemic condition should be on the advice and under the supervision of a physician. As oral iron products interfere with absorption of oral tetracycline antibiotics, these products should not be taken within two hours of each other. As with any drug, if you are pregnant or nursing a baby, seek the advice of a health professional before using this product.
Keep this and all medicines out of reach of children.
Tamper-Evident Packaging.

How Supplied: Blister packages of 30, 60, and child-resistant bottles of 100. Do Not Store Above 86°F. Protect From Moisture.

Shown in Product Identification Guide, page 507

SLOW FE WITH FOLIC ACID   OTC
(Slow Release Iron, Folic Acid)

Description: Slow Fe + Folic Acid delivers 50 mg. elemental iron (160 mg. dried ferrous sulfate) using the unique wax matrix delivery system described above, plus 400 mcg. folic acid.
Provides women of childbearing potential with the daily target level of folic acid to reduce the risk of neural tube birth defects. These birth defects are rare, but serious, and occur within 28 days of conception, often before a woman knows she's pregnant.

Formula: Each tablet contains: Active Ingredients: 160 mg. dried ferrous sulfate, USP (equivalent to 50 mg. elemental iron) and 400 mcg. folic acid. Inactive Ingredients: cetostearyl alcohol, hydroxypropyl methylcellulose, lactose, magnesium stearate, polysorbate 80, talc, titanium dioxide, yellow iron oxide 17628.

Dosage: ADULTS—One or two tablets once a day or as recommended by a physician. A maximum of two tablets daily may be taken. CHILDREN UNDER 12—Consult a physician. Tablets must be swallowed whole.

Warning: The treatment of any anemic condition should be under the advice and supervision of a physician. As oral iron products interfere with absorption of oral tetracycline antibiotics, these products should not be taken within two hours of each other. Intake of folic acid from all sources should be limited to 1000 mcg. per day to prevent the masking of Vitamin B12 deficiencies. Should you become pregnant while using this product, consult a physician as soon as possible about good prenatal care and the continued use of this product. If you are already pregnant or nursing a baby, seek the advice of a health care professional before using this product. KEEP THIS PRODUCT AND ALL MEDICATIONS OUT OF THE REACH OF CHILDREN:

Contains iron, which can be harmful or fatal to children in large doses. In case of accidental overdose, contact a physician or a poison control center immediately.

How Supplied: Blister packages of 20 supplied in Child-Resistant packaging. Do not store above 86°F. Protect from moisture.

CHILD-RESISTANT
Blister packaged for your protection. Do not use if individual seals are broken.

Distributed by: CIBA Consumer Pharmaceuticals
Woodbridge, NJ 07095
Tablets made in Great Britain
©1994 CIBA Consumer
    Pharmaceuticals
a Division of Ciba-Geigy Corporation
*Shown in Product Identification
Guide, page 507*

SUNKIST® CHILDREN'S CHEWABLE MULTIVITAMINS—REGULAR

Vitamin Ingredients: Each tablet contains:
[See table above.]

Indication: Dietary supplementation.

Dosage and Administration: One chewable tablet daily for adults and children two years and older.

Warning: Phenylketonurics: Contains Phenylalanine

How Supplied: SUNKIST Children's Multivitamins-Regular are supplied in bottles of 60 chewable tablets with child resistant safety caps.
SUNKIST® is a registered trademark of SUNKIST Growers, Inc., Sherman Oaks, CA 91423. ©
*Shown in Product Identification
Guide, page 507*

SUNKIST® CHILDREN'S CHEWABLE MULTIVITAMINS—PLUS EXTRA C

Vitamin Ingredients: Each tablet contains the ingredients of the Regular multivitamin product plus extra Vitamin C (a total of 250 mg).

Indication: Dietary supplementation.

Dosage and Administration: One chewable tablet daily for adults and children two years and older.

Warning: Phenylketonurics: Contains Phenylalanine.

How Supplied: SUNKIST Children's Multivitamins Plus Extra C are supplied in bottles of 60 chewable tablets with child resistant caps.
Sunkist® is a registered trademark of Sunkist Growers, Inc., Sherman Oaks, CA 91423.©
*Shown in Product Identification
Guide, page 507*

SUNKIST® CHILDREN'S
CHEWABLE MULTIVITAMINS-REGULAR

VITAMINS	QUANTITY PER TABLET	PERCENT U.S. RDA FOR CHILD. 2 TO 4 YRS OF AGE (1 TABLET)	FOR ADULTS & CHILD. OVER 4 YRS OF AGE (1 TABLET)
Vitamin A (as Palmitate + Beta Carotene)	2500 IU	100	50
Vitamin D-3	400 IU	100	100
Vitamin E	15 IU	150	50
Vitamin C	60 mg	150	100
Folic Acid	0.3 mg	150	75
Niacinamide	13.5 mg	150	68
Vitamin B-6	1.05 mg	150	53
Vitamin B-12	4.5 mcg	150	75
Vitamin B-1	1.05 mg	150	70
Vitamin B-2	1.20 mg	150	71
Vitamin K-1	5 mcg	*	*

*Recognized as essential in human nutrition, but no U.S. RDA established.

SUNKIST® CHILDREN'S CHEWABLE MULTIVITAMINS—PLUS IRON

Vitamin Ingredients: Each tablet contains the vitamins of the Regular multivitamin product plus 15 mg of Iron.

Indication: Dietary supplementation.

Dosage and Administration: One chewable tablet daily for adults and children two years and older.

Warning: Close tightly and keep out of reach of children. Contains iron, which can be harmful or fatal to children in large doses. In case of accidental overdose, seek professional assistance or contact a Poison Control Center immediately.
Phenylketonurics: Contains phenylalanine.

How Supplied: SUNKIST Children's Multivitamins Plus Iron are supplied in bottles of 60 chewable tablets with child resistant safety caps.
Sunkist® is a registered trademark of Sunkist Growers, Inc., Sherman Oaks, CA 91423.©
*Shown in Product Identification
Guide, page 507*

SUNKIST® CHILDREN'S CHEWABLE MULTIVITAMINS—COMPLETE

Vitamin Ingredients: Each tablet contains the following ingredients:
[See table at bottom of next page.]

Indication: Dietary supplementation.

Dosage and Administration: Children ages 2 to 4: one-half chewable tablet daily; One chewable tablet daily for adults and children four years and older.

Warning: Close tightly and keep out of reach of children. Contains iron, which can be harmful or fatal to children in large doses. In case of accidental overdose, seek professional assistance or contact a Poison Control Center immediately.
Phenylketonurics: Contains phenylalanine.

How Supplied: SUNKIST Children's Multivitamins Complete are supplied in bottles of 60 chewable tablets with child resistant safety caps.
Sunkist® is a registered trademark of Sunkist Growers, Inc., Sherman Oaks, CA 91423.©
*Shown in Product Identification
Guide, page 507*

SUNKIST® VITAMIN C
Citrus Complex
Chewable Tablets
Easy to Swallow Caplets

Description: All Sunkist Vitamin C chewable tablets have a delicious orange flavor unlike any other Vitamin C tablet. Each 60 mg chewable tablet contains 100% of the U.S. RDA* of Vitamin C. Each 250 mg chewable tablet contains 417% of the U.S. RDA* of Vitamin C. Each 500 mg chewable tablet contains 833% of the U.S. RDA* of Vitamin C.

Each 500 mg easy to swallow caplet contains 833% of the U.S. RDA* of Vitamin C.

Sunkist Vitamin C chewable tablets and easy to swallow caplets do not contain artificial flavors or colors.

*U.S. Recommended Daily Allowance for adults and children over 4 years of age.

Indication: Dietary supplementation.

How Supplied: 60 mg Chewable Tablets—Rolls of 11.
250 mg and 500 mg Chewable Tablets—Bottles of 60.
500 mg Easy to Swallow Caplets—Bottles of 60.

Sunkist® is a registered trademark of Sunkist Growers, Inc., Sherman Oaks, CA 91423.©
*Shown in Product Identification
Guide, page 507*

Continued on next page

The full prescribing information for each CIBA Consumer Pharmaceuticals product is contained herein and is that in effect as of December 15, 1994

CIBA Consumer—Cont.

TING® ANTIFUNGAL CREAM, POWDER, SPRAY LIQUID, and SPRAY POWDER

Active Ingredient: Tolnaftate, 1%.

Other Ingredients: *Cream* —BHT, fragrance, polyethylene glycol 400, polyethylene glycol 3350, titanium dioxide. *Powder* —Corn starch, fragrance, talc. *Spray Liquid* —BHT, fragrance, isobutane (propellant), polyethylene glycol 400, SD alcohol 40-B (41% w/w). *Spray Powder* —BHT, fragrance, isobutane (propellant), PPG-12-buteth-16, SD alcohol 40-B (14% w/w), talc.

Indications: Cures athlete's foot and jock itch with a clinically proven ingredient. Relieves itching and burning. Prevents the recurrence of athlete's foot with daily use.

Warnings: Do not use on children under 2 years of age unless directed by a doctor. For external use only. Avoid contact with the eyes. If irritation occurs or if there is no improvement within 4 weeks for athlete's foot or within 2 weeks for jock itch, discontinue use and consult a doctor. **Keep this and all drugs out of the reach of children.** In case of accidental ingestion, seek professional assistance or contact a Poison Control Center immediately. *For Spray Liquid and Spray Powder only* —Avoid inhaling. Avoid contact with the eyes or other mucous membranes. Contents under pressure; do not puncture or incinerate. Flammable mixture, do not use near fire or flame. Do not expose to heat or temperatures above 49°C (120°F). Use only as directed. Intentional misuse by deliberately concentrating and inhaling contents can be harmful or fatal.

Directions: Clean the affected area and dry thoroughly. Apply a thin layer of the product over affected area twice daily (morning and night) or as directed by a doctor. Supervise children in the use of this product. For athlete's foot: pay special attention to the spaces between the toes, wear well-fitting, ventilated shoes, and change shoes and socks at least once daily. For athlete's foot, use daily for 4 weeks; for jock itch, use daily for 2 weeks. If condition persists longer, consult a doctor. This product is not effective on the scalp or nails. To prevent athlete's foot, apply a thin layer of the product to the feet once or twice daily (morning and/or night) following the above directions.

How Supplied: *Cream* —½ oz (14 g) tube, *Powder* —1.5 oz (43 g) shaker container, *Spray Liquid and Spray Powder* —3 oz (85 g) aerosol containers. TING is a registered trademark of Ciba-Geigy Corporation.

Shown in Product Identification Guide, page 507

VITRON–C® TABLETS
[vī'tron c]

Active Ingredients: Each tablet contains
Ferrous fumarate, USP .... 200 mg equivalent to 66 mg elemental iron (365% U.S. RDA)
Ascorbic acid .... 125 mg (200% U.S. RDA)
Present in part as sodium ascorbate, USP

Other Ingredients: Colloidal silicon dioxide, flavor, glycine, hydroxypropyl methylcellulose, iron oxides, magnesium stearate, microcrystalline cellulose, polyethylene glycol, polysorbate 80, povidone, saccharin sodium, talc, titanium dioxide.

Indications: For iron deficiency anemia.

Actions: Ascorbic acid only enhances iron absorption at doses ≤200 mg. Vitron-C, a well-tolerated formula, is especially useful when pregnancy, menstruation, or chronic blood loss increases iron needs.

Warning: Close tightly and keep out of reach of children. Contains iron, which can be harmful or fatal to children in large doses. In case of accidental overdose, seek professional assistance or contact a Poison Control Center immediately.
The treatment of any anemic condition should be under the advice and supervision of a physician. As oral iron products interfere with absorption of oral tetracycline antibiotics, these products should not be taken within two hours of each other. As with any drug, if you are pregnant or nursing a baby, seek the advice of a health professional before using this product.

Directions: Adults—one or two tablets daily or as directed by a physician. Tablet may be swallowed whole, chewed or sucked like a lozenge.

How Supplied: Bottles of 100 tablets with child-resistant safety closure.

Columbia Laboratories, Inc.
**2665 SOUTH BAYSHORE DRIVE
SUITE PH2B
MIAMI, FL 33133**

DIASORB®
[dī'ă-zorb]
Activated Nonfibrous Attapulgite Liquid and Tablets

Description: Diasorb relieves cramps and pain associated with diarrhea. It is available as a pleasant-tasting cola-flavored liquid and as easy-to-swallow tablets. Diasorb is safe for children.

Active Ingredient: Each liquid teaspoonful and tablet contains 750 mg activated nonfibrous attapulgite.

Inactive Ingredients: *Liquid*—Benzoic acid, citric acid, flavor, glycerin, magnesium aluminum silicate, methylparaben, polysorbate, propylene glycol, propylparaben, saccharin, sodium hypochlorite solution, sorbitol, xanthan gum, and water. *Tablet*—D&C Red No. 30 Al Lake, Gelatin, Hydroxypropyl Cellulose, Hydroxypropyl Methylcellulose, Magnesium Stearate, Pharmaceutical Shellac, Polyethylene Glycol, Povidone, Propyl-

---

**SUNKIST® CHILDREN'S
CHEWABLE MULTIVITAMINS**-COMPLETE

VITAMINS	QUANTITY PER TABLET	PERCENT U.S. RDA FOR CHILD. 2 TO 4 YRS OF AGE (½ TABLET)	PERCENT U.S. RDA FOR ADULTS & CHILD. OVER 4 YRS OF AGE (1 TABLET)
Vitamin A (as Palmitate + Beta Carotene)	5000 IU	100	100
Vitamin D-3	400 IU	50	100
Vitamin E	30 IU	150	100
Vitamin C	60 mg	75	100
Folic Acid	0.4 mg	100	100
Biotin	40 mcg	13	13
Pantothenic Acid	10 mg	100	100
Niacinamide	20 mg	111	100
Vitamin B-6	2 mg	143	100
Vitamin B-12	6 mcg	100	100
Vitamin B-1	1.5 mg	107	100
Vitamin B-2	1.7 mg	106	100
Vitamin K-1	10 mcg	*	*
MINERALS			
Iron	18 mg	90	100
Magnesium	20 mg	5	5
Iodine	150 mcg	107	100
Zinc	10 mg	63	67
Manganese	1 mg	*	*
Calcium	100 mg	6	10
Phosphorus	78 mg	5	8
Copper	2 mg	100	100

*Recognized as essential in human nutrition, but no U.S. RDA established.

Age	Initial Dose	Maximum Dose per 24 hours
Adults and children over 12 years	4 tsp or 4 Tablets	12 tsp or 12 Tablets
Children 6–12 years	2 tsp or 2 Tablets	6 tsp or 6 Tablets
Children 3–6 years	1 tsp or 1 Tablet	3 tsp or 3 Tablets
Infants and children under 3 years	Only as directed by a physician	

ene Glycol, Sorbitol, Titanium Dioxide, and Water.

Directions for Use: Take the full recommended starting dose at the first sign of diarrhea, and repeat after each subsequent bowel movement. Do not exceed maximum recommended dose per day. Shake liquid well before using.

Swallow tablets with water. Do not chew.

Caution: Do not use if foil seal around tablet is broken.

Warning: Do not use for more than 2 days or in the presence of fever or in infants or children under 3, unless directed by a physician. In case of accidental overdose, seek professional assistance or contact a poison control center immediately.

Store at room temperature (59° to 86° F) in a dry place.

KEEP THIS AND ALL MEDICATIONS OUT OF THE REACH OF CHILDREN.

Dosage: See Table for recommended dosage for acute diarrhea.
[See table above.]

How Supplied: *Liquid*—In plastic bottles of 4 fl oz (120 mL).
Tablets—Packaged in blister packs of 24.
Shown in Product Identification Guide, page 508

**Advanced Formula
LEGATRIN PM_{TM}**
[leg 'a-trin]
Pain Reliever/Sleep Aid

Advanced Formula Legatrin PM_{TM} a special night-time medicine which combines extra-strength pain reliever to relieve your muscle aches and pains, with an ingredient to help you fall asleep safely.

Advanced Formula Legatrin PM_{TM} caplets are specially coated and shaped for easy swallowing.

Indications: For the occasional relief of sleeplessness and minor muscle aches and pains, such as leg cramps.

Dosage: Adults and Children 12 years of age and older: One caplet at bedtime or as directed by your physician. Do not exceed recommended dosage.

Warnings: Do not give to Children under 12 years of age or use for more than 10 days unless directed by your physician. Consult your physician if symptoms persist or new ones occur, or if fever persists for more than 3 days, or if sleeplessness persists for more than 2 weeks. Insomnia may be a symptom of serious underlying medical illness. Do not take this product if you have asthma, glaucoma, emphysema, chronic pulmonary disease, shortness of breath, difficulty in breathing or difficulty in urination due to enlargement of the prostate gland unless directed by a physician. Avoid alcoholic beverages while taking this product. Do not take if you are taking sedatives or tranquilizers without first consulting your physician.

Active Ingredients (per caplet): Acetaminophen 500 mg and Diphenhydramine HCl 50 mg.

Inactive Ingredients: Dicalcium phosphate, croscarmellose sodium, stearic acid, microcrystalline cellulose, magnesium stearate, FD&C blue No. 2 aluminum lake, FD&C red No. 40 aluminum lake, hydroxypropyl methylcellulose, polyethylene glycol, talc, titanium dioxide.

Caution: This product will cause drowsiness. Do not drive a motor vehicle or operate machinery after use.

How Supplied: Supplied in child resistant bottles of 30 and 50 count caplets.
DO NOT USE IF PRINTED OVERWRAP ON NECK OF THE BOTTLE OR PRINTED FOIL INNER SEAL IS BROKEN. KEEP THIS AND ALL MEDICATIONS OUT OF THE REACH OF CHILDREN. IN CASE OF ACCIDENTAL OVERDOSE, CONTACT A PHYSICIAN OR POISON CONTROL CENTER IMMEDIATELY. AS WITH ANY DRUG, IF YOU ARE PREGNANT OR NURSING A BABY, SEEK THE ADVICE OF A HEALTH PROFESSIONAL BEFORE USING THIS PRODUCT.
Store at room temperature.
See side panel for expiration date.

Distributed by:
Columbia Laboratories, Inc.
Miami, FL 33133
Shown in Product Identification Guide, page 508

Del Pharmaceuticals, Inc.
A Subsidiary of Del Laboratories, Inc.
**163 E. BETHPAGE ROAD
PLAINVIEW, NY 11803**

ARTHRICARE®
Pain Relieving Rubs

Description: **ArthriCare Odor Free** is perfect for daytime use anywhere. Its unique greaseless and stainless formula provides the warming pain relief of medicinal rubs without the embarrassing medicinal odor. This special formula provides temporary relief of minor aches and pains of muscles and joints associated with arthritis, simple back pain, sprains and strains. This unique formulation contains Capsicum Oleoresin (containing Capsaicin 0.025%), a strong, penetrating pain blocker not commonly found in other rubs. In addition, it has two added fast-acting pain relievers to ease stiffness of muscles and joints.
ArthriCare Triple Medicated is specially formulated with three fast acting pain relievers. It's strong medicine that penetrates deep. You don't have to rub it in; just apply gently. ArthriCare Triple-Medicated provides temporary relief of minor aches and pains of muscles and joints associated with arthritis, simple backache, sprains and strains. Perfect for nightime use to help one sleep.

Active Ingredients: ArthriCare Odor Free Menthol 1.25%, Methyl Nicotinate 0.25%, Capsicum Oleoresin (containing Capsaicin 0.025%).
ArthriCare Triple Medicated Methyl Salicylate 30%, Menthol 1.25%, Methyl Nicotinate 0.25%

Inactive Ingredients: ArthriCare Odor Free Aloe Vera Gel, Carbomer 940, Cetyl Alcohol, DMDM Hydantoin, Emulsifying Wax, Glyceryl Stearate SE, Isocatyl Alcohol, Myristyl Propionate, Propylparaben, Purified Water, Stearyl Alcohol, Triethanolamine.
ArthriCare Triple Medicated Carbomer 940, Dioctyl Sodium Sulfosuccinate, FD&C Blue No. 1, Glycerin, Isopropyl Alcohol, Polysorbate 60, Propylene Gycol, Purified Water.

Directions: Adults and children 2 years of age and older: Apply to affected area not more than 3 to 4 times daily. Children under 2 years of age: Consult a physician.

Warnings: For external use only. Avoid contact with the eyes. If condition worsens, or if symptoms persist for more than 7 days or clear up and occur again within a few days, discontinue use of this product and consult a physician. Do not apply to wounds or damaged skin. Do not bandage tightly. Avoid contact with mucous membranes, broken or irritated skin. Do not use with a heating pad, or immediately before or after taking a shower or bath. As part of its warming

Continued on next page

Del—Cont.

action, temporary redness may occur Keep this and all drugs out of the reach of children. In case of accidental ingestion, seek professional assistance or contact a Poison Control Center immediately. Store at room temperature 15–30 C (59–86 F).

Shown in Product Identification Guide, page 508

BABY ORAJEL®
Teething Pain Medicine

Description: Baby Orajel with fast-acting benzocaine (7.5%) relieves teething pain within one minute. It's pleasant tasting and contains no alcohol.

Active Ingredient: Benzocaine 7.5%.

Inactive Ingredients: FD&C Red No. 40, Flavor, Glycerin, Polyethylene Glycols, Purified Water, Sodium Saccharin, Sorbic Acid, Sorbitol.

Indications: For the temporary relief of sore gums due to teething in infants and children 4 months of age and older. Baby Orajel is a safe, soothing, pleasantly flavored product which helps to immediately relieve teething pain by its topical anesthetic effect on the gums.

Actions: Benzocaine is a topical, local anesthetic commonly used for pain, discomfort, or pruritis associated with wounds, mucous membranes and skin irritations.

Warnings: Do not use this product for more than 7 days unless directed by a dentist or physician. If sore mouth symptoms do not improve in 7 days; if irritation, pain or redness persists or worsens; or if swelling, rash or fever develops, see your dentist or physician promptly. Do not exceed recommended dosage. Do not use this product if you have a history of allergy to local anesthetics such as procaine, butacaine, benzocaine, or other "caine" anesthetics. Fever and nasal congestion are not symptoms of teething and may indicate the presence of infection. If these symptoms persist, consult your physician. Keep this and all drugs out of the reach of children. In case of accidental overdose, seek professional assistance or contact a Poison Control Center immediately. Do not use if tube tip is cut prior to opening.

Precaution: For persistent or excessive teething pain, consult your physician.

Directions: Wash hands. Cut open tip of tube on score mark. Use your fingertip or cotton applicator to apply a small pea-size amount of Baby Orajel. Apply to affected area not more than four times daily or as directed by a dentist or physician. For infants under 4 months of age, there is no recommended dosage or treatment except under the advice and supervision of a dentist or physician.

How Supplied: Baby Orajel: Gel in ⅓ oz (9.45 g) tube.
Shown in Product Identification Guide, page 508

BABY ORAJEL® TOOTH & GUM CLEANSER

Description: Baby Orajel Tooth & Gum Cleanser is specifically designed for children under four. Safe to swallow, non-foaming, fluoride- and abrasive-free, it contains Microdent®, which helps remove plaque and fight its build-up. Available in fruit and vanilla flavors.

Active Ingredients: Microdent® (Poloxamer 407 2.0%, Simethicone 0.12%).

Inactive Ingredients: Carboxymethylcellulose Sodium, Citric Acid, Flavor, Glycerin, Methylparaben, Potassium Sorbate, Propylene Glycol, Propylparaben, Purified Water, Sodium Saccharin, Sorbitol.

Indications and Actions: Baby Orajel Tooth & Gum Cleanser is the first oral cleanser specially formulated to remove the plaque-like film on babies' teeth and gums. It's fluoride-free, non-abrasive and does not foam so it's safe to swallow. It's sugar-free and has a flavor babies love. Only Baby Orajel Tooth & Gum Cleanser contains patented Microdent® to help remove plaque and fight its buildup.

Warnings: Keep out of the reach of children. Do not use if tube tip is cut prior to opening.

Dosage and Administration: Wash hands. Cut open tip of tube on score mark. Apply a small amount to baby's gums and teeth with your finger, a gauze pad or a toothbrush. Gently rub or brush the gums and teeth to remove food and plaque-like film. For best results, use in the morning and at bedtime.

How Supplied: Gel in ½ oz. (14.2g) tube and 1 oz. (28.3g) tube. Available in assorted flavors.
Shown in Product Identification Guide, page 508

Maximum Strength ORAJEL®
[ōr 'ah-jel]
Toothache Medicine

Description: Maximum Strength Orajel with 20% benzocaine provides immediate, long lasting toothache pain relief.

Active Ingredient: Benzocaine 20%.

Inactive Ingredients: Clove Oil, Flavor, Polyethylene Glycols, Sodium Saccharin, Sorbic Acid.

Indications: Maximum Strength Orajel is formulated to provide fast, long lasting relief from toothache pain for hours.

Actions: Benzocaine is a topical, local anesthetic commonly used for pain, discomfort, or pruritis associated with wounds, mucous membranes and skin irritation.

Warning: Keep this and all drugs out of the reach of children. Do not use if tube tip is cut prior to opening. Do not use this product if you have a history of allergy to local anesthetics such as procaine, butacaine, benzocaine or other "caine" anesthetics. In case of accidental overdose, seek professional assistance or contact a Poison Control Center immediately.

Precaution: This preparation is intended for use in cases of toothache only as a temporary expedient until a dentist can be consulted. Do not use continuously.

Directions: Remove cap. Cut open tip of tube on score mark. Squeeze a small quantity of Maximum Strength Orajel directly into cavity and around gum surrounding the teeth.

How Supplied: Gel in two sizes— ³⁄₁₆ oz (5.3 g) and ⅓ oz (9.45 g) tubes.
Shown in Product Identification Guide, page 508

ORAJEL® Mouth-Aid®
[ōr 'ah-jel]
Cold/Canker Sore Medicine

Description: Orajel Mouth-Aid is a unique triple-acting medication which provides fast relief from painful minor mouth and lip sores. It has a protective formula that stays on the sore.

Active Ingredients: Benzocaine 20%, Benzalkonium Chloride 0.02%, Zinc Chloride 0.1%.

Inactive Ingredients: Allantoin, Carbomer, Edetate Disodium, Peppermint Oil, Polyethylene Glycol, Polysorbate 60, Propyl Gallate, Propylene Glycol, Purified Water, Povidone, Sodium Saccharin, Sorbic Acid, Stearyl Alcohol.

Indications: For the temporary relief of pain associated with canker sores, cold sores, fever blisters and minor irritation or injury of the mouth and gums.

Actions: Benzocaine is a topical, local anesthetic commonly used for pain, discomfort, or pruritis associated with wounds, mucous membranes and skin irritations. Benzalkonium chloride is a rapidly acting surface disinfectant and detergent. Zinc chloride provides an astringent effect.

Warnings: Do not use this product for more than 7 days unless directed by a dentist or physician. If sore mouth symptoms do not improve in 7 days; if irritation, pain, or redness persists or worsens; or if swelling, rash or fever develops, see your dentist or physician promptly. Do not exceed recommended dosage. Do not use this product if you have a history of allergy to local anesthetics such as procaine, butacaine, benzocaine or other "caine" anesthetics. Keep this and all drugs out of the reach of children. In case of accidental overdose, seek professional assistance or contact a Poison Control Center immediately. Do not use if tube tip is cut prior to opening.

Precaution: If condition persists, discontinue use and consult your physician or dentist. Not for prolonged use.

Directions: Cut open tip of tube on score mark. Adults and children 2 years and older: Apply to the affected area. Use up to 4 times daily or as directed by a dentist or physician. Children under 12 years of age should be supervised in the use of the product. Children under 2 years of age: Consult a dentist or physician.

How Supplied: Gel in 2 sizes—a ⅓ oz (9.45 g) tube and a ³⁄₁₆ oz (5.3 g) tube.
Shown in Product Identification Guide, page 508

ORAJEL®PERIOSEPTIC®

Description: Orajel Perioseptic is an oxygenating saline cleanser for sore and irritated gums. A pleasant tasting alternative to plain salt water rinses, it contains the maximum amount of the active ingredient carbamide peroxide. Developed by a dentist, Orajel Perioseptic is a safe and effective oral antiseptic wound cleanser that can help decrease the number of micro-organisms populating a wound by its oxygenating action.

Active Ingredient: Carbamide Peroxide 15% in anhydrous glycerin.

Inactive Ingredients: Citric Acid, Edetate Disodium, Flavor, Methylparaben, Propylene Glycol, Purified Water, Sodium Chloride, Sodium Saccharin.

Indications: For temporary use in cleansing minor wounds or minor gum inflammation resulting from minor dental procedures, dentures, orthodontic appliances, accidental injury, or other irritations of the mouth or gums. For temporary use to cleanse canker sores.

Warning: Do not use this product for more than 7 days unless directed by a dentist or doctor. If sore mouth symptoms do not improve in 7 days; if irritation, pain, or redness persists or worsens, or if swelling, rash, or fever develops, see your dentist or doctor promptly. Cap bottle tightly. Keep away from heat and direct sunlight.

Dosage and Administration: Adults and children 2 years of age and older: Apply several drops directly to the affected area of the mouth with cotton swab or applicator. Allow the medication to remain in place at least 1 minute and then spit out. Use up to 4 times daily after meals and at bedtime or as directed by a dentist or doctor. Children under 12 years of age should be supervised in the use of this product. Children under 2 years of age: Consult a dentist or doctor.

How Supplied: 0.45 fl. oz. (13.3 ml) bottle

PRONTO® Lice Killing Shampoo & Conditioner in One Kit

Description: Pronto Concentrate Lice Killing Shampoo & Conditioner in One

contains the maximum strength of pyrethrum extract and piperonyl butoxide. In laboratory testing it has been shown to be effective in killing 100% of lice and their eggs. In addition, a conditioner is included in the formulation to reduce tangles, for easy, effective comb-out of lice and eggs.

Active Ingredients: Piperonyl Butoxide 4%, Pyrethrum Extract 0.33%

Inactive Ingredients: Ammonium Laureth Sulfate, Benzyl Alcohol, BHT, Decyl Alcohol, Disodium EDTA, Fragrance, Isopropyl Alcohol, Glycerin, PEG-14M, Poloxamer 183, Purified Water

Indications: For the treatment of head, pubic (crab), and body lice.

Actions: Pronto contains the maximum strength of pyrethrum extract and piperonyl butoxide. Pyrethrum extract acts directly on the nervous system of insects and piperonyl butoxide enhances the neurotoxic effect of pyrethrum extract by inhibiting the oxidative breakdown of pyrethrum extract by the insect's detoxification system. This results in a longer amount of time which the pyrethrum extract may exert its toxic effect on the insect.

Warning: Use with caution on persons allergic to ragweed. For external use only. Do not use near the eyes or permit contact with mucous membranes, such as inside the nose, mouth, or vagina, as irritation may occur. Keep out of eyes when rinsing hair. Adults and children: Close eyes tightly and do not open eyes until product is rinsed out. Also, protect children's eyes with washcloth, towel or other suitable material, or by similar method. If product gets into the eyes, immediately flush with water. If skin irritation or infection is present or develops, discontinue use and consult a doctor. Consult a doctor if infestation of eyebrows or eyelashes occurs. Wash thoroughly with soap and water after handling. Do not exceed two applications within 24 hours.

Directions: Shake well. Apply to affected area until all the hair is thoroughly wet with product. Allow product to remain on area for 10 minutes but no longer. Add sufficient warm water to form a lather and shampoo as usual. Rinse thoroughly. A fine-toothed comb or a special lice/nit-removing comb may be used to help remove dead lice or their eggs (nits) from hair. A second treatment must be done in 7 to 10 days to kill any newly hatched lice. Handy applicator gloves are provided for your convenience in applying the shampoo to avoid contact with lice.

How Supplied: 2 fl. oz. (59 ml) and 4 fl. oz. (118 ml) plastic bottles.
Shown in Product Identification Guide, page 508

TANAC® Medicated Gel
Fever Blister/Cold Sore Treatment

Description: Tanac Medicated Gel treats cold sores with a unique, long lasting maximum strength pain reliever with Dyclonine Hydrochloride (1.0%). It also protects lip sores while it treats them.

Active Ingredients: Dyclonine Hydrochloride 1.0%, Allantoin 0.5%.

Inactive Ingredients: Citric Acid, Flavor, Hydroxylated Lanolin, Petrolatum, Propylene Glycol, Purified Water, PVP/Hexadecene Copolymer, Yellow Wax.

Indications: For the temporary relief of pain and itching associated with fever blisters and cold sores. Relieves dryness and softens cold sores and fever blisters.

Warnings: DO NOT USE IF TIP IS CUT PRIOR TO OPENING. For external use only. Avoid contact with the eyes. If condition worsens, or if symptoms persist for more than 7 days or clear up and occur again within a few days, discontinue use of this product and consult a physician. Keep this and all other drugs out of reach of children. In case of accidental ingestion, seek professional assistance, or contact a Poison Control Center immediately.

Dosage and Administration: Cut open tip of tube on score mark. Adults and children 2 years of age and older: Apply to fever blisters/cold sores not more than 3 to 4 times daily. Children under 2 years of age: consult a physician.

How Supplied: Available in ⅓ oz. (9.45g) plastic tube.
Shown in Product Identification Guide, page 508

TANAC® No Sting Liquid
Canker Sore Medicine

Description: Tanac Liquid provides fast, soothing relief from painful canker sores and other gum irritations because it contains an effective anesthetic plus an antiseptic. It's alcohol-free so it doesn't sting.

Active Ingredients: Benzocaine 10%, Benzalkonium Chloride 0.12%.

Inactive Ingredients: Flavor, Polyethylene Glycol 400, Propylene Glycol, Sodium Saccharin, Tannic Acid.

Indications: For temporary relief of pain from mouth sores, canker sores, fever blisters and gum irritations.

Warnings: If the condition for which this preparation is used persists or if a rash or irritation develops, discontinue use and consult a physician. Use as indicated but not for more than 5 consecutive days. Not for prolonged use. Avoid getting into eyes. Do not use if you have a history of allergy to local anesthetics such as procaine, butacaine, benzocaine,

Continued on next page

Del—Cont.

or other "caine" anesthetics. KEEP OUT OF THE REACH OF CHILDREN. In case of accidental ingestion, seek professional assistance or contact a Poison Control Center immediately. Do not use if imprinted bottle cap safety seal is broken or missing prior to opening.

Dosage and Administration: Apply with cotton or cotton swab to affected area not more than 3 to 4 times daily.

How Supplied: Available in 0.45 fl. oz. (13 ml) glass bottle.

Shown in Product Identification Guide, page 508

EDUCATIONAL MATERIAL

Teething Booklet From Baby Orajel®
Facts parents should know about tooth development and the teething process.
Free to physicians, pharmacists and patients
Fallacy and Fact Booklet From Pronto®
Answers questions about head lice control.
Free to physicians, pharmacists and patients.
Caring For Your Baby's Teeth and Gums
From Baby Orajel® Tooth & Gum Cleanser. Explains the basics of good oral hygiene. Also includes consumer coupons good on Baby Orajel products.
Free to physicians, pharmacists and patients.
We're Shedding New Light on the Relief of Cold Sores and Canker Sores.
Tanac patient information brochure— questions and answers regarding Canker Sores and Cold Sores. Includes a 50¢ coupon good on the purchase of any Tanac product.

Effcon Laboratories, Inc.
P.O. BOX 7509
MARIETTA, GA 30065-1509

PIN-X®
Pinworm Treatment

Description: Each 1 mL of liquid for oral administration contains:
   Pyrantel base .... 50 mg
     (as Pyrantel Pamoate)

Indication: For the treatment of pinworms.

Warnings: Keep this and all drugs out of the reach of children. In case of accidental overdose, seek professional assistance or contact a poison control center immediately.
If you are pregnant or have liver disease, do not take this product unless directed by a doctor.

Directions for Use: Adults and children 2 years to under 12 years of age: oral dosage is a single dose of 5 milligrams of pyrantel base per pound, or 11 milligrams per kilogram, of body weight not to exceed 1 gram. Dosage information is summarized on the following dosing schedule:

Weight	Dosage
	(taken as a single dose)
25 to 37 lbs.	= ½ tsp.
38 to 62 lbs.	= 1 tsp.
63 to 87 lbs.	= 1½ tsp.
88 to 112 lbs.	= 2 tsp.
113 to 137 lbs.	= 2½ tsp.
138 to 162 lbs.	= 3 tsp. (1 tbsp.)
163 to 187 lbs.	= 3½ tsp.
188 lbs. & over	= 4 tsp.

SHAKE WELL BEFORE USING

How Supplied: Pin-X is supplied as a tan to yellowish, caramel-flavored suspension which contains 50 mg of pyrantel base (as pyrantel pamoate) per mL, in bottles of 30 mL (1 fl oz). NDC 55806-024-10
Store at controlled room temperature 15°–30°C (59°–86°F).
Manufactured for:
Effcon Laboratories Inc.
Marietta, GA 30065-1509
Manufactured by:
MIKART, INC.
Atlanta, GA 30318
Rev. 1/89
Code 587A00

Shown in Product Identification Guide, page 508

Fisons Corporation
P.O. BOX 1766
ROCHESTER, NY 14603

DELSYM® Cough Formula
[del 'sĭm]
(dextromethorphan polistirex)
Extended-Release Suspension
12-Hour Cough Relief

Active Ingredient: Each teaspoonful (5 mL) contains dextromethorphan polistirex equivalent to 30 mg dextromethorphan hydrobromide.

Inactive Ingredients: Citric acid, ethylcellulose, FD&C Yellow No. 6, flavor, high fructose corn syrup, methylparaben, polyethylene glycol 3350, polysorbate 80, propylene glycol, propylparaben, purified water, sucrose, tragacanth, vegetable oil, xanthan gum.

Indications: Temporarily relieves cough due to minor throat and bronchial irritation as may occur with the common cold or inhaled irritants.

Warnings: Do not take this product for persistent or chronic cough such as occurs with smoking, asthma, or emphysema, or if cough is accompanied by excessive phlegm (mucus) unless directed by a physician. A persistent cough may be a sign of a serious condition. If cough persists for more than 1 week, tends to recur, or is accompanied by fever, rash, or persistent headache, consult a physician. As with any drug, if you are pregnant or nursing a baby, seek the advice of a health professional before using this product. **Keep this and all drugs out of the reach of children.** In case of accidental overdose, seek professional assistance or contact a Poison Control Center immediately.

Drug Interaction Precaution: Do not use this product if you are now taking a prescription monoamine oxidase inhibitor (MAOI) (certain drugs for depression, psychiatric or emotional conditions, or Parkinson's disease), or for 2 weeks after stopping the MAOI drug. If you are uncertain whether your prescription drug contains an MAOI, consult a health professional before taking this product.

Directions: **Shake Bottle Well Before Using.** Dose as follows or as directed by a physician.
Adults and Children 12 years of age and over: 2 teaspoonfuls every 12 hours, not to exceed 4 teaspoonfuls in 24 hours.
Children 6 to under 12 years of age: 1 teaspoonful every 12 hours, not to exceed 2 teaspoonfuls in 24 hours.
Children 2 to under 6 years of age: ½ teaspoonful every 12 hours, not to exceed 1 teaspoonful in 24 hours.
Children under 2 years of age: Consult a physician.

How Supplied: 89 mL (3 fl oz) bottles NDC 0585-0842-61
Store at 15°–30°C (59°–86°F).
FISONS Pharmaceuticals
Fisons Corporation
Rochester, NY 14623 U.S.A.
DELSYM is a registered trademark of Fisons Corporation.

Fleming & Company
1600 FENPARK DR.
FENTON, MO 63026

CHLOR–3
Medicinal Condiment

Active Ingredients: A troika of sodium chloride (50% 24.3 mEq/half tsp. iodized); potassium chloride (30% 11.5 mEq/half tsp.); magnesium chloride (20% 5.6 mEq/half tsp.).

Indications: The first medicinal condiment to restore needed K^+ & Mg^{++} lost during diuresis, at the expense of Na^+. To restore electrolytes lost by overcooking foods, or to add to diets that lack green vegetables, bananas, etc. And to replace conventional salting of foods in culinary and gourmet arts.

Symptoms and Treatment of Oral Overdosage: Hyperkalemia and hypermagnesemia are not end-stage results of usage.

How Supplied: In 8-oz plastic shaker, tamper-evident bottles.

IMPREGON Concentrate

Active Ingredient: Tetrachlorosalicyl-anilide 2%

Indications: Diaper Rash Relief, 'Staph' control, Mold inhibitor.

Actions: This is a bacteriostatic/fungistatic agent for home usage and hospital usage.

Warnings: Impregon should not be exposed to direct sunlight for long periods after applications.

Precaution: Addition of bleach prior to diaper treatment negates application effects.

Dosage and Administration: One capful (5ml) per gallon of water to impregnate diapers in the diaper pail. Dilutions for many home areas accompany the full package.

Note: For disposable-type diapers, add one teaspoonful to 8 oz of water to a 'Windex-type' sprayer. Spray middle half area of diapers until damp, and allow to dry before using, to prevent rashes.

How Supplied: Four ounce amber plastic bottles.

MAGONATE TABLETS
MAGONATE LIQUID
Magnesium Gluconate (Dihydrate)

Active Ingredients: Each tablet contains magnesium gluconate (dihydrate) 500mg (27mg of Mg^{++}). Each 5cc of Magonate Liquid contains magnesium gluconate (dihydrate) 1000mg (54mg of Mg^{++}).

Indications: For all patients in negative magnesium balance.

Precaution: Excessive dosage may cause loose stools.

Dosage and Administration: Magonate is recommended during and for three weeks after a course in chemotherapy, then monitored regularly.
Adults and children over 12 yrs.—one or two tablets or $1/2$ to 1 teaspoon of liquid t.i.d. Under 12 yrs.—one tablet or $1/2$ teaspoon of liquid t.i.d. Dosage may be increased in severe cases.

How Supplied: Magonate Tablets are supplied in bottles of 100 and 1000 tablets. Magonate Liquid is supplied in pints and gallons.

MARBLEN Suspension and Tablet

Composition: A modified 'Sippy Powder' antacid containing magnesium and calcium carbonates.

Action and Uses: The peach/apricot (pink) antacid suspension is sugar-free and neutralizes 18 mEq acid per teaspoonful with a low sodium content of 18mg per fl. oz. Each pink tablet consumes 18.0 mEq acid.

Administration and Dosage: One teaspoonful rather than a tablespoonful or one tablet to reduce patient cost by $2/3$.

How Supplied: Plastic pints and bottles of 100 and 1000.

NEPHROX SUSPENSION
(aluminum hydroxide)
Antacid Suspension

Composition: A watermelon flavored aluminum hydroxide (320mg as gel)/mineral oil (10% by volume) antacid per teaspoonful.

Action and Uses: A sugar-free/saccharin-free pink suspension containing no magnesium and low sodium (19mg/oz). Extremely palatable and especially indicated in renal patients. Each teaspoon consumes 9 mEq acid.

Administration and Dosage: Two teaspoonfuls or as directed by a physician.

Caution: To be taken only at bedtime. Do not use at any other time or administer to infants, expectant women, and nursing mothers except upon the advice of a physician as this product contains mineral oil.

How Supplied: Plastic pints and gallons.

NICOTINEX Elixir
nicotinic acid

Composition: Contains niacin 50 mg./tsp. in a sherry wine base (amber color).

Action and Uses: Produces flushing when tablets fail. To increase micro-circulation of inner-ear in Meniere's, tinnitus and labyrinthine syndromes. For 'cold hands & feet', and as a vehicle for additives.

Administration and Dosage: One or two teaspoonsful on fasting stomach.

Side Effects: Patients should be warned of dermal flush. Ulcer and gout patients may be affected by 14% alcoholic content.

Contraindications: Severe hypotension and hemorrhage.

How Supplied: Plastic pints and gallons.

OCEAN MIST
(buffered saline)

Composition: A 0.65% special saline made isotonic by a dual preservative system and buffering excipients prevent nasal irritation.

Action and Uses: Rhinitis medicamentosa, rhinitis sicca and atrophic rhinitis. For patients 'hooked on nose drops' and glaucoma patients on diuretics having dry nasal capillaries. OCEAN may also be used as a mist or drop.

Administration and Dosage: One or two squeezes in each nostril P.R.N.

Supplied: Plastic 45cc spray bottles and pints.

PURGE
(flavored castor oil)

Composition: Contains 95% castor oil (USP) in a sweetened lemon flavored base that completely masks the odor and taste of the oil.

Indications: Preparation of the bowel for x-ray, surgery and proctological procedures, IVPs, and constipation.

Dosage: Infants—1–2 teaspoonfuls. Children—adjust between infant and adult dose. Adult—2–4 tablespoonfuls.

Precaution: Not indicated when nausea, vomiting, abdominal pain or symptoms of appendicitis occur. Pregnancy, use only on advice of physician.

Supplied: Plastic 1 oz. & 2 oz. bottles.

Flemming Pharmaceuticals, Inc.
ELEVEN GREENWAY PLAZA, SUITE 1115
HOUSTON, TX 77046

CAPSIN™
Topical Analgesic Lotion
0.025%, 0.075%

Description: CAPSIN lotion is a topical analgesic containing capsaicin in concentrations of 0.025% and 0.075%.

Active Ingredient: Capsaicin (chemical name trans-8-methyl-N-vanillyl-6-nonenamide) is derived from Capsicum Oleoresin, which is found in a number of common chili pepper plant species.

Inactive Ingredients: Benzyl Alcohol, Propylene Glycol, Denatured Alcohol, Dimethyl Isosorbide, D-Limonene.

Major Uses: CAPSIN lotion 0.025% and 0.075% is used in the management of minor pain associated with arthritis, sprains, strains and simple backaches. CAPSIN lotion is packaged with a unique applicator system that allows direct application of the lotion to the affected area. It is designed to reduce the risk of contact with the eyes and mucous membranes and to minimize waste.

Action: The precise mechanism of action is not fully known. However, capsaicin is believed to work by depleting the supply of the neurotransmitter Substance P resulting in a reduction of pain perception.

Safety Information: An initial burning sensation may occur after applica-

Continued on next page

Flemming Pharm.—Cont.

tion, but generally will subside after continued use.

Warnings: FOR EXTERNAL USE ONLY. Avoid contact with eyes, mucous membranes, broken or irritated skin. Do not bandage tightly. If symptoms persist or recur after seven days of continued use, please discontinue and consult a physician. Keep this and all drugs out of the reach of children. In case of accidental ingestion, seek professional assistance.

Directions: Adults and children two years of age and older: Apply CAPSIN lotion to affected areas 3 to 4 times daily. If applied less than 3 to 4 times per day, optimum pain relief may not occur and the burning sensation may persist.

How Supplied: CAPSIN 0.025%: 2 fl. oz. (59ml) NDC 60976-025-02 CAPSIN 0.075%: 2 fl. oz. (59ml) NDC 60976-075-02 Store at room temperature, 15°–30°C (59°–86°F) Patent Pending

---

Gebauer Company
9410 ST. CATHERINE AVENUE CLEVELAND, OH 44104

SALIVART®
[sal ´ĭ-vart] **Saliva Substitute**

Description: Prompt, lasting relief of dryness of the mouth or throat (hyposalivation, xerostomia).

Contains:

	%W/W
Sodium carboxymethyl-cellulose	1.000
Sorbitol	3.000
Sodium chloride	0.084
Potassium chloride	0.120
Calcium chloride, dihydrate	0.015
Magnesium chloride, hexahydrate	0.005
Potassium phosphate, dibasic	0.034

Preservative Free
Propellant: Nitrogen

Indications: For reduced salivary flow, caused by medications, radiation therapy near the mouth or throat, salivary gland infection, mouth or throat inflammation, dental or oral surgery, fever, emotional factors. Also for relieving nasal crusting and bad taste.

Actions: Moistens and lubricates the oral cavity like natural saliva to allow normal eating, swallowing, and talking. Improves adherence of dentures.

Warnings: Avoid spraying in eyes. Keep out of reach of children. Contents under pressure. Do not puncture or incinerate. Protect from direct sunlight and from heat above 50°C (120°F).

Dosage and Administration: Spray Salivart directly into the mouth or throat, for 1 or 2 seconds, using it as often as needed to maintain moistness, or as instructed by physician. Nasal crusting can be relieved by applying Salivart with a cotton swab.

How Supplied:
75 mL   NDC 0386-0009-75
25 mL   NDC 0386-0009-25
Shown in Product Identification Guide, page 508

A.C. Grace Co.
1100 QUITMAN ROAD P.O. BOX 570 BIG SANDY, TX 75755

UNIQUE E™ Vitamin E

Description: Each beef gelatin 400 I.U. Softgel Capsule contains All-Natural *Un*esterified Extra-High Antioxidant Concentrated Mixed Tocopherols. Not esterified acetate, succinate, *ordinary* Mixed Tocopherols nor d*l* synthetic. Contains *NO* SOY OIL, WHEAT GERM OIL or *ANY* OTHER OIL *DILUENT* which will turn rancid causing harmful free radical pathology. NO ALLERGENS, PRESERVATIVES, COLORS OR FLAVORS. Minimum shelf life FIVE YEARS.

All known natural related tocopherols for extra-high antioxidant function *PLUS* full biological activity and synergistic benefits of the complete all-natural Vitamin E Complex. The *ONLY* form providing all known vital functions of Vitamin E.

Unlike *ordinary* Mixed Tocopherols which can vary in the important d-alpha tocopherol potency, UNIQUE E Softgel capsules are stabilized and Certified by Assay to provide 400 I.U. (International Units) of d-alpha tocopherol *PLUS* all vital antioxidant factors.

Dosage: One or more capsules as directed by physician. Take *ENTIRE* daily dosage just before or with morning meal.

How Supplied: Bottles of 180 and 90 Softgel Capsules in safety-sealed, light protected plastic bottles.

UNKNOWN DRUG?
Consult the
Product Identification Guide
(Gray Pages)
for full-color photos of
leading over-the-counter
medications

Hogil Pharmaceutical Corp.
ONE BYRAM BROOK PLACE ARMONK, NY 10504

A•200
Lice Control Spray

Description: A•200 Spray contains the synthetic pyrethroid permithrin.
Active Ingredients:

*Permithrin	0.50%
Inert Ingredients	99.50%
	100.00%

*(3-phenoxyphenyl) methyl (+/−) cis/trans 3-(2,2-dichloroethenyl) 2,2- dimethylcyclopropanecarboxylate. Cis/ trans ratio: Min. 35% (+/−) cis and max. 65% (+/−) trans.

Indications: A•200 Lice Control Spray is indicated to for use only on garments, bedding, furniture, carpeting, upholstery and other inanimate objects infested with lice. Also for control of fleas and ticks on dogs.

Actions: Permethrin, a highly active synthetic pyrethroid, acts on nerve cell membranes to disrupt polarization creating paralysis of the insect.

Warnings: PRECAUTIONARY STATEMENTS: HAZARDS TO HUMANS AND DOMESTIC ANIMALS-CAUTION: Avoid spraying in the eyes. Avoid breathing spray mist. Avoid contact with skin, wash hands thoroughly after use. Vacate room after treatment and ventilate before reoccupying. Avoid contamination of feed and foodstuffs. Cover or remove fishbowls. This product is not for use on humans. If lice infestations should occur on humans, consult either your physician or pharmacist for a product for use on humans. **Animals:** Do not spray directly in/on eyes, mouth or genitalia. Do not cause exposure to puppies less than four weeks old.
STATEMENT OF PRACTICAL TREATMENT:
IF INHALED: Remove affected person to fresh air. Apply artificial respiration if indicated. IF IN EYES: Flush with plenty of water. Contact a physician if irritation persists. IF ON SKIN: Wash affected areas immediately with soap and water. Get medical attention if irritation persists.

Physical or Chemical Hazards: Contents under pressure. Do not use or store near heat or open flame. Do not puncture or incinerate container. Exposure to temperatures above 130°F may cause bursting.

Directions for Use: It is a violation of Federal law to use this product in a manner inconsistent with its labeling. Do not use in the edible product areas of food/feed processing plants, restaurants or other areas where food/feed is commercially prepared or served. Do not use in serving areas while food is exposed. Do not use on electrical equipment. SHAKE WELL BEFORE USING. Remove protective cap, hold container upright and spray from a distance of 12 to 15 inches. Remove birds and cover fish aquariums before spraying.

To Kill Lice and Louse Eggs: Spray in an inconspicuous area to test for possible staining or discoloration. Inspect again after drying, then proceed to spray entire area to be treated. Hold container upright with nozzle away from you. Depress valve and spray from a distance of 8 to 10 inches. Spray each square foot for three seconds. Spray only those garments and parts of bedding, including mattresses and furniture that can not be either laundered or dry cleaned. Allow all sprayed articles to dry thoroughly before use.

Storage and Disposal: Do not transport or store below 32°F. Storage: Store in a cool dry place away from heat or open flame. Disposal: Do not reuse empty container. Replace cap, wrap container and put out in trash collection. Do not incinerate or puncture.

How Supplied: 6 Oz. aerosol can. Also available in combination with A•200 Lice Treatment Kit.
Shown in Product Identification Guide, page 508

A•200®
LICE KILLING SHAMPOO

Description: A•200 Pediculicide, a synergized pyrethrum extract contains:
Active Ingredients:
Pyrethrum Extract 0.33%
Piperonyl Butoxide 4.0%
Other Ingredients:
Alcohol, $C_{13}C_{14}$Isoparaffin, Polyoxyethylene (1, 1, 3, 3-tetra-methylbutyl) ether, Water.

Indications: A•200 is indicated for the treatment of head and body lice.

Actions: Pyrethrum Extract disrupts nervous transmission in lice resulting in paralysis and death. Piperonyl Butoxide is a synergist that potentiates the lethal actions of pyrethrum extract by blocking detoxification of the drug by the lice. Pyrethrum extract is poorly absorbed through the skin.

Warning: Should be used with caution on persons allergic to ragweed.

Precautions: For external use only. Do not use near the eyes or permit contact with mucous membranes, such as inside the nose, mouth or vagina, as irritation may occur. Keep out of eyes when rinsing hair. Adults and children: Close eyes tightly and do not open until product is rinsed out. Also protect children's eyes with washcloth, towel or other suitable material, or by a similar method. If product gets in the eyes: immediately flush with water. If skin irritation or infection is present or develops, discontinue use and consult a physician. Consult a physician if infestation of eyebrows or eyelashes occurs. In case of accidental ingestion, seek professional assistance or call a poison control center. If pregnant

or nursing a baby, seek advice from a health professional before using this product.

Storage and Disposal: Do not contaminate water, food or feed by storage or disposal. Do not reuse container. Wrap and put in trash collection. Do not transport or store below 32°F (0°C).

Directions for Use: Important—Read warnings before using. Shake well before using. Apply to the affected area until all the hair is thoroughly wet with product. Allow product to remain on the area for 10 minutes but no longer. Then add sufficient warm water to form a lather and shampoo as usual. Rinse thoroughly. Use the special A•200 Lice/Nit comb supplied to help remove the dead lice and their eggs(nits) from the hair. A second treatment must be done in 7 to 10 days to kill any newly hatched lice.

How Supplied: In 2 and 4 oz. unbreakable plastic bottles. A special patented A•200 Lice/Nit Comb for lice and egg (nit) removal and a patient insert in both English and Spanish are included.
Shown in Product Identification Guide, page 508

INNOGel PLUS®
Pubic(Crab) Lice Treatment Gel

Description: Active Ingredients:
Pyrethrum Extract 0.30%
Piperonyl Butoxide 3.0%
Other Ingredients:
Carbomer-934, D&C Red# 33, FD&C Blue# 1, Petroleum Distillate, Triethanolamine, Water.

Indications: InnoGel Plus is indicated for the treatment of pubic(crab) and body lice.

Actions: Pyrethrum extract disrupts nervous transmission in lice resulting in paralysis and death. Piperonyl Butoxide is a synergist that potentiates the lethal actions of pyrethum extract by blocking detoxification of the drug by the lice. Pyrethrum extract is poorly absorbed through the skin.

Warning: Should be used with caution on persons allergic to ragweed.

Precautions: For external use only. Do not use near the eyes or permit contact with mucous membranes, such as inside the nose, mouth or vagina, as irritation may occur. Keep out of eyes when rinsing hair. Adults and children: Close eyes tightly and do not open until product is rinsed out. Also protect children's eyes with washcloth, towel or other suitable material, or by a similar method. If product gets in the eyes: immediately flush with water. If skin irritation or infection is present or develops, discontinue use and consult a physician. Consult a physician if infestation of eyebrows or eyelashes occurs. In case of accidental ingestion, seek professional assistance or call a poison control center. If pregnant or nursing a baby, seek advice from a

health professional before using this product.

Directions for Use: Apply InnoGel Plus to affected area until hair is thoroughly covered with product. Allow product to remain on the area for 10 minutes but no longer. Wash area thoroughly with warm water and soap or shampoo. Use the special InnoGel Plus Lice/Nit Comb supplied to remove dead lice and their eggs(nits) from the hair. A second treatment must be done in 7 to 10 days to kill any newly hatched lice.

How Supplied: Consumer package containing 3-4 gram pre-dosed gel packettes and a special InnoGel Lice/Nit Comb.
Shown in Product Identification Guide, page 508

EDUCATIONAL MATERIAL

The Contemporary Approach to the Control of Head Lice in Schools and communities. (A comprehensive training Manual for health Professionals)
Head Lice: Differential Diagnosis Cards

Immunostics, Inc.
3505 SUNSET AVENUE
OCEAN, NJ 07712

IMMUNO HCG Detector
Pregnancy Test

HOW TO PERFORM THE TEST

1. Remove the test device from its protective pouch (bring the device to room temperature before opening the pouch to avoid condensation of the moisture on the membrane).
2. Dispense five drops of specimen into the sample well. Wait for colored bands to appear. Depending on the concentration of HCG, positive results may be observed in as short as one minute. However, to confirm negative results, the complete reaction time (five minutes) is required. DO NOT INTERPRET RESULT AFTER 10 MINUTES.

INTERPRETATION OF RESULTS

1. Negative: Only one colored band appears on the control region. No apparent band on the test region.
2. Positive: In addition to the control band, a distinct colored band also appears on the test region.
3. When neither test band nor control appears on the membrane, the test should be voided since improper test procedure or deterioration of reagents probably occurred.

To order please call Customer Service at 1-800-633-4750

Inter-Cal Corporation
533 MADISON AVENUE
PRESCOTT, AZ 86301

ESTER–C®
(Calcium Ascorbate)

Description: Each Ester-C tablet & caplet contains 500 mg Vitamin C in the form of Calcium Ascorbate 550 mg, vegetable-derived cellulose, stearic acid, and magnesium stearate. Ester-C contains no preservatives, sugars, artificial colorings, or flavorings.

As the calcium salt of L-ascorbic acid, calcium ascorbate, the primary constituent of Ester-C, has an empirical formula of $CaC_{12}H_{14}O_{12}$ and a formula weight of 390.3. The water-based neutralization process yields natural C metabolites, including dehydroascorbate and the calcium salt of threonic acid, which make up the balance of the patented Ester-C complex.

Actions: Vitamin C has been found to be essential for the prevention of scurvy. In humans, an exogenous source of the vitamin is required for collagen formation and tissue repair. Ascorbate ion is reversibly oxidized to dehydroascorbate ion in the body. Both of these are active forms of the vitamin and are considered to play important roles in biochemical oxidation-reduction reactions. Other C metabolites have demonstrated absorption enhancing properties. The vitamin is involved in tyrosine metabolism, carbohydrate metabolism, iron metabolism, folic acid-folinic acid conversion, synthesis of lipids and proteins, resistance to infections, and cellularrespiration.

Indications and Usage: Vitamin C and its salts, such as Calcium Ascorbate, are recommended as nutritional supplements in the prevention of scurvy. In scurvy, collagenous structures are primarily affected, and lesions develop in blood vessels and bones. Symptoms of mild deficiency may include faulty development of teeth and bones, bleeding gums, gingivitis, and loose teeth. An increased need for the vitamin exists in febrile states, chronic illness and infection, e.g., rheumatic fever, pneumonia, tuberculosis, whooping cough, diphtheria, sinusitis, etc. Additional increases in the daily intake of ascorbate are indicated in burns, delayed healing of bone fractures and wounds, and hemovascular disorders. Immature and premature infants require relatively larger amounts of Vitamin C.

Contraindications: Because of its calcium content, Ester-C is contraindicated in hypercalcemic states, e.g., from dosing with parathyroid hormone or overdosage of Vitamin D.

Adverse Reactions: There are no known adverse reactions following ingestion of Ester-C tablets, caplets & powder. The gastric disturbances characteristic of large doses of ascorbic acid are absent or greatly diminished when the pH-neu-tral form of calcium ascorbate present in Ester-C tablets, caplets & powder are utilized as the source of Vitamin C supplementation.

Dosage and Administration: The minimum U.S. Recommended Daily Allowance for Vitamin C for the prevention of diseases such as scurvy is 60 mg per day. Optimum daily allowances, e.g., for the maintenance of increased plasma and cellular reserves, are significantly greater. For adults, the recommended average preventive dose of the vitamin is 70 to 150 mg daily. The recommended average optimum dose of Ester-C is 550 to 1650 mg (1 to 3 tablets or caplets) daily.

For frank scurvy, doses of 300 mg to one gram of Vitamin C daily have been recommended. Normal adults, however, have received as much as six grams of the vitamin without evidence of toxicity.

For enhancement of wound healing, doses of the vitamin approximating two Ester-C tablets, caplets and powder daily for a week or ten days both preoperatively and postoperatively are generally considered adequate, although considerably larger amounts may be recommended. In the treatment of burns, the daily number of Ester-C tablets, caplets and powder recommended is governed by the extent of tissue injury. For severe burns, daily doses of 2 to 4 tablets or caplets (approximately one to two grams of Vitamin C) are recommended.

In other conditions in which the need for increased Vitamin C is recognized, three to five times the optimum allowance appears to be adequate.

How Supplied: 550 mg tablets and caplets of Ester-C in bottles. Capsules, tablets and powders in varying potencies, formulations, and packages are available. Used as a food fortifier, preservative, flavor enhancer, and cosmetic ingredient. Also available as magnesium, potassium, sodium and zinc salts.

Store at room temperature.

U.S. Patent granted April 18, 1989; No. 4,822,816.

Literature revised: September 1994.
Mfd. by Inter-Cal Corp.
Prescott, AZ 86301

UNKNOWN DRUG?
Consult the
Product Identification Guide
(Gray Pages)
for full-color photos of
leading over-the-counter
medications

Jamol Laboratories, Inc.
13 ACKERMAN AVENUE
EMERSON, NEW JERSEY 07630

PONARIS   OTC
Nasal Mucosal Emollient

Composition: Essential oils of Pine, Eucalyptus, Peppermint, Cajeput, and Cottonseed as specailly prepared iodized organic oils. Total Iodine 0.5%–0.7% Assimilable hence NON-lipoid potential.

Indications and Uses: For relief of nasal congestion due to colds, nasal irritations, Atrophic Rhinitis, (dry inflamed nasal passages), nasal mucosal encrustations, and allergy manifestations (Rose and Hay Fever).

Nasal intubations and sterile gauze impregnated for epistaxis packing.

Administration and Dosage: Half dropperful each application as needed or as directed by a physician. May be used in a compressed air neubulizer or a De Vilbiss nebulizer No. 15.

Children's Dosage: As directed by physician.

How Supplied: One ounce bottle with dropper.

Johnson & Johnson Consumer Products, Inc.
GRANDVIEW RD
SKILLMAN, NJ 08558

K-Y® BRAND JELLY PERSONAL LUBRICANT

Description: K-Y® Brand Jelly Personal Lubricant is a greaseless, water-soluble jelly which is clear, spreads easily, is non-irritating, and is safe to use with latex products.

Indications: K-Y® Jelly provides vaginal moisture, lubricates condoms and helps ease insertion of tampons, rectal thermometers, enemas, douches and other devices inserted into body cavities. K-Y® Jelly will not harm rubber, plastic, diaphragms or glass surfaces.

Actions: Helps lubricate body cavities for easier insertion. When used as a sexual lubricant, K-Y® Jelly helps overcome vaginal dryness from sexual intercourse, menopause, childbirth, lactation or stressful periods.

Directions: Squeeze tube to obtain desired amount of lubricant (a 1–2 inch strip should be sufficient). Reapply as needed.

Ingredients: Chlorhexidine Gluconate, Glucono Delta Lactone, Glycerin, Hydroxyethyl Cellulose, Methylparaben, Purified Water, Sodium Hydroxide

THIS PRODUCT IS NOT A CONTRACEPTIVE AND DOES NOT CONTAIN A SPERMICIDE. Store at room temperature.

How Supplied: K-Y® Jelly is available in 2 and 4 oz. tubes and a convenient 3-pack (containing 0.4 oz. tubes).

Shown in Product Identification Guide, page 508

K-Y® PLUS
VAGINAL CONTRACEPTIVE AND PERSONAL LUBRICANT

Description: K-Y® PLUS Spermicidal Lubricant jelly with Nonoxynol-9 provides the same safe, water-soluble personal lubrication found in K-Y® Brand Jelly plus the added protection of the fast-acting vaginal contraceptive nonoxynol-9.

Active Ingredient: Nonoxynol-9 (2.2%)

Other Ingredients: Cremophor, Hydroxyethyl Cellulose, Methylparaben, Propylene Glycol, Purified Water, Sorbic Acid

Indications: K-Y® PLUS is an effective lubricant and provides effective protection against pregnancy. Provides protection for women who forget to take one or more contraceptive pills or who find other methods of contraception unacceptable.

Actions: K-Y® PLUS, when used in combination with condoms, provides even more protection against unplanned pregnancy. Its jelly formula provides effective personal lubrication plus protection against unplanned pregnancy. K-Y® PLUS is especially beneficial when used with condoms because, unlike oil-based lubricants which can break down the latex in condoms, its water-soluble lubrication may actually reduce friction to help prevent condoms from breaking during use. K-Y® Plus is hormone free and does not have the side effects associated with oral contraceptives. K-Y® PLUS can be inserted up to an hour before intercourse.

Directions: Remove cap from tube, puncture safety seal and attach applicator by turning applicator clockwise. Fill the applicator until the plunger is pushed out as far as it will go and the barrel is completely filled. After detaching from tube, hold the filled applicator by the barrel and gently insert into the vagina as far as it will comfortably go. Press the plunger, and, with the plunger still depressed, remove the applicator, holding it by the barrel. Intercourse should occur within 1 hour after insertion. Repeat prior to each additional act of intercourse. This method of contraception must be used each and every time intercourse takes place, regardless of time of month. Wash the applicator in mild soap and water and rinse thoroughly after each use. For extra lubrication, squeeze desired amount of K-Y® PLUS Brand Spermicidal Lubricant (1–2 inch strip) and apply externally to genital area or directly on condom. Reapply as needed.

Cautions: Keep this and all drugs out of the reach of children. If you or your partner experience irritation, discontinue use. If irritation persists, consult your doctor. In case of accidental ingestion, call a Poison Control Center, emergency medical facility, or a doctor. If your physician has told you that you should not become pregnant, ask your physician if you can use this product for contraception. PLEASE NOTE: No method of birth control can absolutely guarantee against pregnancy. For maximum protection, all methods - including K-Y® PLUS - must be used according to directions.

Storage Conditions: Keep away from excessive heat. Store at controlled room temperature: 15–30 degrees C (59–86 degrees F).

How Supplied: K-Y® PLUS Brand of Spermicidal Lubricant is available in 4 oz. tubes. Sold with reusable applicator.

Shown in Product Identification Guide, page 508

Johnson & Johnson •
MERCK
Consumer Pharmaceuticals Co.
CAMP HILL ROAD
FORT WASHINGTON, PA 19034

ALternaGEL™   OTC
[al-tern 'a-jel]
Liquid
High-Potency Aluminum Hydroxide Antacid

Description: ALternaGEL is available as a white, pleasant-tasting, high-potency aluminum hydroxide liquid antacid.

Ingredients: Each 5 mL teaspoonful contains: Active: 600 mg aluminum hydroxide (equivalent to dried gel, USP) providing 16 milliequivalents (mEq) of acid-neutralizing capacity (ANC), and less than 2.5 mg (0.109 mEq) of sodium and no sugar. Inactive: butylparaben, flavors, propylparaben, purified water, simethicone, and other ingredients.

Indications: ALternaGEL is indicated for the symptomatic relief of hyperacidity associated with peptic ulcer, gastritis, peptic esophagitis, gastric hyperacidity, hiatal hernia, and heartburn.
ALternaGEL will be of special value to those patients for whom magnesium-containing antacids are undesirable, such as patients with renal insufficiency, patients requiring control of attendant GI complications resulting from steroid or other drug therapy, and patients experiencing the laxation which may result from magnesium or combination antacid regimens.

Directions: One to two teaspoonfuls, as needed, between meals and at bedtime, or as directed by a physician: May be followed by a sip of water if desired. Concentrated product. Shake well before using. Keep tightly closed.

Warnings: Keep this and all drugs out of the reach of children. ALternaGEL may cause constipation.
Except under the advice and supervision of a physician: do not take more than 18 teaspoonfuls in a 24-hour period, or use the maximum dose of ALternaGEL for more than two weeks. ALternaGEL may cause constipation.
Prolonged use of aluminum-containing antacids in patients with renal failure may result in or worsen dialysis osteomalacia. Elevated tissue aluminum levels contribute to the development of the dialysis encephalopathy and osteomalacia syndromes. Small amounts of aluminum are absorbed from the gastrointestinal tract and renal excretion of aluminum is impaired in renal failure. Aluminum is not well removed by dialysis because it is bound to albumin and transferrin, which do not cross dialysis membranes. As a result, aluminum is deposited in bone, and dialysis osteomalacia may develop when large amounts of aluminum are ingested orally by patients with imparied renal function.
Aluminum forms insoluble complexes with phosphate in the gastrointestinal tract, thus decreasing phosphate absorption. Prolonged use of aluminum-containing antacids by normophosphatemic patients may result in hypophosphatemia if phosphate intake is not adequate. In its more severe forms, hypophosphatemia can lead to anorexia, malaise, muscle weakness, and osteomalacia.

Drug Interaction Precaution: Antacids may interact with certain prescription drugs. If you are presently taking a prescription drug, do not take this product without checking with your physician or other health professional.

How Supplied: ALternaGEL is available in bottles of 12 fluid ounces and 1 fluid ounce hospital unit doses. NDC 16837-860.

Shown in Product Identification Guide, page 508

DIALOSE® Tablets   OTC
[di 'a-lose]
Stool Softener Laxative

Description: DIALOSE is a very low sodium, nonhabit forming, stool softener containing 100 mg docusate sodium per tablet.
The docusate in DIALOSE is a highly efficient surfactant which facilitates absorption of water by the stool to form a soft, easily evacuated mass. Unlike stimulant laxatives, DIALOSE does not interfere with normal peristalsis, neither does it cause griping nor sensations of urgency.

Ingredients: Active: Docusate Sodium, 100 mg per tablet
Inactive: Colloidal Silicone Dioxide, Dextrates, Flavors, Hydroxypropyl Methylcellulose, Magnesium Stearate,

Continued on next page

J&J • Merck—Cont.

Microcrystalline Cellulose, Polyethylene Glycol, Polysorbate 80, Pregelatinized Starch, Propylene Glycol, Sodium Starch Glycolate, Titanium Dioxide, D&C Red No. 28, D&C Red No. 27 Aluminum Lake, FD&C Blue No. 1, FD&C Blue No. 1 Aluminum Lake, FD&C Red No. 40.

Indications: DIALOSE is indicated for the relief of occasional constipation (irregularity).

DIALOSE is an effective aid to soften or prevent formation of hard stools in a wide range of conditions that may lead to constipation. DIALOSE helps to eliminate straining associated with obstetric, geriatric, cardiac, surgical, anorectal, or proctologic conditions. In cases of mild constipation, the fecal softening action of DIALOSE can prevent constipation from progressing and relieve painful defecation.

Directions: *Adults:* One tablet, one to three times daily; adjust dosage as needed.
Children 6 to under 12 years: One tablet daily as needed.
Children under 6 years: As directed by physician.
It is helpful to increase the daily intake of fluids by taking a glass of water with each dose.

Warnings: Unless directed by a physician: Do not use when abdominal pain, nausea, or vomiting are present. Do not use for a period longer than one week. Do not take this product if you are presently taking a prescription drug or mineral oil. As with any drug, if you are pregnant or nursing a baby, seek the advice of a health professional before using this product. Keep out of the reach of children.

How Supplied: Bottles of 100 pink tablets. Also available in 100 tablet unit dose boxes (10 strips of 10 tablets each). NDC-16837-870.
Shown in Product Identification Guide, page 508

DIALOSE® PLUS Tablets   OTC
[*di'a-lose Plus*]
Stool Softener/Stimulant Laxative

Description: DIALOSE PLUS provides a very low sodium tablet formulation of 100 mg docusate sodium and 65 mg yellow phenolphthalein.

Ingredients: Each tablet contains: Actives: Docusate Sodium, 100 mg., yellow phenolphthalein, 65 mg.
Inactive: Dextrates, Dibasic Calcium Phosphate Dihydrate, Flavors, Hydroxypropyl Methylcellulose, Magnesium Stearate, Microcrystalline Cellulose, Polydextrose, Polythylene Glycol, Polysorbate 80, Propylene Glycol, Sodium Starch Glycolate, Titanium Dioxide, Triacetin, D&C Yellow NO. 10 Aluminum Lake, D&C Red NO. 28, FD&C Blue NO. 1, FD&C Red NO. 40, FD&C Red NO. 40 Aluminum Lake.

Indications: DIALOSE PLUS is indicated for the treatment of constipation characterized by lack of moisture in the intestinal contents, resulting in hardness of stool and decreased intestinal motility. DIALOSE PLUS combines the advantages of the stool softener, docusate sodium, with the peristaltic activating effect of yellow phenolphthalein.

Directions: *Adults:* One or two tablets daily as needed, at bedtime or on arising
Children 6 to under 12 years: One tablet daily as needed
Children under 6 years: As directed by physician.
It is helpful to increase the daily intake of fluids by taking a glass of water with each dose.

Warnings: Unless directed by a physician: Do not use when abdominal pain, nausea, or vomiting are present. Do not use for a period longer than one week. If skin rash appears do not use this product or any other preparation containing phenolphthalein. Frequent or prolonged use may result in dependence on laxatives. Do not take this product if you are presently taking a prescription drug or mineral oil.
As with any drug, if you are pregnant or nursing a baby, seek the advice of a health professional before using this Keep out of the reach of children.

How Supplied: Bottles of 100 yellow tablets. Also available in100 capsule unit dose boxes (10 strips of 10 capsules each). NDC 16837-871.
Shown in Product Identification Guide, page 508

INFANTS' MYLICON® Drops   OTC
[*my'li-con*]
Antiflatulent

Ingredients: Each 0.6 mL of drops contains: Active: simethicone, 40 mg. Inactive: carbomer 934P, citric acid, flavors, hydroxypropyl methylcellulose, purified water, Red 3, saccharin calcium, sodium benzoate, sodium citrate.

Indications: For relief of the painful symptoms of excess gas in the digestive tract. Such gas is frequently caused by excessive swallowing of air or by eating foods that disagree. The defoaming action of INFANTS' MYLICON® Drops relieves flatulence by dispersing and preventing the formation of mucus-surrounded gas pockets in the gastrointestinal tract. INFANTS' MYLICON® Drops act in the stomach and intestines to change the surface tension of gas bubbles enabling them to coalesce, thereby freeing and eliminating the gas more easily by belching or passing flatus.

Directions: Infants (under 2 years): 0.3 ml four times daily after meals and at bedtime, or as directed by a physician. The dosage can also be mixed with 1 oz of cool water, infant formula or other suitable liquids to ease administration.

Adults and children: 0.6 ml four times daily, after meals and at bedtime, or as directed by a physician.

Warnings: Do not exceed 12 doses per day except under the advice and supervision of a physician. Keep this and all drugs out of the reach of chldren.

How Supplied: INFANTS' MYLICON® Drops are available in bottles of 15 ml (0.5 fl oz) and 30 ml (1.0 fl oz) pink, pleasant tasting liquid. NDC 16837-630.
Shown in Product Identification Guide, page 509

MYLANTA® AND   OTC
MYLANTA® DOUBLE STRENGTH
[*my-lan'ta*]
Aluminum, Magnesium and Simethicone
Liquid and Tablets
Antacid/Anti-Gas

Description: MYLANTA® and MYLANTA® Double Strength are well-balanced, pleasant-tasting, antacid/anti-gas medications that provide consistent, effective relief of symptoms associated with gastric hyperacidity and excess gas. Non-constipating and considered dietetically low sodium or sodium free, MYLANTA® and MYLANTA® Double Strength contain two proven antacids, aluminum hydroxide and magnesium hydroxide, plus simethicone for gas relief.

Active Ingredients: Each 5 mL teaspoon or one chewable tablet contains:

	MYLANTA®	MYLANTA® Double Strength
Aluminum Hydroxide	200 mg	400 mg
Magnesium Hydroxide	200 mg	400 mg
Simethicone	20 mg	40 mg

Inactive Ingredients:
TABLETS:
Colloidal silicon dioxide, dextrates, flavors, magnesium stearate, mannitol, saccharin sodium, sorbitol, FD & C Blue 1 or FD & C Yellow 10.
LIQUIDS:
Butylparaben, carboxymethylcellulose sodium, flavors, hydroxypropyl methylcellulose, microcrystalline cellulose, propylparaben, purified water, saccharin sodium, and sorbitol.

Sodium Content: Each 5 mL teaspoon or one chewable tablet contains the following amount of sodium:

	MYLANTA®	MYLANTA® Double Strength
Tablets	0.77 mg (0.33 mEq)*	1.3 mg (0.06 mEq)†
Liquid	0.68 mg (0.03 mEq)*	1.14 mg (0.05 mEq)*

* considered dietetically sodium free
† considered dietetically low sodium

Acid Neutralizing Capacity: Two teaspoonfuls or two chewable tablets have the following acid neutralizing capacity:

	MYLANTA®	MYLANTA® Double Strength
Tablets	23.0 mEq	46.0 mEq
Liquid	25.4 mEq	50.8 mEq

Indications: MYLANTA® and MYLANTA® Double Strength are indicated for the relief of acid indigestion, heartburn, sour stomach, and symptoms of gas and upset stomach associated with those conditions. MYLANTA® and MYLANTA® Double Strength are also indicated as antacids for the symptomatic relief of hyperacidity associated with the diagnosis of peptic ulcer, gastritis, peptic esophagitis, heartburn and hiatal hernia and as antiflatulents to alleviate the symptoms of mucus-entrapped gas, including postoperative gas pain.

Advantages: MYLANTA® and MYLANTA® Double Strength are homogenized for a smooth, creamy taste. The choice of three pleasant-tasting liquid flavors and the non-constipating formula encourage patient acceptance, thereby minimizing the skipping of prescribed doses. MYLANTA® and MYLANTA® Double Strength are also available in tablets, and both the liquid and tablet forms are considered dietetically low sodium or sodium free. MYLANTA® and MYLANTA® Double Strength provide consistent relief in patients suffering from distress associated with hyperacidity, mucus-entrapped gas, or swallowed air.

Directions:
Liquid:
Shake well. 2-4 teaspoonfuls between meals and at bedtime, or as directed by a physician.
Tablets:
2-4 tablets, well chewed, between meals and at bedtime, or as directed by physician.

Warnings: Keep this and all drugs out of the reach of children. Do not take more than 24 tsps/tablets of MYLANTA® or 12 tsps/tablets of MYLANTA® Double Strength in a 24-hour period or use the maximum dose of this product for more than two weeks, except under the advice and supervison of a physician. Do not use this product if you have kidney disease. Prolonged use of aluminum-containing antacids in patients with renal failure may result in or worsen dialysis osteomalacia. Elevated tissue aluminum levels contribute to the development of the dialysis encephalopathy and osteomalacia syndromes. Small amounts of aluminum are absorbed from the gastrointestinal tract and renal excretion of aluminum is impaired in renal failure. Aluminum is not well removed by dialysis because it is bound to albumin and transferrin, which do not cross dialysis membranes. As a result, aluminum is deposited in bone, and dialysis osteomalacia may develop when large amounts of aluminum are ingested orally by patients with impaired renal function.

Aluminum forms insoluble complexes with phosphate in the gastrointestinal tract, thus decreasing phosphate absorption. Prolonged use of aluminum-containing antacids by normophosphatemic patients may result in hypophosphatemia if phosphate intake is not adequate. In its more severe forms, hypophosphatemia can lead to anorexia, malaise, muscle weakness, and osteomalacia.

Drug Interaction Precaution: Antacids may interact with certain prescription drugs. If you are presently taking a prescription drug, do not take this product without checking with your physician or other health professional.

How Supplied: MYLANTA® and MYLANTA® Double Strength are available as white liquid suspensions in pleasant-tasting flavors, Original, Cherry Creme and Cool Mint Creme, and as two-layer green and white Cool Mint Creme and two-layer pink and white Cherry Creme chewable tablets. Tablets are identified as either MYLANTA® or MYLANTA® DS. Liquids are supplied in bottles of 5 oz, 12 oz, and 24 oz. MYLANTA® tablets are supplied in bottles of 48 and 100 count sizes and in 12 tablet roll packs. MYLANTA® Double Strength tablets are supplied in bottles of 30 and 60 count sizes and in 8 tablet roll packs. Also available for hospital use in liquid unit dose bottles of 1 oz and bottles of 5 oz.

MYLANTA®
NDC 16837-610 ORIGINAL LIQUID
NDC 16837-629 COOL MINT CREME LIQUID
NDC 16837-621 CHERRY CREME LIQUID
NDC 16837-628 CHERRY CREME TABLETS
NDC 16837-620 COOL MINT CREME TABLETS
MYLANTA® Double Strength
NDC 16837-652 ORIGINAL LIQUID
NDC 16837-624 COOL MINT CREME LIQUID
NDC 16837-622 CHERRY CREME LIQUID
NDC 16837-627 CHERRY CREME TABLETS
NDC 16837-651 COOL MINT CREME TABLETS
Professional Labeling
Indications: Stress-induced upper gastrointestinal hemorrhage: MYLANTA DOUBLE STRENGTH is indicated for the prevention of stress-induced upper gastrointestinal hemorrhage. Hyperacidic conditions: As an antacid, for the symptomatic relief of hyperacidity associated with the diagnosis of peptic ulcer and other gastrointestinal conditions where a high degree of acid neutralization is desired.

Directions: Prevention of stress-induced upper gastrointestinal hemorrhage: 1) Aspirate stomach via nasogastric tube* and record pH. 2) Instill 10 mL of MYLANTA DOUBLE STRENGTH followed by 30 mL of water via nasogastric tube. Clamp tube. 3) Wait one hour. Aspirate stomach and record pH. 4a) If pH equals or exceeds 4.0, apply drainage or intermittent suction for one hour, then repeat the cycle. 4b) If pH is less than 4.0, instill double (20 mL) MYLANTA DOUBLE STRENGTH followed by 30 mL of water. Clamp tube. 5) Wait one hour. If pH equals or exceeds 4.0, see number 7, if pH is still less than 4.0, instill double (40 mL) MYLANTA DOUBLE STRENGTH followed by 30 mL of water. Clamp tube. 6) Wait one hour. If pH equals or exceeds 4.0, see number 7. If pH is still less than 4.0, instill double (80 mL)† MYLANTA DOUBLE STRENGTH followed by 30 mL of water. 7) Drain for one hour and repeat cycle with the effective dosage of MYLANTA DOUBLE STRENGTH.

In hyperacid states for symptomatic relief: One or two teaspoonfuls as needed between meals and at bedtime or as directed by a physician. Higher dosage regimens may be employed under the direct supervision of a physician in the treatment of active peptic ulcer disease.

Precaution: Aluminum-magnesium hydroxide containing antacids should be used with caution in patients with renal impairment.

Adverse Effects: Occasional regurgitation and mild diarrhea have been reported with the dosage recommended for the prevention of stress-induced upper gastrointestinal hemorrhage.

References: 1. Zinner MJ, Zuidema GD, Smigh PL, Mignosa M: The prevention of upper gastrointestinal tract bleeding in patients in an intensive care unit. *Surg Gynecol Obster* 153:214–220, 1981. 2. Lucas CE, Sugawa C, Riddle J, et al.: Natural history and surgical dilemma of "stress" gastric bleeding. *Arch Surg* 102:266–273, 1971. 3. Hastings PR, Skillman JJ, Bushnell LS, Silen W: Antacid titration in the prevention of acute gastrointestinal bleeding: a controlled, randomized trial in 100 critically ill patients. *N Engl J Med* 298:1042–1045, 1978. 4. Day SB, MacMillan BG, Altemeier WA: *Curling's Ulcer, An Experience of Nature.* Springfield, IL, Charles C Thomas Co., 1972, p. 205. 5. Skillman JJ, Bushnell LS, Goldman H, Silen W: Respiratory failure, hypotension, sepsis, and jaundice. A clinical syndrome associated with lethal hemorrhage from acute stress ulceration of the stomach. *Am J Surg* 117:523–530, 1969. 6. Priebe HJ,

*If nasogastric tube is not in place, administer 20 mL of MYLANTA DOUBLE STRENGTH orally q2h.
†In a recent clinical study[1] 20 mL of MYLANTA DOUBLE STRENGTH, q2h, was sufficient in more than 85 percent of the patients. No patient studied required more than 80 mL of MYLANTA DOUBLE STRENGTH q2h.

Continued on next page

J&J • Merck—Cont.

Skillman J, Bushnell LS, et al. Antacid versus cimetidine in preventing acute gastrointestinal bleeding. *N Engl J Med* 302:426–430, 1980. 7. Silen W: The prevention and management of stress ulcers. *Hosp Pract* 15:93–97, 1980. 8. Herrmann V, Kaminski DL: Evaluation of intragastric pH in acutely ill patients. *Arch Surg* 114:511–514, 1979. 9. Martin LF, Staloch DK, Simonowitz DA, et al.: Failure of cimetidine prophylaxis in the critically ill. *Arch Surg* 114:492–496, 1979. 10. Zinner MJ, Turtinen L, Gurll NJ, Reynolds DG: The effect of metiamide on gastric mucosal injury in rat restraint. *Clin Res* 23:484A, 1975. 11. Zinner M, Turtinen BA, Gurll NJ: The role of acid and ischemia in production of stress ulcers during canine hemorrhagic shock. *Surgery* 77:807–816, 1975. 12. Winans CS: Prevention and treatment of stress ulcer bleeding: Antacids or cimetidine? *Drug Ther Bull* (hospital) 12:37–45, 1981.

Shown in Product Identification Guide, page 509

MYLANTA® GAS Relief Tablets
Maximum Strength MYLANTA®
GAS Relief Tablets
[*My-lan'-ta*]
Antiflatulent

Active Ingredients:
Each chewable tablet contains:

	Simethicone
MYLANTA® GAS Relief	80 mg
Maximum Strength MYLANTA® GAS Relief	125 mg

Inactive Ingredients: Dextrates, flavor, sorbitol, stearic acid, tricalcium phosphate. Cherry: Red 7.

Indications: For relief of the painful symptoms of excess gas in the digestive tract. Such gas is frequently caused by excessive swallowing of air or by eating foods that disagree. MYLANTA® GAS Relief, and Maximum Strength MYLANTA® GAS Relief Tablets are high capacity antiflatulents for adjunctive treatment of many conditions in which the retention of gas may be a problem, such as the following: air swallowing, postoperative gaseous distention, peptic ulcer, spastic or irritable colon, diverticulosis. If condition persists, consult your physician.
MYLANTA® GAS Relief, and Maximum Strength MYLANTA®GAS Relief Tablets have a defoaming action that relieves flatulence by dispersing and preventing the formation of mucus-surrounded gas pockets in the gastrointestinal tract. MYLANTA® GAS Relief, and Maximum Strength MYLANTA® GAS Relief Tablets act in the stomach and intestines to change the surface tension of gas bubbles enabling them to coalesce, thereby freeing and eliminating the gas more easily by belching or passing flatus.

Directions:
MYLANTA® GAS Relief Tablets
One tablet four times daily after meals and at bedtime. May also be taken as needed up to six tablets daily or as directed by a physician.
Maximum Strength MYLANTA® GAS Relief Tablets
One tablet four times daily after meals and at bedtime or as directed by a physician.

TABLETS SHOULD BE CHEWED THOROUGHLY

Warnings: Keep this and all drugs out of the reach of children.

How Supplied: 100 tablet unit dose boxes (10 strips of 10 tablets each). NDC 16837-450.
MYLANTA® GAS Relief Tablets are available as white (mint) or pink (cherry) scored, chewable tablets identified "MYL GAS 80." Mint flavor is available in bottles of 60 and 100 tablets and individually wrapped 12 and 30 tablet packages. Cherry flavor is available in packages of 12 individually wrapped tablets. Mint NDC 16837-858. Cherry NDC 16837-859. Maximum Strength MYLANTA® GAS Relief Tablets are available as white, scored, chewable tablets identified "MYL GAS 125" in individually wrapped 12 and 24 tablet packages and economical 48 tablet bottles. NDC 16837-455.
Shown in Product Identification Guide, page 509

MYLANTA® GELCAPS   **OTC**
[*my-lan'ta*]
Antacid

Description: MYLANTA® GELCAPS are an easy-to-swallow, non-chalky alternative to liquid and tablet antacids. The gelcaps contain two antacid ingredients, calcium carbonate, and magnesium carbonate, have no chalky taste, are low in sodium and provide fast, effective acid pain relief.

Ingredients: Each gelcap contains:
Active: Calcium Carbonate 311 mg and Magnesium Carbonate 232 mg. **Inactive:** Benzyl Alcohol, Butylparaben, Castor Oil, D&C Yellow 10, Disodium Calcium Edetate, FD&C Blue 1, Gelatin, Hydroxypropyl Cellulose, Magnesium Stearate, Methylparaben, Microcrystalline Cellulose, Propylparaben, Sodium Croscarmellose, Sodium Lauryl Sulfate, Sodium Propionate, Titanium Dioxide.
Sodium Content: MYLANTA® GELCAPS contain a very low amount of sodium per daily dose. Typical value is 2.5 mg (.1087 mEq) sodium per gelcap.
Acid Neutralizing Capacity: Two MYLANTA® GELCAPS have an acid neutralizing capacity of 23.0 mEq.

Indications: For the relief of acid indigestion, heartburn, sour stomach and upset stomach associated with these symptoms.

Advantages: MYLANTA® GELCAPS are easy to swallow, provide fast, effective relief, eliminate antacid taste and are low in sodium. Convenience of dosage in the unique gelcap form can promote patient compliance.

Directions: 2–4 gelcaps as needed or as directed by a physician.

Warnings: Keep this and all other drugs out of the reach of children. Do not take more than 24 gelcaps in a 24-hour period or use the maximum dosage for more than two weeks or use if you have kidney disease, except under the advice and supervision of a physician.

Drug Interaction Precaution: Antacids may interact with certain prescription drugs. If you are presently taking a prescription drug, do not take this product without checking with your physician or other health professional.

How Supplied: MYLANTA® GELCAPS are available as a blue and white gelcap in convenient blister packs in boxes of 24 solid gelcaps or in bottles of 50 and 100 solid gelcaps.
NDC 16837-850   1/93
Shown in Product Identification Guide, page 509

MYLANTA NATURAL FIBER **OTC**
SUPPLEMENT
[*my-lan'ta*]
Natural Fiber Bulking Agent

Description: MYLANTA NATURAL FIBER SUPPLEMENT is an ultra smooth bulk laxative powder. Each rounded tablespoon (sugar) or teaspoon (sugar free) contains approximately 3.4 grams of psyllium hydrophilic mucilloid fiber. MYLANTA NATURAL FIBER SUPPLEMENT contains no chemical stimulants and is nonaddictive.

Ingredients: Active: Each dose contains approximately 3.4 grams of psyllium hydrocolloid mucilloid fiber per dose.
Inactives:
Sugar: ascorbic acid, citric acid, gum arabic (acacia gum), natural orange flavor, silicone dioxide, sucrose, D&C yellow no. 10, FD&C yellow no.6.
Sugar-free: ascorbic acid, aspartame, citric acid, gum arabic (acacia gum), maltodextrin, natural orange flavor, silicone dioxide, D&C yellow no. 10, FD&C yellow no.6.

Indications: MYLANTA NATURAL FIBER SUPPLEMENT is indicated to restore normal bowel habits in chronic constipation, to promote normal elimination in irritable bowel syndrome, and to ease the passage of stools in presence of anorectal disorders. MYLANTA NATURAL FIBER SUPPLEMENT produces a soft, lubricating bulk which promotes natural elimination. MYLANTA NATURAL FIBER SUPPLEMENT is not a one-dose, fast-acting bowel regulator. Administration for several days may be needed to establish regularity.

Directions: *Adults:* One rounded tablespoon of the sugar-containing product or one rounded teaspoon of the sugar-free product, in a glass of water one to three times a day, or as directed by a physician. *Children:* Consult your doctor.
MIX THIS PRODUCT (CHILD OR ADULT DOSE) WITH AT LEAST 8 OUNCES (A FULL GLASS) OF WATER OR OTHER FLUID. TAKING THIS PRODUCT WITHOUT ENOUGH LIQUID MAY CAUSE CHOKING. SEE WARNINGS.

Instructions: Pour MYLANTA NATURAL FIBER SUPPLEMENT into a *dry* glass, add approximately 8 oz. of water and stir briskly. Replace cap tightly. Keep in a dry place.

Warning: TAKING THIS PRODUCT WITHOUT ADEQUATE FLUID MAY CAUSE IT TO SWELL AND BLOCK YOUR THROAT OR ESOPHAGUS AND MAY CAUSE CHOKING. DO NOT TAKE THIS PRODUCT IF YOU HAVE DIFFICULTY IN SWALLOWING. IF YOU EXPERIENCE CHEST PAIN, VOMITING, OR DIFFICULTY IN SWALLOWING OR BREATHING AFTER TAKING THIS PRODUCT, SEEK IMMEDIATE MEDICAL ATTENTION. Avoid inhalation. May cause a potentially severe reaction when inhaled by persons sensitive to psyllium powder or suffering from respiratory disorders. As with all medications, keep out of the reach of children.

How Supplied: Bottles of 13 oz (sugar) and 10 oz (sugar-free) tan, granular instant mix powder.
NDC 16837-881 (sugar-free)
NDC 16837-880 (sugar)
Shown in Product Identification Guide, page 509

MYLANTA® SOOTHING LOZENGES
[*mi-lan 'ta*]
ANTACID

Description: MYLANTA® SOOTHING LOZENGES are a dietically sodium free calcium rich antacid which dissolve in your mouth to quickly soothe your heartburn pain or acid indigestion.

Ingredients: Each MYLANTA® SOOTHING LOZENGE contains:

Active: Calcium Carbonate, 600 mg

Inactive: Citric Acid, Corn Syrup, FD&C Red 40, Flavor, Propylene Glycol, Soybean Oil, Sucrose, Titanium Dioxide

Indications: For the relief of heartburn, acid indigestion, sour stomach and upset stomach associated with these symptoms.

Acid Neutralizing Capacity: Each MYLANTA® SOOTHING LOZENGE has an acid neutralizing capacity of 11.4 mEq.

Directions: Allow 1 lozenge to dissolve in your mouth and if necessary, follow with a second. Repeat as needed or as directed by a physician.

Warnings: Keep this and all other drugs out of the reach of children. Do not take more than 12 lozenges in a 24-hour period or use the maximum dosage for more than two weeks, except under the advice and supervision of a physician.

Drug Interaction Precaution: Antacids may interact with certain prescription drugs. If you are presently taking a prescription drug, do not take this product without checking with your physician or other health professional.

How Supplied: MYLANTA® SOOTHING LOZENGES are available as green Cool Mint Creme flavored lozenges, and as pink Cherry Creme flavored lozenges identified as "M". Lozenges supplied in 18 count boxes and 50 count bottles.
NDC 16837-876 (Cherry Creme)
NDC 16837-875 (Cool Mint Creme)
Shown in Product Identification Guide, page 509

THE STUART FORMULA®   OTC
Tablets
Multivitamin/Multimineral Supplement
ONE TABLET DAILY PROVIDES:
VITAMINS: US RDA*

A	100%	5,000 IU
D	100%	400 IU
E	33%	10 IU
C	83%	50 mg
Folic Acid	25%	100 mcg
B_1 (thiamin)	100%	1.5 mg
B_2 (riboflavin)	100%	1.7 mg
Niacin	100%	20 mg
B_6	50%	1.0 mg
(pyridoxine hydrochloride)		
B_{12}	50%	3 mcg
(cyanocobalamin)		

MINERALS: US RDA

Calcium	12.5%	125 mg
Copper	50%	1 mg
Iodine	100%	150 mcg
Iron	27.8%	5 mg

*Percentage of US Recommended Daily Allowances for adults and children 4 or more years of age.

Ingredients: Dibasic Calcium Phosphate, Microcrystalline Cellulose, Ascorbic Acid, Ferrous Fumerate, Niacinamide, dl-alpha Tocopheryl Acetate, Sodium Starch Glycolate, Magnesium Stearate, Vitamin A Acetate, Hydroxypropyl Methylcellulose, Colloidal Silicon Dioxide, Vitamin D3, Copper Sulfate, Thiamine Mononitrate, Riboflavin, Pyridoxine Hydrochloride, Cyanocobalamin, Iodine, Folic Acid, Carnauba Wax, Flavors, FD&C Red #40.

May Also Contain: Propylene Glycol, Polysorbate 80

Indications: The STUART FORMULA tablet provides a well-balanced multivitamin/multimineral formula intended for use as a daily dietary supplement for adults and children over age four.

Directions: One tablet daily or as directed by physician.

Warnings: Keep this and all drugs out of the reach of children. In case of accidental overdose, seek professional assistance or contact a Poison Control Center immediately.

How Supplied: Bottles of 100 white, round tablets. Child-resistant safety caps are standard on both bottles as a safeguard against accidental ingestion by children.
NDC 16837-866.
Shown in Product Identification Guide, page 509

Konsyl Pharmaceuticals, Inc.
**4200 S. HULEN
FORT WORTH, TX 76109**

**KONSYL Fiber Tablets
(Calcium Polycarbophil 625mg)**

Description: KONSYL Fiber Tablets is a bulk forming fiber laxative for restoring and maintaining regularity. Promotes normal function of the bowel by increasing bulk volume and water content of stool. KONSYL Fiber Tablets contain 625 mg calcium polycarbophil equivalent to 500 mg polycarbophil.

Inactive Ingredients: Caramel, Crospovidone, Ethycellulose, Hydroxypropyl Methylcellulose, Magnesium Stearate, Microcrystalline Cellulose, Polyethylene Glycol, Povidone, Silicon Dioxide.

Actions: KONSYL Fiber Tablets provide bulk that promotes normal elimination. KONSYL Fiber Tablets provide convenience of a bulk forming laxative in a tablet form. The product is easy-to-swallow and non-irritative in the gastrointestinal tract.

Indications: KNOSYL Fiber Tablets are indicated in the management of chronic constipation, irritable bowel syndrome, as adjunctive therapy in the constipation of diverticular disease, bowel management of patients with hemorrhoids, and for constipation during pregnancy, convalescence, and senility. KONSYL Fiber Tablets are also used for other indications as prescribed by physician.

Contraindications: Intestinal obstruction, fecal impaction.

WARNINGS: KEEP THIS AND ALL DRUGS OUT OF THE REACH OF CHILDREN. TAKING THIS PRODUCT WITHOUT ADEQUATE FLUID MAY CAUSE IT TO SWELL AND BLOCK YOUR THROAT OR ESOPHAGUS AND MAY CAUSE CHOKING. DO NOT TAKE THIS PRODUCT IF YOU HAVE DIFFICULTY IN SWALLOWING. IF YOU EXPERIENCE CHEST PAIN, VOMITING, OR DIFFICULTY IN

Continued on next page

Konsyl—Cont.

SWALLOWING OR BREATHING AFTER TAKING THIS PRODUCT, SEEK IMMEDIATE MEDICAL ATTENTION.

Interaction Precaution: Contains calcium. If you are taking any form of tetracycline antibiotic, this product should be taken at least 1 hour before or 2 hours after you have taken the antibiotic. Store at controlled room temperature 59°–86°F (15°–30°C). Protect from moisture.

Dosage and Administration: TAKE THIS PRODUCT (CHILD OR ADULT DOSE) WITH AT LEAST 8 OUNCES (A FULL GLASS) OF WATER OR OTHER FLUID. TAKING THIS PRODUCT WITHOUT ENOUGH LIQUID MAY CAUSE CHOKING. SEE WARNINGS. **ADULTS:** 2 TABLETS 1 TO 4 TIMES A DAY. **CHILDREN** (6 TO 12 YEARS OLD): 1 TABLET 1 TO 3 TIMES A DAY. CHILDREN UNDER 6 YEARS CONSULT A PHYSICIAN. DOSAGE WILL VARY ACCORDING TO DIET, EXERCISE, PREVIOUS LAXATIVE USE OR SEVERITY OF CONSTIPATION. THE RECOMMENDED ADULT STARTING DOSE IS 2 TO 4 TABLETS DAILY. MAY BE INCREASED UP TO 8 TABLETS DAILY.

How Supplied: Tablets, containers of 90 tablets.
Is this product OTC? Yes

KONSYL® POWDER
(psyllium hydrophilic mucilloid)
Sugar Free, Sugar Substitute Free.
6.0 grams of psyllium per
TEASPOON

Description: Konsyl is a bulk-forming natural therapeutic fiber for restoring and maintaining regularity. Konsyl contains 100% psyllium hydrophilic mucilloid, a highly efficient dietary fiber derived from the husk of the psyllium seed. Konsyl contains no chemical stimulants and is non-addictive. Each dose contains 6.0 grams of psyllium compared to 3.4 grams of psyllium in most other products.

Inactive Ingredients: None. Each 6 gram dose provides 3 calories. Konsyl is sodium free. Since Konsyl is sugar free, it is excellent for diabetics who require a bowel normalizer.

Actions: Konsyl provides bulk that promotes normal elimination. The product is uniform, instantly miscible, palatable, and non-irritative in the gastrointestinal tract.

Indications: Konsyl is indicated in the management of chronic constipation, irritable bowel syndrome, as adjunctive therapy in the constipation of diverticular disease, bowel management of patients with hemorrhoids, and for constipation during pregnancy, convalescence, and senility. Konsyl is also indicated for other indications as prescribed by physician.

Contraindications: Intestinal obstruction, fecal impaction.

Warnings: KEEP THIS AND ALL DRUGS OUT OF THE REACH OF CHILDREN. TAKING THIS PRODUCT WITHOUT ADEQUATE FLUID MAY CAUSE IT TO SWELL AND BLOCK YOUR THROAT OR ESOPHAGUS AND MAY CAUSE CHOKING. DO NOT TAKE THIS PRODUCT IF YOU HAVE DIFFICULTY IN SWALLOWING. IF YOU EXPERIENCE CHEST PAIN, VOMITING OR DIFFICULTY IN SWALLOWING OR BREATHING AFTER TAKING THIS PRODUCT, SEEK IMMEDIATE MEDICAL ATTENTION.

Precautions: May cause allergic reaction in people sensitive to inhaled or ingested psyllium powder.

Dosage and Administration:
MIX THIS PRODUCT (CHILD OR ADULT DOSE) WITH AT LEAST 8 OUNCES OF WATER OR OTHER FLUID. TAKING THIS PRODUCT WITHOUT ENOUGH LIQUID MAY CAUSE CHOKING. SEE WARNINGS. **ADULTS:** Place one rounded teaspoon (6.0 grams) into a dry shaker cup or container that can be closed. Add 8 oz. of juice, cold water or your favorite beverage. Shake, don't stir, for 3–5 seconds. Drink promptly. If mixture thickens, add more liquid and shake. Follow with an 8 oz. glass of juice or water to aid product action. Konsyl can be taken one to three times daily, depending on need and response. Konsyl generally produces results within 12–72 hours. Take Konsyl at any convenient time, morning or evening; before or after meals. When taking Konsyl, one should drink several 8 oz. glasses of water a day to aid product action.
CHILDREN: (6–12 years old) Use ½ adult dose in 8 oz. of liquid, 1–3 times daily.

New Users: Easy Does It. Medical research shows that higher fiber intake is important for good digestive health. To help the body adjust and avoid minor gas and bloating sometimes associated with high fiber intake, it may be necessary to take one half dose over several days and then slowly increase the dosage over several days. Always follow with 8 oz. of liquid.

How Supplied: Powder, containers of 10.6 oz. (300 g), 15.9 oz. (450 g) and 30 single dose (6.0 g) packets.

Is this product OTC? Yes.

KONSYL-D® POWDER
(Psyllium hydrophilic mucilloid)
3.4 grams of psyllium per
TEASPOON with dextrose added

Description: Konsyl-D is a bulk-forming natural therapeutic fiber for restoring and maintaining regularity. Konsyl-D contains 3.4 grams of psyllium hydrophilic mucilloid, a highly efficient dietary fiber derived from the husk of the psyllium seed. Konsyl-D contains no chemical stimulants and is non-addictive. Each teaspoon dose contains 3.4 grams of psyllium which is unflavored and can be mixed with a variety of juices.

Inactive Ingredients: Dextrose. Each 6.5 gram dose provides 14 calories. Konsyl-D is sodium free.

Actions: See Konsyl description of Actions.

Indications: See Konsyl description of Indications.

Contraindications: Intestinal obstruction, fecal impaction.

Warnings: See Konsyl description of Warnings.

Precaution: May cause allergic reaction in people sensitive to inhaled or ingested psyllium powder.

Dosage and Administration:
MIX THIS PRODUCT (CHILD OR ADULT DOSE) WITH AT LEAST 8 OUNCES (A FULL GLASS) OF WATER OR OTHER FLUID. TAKING THIS PRODUCT WITHOUT ENOUGH LIQUID MAY CAUSE CHOKING. SEE WARNINGS. **ADULTS:** Place one rounded teaspoon (6.5 grams) into a dry glass. Add 8 oz. of juice or other beverage. Stir for 3–5 seconds. Drink promptly. Follow with an 8 oz. glass of juice or water to aid product action. Konsyl-D can be taken one to three times daily, depending on need and response. Konsyl-D generally produces results within 12–72 hours. Take Konsyl-D at any convenient time, morning or evening; before or after meals. When taking Konsyl-D, one should drink several 8 oz. glasses of water a day to aid product action.
CHILDREN: (6–12 years old) ½ adult dose in 8 oz. of liquid, 1–3 times daily.

New Users: See Konsyl instructions for New Users.

How Supplied: Powder, containers of 11.5 oz (325 g), 17.6 oz (500 g) and 30 single dose (6.5 g) packets.

Is the Product OTC? Yes.

KONSYL®-ORANGE POWDER
(psyllium hydrophilic mucilloid)
Ultra Fine Texture ... Easy to Mix
Formula
3.4 grams of psyllium per
TABLESPOON

Description: Konsyl-Orange is a bulk-forming natural therapeutic fiber for restoring and maintaining regularity. Konsyl-Orange contains 3.4 grams of psyllium hydrophilic mucilloid, a highly efficient dietary fiber derived from the husk of the psyllium seed. Konsyl-Orange contains no chemical stimulants and is non-addictive. Each TABLESPOON dose contains 3.4 grams of psyllium which is ultrafine texture for easy mixing.

Inactive Ingredients: Sucrose, citric acid, FD&C Yellow #6 and D&C Yellow #10 and flavoring. Each 12 gram dose provides 35 calories. Konsyl-Orange is sodium free.

Actions: See Konsyl description of Actions.

Indications: See Konsyl description of Indication.

Contraindications: Intestinal obstruction, fecal impaction.

Precaution: May cause allergic reaction in people sensitive to inhaled or ingested psyllium powder.

Warnings: See Konsyl description of Warnings.

Dosage and Administration:
MIX THIS PRODUCT (CHILD OR ADULT DOSE) WITH AT LEAST 8 OUNCES (A FULL GLASS) OF WATER OR OTHER FLUID. TAKING THIS PRODUCT WITHOUT ENOUGH LIQUID MAY CAUSE CHOKING. SEE WARNINGS.
ADULTS: Place one rounded tablespoon (12.0 grams) into a dry glass. Add 8 oz. of water or other beverage. Stir for 3–5 seconds. Drink promptly. Follow with an 8 oz. glass of water to aid product action. Konsyl-Orange can be taken one to three times daily, depending on need and response. Konsyl Orange generally produces results within 12–72 hours. Take Konsyl Orange at any convenient time, morning or evening; before or after meals. When taking Konsyl-Orange, one should drink several 8 oz. glasses of water daily to aid product action.
CHILDREN: (6–12 years old) ½ adult dose in 8 oz. of liquid, 1–3 times daily.

New Users: See Konsyl instructions for New Users.

How Supplied: Ultra fine powder container of 19 oz (538 g) and 30 single dose (12.0 g) packets.

Is the product OTC? Yes.

Lavoptik Company, Inc.
661 WESTERN AVENUE N.
ST. PAUL, MN 55103

LAVOPTIK® Eye Cups

Description: Device—Sterile disposable eye cups.

How Supplied: Individually bagged eye cups are packed 12 per box, NDC 10651-01004.

LAVOPTIK® Eye Wash

Description: Isotonic LAVOPTIK Eye Wash is a buffered solution designed to help physically remove contaminants from the surface of the eye and lids. Formulated to buffer contaminants toward

the safe range and help restore normal salts and water ratios in the tears.

Contents: Each 100 ml
Sodium Chloride	0.49	gram
Sodium Biphosphate	0.40	gram
Sodium Phosphate	0.45	gram
Preservative Agent		
Benzalkonium Chloride	0.005	gram

Precautions: If you experience severe eye pain, headache, rapid change in vision (side or straight ahead); sudden appearance of floating objects, acute redness of the eyes, pain on exposure to light or double vision consult a physician at once. If symptoms persist or worsen after use of this product, consult a physician. If solution changes color or becomes cloudy do not use. Keep this and all medicines out of reach of children. Keep container tightly closed. Do not use if safety seal is broken at time of purchase.

Administration: 6 ounce size with Eye Cup.
Rinse cup with clean water immediately before and after each use, avoid contamination of rim and inside surfaces of cup. Apply cup, half-filled with LAVOPTIK Eye Wash tightly to the eye. Tilt head backward. Open eyelids wide, rotate eyeball and blink several times to insure thorough washing. Discard washings. Repeat other eye. Tightly cap bottle.
32 ounce size.
Break seal as you remove cap and pour directly on contaminated area.

How Supplied: 6 ounce bottle with eyecup, NDC 10651-01040.
32 ounce bottle, NDC 10651-01019.

Lederle Laboratories
A Division of American Cyanamid Co.
ONE CYANAMID PLAZA
WAYNE, NJ 07470

LEDERMARK®
Product Identification Code

Many Lederle tablets and capsules bear an identification code. A current listing appears in the Product Information Section of the 1995 PDR for prescription drugs.

CALTRATE® 600
[căl-trāte]
High Potency Calcium Supplement
Nature's Most Concentrated Form of Calcium®
No Sugar, No Salt, No Lactose, No Preservatives, Tablet Shape Specially Designed for Easier Swallowing

Inactive Ingredients: Maltodextrin, Cellulose, Mineral Oil, Hydroxypropyl Methylcellulose, Titanium Dioxide, Sodium Lauryl Sulfate, Gelatin, Crospovidone, Stearic Acid, Magnesium Stearate

EACH TABLET CONTAINS:
		% Daily Value
Calcium	600 mg	60%

Recommended Intake: One or two tablets daily or as directed by your physician.

Warning: Keep out of reach of children.

How Supplied: Bottle of 60—
NDC 0005-5510-19
Store at Room Temperature.

P40946-94
LCH1

Shown in Product Identification Guide, page 509

CALTRATE® 600 + D
[căl-trāte]
High Potency Calcium Supplement With Vitamin D
Nature's Most Concentrated Form of Calcium®
No Sugar, No Salt, No Lactose, No Preservatives, Tablet Shape Specially Designed for Easier Swallowing

Inactive Ingredients: Maltodextrin, Cellulose, Mineral Oil, Hydroxypropyl Methylcellulose, Titanium Dioxide, Sodium Lauryl Sulfate, FD&C Yellow No. 6, Gelatin, Crospovidone, Stearic Acid, Magnesium Stearate

EACH TABLET CONTAINS:
		% Daily Value
Vitamin D	200 IU	50%
Calcium	600 mg	60%

Recommended Intake: One or two tablets daily or as directed by your physician.

Warning: Keep out of reach of children.

How Supplied: Bottle of 60—
NDC 0005-5509-19
Store at Room Temperature.
© 1990
P40944-94
LCH1

Shown in Product Identification Guide, page 509

CALTRATE® PLUS
[căl-trāte]
High Potency Calcium Supplement With Vitamin D & Minerals
Nature's Most Concentrated Form of Calcium®
No Sugar, No Salt, No Lactose, No Preservatives, Tablet Shape Specially Designed for Easier Swallowing

Inactive Ingredients: Maltodextrin, Cellulose, Mineral Oil, Hydroxypropyl Methylcellulose, Titanium Dioxide, Sodium Lauryl Sulfate, FD&C Red No. 40, FD&C Yellow No. 6, FD&C Blue No. 1, Gelatin, Crospovidone, Stearic Acid, Magnesium Stearate.

Continued on next page

Lederle—Cont.

EACH TABLET CONTAINS

	% Daily Value
Vitamin D 200 IU	50%
Calcium 600 mg	60%
Magnesium 40 mg	10%
Zinc 7.5 mg	50%
Copper 1 mg	50%
Manganese 1.8 mg	*

OTHER IMPORTANT NUTRIENTS*
Boron 250 mcg

* Daily Value Not Established

Recommended Intake: One or two tablets daily or as directed by your physician.

Warning: Keep out of reach of children.

How Supplied: Bottle of 60—
NDC 0005-5556-19
Store at Room Temperature.

P40948-94
LCH1

Shown in Product Identification Guide, page 509

CENTRUM®
[sĕn-trŭm]
**High Potency
Multivitamin-Multimineral Formula,
Advanced Formula
From A to Zinc®**

Each tablet contains:

	For Adults—Percentage of US Recommended Daily Allowance (US RDA)
VITAMINS	
Vitamin A	5000 IU (100%)
(as Acetate and Beta Carotene)	
Vitamin D	400 IU (100%)
Vitamin E	30 IU (100%)
Vitamin K₁	25 mcg*
Vitamin C	60 mg (100%)
Folic Acid	400 mcg (100%)
Vitamin B₁	1.5 mg (100%)
Vitamin B₂	1.7 mg (100%)
Niacinamide	20 mg (100%)
Vitamin B₆	2 mg (100%)
Vitamin B₁₂	6 mcg (100%)
Pantothenic Acid	10 mg (100%)
Biotin	30 mcg (10%)
MINERALS	
Calcium	162 mg (16%)
Phosphorus	109 mg (11%)
Iodine	150 mcg (100%)
Iron	18 mg (100%)
Magnesium	100 mg (25%)
Copper	2 mg (100%)
Zinc	15 mg (100%)
Manganese	2.5 mg*
Potassium	40 mg*

Chloride	36.3 mg*
Chromium	25 mcg*
Molybdenum	25 mcg*
Selenium	20 mcg*
Nickel	5 mcg*
Tin	10 mcg*
Silicon	2 mg*
Vanadium	10 mcg*
Boron	150 mcg*

*No US RDA established.

Inactive Ingredients: FD&C Yellow No. 6, Hydroxypropyl Methylcellulose, Lactose, Magnesium Stearate, Microcrystalline Cellulose, Polysorbate 80, Polyvinylpyrrolidone, Stearic Acid, Titanium Dioxide, and Triethyl Citrate.

Recommended Intake: Adults, 1 tablet daily.

How Supplied:
Light peach, engraved CENTRUM C1.
Bottle of 60—NDC 0005-4239-19
Combopack†—NDC 0005-4239-30
†Bottles of 100 plus 30
Store at Room Temperature.

22513-92
D38

Shown in Product Identification Guide, page 509

**CENTRUM® Liquid
High Potency
Multivitamin-Multimineral Formula
Advanced Formula**

Each 15 mL (1 tablespoon) contains:

	For Adults—Percentage of US Recommended Daily Allowance (US RDA)	
Vitamin A	2500 IU	(50%)
(as Palmitate)		
Vitamin E	30 IU	(100%)
(as dl-Alpha Tocopheryl Acetate)		
Vitamin C	60 mg	(100%)
(as Ascorbic Acid)		
Vitamin B₁	1.5 mg	(100%)
(as Thiamine Hydrochloride)		
Vitamin B₂	1.7 mg	(100%)
(as Riboflavin)		
Niacinamide	20 mg	(100%)
Vitamin B₆	2 mg	(100%)
(as Pyridoxine Hydrochloride)		
Vitamin B₁₂	6 mcg	(100%)
(as Cyanocobalamin)		
Vitamin D₂	400 IU	(100%)
Biotin	300 mcg	(100%)
Pantothenic Acid	10 mg	(100%)
(as Panthenol)		
Iodine	150 mcg	(100%)
(as Potassium Iodide)		
Iron	9 mg	(50%)
(as Ferrous Gluconate)		
Zinc	3 mg	(20%)
(as Zinc Gluconate)		
Manganese	2.5 mg	*
(as Manganese Chloride)		
Chromium	25 mcg	*
(as Chromium Chloride)		
Molybdenum	25 mcg	*
(as Sodium Molybdate)		

*No US RDA established.

Inactive Ingredients: Alcohol 6.7%, Artificial and Natural Flavors, BHA, Citric Acid, Edetic Acid, Glycerin, Polysorbate 80, Sodium Benzoate, and Sucrose.

Recommended Intake: Adults, 1 tablespoonful (15 mL) daily.

Warning: Keep this and all medication out of the reach of children.

How Supplied: 8 oz Bottle—
NDC 0005-4343-61
Store at Controlled Room Temperature 15°–30°C (59°–86°F).
PROTECT FROM FREEZING.

32537-93
D6

Shown in Product Identification Guide, page 509

CENTRUM, JR.®
[sĕn-trŭm]
**Shamu and his Crew™
+ EXTRA C
Children's Chewable
Vitamin/Mineral Formula
Nutritional Support From Head to Toe®**

[See table at top of next page.]

Inactive Ingredients: Artificial Flavorings, Aspartame,† Blue 2, Citric Acid, FD&C Yellow No. 6, Lactose, Magnesium Stearate, Microcrystalline Cellulose, Pregelatinized Starch, Red 40, Silica Gel, Sorbitol, Stearic Acid, and Sucrose.

† **Phenylketonurics: Contains Phenylalanine.**

Warnings: CONTAINS IRON, WHICH CAN BE HARMFUL IN LARGE DOSES. CLOSE TIGHTLY AND KEEP OUT OF THE REACH OF CHILDREN. IN CASE OF ACCIDENTAL OVERDOSE, CONTACT A PHYSICIAN OR POISON CONTROL CENTER IMMEDIATELY.

Recommended Intake: Children 2 to 4 years of age: Chew approximately one-half tablet daily. Children over 4 years of age: Chew one tablet daily.

How Supplied: Bottle of 60—
NDC 0005-4249-19

Tamper Resistant Feature: Bottle sealed with clear band printed LEDERSEAL®. Do not accept if band is not below the label panel or if it is missing or broken.
Store at Room Temperature.
© 1993
32302-93
D11
Sea World Characters ©1993 Sea World, Inc. All Rights Reserved.
Shamu and his Crew™ are trademarks and copyrights of Sea World, Inc.
CENTRUM, JR.®, The Spectrum Design and all other marks and indicia are trademarks and copyrights of Lederle.

Shown in Product Identification Guide, page 510

CENTRUM, JR.® + EXTRA C
Children's Chewable Vitamin/Mineral Formula

	Quantity per tablet	Percentage of US Recommended Daily Allowance (US RDA)	
		For Children 2 to 4 (½ tablet)	For Children Over 4 (1 tablet)
EACH TABLET CONTAINS:			
VITAMINS			
Vitamin A (as Acetate and Beta Carotene)	5,000 IU	(100%)	(100%)
Vitamin D	400 IU	(50%)	(100%)
Vitamin E	30 IU	(150%)	(100%)
Vitamin C	300 mg	(375%)	(500%)
Folic Acid	400 mcg	(100%)	(100%)
Biotin	45 mcg	(15%)	(15%)
Thiamine	1.5 mg	(107%)	(100%)
Pantothenic Acid	10 mg	(100%)	(100%)
Riboflavin	1.7 mg	(107%)	(100%)
Niacinamide	20 mg	(111%)	(100%)
Vitamin B_6	2 mg	(143%)	(100%)
Vitamin B_{12}	6 mcg	(100%)	(100%)
Vitamin K_1	10 mcg*		
MINERALS			
Iron	18 mg	(90%)	(100%)
Magnesium	40 mg	(10%)	(10%)
Iodine	150 mcg	(107%)	(100%)
Copper	2 mg	(100%)	(100%)
Phosphorus	50 mg	(3.12%)	(5.0%)
Calcium	108 mg	(6.75%)	(10.8%)
Zinc	15 mg	(93%)	(100%)
Manganese	1 mg*		
Molybdenum	20 mcg*		
Chromium	20 mcg*		

*Recognized as essential in human nutrition but no US RDA established.

CENTRUM, JR.®
[sĕn-trŭm]
Shamu and his Crew™
+EXTRA CALCIUM
Children's Chewable Vitamin/Mineral Formula
Nutritional Support From Head to Toe®

[See table below.]

Inactive Ingredients: Artificial Flavorings, Aspartame,† Blue 2, Citric Acid, FD&C Yellow No. 6, Lactose, Magnesium Stearate, Microcrystalline Cellulose, Pregelatinized Starch, Red 40, Silica Gel, Sorbitol, Stearic Acid, and Sucrose.

† **Phenylketonurics: Contains Phenylalanine.**

Warnings: CONTAINS IRON, WHICH CAN BE HARMFUL IN LARGE DOSES. CLOSE TIGHTLY AND KEEP OUT OF THE REACH OF CHILDREN. IN CASE OF ACCIDENTAL OVERDOSE, CONTACT A PHYSICIAN OR POISON CONTROL CENTER IMMEDIATELY.

Recommended Intake: Children 2 to 4 years of age: chew approximately one-half tablet daily. Children over 4 years of age: chew one tablet daily.

CENTRUM, JR.®+EXTRA CALCIUM
Children's Chewable Vitamin/Mineral Formula

	Quantity per tablet	Percentage of US Recommended Daily Allowance (US RDA)	
		For Children 2 to 4 (½ tablet)	For Children Over 4 (1 tablet)
EACH TABLET CONTAINS:			
VITAMINS			
Vitamin A (as Acetate and Beta Carotene)	5,000 IU	(100%)	(100%)
Vitamin D	400 IU	(50%)	(100%)
Vitamin E	30 IU	(150%)	(100%)
Vitamin C	60 mg	(75%)	(100%)
Folic Acid	400 mcg	(100%)	(100%)
Biotin	45 mcg	(15%)	(15%)
Thiamine	1.5 mg	(107%)	(100%)
Pantothenic Acid	10 mg	(100%)	(100%)
Riboflavin	1.7 mg	(107%)	(100%)
Niacinamide	20 mg	(111%)	(100%)
Vitamin B_6	2 mg	(143%)	(100%)
Vitamin B_{12}	6 mcg	(100%)	(100%)
Vitamin K_1	10 mcg*		
MINERALS			
Iron	18 mg	(90%)	(100%)
Magnesium	40 mg	(10%)	(10%)
Iodine	150 mcg	(107%)	(100%)
Copper	2 mg	(100%)	(100%)
Phosphorus	50 mg	(3.12%)	(5.0%)
Calcium	160 mg	(10%)	(16%)
Zinc	15 mg	(93%)	(100%)
Manganese	1 mg*		
Molybdenum	20 mcg*		
Chromium	20 mcg*		

*Recognized as essential in human nutrition but no US RDA established.

Continued on next page

Lederle—Cont.

How Supplied: Bottle of 60—NDC 0005-4222-19

Tamper Resistant Feature: Bottle sealed with clear band printed LEDER-SEAL®. Do not accept if band is not below the label panel or if it is missing or broken.

Store at Room Temperature.

© 1993   32303-93
                              D9

Sea World Characters ©1993 Sea World, Inc. All Rights Reserved.

Shamu and his Crew™ are trademarks and copyrights of Sea World, Inc. CENTRUM, JR.®, The Spectrum Design and all other marks and indicia are trademarks and copyrights of Lederle.

Shown in Product Identification Guide, page 510

CENTRUM, JR.®

[sĕn-trŭm]

Shamu and his Crew™
+ IRON
Children's Chewable
Vitamin/Mineral Formula
Nutritional Support From Head to Toe®

[See table below.]

Inactive Ingredients: Artificial Flavorings, Aspartame,† Blue 2, Citric Acid, FD&C Yellow No. 6, Lactose, Magnesium Stearate, Microcrystalline Cellulose, Pregelatinized Starch, Red 40, Silica Gel, Sorbitol, Stearic Acid, and Sucrose.

† **Phenylketonurics: Contains Phenylalanine.**

Warnings: CONTAINS IRON, WHICH CAN BE HARMFUL IN LARGE DOSES. CLOSE TIGHTLY AND KEEP OUT OF THE REACH OF CHILDREN. IN CASE OF ACCIDENTAL OVERDOSE, CONTACT A PHYSICIAN OR POISON CONTROL CENTER IMMEDIATELY.

Recommended Intake: Children 2 to 4 years of age: Chew approximately one-half tablet daily. Children over 4 years of age: Chew one tablet daily.

How Supplied: Assorted Flavors—Uncoated Tablet—Partially Scored—Engraved Lederle C2 and CENTRUM, JR. Bottle of 60—NDC 0005-4234-19

Tamper Resistant Feature: Bottle sealed with clear band printed LEDER-SEAL®. Do not accept if band is not below the label panel or if it is missing or broken.

Store at Room Temperature.

© 1993   32304-93
                              D12

Sea World Characters ©1993 Sea World, Inc. All Rights Reserved.

Shamu and his Crew™ are trademarks and copyrights of Sea World, Inc. CENTRUM, JR.®, The Spectrum Design and all other marks and indicia are trademarks and copyrights of Lederle.

Shown in Product Identification Guide, page 510

CENTRUM® SILVER®
Specially Formulated
Multivitamin-Multimineral for Adults 50+
Complete
From A to Zinc®

Each tablet contains:

		For Adults—Percentage of US Recommended Daily Allowance (US RDA)
Vitamin A	6000 IU	(120%)
(as Acetate and Beta Carotene)†		
Vitamin B$_1$	1.5 mg	(100%)
Vitamin B$_2$	1.7 mg	(100%)
Vitamin B$_6$	3 mg	(150%)
Vitamin B$_{12}$	25 mcg	(416%)
Biotin	30 mcg	(10%)
Folic Acid	200 mcg	(50%)
Niacinamide	20 mg	(100%)
Pantothenic Acid	10 mg	(100%)
Vitamin C†	60 mg	(100%)
Vitamin D	400 IU	(100%)
Vitamin E†	45 IU	(150%)
Vitamin K$_1$	10 mcg	*
Calcium	200 mg	(20%)
Copper†	2 mg	(100%)
Iodine	150 mcg	(100%)
Iron	9 mg	(50%)
Magnesium	100 mg	(25%)
Phosphorus	48 mg	(5%)
Zinc†	15 mg	(100%)
Chloride	72 mg	*
Chromium	100 mcg	*
Manganese†	2.5 mg	*

CENTRUM, JR.® +IRON
Children's Chewable
Vitamin/Mineral Formula

EACH TABLET CONTAINS:	Quantity per tablet	Percentage of US Recommended Daily Allowance (US RDA) For Children 2 to 4 (½ tablet)	For Children Over 4 (1 tablet)
VITAMINS			
Vitamin A (as Acetate and Beta Carotene)	5,000 IU	(100%)	(100%)
Vitamin D	400 IU	(50%)	(100%)
Vitamin E	30 IU	(150%)	(100%)
Vitamin C	60 mg	(75%)	(100%)
Folic Acid	400 mcg	(100%)	(100%)
Biotin	45 mcg	(15%)	(15%)
Thiamine	1.5 mg	(107%)	(100%)
Pantothenic Acid	10 mg	(100%)	(100%)
Riboflavin	1.7 mg	(107%)	(100%)
Niacinamide	20 mg	(111%)	(100%)
Vitamin B$_6$	2 mg	(143%)	(100%)
Vitamin B$_{12}$	6 mcg	(100%)	(100%)
Vitamin K$_1$	10 mcg*		
MINERALS			
Iron	18 mg	(90%)	(100%)
Magnesium	40 mg	(10%)	(10%)
Iodine	150 mcg	(107%)	(100%)
Copper	2 mg	(100%)	(100%)
Phosphorus	50 mg	(3.12%)	(5.0%)
Calcium	108 mg	(6.75%)	(10.8%)
Zinc	15 mg	(93%)	(100%)
Manganese	1 mg*		
Molybdenum	20 mcg*		
Chromium	20 mcg*		

*Recognized as essential in human nutrition but no US RDA established.

Molybdenum	25 mcg	*
Nickel	5 mcg	*
Potassium	80 mg	*
Selenium†	20 mcg	*
Silicon	10 mcg	*
Vanadium	10 mcg	*
Boron	150 mcg	*

* No US RDA established.
† Included in the Complete Antioxidant Group.

Inactive Ingredients: Blue 2, Crospovidone, FD&C Yellow No. 6, Hydroxypropyl Methylcellulose, Lactose, Magnesium Stearate, Microcrystalline Cellulose, Polyethylene Glycol, Polysorbate 80, Red 40, Silica Gel, Stearic Acid, and Titanium Dioxide.

Recommended Intake:
Adults, 1 tablet daily.

How Supplied: Bottle of 60—
NDC 0005-4177-19
Bottle of 100—NDC 0005-4177-23
Store at Room Temperature.
© 1992   32494-93
                                              D4

Shown in Product Identification Guide, page 510

CENTRUM® SINGLES®
[sĕn-trŭm]
BETA CAROTENE
For extra nutritional support™
Low sodium; no sugar, preservatives or artificial flavors.

Each softgel contains:

	For Adults— Percentage of US Recommended Daily Allowance (USRDA)
Vitamin Beta Carotene	25,000 IU (500%)

Inactive Ingredients: Gelatin, Glycerin, Lecithin, Purified Water, Vegetable Oil, Vegetable Shortening and Yellow Wax.

Recommended Intake: Adults—one softgel daily as a dietary supplement.

How Supplied: Bottle of 75—
NDC 0005-4080-40
Store at room temperature.

Warning: Keep out of the reach of children.

                                              32411-93
                                              LCH1

Shown in Product Identification Guide, page 510

CENTRUM® SINGLES®
[sĕn-trŭm]
CALCIUM
For extra nutritional support™
No sugar, salt, preservatives or artificial flavors.

Each tablet contains:

	For Adults— Percentage of US Recommended Daily Allowance (USRDA)
Mineral Calcium (as Calcium Carbonate)	500 mg (50%)

Inactive Ingredients: Cellulose, Crospovidone, Hydroxypropyl Methylcellulose, Maltodextrin, Mineral Oil, Silica, Soy Polysaccharide, Stearic Acid and Titanium Dioxide.

Recommended Intake: Adults—one or two tablets daily as a dietary supplement.

How Supplied: Bottle of 60—
NDC 0005-4084-19
Store at room temperature.

Warning: Keep out of the reach of children.

                                              32414-93
                                              LCH1

Shown in Product Identification Guide, page 510

CENTRUM® SINGLES®
[sĕn-trŭm]
VITAMIN C
For extra nutritional support™
No sugar, salt, preservatives or artificial flavors.

Each tablet contains:

	For Adults— Percentage of US Recommended Daily Allowance (USRDA)
Vitamin C	500 mg (833%)

Inactive Ingredients: Alpha Cellulose, Cellulose, Crospovidone, Hydroxypropyl Methylcellulose, Mineral Oil, Povidone, Sodium Lauryl Sulfate, Starch and Stearic Acid.

Recommended Intake: Adults—one tablet daily as a dietary supplement.

How Supplied: Bottle of 75—
NDC 0005-4082-40
Store at room temperature.

Warning: Keep out of the reach of children.

                                              32412-93
                                              LCH1

Shown in Product Identification Guide, page 510

CENTRUM® SINGLES®
[sĕn-trŭm]
VITAMIN E
For extra nutritional support™
Low sodium; no sugar, preservatives or artificial flavors.

Each softgel contains:

	For Adults— Percentage of US Recommended Daily Allowance (USRDA)
Vitamin E	400 IU (1333%)

Inactive Ingredients: Gelatin, Glycerin and Purified Water.

Recommended Intake: Adults—one or two tablets daily as a dietary supplement.

How Supplied: Bottle of 75—
NDC 0005-4081-40
Store at room temperature.

Warning: Keep out of the reach of children.

                                              32413-93
                                              LCH1

Shown in Product Identification Guide, page 510

FERRO–SEQUELS®
[fer "rō-sē 'quls]
High potency, time-release iron supplement.
Specially formulated to minimize iron-induced constipation.
Easy to swallow tablets.
Low sodium, no sugar.

Description: Each FERRO-SEQUELS tablet contains 150 mg of ferrous fumarate, equivalent to 50 mg of elemental iron and 100 mg of docusate sodium (DSS). FERRO-SEQUELS is a high potency iron supplement that employs a time release system to deliver iron slowly to maximize absorption, and to reduce the irritation associated with iron tablets.
Inactive Ingredients: Blue 1, Corn Starch, Crospovidone, Hydroxypropyl Methylcellulose, Lactose, Magnesium Stearate, Microcrystalline Cellulose, Modified Food Starch, Povidone, Silica Gel, Sodium Lauryl Sulfate, Titanium Dioxide, and Yellow 10.

Indications: As a supplement to treat simple iron deficiency and iron deficiency anemia.

Recommended Intake: One tablet, once or twice daily, or as directed by a health care professional.

Warnings: Keep out of reach of children. Contains iron, which can be harmful or fatal to children in large doses. In case of accidental overdose, seek profes-

Continued on next page

Lederle—Cont.

sional assistance or contact a Poison Control Center immediately. As with any supplement, if you are pregnant or nursing a baby, seek the advice of a health care professional before using this product.

How Supplied: Box of 30 tablets, NDC 0005-5267-68
Bottle of 30 tablets, NDC 0005-5267-13
Bottle of 100 tablets, NDC 0005-5267-23
Unit Dose Package 10 × 10, NDC 0005-5267-60
Bottle of 1,000 tablets, NDC 0005-5267-34
Store at Controlled Room Temperature 15°–30°C (59°–86°F)
LEDERLE CONSUMER HEALTH DIVISION
American Cyanamid Company
Pearl River, NY 10965
MADE IN USA

40631-94

Shown in Product Identification Guide, page 510

FIBERCON®

[fĭ-bĕr-cŏn]
Calcium Polycarbophil
Bulk-Forming Fiber Laxative

Film-coated for easy swallowing.
Contains 200 mg calcium per 2 caplet dose. No chemical stimulants.
Non-habit forming.
Less than one calorie per caplet.
Sodium and Preservative-free.

Description: FIBERCON is a bulk-forming fiber which comes in an easy-to-swallow caplet form.

Active Ingredient: Each caplet contains 625 mg calcium polycarbophil equivalent to 500 mg polycarbophil.

Inactive Ingredients: Calcium Carbonate, Caramel, Crospovidone, Hydroxypropyl Methylcellulose, Magnesium Stearate, Microcrystalline Cellulose, Mineral Oil, Povidone, Silica Gel, and Sodium Lauryl Sulfate.

Indications: Relief of constipation. FIBERCON restores and maintains regularity and promotes normal function of the bowel. FIBERCON is indicated for the relief of constipation and constipation associated with other bowel disorders such as irritable bowel syndrome, diverticular disease, hemorrhoids, convalescence, senility and for occasional constipation during pregnancy, postpartum, and postsurgical periods when under the care of a physician.

Directions: FIBERCON dosage will vary according to diet, exercise, previous laxative use, or severity of constipation. FIBERCON works naturally so continued use for one to three days is normally required to promote full benefit. **TAKE THIS PRODUCT (CHILD OR ADULT DOSE) WITH AT LEAST 8 OUNCES (A FULL GLASS) OF WATER OR OTHER FLUID. TAKING THIS PRODUCT WITHOUT ENOUGH LIQUID**

MAY CAUSE CHOKING. SEE WARNINGS.
For Adult Patients Not Currently Using a Laxative: Two caplets once per day. May be increased up to two caplets 4 times per day as needed for regularity.
For Adult Patients Switching from Another Laxative: Two caplets 4 times per day, decreasing down to two caplets 3, 2 or 1 time per day as needed for regularity.
For Children 6–12 Years: One caplet 1 to 3 times a day.
For Children Under 6 Years: Consult a physician.

Warnings: Any sudden change in bowel habits may indicate a more serious condition than constipation. Consult your physician if symptoms such as nausea, vomiting, abdominal pain, or rectal bleeding occur or if this product has no effect within one week. For chronic or continued constipation consult your physician. **TAKING THIS PRODUCT WITHOUT ADEQUATE FLUID MAY CAUSE IT TO SWELL AND BLOCK YOUR THROAT OR ESOPHAGUS AND MAY CAUSE CHOKING. DO NOT TAKE THIS PRODUCT IF YOU HAVE DIFFICULTY IN SWALLOWING. IF YOU EXPERIENCE CHEST PAIN, VOMITING, OR DIFFICULTY IN SWALLOWING OR BREATHING AFTER TAKING THIS PRODUCT, SEEK IMMEDIATE MEDICAL ATTENTION.**

Interaction Precaution: If you are taking any form of tetracycline antibiotic, FIBERCON should be taken at least 1 hour before or 2 hours after you have taken the tetracycline antibiotic.
KEEP THIS AND ALL MEDICINES OUT OF THE REACH OF CHILDREN. STORE AT CONTROLLED ROOM TEMPERATURE 15°–30°C (59°–86°F). PROTECT CONTENTS FROM MOISTURE.

How Supplied:
Film-coated caplets, scored, engraved LL and F66.
Package of 36 caplets, NDC 0005-2500-02
Package of 60 caplets, NDC 0005-2500-86
Package of 90 caplets, NDC 0005-2500-33
Bottle of 150 caplets, NDC 0005-2500-58
Bottle of 500 caplets, NDC 0005-2500-31
Unit dose package of 200 caplets, NDC 0005-2500-28
LEDERLE CONSUMER HEALTH DIVISION
American Cyanamid Company
Pearl River, NY 10965

Rev. 8/94
40907-94

Shown in Product Identification Guide, page 510

GEVRABON®

[jĕv-ra băn]
Vitamin-Mineral Supplement

Composition: Each fluid ounce (30 mL) contains:

For Adults—Percentage of US Recommended Daily Allowance (US RDA)		
Vitamin B$_1$ (as Thiamine Hydrochloride)	5 mg	(333%)
Vitamin B$_2$ (as Riboflavin-5-Phosphate Sodium)	2.5 mg	(147%)
Niacinamide	50 mg	(250%)
Vitamin B$_6$ (Pyridoxine Hydrochloride)	1 mg	(50%)
Vitamin B$_{12}$ (as Cyanocobalamin)	1 mcg	(17%)
Pantothenic Acid (as D-Pantothenyl Alcohol)	10 mg	(100%)
Iodine (as Potassium Iodide)	100 mcg	(67%)
Iron (as Ferrous Gluconate)	15 mg	(83%)
Magnesium (as Magnesium Chloride)	2 mg	(0.5%)
Zinc (as Zinc Chloride)	2 mg	(13%)
Choline (as Tricholine Citrate)	100 mg*	
Manganese (as Manganese Chloride)	2 mg*	

*Recognized as essential in human nutrition but no U.S. RDA established.
| Alcohol | 18% |

Inactive Ingredients: Alcohol, Citric Acid, Glycerin, Sherry Wine, Sucrose.

Indications: For use as a nutritional supplement. Shake well.

Warnings: As with any drug, if you are pregnant or nursing a baby, seek the advice of a health professional before using this product. Keep this preparation out of the reach of children.

Administration and Dosage: Adult: One ounce (30 mL) daily or as prescribed by the physician as a nutritional supplement.

Important Note: In time a slight natural deposit, characteristic of the sherry wine base, may occur. This does not indicate in any way a loss of quality.

How Supplied: Syrup (sherry flavor) decanters of 16 fl oz—NDC 0005-5250-35
Keep Out of Direct Sunlight.
Store at Room Temperature, 15°–30°C (59°–86°F).
DO NOT FREEZE.

16520
D4

PROTEGRA®

[prŏ-tĕg-ră]
Antioxidant Vitamin & Mineral Supplement

Each softgel contains:

	For Adults—Percentage of US Recommended Daily Allowance (US RDA)	
Vitamin E	200 IU	667%
Vitamin C	250 mg	417%
Beta Carotene	3 mg	100%*
Zinc	7.5 mg	50%
Copper	1 mg	50%

Selenium	15 mcg	**
Manganese	1.5 mg	**

*US RDA for Vitamin A.
**No US RDA established but essential.

Inactive Ingredients: Gelatin, Cottonseed Oil, Glycerin, Dibasic Calcium Phosphate, Lecithin, Partially Hydrogenated Cottonseed and Soybean Oils, Beeswax, Titanium Dioxide, FD&C Yellow #6, and FD&C Red #40.

Recommended Intake: Adults: One softgel daily or as directed by your physician. PROTEGRA® can be taken by itself or with a multiple vitamin.

How Supplied: Bottle of 50—NDC-0005-4377-18
Store at Controlled Room Temperature 15°–30°C (59°–86°F)

Warning: Keep out of the reach of children.

20156-92

Shown in Product Identification Guide, page 510

STRESSTABS®

[strĕss-tăbs]
High Potency
Stress Formula Vitamins

Each tablet contains:

**For Adults—
Percentage of US
Recommended Daily
Allowance (US RDA)**

Vitamin E	30 IU	(100%)
Vitamin C	500 mg	(833%)
B VITAMINS		
Folic Acid	400 mcg	(100%)
Vitamin B₁	10 mg	(667%)
Vitamin B₂	10 mg	(588%)
Niacinamide	100 mg	(500%)
Vitamin B₆	5 mg	(250%)
Vitamin B₁₂	12 mcg	(200%)
Biotin	45 mcg	(15%)
Pantothenic Acid	20 mg	(200%)

Inactive Ingredients: Calcium Carbonate, FD&C Yellow No. 6, Magnesium Stearate, Microcrystalline Cellulose, Modified Food Starch, Silica Gel and Stearic Acid.

Recommended Intake: Adults, 1 tablet daily or as directed by the physician.

How Supplied: Capsule-shaped tablet (film coated, orange, scored). Engraved LL and S1.
Bottle of 60—NDC 0005-4124-19
Store at Room Temperature.
LEDERLE CONSUMER HEALTH DIVISION
American Cyanamid Company
Peal River, NY 10965

32557-93
D22

Shown in Product Identification Guide, page 510

STRESSTABS® + IRON

[strĕss-tăbs]
High Potency
Stress Formula Vitamins

Each tablet contains:

**For Adults—
Percentage of US
Recommended Daily
Allowance (US RDA)**

Vitamin E	30 IU	(100%)
Vitamin C	500 mg	(833%)
B VITAMINS		
Folic Acid	400 mcg	(100%)
Vitamin B₁	10 mg	(667%)
Vitamin B₂	10 mg	(588%)
Niacinamide	100 mg	(500%)
Vitamin B₆	5 mg	(250%)
Vitamin B₁₂	12 mcg	(200%)
Biotin	45 mcg	(15%)
Pantothenic Acid	20 mg	(200%)
Iron	18 mg	(100%)

Inactive Ingredients: Calcium Carbonate, FD&C Yellow No. 6, Magnesium Stearate, Microcrystalline Cellulose, Modified Food Starch, Red 40, Silica Gel and Stearic Acid.

Recommended Intake: Adults, 1 tablet daily or as directed by the physician.

WARNING: Always replace poplock top, close tightly, and keep out of reach of children. Contains iron, which can be harmful or fatal to children in large doses. In case of accidental overdose, seek professional assistance or contact a Poison Control Center immediately. As with any supplement, if you are pregnant or nursing a baby, seek the advice of a health professional before using this product.

How Supplied: Capsule-shaped tablets (film coated, orange red, scored). Engraved LL and S2.
Bottle of 60—NDC 0005-4126-19
Store at Room Temperature.
LEDERLE CONSUMER HEALTH DIVISION
American Cyanamid Company
Pearl River, NY 10965

32559-93
D20

Shown in Product Identification Guide, page 510

STRESSTABS® + ZINC

[strĕss tăbs]
High Potency
Stress Formula Vitamins

Each tablet contains:

**For Adults—
Percentage of US
Recommended Daily
Allowance (US RDA)**

Vitamin E	30 IU	(100%)
Vitamin C	500 mg	(833%)

B VITAMINS

Folic Acid	400 mcg	(100%)
Vitamin B₁	10 mg	(667%)
Vitamin B₂	10 mg	(588%)
Niacinamide	100 mg	(500%)
Vitamin B₆	5 mg	(250%)
Vitamin B₁₂	12 mcg	(200%)
Biotin	45 mcg	(15%)
Pantothenic Acid	20 mg	(200%)
Copper	3 mg	(150%)
Zinc	23.9 mg	(159%)

Inactive Ingredients: Calcium Carbonate, FD&C Yellow No. 6, Magnesium Stearate, Microcrystalline Cellulose, Modified Food Starch, Silica Gel and Stearic Acid.

Recommended Intake: Adults, 1 tablet daily or as directed by the physician.

How Supplied: Capsule-shaped tablet (film coated, peach color, scored). Engraved LL and S3.
Bottle of 60—NDC 0005-4125-19
Store at Room Temperature.
LEDERLE CONSUMER HEALTH DIVISION
American Cyanamid Company
Pearl River, NY 10965

32558-93
D22

Shown in Product Identification Guide, page 511

ZINCON®

[zinc-ŏn]
Dandruff Shampoo

Contains: Pyrithione Zinc (1%), Deionized Water, Sodium Lauryl Sulfate, Sodium Laureth Sulfate, Cocamide MEA, Glycol Distearate, Magnesium Aluminum Silicate, Propylene Glycol, Citric Acid, Sodium Chloride, Fragrance, Methylchloroisothiazolinone, Methylisothiazolinone, FD&C Blue No. 1

Indications: Relieves the itching and scalp flaking associated with dandruff. Also relieves the itching, irritation, and skin flaking associated with seborrheic dermatitis of the scalp.

Directions: Shake well before using. For best results use twice a week. Wet hair, apply to scalp and massage vigorously. Rinse and repeat.

Warnings: Keep this and all drugs out of the reach of children. For external use only. Avoid contact with the eyes—if this happens, rinse thoroughly with water. If condition worsens, covers a large area of the body, or does not improve after regular use of this product as directed, consult a doctor. Do not use on children under 2 years of age except as directed by a doctor.

How Supplied:
4 oz Bottle—NDC 0005-5455-58
8 oz Bottle—NDC 0005-5455-61

32484-93
LCH1

Shown in Product Identification Guide, page 511

Continued on next page

Lederle—Cont.

If desired, additional information on any Lederle product will be provided by contacting Lederle Professional Services Dept.

| EDUCATIONAL MATERIAL |

Everyone Needs to Know About Antioxidant Nutrients
6-page pamphlet explaining the importance of antioxidants in a healthy diet and good sources of antioxidants in food and vitamin supplements.
Write to: Lederle Promotional Center
2200 Bradley Hill Road
Blauvelt, NY 10913

Lever Brothers Company
**390 PARK AVENUE
NEW YORK, NY 10022**

DOVE® BAR AND LIQUID DOVE® BEAUTY WASH

Active Ingredients: Sodium Cocoyl Isethionate, Stearic Acid, Sodium Tallowate, Water, Sodium Isethionate, Coconut Acid, Sodium Stearate, Sodium Dodecylbenzenesulfonate, Sodium Cocoate, Fragrance, Sodium Chloride, Titanium Dioxide.

Actions and Uses: Dove is specially formulated to be predictably gentle to all kinds of skin including those with common dermatoses. The mildness of Dove is suitable for Acne and Rosacea patients on drying topical medications and Dove is non-acnegenic, non-comedogenic and oil-free.
Dove is also available in a NEW Sensitive Skin Formula that provides clinically proven superior mildness in a nonsensitizing 100% fragrance-free formula.

Directions: Instruct patients to use Dove as they would any other cleanser.

How Supplied: Original Dove 3.5 oz. and 4.75 bars; Unscented Dove 4.75 oz.; Sensitive Skin Formula Dove 4.25 oz. bars. 6 oz. pump dispenser—Liquid Dove beauty wash.
Shown in Product Identification Guide, page 511

LEVER 2000®

Active Ingredients: Triclosan. Other ingredients: Sodium tallowate, sodium cocoyl isethionate, sodium cocoate, water, sodium isethionate, stearic acid, coconut fatty acid, fragrance, titanium dioxide, sodium chloride, tetrasodium EDTA, disodium phosphate, trisodium etidronate, BHT.

Actions and Uses: Lever 2000® is the mildest antibacterial bar soap available. Lever 2000® offers broad spectrum antibacterial activity against both gram-neg-
ative and gram-positive pathogens. It is a useful adjunct to any therapeutic regimen that fights topical bacterial infection. It is also milder to the skin than any other antibacterial or deodorant bar soap. Lever 2000® has been proven mild enough for children's tender skin as young as 18 months and can also be used by adolescents and adults.

Directions: Instruct patients to use Lever 2000® as they would any other mild antibacterial or deodorant soap.

How Supplied: Original Lever 2000 3.5 oz, 5.0 oz bars; Liquid Lever 2000 7 oz pump, 14 oz and 64 oz refills; 28 oz Wall Dispenser; Unscented Lever 2000 5.0 oz bar.
Shown in Product Identification Guide, page 511

3M
**BUILDING 270-3N-07
ST PAUL, MN 55144-1000**

TITRALAC™ REGULAR AND EXTRA STRENGTH
[*T ī' tră lăc*]

Active Ingredients: Calcium Carbonate: *Regular:* 420mg./tablet (168 mg. elemental calcium). *Extra Strength:* 750mg/tablet (300 mg. elemental calcium).

Inactive Ingredients: Glycine, Magnesium Stearate, Saccharin, Spearmint Oil, Starch.

Indications: A spearmint flavored non-chalky antacid tablet which quickly relieves heartburn, sour stomach, acid indigestion and upset stomach associated with these symptoms.

Dosage and Administration: *Regular:* Two tablets every two or three hours as symptoms occur or as directed by a physician. Tablets can be chewed, swallowed or allowed to melt in the mouth. *Extra Strength:* One or two tablets every two or three hours as symptoms occur or as directed by a physician. Tablets can be chewed or allowed to melt in the mouth.

Warnings: *Regular:* Do not take more than 19 tablets in a 24-hour period or use maximum dosage for more than two weeks, except under the advise and supervision of a physician. *Extra Strength:* Do not take more than ten tablets in a 24-hour period or use maximum dosage for more than two weeks, except under the advice and supervision of a physician. **Keep this and all medication out of the reach of children**

Dietary Guidelines: Titralac™ Antacid is sodium free and sugar free. Also aluminum free.

How Supplied: *Regular:* Available in bottles of 40, 100, 1000 tablets. *Extra Strength:* Available in bottles of 100 tablets.
Shown in Product Identification Guide, page 511

TITRALAC PLUS ANTACID
[*T ī 'tră lăc*]
TITRALAC PLUS™ LIQUID AND TABLETS

Active Ingredients: *Tablets:* Calcium Carbonate: 420 mg/tablet (168 mg elemental calcium), Simethicone: 21 mg/tablet. *Liquid:* Calcium Carbonate: 1000 mg/2 teaspoons (10 ml.) (400 mg elemental calcium), Simethicone: 40 mg/2 teaspoons (10 ml.)

Inactive Ingredients: *Tablets:* Glycine, Magnesium Stearate, Saccharin, Spearmint Oil, Starch. May also contain Croscarmellose Sodium. *Liquid:* Benzyl Alcohol, Colloidal Silicon Dioxide, Glyceryl Laurate, Methylparaben, Potassium Benzoate, Propylparaben, Saccharin, Sorbitol, Spearmint Flavor, Water, Xanthan Gum.

Indications: A spearmint flavored non-chalky antacid which quickly relieves heartburn, sour stomach, acid indigestion, and accompanying gas often associated with these symptoms.

Dosage and Administration: *Tablets:* Two tablets every two or three hours as symptoms occur or as directed by a physician. Tablets can be chewed, swallowed or allowed to melt in the mouth. *Liquid:* Two teaspoons, between meals and at bedtime or as directed by a physician. Shake well before using.

Warnings: *Tablets:* Do not take more than 19 tablets in a 24-hour period or use maximum dosage for more than two weeks, except under the advice and supervision of a physician. *Liquid:* do not take more than 16 teaspoons in a 24-hour period, or use maximum dosage for more than two weeks, except under the advice and supervision of a physician. Keep this and all medication out of the reach of children.

Dietary Guidelines: Tablets and liquid are sodium free, sugar free, and aluminum free.

How Supplied: *Tablets:* Available in bottles of 100 tablets. *Liquid:* Available in 12 fl. oz. bottles.
Shown in Product Identification Guide, page 511

UNKNOWN DRUG?
Consult the
Product Identification Guide
(Gray Pages)
for full-color photos of
leading over-the-counter
medications

Marlyn Nutraceuticals
14851 N. SCOTTSDALE RD
SCOTTSDALE, AZ 85254

MARLYN FORMULA 50®

PRODUCT OVERVIEW

Key Facts: MARLYN FORMULA 50 is a combination of amino acids and B6 in a gelatin capsule which provides protein "building blocks" important to growth and development of all protein containing tissue including nails, hair and skin.

Major Uses: Dermatologists recommend Formula 50 not only for splitting, peeling nails but also prescribe it in conjunction with their favorite topical cream for control of nail fungus. OB-Gyn's recommend it for help in controlling excessive hair fall-out after child birth.
The recommended daily dose is six capsules daily.

Safety Information: There are no known contraindications or adverse reactions.

PRESCRIBING INFORMATION

MARLYN FORMULA 50®

Composition: Each capsule contains:
Amino Acids.....................0.3 Gm*
Vitamin B6 (pyridoxine HCl).....1.0 mg.
*Approximate analysis of the amino acids: indispensable amino acids (lysine, tryptophan, phenylalanine, methionine, threonine, leucine, isoleucine, valine), 35.30%; semi-dispensable amino acids (arginine, histidine, tyrosine, cystine, glycine), 19.18%; dispensable amino acids (glutamic acid, alanine, aspartic acid, serine, proline), 45.56%.
Amino acids: Protein "building blocks" important to growth and development of all protein containing tissue including nails, hair, and skin.

Dosage and Administration: The recommended daily dose is 6 capsules daily.

Supply: Bottles of 100, 250.

WOBENZYM N™
[wō-běn-zy-m]

Manufactured by Mucos Pharma GMbH in Germany. Exclusively distributed by Marlyn Co., Scottsdale, AZ USA.

Description: Each enteric coated Wobenzym N tablet contains:

Pancreatin 8 NF	100 mg
Trypsin 720 FIP-U	24 mg
Chymotrypsin 300 FIP-U	1 mg
Bromelain 225 FIP-U	45 mg
Papain 164 FIP-U	60 mg
Rutosid 3 H$_2$O	50 mg

Dosage and Administration: Take 2 (two) tablets 3 (three) times daily after each meal.

How Supplied: Tamper-resistant blister packs of either 40 enteric coated tablets or 200 enteric coated tablets. Available without a prescription.

McNeil Consumer Products Company
Division of McNeil-PPC, Inc.
FORT WASHINGTON, PA 19034

Maximum Strength   OTC
ARTHRITIS FOUNDATION™
Aspirin Free
Pain Reliever

Description: Each Arthritis Foundation™ Aspirin Free Caplet contains acetaminophen 500 mg.

Actions: Acetaminophen is a clinically proven analgesic and antipyretic. Acetaminophen produces analgesia by elevation of the pain threshold and antipyresis through action on the hypothalmic heat-regulating center. Acetaminophen may be used safely by most persons with peptic ulcers, when taken as directed for recommended conditions. Since Arthritis Foundation™ Aspirin Free Pain Reliever contains no aspirin, it is not likely to cause a reaction in those who are allergic to aspirin.

Indications: For the temporary relief of minor aches, pains, headaches, fever and minor pain or arthritis.

Precautions: If a rare sensitivity reaction occurs, the drug should be discontinued.

Directions: Adults and Children 12 years of Age and Older: Take two caplets every 4 to 6 hours. No more than a total of 8 caplets in any 24 hours period, or as directed by a doctor. Not for use in children under 12 years of age.

Warnings: Do not use if carton is opened or printed neck wrap or printed foil inner seal is broken. Do not take for pain for more than 10 days or for fever for more than 3 days unless directed by a physician. Severe or recurrent pain or high or continued fever may be indicative of serious illness. Under these conditions, consult a physician. Keep this and all medication out of the reach of children. As with any drug, if you are pregnant or nursing a baby, seek the advice of a health professional before using this product. In the case of accidental overdose, contact a physician or poison control center immediately. Prompt medical attention is critical for adults as well as for children even if you do not notice any signs or symptoms. Do not use with other products containing acetaminophen.

Alcohol Warning: If you generally consume 3 or more alcohol-containing drinks per day, you should consult your physician for advice on when and how you should take ARTHRITIS FOUNDATION™ Aspirin Free and other pain relievers.

Overdosage Information: Acetaminophen in massive overdosage may cause hepatic toxicity in some patients. In adults and adolescents, hepatic toxicity has rarely been reported following inges-

tion of acute overdoses of less than 10 grams. Fatalities are infrequent (less than 3–4% of untreated cases) and have rarely been reported with overdoses of less than 15 grams. In children, an acute overdosage of less than 150 mg/kg has not been associated with hepatic toxicity. Early symptoms following a potentially hepatotoxic overdose may include: nausea, vomiting, diaphoresis and general malaise. Clinical and laboratory evidence of hepatic toxicity may not be apparent until 48 to 72 hours postingestion. In adults and adolescents, regardless of the quantity of acetaminophen reported to have been ingested, administer acetylcysteine immediately if 24 hours or less have elapsed from the reported time of ingestion. For full prescribing information, refer to the acetylcysteine package insert. Do not await results of assays for plasma acetaminophen level before initiating treatment with acetylcysteine. The following additional procedures are recommended. The stomach should be emptied promptly by lavage or by induction of emesis with syrup of ipecac. A plasma acetaminophen assay should be obtained as early as possible, but no sooner than four hours following ingestion. If plasma level falls above the lower treatment line on the acetaminophen overdose nomogram, acetylcysteine therapy should be continued. Liver function studies should be obtained initially and repeated at 24-hour intervals.

Serious toxicity or fatalities are extremely infrequent in children, possibly due to differences in the way they metabolize acetaminophen. In children, the maximum potential amount ingested can be more easily estimated. If more than 150 mg/kg or an unknown amount was ingested, obtain a plasma acetaminophen level. The plasma acetaminophen level should be obtained as soon as possible, but no sooner than 4 hours following the ingestion. If plasma level falls above the lower treatment line on the acetaminophen overdose nomogram, the acetylcysteine therapy should be initiated and continued for a full course of therapy. If plasma acetaminophen assay capability is not available, and the estimated acetaminophen ingestion exceeds 150 mg/kg, acetylcysteine therapy should be initiated and continued for a full course of therapy.

For additional emergency information, call your regional poison center or call the Rocky Mountain Poison Center toll-free (1-800-525-6115).

Alcohol Information: Chronic heavy alcohol abusers may be at increased risk of liver toxicity from excessive acetaminophen use, although reports of this event are rare. Reports almost invariably involve cases of severe chronic alcoholics and the dosages of acetaminophen most often exceed recommended doses and often involve substantial overdose. Professionals should alert their patients who regularly consume large amounts of

Continued on next page

McNeil Consumer—Cont.

alcohol not to exceed recommended doses of acetaminophen.

Inactive Ingredients: Cellulose, Cornstarch, Hydroxypropyl Methylcellulose, Magnesium Stearate, Polyethylene Glycol, Sodium Starch Glycolate and Red No. 40.

How Supplied: Caplets (colored white, imprinted with Arthritis Foundation™ logo and "AF" in red) in tamper resistant bottles of 50 and FastCap easy open packages of 100.

Shown in Product Identification Guide, page 511

ARTHRITIS FOUNDATION™ OTC
Ibuprofen
Pain Reliever/Fever Reducer

Description: Each Arthritis Foundation™ Ibuprofen Tablet contains ibuprofen 200 mg.

Actions: Ibuprofen is a nonsteroidal anti-inflammatory drug (NSAID) that possesses analgesic and antipyretic activity. Its mode of action, like that of other NSAIDs, is not completely understood, but may be related to prostaglandin synthetase inhibition. In clinical studies, ibuprofen has been shown to be comparable to aspirin in controlling pain, though causing fewer of the mild gastrointestinal side effects.

Indications: For the temporary relief of minor aches and pains associated with the common cold, headache, toothache, muscular aches, backache, for the minor pain of arthritis, for the pain of menstrual cramps and for reduction of fever.

Directions: Adults: Take 1 tablet every 4 to 6 hours while symptoms persist. If pain or fever does not respond to 1 tablet, 2 tablets may be used but do not exceed 6 tablets in 24 hours, unless directed by a doctor. The smallest effective dose should be used. Take with food or milk if occasional and mild heartburn, upset stomach, or stomach pain occurs with use. Consult a doctor if these symptoms are more than mild or if they persist. **Children:** Do not give this product to children under 12 except under the advice and supervision of a doctor.

Warnings: Do not take for pain for more than 10 days or for fever for more than 3 days unless directed by a doctor. If pain or fever persists or gets worse, if new symptoms occur, or if the painful area is red or swollen, consult a doctor. These could be signs of serious illness. If you are under a doctor's care for any serious condition, consult a doctor before taking this product. As with aspirin and acetaminophen, if you have any condition which requires you to take prescription drugs or if you have had any problems or serious side effects from taking any non-prescription pain reliever, do not take ibuprofen tablets without first discussing it with your doctor. If you experience any symptoms which are unusual or seem unrelated to the condition for which you took ibuprofen, consult a doctor before taking any more of it. Although ibuprofen is indicated for the same conditions as aspirin and acetaminophen, it should not be taken with them except under a doctor's direction. Do not combine this product with any other ibuprofen-containing product. As with any drug, if you are pregnant or nursing a baby, seek the advice of a health professional before using this product. IT IS ESPECIALLY IMPORTANT NOT TO USE IBUPROFEN DURING THE LAST 3 MONTHS OF PREGNANCY UNLESS SPECIFICALLY DIRECTED TO DO SO BY A DOCTOR BECAUSE IT MAY CAUSE PROBLEMS IN THE UNBORN CHILD OR COMPLICATIONS DURING DELIVERY. Keep this and all drugs out of the reach of children. In case of accidental overdose, seek professional assistance or contact a poison control center immediately. Do not use if imprinted foil seal under the cap is broken or missing.

Warning: ASPIRIN SENSITIVE PATIENTS: Do not take this product if you have had a severe allergic reaction to aspirin, e.g.,—asthma, swelling, shock or hives, because even though this product contains no aspirin or salicylates, cross-reactions may occur in patients allergic to aspirin.

Inactive Ingredients: Carnauba Wax, Microcrystalline Cellulose, Croscarmellose Sodium, Hydroxypropyl Methylcellulose, Polyethylene Glycol, Polysorbate 80, Povidone, Silicon Dioxide, Sodium Starch Glycolate, Pregelatinized Starch, Stearic Acid, Titanium Dioxide.

How Supplied: Tablets (colored white, imprinted or debossed with Arthritis Foundation logo) in tamper resistant bottles of 50 and 100. Store at room temperature; avoid excessive heat 40 degrees C (104 degrees F).

Shown in Product Identification Guide, page 511

Maximum Strength OTC
ARTHRITIS FOUNDATION™
Nighttime
Pain Reliever/Nighttime Sleep Aid

Description: Each Arthritis Foundation™ Nighttime Caplet contains acetaminophen 500 mg and diphenhydramine HCl 25 mg.

Actions: Arthritis Foundation™ Nighttime Caplets contain a clinically proven analgesic-antipyretic and an antihistamine. Maximum allowable non-prescription levels of acetaminophen and diphenhydramine provide temporary relief of occasional headaches and minor aches and pains accompanying sleeplessness. Acetaminophen produces analgesia by elevation of the pain threshold. Diphenhydramine HCl is an antihistamine with sedative properties.

Indications: For the temporary relief of occasional headaches, minor aches, pains and minor pain of arthritis with accompanying sleeplessness.

Precautions: If a rare sensitivity reaction occurs, the drug should be discontinued.

Directions: Adults and Children 12 years of Age and Older: Take two caplets at bedtime or as directed by physician. Do not exceed recommended dosage. Not for use in children under 12 years of age.

Warnings: Do not use for more than 10 days unless directed by a physician. Consult your physician if symptoms persist or new ones occur, or if fever persists for more than 3 days, or if sleeplessness persists continuously for more than 2 weeks. Insomnia may be a symptom of serious underlying medical illness. Do not take this product unless directed by a doctor, if you have a breathing problem such as emphysema or chronic bronchitis, or if you have glaucoma or difficulty in urination due to enlargement of the prostate gland. Avoid alcoholic beverages while taking this product. Do not take if you are taking sedatives or tranquilizers without first consulting your physician. Do not use if carton is opened or printed neck wrap or printed foil inner seal is broken. Keep this and all medication out of the reach of children. In the case of accidental overdose, contact a physician or poison control center immediately. Prompt medical attention is critical for adults as well as for children even if you do not notice any signs or symptoms. As with any drug, if you are pregnant or nursing a baby, seek the advice of a health professional before using this product. Do not use with other products containing acetaminophen.

Alcohol Warning: If you generally consume 3 or more alcohol-containing drinks per day, you should consult your physician for advice on when and how you should take ARTHRITIS FOUNDATION™ Nighttime and other pain relievers.

Caution: This Product will cause drowsiness. Do not drive a motor vehicle or operate machinery after use.

Overdosage Information: Acetaminophen in massive overdosage may cause hepatic toxicity in some patients. In adults and adolescents, hepatic toxicity has rarely been reported following ingestion of acute overdoses of less than 10 grams. Fatalities are infrequent (less than 3–4% of untreated cases) and have rarely been reported with overdoses of less than 15 grams. In children, an acute overdosage of less than 150 mg/kg has not been associated with hepatic toxicity. Early symptoms following a potentially hepatotoxic overdose may include nausea, vomiting, diaphoresis and general malaise. Clinical and laboratory evidence of hepatic toxicity may not be apparent until 48 to 72 hours postingestion. In adults and adolescents, regardless of the quantity of acetaminophen reported to have been ingested, administer acetylcysteine immediately if 24 hours or less have elapsed from the reported time of ingestion. For full prescribing information, refer to the acetylcysteine package insert. Do not await results of assays for plasma acetaminophen level before initiating treatment with acetylcysteine. The following additional procedures are recommended: The stomach should be emptied promptly by lavage or by induction of emesis with syrup of ipecac. A plasma acetaminophen assay should be obtained as early as possible, but no sooner than four hours following ingestion. If plasma level falls above the lower treatment line on the acetaminophen overdose nomogram, acetylcysteine therapy should be continued. Liver function studies should be obtained initially and repeated at 24-hour intervals.

Serious toxicity or fatalities are extremely infrequent in children, possibly due to differences in the ways they metabolize acetaminophen. In children, the maximum potential amount ingested can be more easily estimated. If more than 150 mg/kg or an unknown amount was ingested, obtain a plasma acetaminophen level. The plasma acetaminophen level should be obtained as soon as possible, but no sooner than 4 hours following the ingestion. If plasma level falls above the lower treatment line on the acetaminophen overdose nomogram, the acetylcysteine therapy should be initiated and continued for a full course of therapy. If plasma acetaminophen assay capability is not available, and the estimated acetaminophen ingestion exceeds 150 mg/kg, acetylcysteine therapy should be initiated and continued for a full course of therapy.

For additional emergency information, call your regional poison center or call the Rocky Mountain Poison Center toll-free (1-800-525-6115).

Diphenhydramine toxicity should be treated as you would an antihistamine/anticholinergic overdose and is likely to be present within a few hours after acute ingestion.

Alcohol Information: Chronic heavy alcohol abusers may be at increased risk of liver toxicity from excessive acetaminophen use, although reports of this event are rare. Reports almost invariably involve cases of severe chronic alcoholics and the dosages of acetaminophen most often exceed recommended doses and often involve substantial overdose. Professionals should alert their patients who regularly consume large amounts of alcohol not to exceed recommended doses of acetaminophen.

Inactive Ingredients: Cellulose, Cornstarch, Hydroxypropyl Methylcellulose, Magnesium Stearate, Polyethylene Glycol, Sodium Starch Glycolate and Red No. 40.

How Supplied: Caplets (colored blue, imprinted with Arthritis Foundation logo and "NT" in blue) in tamper resistant bottles of 50 and FastCap easy open packages of 100.

Shown in Product Identification Guide, page 511

Maximum Strength   OTC
ARTHRITIS FOUNDATION™
Safety Coated Aspirin
Pain Reliever

Description: Each Arthritis Foundation™ Safety Coated Aspirin Tablet contains aspirin 500 mg.

Actions: Aspirin is a clinically proven analgesic for fast, effective relief of minor pain of arthritis. Arthritis Foundation™ Safety Coated Aspirin Tablets are safety coated to help protect against stomach upset caused by aspirin.

Indications: For the temporary relief of minor pain of arthritis while protecting against stomach irritation.

Directions: Adults and Children 12 years of Age and Older: Take two tablets every 6 hours, as needed. Do not exceed 8 tablets in 24 hours unless directed by a doctor. Children: Do not give this product to children uner 12 except under the advice and supervision of a doctor.

Warnings: Children and teenagers should not use this medicine for chicken pox or flu symptoms before a doctor is consulted about Reye Syndrome, a rare but serious illness reported to be associated with aspirin. Do not take this product for pain for more than 10 days or for fever for more than 3 days unless directed by a doctor. If pain or fever persists or gets worse, if new symptoms occur, or if redness or swelling is present, consult a doctor because these could be signs of a serious condition. Do not take this product if you are allergic to aspirin, have asthma, have stomach problems (such as heartburn, upset stomach or stomach pain) that persist or recur, or if you have ulcers or bleeding problems unless directed by a doctor. If ringing in the ears or a loss of hearing occurs, consult a doctor before taking any more of this product. Do not use if carton is opened or printed neck wrap or printed foil inner seal is broken. Keep this and all drugs out of the reach of children. In case of accidental overdose, contact a doctor or poison control center immediately. As with any drug, if you are pregnant or nursing a baby, seek the advice of a health professional before using this product. IMPORTANT: IT IS ESPECIALLY IMPORTANT NOT TO USE ASPIRIN DURING THE LAST 3 MONTHS OF PREGNANCY UNLESS SPECIFICALLY DIRECTED TO DO SO BY A DOCTOR BECAUSE IT MAY CAUSE PROBLEMS IN THE UNBORN CHILD OR COMPLICATIONS DURING DELIVERY.

Drug Interaction Precaution: Do not take this product if you are taking a pre-scription drug for anticoagulation (thinning the blood), diabetes, gout or arthritis unless directed by a doctor.

Inactive Ingredients: Carnauba Wax, Cornstarch, Hydroxypropyl Methylcellulose, Methacrylic Acid Copolymer, Microcrystalline Cellulose, Polyethylene Glycol, Polysorbate 80, Sodium Lauryl Sulfate, Talc, Titanium Dioxide, Triacetin, Yellow No. 6, Yellow No. 10. May contain Blue No. 1 and Blue No. 2 or Iron Oxide Black.

How Supplied: Tablets (colored orange, imprinted with Arthritis Foundation logo in dark blue) in tamper resistant bottles of 50 and FastCap easy open packages of 100.
Keep tightly closed in a dry place. Do not expose to excessive heat.

Shown in Product Identification Guide, page 511

IMODIUM® A-D   OTC
(loperamide hydrochloride)

Description: Each 5 ml (teaspoon) of Imodium A-D liquid contains loperamide hydrochloride 1 mg. Imodium A-D liquid is stable, cherry flavored, and clear in color.
Each caplet of Imodium AD contains 2 mg of loperamide and is scored and colored green.

Actions: Imodium A-D contains a clinically proven antidiarrheal medication. Loperamide HCl acts by slowing intestinal motility and by affecting water and electrolyte movement through the bowel.

Indications: Imodium A-D is indicated for the control and symptomatic relief of acute nonspecific diarrhea, including travelers' diarrhea.

Usual Dosage: Adults: Take four teaspoonfuls or two caplets after first loose bowel movement. If needed, take two teaspoonfuls or one caplet after each subsequent loose bowel movement. Do not exceed eight teaspoonfuls or four caplets in any 24 hour period, unless directed by a physician.
9–11 years old (60–95 lbs.): Two teaspoonfuls or one caplet after first loose bowel movement, followed by one teaspoonful or one-half caplet after each subsequent loose bowel movement. Do not exceed six teaspoonfuls or three caplets a day.
6–8 years old (48–59 lbs.): Two teaspoonfuls or one caplet after first loose bowel movement, followed by one teaspoonful or one-half caplet after each subsequent loose bowel movement. Do not exceed four teaspoonfuls or two caplets a day.
Professional Dosage Schedule for children two-five years old (24–47 lbs): one teaspoon after first loose bowel movement, followed by one after each subsequent loose bowel movement. Do not exceed three teaspoonfuls a day.
Warnings: KEEP THIS AND ALL DRUGS OUT OF THE REACH OF CHILDREN. Do not use for more than

Continued on next page

McNeil Consumer—Cont.

two days unless directed by a physician. Do not use if diarrhea is accompanied by high fever (greater than 101°F), or if blood or mucus is present in the stool, or if you have had a rash or other allergic reaction to loperamide HCl. If you are taking antibiotics or have a history of liver disease, consult a physician before using this product. As with any drug, if you are pregnant or nursing a baby, seek the advice of a physician before using this product. In case of accidental overdose, seek professional assistance or contact a poison control center immediately. Store at room temperature.

Overdosage: Overdosage of loperamide HCl in man may result in constipation, CNS depression and nausea. A slurry of activated charcoal administered promptly after ingestion of loperamide hydrochloride can reduce the amount of drug which is absorbed. If vomiting occurs spontaneously upon ingestion, a slurry of 100 grams of activated charcoal should be administered orally as soon as fluids can be retained. If vomiting has not occurred, and CNS depression is evident, gastric lavage should be performed followed by administration of 100 gms of the activated charcoal slurry through the gastric tube. In the event of overdosage, patients should be monitored for signs of CNS depression for at least 24 hours. Children may be more sensitive to central nervous system effects than adults. If CNS depression is observed, naloxone may be administered. If responsive to naloxone, vital signs must be monitored carefully for recurrence of symptoms of drug overdose for at least 24 hours after the last dose of naloxone.

Inactive Ingredients: Liquid: Alcohol (5.25%), citric acid, flavors, glycerin, methylparaben, propylparaben and purified water.
Caplets: Corn starch, lactose, magnesium stearate, microcrystalline cellulose, FD&C Blue #1 and D&C Yellow #10.

How Supplied: Cherry flavored liquid (clear) 2 fl. oz., 3 fl. oz., and 4 fl. oz. tamper resistant bottles with child resistant safety caps and special dosage cups. Green Scored caplets in 6's and 12's and 18's blister packaging which is tamper resistant and child resistant.

Shown in Product Identification Guide, page 511

LACTAID® Caplets
(lactase enzyme)

PRODUCT OVERVIEW

Key Facts: Lactaid® is the original dairy digestive supplement that makes milk and dairy foods more digestible. Lactaid® lactase enzyme hydrolyzes lactose into two digestible simple sugars: glucose and galactose. Lactaid Caplets are taken orally for *in vivo* hydrolysis of lactose.

Major Uses: Lactose intolerance, suspected from gastrointestinal discomfort (ie, gas, bloating, cramps, and diarrhea) after drinking milk or ingesting other dairy foods such as cheese and ice cream.

PRESCRIBING INFORMATION

Description: Each Lactaid Caplet contains 3000 FCC (Food Chemical Codex) units of lactase enzyme (derived from *Aspergillus oryzae*).

Action: Lactaid Caplets work to naturally replenish lactase enzyme that aids in dairy food digestion. Lactase enzyme hydrolyzes lactose sugar (a double sugar) into its simple sugar components, glucose and galactose.

Indications: Lactose intolerance, suspected from gastrointestinal discomfort (ie, gas, bloating, flatulence, cramps, and diarrhea) after drinking milk or ingesting other dairy foods such as cheese and ice cream.

Usual Dosage: These convenient, portable caplets are easy to swallow or chew and can be used with milk or any dairy food. We recommend swallowing or chewing 3 caplets with the first bite of dairy food. Take no more than 6 caplets at a time. Don't be discouraged if at first Lactaid does not work to your satisfaction. Because the degree of enzyme deficiency naturally varies from person to person and from food to food, you may have to adjust the number of caplets up or down to find your own level of comfort. Since Lactaid Caplets work only on the food as you eat it, use them every time you enjoy dairy foods.

Warning: If you experience any symptoms which are unusual or seem unrelated to the condition for which you took this product, consult a physician before taking any more of it. Do not use if carton is opened or if printed plastic neckwrap is broken.

Inactive Ingredients: Dextrates, Dibasic Calcium Phosphate, Microcrystalline Cellulose, Croscarmellose Sodium, Hydrogenated Vegetable Oil, Cornstarch. Dextrose and Sodium Citrate.

Nutritional Information: Serving size: 3 Caplets. Servings per container: 4. Calories: 4. Protein: less than 1 g. Carbohydrate: less than 1 g. Fat: less than 1 g. Sodium: 10 mg. Percentage of U.S. Recommended Daily Allowances (U.S. RDA): Contains less than 2% of the U.S. RDA of Protein, Vitamin A, Vitamin C and Thiamine.

How Supplied: Lactaid Caplets are available in bottles of 12, 50, and 100 counts. Store at or below room temperature (below 77°F) but do not refrigerate. Keep away from heat.
Lactaid Caplets are certified kosher from the Orthodox Union.

Shown in Product Identification Guide, page 511

LACTAID® Drops
(lactase enzyme)

PRODUCT OVERVIEW

Key Facts: Lactaid® is the original dairy digestive supplement that makes milk more digestible. Lactaid® lactase enzyme hydrolyzes lactose into two digestible simple sugars: glucose and galactose. Lactaid Drops are added to milk for *in vitro* hydrolysis of lactose.

Major Uses: Lactose intolerance, suspected from gastrointestinal discomfort (ie, gas, bloating, cramps, and diarrhea) after drinking milk.

PRESCRIBING INFORMATION

Description: Lactaid drops contain sufficient lactase enzyme (derived from *Kluyveromyces lactis*) to hydrolyze lactose in milk.

Action: Lactaid Drops are a liquid form of the natural lactase enzyme that makes milk more digestible. The lactase enzyme hydrolyzes the lactose sugar (a double sugar) into its simple sugar components, glucose and galactose.

Indications: Lactose intolerance, suspected from gastrointestinal discomfort (ie, gas, bloating, cramps, and diarrhea) after drinking milk.

Usual Dosage: Lactaid drops are a liquid form of the natural lactase enzyme that makes milk more digestible. To use, add Lactaid drops to a quart of milk, shake gently and refrigerate for 24 hours. We recommend starting with 5-7 drops per quart of milk but because sensitivity to lactose can vary you may have to adjust the number of drops you use. If you are still experiencing discomfort after consuming milk with 5-7 Lactaid drops per quart, you may want to add 10 drops per quart or even 15 drops per quart. 15 drops per quart should remove nearly all of the lactose in the milk. Lactaid can be used with any kind of milk: whole, 1%, 2%, non-fat, skim, powdered and chocolate milk.

Warning: If you experience any symptoms which are unusual or seem unrelated to the condition for which you took this product, consult a doctor before taking any more of it. Do not use if carton is opened or if printed plastic bodywrap is broken.

Inactive Ingredients: Glycerin, Water

Nutritional Facts: 16 mL size
Serv. Size: 5-7 drops (0.2 mL). Servings Approx. 75.
Calories 0.

Amount/Serving	%DV*
Total Fat 0g	0%
Sodium 0mg	0%
Total Carb. 0g	0%
Sugars 0g	
Protein 0g	0%

*Percent Daily Values (DV) are based on 2,000 calorie diet.

How Supplied: Lactaid Drops are available in .22 fl. oz. (7 mL), and .53 fl.

oz. (16 mL) (30 and 75 quart supply, respectively). Store at or below room temperature (below 77°F). Refrigerate after opening.

Lactaid Drops are certified kosher from the Orthodox Union.

Shown in Product Identification Guide, page 511

**PEDIACARE® Cold-Allergy
Chewable Tablets
PEDIACARE® Cough-Cold Liquid
and Chewable Tablets
PEDIACARE® NightRest
Cough-Cold Liquid
PEDIACARE® Infants'
Decongestant Drops**

Description: Each PEDIACARE Cold-Allergy Chewable Tablet contains chlorpheniramine maleate 1 mg and pseudoephedrine hydrochloride 15 mg. Each 5 ml of PEDIACARE Cough-Cold Liquid contains pseudoephedrine hydrochloride 15 mg, chlorpheniramine maleate 1 mg and dextromethorphan hydrobromide 5 mg. Each Pediacare Cough-Cold Formula Chewable Tablet contains pseudoephedrine hydrochloride 15 mg, chlorpheniramine maleate 1 mg and dextromethorphan hydrobromide 5 mg. Each 0.8 ml oral dropper of PEDIACARE Infants' Oral Decongestant Drops contains pseudoephedrine hydrochloride 7.5 mg. PEDIACARE NightRest Cough-Cold liquid contains pseudoephedrine hydrochloride 15 mg, chlorpheniramine maleate 1 mg and dextromethorphan hydrobromide 7.5 mg per 5 ml. PEDIACARE Cough-Cold Liquid and Infants' Drops are stable, cherry flavored and red in color. PEDIACARE Cold-Allergy Chewable Tablets are fruit flavored and pink in color. PEDIACARE Cough-Allergy Chewable Tablets are fruit flavored and pink in color.

Actions: PEDIACARE Products are available in four different formulas, allowing you to select the ideal product to temporarily relieve the patient's symptoms. PEDIACARE Cold-Allergy Chewable Tablets contain an antihistamine and a nasal decongestant to relieve children's cold and allergy symptoms. PEDIACARE Cough-Cold Liquid and Chewable Tablets contain both of the above ingredients plus a cough suppressant, dextromethorphan hydrobromide, to provide temporary relief of nasal congestion, runny nose, sneezing and coughing due to the common cold, hay fever or other upper respiratory allergies. PEDIACARE NightRest Cough-Cold Liquid contains a decongestant, pseudoephedrine hydrochloride, an antihistamine, chlorpheniramine maleate, and a cough suppressant, dextromethorphan hydrobromide, to provide temporary relief of coughs, nasal congestion, runny nose and sneezing due to the common cold. PEDIACARE NightRest may be used day or night to relieve cough and cold symptoms. PEDIACARE Infants' Oral Decongestant Drops contain a decongestant, pseudoephedrine hydrochloride, to provide temporary relief of nasal congestion due to the common cold, hay fever or other upper respiratory allergies.

Professional Dosage: A calibrated dosage cup is provided for accurate dosing of the PEDIACARE Liquid formulas. A calibrated oral dropper is provided for accurate dosing of PEDIACARE Infants' Drops. All doses of PEDIACARE Cold-Allergy Chewable Tablets, PEDIACARE Cough-Cold Liquid and Chewable Tablets, as well as PEDIACARE Infants' Drops may be repeated every 4–6 hours, not to exceed 4 doses in 24 hours. PEDIACARE NightRest Liquid may be repeated every 6–8 hrs, not to exceed 4 doses in 24 hours.

[See table below.]

WARNINGS: DO NOT USE IF CARTON IS OPENED, OR IF PRINTED PLASTIC BOTTLE WRAP OR FOIL INNER SEAL IS BROKEN. KEEP THIS AND ALL MEDICATION OUT OF THE REACH OF CHILDREN. IN CASE OF ACCIDENTAL OVERDOSAGE, CONTACT A PHYSICIAN OR POISON CONTROL CENTER IMMEDIATELY.

The following information appears on the appropriate package labels:

PEDIACARE Cold-Allergy Chewable Tablets: PHENYLKETONURICS: CONTAINS PHENYALANINE 8MG PER TABLET. Do not exceed recommended dosage because at higher doses nervousness, dizziness or sleeplessness may occur. Do not give this product to children for more than 7 days. If symptoms do not improve, or are accompanied by fever, consult a physician. May cause excitability, especially in children. May cause drowsiness. Sedatives and tranquilizers may increase the drowsiness effect. Do not give this product to children who are taking sedatives or tranquilizers, without first consulting the child's physician. Do not give this product to children who have a breathing problem such as chronic bronchitis, or who have glaucoma, heart disease, high blood pressure, thyroid disease, or diabetes, without first consulting the child's physician.

PEDIACARE Cough-Cold Chewable Tablets:
PHENYLKETONURICS: CONTAINS PHENYLALANINE 6MG PER TABLET.

PEDIACARE Cough-Cold Liquid, Night Rest Cough-Cold Liquid, and Chewable Tablets: Do not exceed recommended dosage because at higher doses nervousness, dizziness or sleeplessness may occur. Do not give this product to children for more than 7 days. If symptoms do not improve, or are accompanied by fever, consult a physician. A persistent cough may be a sign of a serious condition. If cough persists for more than one week, tends to recur or is accompanied by fever, rash, or persistent headache, consult a physician. Do not give this product for persistent or chronic cough such as occurs with asthma or if cough is accompanied by excessive phlegm (mucus) unless directed by a physician. May cause excitability especially in children. [May cause drowsiness. Sedatives and tranquilizers may increase the drowsiness effect. Do not give this product to children who are taking sedatives or tranquilizers without first consulting the child's physician.] Do not give this product to children who have a breathing problem such as chronic bronchitis, or who have glaucoma, heart disease, high blood pressure, thyroid disease or diabetes, without first consulting the child's physician.

Age Group	0–3 mos	4–11 mos	12–23 mos	2–3 yrs	4–5 yrs	6–8 yrs	9–10 yrs	11 yrs	Dosage
Weight (lbs)	6–11 lb	12–17 lb	18–23 lb	24–35 lb	36–47 lb	48–59 lb	60–71 lb	72–95 lb	
PEDIACARE Infants' Drops*	½ dropper (0.4 ml)	1 dropper (0.8 ml)	1½ droppers (1.2 ml)	2 droppers (1.6 ml)					q4–6h
PEDIACARE Cold-Allergy Chewable Tablets**				1 tabs	1½ tabs	2 tabs	2½ tabs	3 tabs	q4–6h
PEDIACARE Cough-Cold Liquid** and Chewable Tablets**				1 tsp / 1 tabs	1½ tsp / 1½ tabs	2 tsp / 2 tabs	2½ tsp / 2½ tabs	3 tsp / 3 tabs	q4–6h / q4–6h
PEDIACARE NightRest Liquid**				1 tsp	1½ tsp	2 tsp	2½ tsp	3 tsp	q6–8h

*Administer to children under 2 years only on the advice of a physician.
**Administer to children under 6 years only on the advice of a physician.

Continued on next page

McNeil Consumer—Cont.

DRUG INTERACTION PRECAUTION: Do not give this product to a child who is taking a prescription drug for high blood pressure or to a child who is taking a prescription containing an oxidase inhibitor (MAOI) (certain drugs for depression, psychiatric or emotional conditions) or for 2 weeks after stopping the MAOI drug. If you are uncertain whether your child's prescription drug contains an MAOI consult a health professional before giving this drug.

PEDIACARE Infants' Oral Decongestant Drops: Do not exceed the recommended dosage because at higher doses nervousness, dizziness or sleeplessness may occur. Do not give this product to children who have heart disease, high blood pressure, thyroid disease or diabetes unless directed by a physician. Do not give this product to children for more than seven days. If symptoms do not improve or are accompanied by fever, consult a physician. Do not give this product to children who are taking a prescription drug for high blood pressure or depression without first consulting a physician. Take by mouth only. Not for nasal use.

INACTIVE INGREDIENTS:
PEDIACARE Cold-Allergy Chewable Tablets: Aspartame, Cellulose, Citric Acid, Corn Starch, Flavors, Mannitol, Colloidal Silicon Dioxide, Stearic Acid, and Red #7."
PEDIACARE Cough-Cold Liquid: Citric acid, corn syrup, flavors, glycerin, propylene glycol, sodium benzoate, sodium carboxymethylcellulose, sorbitol, purified water and Red #40.
PEDIACARE NightRest Cough-Cold Liquid: Citric acid, corn syrup, flavors, glycerin, propylene glycol, sodium benzoate, sodium carboxymethylcellulose, sorbitol, purified water and Red #40.
PEDIACARE Cough-Cold Chewable Tablets: Aspartame, cellulose, citric acid, flavors, magnesium stearate, magnesium trisilicate, mannitol, corn starch and Red #7."
PEDIACARE Infants' Oral Decongestant Drops: Benzoic acid, citric acid, flavors, glycerin, polyethylene glycol, propylene glycol, purified water, sodium benzoate, sorbitol, sucrose and Red #40.

Overdosage: Acute dextromethorphan overdose usually does not result in serious signs and symptoms unless massive amounts have been ingested. Signs and symptoms of a substantial overdose may include nausea and vomiting, visual disturbances, CNS disturbances, and urinary retention. Symptoms from pseudoephedrine overdose consist most often of mild anxiety, tachycardia and/or mild hypertension. Symptoms usually appear within 4 to 8 hours of ingestion and are transient, usually requiring no treatment. Chlorpheniramine toxicity should be treated as you would an antihistamine/anticholinergic overdose and is likely to be present within a few hours after acute ingestion. Symptoms from pseudoephedrine overdose consist often

of mild anxiety, tachycardia and/or mild hypertension. Symptoms usually appear within 4 to 8 hours of ingestion and are transient, usually requiring no treatment.

How Supplied: PEDIACARE Cough-Cold Liquid and NightRest Cough-Cold Liquid (colored red)—bottles of 4 fl. oz. (120 ml) with child-resistant safety cap and calibrated dosage cup. PEDIACARE Cold-Allergy Chewable Tablets (pink, scored)—blister packs of 16. PEDIACARE Cough-Cold Chewable Tablets (pink, scored)—blister packs of 16. PEDIACARE Infants' Drops (colored red)—bottles of ½ fl. oz (15 ml) with calibrated dropper.

Shown in Product Identification Guide, page 511 and 512

IBUPROFEN STRENGTH SINE-AID® IB CAPLETS   OTC

Description: Each Ibuprofen-Strength SINE-AID® IB Caplet contains Ibuprofen 200mg and Pseudoephedrine Hydrochloride 30mg.

Indications: SINE-AID® IB provides effective temporary relief of symptoms associated with the common cold, sinusitis or flu including nasal congestion, headache, fever, body aches, and pains.

Precautions: Although pseudoephedrine is virtually without pressor effect in normotensive patients, it should be used with caution in hypertensives.

Directions: Adults and Children 12 Years of Age and Older: Take 1 caplet every 4 to 6 hours while symptoms persist. If symptoms do not respond to 1 caplet, 2 caplets may be used but do not exceed 6 caplets in 24 hours, unless directed by a doctor. The smallest effective dose should be used. Take with food or milk if occasional and mild heartburn, upset stomach, or stomach pain occurs with use. Consult a doctor if these symptoms are more than mild or if they persist. *Children:* Do not give this product to children under 12 years of age except under the advice and supervision of a doctor.

Warnings: Do not take for colds for more than 7 days or for fever for more than 3 days unless directed by a doctor. If the cold or fever persists or gets worse or if new symptoms occur, consult a doctor. These could be signs of serious illness. As with aspirin and acetaminophen, if you have any condition which requires you to take prescription drugs or if you have had any problems or serious side effects from taking any non-prescription pain reliever, do not take this product without first discussing it with your doctor. **IF YOU EXPERIENCE ANY SYMPTOMS WHICH ARE UNUSUAL OR SEEM UNRELATED TO THE CONDITION FOR WHICH YOU TOOK THIS PRODUCT, CONSULT A DOCTOR BEFORE TAKING ANY MORE OF IT.**

If you are under a doctor's care for any serious condition, consult a doctor before taking this product. Do not exceed recommended dosage because at higher doses nervousness, dizziness or sleeplessness may occur. Do not take this product if you have high blood pressure, heart disease, diabetes, thyroid disease or difficulty in urination due to enlargement of the prostate gland, except under the advice and supervision of a doctor.
As with any drug, if you are pregnant or nursing a baby, seek the advice of a health professional before using this product. **IT IS ESPECIALLY IMPORTANT NOT TO USE THIS PRODUCT DURING THE LAST 3 MONTHS OF PREGNANCY UNLESS SPECIFICALLY DIRECTED TO DO SO BY A DOCTOR BECAUSE IT MAY CAUSE PROBLEMS IN THE UNBORN CHILD OR COMPLICATIONS DURING DELIVERY.**Keep this and all drugs out of the reach of children. In case of accidental overdose, seek professional assistance or contact a poison control center immediately.

Warning: ASPIRIN SENSITIVE PATIENTS: Do not take this product if you have had a severe allergic reaction to aspirin—e.g., asthma, swelling, shock or hives—because, even though this product contains no aspirin or salicylates, cross-reactions may occur in patients allergic to aspirin.

Drug Interaction Precaution: Do not take this product if you are presently taking a prescription drug for high blood pressure or depression without first consulting your doctor. Do not combine this product with other non-prescription pain relievers. Do not combine this product with any other Ibuprofen-containing product.

Overdosage: Symptoms from pseudoephedrine overdose consist most often of mild anxiety, tachycardia and/or hypertension. Symptoms usually appear within 4 to 8 hours of ingestion and are transient, usually requiring no treatment.

Inactive Ingredients: Caplets: Cellulose, Corn Starch, Glyceryl Triacetate, Hydroxypropyl Methylcellulose, Silicon Dioxide, Sodium Lauryl Sulfate, Sodium Starch Glycolate, Stearic Acid, Titanium Dioxide, Red #40 Aluminum Lake, Yellow #10 Aluminum Lake.

How Supplied: Caplets (bright yellow, imprinted "SINE-AID IB")—Child-resistant blister packs of 10.
Shown in Product Identification Guide, page 512

MAXIMUM STRENGTH SINE-AID®   OTC
Sinus Headache Gelcaps, Caplets and Tablets

Description: Each Maximum Strength SINE-AID® Gelcap, Caplet or Tablet contains acetaminophen 500 mg and pseudoephedrine hydrochloride 30 mg.

Actions: Maximum Strength SINE-AID® Gelcaps, Caplets and Tablets contain a clinically proven analgesic-antipyretic and a decongestant. Maximum allowable non-prescription levels of acetaminophen and pseudophedrine provide temporary relief of sinus congestion and pain. Acetaminophen is equal to aspirin in analgesic and antipyretic effectiveness and it is unlikely to produce many of the side effects associated with aspirin and aspirin-containing products. Acetaminophen produces analgesia by elevation of the pain threshold and antipyresis through action on the hypothalamic heat-regulating center. Pseudoephedrine hydrochloride is a sympathomimetic amine that promotes sinus cavity drainage by reducing nasopharyngeal mucosal congestion.

Indications: Maximum Strength SINE-AID® Gelcaps, Caplets and Tablets provide effective symptomatic relief from sinus headache pain and congestion. SINE-AID® is particularly well-suited in patients with aspirin allergy, hemostatic disturbances (including anticoagulant therapy), and bleeding diatheses (e.g. hemophilia) and upper gastrointestinal disease (e.g. ulcer, gastritis, hiatus hernia).

Precautions: If a rare sensitivity occurs, the drug should be discontinued. Although pseudoephedrine is virtually without pressor effect in normotensive patients, it should be used with caution in hypertensives.

Directions: Adults & children 12 years of age and older: Two gelcaps, caplets or tablets every four to six hours. Do not exceed eight gelcaps, caplets or tablets in any 24 hour period. Not for use in children under 12 years of age.

Warning: Do not exceed the recommended dosage because at higher doses nervousness, dizziness or sleeplessness may occur. Do not take this product for more than 7 days. If symptoms do not improve or are accompanied by a fever, consult a physician. Do not take this product if you have heart disease, high blood pressure, thyroid disease, diabetes or difficulty in urination due to enlargement of the prostate gland unless directed by a doctor. Do not use with other products containing acetaminophen.

Do not use if carton is open or if blister unit is broken, or if printed neck wrap or printed foil inner seal is broken. Keep this and all medication out of the reach of children. As with any drug, if you are pregnant or nursing a baby, seek the advice of a health professional before using this product. In case of accidental overdosage, contact a doctor or poison control center immediately. Prompt medical attention is critical for adults as well as for children even if you do not notice any signs or symptoms.

Alcohol Warning: If you generally consume 3 or more alcohol-containing drinks per day, you should consult your physician for advice on when and how you should take Maximum Strength SINE-AID and other pain relievers.

Drug Interaction Precaution: Do not take this product if you are presently taking a prescription drug for high blood pressure or depression without first consulting your doctor.

Overdosage Information: Acetaminophen in massive overdosage may cause hepatic toxicity in some patients. In adults and adolescents, hepatic toxicity has rarely been reported following ingestion of acute overdoses of less than 10 grams. Fatalities are infrequent (less than 3–4% of untreated cases) and have rarely been reported with overdoses of less than 15 grams. In children, an acute overdosage of less than 150 mg/kg has not been associated with hepatic toxicity. Early symptoms following a potentially hepatotoxic overdose may include: nausea, vomiting, diaphoresis and general malaise. Clinical and laboratory evidence of hepatic toxicity may not be apparent until 48 to 72 hours postingestion. In adults and adolescents, regardless of the quantity of acetaminophen reported to have been ingested, administer acetylcysteine immediately if 24 hours or less have elapsed from the reported time of ingestion. For full prescribing information, refer to the acetylcysteine package insert. Do not await results of assays for plasma acetaminophen level before initiating treatment with acetylcysteine. The following additional procedures are recommended: The stomach should be emptied promptly by lavage or by induction of emesis with syrup of ipecac. A plasma acetaminophen assay should be obtained as early as possible, but no sooner than four hours following ingestion. If plasma level falls above the lower treatment line on the acetaminophen overdose nomogram, acetylcysteine therapy should be continued. Liver function studies should be obtained initially and repeated at 24-hour intervals.

Serious toxicity or fatalities are extremely infrequent in children, possibly due to differences in the way they metabolize acetaminophen. In children, the maximum potential amount ingested can be more easily estimated. If more than 150 mg/kg or an unknown amount was ingested, obtain an plasma acetaminophen level. The plasma acetaminophen level should be obtained as soon as possible, but no sooner than 4 hours following the ingestion. If plasma level falls above the lower treatment line on the acetaminophen overdose nomogram, the acetylcysteine therapy should be initiated and continued for a full course of therapy. If plasma acetaminophen assay capability is not available, and the estimated acetaminophen ingestion exceeds 150 mg/kg, acetylcysteine therapy should be initiated and continued for a full course of therapy.

For additional emergency information, call your regional poison center or call the Rocky Mountain Poison Center toll-free, (1-800-525-6115).

Symptoms from pseudoephedrine overdose consist most often of mild anxiety, tachycardia and/or mild hypertension. Symptoms usually appear within 4 to 8 hours of ingestion and are transient, usually requiring no treatment.

Alcohol Information: Chronic heavy alcohol abusers may be at increased risk of liver toxicity from excessive acetaminophen use, although reports of this event are rare. Reports almost invariably involve cases of severe chronic alcoholics and the dosages of acetaminophen most often exceed recommended doses and often involve substantial overdose. Professionals should alert their patients who regularly consume large amounts of alcohol not to exceed recommended doses of acetaminophen.

Inactive Ingredients: Gelcaps: Benzyl Alcohol, Butylparaben, Castor Oil, Cellulose, Corn Starch, Edetate Calcium Disodium, Gelatin, Hydroxypropyl Methylcellulose, Iron Oxide Black, Magnesium Stearate, Methylparaben, Propylparaben, Sodium Lauryl Sulfate, Sodium Propionate, Sodium Starch Glycolate, Titanium Dioxide, FD&C Red #40.
Caplets: Cellulose, Corn Starch, Hydroxypropyl Methylcellulose, Magnesium Stearate, Polyethylene Glycol, Sodium Starch Glycolate, Titanium Dioxide, Blue #1 and Red #40.
Tablets: Cellulose, Corn Starch, Magnesium Stearate and Sodium Starch Glycolate.

How Supplied: Gelcaps (colored red and white imprinted "SINE-AID")—blister package of 20 and tamper resistant bottle of 40.
Caplets (colored white imprinted "Maximum SINE-AID")—blister package of 24 and tamper resistant bottle of 50.
Tablets (colored white embossed "Sine-Aid")—blister package of 24 and tamper resistant bottle of 50.
Shown in Product Identification Guide, page 512

CHILDREN'S TYLENOL®   OTC
acetaminophen
Chewable Tablets, Elixir, Drops
Suspension Liquid, Drops

Description: Infants' TYLENOL acetaminophen Drops are stable, alcohol-free, fruit-flavored and orange in color. Infants' TYLENOL Suspension Drops are alcohol-free, grape-flavored and purple in color. Each 0.8 ml (one calibrated dropperful) contains 80 mg acetaminophen. Children's TYLENOL Elixir is stable and alcohol-free, cherry-flavored, and red in color or grape-flavored, and purple in color. Children's TYLENOL Suspension Liquid is alcohol-free, cherry-flavored, and red in color or bubble gum flavored, and pink in color. Each 5 ml con-

Continued on next page

McNeil Consumer—Cont.

tains 160 mg acetaminophen. Each Children's TYLENOL Chewable Tablet contains 80 mg acetaminophen in a grape, fruit, or bubble gum flavored tablet.

Actions: Acetaminophen is a clinically proven analgesic/antipyretic. Acetaminophen produces analgesia by elevation of the pain threshold and antipyresis through action on the hypothalamic heat regulating center. Acetaminophen is equal to aspirin in analgesic and antipyretic effectiveness and it is unlikely to produce many of the side effects associated with aspirin and aspirin containing products.

Indications: Children's TYLENOL Chewable Tablets, Elixir, Drops, Suspension Liquid and Suspension Drops are designed for treatment of infants and children with conditions requiring temporary relief of fever and discomfort due to colds and "flu," and of simple pain and discomfort due to teething, immunizations and tonsillectomy.

Precautions: If a rare sensitivity reaction occurs, the drug should be discontinued.

Directions: All dosages may be repeated every 4 hours, but not more than 5 times daily. Administer to children under 2 years only on the advice of a physician. Children's TYLENOL Chewable Tablets: 2–3 years: two tablets, 4–5 years: three tablets, 6–8 years: four tablets, 9–10 years: five tablets, 11–12 years: six tablets.
Children's TYLENOL Elixir and Suspension Liquid: (special cup for measuring dosage is provided) 4–11 months: one-half teaspoon, 12–23 months: three-quarters teaspoon, 2–3 years: one teaspoon, 4–5 years: one and one-half teaspoons, 6–8 years: 2 teaspoons, 9–10 years: two and one-half teaspoons, 11–12 years: three teaspoons.
Infants' TYLENOL Drops and Suspension Drops: 0–3 months: 0.4 ml. 4–11 months: 0.8 ml, 12–23 months: 1.2 ml, 2–3 years: 1.6 ml, 4–5 years: 2.4 ml.

Warning: Keep this and all medication out of reach of children. In case of accidental overdosage, contact a physician or poison control center immediately. Prompt medical attention is critical for adults as well as for children even if you do not notice any signs or symptoms. Consult your physician if fever persists for more than 3 days or if pain continues for more than 5 days. Do not use with other products containing acetaminophen. Store at room temperature.
NOTE: In addition to the above:
Infants' TYLENOL® Drops and Suspension Drops—Do not use if printed carton overwrap or printed plastic bottle wrap is broken or missing or if carton is opened.
Children's TYLENOL Elixir and Suspension Liquid—Do not use if printed carton overwrap is broken or missing or if car-

ton is opened. Do not use if printed plastic bottle wrap or printed foil inner seal is broken. Not a USP elixir.
Children's TYLENOL Chewables—Do not use if carton is opened or if printed plastic bottle wrap or printed foil inner seal is broken. Phenylketonurics: contains phenylalanine 3 mg per tablet.

Overdosage Information: Acetaminophen in massive overdosage may cause hepatic toxicity in some patients. In adults and adolescents, hepatic toxicity has rarely been reported following ingestion of acute overdoses of less than 10 grams. Fatalities are infrequent (less than 3–4% of untreated cases) and have rarely been reported with overdoses of less than 15 grams. In children, an acute overdosage of less than 150 mg/kg has not been associated with hepatic toxicity. Early symptoms following a potentially hepatotoxic overdose may include: nausea, vomiting, diaphoresis and general malaise. Clinical and laboratory evidence of hepatic toxicity may not be apparent until 48 to 72 hours postingestion. In adults and adolescents, regardless of the quantity of acetaminophen reported to have been ingested, administer acetylcysteine immediately if 24 hours or less have elapsed from the reported time of ingestion. For full prescribing information, refer to the acetylcysteine package insert. Do not await results of assays for plasma acetaminophen level before initiating treatment with acetylcysteine. The following additional procedures are recommended: The stomach should be emptied promptly by lavage or by induction of emesis with syrup of ipecac. A plasma acetaminophen assay should be obtained as early as possible, but no sooner than four hours following ingestion. If plasma level falls above the lower treatment line on the acetaminophen overdose nomogram, acetylcysteine therapy should be continued. Liver function studies should be obtained initially and repeated at 24-hour intervals.
Serious toxicity or fatalities are extremely infrequent in children, possibly due to differences in the way they metabolize acetaminophen. In children, the maximum potential amount ingested can be more easily estimated. If more than 150 mg/kg or an unknown amount was ingested, obtain a plasma acetaminophen level. The plasma acetaminophen level should be obtained as soon as possible, but no sooner than 4 hours following the ingestion. If plasma level falls above the lower treatment line on the acetaminophen overdose nomogram, the acetylcysteine therapy should be initiated and continued for a full course of therapy. If plasma acetaminophen assay capability is not available, and the estimated acetaminophen ingestion exceeds 150 mg/kg, acetylcysteine therapy should be initiated and continued for a full course of therapy.
For additional emergency information, call your regional poison center or call the Rocky Mountain Poison Center toll free, (1-800-525-6115).

Inactive Ingredients: Children's TYLENOL Fruit Flavored Chewable Tablets—Aspartame, Cellulose, Citric Acid, Cornstarch, Ethylcellulose, Flavors, Magnesium Stearate, mannitol, and Red #7.
Children's TYLENOL Grape Flavored Chewable Tablets-Aspartame, Cellulose, Cellulose Acetate, Citric Acid, Cornstarch, Flavors, Magnesium Stearate, Mannitol, Povidone. Blue #1, Red #7, and Red #30.
Children's TYLENOL Bubble Gum Flavored Chewable Tablets-Aspartame, Cellulose, Cellulose Acetate, Cornstarch, Flavors, Magnesium Stearate, Mannitol, Povidone and red #7.
Children's TYLENOL Elixir—Benzoic Acid, Citric Acid, Flavors, Glycerin, Polyethylene Glycol, Propylene Glycol, Sodium Benzoate, Sorbitol, Sucrose, Purified Water, Red #40. In addition to the above ingredients cherry flavored elixir contains Red #33 and grape flavored elixir contains malic acid and Blue #1.
Children's TYLENOL Suspension Liquid—Butylparaben, Cellulose, Citric Acid, Corn Syrup, Flavors, Glycerin, Propylene Glycol, Purified Water, Sodium Benzoate, Sorbitol, Xanthan Gum, FD&C Red #40. In addition to the above ingredients bubble gum flavored suspension contains D&C Red #33.
Infant's TYLENOL Drops—Butylparaben, Citric Acid, Flavors, Glycerin, Polyethylene Glycol, Propylene Glycol, Saccharin, Sodium Citrate, Purified water and Yellow #6.
Infant's TYLENOL Suspension Drops—Butylparaben, Cellulose, Citric Acid, Corn Syrup, Flavors, Glycerin, Propylene Glycol, Purified Water, Sodium Benzoate, Sorbitol, Xanthan Gum, D&C Red #33 and D&C Blue #1.

How Supplied: Chewable Tablets (pink colored fruit, purple colored grape, pink colored bubble gum, scored, imprinted "TYLENOL")—Bottles of 30 and child resistant blister packs of 48 (fruit only). Elixir (cherry colored red and grape colored purple). Suspension liquid (cherry flavored colored red)—bottles of 2 and 4 fl. oz. (bubble gum flavored colored pink)—bottle of 4 fl. oz. Drops (colored orange)—bottles of ½ oz. (15 ml) and 1 oz. (30 ml) with calibrated plastic dropper. Suspension drops (grape flavored colored purple)—bottles of ½ oz (15 ml) with calibrated plastic dropper. All packages listed above have child-resistant safety caps.
Shown in Product Identification Guide, page 512

CHILDREN'S TYLENOL COLD®OTC
Multi Symptom Chewable Tablets and Liquid

Description: Each CHILDREN'S TYLENOL COLD Multi Symptom Chewable Grape-Flavored Tablet contains acetaminophen 80 mg, chlorpheniramine maleate 0.5 mg and pseudoephedrine hydrochloride 7.5 mg. CHILDREN'S TYLE-

NOL COLD Multi Symptom Liquid is grape flavored and contains no alcohol. Each teaspoon (5 ml) contains acetaminophen 160 mg, chlorpheniramine maleate 1 mg, and pseudoephedrine hydrochloride 15 mg.

Actions: CHILDREN'S TYLENOL COLD Multi Symptom Chewable Tablets and Liquid combine the analgesic-antipyretic acetaminophen with the decongestant pseudoephedrine hydrochloride and the antihistamine chlorpheniramine maleate to help relieve nasal congestion, dry runny noses and prevent sneezing as well as to relieve the fever, aches, pains and general discomfort associated with colds and upper respiratory infections. Acetaminophen is equal to aspirin in analgesic and antipyretic effectiveness and it is unlikely to produce the side effects often associated with aspirin or aspirin-containing products.

Indications: Provides fast, effective temporary relief of nasal congestion, runny nose, sore throat, sneezing, minor aches and pains, headaches and fever due to the common cold, hay fever or other upper respiratory allergies.

Precautions: If a rare sensitivity reaction occurs, the drug should be discontinued.

Directions: All doses may be repeated every 4–6 hours, not to exceed 4 doses in 24 hours.
Administer to children under 6 years only on the advice of a physician. Children's Tylenol Cold Chewable Tablets: 2–5 years—2 tablets: 6–11 years—4 tablets.
Children's Tylenol Cold Liquid Formula: 2–5 years—1 teaspoonful; 6–11 years—2 teaspoonful. Measuring cup is provided and marked for accurate dosing.

Warning: KEEP THIS AND ALL MEDICATION OUT OF THE REACH OF CHILDREN. IN CASE OF ACCIDENTAL OVERDOSAGE, CONTACT A PHYSICIAN OR POISON CONTROL CENTER IMMEDIATELY. PROMPT MEDICAL ATTENTION IS CRITICAL FOR ADULTS AS WELL AS FOR CHILDREN EVEN IF YOU DO NOT NOTICE ANY SIGNS OR SYMPTOMS. Do not exceed recommended dosage because at higher doses nervousness, dizziness or sleeplessness may occur. Do not give this product to children for more than 7 days. If fever persists for more than 3 days, or if symptoms do not improve or new ones occur within 5 days or are accompanied by fever, consult a physician before continuing use. If sore throat is severe, persists for more than 2 days, is accompanied or followed by fever, headache, rash, nausea or vomiting, consult a physician promptly. May cause excitability especially in children. Do not give this product to children who have a breathing problem such as chronic bronchitis, or who have glaucoma, heart disease, high blood pressure, thyroid disease or diabetes without first consulting the

child's physician. May cause drowsiness. Sedatives and tranquilizers may increase the drowsiness effect. Do not give this product to children who are taking sedatives or tranquilizers, without first consulting the child's physician. Do not use with other products containing acetaminophen.
NOTE: In addition to the above:
Children's TYLENOL COLD Chewables—DO NOT USE IF CARTON IS OPENED, OR IF PRINTED NECK WRAP OR PRINTED FOIL INNER SEAL IS BROKEN. PHENYLKETONURICS: CONTAINS PHENYLALANINE 4 MG PER TABLET.
Children's TYLENOL COLD Liquid—DO NOT USE IF CARTON IS OPENED, OR IF PRINTED PLASTIC BOTTLE WRAP OR PRINTED FOIL INNER SEAL IS BROKEN.

Drug Interaction Precaution: Do not give this product to a child who is taking a prescription drug for high blood pressure or depression without first consulting the child's physician.

Overdosage Information: Acetaminophen in massive overdosage may cause hepatic toxicity in some patients. In adults and adolescents, hepatic toxicity has rarely been reported following ingestion of acute overdosage of less than 10 grams. Fatalities are infrequent (less than 3–4% of untreated cases) and have rarely been reported with overdoses of less than 15 grams. In children, an acute overdosage of less than 150 mg/kg has not been associated with hepatic toxicity. Early symptoms following a potentially hepatotoxic overdose may include: nausea, vomiting, diaphoresis and general malaise. Clinical and laboratory evidence of hepatic toxicity may not be apparent until 48 to 72 hours postingestion. In adults and adolescents, regardless of the quantity of acetaminophen reported to have been ingested, administer acetylcysteine immediately if 24 hours or less have elapsed from the reported time of ingestion. For full prescribing information, refer to the acetylcysteine package insert. Do not await the results of assays for plasma acetaminophen level before initiating treatment with acetylcysteine. The following additional procedures are recommended: The stomach should be emptied promptly by lavage or by induction of emesis with syrup of ipecac. A plasma acetaminophen assay should be obtained as early as possible, but no sooner than four hours following ingestion. If plasma level falls above the lower treatment line on the acetaminophen overdose nomogram, acetylcysteine therapy should be continued. Liver function studies should be obtained initially and repeated at 24-hour intervals.
Serious toxicity or fatalities are extremely infrequent in children, possibly due to differences in the way they metabolize acetaminophen. In children, the maximum potential amount ingested can be more easily estimated. If more than 150 mg/kg or an unknown amount was ingested, obtain an plasma acetami-

nophen level. The plasma acetaminophen level should be obtained as soon as possible, but no sooner than 4 hours following the ingestion. If the plasma level falls above the lower treatment line on the acetaminophen overdose nomogram, the acetylcysteine therapy should be initiated and continued for a full course of therapy. If plasma acetaminophen assay capability is not available, and the estimated acetaminophen ingestion exceeds 150 mg/kg, acetylcysteine therapy should be initiated and continued for a full course of therapy.
For additional emergency information, call your regional poison center or call the Rocky Mountain Poison Center toll-free, (1-800-525-6115).
Chlorpheniramine toxicity should be treated as you would an antihistamine/anticholinergic overdose and is likely to be present within a few hours after acute ingestion.
Symptoms from pseudoephedrine overdose consist most often of mild anxiety, tachycardia and/or mild hypertension. Symptoms usually appear within 4 to 8 hours of ingestion and are transient, usually requiring no treatment.

Inactive Ingredients: Chewable Tablets—Aspartame, citric acid, ethylcellulose, flavors, magnesium stearate, mannitol, microcrystalline cellulose, pregelatinized starch, sucrose, Blue #1 and Red #7.
Liquid—Benzoic acid, citric acid, flavors, glycerin, malic acid, polyethylene glycol, propylene glycol, sodium benzoate, sorbitol, sucrose, purified water, Blue #1 and Red #40.

How Supplied: Chewable Tablets (colored purple, scored, imprinted "Tylenol Cold" on one side and "TC" on opposite side)—bottles of 24. Liquid (colored purple)—bottles of 4 fl. oz.
Shown in Product Identification Guide, page 512

CHILDREN'S TYLENOL® COLD PLUS COUGH OTC
Multi Symptom Chewable Tablets and Liquid

Description: Each CHILDREN'S TYLENOL COLD Multi Symptom PLUS COUGH Chewable Cherry-Flavored Tablet contains:
acetaminophen 80 mg
chlorpheniramine maleate 0.5 mg
dextromethorphan hydrobromide 2.5 mg
pseudoephedrine hydrochloride 7.5 mg
CHILDREN'S TYLENOL COLD Multi Symptom PLUS COUGH Liquid is cherry flavored and contains no alcohol. Each teaspoon (5 ml) contains acetaminophen 160 mg, chlorpheniramine maleate 1 mg, dextromethorphan hydrobromide 5 mg and pseudoephedrine hydrochloride 15 mg.

Actions: CHILDREN'S TYLENOL COLD Multi Symptom PLUS COUGH

Continued on next page

McNeil Consumer—Cont.

Chewable Tablets and Liquid combines the analgesic-antipyretic acetaminophen with the decongestant pseudoephedrine hydrochloride, the cough suppressant dextromethorphan hydrobromide, and the antihistamine chlorpheniramine maleate to help relieve coughs, nasal congestion, and sore throat, dry runny noses, and prevent sneezing as well as to relieve the fever, aches, pains and general discomfort associated with colds and upper respiratory infections.

Acetaminophen is equal to aspirin in analgesic and antipyretic effectiveness and it is unlikely to produce the side effects often associated with aspirin or aspirin-containing products.

Indications: Provides fast, effective temporary relief of coughs, nasal congestion, runny nose, sore throat, sneezing, minor aches and pains, headaches and fever due to the common cold, hay fever or other upper respiratory allergies.

Precaution: If a rare sensitivity reaction occurs, the drug should be discontinued.

Directions: All doses may be repeated every 4–6 hours, not to exceed 4 doses in 24 hours.

Administer to children under 6 years only on the advice of a physician.

Children's Tylenol Cold Plus Cough Chewable Tablets: 2–5 years—2 tablets, 6–11 years—4 tablets.

Children's Tylenol Cold Plus Cough Liquid Formula: 2–5 years—1 teaspoonful, 6–11 years—2 teaspoonfuls. Measuring cup is provided and marked for accurate dosing.

Warning: KEEP THIS AND ALL MEDICATION OUT OF THE REACH OF CHILDREN. IN CASE OF ACCIDENTAL OVERDOSAGE, CONTACT A PHYSICIAN OR POISON CONTROL CENTER IMMEDIATELY. PROMPT MEDICAL ATTENTION IS CRITICAL FOR ADULTS AS WELL AS FOR CHILDREN EVEN IF YOU DO NOT NOTICE ANY SIGNS OR SYMPTOMS. Do not exceed recommended dosage because at higher doses nervousness, dizziness or sleeplessness may occur. Do not give this product to children for more than 7 days. If fever persists for more than 3 days, or if symptoms do not improve or new ones occur within 5 days or are accompanied by fever, consult a physician before continuing use. If sore throat is severe, persists for more than 2 days, is accompanied or followed by fever, headache, rash, nausea or vomiting, consult physician promptly. May cause excitability especially in children. Do not give this product to children who have a breathing problem such as chronic bronchitis, or who have glaucoma, heart disease, high blood pressure, thyroid disease or diabetes without first consulting the child's physician.

May cause drowsiness. Sedatives and tranquilizers may increase the drowsiness effect. Do not give this product to children who are taking sedatives or tranquilizers, without first consulting the child's physician. A persistent cough may be a sign of a serious condition. If cough persists for more than 1 week, tends to recur, or is accompanied by fever, rash or persistent headache, consult a physician. Do not give this product for persistent or chronic cough such as occurs with asthma or if cough is accompanied by excessive phlegm (mucus) unless directed by a physician. Do not use with other products containing acetaminophen.
NOTE: In addition to the above:
Chewable Tablets—DO NOT USE IF CARTON IS OPENED, OR IF PRINTED NECK WRAP OR PRINTED FOIL INNER SEAL IS BROKEN. PHENYLKETONURICS: CONTAINS PHENYLALANINE 4 MG PER TABLET.
Liquid—DO NOT USE IF CARTON IS OPENED, OR IF PRINTED PLASTIC BOTTLE WRAP OR PRINTED FOIL INNER SEAL IS BROKEN.

Drug Interaction Precaution: Do not give this product to a child who is taking a prescription drug for high blood pressure or to a child who is taking a prescription monoamine oxidase inhibitor (MAOI) (certain drugs for depression, psychiatric or emotional conditions), or for 2 weeks after stopping the MAOI drug. If you are uncertain whether your child's prescription drug contains an MAOI, consult a health professional before giving this product.

Overdosage Information: Acetaminophen in massive overdosage may cause hepatic toxicity in some patients. In adults and adolescents, hepatic toxicity has rarely been reported following ingestion of acute overdoses of less than 10 grams. Fatalities are infrequent (less than 3–4% of untreated cases) and have rarely been reported with overdoses of less than 15 grams. In children, an acute overdosage of less than 150 mg/kg has not been associated with hepatic toxicity. Early symptoms following a potentially hepatotoxic overdose may include: nausea, vomiting, diaphoresis and general malaise. Clinical and laboratory evidence of hepatic toxicity may not be apparent until 48 to 72 hours postingestion. In adults and adolescents, regardless of the quantity of acetaminophen reported to have been ingested, administer acetylcysteine immediately if 24 hours or less have elapsed from the reported time of ingestion. For full prescribing information, refer to the acetylcysteine package insert. Do not await the results of assays for plasma acetaminophen level before initiating treatment with acetylcysteine. The following additional procedures are recommended: The stomach should be emptied promptly by lavage or by induction of emesis with syrup of ipecac. A plasma acetaminophen assay should be obtained as early as possible, but no

sooner than four hours following ingestion. If plasma level falls above the lower treatment line on the acetaminophen overdose nomogram, acetylcysteine therapy should be continued. Liver function studies should be obtained initially and repeated at 24-hour intervals.

Serious toxicity or fatalities are extremely infrequent in children, possibly due to differences in the way they metabolize acetaminophen. In children, the maximum potential amount ingested can be more easily estimated. If more than 150 mg/kg or an unknown amount was ingested, obtain an plasma acetaminophen level. The plasma acetaminophen level should be obtained as soon as possible, but no sooner than 4 hours following the ingestion. If plasma level falls above the lower treatment line on the acetaminophen overdose nomogram, the acetylcysteine therapy should be initiated and continued for a full course of therapy. If plasma acetaminophen assay capability is not available, and the estimated acetaminophen ingestion exceeds 150 mg/kg, acetylcysteine therapy should be initiated and continued for a full course of therapy.

For additional emergency information, call your regional poison center or call the Rocky Mountain Poison Center toll-free, (1-800-525-6115).

Chlorpheniramine toxicity should be treated as you would an antihistamine/anticholinergic overdose and is likely to be present within a few hours after acute ingestion.

Symptoms from pseudoephedrine overdose consist most often of mild anxiety, tachycardia and/or mild hypertension. Symptoms usually appear within 4 to 8 hours of ingestion and are transient, usually requiring no treatment.

Acute dextromethorphan overdose usually does not result in serious signs and symptoms unless massive amounts have been ingested. Signs and symptoms of a substantial overdose may include nausea and vomiting, visual disturbances, CNS disturbances, and urinary retention.

Inactive Ingredients: Chewable Tablets—Aspartame, Basic Polymethacrylate, Cellulose Acetate, Colloidal Silicon Dioxide, Flavors, Hydroxypropyl Methylcellulose, Mannitol, Microcrystalline Cellulose, Stearic Acid and Red #7.
Liquid-Citric Acid, Corn Syrup, Flavors, Polyethylene Glycol, Propylene Glycol, Sodium Benzoate, Sodium Carboxymethylcellulose, Sorbitol, Purified Water, Red #33 and Red #40.

How Supplied: Chewable Tablets (colored pink, imprinted "TYLENOL C/C" on one side and "TC/C" on the opposite side)—bottles of 24.
Liquid Formula—(red colored) bottles of 4 fl. oz.

Shown in Product Identification Guide, page 513

TYLENOL® OTC
Cold Multi-Symptom
Hot Medication Liquid
Packets

Description: Each packet of TYLENOL Cold Multi-Symptom Hot Medication contains acetaminophen 650 mg, chlorpheniramine maleate 4 mg, pseudoephedrine hydrochloride 60 mg and dextromethorphan hydrobromide 30 mg.

Actions: TYLENOL Cold Multi-Symptom Hot Medication contains a clinically proven analgesic-antipyretic, decongestant, cough suppressant and antihistamine. Acetaminophen produces analgesia by elevation of the pain threshold and antipyresis through action on the hypothalamic heat-regulating center. Acetaminophen is equal to aspirin in analgesic and antipyretic effectiveness and it is unlikely to produce many of the side effects associated with aspirin and aspirin-containing products. Pseudoephedrine hydrochloride is a sympathomimetic amine which provides temporary relief of nasal congestion. Dextromethorphan is a cough suppressant which provides temporary relief of coughs due to minor throat irritations that may occur with the common cold. Chlorpheniramine is an antihistamine which helps provide temporary relief of runny nose, sneezing and watery and itchy eyes.

Indications: TYLENOL Cold Multi-Symptom Hot Medication provides effective temporary relief of runny nose, sneezing, watery and itchy eyes, nasal congestion, coughing, and body aches, pains, headache, sore throat and fever due to a cold or "flu."

Precautions: If a rare sensitivity reaction occurs, the drug should be discontinued. Although pseudoephedrine is virtually without pressor effect in normotensive patients, it should be used with caution in hypertensives.

Directions: Adults (12 years and older): Dissolve one packet in 6 oz. cup of hot water. Sip while hot. Sweeten to taste, if desired. May repeat every 6 hours, not to exceed 4 doses in 24 hours. Not for use in children under 12 years of age.

Warnings: Do not take this product for more than 7 days or for fever for more than 3 days unless directed by a doctor. If symptoms do not improve or are accompanied by fever, consult a doctor. If sore throat is severe, persists for more than 2 days, is accompanied or followed by fever, headache, rash, nausea or vomiting, consult a doctor promptly. A persistent cough may be a sign of a serious condition. If cough persists for more than 1 week, tends to recur or is accompanied by fever, rash or persistent headache, consult a doctor. Do not take this product for persistent or chronic cough such as occurs with smoking, asthma, emphysema or if cough is accompanied by excessive phlegm (mucus) unless directed by a doctor. Do not exceed recommended dosage because at higher doses, nervousness, dizziness or sleeplessness my occur. May cause excitability especially in children. Do not take this product, unless directed by a doctor, if you have a breathing problem such as emphysema or chronic bronchitis, or if you have glaucoma or difficulty in urination due to enlargement of the prostate gland. Do not take this product if you have heart disease, high blood pressure, thyroid disease or diabetes unless directed by a doctor. May cause drowsiness; alcohol, sedatives and tranquilizers may increase the drowsiness effect. Avoid alcoholic beverages while taking this product. Do not take this product if you are taking sedatives or tranquilizers without first consulting your doctor. Use caution when driving a motor vehicle or operating machinery. Do not use with other products containing acetaminophen.

DO NOT USE IF PRINTED CARTON OVERWRAP IS BROKEN OR MISSING OR IF FOIL PACKET IS TORN OR BROKEN. KEEP THIS AND ALL MEDICATION OUT OF THE REACH OF CHILDREN. AS WITH ANY DRUG, IF YOU ARE PREGNANT OR NURSING A BABY, SEEK THE ADVICE OF A HEALTH PROFESSIONAL BEFORE USING THIS PRODUCT. IN CASE OF ACCIDENTAL OVERDOSE, CONTACT A DOCTOR OR POISON CONTROL CENTER IMMEDIATELY. PROMPT MEDICAL ATTENTION IS CRITICAL FOR ADULTS AS WELL AS FOR CHILDREN EVEN IF YOU DO NOT NOTICE ANY SIGNS OR SYMPTOMS.

PHENYLKETONURICS: CONTAINS PHENYLALANINE 11 MG PER PACKET.

Alcohol Warning: If you generally consume 3 or more alcohol-containing drinks per day, you should consult your physician for advice on when and how you should take TYLENOL® Cold Multi-Symptom Hot Medication Liquid and other pain relievers.

Drug Interaction Precaution: Do not take this product if you are presently taking a prescription drug for high blood pressure or you are now taking a prescription monoamine oxidase inhibitor (MAOI) (certain drugs for depression, psychiatric or emotional conditions, or Parkinson's disease), or for 2 weeks after stopping the MAOI drug. If you are uncertain whether your prescription drug contains an MAOI, consult a health professional before taking this product.

Overdosage Information: Acetaminophen in massive overdosage may cause hepatic toxicity in some patients. In adults and adolescents, hepatic toxicity has rarely been reported following ingestion of acute overdoses of less than 10 grams. Fatalities are infrequent (less than 3–4% of untreated cases) and have rarely been reported with overdoses of less than 15 grams. In children, an acute overdosage of less than 150 mg/kg has not been associated with hepatic toxicity. Early symptoms following a potentially hepatotoxic overdose may include: nausea, vomiting, diaphoresis and general malaise. Clinical and laboratory evidence of hepatic toxicity may not be apparent until 48 to 72 hours postingestion. In adults and adolescents, regardless of the quantity of acetaminophen reported to have been ingested, administer acetylcysteine immediately if 24 hours or less have elapsed from the reported time of ingestion. For full prescribing information, refer to the acetylcysteine package insert. Do not await results of assays for plasma acetaminophen level before initiating treatment with acetylcysteine. The following additional procedures are recommended: The stomach should be emptied promptly by lavage or by induction of emesis with syrup of ipecac. A plasma acetaminophen assay should be obtained as early as possible, but no sooner than four hours following ingestion. If plasma level falls above the lower treatment line on acetaminophen overdose nomogram, acetylcysteine therapy should be continued. Liver function studies should be obtained initially and repeated at 24-hour intervals.

Serious toxicity or fatalities are extremely infrequent in children, possibly due to differences in the way they metabolize acetaminophen. In children, the maximum potential amount ingested can be more easily estimated. If more than 150 mg/kg or an unknown amount was ingested, obtain an acetaminophen level. The plasma acetaminophen level should be obtained as soon as possible, but no sooner than 4 hours following the ingestion. If plasma level falls above the lower treatment line on the acetaminophen overdose nomogram, the acetylcysteine therapy should be initiated and continued for a full course of therapy. If plasma acetaminophen assay capability is not available, and the estimated acetaminophen ingestion exceeds 150 mg/kg, acetylcysteine therapy should be initiated and continued for a full course of therapy.

For additional emergency information, call your regional poison center or call the Rocky Mountain Poison Center toll-free, (1-800-525-6115).

Symptoms from pseudoephedrine overdose consist most often of mild anxiety, tachycardia and/or mild hypertension. Symptoms usually appear within 4 to 8 hours of ingestion and are transient, usually requiring no treatment.

Acute dextromethorphan overdose usually does not result in serious signs and symptoms unless massive amounts have been ingested. Signs and symptoms of a substantial overdose may include nausea and vomiting, visual disturbances, CNS disturbances, and urinary retention.

Chlorpheniramine toxicity should be treated as you would an antihistamine/anticholinergic overdose and is likely to be present within a few hours after acute ingestion.

Alcohol Information: Chronic heavy alcohol abusers may be at increased risk

Continued on next page

McNeil Consumer—Cont.

of liver toxicity from excessive acetaminophen use, although reports of this event are rare. Reports almost invariably involve cases of severe chronic alcoholics and the dosages of acetaminophen most often exceed recommended doses and often involve substantial overdose. Professionals should alert their patients who regularly consume large amounts of alcohol not to exceed recommended doses of acetaminophen.

Inactive Ingredients: Aspartame, Citric Acid, Corn Starch, Sodium Citrate, Sucrose, Red #40 and Yellow #10.

How Supplied: Packets of powder (yellow colored) in cartons of 6 tamper-resistant foil packets.
Shown in Product Identification Guide, page 513

TYLENOL® Extended Relief acetaminophen extended release Caplets

Description: Each TYLENOL Extended Relief Caplet contains acetaminophen 650 mg.

Actions: Acetaminophen is a clinically proven analgesic and antipyretic. Acetaminophen produces analgesia by elevation of the pain threshold and antipyresis through action on the hypothalamic heat-regulating center. Acetaminophen is equal to aspirin in analgesic and antipyretic effectiveness and it is unlikely to produce many of the side effects associated with aspirin and aspirin-containing products. Tylenol Extended Relief uses a unique, patented bilayer caplet. The first layer dissolves quickly to provide prompt relief while the second layer is time released to provide up to 8 hours of relief.

Indications: For the temporary relief of minor aches and pains associated with the common cold, headache, toothache, muscular aches, back ache, for the minor pain of arthritis, for the pain of menstrual cramps and for the reduction of fever.

Precautions: If a rare sensitivity reaction occurs, the drug should be discontinued.

Directions: Adults and Children 12 years of Age and Older: Take two caplets every 8 hours, not to exceed 6 caplets in any 24-hour period. TAKE TWO CAPLETS WITH WATER, SWALLOW EACH CAPLET WHOLE. DO NOT CRUSH, CHEW, OR DISSOLVE THE CAPLET. Not for use in children under 12 years of age.

Warnings: DO NOT USE IF CARTON IS OPENED OR PRINTED RED NECK WRAP OR PRINTED FOIL INNER SEAL IS BROKEN. DO NOT TAKE FOR PAIN FOR MORE THAN 10 DAYS OR FOR FEVER FOR MORE THAN 3 DAYS UNLESS DIRECTED BY A PHYSICIAN. IF PAIN OR FEVER PERSISTS, OR GETS WORSE, IF NEW SYMPTOMS OCCUR, OR IF REDNESS OR SWELLING IS PRESENT, CONSULT A PHYSICIAN BECAUSE THESE COULD BE SIGNS OF A SERIOUS CONDITION. AS WITH ANY DRUG, IF YOU ARE PREGNANT OR NURSING A BABY, SEEK THE ADVICE OF A HEALTH PROFESSIONAL BEFORE USING THIS PRODUCT. KEEP THIS AND ALL DRUGS OUT OF THE REACH OF CHILDREN. IN CASE OF ACCIDENTAL OVERDOSE, CONTACT A PHYSICIAN OR POISON CONTROL CENTER IMMEDIATELY. PROMPT MEDICAL ATTENTION IS CRITICAL FOR ADULTS AS WELL AS FOR CHILDREN EVEN IF YOU DO NOT NOTICE ANY SIGNS OR SYMPTOMS. DO NOT USE WITH OTHER PRODUCTS CONTAINING ACETAMINOPHEN.

Alcohol Warning: If you generally consume 3 or more alcohol-containing drinks per day, you should consult your physician for advice on when and how you should take TYLENOL® Extended Relief and other pain relievers.

Overdosage Information: Acetaminophen in massive overdosage may cause hepatic toxicity in some patients. In adults and adolescents, hepatic toxicity has rarely been reported following ingestion of acute overdoses of less than 10 grams. Fatalities are infrequent (less than 3–4% of untreated cases) and have rarely been reported with overdoses of less than 15 grams. In children, an acute overdosage of less than 150 mg/kg has not been associated with hepatic toxicity. Early symptoms following a potentially hepatotoxic overdose may include: nausea, vomiting, diaphoresis and general malaise. Clinical and laboratory evidence of hepatic toxicity may not be apparent until 48 to 72 hours postingestion. In adults and adolescents, regardless of the quantity of acetaminophen reported to have been ingested, administer acetylcysteine immediately if 24 hours or less have elapsed from the reported time of ingestion. For full prescribing information, refer to the acetylcysteine package insert. Do not await results of assays for plasma acetaminophen level before initiating treatment with acetylcysteine. The following additional procedures are recommended. The stomach should be emptied promptly by lavage or by induction of emesis with syrup of ipecac. A plasma acetaminophen assay should be obtained as early as possible, but no sooner than four hours following ingestion. If an acetaminophen extended release product is involved, it may be appropriate to obtain an additional plasma acetaminophen level 4–6 hours following the initial plasma acetaminophen level. If either plasma level falls above the lower treatment line on the acetaminophen overdose nomogram, acetylcysteine therapy should be continued. Liver function studies should be obtained initially and repeated at 24-hour intervals.

Serious toxicity or fatalities are extremely infrequent in children, possibly due to differences in the way they metabolize acetaminophen. In children, the maximum potential amount ingested can be more easily estimated. If more than 150 mg/kg or an unknown amount was ingested, obtain a plasma acetaminophen level. The plasma level should be obtained as soon as possible, but no sooner than 4 hours following the ingestion. If an acetaminophen extended release product is involved, it may be appropriate to obtain and additional plasma acetaminophen level 4–6 hours following the initial plasma acetaminophen level. If either plasma level falls above the lower treatment line on the acetaminophen overdose nomogram, the acetylcysteine therapy should be initiated and continued for a full course of therapy. If plasma acetaminophen assay capability is not available, and the estimated acetaminophen ingestion exceeds 150 mg/kg, acetylcysteine therapy should be initiated and continued for a full course of therapy.

For additional emergency information, call your regional poison center or call the Rocky Mountain Poison Center toll-free (1-800-525-6115).

Alcohol Information: Chronic heavy alcohol abusers may be at increased risk of liver toxicity from excessive acetaminophen use, although reports of this event are rare. Reports almost invariably involve cases of severe chronic alcoholics and the dosages of acetaminophen most often exceed recommended doses and often involve substantial overdose. Professionals should alert their patients who regularly consume large amounts of alcohol not to exceed recommended doses of acetaminophen.

Inactive Ingredients: Corn Starch, Hydroxyethyl Cellulose, Hydroxypropyl Methylcellulose, Magnesium Stearate, Microcrystalline Cellulose, Povidone, Powdered Cellulose, Pregelatinized Starch, Sodium Starch Glycolate, Titanium Dioxide, Triacetin.

How Supplied: Caplets (colored white, engraved "TYLENOL ER") tamper-resistant bottles of 24, 50, and 100's.
Shown in Product Identification Guide, page 513

Extra-Strength TYLENOL® acetaminophen Adult Liquid Pain Reliever   OTC

Description: Each 15 ml (½ fl oz or one tablespoonful) of Extra-Strength TYLENOL® acetaminophen Adult Liquid Pain Reliever contains 500 mg. acetaminophen (alcohol 7%).

Actions: Acetaminophen is a clinically proven analgesic and antipyretic. Acetaminophen produces analgesia by elevation of the pain threshold and antipyresis through action on the hypothalamic heat-regulating center. Acetaminophen is equal to aspirin in analgesic and antipyretic effectiveness and it is unlikely to produce many of the side effects associated with aspirin and aspirin-containing products. Tylenol Extended Relief uses a unique, patented bilayer caplet. The first layer dissolves quickly to provide prompt relief while the second layer is time released to provide up to 8 hours of relief.

Indications: For the temporary relief of minor aches and pains associated with the common cold, headache, toothache, muscular aches, back ache, for the minor pain of arthritis, for the pain of menstrual cramps and for the reduction of fever.

Precautions: If a rare sensitivity reaction occurs, the drug should be discontinued.

Directions: Adults and Children 12 years of Age and Older: Fill measuring cup once to 2-tablespoon line (1,000 mg) which is equivalent to two 500 mg Extra Strength TYLENOL® Caplets or Tablets. Take every 4–6 hours. No more than 4 doses in any 24-hour period, or as directed by a doctor. Not for use in children under 12 years of age.

Warnings: DO NOT USE IF CARTON IS OPENED OR PRINTED RED NECK WRAP OR PRINTED FOIL INNER SEAL IS BROKEN. DO NOT TAKE FOR PAIN FOR MORE THAN 10 DAYS OR FOR FEVER FOR MORE THAN 3 DAYS UNLESS DIRECTED BY PHYSICIAN. IF PAIN OR FEVER PERSISTS, OR GETS WORSE, IF NEW SYMPTOMS OCCUR, OR IF REDNESS OR SWELLING IS PRESENT, CONSULT A PHYSICIAN BECAUSE THESE COULD BE SIGNS OF A SERIOUS CONDITION. AS WITH ANY DRUG, IF YOU ARE PREGNANT OR NURSING A BABY, SEEK THE ADVICE OF A HEALTH PROFESSIONAL BEFORE USING THIS PRODUCT. KEEP THIS AND ALL DRUGS OUT OF THE REACH OF CHILDREN. IN CASE OF ACCIDENTAL OVERDOSE, CONTACT A PHYSICIAN OR POISON CONTROL CENTER IMMEDIATELY. PROMPT MEDICAL ATTENTION IS CRITICAL FOR ADULTS AS WELL AS FOR CHILDREN EVEN IF YOU DO NOT NOTICE ANY SIGNS OR SYMPTOMS. DO NOT USE WITH OTHER PRODUCTS CONTAINING ACETAMINOPHEN.

Alcohol Warning: If you generally consume 3 or more alcohol-containing drinks per day, you should consult your physician for advice on when and how you should take Extra Strength TYLENOL® Liquid and other pain relievers.

Overdosage Information: Acetaminophen in massive overdosage may cause hepatic toxicity in some patients. In adults and adolescents, hepatic toxicity has rarely been reported following ingestion of acute overdoses of less than 10 grams. Fatalities are infrequent (less than 3–4% of untreated cases) and have rarely been reported with overdoses of less than 15 grams. In children, an acute overdosage of less than 150 mg/kg has not been associated with hepatic toxicity. Early symptoms following a potentially hepatotoxic overdose may include: nausea, vomiting, diaphoresis and general malaise. Clinical and laboratory evidence of hepatic toxicity may not be apparent until 48 to 72 hours postingestion. In adults and adolescents, regardless of the quantity of acetaminophen reported to have been ingested, administer acetylcysteine immediately if 24 hours or less have elapsed from the reported time of ingestion. For full prescribing information, refer to the acetylcysteine package insert. Do not await the results of assays for plasma acetaminophen level before initiating treatment with acetylcysteine. The following additional procedures are recommended: The stomach should be emptied promptly by lavage or by induction of emesis with syrup of ipecac. A plasma acetaminophen assay should be obtained as early as possible, but no sooner than four hours following ingestion. If plasma level falls above the lower treatment line on the acetaminophen overdose nomogram, acetylcysteine therapy should be continued. Liver function studies should be obtained initially and repeated at 24-hour intervals.

Serious toxicity or fatalities are extremely infrequent in children, possibly due to differences in the way they metabolize acetaminophen. In children, the maximum potential amount ingested can be more easily estimated. If more than 150 mg/kg or an unknown amount was ingested, obtain a plasma acetaminophen level. The plasma acetaminophen level should be obtained as soon as possible, but no sooner than 4 hours following the ingestion. If plasma level falls above the lower treatment line on the acetaminophen overdose nomogram, the acetylcysteine therapy should be initiated and continued for a full course of therapy. If plasma acetaminophen assay capability is not available, and the estimated acetaminophen ingestion exceeds 150 mg/kg, acetylcysteine therapy should be initiated and continued for a full course of therapy.

For additional emergency information, call your regional poison center or call the Rocky Mountain Poison Center toll-free (1-800-525-6115).

Alcohol Information: Chronic heavy alcohol abusers may be at increased risk of liver toxicity from excessive acetaminophen use, although reports of this event are rare. Reports almost invariably involve cases of severe chronic alcoholics and the dosages of acetaminophen most often exceed recommended doses and often involve substantial overdose. Professionals should alert their patients who regularly consume large amounts of alcohol not to exceed recommended doses of acetaminophen.

Inactive Ingredients: Alcohol (7%), Citric Acid, Flavors, Glycerin, Polyethylene Glycol, Purified Water, Sodium Benzoate, Sorbitol, Sucrose, Yellow #6 (Sunset Yellow), Yellow #10 and Blue #1.

How Supplied: Mint-flavored liquid (colored green), 8 fl. oz. tamper-resistant bottle with child resistant safety cap and special dosage cup.

EXTRA STRENGTH TYLENOL®   OTC
Headache Plus
Pain Reliever with Antacid Caplets

Description: Each Extra Strength TYLENOL® Headache Plus Pain Reliever with Antacid caplet contains acetaminophen 500 mg. and calcium carbonate 250 mg.

Actions: TYLENOL® Headache Plus contains a clinically proven analgesic and antacid. Acetaminophen produces analgesia by elevation of the pain threshold. Acetaminophen is equal to aspirin in analgesic effectiveness, and it is unlikely to produce many of the side effects associated with aspirin and aspirin-containing products. The antacid, calcium carbonate, provides fast relief of heartburn or acid indigestion and upset stomach associated with these symptoms.

Indications: TYLENOL® Headache Plus provides temporary relief of minor aches and pains with heartburn or acid indigestion and upset stomach associated with these symptoms.

Directions: Adults and children 12 years of age and older: Two caplets every 6 hours. No more than a total of 8 caplets in any 24 hour period or as directed by a physician. Not for use in children under 12 years of age.

Precautions: If a rare sensitivity reaction occurs, the drug should be stopped.

Warnings: Do not use the maximum dosage of this product for more than 10 days except under the advice and supervision of a physician. Do not take the product for pain for more than 10 days, or for fever for more than 3 days unless directed by a physician. If pain or fever persists or gets worse, if new symptoms occur, or if redness or swelling is present, consult a physician because these could be signs of a serious condition. Do not use with other products containing acetaminophen. DO NOT USE IF CARTON IS OPENED, OR IF PRINTED NECK WRAP OR PRINTED FOIL SEAL IS BROKEN. KEEP THIS AND ALL MEDICATION OUT OF THE REACH OF CHILDREN. AS WITH ANY DRUG, IF YOU ARE PREGNANT OR NURSING A BABY, SEEK THE ADVICE OF A HEALTH PROFESSIONAL BEFORE USING THIS PRODUCT. IN THE CASE OF ACCIDENTAL OVERDOSE, CONTACT A DOCTOR OR A POISON CONTROL CENTER IMMEDIATELY. PROMPT MEDICAL ATTENTION IS CRITICAL FOR ADULTS AS WELL AS FOR CHILDREN EVEN IF

Continued on next page

McNeil Consumer—Cont.

YOU DO NOT NOTICE ANY SIGNS OR SYMPTOMS.

Alcohol Warning: If you generally consume 3 or more alcohol-containing drinks per day, you should consult your physician for advice on when and how you should take Extra Strength TYLENOL® Headache Plus and other pain relievers.

Drug Interaction Precaution: Antacids may interact with certain prescription drugs. If you are presently taking a prescription drug, do not take this product without checking with your physician or other health professional.

Overdosage Information: Acetaminophen in massive overdosage may cause hepatic toxicity in some patients. In adults and adolescents, hepatic toxicity has rarely been reported following ingestion of acute overdosage of less than 10 grams. Fatalities are infrequent (less than 3–4% of untreated cases) and have rarely been reported with overdoses of less than 15 grams. In children, an acute overdosage of less than 150 mg/kg has not been associated with hepatic toxicity. Early symptoms following a potentially hepatotoxic overdose may include: nausea, vomiting, diaphoresis and general malaise. Clinical and laboratory evidence of hepatic toxicity may not be apparent until 48 to 72 hours postingestion. In adults and adolescents, regardless of the quantity of acetaminophen reported to have been ingested, administer acetylcysteine immediately if 24 hours or less have elapsed from the reported time of ingestion. For full prescribing information, refer to the acetylcysteine package insert. Do not await results of assays for plasma acetaminophen level before initiating treatment with acetylcysteine. The following additional procedures are recommended. The stomach should be emptied promptly by lavage or by induction of emesis with syrup of ipecac. A plasma acetaminophen assay should be obtained as early as possible, but no sooner than four hours following ingestion. If plasma level falls above the lower treatment line on the acetaminophen overdose nomogram, acetylcysteine therapy should be continued. Liver function studies should be obtained initially and repeated at 24-hour intervals. Serious toxicity or fatalities are extremely infrequent in children, possibly due to differences in the way they metabolize acetaminophen. In children, the maximum potential amount ingested can be more easily estimated. If more than 150 mg/kg or an unknown amount was ingested, obtain a plasma acetaminophen level. The plasma acetaminophen level should be obtained as soon as possible, but no sooner than 4 hours following the ingestion. If the plasma level falls above the lower treatment line on the acetaminophen overdose nomogram, the acetylcysteine therapy should be initiated and continued for a full course of therapy. If plasma acetaminophen, assay capability is not available, and the estimated acetaminophen ingestion exceeds 150 mg/kg, acetylcysteine therapy should be initiated and continued for a full course of therapy.

For additional emergency information, call your regional poison center or call the Rocky Mountain Poison Center toll-free (1-800-525-6115).

Alcohol Information: Chronic heavy alcohol abusers may be at increased risk of liver toxicity from excessive acetaminophen use, although reports of this event are rare. Reports almost invariably involve cases of severe chronic alcoholics and the dosages of acetaminophen most often exceed recommended doses and often involve substantial overdose. Professionals should alert their patients who regularly consume large amounts of alcohol not to exceed recommended doses of acetaminophen.

Inactive Ingredients: Acacia, Cellulose, Corn Starch, Croscarmellose Sodium, Hydroxypropyl Methylcellulose, Magnesium Stearate, Maltodextrin, Propylene Glycol, Sodium Starch Glycolate, Titanium Dioxide, Triacetin, Blue #1 and Blue #2.

How Supplied: Caplets (white with royal blue imprinted "TYLENOL Headache Plus"). Tamper resistant bottles of 24 and 50.

Shown in Product Identification Guide, page 514

EXTRA STRENGTH TYLENOL® PM   OTC
Pain Reliever/Sleep Aid Gelcaps, Caplets and Geltabs

Description: Each EXTRA STRENGTH TYLENOL® PM Gelcap, Caplet or Geltab contains acetaminophen 500 mg and diphenhydramine HCl 25 mg.

Actions: EXTRA STRENGTH TYLENOL® PM Gelcaps, Caplets and Geltabs contain a clinically proven analgesic-antipyretic and an antihistamine. Maximum allowable non-prescription levels of acetaminophen and diphenhydramine provide temporary relief of occasional headaches and minor aches and pains accompanying sleeplessness. Acetaminophen is equal to aspirin in analgesic and antipyretic effectiveness and it is unlikely to produce many of the side effects associated with aspirin containing products. Acetaminophen produces analgesia by elevation of the pain threshold. Diphenhydramine HCl is an antihistamine with sedative properties.

Indications: EXTRA STRENGTH TYLENOL® PM Gelcaps, Caplets and Geltabs provide temporary relief of occasional headaches and minor aches and pains with accompanying sleeplessness.

Precautions: If a rare sensitivity reaction occurs, the drug should be discontinued.

Directions: Adults and Children 12 years of Age and Older: Two gelcaps, caplets or geltabs at bedtime or as directed by physician. Do not exceed recommended dosage. Not for use in children under 12 years of age.

Warnings: Do not use for more than 10 days unless directed by a physician. Consult your physician if symptoms persist or new ones occur, or if fever persists for more than 3 days, or if sleeplessness persists continuously for more than 2 weeks. Insomnia may be a symptom of serious underlying medical illness. Do not take this product, unless directed by a doctor, if you have a breathing problem such as emphysema or chronic bronchitis, or if you have glaucoma or difficulty in urination due to enlargement of the prostate gland. Avoid alcoholic beverages while taking this product. Do not take if you are taking sedatives or tranquilizers without first consulting your physician. **DO NOT USE IF CARTON IS OPEN OR IF PRINTED NECK WRAP OR PRINTED FOIL INNER SEAL IS BROKEN. KEEP THIS AND ALL MEDICATIONS OUT OF THE REACH OF CHILDREN. IN CASE OF ACCIDENTAL OVERDOSE, CONTACT A PHYSICIAN OR POISON CONTROL CENTER IMMEDIATELY. PROMPT MEDICAL ATTENTION IS CRITICAL FOR ADULTS AS WELL AS FOR CHILDREN EVEN IF YOU DO NOT NOTICE ANY SIGNS OR SYMPTOMS. AS WITH ANY DRUG, IF YOU ARE PREGNANT OR NURSING A BABY, SEEK THE ADVISE OF A HEALTH PROFESSIONAL BEFORE USING THIS PRODUCT. DO NOT USE WITH OTHER PRODUCTS CONTAINING ACETAMINOPHEN.**

Alcohol Warning: If you generally consume 3 or more alcohol-containing drinks per day, you should consult your physician for advice on when and how you should take Extra Strength TYLENOL® PM and other pain relievers.

Caution: This product will cause drowsiness. Do not drive a motor vehicle or operate machinery after use.

Overdosage Information: Acetaminophen in massive overdosage may cause hepatic toxicity in some patients. In adults and adolescents, hepatic toxicity has rarely been reported following ingestion of acute overdoses of less than 10 grams. Fatalities are infrequent (less than 3–4% of untreated cases) and have rarely been reported with overdoses of less than 15 grams. In children, an acute overdosage of less than 150 mg/kg has not been associated with hepatic toxicity. Early symptoms following a potentially hepatotoxic overdose may include: nausea, vomiting, diaphoresis and general malaise. Clinical and laboratory evidence of hepatic toxicity may not be apparent until 48 to 72 hours postingestion. In adults and adolescents, regardless of the quantity of acetaminophen reported to have been ingested, administer acetylcysteine immediately if 24 hours or less have elapsed from the reported time of ingestion. For full prescribing information, refer to the acetylcysteine package insert. Do not await results of assays for plasma acetaminophen level before initiating treatment with acetylcysteine. The following additional procedures are recommended. The stomach should be emptied promptly by lavage or by induction of emesis with syrup of ipecac. A plasma acetaminophen assay should be obtained as early as possible, but no sooner than four hours following ingestion. If plasma level falls above the lower treatment line on the acetaminophen overdose nomogram, acetylcysteine therapy should be continued. Liver function studies should be obtained initially and repeated at 24-hour intervals.

Serious toxicity or fatalities are extremely infrequent in children, possibly due to differences in the way they metabolize acetaminophen. In children, the maximum potential amount ingested can be more easily estimated. If more than 150 mg/kg or an unknown amount was ingested, obtain a plasma acetaminophen level. The plasma acetaminophen level should be obtained as soon as possible, but no sooner than 4 hours following the ingestion. If the plasma level falls above the lower treatment line on the acetaminophen overdose nomogram, the acetylcysteine therapy should be initiated and continued for a full course of therapy. If plasma acetaminophen assay capability is not available, and the estimated acetaminophen ingestion exceeds 150 mg/kg, acetylcysteine therapy should be initiated and continued for a full course of therapy.

For additional emergency information, call your regional poison center or call the Rocky Mountain Poison Center toll-free, (1-800-525-6115).

Diphenhydramine toxicity should be treated as you would an antihistamine/anticholinergic overdose and is likely to be present within a few hours after acute ingestion.

Alcohol Information: Chronic heavy alcohol abusers may be at increased risk of liver toxicity from excessive acetaminophen use, although reports of this event are rare. Reports almost invariably involve cases of severe chronic alcoholics and the dosages of acetaminophen most often exceed recommended doses and often involve substantial overdose. Professionals should alert their patients who regularly consume large amounts of alcohol not to exceed recommended doses of acetaminophen.

Inactive Ingredients: Geltabs/Gelcaps: Benzyl Alcohol, Butylparaben, Castor Oil, Cellulose, Cornstarch, Edetate Calcium Disodium, Gelatin, Hydroxypropyl Methylcellulose, Magnesium Stearate, Propylparaben, Sodium Lauryl Sulfate, Sodium Citrate, Sodium Propionate, Sodium Starch Glycolate, Titanium Dioxide, Blue #1 and Red #28.
Caplets: Cellulose, Cornstarch, Hydroxypropyl Methylcellulose, Magnesium Stearate or Stearic Acid and Colloidal Silicon Dioxide, Polyethylene Glycol, Polysorbate 80, Sodium Citrate, Sodium Starch Glycolate, Titanium Dioxide, Blue #1 and Blue #2.

How Supplied: Geltabs/Gelcaps (colored blue and white imprinted "TYLENOL PM") tamper-resistant bottles of 24, 50, and 100.
Caplets (colored light blue imprinted "Tylenol PM") tamper-resistant bottles of 24, 50, and 100.

Shown in Product Identification Guide, page 514

Extra Strength   OTC
TYLENOL® acetaminophen
Gelcaps, Geltabs; Caplets, Tablets

Description: Each Extra Strength TYLENOL Gelcap, Geltabs, Caplet, or Tablet contains acetaminophen 500 mg.

Actions: Acetaminophen is a clinically proven analgesic and antipyretic. Acetaminophen produces analgesia by elevation of the pain threshold and antipyresis through action on the hypothalamic heat-regulating center. Acetaminophen is equal to aspirin in analgesic and antipyretic effectiveness and it is unlikely to produce many of the side effects associated with aspirin and aspirin-containing products.

Indications: For the temporary relief of minor aches and pains associated with the common cold, headache, toothache, muscular aches, back ache, for the minor pain of arthritis, for the pain of menstrual cramps and for the reduction of fever.

Precautions: If a rare sensitivity reaction occurs, the drug should be discontinued.

Directions: Adults and Children 12 years of Age and Older: Take two gelcaps, geltabs, caplets, or tablets every 4 to 6 hours. Not to exceed 8 gelcaps, geltabs, caplets, or tablets in any 24-hour period. Not for use in children under 12 years of age.

Warnings: DO NOT USE IF CARTON IS OPENED OR PRINTED RED NECK WRAP OR PRINTED FOIL INNER SEAL IS BROKEN. DO NOT TAKE FOR PAIN FOR MORE THAN 10 DAYS OR FOR FEVER FOR MORE THAN 3 DAYS UNLESS DIRECTED BY A PHYSICIAN. IF PAIN OR FEVER PERSISTS, OR GETS WORSE, IF NEW SYMPTOMS OCCUR, OR IF REDNESS OR SWELLING IS PRESENT, CONSULT A PHYSICIAN BECAUSE THESE COULD BE SIGNS OF A SERIOUS CONDITION. AS WITH ANY DRUG, IF YOU ARE PREGNANT OR NURSING A BABY, SEEK THE ADVICE OF A HEALTH PROFESSIONAL BEFORE USING THIS PRODUCT. KEEP THIS AND ALL DRUGS OUT OF THE REACH OF CHILDREN. IN CASE OF ACCIDENTAL OVERDOSE, CONTACT A PHYSICIAN OR POISON CONTROL CENTER IMMEDIATELY. PROMPT MEDICAL ATTENTION IS CRITICAL FOR ADULTS AS WELL AS FOR CHILDREN EVEN IF YOU DO NOT NOTICE ANY SIGNS OR SYMPTOMS. DO NOT USE WITH OTHER PRODUCTS CONTAINING ACETAMINOPHEN.

Alcohol Warning: If you generally consume 3 or more alcohol-containing drinks per day, you should consult your physician for advice on when and how you should take Extra Strength TYLENOL® and other pain relievers.

Overdosage Information: Acetaminophen in massive overdosage may cause hepatic toxicity in some patients. In adults and adolescents, hepatic toxicity has rarely been reported following ingestion of acute overdoses of less than 10 grams. Fatalities are infrequent (less than 3–4% of untreated cases) and have rarely been reported with overdoses of less than 15 grams. In children, an acute overdosage of less than 150 mg/kg has not been associated with hepatic toxicity. Early symptoms following a potentially hepatotoxic overdose may include: nausea, vomiting, diaphoresis and general malaise. Clinical and laboratory evidence of hepatic toxicity may not be apparent until 48 to 72 hours postingestion. In adults and adolescents, regardless of the quantity of acetaminophen reported to have been ingested, administer acetylcysteine immediately if 24 hours or less have elapsed from the reported time of ingestion. For full prescribing information, refer to the acetylcysteine package insert. Do not await results of assays for plasma acetaminophen level before initiating treatment with acetylcysteine. The following additional procedures are recommended: The stomach should be emptied promptly by lavage or by induction of emesis with syrup of ipecac. A plasma acetaminophen assay should be obtained as early as possible, but no sooner than four hours following ingestion. If plasma level falls above the lower treatment line on the acetaminophen overdose nomogram, acetylcysteine therapy should be continued. Liver function studies should be obtained initially and repeated at 24-hour intervals.

Serious toxicity or fatalities are extremely infrequent in children, possibly due to differences in the way they metabolize acetaminophen. In children, the maximum potential amount ingested can be more easily estimated. If more than 150 mg/kg or an unknown amount was ingested, obtain a plasma acetaminophen level. The plasma acetaminophen level should be obtained as soon as possible, but no sooner than 4 hours following the ingestion. If plasma level falls above the lower treatment line on the acetaminophen overdose nomogram, the acetylcysteine therapy should be initiated and continued for a full course of therapy. If plasma acetaminophen assay capability is not available, and the esti-

Continued on next page

McNeil Consumer—Cont.

mated acetaminophen ingestion exceeds 150 mg/kg, acetylcysteine therapy should be initiated and continued for a full course of therapy.

For additional emergency information, call your regional poison center or call the Rocky Mountain Poison Center toll-free, (1-800-525-6115).

Alcohol Information: Chronic heavy alcohol abusers may be at increased risk of liver toxicity from excessive acetaminophen use, although reports of this event are rare. Reports almost invariably involve cases of severe chronic alcoholics and the dosages of acetaminophen most often exceed recommended doses and often involve substantial overdose. Professionals should alert their patients who regularly consume large amounts of alcohol not to exceed recommended doses of acetaminophen.

Inactive Ingredients: Tablets—Magnesium Stearate, Cellulose, Sodium Starch Glycolate and Starch.
Caplets—Cellulose, Cornstarch, Hydroxypropyl Methylcellulose, Magnesium Stearate, Polyethylene Glycol, Sodium Starch Glycolate, and Red #40.
Gelcaps—Benzyl Alcohol, Butylparaben, Castor Oil, Cellulose, Edetate Calcium Disodium, Gelatin, Hydroxypropyl Methylcellulose, Magnesium Stearate, Methylparaben, Propylparaben, Sodium Lauryl Sulfate, Sodium Propionate, Sodium Starch Glycolate, Starch, Titanium Dioxide, Blue #1 and #2, Red #40 and Yellow #10.
Geltabs—Benzyl Alcohol, Butylparaben, Castor Oil, Cellulose, Corn Starch, Edetate Calcium Disodium, Gelatin, Hydroxypropyl Methylcellulose, Magnesium Stearate, Methylparaben, Propylparaben, Sodium Lauryl Sulfate, Sodium Propionate, Sodium Starch Glycolate, Titanium Dioxide, Blue #1 and #2, Red #40, and Yellow #10.

How Supplied: Tablets (colored white, imprinted "TYLENOL" and "500")—vials of 10 and tamper-resistant bottles of 30, 60, 100, and 200. Caplets (colored white, imprinted "TYLENOL 500 mg")—vials of 10 and tamper-resistant bottles of 24, 50, 100, 175, and 250's. Gelcaps (colored yellow and red, imprinted "Tylenol 500") tamper-resistant bottles of 24, 50, 100, and 150 and Fast Cap Package of 72. Geltabs (colored yellow and red, imprinted "Tylenol 500") tamper-resistant bottles of 24, 50, and 100. For adults who prefer liquids or can't swallow solid medication, Extra-Strength TYLENOL® Adult Liquid Pain Reliever, mint flavored, is also available (colored green; 1 fl. oz. = 1000 mg.).

Shown in Product Identification Guide, page 513

Junior Strength TYLENOL® OTC
acetaminophen
Coated Caplets and Chewable Tablets

Description: Each Junior Strength Tylenol Coated Caplet or Chewable tablet contains 160 mg acetaminophen in a small, coated, capsule shaped tablet or grape or fruit chewable tablet.

Actions: Acetaminophen is a clinically proven analgesic/antipyretic. Acetaminophen produces analgesia by elevation of the pain threshold and antipyresis through action on the hypothalamic heat-regulating center. Acetaminophen is equal to aspirin in analgesic and antipyretic effectiveness and it is unlikely to produce many of the side effects associated with aspirin and aspirin-containing products.

Indications: Junior Strength TYLENOL Caplets are designed for easy swallowability in older children and young adults. Both Junior Strength TYLENOL Caplets and Junior Strength Chewable Tablets provide fast, effective temporary relief of fever and discomfort due to colds and "flu," and pain and discomfort due to simple headaches, minor muscle aches, sprains and overexertion.

Precautions: If a rare sensitivity reaction occurs, the drug should be stopped.

Directions: Caplets should be taken with liquid. Chewable tablets should be well chewed. All dosages may be repeated every 4 hours, but not more than 5 times daily. For ages: 6–8 years: two caplets or tablets, 9–10 years: two and one-half caplets or tablets, 11 years: three caplets or tablets, 12 years: four caplets or tablets.

Warning: **Do not use if carton is opened or if a blister unit is broken.** Keep this and all medications out of the reach of children. In case of accidental overdosage, contact a physician or poison control center immediately. Prompt medical attention is critical for adults as well as for children even if you do not notice any signs or symptoms. Consult your physician if fever persists for more than three days or if pain continues for more than five days. Do not use with other products containing acetaminophen. As with any drug, if you are pregnant or nursing a baby, seek the advice of a health professional before using this product. In addition the caplet package states: Not for children who have difficulty swallowing tablets. In addition the chewable tablet package states: Phenylketonurics: contains phenylalanine 6 mg per tablet.

Overdosage Information: Acetaminophen in massive overdosage may cause hepatic toxicity in some patients. In adults and adolescents, hepatic toxicity has rarely been reported following ingestion of acute overdosage of less than 10 grams. Fatalities are infrequent (less than 3–4% of untreated cases) and have rarely been reported with overdoses of less than 15 grams. In children, an acute overdosage of less than 150 mg/kg has not been associated with hepatic toxicity. Early symptoms following a potentially hepatotoxic overdose may include: nausea, vomiting, diaphoresis and general malaise. Clinical and laboratory evidence of hepatic toxicity may not be apparent until 48 to 72 hours postingestion. In adults and adolescents, regardless of the quantity of acetaminophen reported to have been ingested, administer acetylcysteine immediately if 24 hours or less have elapsed from the reported time of ingestion. For full prescribing information, refer to the acetylcysteine package insert. Do not await results of assays for plasma acetaminophen level before initiating treatment with acetylcysteine. The following additional procedures are recommended. The stomach should be emptied promptly by lavage or by induction of emesis with syrup of ipecac. A plasma acetaminophen assay should be obtained as early as possible, but no sooner than four hours following ingestion. If plasma level falls above the lower treatment line on the acetaminophen overdose nomogram, acetylcysteine therapy should be continued. Liver function studies should be obtained initially and repeated at 24-hour intervals.

Serious toxicity or fatalities are extremely infrequent in children, possibly due to differences in the way they metabolize acetaminophen. In children, the maximum potential amount ingested can be more easily estimated. If more than 150 mg/kg or an unknown amount was ingested, obtain a plasma acetaminophen level. The plasma acetaminophen level should be obtained as soon as possible, but no sooner than 4 hours following the ingestion. If plasma level falls above the lower treatment line on the acetaminophen overdose nomogram, the acetylcysteine therapy should be initiated and continued for a full course of therapy. If plasma acetaminophen assay capability is not available, and the estimated acetaminophen ingestion exceeds 150 mg/kg, acetylcysteine therapy should be initiated and continued for a full course of therapy.

For additional emergency information, call your regional poison center or call the Rocky Mountain Poison Center toll-free (1-800-525-6115).

Inactive Ingredients: Junior Strength Caplets: Cellulose, Cornstarch, Ethylcellulose, Magnesium Stearate, Sodium Lauryl Sulfate, Sodium Starch Glycolate, Junior Strength Fruit Chewable Tablets: Aspartame, Cellulose, Citric acid, Cornstarch, Ethylcellulose, Flavors, Magnesium stearate, Mannitol, and Red #7.
Junior Strength Grape Flavored Chewable Tablets: Aspartame Cellulose, Cellulose Acetate, Citric Acid, Cornstarch, Flavors, Magnesium Stearate, Mannitol, Povidone, Blue #1, Red #7 and Red #30.

How Supplied: Coated Caplets, (colored white, coated, scored, imprinted "TYLENOL 160") Package of 30. Chewable tablets (colored purple or pink, imprinted "TYLENOL 160") Package of 24. All packages are safety sealed and use child resistant blister packaging.

Shown in Product Identification Guide, page 512

Maximum-Strength   **OTC**
TYLENOL® Allergy Sinus
Medication Caplets, Gelcaps

Description: Each Maximum Strength TYLENOL® Allergy Sinus Caplet or Gelcap contains acetaminophen 500 mg, chlorpheniramine maleate 2 mg, and pseudoephedrine hydrochloride 30 mg.

Actions: Maximum Strength TYLENOL® Allergy Sinus Caplets or Gelcaps contain a clinically proven analgesic-antipyretic, decongestant, and antihistamine. Acetaminophen produces analgesia by elevation of the pain threshold and antipyresis through action on the hypothalamic heat-regulating center. Acetaminophen is equal to aspirin in analgesic and antipyretic effectiveness, and is unlikely to produce many of the side effects associated with aspirin and aspirin-containing products. Pseudoephedrine hydrochloride is a sympathomimetic amine which provides temporary relief of nasal congestion. Chlorpheniramine is an antihistamine which helps provide temporary relief of runny nose, sneezing and watery and itchy eyes.

Indications: TYLENOL® Allergy Sinus provides effective temporary relief of these upper respiratory allergy, hay fever and sinusitis symptoms: sneezing, itchy, watery eyes, runny nose, itching of the nose or throat, nasal and sinus congestion and sinus pain and headaches.

Precautions: If a rare sensitivity reaction occurs, the drug should be stopped. Although pseudoephedrine is virtually without pressor effect in normotensive patients, it should be used with caution in hypertensives.

Directions: Adults and children 12 years of age and older: Two caplets or gelcaps every 6 hours, not to exceed 8 caplets or gelcaps in 24 hours. Not for use in children under 12 years of age.

Warnings: Do not exceed the recommended dosage because at higher doses, nervousness, dizziness or sleeplessness may occur. May cause excitability, especially in children. Do not take this product for more than 7 days. If symptoms do not improve or are accompanied by fever, consult a doctor. Do not take this product unless directed by a doctor, if you have a breathing problem such as emphysema or chronic bronchitis, or if you have glaucoma or difficulty in urination due to enlargement of the prostate gland. Do not take this product if you have heart disease, high blood pressure, thyroid disease or diabetes. May cause drowsiness; alcohol, sedatives and tranquilizers may increase the drowsiness effect. Avoid alcoholic beverages when taking this product. Do not take this product if you are taking sedatives or tranquilizers, without first consulting your doctor. Use caution when driving a motor vehicle or operating machinery. Do not use with other products containing acetaminophen. DO NOT USE IF CARTON IS OPEN OR IF GREEN NECK WRAP OR PRINTED FOIL INNER SEAL IS BROKEN. KEEP THIS AND ALL MEDICATION OUT OF THE REACH OF CHILDREN. AS WITH ANY DRUG, IF YOU ARE PREGNANT OR NURSING A BABY, SEEK THE ADVICE OF A HEALTH PROFESSIONAL BEFORE USING THIS PRODUCT. IN CASE OF ACCIDENTAL OVERDOSE, CONTACT A DOCTOR OR POISON CONTROL CENTER IMMEDIATELY. PROMPT MEDICAL ATTENTION IS CRITICAL FOR ADULTS AS WELL AS FOR CHILDREN EVEN IF YOU DO NOT NOTICE ANY SIGNS OR SYMPTOMS.

Alcohol Warning: If you generally consume 3 or more alcohol-containing drinks per day, you should consult your physician for advice on when and how you should take Maximum Strength TYLENOL Allergy Sinus Medication and other pain relievers.

Drug Interaction Precaution: Do not take this product if you are presently taking a prescription drug for high blood pressure or depression without first consulting your doctor.

Overdosage Information: Acetaminophen in massive overdosage may cause hepatic toxicity in some patients. In adults and adolescents, hepatic toxicity has rarely been reported following ingestion of acute overdoses of less than 10 grams. Fatalities are infrequent (less than 3–4% of untreated cases) and have rarely been reported with overdoses of less than 15 grams. In children, an acute overdosage of less than 150 mg/kg has not been associated with hepatic toxicity. Early symptoms following a potentially hepatotoxic overdose may include: nausea, vomiting, diaphoresis and general malaise. Clinical and laboratory evidence of hepatic toxicity may not be apparent until 48 to 72 hours postingestion. In adults and adolescents, regardless of the quantity of acetaminophen reported to have been ingested, administer acetylcysteine immediately if 24 hours or less have elapsed from the reported time of ingestion. For full prescribing information, refer to the acetylcysteine package insert. Do not await results of assays for plasma acetaminophen level before initiating treatment with acetylcysteine. The following additional procedures are recommended: The stomach should be emptied promptly by lavage or by induction of emesis with syrup of ipecac. A plasma acetaminophen assay should be obtained as early as possible, but no sooner than four hours following ingestion. If plasma level falls above the lower treatment line on the acetaminophen overdose nomogram, acetylcysteine therapy should be continued. Liver function studies should be obtained initially and repeated at 24-hour intervals.

Several toxicity or fatalities are extremely infrequent in children, possibly due to differences in the way they metabolize acetaminophen. In children, the maximum potential amount ingested can be easily estimated. If more than 150 mg/kg or an unknown amount was ingested, obtain a plasma acetaminophen level. The plasma acetaminophen level should be obtained as soon as possible, but no sooner than 4 hours following ingestion. If plasma level falls above the lower treatment line on the acetaminophen overdose nomogram, the acetylcysteine therapy should be initiated and continued for a full course of therapy. If plasma acetaminophen assay capability is not available, and the estimated acetaminophen ingestion exceeds 150 mg/kg, acetylcysteine therapy should be initiated and continued for a full course of therapy.

For additional emergency information, call your regional poison center or call the Rocky Mountain Poison Control Center toll-free, (1-800-525-6115).

Chlorpheniramine toxicity should be treated as you would an antihistamine/anticholinergic overdose and is likely to be present within a few hours after acute ingestion.

Symptoms from pseudophedrine overdose consist most often of mild anxiety, tachycardia and/or hypertension. Symptoms usually appear within 4 to 8 hours of ingestion and are transient, usually requiring no treatment.

Alcohol Information: Chronic heavy alcohol abusers may be at increased risk of liver toxicity from excessive acetaminophen use, although reports of this event are rare. Reports almost invariably involve cases of severe chronic alcoholics and the dosages of acetaminophen most often exceed recommended doses and often involve substantial overdose. Professionals should alert their patients who regularly consume large amounts of alcohol not to exceed recommended doses of acetaminophen.

Inactive Ingredients: Caplets: Cannuba Wax, Cellulose, Cornstarch, Hydroxypropyl Cellulose, Hydroxypropyl Methylcellulose, Iron Oxide Black, Magnesium Stearate, Polyethylene Glycol, Sodium Starch Glycolate, Titanium Dioxide, Blue #1, Yellow #6, Yellow #10. Gelcaps: Benzyl Alcohol, Butylparaben, Castor oil, Cellulose, Cornstarch, Edetate Calcium Disodium, Gelatin, Hydroxypropyl Methylcellulose, Magnesium Stearate, Methylparaben, Propylparaben, Sodium Lauryl Sulfate, Sodium Propionate, Sodium Starch Gly-

Continued on next page

McNeil Consumer—Cont.

colate, Titanium Dioxide, Blue #1 and #2 and Yellow #10.

How Supplied: Caplets: (dark yellow, imprinted "TYLENOL Allergy Sinus")—Blister packs of 24 and tamper-resistant bottles of 60.
Gelcaps: (dark green and dark yellow, imprinted "TYLENOL A/S")—Blister packs of 24 and tamper-resistant bottles of 60.

Shown in Product Identification Guide, page 513

MAXIMUM STRENGTH OTC TYLENOL® ALLERGY SINUS NIGHTTIME MEDICATION CAPLETS

Description: Each Maximum Strength TYLENOL® Allergy Sinus NightTime Caplet contains Acetaminophen 500mg, Pseudoephedrine Hydrochloride 30mg, and Diphenhydramine Hydrochloride 25mg.

Actions: Maximum Strength TYLENOL® Allergy Sinus NightTime Medication contains a clinically proven analgesic-antipyretic, decongestant, and antihistamine. Acetaminophen produces analgesia by elevation of the pain threshold and antipyresis through action on the hypothalamic heat-regulating center. Acetaminophen is equal to aspirin in analgesic and antipyretic effectiveness, and it is unlikely to produce many of the side effects associated with aspirin and aspirin-containing products. Pseudoephedrine Hydrochloride is a sympathomimetic amine which provides temporary relief of nasal congestion. Diphenhydramine Hydrochloride is an antihistamine with sedative properties which helps provide temporary relief of runny nose, sneezing and watery and itchy eyes.

Indications: TYLENOL® Allergy Sinus NightTime provides effective temporary relief of these upper respiratory allergy, hay fever and sinusitis symptoms: sneezing, itchy, watery eyes, runny nose, itching of the nose or throat, nasal and sinus congestion, and sinus pain and headaches.

Precautions: If a rare sensitivity reaction occurs, the drug should be stopped. Although psuedoephedrine is virtually without pressor effect in normotensive patients, it should be used with caution in hypertensives.

Directions: Adults and children 12 years of age and older: Two caplets at bedtime. Not for use in children under 12 years of age.

Warnings: Do not exceed the recommended dosage because nervousness, dizziness or sleeplessness may occur. Do not take this product for more than 7 days or for fever for more than 3 days unless directed by a doctor. If symptoms do not improve or are accompanied by fever, consult a doctor. May cause excitability, especially in children. Do not take this product, unless directed by a doctor, if you have a breathing problem such as emphysema or chronic bronchitis, or if you have glaucoma or difficulty in urination due to enlargement of the prostate gland. Do not take this product if you have heart disease, high blood pressure, thyroid disease or diabetes unless directed by a doctor. May cause marked drowsiness; alcohol, sedatives and tranquilizers may increase the drowsiness effect. Avoid alcoholic beverages while taking this product. Do not take this product if you are taking sedatives or tranquilizers, without first consulting your doctor. Use caution when driving a motor vehicle or operating machinery. Do not use with other products containing acetaminophen. **DO NOT USE IF CARTON IS OPEN OR IF A BLISTER UNIT IS BROKEN. KEEP THIS AND ALL MEDICATION OUT OF THE REACH OF CHILDREN. AS WITH ANY DRUG, IF YOU ARE PREGNANT OR NURSING A BABY, SEEK THE ADVICE OF A HEALTH PROFESSIONAL BEFORE USING THIS PRODUCT. IN CASE OF ACCIDENTAL OVERDOSE, CONTACT A DOCTOR OR POISON CONTROL CENTER IMMEDIATELY. PROMPT MEDICAL ATTENTION IS CRITICAL FOR ADULTS AS WELL AS FOR CHILDREN EVEN IF YOU DO NOT NOTICE ANY SIGNS OR SYMPTOMS.**

Alcohol Warning: If you generally consume 3 or more alcohol-containing drinks per day, you should consult your physician for advice on when and how you should take Maximum Strength TYLENOL® Allergy Sinus NightTime and other pain relievers.

Drug Interaction Precaution: Do not take this product if you are presently taking a prescription drug for high blood pressure or depression without first consulting your doctor.

Overdosage Information: Acetaminophen in massive overdosage may cause hepatic toxicity in some patients. In adults and adolescents, hepatic toxicity has rarely been reported following ingestion of acute overdose of less than 10 grams. Fatalities are infrequent (less than 3–4% of untreated cases) and have rarely been reported with overdoses of less than 15 grams. In children, an acute overdoses of less than 150 mg/kg has not been associated with hepatic toxicity. Early symptoms following a potentially hepatotoxic overdose may include: nausea, vomiting, diaphoresis and general malaise. Clinical and laboratory evidence of hepatic toxicity may not be apparent until 48 to 72 hours postingestion. In adults and adolescents, regardless of the quantity of acetaminophen reported to have been ingested, administer acetylcysteine immediately if 24 hours or less have elapsed from the reported time of ingestion. For full prescribing information, refer to the acetylcysteine package insert. Do not await results of assays for plasma acetaminophen level before initiating treatment with acetylcysteine. The following additional procedures are recommended: The stomach should be emptied promptly by lavage or by induction of emesis with syrup of ipecac. A plasma acetaminophen assay should be obtained as early as possible, but no sooner than four hours following ingestion. If plasma level falls above the lower treatment line on the acetaminophen overdose nomogram, acetylcysteine therapy should be continued. Liver function studies should be obtained initially and repeated at 24-hour intervals.

Serious toxicity or fatalities are extremely infrequent in children, possibly due to differences in the way they metabolize acetaminophen. In children, the maximum potential amount ingested can be more easily estimated. If more than 150 mg/kg or an unknown amount was ingested, obtain an plasma acetaminophen level. The plasma acetaminophen level should be obtained as soon as possible, but no sooner than 4 hours following ingestion. If plasma level falls above the lower treatment line on the acetaminophen overdose nomogram, the acetylcysteine therapy should be initiated and continued for a full course of therapy. If plasma acetaminophen assay capability is not available, and the estimated acetaminophen ingestion exceeds 150 mg/kg, acetylcysteine therapy should be initiated and continued for a full course of therapy.

For additional emergency information, call your regional poison control center or call the Rocky Mountain Poison Control Center toll-free, at (1-800-525-6115). Symptoms for pseudoephedrine overdose consist most often of mild anxiety, tachycardia and/or hypertension. Symptoms usually appear within 4 to 8 hours of ingestion and are transient, usually requiring no treatment.

Diphenhydramine toxicity should be treated as you would an antihistamine/anticholinergic overdose and is likely to be present within a few hours after acute ingestion.

Alcohol Information: Chronic heavy alcohol abusers may be at increased risk of liver toxicity from excessive acetaminophen use, although reports of this event are rare. Reports almost invariably involve cases of severe chronic alcoholics and the dosages of acetaminophen most often exceed recommended doses and often involve substantial overdose. Professionals should alert their patients who regularly consume large amounts of alcohol not to exceed recommended doses of acetaminophen.

Inactive Ingredients: Caplet: Cellulose, Corn Starch, Hydroxypropyl Methylcellulose, Iron Oxide Black, Magnesium Stearate, Polyethylene Glycol, Polysorbate 80, Sodium Citrate, Sodium Starch Glycolate, Titanium Dioxide, Blue #1, Yellow #10.

How Supplied: Caplets (light blue, imprinted "TYLENOL A/S Night Time")—Child-resistant blister packs of 24.

Shown in Product Identification Guide, page 513

MULTI-SYMPTOM TYLENOL®   OTC
COUGH MEDICATION WITH DECONGESTANT

Description: Each 15 ml (3 tsp.) adult dose contains dextromethorphan HBr 30 mg., acetaminophen 650mg, and pseudoephedrine HCl 60mg.

Actions: Multi-Symptom TYLENOL® COUGH Medication with Decongestant Liquid contains a clinically proven cough suppressant, an analgesic-antipyretic, and decongestant. Acetaminophen produces analgesia by elevation of the pain threshold and antipyresis through action on the hypothalamic heat-regulating center. Dextromethorphan is a cough suppressant which provides temporary relief of coughs due to minor throat irritations that may occur with the common cold. Pseudoephedrine hydrochloride is a sympathomimetic amine which provides temporary relief of nasal congestion.

Indications: Multi-Symptom TYLENOL® COUGH Medication with Decongestant provides effective, temporary relief of coughing, nasal congestion and the aches, pains and sore throat that may accompany a cough due to a cold.

Precautions: If a rare sensitivity reaction occurs, the drug should be discontinued. Although pseudoephedrine is virtually without pressor effect in normotensive patients, it should be used with caution in hypertensives.

Directions: Adults: (12 years and older): 1 tablespoon or 3 teaspoons every 6–8 hours, not to exceed 4 doses in 24 hours. Children: (ages 6–11) 1 1/2 teaspoons every 6–8 hours, not to exceed 4 doses in 24 hours. Not for use in children under 6 years of age.

Warning: Do not take this product for more than 7 days or for fever for more than 3 days unless directed by a doctor. If symptoms do not improve or are accompanied by fever, consult a doctor. A persistent cough may be a sign of a serious condition. If cough persists for more than 1 week, tends to recur or is accompanied by fever, rash or persistent headache, consult a doctor. Do not take this product for persistent or chronic cough such as occurs with smoking, asthma, emphysema, or if cough is accompanied by excessive phlegm (mucus) unless directed by a doctor. Do not exceed the recommended dosage because at higher doses nervousness, dizziness or sleeplessness may occur. Do not take this product if you have heart disease, high blood pressure, thyroid disease, diabetes or difficulty in urination due to enlargement of the prostate gland unless directed by a doctor. If sore throat is severe, persists for more than 2 days, is accompanied or followed by fever, headache, rash, nausea or vomiting, consult a doctor promptly. Do not use with other products containing acetaminophin.

DO NOT USE IF PRINTED PLASTIC BOTTLE WRAP OR PRINTED FOIL INNER SEAL IF BROKEN. Keep this and all medication out of the reach of children. As with any drug, if you are pregnant or nursing a baby, seek the advice of a health professional before using this product. In case of accidental overdosage, contact a doctor or poison control center immediately. Prompt medical attention is critical for adults as well as for children even if you do not notice any signs or symptoms.

Alcohol Warning: If you generally consume 3 or more alcohol-containing drinks per day, you should consult your physician for advice on when and how you should take Multi-Symptom TYLENOL® Cough Medication with Decongestant and other pain relievers.

Drug Interaction Precaution: Do not use this product if you are presently taking a prescription drug for high blood pressure or you are now taking a prescription monoamine oxidase inhibitor (MAOI) (certain drugs for depression, psychiatric or emotional conditions, or Parkinson's Disease), or for 2 weeks after stopping the MAOI drug. If you are uncertain whether your prescription drug contains an MAOI, consult a health professional before taking this product.

Overdosage Information: Acetaminophen in massive overdosage may cause hepatic toxicity in some patients. In adults and adolescents, hepatic toxicity has rarely been reported following ingestion of acute overdoses of less than 10 grams. Fatalities are infrequent (less than 3–4% of untreated cases) and have rarely been reported with overdoses of less than 15 grams. In children, an acute overdosage of less than 150mg/kg has not been associated with hepatic toxicity. Early symptoms following a potentially hepatotoxic overdose may include: nausea, vomiting, diaphoresis and general malaise. Clinical and laboratory evidence of hepatic toxicity may not be apparent until 48 to 72 hours postingestion. In adults and adolescents, regardless of the quantity of acetaminophen reported to have been ingested, administer acetylcysteine immediately if 24 hours or less have elapsed from the reported time of ingestion. For full prescribing information, refer to the acetylcysteine package insert. Do not await results of assays for acetaminophen level before initiating treatment with acetylcysteine. The following additional procedures are recommended: The stomach should be emptied by lavage or by induction of emesis with syrup of ipecac. A plasma acetaminophen assay should be obtained as early as possible, but no sooner than four hours following ingestion. If plasma level falls above the lower treatment line on the acetaminophen overdose nomogram, ace-

tylcysteine therapy should be continued. Liver function studies should be obtained initially and repeated at 24-hour intervals.

Serious toxicity or fatalities are extremely infrequent in children, possibly due to differences in the way they metabolize acetaminophen. In children, the maximum potential amount ingested can be more easily estimated. If more than 150 mg/kg or an unknown amount was ingested, obtain a plasma acetaminophen level. The plasma acetaminophen level should be obtained as soon as possible, but no sooner than 4 hours following the ingestion. If plasma level falls above the lower treatment line on the acetaminophen overdose nomogram, the acetylcysteine therapy should be initiated and continued for a full course of therapy. If plasma acetaminophen assay capability is not available, and the estimated acetaminophen ingestion exceeds 150 mg/kg, acetycysteine therapy should be initiated and continued for a full course of therapy.

For additional emergency information, call your regional poison center or call the Rocky Mountain Poison Center toll-free (1-800-526-6115).

Acute dextromethorphan overdose usually does not result in serious signs and symptoms unless massive amounts have been ingested. Signs and symptoms of a substantial overdose may include nausea and vomiting, visual disturbances, CNS disturbances, and urinary retention.

Symptoms from pseudoephedrine overdose consist most often of mild anxiety, tachycardia and/or mild hypertension. Symptoms usually appear within 4 to 8 hours of ingestion and are transient, usually requiring no treatment.

Alcohol Information: Chronic heavy alcohol abusers may be at increased risk of liver toxicity from excessive acetaminophen use, although reports of this event are rare. Reports almost invariably involve cases of severe chronic alcoholics and the dosages of acetaminophen most often exceed recommended doses and often involve substantial overdose. Professionals should alert their patients who regularly consume large amounts of alcohol not to exceed recommended doses of acetaminophen.

Inactive Ingredients: Alcohol (5%), Citric Acid, Flavors, High Fructose Corn Syrup, Polyethylene Glycol, Propylene Glycol, Purified Water, Sodium Benzoate, Sodium Carboxymethylcellulose, Sodium Saccharin, Sorbitol, Sucrose, Blue #1, Red #40.

How Supplied: Multi-Symptom TYLENOL COUGH with Decongestant is available in a 4 oz. bottle with child-resistant safety cap, and tamper resistant packaging.

Shown in Product Identification Guide, page 513

Continued on next page

McNeil Consumer—Cont.

**Maximum Strength
TYLENOL Flu**   OTC
**Medication
No Drowsiness Formula
Gelcaps**

Description: Each Maximum Strength TYLENOL Flu Medication No Drowsiness Formula Gelcap contains acetaminophen 500 mg., pseudoephedrine hydrochloride 30 mg., and dextromethorphan hydrobromide 15 mg.

Actions: Maximum Strength TYLENOL Flu Medication No Drowsiness Formula Gelcaps contain a clinically proven analgesic-antipyretic, decongestant and cough suppressant. Acetaminophen produces analgesia by elevation of the pain threshold and antipyresis through action on the hypothalamic heat-regulating center. Acetaminophen is equal to aspirin in analgesic and antipyretic effectiveness and it is unlikely to produce many of the side effects associated with aspirin and aspirin-containing products. Pseudoephedrine hydrochloride is a sympathomimetic amine which provides temporary relief of nasal congestion. Dextromethorphan is a cough suppressant which provides temporary relief of coughs due to minor throat irritations that may occur with the common cold.

Indications: Maximum Strength TYLENOL Flu Medication No Drowsiness Formula provides effective temporary relief of body aches, headaches, fever, sore throat, coughing and nasal congestion due to a cold or "flu."

Precautions: If a rare sensitivity reaction occurs, the drug should be stopped. Although pseudoephedrine is virtually without pressor effect in normotensive patients, it should be used with caution in hypertensives.

Directions: Adults (12 Years and older): Two gelcaps every 6 hours, not to exceed 8 gelcaps in 24 hours. Not for use in children under 12 years of age.

Warnings: Do not take this product for more than 7 days or for fever for more than 3 days unless directed by a doctor. If symptoms do not improve or are accompanied by fever, consult a doctor. A persistent cough may be a sign of a serious condition. If cough persists for more than 1 week, tends to recur or is accompanied by fever, rash or persistent headache, consult a doctor. Do not take this product for persistent or chronic cough such as occurs with smoking, asthma, emphysema or if cough is accompanied by excessive phlegm (mucus) unless directed by a doctor. If sore throat is severe, persists for more than 2 days, is accompanied or followed by fever, headache, rash, nausea or vomiting, consult a doctor promptly. Do not exceed recommended dosage because at higher doses, nervousness, dizziness or sleeplessness may occur. Do not take this product if you have heart disease, high blood pressure, thyroid disease, diabetes, or difficulty in urination due to enlargement of the prostate gland unless directed by a doctor. Do not use with other products containing acetaminophen.

DO NOT USE IF CARTON IS OPENED OR IF A BLISTER UNIT IS BROKEN. KEEP THIS AND ALL MEDICATION OUT OF THE REACH OF CHILDREN. AS WITH ANY DRUG, IF YOU ARE PREGNANT OR NURSING A BABY, SEEK THE ADVICE OF A HEALTH PROFESSIONAL BEFORE USING THIS PRODUCT. IN CASE OF ACCIDENTAL OVERDOSE, CONTACT A DOCTOR OR POISON CONTROL CENTER IMMEDIATELY. PROMPT MEDICAL ATTENTION IS CRITICAL FOR ADULTS AS WELL AS CHILDREN EVEN IF YOU DO NOT NOTICE ANY SIGNS OR SYMPTOMS.

Alcohol Warning: If you generally consume 3 or more alcohol-containing drinks per day, you should consult your physician for advice on when and how you should take Maximum Strength TYLENOL® Flu Medication No Drowsiness Formula and other pain relievers.

Drug Interaction Precaution: Do not take this product if you are presently taking a prescription drug for high blood pressure or you are now taking a prescription monoamine oxidase inhibitor (MAOI) (certain drugs for depression, psychiatric or emotional conditions, or Parkinson's disease), or for 2 weeks after stopping the MAOI drug. If you are uncertain whether your prescription drug contains an MAOI, consult a health professional before taking this product.

Overdosage Information: Acetaminophen in massive overdosage may cause hepatic toxicity in some patients. In adults and adolescents, hepatic toxicity has rarely been reported following ingestion of acute overdoses of less than 10 grams. Fatalities are infrequent (less than 3–4% of untreated cases) and have rarely been reported with overdosage of less than 15 grams. In children, an acute overdosage of less than 150 mg/kg has not been associated with hepatic toxicity. Early symptoms following a potentially hepatotoxic overdose may include: nausea, vomiting, diaphoresis and general malaise. Clinical and laboratory evidence of hepatic toxicity may not be apparent until 48 to 72 hours postingestion. In adults and adolescents, regardless of the quantity of acetaminophen reported to have been ingested, administer acetylcysteine immediately if 24 hours or less have elapsed from the reported time of ingestion. For full prescribing information, refer to the acetylcysteine package insert. Do not await results of assays for plasma acetaminophen level before initiating treatment with acetyleysteine. The following additional procedures are recommended: The stomach should be emptied promptly by lavage or by induction of emesis with syrup of ipecac. A plasma acetaminophen assay should be obtained as early as possible, but not sooner than four hours following ingestion. If plasma level falls above the lower treatment line on the acetaminophen overdose nomogram, acetylcysteine therapy should be continued. Liver function studies should be obtained initially and repeated at 24-hour intervals.

Serious toxicity or fatalities are extremely infrequent in children, possibly due to differences in the way they metabolize acetaminophen. In children, the maximum potential amount ingested can be more easily estimated. If more than 150 mg/kg or an unknown amount was ingested, obtain an plasma acetaminophen level. The plasma acetaminophen level should be obtained as soom as possible, but no sooner than 4 hours following the ingestion. If plasma level falls above the lower treatment line on the acetaminophen overdose nomogram, the acetylcysteine therapy should be initiated and continued for a full course of therapy. If plasma acetaminophen assay capability is not available, and the estimated acetaminophen ingestion exceeds 150 mg/kg, acetyleysteine therapy should be initiated and continued for a full course of therapy.

For additional emergency information, call your regional poison center or call the Rocky Mountain Poison Center toll-free, (1-800-525-6115).

Symptoms of pseudoephedrine overdose consist most often of mild anxiety, tachycardia and/or mild hypertension.

Symptoms usually appear within 4 to 8 hours of ingestion and are transient, usually requiring no treatment.

Acute dextromethorphan overdose usually does not result in serious signs and symptoms unless massive amounts have been ingested. Signs and symptoms of a substantial overdose may include nausea and vomiting, visual disturbances, CNS disturbances, and urinary retention.

Alcohol Information: Chronic heavy alcohol abusers may be at increased risk of liver toxicity from excessive acetaminophen use, although reports of this event are rare. Reports almost invariably involve cases of severe chronic alcoholics and the dosages of acetaminophen most often exceed recommended doses and often involve substantial overdose. Professionals should alert their patients who regularly consume large amounts of alcohol not to exceed recommended doses of acetaminophen.

Inactive Ingredients: Benzyl Alcohol, Butylparaben, Castor Oil, Cellulose, Corn Starch, Edetate Calcium Disodium, Gelatin, Hydroxypropyl Methylcellulose, Iron Oxide Black, Magnesium Stearate, Methylparaben, Propylparaben, Sodium Lauryl Sulfate, Sodium Propionate, Sodium Starch Glycolate, Titanium Dioxide, Red #40 and Blue #1.

How Supplied: Gelcaps (colored burgundy and white, imprinted "TYLENOL FLU") in blister packs of 10 and 20.

Shown in Product Identification Guide, page 513

Maximum Strength TYLENOL® Flu NightTime Hot Medication Packets OTC

Description: Each packet of Maximum Strength TYLENOL Flu NightTime contains acetaminophen 1000 mg., pseudoephedrine hydrochloride 60 mg and diphenhydramine hydrochloride 50 mg.

Actions: Maximum Strengh TYLENOL Flu NightTime Hot Medication contains a clinically proven analgesic-antipyretic, decongestant, and antihistamine. Acetaminophen produces analgesia by elevation of the pain threshold and antipyresis through action on the hypothalamic heat-regulating center. Acetaminophen is equal to aspirin in analgesic and antipyretic effectiveness and it is unlikely to produce many of the side effects associated with aspirin and aspirin-containing products. Pseudoephedrine hydrochloride is a sympathomimetic amine which provides temporary relief of nasal congestion. Diphenhydramine is an antihistamine which helps provide temporary relief of runny nose and sneezing.

Indications: Maximum Strength TYLENOL Flu NightTime Hot Medication provides effective temporary relief of body aches, headaches, fever, sore throat, nasal congestion, and runny nose/sneezing due to a cold or "flu" so you can rest.

Precautions: If a rare sensitivity reaction occurs, the drug should be stopped. Although pseudoephedrine is virtually without pressor effect in normotensive patients, it should be used with caution in hypertensives.

Directions: Adults (12 years and older): Dissolve one packet in 6 oz. cup of hot water. Sip while hot. Sweeten to taste, if desired. May repeat every 6 hours, not to exceed 4 doses in 24 hours. Not for use in children under 12 years of age.

Warnings: Do not exceed the recommended dosage because at higher doses, nervousness, dizziness or sleeplessness may occur. Do not take this product for more than 7 days or for fever for more than 3 days unless directed by a doctor. If symptoms do not improve or are accompanied by fever, consult a doctor. If sore throat is severe, persists for more than 2 days, is accompanied or followed by fever, headache, rash, nausea or vomiting, consult a doctor promptly. May cause excitability especially in children. Do not take this product, unless directed by a doctor, if you have a breathing problem such as emphysema or chronic bronchitis, or if you have glaucoma or difficulty in urination due to enlargement of the prostate gland. Do not take this product if you have heart disease, high blood pressure, thyroid disease or diabetes unless directed by a doctor. May cause marked drowsiness; alcohol, sedatives and tranquilizers may increase the drowsiness effect. Avoid alcoholic beverages while taking this product. Do not take this product if you are taking sedatives or tranquilizers, without first consulting your doctor. Use caution when driving a motor vehicle or operating machinery. Do not use with other products containing acetaminophen.

DO NOT USE IF PRINTED CARTON OVERWRAP IS BROKEN OR MISSING OR IF CARTON IS OPENED OR FOIL PACKET IS TORN OR BROKEN. KEEP THIS AND ALL MEDICATION OUT OF THE REACH OF CHILDREN. AS WITH ANY DRUG, IF YOU ARE PREGNANT OR NURSING A BABY, SEEK THE ADVICE OF A HEALTH PROFESSIONAL BEFORE USING THIS PRODUCT. IN CASE OF ACCIDENTAL OVERDOSE, CONTACT A DOCTOR OR POISON CONTROL CENTER IMMEDIATELY. PROMPT MEDICAL ATTENTION IS CRITICAL FOR ADULTS AS WELL AS FOR CHILDREN EVEN IF YOU DO NOT NOTICE ANY SIGNS OR SYMPTOMS.

Phenylketonurics: CONTAINS PHENYLALANINE 67 MG PER PACKET.

Alcohol Warning: If you generally consume 3 or more alcohol-containing drinks per day, you should consult your physician for advice on when and how you should take Maximum Strength TYLENOL® Flu NightTime Hot Medication and other pain relievers.

Drug Interaction Precautions: Do not take this product if you are presently taking a prescription drug for high blood pressure or depression without first consulting your doctor.

Overdosage Information: Acetaminophen in massive overdosage may cause hepatic toxicity in some patients. In adults and adolescents, hepatic toxicity has rarely been reported following ingestion of acute overdoses of less than 10 grams. Fatalities are infrequent (less than 3–4% of untreated cases) and have rarely been reported with overdoses of less than 15 grams. In children, an acute overdosage of less than 150 mg/kg has not been associated with hepatic toxicity. Early symptoms following a potentially hepatotoxic overdose may include: nausea, vomiting, diaphoresis and general malaise. Clinical and laboratory evidence of hepatic toxicity may not be apparent until 48 to 72 hours postingestion. In adults and adolescents, regardless of the quantity of acetaminophen reported to have been ingested, administer acetylcysteine immediately if 24 hours or less have elapsed from the reported time of ingestion. For full prescribing information, refer to the plasma acetylcysteine package insert. Do not await results of assays for plasma acetaminophen level before initiating treatment with acetylcysteine. The following additional procedures are recommended. The stomach should be emptied promptly by lavage or by induction of emesis with syrup of ipecac. A plasma acetaminophen assay should be obtained as early as possible, but no sooner than four hours following ingestion. If plasma level falls above the lower treatment line on the acetaminophen overdose nomogram, acetylcysteine therapy should be continued. Liver function studies should be obtained initially and repeated at 24-hour intervals.

Serious toxicity or fatalities are extremely infrequent in children, possibly due to differences in the way they metabolize acetaminophen. In children, the maximum potential amount ingested can be more easily estimated. If more than 150 mg/kg or an unknown amount was ingested, obtain a plasma acetaminophen level. The plasma acetaminophen level should be obtained as soon as possible, but not sooner than 4 hours following the ingestion. If plasma level falls above the lower treatment line on the acetaminophen overdose nomogram, the acetylcysteine therapy should be initiated and continued for a full course of therapy. If plasma acetaminophen assay capability is not available, and the estimated acetaminophen ingestion exceeds 150 mg/kg, acetylcysteine therapy should be initiated and continued for a full course of therapy.

For additional emergency information, call your regional poison center or call the Rocky Mountain Poison Control toll-free, (1-800-525-6115).

Symptoms of pseudoephedrine overdose consist most often of mild anxiety, tachycardia and/or mild hypertension. Symptoms usually appear within 4 to 8 hours of ingestion and are transient, usually requiring no treatment.

Diphenhydramine toxicity should be treated as you would an antihistamine/anticholinergic overdose and is likely to be present within a few hours after acute ingestion.

Alcohol Information: Chronic heavy alcohol abusers may be at increased risk of liver toxicity from excessive acetaminophen use, although reports of this event are rare. Reports almost invariably involve cases of severe chronic alcoholics and the dosages of acetaminophen most often exceed recommended doses and often involve substantial overdose. Professional should alert their patients who regularly consume large amounts of alcohol not to exceed recommended doses of acetaminophen.

Inactive Ingredients: Ascorbic Acid (Vitamin C), Aspartame, Citric Acid, Flavors, Sodium Citrate, Sucrose. Yellow #10, Blue #1, Red #40, Yellow #6. May also contain: Silicon Dioxide.

How Supplied: Packets of powder (yellow colored) in cartons of 6 tamper-resistant foil packets.

Shown in Product Identification Guide, page 513

Continued on next page

McNeil Consumer—Cont.

Maximum Strength TYLENOL Flu NightTime Medication Gelcaps   OTC

Description: Each Maximum Strength TYLENOL Flu NightTime Medication Gelcap contains acetaminophen 500 mg., pseudoephedrine hydrochloride 30 mg., and diphenhydramine hydrochloride 25 mg.

Actions: Maximum Strength TYLENOL Flu NightTime Medication Gelcaps contain a clinically proven analgesic-antipyretic, decongestant and antihistamine. Acetaminophen produces analgesia by elevation of the pain threshold and antipyresis through action on the hypothalamic heat-regulating center. Acetaminophen is equal to aspirin in analgesic and antipyretic effectiveness and it is unlikely to produce many of the side effects associated with aspirin and aspirin-containing products. Pseudoephedrine hydrochloride is a sympathomimetic amine which provides temporary relief of nasal congestion. Diphenhydramine is an antihistamine which helps provide temporary relief of runny nose and sneezing.

Indications: Maximum Strength TYLENOL Flu NightTime Medication provides effective temporary relief of body aches, headaches, fever, sore throat, nasal congestion and runny nose/sneezing due to a cold or "flu" so you can rest.

Precautions: If a rare sensitivity reaction occurs, the drug should be stopped. Although pseudoephedrine is virtually without pressor effect in normotensive patients, it should be used with caution in hypertensives.

Directions: Adults (12 Years and older): Two gelcaps at bedtime. May repeat every 6 hours, not to exceed 8 gelcaps in 24 hours. Not for use in children under 12 years of age.

Warnings: Do not exceed the recommended dosage, because at higher doses, nervousness, dizziness or sleeplessness may occur. Do not take this product for more than 7 days or for fever for more than 3 days unless directed by a doctor. If symptoms do not improve or are accompanied by fever, consult a doctor. If sore throat is severe, persists for more than 2 days, is accompanied or followed by fever, headache, rash, nausea or vomiting, consult a doctor promptly. May cause excitability, especially in children. Do not take this product, unless directed by a doctor, if you have a breathing problem such as emphysema or chronic bronchitis, or if you have glaucoma or difficulty in urination due to enlargement of the prostate gland. Do not take this product if you have heart disease, high blood pressure, thyroid disease, or diabetes unless directed by a doctor. May cause marked drowsiness; alcohol, sedatives and tranquilizers may increase the drow-siness effect. Avoid alcoholic beverages while taking this product. Do not take this product if you are taking sedatives or tranquilizers without first consulting your doctor. Use caution when driving a motor vehicle or operating machinery. Do not use with other products containing acetaminophen.

DO NOT USE IF CARTON IS OPENED OR IF A BLISTER UNIT IS BROKEN. KEEP THIS AND ALL MEDICATION OUT OF THE REACH OF CHILDREN. AS WITH ANY DRUG, IF YOU ARE PREGNANT OR NURSING A BABY, SEEK THE ADVICE OF A HEALTH PROFESSIONAL BEFORE USING THIS PRODUCT. IN CASE OF ACCIDENTAL OVERDOSE, CONTACT A DOCTOR OR POISON CONTROL CENTER IMMEDIATELY. PROMPT MEDICAL ATTENTION IS CRITICAL FOR ADULTS AS WELL AS CHILDREN EVEN IF YOU DO NOT NOTICE ANY SIGNS AND SYMPTOMS.

Alcohol Warning: If you generally consume 3 or more alcohol-containing drinks per day, you should consult your physician for advice on when and how you should take Maximum Strength TYLENOL® Flu NightTime Medication and other pain relievers.

Drug Interaction Precaution: Do not take this product if you are presently taking a prescription drug for high blood pressure or depression without first consulting your physician.

Overdosage Information: Acetaminophen in massive overdosage may cause hepatic toxicity in some patients. In adults and adolescents, hepatic toxicity has rarely been reported following ingestion of acute overdoses of less than 10 grams. Fatalities are infrequent (less than 3–4% of untreated cases) and have rarely been reported with overdosage of less than 15 grams. In children, an acute overdosage of less than 150 mg/kg has not been associated with hepatic toxicity. Early symptoms following a potentially hepatotoxic overdose may include: nausea, vomiting, diaphoresis and general malaise. Clinical and laboratory evidence of hepatic toxicity may not be apparent until 48 to 72 hours postingestion. In adults and adolescents, regardless of the quantity of acetaminophen reported to have been ingested, administer acetylcysteine immediately if 24 hours or less have elapsed from the reported time of ingestion. For full prescribing information, refer to the acetylcysteine package insert. Do not await results of assays for plasma acetaminophen level before initiating treatment with acetylcysteine. The following additional procedures are recommended: The stomach should be emptied promptly by lavage or by induction of emesis with syrup of ipecac. A plasma acetaminophen assay should be obtained as early as possible, but not sooner than four hours following ingestion. If plasma level falls above the lower treatment line on the acetaminophen overdose nomogram, acetylcysteine ther-apy should be continued. Liver function studies should be obtained initially and repeated at 24-hour intervals.

Serious toxicity or fatalities are extremely infrequent in children, possibly due to differences in the way they metabolize acetaminophen. In children, the maximum potential amount ingested can be more easily estimated. If more than 150 mg/kg or an unknown amount was ingested, obtain a plasma acetaminophen level. The plasma acetaminophen level should be obtained as soon as possible, but no sooner than 4 hours following the ingestion. If plasma level falls above the lower treatment line on the acetaminophen overdose nomogram, the acetylcysteine therapy should be initiated and continued for a full course of therapy. If plasma acetaminophen assay capability is not available, and the estimated acetaminophen ingestion exceeds 150 mg/kg, acetylcysteine therapy should be initiated and continued for a full course of therapy.

For additional emergency information, call your regional poison center or call the Rocky Mountain Poison Center toll-free, (1-800-525-6115).

Symptoms from pseudoephedrine overdose consist most often of mild anxiety, tachycardia and/or mild hypertension. Symptoms usually appear within 4 to 8 hours of ingestion and are transient, usually requiring no treatment.

Diphenhydramine toxicity should be treated as you would an antihistamine/anticholinergic overdose and is likely to be present within a few hours after acute ingestion.

Alcohol Information: Chronic heavy alcohol abusers may be at increased risk of liver toxicity from excessive acetaminophen use, although reports of this event are rare. Reports almost invariably involve cases of severe chronic alcoholics and the dosages of acetaminophen most often exceed recommended doses and often involve substantial overdose. Professionals should alert their patients who regularly consume large amounts of alcohol not to exceed recommended doses of acetaminophen.

Inactive Ingredients: Benzyl Alcohol, Butylparaben, Castor Oil, Cellulose, Corn Starch, Edetate Calcium Disodium, Gelatin, Hydroxypropyl Methylcellulose, Iron Oxide Black, Magnesium Stearate, Methylparaben, Propylparaben, Sodium Citrate, Sodium Lauryl Sulfate, Sodium Propionate, Sodium Starch Glycolate, Titanium Dioxide, Red #28 and Blue #1.

How Supplied: Gelcaps (colored blue and white, imprinted "TYLENOL FLU NT") in blister packs of 10 and 20.

Shown in Product Identification Guide, page 513

TYLENOL® Severe Allergy Medication Caplets   OTC

Description: Each TYLENOL® Severe Allergy Caplet contains acetaminophen 500 mg. and Diphenhydramine HCl 12.5 mg.

Actions: TYLENOL® Severe Allergy Caplets contain a clinically proven analgesic-antipyretic, and antihistamine. Acetaminophen produces analgesia by elevation of the pain threshold and antipyresis through action on the hypothalamic heat-regulating center. Acetaminophen is equal to aspirin in analgesic and antipyretic effectiveness, and it is unlikely to produce many of the side effects associated with aspirin and aspirin-containing products. Diphenhydramine is an antihistamine which helps provide temporary relief itchy, watery eyes, runny nose, sneezing, itching of the nose or throat due to hay fever or other respiratory allergies.

Indications: TYLENOL® Severe Allergy provides effective temporary relief of itchy, watery eyes, runny nose, sneezing, sore or scratchy throat and itching of the nose or throat due to hay fever or other upper respiratory allergies.

Precautions: If a rare sensitivity reaction occurs, the drug should be stopped.

Directions: Adults and children 12 years of age and older: Two caplets every 4 to 6 hours, do not exceed 8 caplets in any 24 hours period. Not for use in children under 12 years of age.

Warnings: DO NOT USE IF CARTON IS OPEN OR IF A BLISTER UNIT IS BROKEN. Do not take for pain for more than 10 days or for fever for more than 3 days unless directed by a doctor if pain or fever persists, or gets worse, if new symptoms occur, or if redness or swelling is present, consult a doctor because these could be signs of a serious condition. If sore throat is severe, persists for more than 2 days, is accompanied or followed by fever, headache, rash, nausea or vomiting, consult a doctor promptly. May cause excitability especially in children. Do not take this product, unless directed by a doctor if you have a breathing problem such as emphysema or chronic bronchitis or if you have glaucoma or difficulty in urination due to enlargement of the prostate gland. May cause marked drowsiness, alcohol, sedatives and tranquilizers may increase the drowsiness effect. Avoid alcoholic beverages while taking this product. Do not take this product if you are taking sedatives or tranquilizers without first consulting your doctor. Use caution when driving a motor vehicle or operating machinery. As with any drug, if you are pregnant or nursing a baby, seek the advice of a health professional before using this product. Keep this and all drugs out of reach of children. In case of accidental overdose, contact a doctor or poison control center immediately. Prompt medical attention is critical for adults as well as for children even if you do not notice any signs or symptoms. Do not use with other products containing acetaminophen.

Alcohol Warning: If you generally consume 3 or more alcohol-containing drinks per day, you should consult your physician for advice on when and how you should take Tylenol® Severe Allergy Caplets and other pain relievers.

Overdosage Information: Acetaminophen in massive overdosage may cause hepatic toxicity in some patients. In adults and adolescents, hepatic toxicity has rarely been reported following ingestion of acute overdoses of less than 10 grams. Fatalities are infrequent (less than 3-4% of untreated cases) and have rarely been reported with overdoses of less than 15 grams. In children, an acute overdosage of less than 150 mg/kg has not been associated with hepatic toxicity. Early symptoms following a potentially hepatotoxic overdose may include: nausea, vomiting, diaphoresis and general malaise. Clinical and laboratory evidence of hepatic toxicity may not be apparent until 48 to 72 hours postingestion. In adults and adolescents, regardless of the quantity of acetaminophen reported to have been ingested, administer acetylcysteine immediately if 24 hours or less have elapsed from the reported time of ingestion. For full prescribing information, refer to the acetylcysteine package insert. Do not await results of assays for plasma acetaminophen level before initiating treatment with acetylcysteine. The following additional procedures are recommended. The stomach should be emptied promptly by lavage or by induction of emesis with syrup of ipecac. A plasma acetaminophen assay should be obtained as early as possible, but no sooner than four hours following ingestion. If plasma level falls above the lower treatment line on the acetaminophen overdose nomogram, acetylcysteine therapy should be continued. Liver function studies should be obtained initially and repeated at 24-hour intervals.

Serious toxicity or fatalities are extremely infrequent in children, possibly due to differences in the way they metabolize acetaminophen. In children, the maximum potential amount ingested can be more easily estimated. If more than 150 mg/kg or an unknown amount was ingested, obtain a plasma acetaminophen level. The plasma acetaminophen level should be obtained as soon as possible, but no sooner than 4 hours following the ingestion. If plasma level falls above the lower treatment line on the acetaminophen overdose nomogram, the acetylcysteine therapy should be initiated and continued for a full course of therapy. If plasma acetaminophen assay capability is not available, and the estimated acetaminophen ingestion exceeds 150 mg/kg, acetylcysteine therapy should be initiated and continued for a full course of therapy.

For additional emergency information, call your regional poison center or call the Rocky Mountain Poison Center toll-free (1-800-525-6115).

Diphenhydramine toxicity should be treated as you would an antihistamine/anticholinergic overdose and is likely to be present within a few hours after acute ingestion.

Alcohol Information Chronic heavy alcohol abusers may be at increased risk of liver toxicity from excessive acetaminophen use, although reports of this event are rare. Reports almost invariably involve cases of severe chronic alcoholics and the dosages of acetaminophen most often exceed recommended doses and often involve substantial overdose. Professionals should alert their patients who regularly consume large amounts of alcohol not to exceed recommended doses of acetaminophen.

Inactive Ingredients: Cellulose, Corn Starch, Hydroxypropyl Cellulose, Hydroxypropyl Methylcellulose, Iron Oxide Black, Magnesium Stearate, Polyethylene Glycol, Sodium Citrate, Sodium Starch Glycolate, Titanium Dioxide, Yellow #6, Yellow #10.

How Supplied: Caplets: dark yellow, imprinted "TYLENOL Severe Allergy"–Blister packs of 12 and 24.

Shown in Product Identification Guide, page 513

Maximum-Strength TYLENOL® Sinus Medication Geltabs, Gelcaps, Caplets and Tablets   OTC

Description: Each Maximum-Strength TYLENOL® Sinus Medication Geltab, Gelcap, Caplet or Tablet contains acetaminophen 500 mg and pseudoephedrine hydrochloride 30 mg.

Actions: Maximum-Strength TYLENOL Sinus Medication contains a clinically proven analgesic-antipyretic and a decongestant. Maximum allowable nonprescription levels of acetaminophen and pseudoephedrine provide temporary relief of sinus headache and congestion. Acetaminophen is equal to aspirin in analgesic and antipyretic effectiveness and it is unlikely to produce many of the side effects associated with aspirin and aspirin-containing products.

Acetaminophen produces analgesia by elevation of the pain threshold and antipyresis through action on the hypothalamic heat-regulating center. Pseudoephedrine hydrochloride is a sympathomimetic amine which promotes sinus cavity drainage by reducing nasopharyngeal mucosal congestion.

Indications: Maximum-Strength TYLENOL Sinus Medication provides for the temporary relief of nasal and sinus congestion and sinus pain and headaches. Maximum-Strength TYLENOL Sinus Medication is particularly well-suited in patients with aspirin allergy, hemostatic disturbances (including anticoagulant therapy), and bleeding diatheses (e.g., hemophilia) and upper gastroin-

Continued on next page

McNeil Consumer—Cont.

testinal disease (e.g., ulcer, gastritis, hiatus hernia).

Precautions: If a rare sensitivity occurs, the drug should be discontinued. Although pseudoephedrine is virtually without pressor effect in normotensive patients, it should be used with caution in hypertensives.

Directions: Adults and Children 12 years of Age and Older: Two Tablets, Caplets, Geltabs, or Gelcaps every 4–6 hours. Do not exceed eight Tablets, Caplets, Geltabs, or Gelcaps in any 24-hour period. Not for use in children under 12 years of age.

Warnings: Do not exceed the recommended dosage because at higher doses nervousness, dizziness, or sleeplessness may occur. Do not take this product for more than 7 days. If symptoms do not improve or are accompanied by fever, consult a physician. Do not take this product if you have heart disease, high blood pressure, thyroid disease, diabetes, or difficulty in urination due to enlargement of the prostate gland unless directed by a doctor. Do not use with other products containing acetaminophen. **DO NOT USE IF CARTON IS OPENED OR IF BLISTER UNIT IS BROKEN OR IF PRINTED GREEN NECK WRAP OR PRINTED FOIL INNER SEAL IS BROKEN. Keep this and all medication out of the reach of children. As with any drug, if you are pregnant or nursing a baby, seek the advice of a health professional before using this product. In case of accidental overdosage, contact a doctor or poison control center immediately. Prompt medical attention is critical for adults as well as for children even if you do not notice any signs or symptoms.**

Alcohol Warning: If you generally consume 3 or more alcohol-containing drinks per day, you should consult your physician for advice on when and how you should take Maximum-Strength TYLENOL® Sinus Medication and other pain relievers.

Drug Interaction Precaution: Do not take this product if you are presently taking a prescription drug for high blood pressure or depression without first consulting your doctor.

Overdosage Information: Acetaminophen in massive overdosage may cause hepatic toxicity in some patients. In adults and adolescents, hepatic toxicity has rarely been reported following ingestion of acute overdoses age of less than 10 grams. Fatalities are infrequent (less than 3–4% of untreated cases) and have rarely been reported with overdoses of less than 15 grams. In children, an acute overdosage of less than 150 mg/kg has not been associated with hepatic toxicity. Early symptoms following a potentially hepatotoxic overdose may include: nausea, vomiting, diaphoresis and general

malaise. Clinical and laboratory evidence of hepatic toxicity may not be apparent until 48 to 72 hours postingestion. In adults and adolescents, regardless of the quantity of acetaminophen reported to have been ingested, administer acetylcysteine immediately if 24 hours or less have elapsed from the reported time of ingestion. For full prescribing information, refer to the acetylcysteine package insert. Do not await results of assays for plasma acetaminophen level before initiating treatment with acetylcysteine. The following additional procedures are recommended. The stomach should be emptied promptly by lavage or by induction of emesis with syrup of ipecac. A plasma acetaminophen assay should be obtained as early as possible, but no sooner than four hours following ingestion. If plasma level falls above the lower treatment line on the acetaminophen overdose nomogram, acetylcysteine therapy should be continued. Liver function studies should be obtained initially and repeated at 24-hour intervals.

Serious toxicity or fatalities are extremely infrequent in children, possibly due to differences in the way they metabolize acetaminophen. In children, the maximum potential amount ingested can be more easily estimated. If more than 150 mg/kg or an unknown amount was ingested, obtain a plasma acetaminophen level. The plasma acetaminophen level should be obtained as soon as possible, but no sooner than 4 hours following the ingestion. If plasma level falls above the lower treatment line on the acetaminophen overdose nomogram, the acetylcysteine therapy should be initiated and continued for a full course of therapy. If plasma acetaminophen assay capability is not available, and the estimated acetaminophen ingestion exceeds 150 mg/kg, acetylcysteine therapy should be initiated and continued for a full course of therapy.

For additional emergency information, call your regional poison center or call the Rocky Mountain Poison Center toll-free (1-800-525-6115).

Symptoms from pseodoephedrine overdose consist most often of mild anxiety, tachycardia and/or mild hypertension. Symptoms usually appear within 4 to 8 hours after ingestion and are transient, usually requiring no treatment.

Alcohol Information: Chronic heavy alcohol abusers may be at increased risk of liver toxicity from excessive acetaminophen use, although reports of this event are rare. Reports almost invariably involve cases of severe chronic alcoholics and the dosages of acetaminophen most often exceed recommended doses and often involve substantial overdose. Professionals should alert their patients who regularly consume large amounts of alcohol not to exceed recommended doses of acetaminophen.

Inactive Ingredients: Caplets—Cannuba Wax, Cellulose, Corn Starch, Hydroxypropyl Methylcellulose, Magnesium Stearate, Polyethylene Glycol,

Polysorbate 80, Sodium Starch Glycolate, Titanium Dioxide, Blue #1, Red #40, Yellow #10.

Tablets—Cellulose, Corn Starch, Magnesium Stearate, Sodium Starch Glycolate, Blue #1, Yellow #6, and Yellow #10.

Gelcaps—Benzyl Alcohol, Butylparaben, Castor Oil, Cellulose, Corn Starch, Edetate Calcium Disodium, Gelatin, Hydroxypropyl Methylcellulose, Iron Oxide Black, Magnesium Stearate, Methylparaben, Propylparaben, Sodium Lauryl Sulfate, Sodium Propionate, Sodium Starch Glycolate, Titanium Dioxide, Blue #1 and Yellow #10.

Geltabs—Benzyl Alcohol, Butylparaben, Castor Oil, Cellulose, Corn Starch, Edetate Calcium Disodium, Gelatin, Hydroxypropyl Methylcellulose, Iron Oxide Black, Magnesium Stearate Methylparaben, Propylparaben, Sodium Lauryl Sulfate, Sodium Propionate, Sodium Starch Glycolate, Titanium Dioxide, D&C Yellow #10, FD&C Blue #1.

How Supplied: Tablets (colored light green, imprinted "Maximum-Strength TYLENOL Sinus")—in blister packs of 24 and tamper-resistant bottles of 50.

Caplets (light green coating, printed "TYLENOL Sinus" in dark green) in blister packs of 24 and tamper-resistant bottles of 60.

Gelcaps (colored green and white), printed "TYLENOL Sinus" in blister packs of 24 and tamper-resistant bottles of 60.

Geltabs (colored green and white), printed "TYLENOL Sinus" in blister packs of 24 and tamper-resistant bottles of 60.

Shown in Product Identification Guide, page 514

**Multisymptom Formula   OTC
TYLENOL® COLD Medication
Tablets and Caplets**

Description: Each Multi-Symptom Formula TYLENOL COLD Tablet or Caplet contains acetaminophen 325 mg, chlorpheniramine maleate 2 mg, pseudoephedrine hydrochloride 30 mg and dextromethorphan hydrobromide 15 mg.

Actions: Multi-Symptom Formula TYLENOL COLD Medication Tablets and Caplets contain a clinically proven analgesic-antipyretic, decongestant, cough suppressant and antihistamine. Acetaminophen produces analgesia by elevation of the pain threshold and antipyresis through action on the hypothalamic heat-regulating center. Acetaminophen is equal to aspirin in analgesic and antipyretic effectiveness and it is unlikely to produce many of the side effects associated with aspirin and aspirin-containing products. Pseudoephedrine hydrochloride is a sympathomimetic amine which provides temporary relief of nasal congestion. Dextromethorphan is a cough suppressant which provides temporary relief of coughs due to minor throat irritations that may occur with the common cold. Chlorpheniramine is an antihistamine which helps provide temporary relief of runny nose, sneezing and watery and itchy eyes.

Indications: Multi-Symptom Formula TYLENOL COLD Medication provides effective temporary relief of runny nose, sneezing, watery and itchy eyes, nasal congestion, coughing, and body aches, pains, headache, sore throat and fever due to a cold or "flu."

Precautions: If a rare sensitivity reaction occurs, the drug should be stopped. Although pseudoephedrine is virtually without pressor effect in normotensive patients, it should be used with caution in hypertensives.

Directions: Adults (12 years and older): Two tablets or caplets every 6 hours, not to exceed 8 tablets or caplets in 24 hours. Children (6–11 years): One tablet or caplet every 6 hours, not to exceed 4 tablets or caplets in 24 hours. Not for use in children under 6 years of age.

Warning: Do not take this product for more than 7 days or for fever for more than 3 days unless directed by a doctor. If symptoms do not improve or are accompanied by fever, consult a doctor. If sore throat is severe, persists for more than 2 days, is accompanied or followed by fever, headache, rash, nausea or vomiting, consult a doctor promptly. A persistent cough may be a sign of a serious condition. If cough persists for more than 1 week, tends to recur or is accompanied by fever, rash or persistent headache, consult a doctor. Do not take this product for persistent or chronic cough such as occurs with smoking, asthma, emphysema or if cough if accompanied by excessive phlegm (mucus) unless directed by a doctor. Do not exceed recommended dosage because at higher doses, nervousness, dizziness or sleeplessness may occur. May cause excitability especially in children. Do not take this product, unless directed by a doctor, if you have a breathing problem such as emphysema or chronic bronchitis, or if you have glaucoma or difficulty in urination due to enlargement of the prostate gland. Do not take this product if you have heart disease, high blood pressure, thyroid disease or diabetes unless directed by a doctor. May cause drowsiness; alcohol, sedatives and tranquilizers may increase the drowsiness effect. Avoid alcoholic beverages while taking this product. Do not take this product if you are taking sedatives or tranquilizers without first consulting your doctor. Use caution when driving a motor vehicle or operating machinery. Do not use with other products containing acetaminophen.

DO NOT USE IF CARTON IS OPENED OR IF A BLISTER UNIT IS BROKEN. KEEP THIS AND ALL MEDICATION OUT OF THE REACH OF CHILDREN. AS WITH ANY DRUG, IF YOU ARE PREGNANT OR NURSING A BABY, SEEK THE ADVICE OF A HEALTH PROFESSIONAL BEFORE USING THIS PRODUCT. IN CASE OF ACCIDENTAL OVERDOSE, CONTACT A DOCTOR OR POISON CONTROL CENTER IMMEDIATELY. PROMPT MEDICAL ATTENTION IS CRITICAL FOR ADULTS AS WELL AS FOR CHILDREN EVEN IF YOU DO NOT NOTICE ANY SIGNS OR SYMPTOMS.

Alcohol Warning: If you generally consume 3 or more alcohol-containing drinks per day, you should consult your physician for advice on when and how you should take Multi-Symptom Formula TYLENOL® Cold Medication and other pain relievers.

Drug Interaction Precaution: Do not take this product if you are presently taking a prescription drug for high blood pressure or you are now taking a prescription monoamine oxidase inhibitor (MAOI) (certain drugs for depression, psychiatric or emotional conditions, or Parkinson's disease), or for 2 weeks after stopping the MAOI drug. If you are uncertain whether your prescription drug contains an MAOI, consult a health professional before taking this product.

Overdosage Information: Acetaminophen in massive overdosage may cause hepatic toxicity in some patients. In adults and adolescents, hepatic toxicity has rarely been reported following ingestion of acute overdoses of less than 10 grams. Fatalities are infrequent (less than 3–4% of untreated cases) and have rarely been reported with overdoses of less than 15 grams. In children, an acute overdosage of less than 150 mg/kg has not been associated with hepatic toxicity. Early symptoms following a potentially hepatotoxic overdose may include: nausea, vomiting, diaphoresis and general malaise. Clinical and laboratory evidence of hepatic toxicity may not be apparent until 48 to 72 hours postingestion. In adults and adolescents, regardless of the quantity of acetaminophen reported to have been ingested, administer acetylcysteine immediately if 24 hours or less have elapsed from the reported time of ingestion. For full prescribing information, refer to the acetylcysteine package insert. Do not await results of assays for plasma acetaminophen level before initiating treatment with acetylcysteine. The following additional procedures are recommended. The stomach should be emptied promptly by lavage or by induction of emesis with syrup of ipecac. A plasma acetaminophen assay should be obtained as early as possible, but no sooner than four hours following ingestion. If plasma level falls above the lower treatment line on the acetaminophen overdose nomogram, acetylcysteine therapy should be continued. Liver function studies should be obtained initially and repeated at 24-hour intervals. Serious toxicity or fatalities are extremely infrequent in children, possibly due to differences in the way they metabolize acetaminophen. In children, the maximum potential amount ingested can be more easily estimated. If more than 150 mg/kg or an unknown amount was ingested, obtain a plasma acetaminophen plasma level. The plasma acetaminophen level should be obtained as soon as possible, but no sooner than 4 hours following the ingestion. If plasma level falls above the lower treatment line on the acetaminophen overdose nomogram, the acetylcysteine therapy should be initiated and continued for a full course of therapy. If plasma acetaminophen assay capability is not available, and the estimated acetaminophen ingestion exceeds 150 mg/kg, acetylcysteine therapy should be initiated and continued for a full course of therapy.

For additional emergency information, call your regional poison center or call the Rocky Mountain Poison Center toll-free (1-800-525-6115).

Chlorpheniramine toxicity should be treated as you would an antihistamine/anticholinergic overdose and is likely to be present within a few hours after acute ingestion.

Symptoms from pseudoephedrine overdose consist most often of mild anxiety, tachycardia and/or mild hypertension. Symptoms usually appear within 4 to 8 hours of ingestion and are transient, usually requiring no treatment.

Acute dextromethorphan overdose usually does not result in serious signs and symptoms unless massive amounts have been ingested. Signs and symptoms of a substantial overdose may include nausea and vomiting, visual disturbances, CNS disturbances, and urinary retention.

Alcohol Information: Chronic heavy alcohol abusers may be at increased risk of liver toxicity from excessive acetaminophen use, although reports of this event are rare. Reports almost invariably involve cases of severe chronic alcoholics and the dosages of acetaminophen most often exceed recommended doses and often involve substantial overdose. Professionals should alert their patients who regularly consume large amounts of alcohol not to exceed recommended doses of acetaminophen.

Inactive Ingredients: Tablets: Cellulose, Corn Starch, Magnesium Stearate, Yellow #6 and Yellow #10. Caplets: Cellulose, Corn Starch, Glyceryl Triacetate, Hydroxypropyl Methylcellulose, Iron Oxide Black, Magnesium Stearate, Sodium Starch Glycolate, Titanium Dioxide, Blue #1 and Yellow #6 & #10.

How Supplied: Tablets (colored yellow, imprinted "TYLENOL Cold")—blister packs of 24 and tamper-resistant bottles of 50. Caplets (light yellow, imprinted "TYLENOL Cold")—blister packs of 24 and tamper-resistant bottles of 50.

Shown in Product Identification Guide, page 513

Continued on next page

McNeil Consumer—Cont.

MULTI-SYMPTOM TYLENOL®OTC COUGH MEDICATION

Description: Each 15 ml (3 tsp.) dose contains dextromethorphan HBr 30 mg., and acetaminophen 650mg.

Actions: Multi-Symptom TYLENOL® COUGH Medication Liquid contains a clinically proven cough suppressant and analgesic-antipyretic. Acetaminophen produces analgesia by elevation of the pain threshold and antipyresis through action on the hypothalamic heat-regulating center. Dextromethorphan is a cough suppressant which provides temporary relief of coughs due to minor throat irritations that may occur with the common cold.

Indications: Multi-Symptom TYLENOL® COUGH Medication provides effective, temporary relief of coughing, and the aches, pains and sore throat that may accompany a cough due to a cold.

Precautions: If a rare sensitivity reaction occurs, the drug should be discontinued.

Directions: Adults (12 years and older): 1 tablespoon or 3 teaspoons every 6–8 hours, not to exceed 4 doses in 24 hours. Children: (ages 6–11) 1 1/2 teaspoons every 6–8 hours, not to exceed 4 doses in 24 hours. Not for use in children under 6 years of age.

Warning: Do not take this product for more than 10 days or for fever for more than 3 days unless directed by a physician. Severe or recurrent pain or high or continued fever may be indicative of serious illness. Under these conditions, consult a doctor. A persistent cough may be a sign of a serious condition. If cough persists for more than 1 week, tends to recur or is accompanied by fever, rash or persistent headache, consult a doctor. Do not take this product for persistent or chronic cough such as occurs with smoking, asthma, emphysema, or if cough is accompanied by excessive phlegm (mucus) unless directed by a doctor. If sore throat is severe, persists for more than 2 days, is accompanied or followed by fever, headache, rash, nausea or vomiting, consult a doctor promptly. Do not use with other products containing acetaminophen.
DO NOT USE IF PRINTED PLASTIC BOTTLE WRAP OR PRINTED FOIL INNER SEAL IS BROKEN. Keep this and all medication out of the reach of children. As with any drug, if you are pregnant or nursing a baby, seek the advice of a health professional before using this product. In case of accidental overdosage, contact a doctor or poison control center immediately. Prompt medical attention is critical for adults as well as children even if you do not notice any signs or symptoms.

Alcohol Warning: If you generally consume 3 or more alcohol-containing drinks per day, you should consult your physician for advice on when and how you should take Multi-Symptom TYLENOL® Cough Medication and other pain relievers.

Drug Interaction Precaution: Do not use this product if you are taking a prescription drug containing a monoamine oxidase inhibitor (MAOI) (certain drugs for depression or psychiatric or emotional conditions), without first consulting your doctor. If you are uncertain whether your prescription drug contains an MAOI, consult a health professional before taking this product.

Overdosage Information: Acetaminophen in massive dosage may cause hepatic toxicity in some patients. In adults and adolescents, hepatic toxicity has rarely been reported following ingestion of acute overdosage of less than 10 grams. Fatalities are infrequent (less than 3–4% of untreated cases) and have rarely been reported with overdoses of less than 15 grams. In children, an acute overdosage of less than 150mg/kg has not been associated with hepatic toxicity. Early symptoms following a potentially hepatotoxic overdose may include: nausea, vomiting, diaphoresis and general malaise. Clinical and laboratory evidence of hepatic toxicity may not be apparent until 48 to 72 hours postingestion. In adults and adolescents, regardless of the quantity of acetaminophen reported to have been ingested, administer acetylcysteine immediately if 24 hours or less have elapsed from the reported time of ingestion. For full prescribing information, refer to the acetylcysteine package insert. Do not await results of assays for plasma acetaminophen level before initiating treatment with acetylcysteine. The following additional procedures are recommended: The stomach should be emptied by lavage or by induction of emesis with syrup of ipecac. A plasma acetaminophen assay should be obtained as early as possible, but no sooner than four hours following ingestion. If plasma level falls above the lower treatment line on the acetaminophen overdose nomogram, acetylcysteine therapy should be continued. Liver function studies should be obtained initially and repeated at 24-hour intervals.
Serious toxicity or fatalities are extremely infrequent in children, possibly due to differences in the way they metabolize acetaminophen. In children, the maximum potential amount ingested can be more easily estimated. If more than 150mg/kg or an unknown amount was ingested, obtain a plasma acetaminophen level. The plasma acetaminophen level should be obtained as soon as possible, but no sooner than 4 hours following the ingestion. If the plasma level falls above the lower treatment line on the acetaminophen overdose nomogram, the acetylcysteine therapy should be initiated and continued for a full course of therapy. If plasma acetaminophen assay capability is not available, and the estimated acetaminophen ingestion exceeds 150mg/kg, acetycysteine therapy should be initiated and continued for a full course of therapy.
For additional emergency information, call your regional poison center or call the Rocky Mountain Poison Center toll free (1-800-525-6115).
Acute dextromethorphan overdose usually does not result in serious signs and symptoms unless massive amounts have been ingested. Signs and symptoms of a substantial overdose may include nausea and vomiting, visual disturbances, CNS disturbances, and urinary retention.

Alcohol Information: Chronic heavy alcohol abusers may be at increased risk of liver toxicity from excessive acetaminophen use, although reports of this event are rare. Reports almost invariably involve cases of severe chronic alcoholics and the dosages of acetaminophen most often exceed recommended doses and often involve substantial overdose. Professionals should alert their patients who regularly consume large amounts of alcohol not to exceed recommended doses of acetaminophen.

Inactive Ingredients: Alcohol (5%), Citric Acid, Flavors, High Fructose Corn Syrup, Polyethylene Glycol, Propylene Glycol, Purified Water, Sodium Benzoate, Sodium Carboxymethylcellulose, Sodium Saccharin, Sorbitol, Red #40.

How Supplied: Multi-Symptom TYLENOL® COUGH is available in a 4 oz. bottle with child-resistant safety cap and tamper resistant packaging.
Shown in Product Identification Guide, page 513

TYLENOL® COLD Medication OTC No Drowsiness Formula Caplets and Gelcaps

Description: Each TYLENOL COLD Medication No Drowsiness Formula Caplet and Gelcap contains acetaminophen 325 mg., pseudoephedrine hydrochloride 30 mg. and dextromethorphan hydrobromide 15 mg.

Actions: TYLENOL COLD Medication No Drowsiness Formula Caplets and Gelcaps contain a clinically proven analgesic-antipyretic, decongestant and cough suppressant. Acetaminophen produces analgesia by elevation of the pain threshold and antipyresis through action on the hypothalamic heat-regulating center.

Acetaminophen is equal to aspirin in analgesic and antipyretic effectiveness and it is unlikely to produce many of the side effects associated with aspirin and aspirin-containing products. Pseudoephedrine hydrochloride is a sympathomimetic amine which provides temporary relief of nasal congestion. Dextromethorphan is a cough suppressant which provides temporary relief of coughs due to minor throat irritations that may occur with the common cold.

Indications: TYLENOL COLD Medication No Drowsiness Formula provides effective temporary relief of the nasal congestion, coughing, and body aches, pains, headache, sore throat and fever due to a cold or "flu."

Precautions: If a rare sensitivity reaction occurs, the drug should be stopped. Although pseudoephedrine is virtually without pressor effect in normotensive patients, it should be used with caution in hypertensives.

Directions: Adults (12 years and older): Two caplets or gelcaps every 6 hours, not to exceed 8 caplets or gelcaps in 24 hours. Children (6–11 years): One caplet or gelcap every 6 hours, not to exceed 4 caplets or gelcaps in 24 hours. Not for use in children under 6 years of age.

Warning: Do not take this product for more than 7 days or for fever for more than 3 days unless directed by a doctor. If symptoms do not improve or are accompanied by fever, consult a doctor. If sore throat is severe, persists for more than 2 days, is accompanied or followed by fever, headache, rash, nausea or vomiting, consult a doctor promptly. A persistent cough may be a sign of a serious condition. If cough persists for more than 1 week, tends to recur or is accompanied by fever, rash or persistent headache, consult a doctor. Do not take this product for persistent or chronic cough such as occurs with smoking, asthma, emphysema or if cough is accompanied by excessive phlegm (mucus) unless directed by a doctor. Do not exceed recommended dosage because at higher doses, nervousness, dizziness or sleeplessness may occur. Do not take this product if you have heart disease, high blood pressure, thyroid disease, diabetes or difficulty in urination due to enlargment of the prostate gland unless directed by a doctor. Do not use with other products containing acetaminophen.
DO NOT USE IF CARTON IS OPENED OR IF A BLISTER UNIT IS BROKEN. KEEP THIS AND ALL MEDICATION OUT OF THE REACH OF CHILDREN. AS WITH ANY DRUG, IF YOU ARE PREGNANT OR NURSING A BABY, SEEK THE ADVICE OF A HEALTH PROFESSIONAL BEFORE USING THIS PRODUCT. IN CASE OF ACCIDENTAL OVERDOSE CONTACT A DOCTOR OR POISON CONTROL CENTER IMMEDIATELY. PROMPT MEDICAL ATTENTION IS CRITICAL FOR ADULTS AS WELL AS CHILDREN EVEN IF YOU DO NOT NOTICE ANY SIGNS OR SYMPTOMS.

Alcohol Warning: If you generally consume 3 or more alcohol-containing drinks per day, you should consult your physician for advice on when and how you should take TYLENOL® COLD Medication No Drowsiness Formula and other pain relievers.

Drug Interaction Precaution: Do not take this product if you are presently taking a prescription drug for high blood pressure or if you are now taking a prescription monoamine oxidase inhibitor (MAOI) (certain drugs for depression, psychiatric or emotional conditions, or Parkinson's disease), or for 2 weeks after stopping the MAOI drug. If you are uncertain whether your prescription drug contains an MAOI, consult a health professional before taking this product.

Overdosage Information: Acetaminophen in massive overdosage may cause hepatic toxicity in some patients. In adults and adolescents, hepatic toxicity has rarely been reported following ingestion of acute overdosage of less than 10 grams. Fatalities are infrequent (less than 3–4% of untreated cases) and have rarely been reported with overdosage of less than 15 grams. In children, an acute overdosage of less than 150 mg/kg has not been associated with hepatic toxicity. Early symptoms following a potentially hepatotoxic overdose may include: nausea, vomiting, diaphoresis and general malaise. Clinical and laboratory evidence of hepatic toxicity may not be apparent until 48 to 72 hours postingestion. In adults and adolescents, regardless of the quantity of acetaminophen reported to have been ingested, administer acetylcysteine immediately if 24 hours or less have elapsed from the reported time of ingestion. For full prescribing information, refer to the acetylcysteine package insert. Do not await results of assays for plasma acetaminophen level before initiating treatment with acetylcysteine. The following additional procedures are recommended: The stomach should be emptied promptly by lavage or by induction of emesis with syrup of ipecac. A plasma acetaminophen assay should be obtained as early as possible, but no sooner than four hours following ingestion. If plasma level falls above the lower treatment line on the acetaminophen overdose nomogram, acetylcysteine therapy should be continued. Liver function studies should be obtained initially and repeated at 24–hour intervals.
Serious toxicity or fatalities are extremely infrequent in children, possibly due to differences in the way they metabolize acetaminophen. In children, the maximum potential amount ingested can be more easily estimated. If more than 150 mg/kg or an unknown amount was ingested, obtain a plasma acetaminophen level. The plasma acetaminophen level should be obtained as soon as possible, but no sooner than 4 hours following the ingestion. If the plasma level falls above the lower treatment line on the acetaminophen overdose nomogram, the acetylcysteine therapy should be initiated and continued for a full course of therapy. If plasma acetaminophen assay capability is not available, and the estimated acetaminophen ingestion exceeds 150 mg/kg. acetylcysteine therapy should be initiated and continued for a full course of therapy.
For additional emergency information, call your regional poison center or call the Rocky Mountain Poison Center toll-free, (1-800-525-6115).
Symptoms from pseudoephedrine overdose consist most often of mild anxiety, tachycardia and/or mild hypertension. Symptoms usually appear within 4 to 8 hours of ingestion and are transient, usually requiring no treatment.
Acute dextromethorphan overdose usually does not result in serious signs and symptoms unless massive amounts have been ingested. Signs and symptoms of a substantial overdose may include nausea and vomiting, visual disturbances, CNS disturbances, and urinary retention.

Alcohol Information: Chronic heavy alcohol abusers may be at increased risk of liver toxicity from excessive acetaminophen use, although reports of this event are rare. Reports almost invariably involve cases of severe chronic alcoholics and the dosages of acetaminophen most often exceed recommended doses and often involve substantial overdose. Professionals should alert their patients who regular consume large amounts of alcohol not to exceed recommended doses of acetaminophen.

Inactive Ingredients: Caplet: Cellulose, Corn Starch, Glyceryl Triacetate, Hydroxypropyl Methylcellulose, Iron Oxide Black, Magnesium Stearate, Sodium Starch Glycolate, Titanium Dioxide, Blue #1 and Yellow #10.
Gelcap: Benzyl Alcohol, Butylparaben, Castor Oil, Cellulose, Corn Starch, Edetate Calcium Disodium, Gelatin, Hydroxypropyl Methylcellulose, Magnesium Stearate, Methylparaben, Propylparaben, Sodium Propionate, Sodium Lauryl Sulfate, Sodium Starch Glycolate, Titanium Dioxide, Red #40 and Yellow #10.

How Supplied: Caplets (colored white, imprinted "TYLENOL COLD")—blister packs of 24 and tamper-resistant bottles of 50.
Gelcaps (colored red and tan, imprinted "TYLENOL COLD")—blister packs of 20 and tamper-resistant bottles of 40.

Shown in Product Identification Guide, page 513

**Regular Strength
TYLENOL® acetaminophen
Caplets and Tablets**

Description: Each Regular Strength TYLENOL Caplet or Tablet contains acetaminophen 325 mg

Continued on next page

McNeil Consumer—Cont.

Actions: Acetaminophen is a clinically proven analgesic and antipyretic. Acetaminophen produces analgesia by elevation of the pain threshold and antipyresis through action on the hypothalamic heat-regulating center. Acetaminophen is equal to aspirin in analgesic and antipyretic effectiveness and it is unlikely to produce many of the side effects associated with aspirin and aspirin-containing products.

Indications: For the temporary relief of minor aches and pains associated with the common cold, headache, toothache, muscular aches, back ache, for the minor pain of arthritis, for the pain of menstrual cramps and for the reduction of fever.

Precautions: If a rare sensitivity reaction occurs, the drug should be discontinued.

Directions: Adults and Children 12 years of Age and Older: Take two caplets or tablets every 4 to 6 hours. No more than a total of 12 caplets or tablets in any 24-hour period, or as directed by a doctor. Children (6-11): ½ to 1 caplet or tablet every 4 to 6 hours, not to exceed 5 doses in 24 hours. Consult a physician for use by children under 6 years of age.

Warnings: Do not use if carton is opened or printed red neck wrap or printed foil inner seal is broken. Do not take for pain for more than 10 days or for fever for more than 3 days unless directed by a physician. If pain or fever persists, or gets worse, if new symptoms occur, or if redness or swelling is present, consult a physician because these could be signs of a serious condition. As with any drug, if your are pregnant or nursing a baby, seek the advice of a health professional before using this product. Keep this and all drugs out of the reach of children. In case of accidental overdose, contact a physician or poison control center immediately. Prompt medical attention is critical for adults as well as for children even if you do not notice any signs or symptoms. Do not use with other products containing acetaminophen.

Alcohol Warning: If you generally consume 3 or more alcohol-containing drinks per day, you should consult your physician for advice on when and how you should take Regular Strength TYLENOL® and other pain relievers.

Overdosage Information: Acetaminophen in massive overdosage may cause hepatic toxicity in some patients. In adults and adolescents, hepatic toxicity has rarely been reported following ingestion of acute overdoses of less than 10 grams. Fatalities are infrequent (less than 3-4% of untreated cases) and have rarely been reported with overdoses of less than 15 grams. In children, an aucte overdosage of less than 150 mg/kg has not been associated with hepatic toxicity. Early symptoms following a potentially hepatotoxic overdose may include: nausea, vomiting, diaphoresis and general malaise. Clinical and laboratory evidence of hepatic toxicity may not be apparent until 48 to 72 hours postingestion. In adults and adolescents, regardless of the quantity of acetaminophen reported to have been ingested, administer acetylcysteine immediately if 24 hours or less have elapsed from the reported time of ingestion. For full prescribing information, refer to the acetylcysteine package insert. Do not await results of assays for plasma acetaminophen level before initiating treatment with acetylcysteine. The following additional procedures are recommended. The stomach should be emptied promptly by lavage or by induction of emesis with syrup of ipecac. A plasma acetaminophen assay should be obtained as early as possible, but no sooner than four hours following ingestion. If plasma level falls above the lower treatment line on the acetaminophen overdose nomogram, acetylcysteine therapy should be continued. Liver function studies should be obtained initially and repeated at 24-hour intervals.

Serious toxicity or fatalities are extremely infrequent in children, possibly due to differences in the way they metabolize acetaminophen. In children, the maximum potential amount ingested can be more easily estimated. If more than 150 mg/kg or an unknown amount was ingested, obtain a plasma acetaminophen level. The plasma acetaminophen level should be obtained as soon as possible, but no sooner than 4 hours following the ingestion. If plasma level falls above the lower treatment line on the acetaminophen overdose nomogram, the acetylcysteine therapy should be initiated and continued for a full course of therapy. If plasma acetaminophen assay capability is not available, and the estimated acetaminophen ingestion exceeds 150 mg/kg, acetylcysteine therapy should be initiated and continued for a full course of therapy.

For additional emergency information, call your regional poison center or call the Rocky Mountain Poison Center toll-free (1-800-525-6115).

Alcohol Information

Chronic heavy alcohol abusers may be at increased risk of liver toxicity from excessive acetaminophen use, although reports of this event are rare. Reports almost invariably involve cases of severe chronic alcoholics and the dosages of acetaminophen most often exceed recommended doses and often involve substantial overdose. Professionals should alert their patients who regularly consume large amounts of alcohol not to exceed recommended doses of acetaminophen.

Inactive Ingredients: Tablets - Magnesium Stearate, Cellulose, Sodium Starch Glycolate and Starch. Caplets - Cellulose, Hydroxypropyl Methylcellulose, Magnesium Stearate, Polyethylene Glycol, Sodium Starch Glycolate, Starch and Red #40.

How Supplied: Tablets (colored white, scored, imprinted "TYLENOL") - tins of 12, and tamper-resistant bottles of 24, 50, 100 and 200. Caplets (colored white, "TYLENOL") - tamper-resistant bottles of 24, 50, 100. For additional pain relief, Extra Strength TYLENOL® Gelcaps, Geltabs, Caplets, and Tablets, 500 mg, and Extra Strength TYLENOL® Adult Liquid Pain Reliever are available (colored green; 1 fl. oz = 1000 mg)

Shown in Product Identification Guide, page 513

Mead Johnson Nutritionals

Mead Johnson & Company
A Bristol-Myers Squibb Company
2400 W. LLOYD EXPRESSWAY
EVANSVILLE, IN 47721

Enfamil® Infant Formula[1]
Enfamil® With Iron Infant Formula[1]
Enfamil® Infant Formula Nursette®
Enfamil® Premature Formula
Enfamil® Premature Formula With Iron
Enfamil® Human Milk Fortifier
Enfamil® Next Step® Toddler Formula[1]
Fer-In-Sol® Iron Supplement Drops, Syrup, Capsules
Lactofree® Milk-Based, Lactose-Free Formula for Baby's 1st year & beyond.[1]
Nutramigen® Hypoallergenic Protein Hydrolysate Formula[1]
Poly-Vi-Sol® Vitamins, Chewable Tablets and Drops (without Iron)
Poly-Vi-Sol® Vitamins, Peter Rabbit[2] Shaped Chewable Tablets (without Iron)
Poly-Vi-Sol® Vitamins with Iron, Peter Rabbit[2] Shaped Chewable Tablets
Poly-Vi-Sol® Vitamins with Iron, Drops
ProSobee® Soy Formula[1]
ProSobee® Soy Formula Nursette®

[1] Concentrated liquid, powder, and ready to use

[2] Registered trademark of F. Warne & Co., Inc.

Special Metabolic Diets:
Lofenalac® Iron Fortified Low Phenylalanine Diet Powder
Product 3200K Low Methionine Diet Powder
Product 3200AB Low PHE/TYR Diet Powder
Moducal® Dietary Carbohydrate Powder

Product 3232A Mono- and Disaccharide-Free Diet Powder

MSUD Diet Powder

Phenyl-Free® Phenylalanine-Free Diet Powder

Portagen® Iron Fortified Powder with Medium Chain Triglycerides

Pregestimil® Iron Fortified Protein Hydrolysate Formula with Medium Chain Triglycerides

Infalyte® Oral Electrolyte Maintenance Solution Made With Rice Syrup Solids

Special Metabolic Modules:

HIST 1
HIST 2
HOM 1
HOM 2
LYS 1
LYS 2
MSUD 1
MSUD 2
OS 1
OS 2
PKU 1
PKU 2
PKU 3
Protein-Free Diet Powder (Product 80056)
TYR 1
TYR 2
UCD 1
UCD 2

Tempra® 1 Acetaminophen Infant Drops

Tempra® 2 Acetaminophen Toddlers Syrup

Tempra® 3 Chewable Tablets, Regular or Double-Strength

Tri-Vi-Sol® Vitamin Drops

Tri-Vi-Sol® Vitamin Drops with Iron

Detailed information may be obtained by contacting Mead Johnson Nutritionals Medical Affairs Department at (812) 429-5599.

Miles Inc.
P. O. BOX 340
ELKHART, IN 46515

ALKA–MINTS® Chewable Antacid Rich in Calcium

Active Ingredient: Each ALKA-MINTS Chewable Antacid tablet contains calcium carbonate 850 mg (340 mg of elemental calcium). Each tablet contains less than .5 mg sodium per tablet, and is dietarily sodium free.

Inactive Ingredients: Dioctyl sodium sulfosuccinate, flavor, hydrolyzed cereal solids, magnesium stearate, polyethylene glycol, sorbitol, sugar (compressible).

Indications: ALKA-MINTS is an antacid for occasional use for relief of acid indigestion, heartburn and sour stomach.

Actions: ALKA-MINTS has a natural, clean, spearmint taste that leaves the mouth feeling refreshed. Measured by the in-vitro standard established by the Food and Drug Administration, one ALKA-MINTS tablet neutralizes 15.9 mEq of acid.

Warnings: Do not take more than 9 tablets in a 24 hour period, or use the maximum dosage of this product for more than 2 weeks, except under the advice and supervision of a physician. May cause constipation. As with any drug, if you are pregnant or nursing a baby, seek the advice of a health professional before using this product. Keep this and all drugs out of the reach of children.

Drug Interaction Precaution: Antacids may interact with certain prescription drugs. If you are presently taking a prescription drug, do not take this product without checking with your doctor or other health professional.

Dosage and Administration: Chew 1 or 2 tablets every 2 hours or as directed by a physician.

How Supplied: Bottles of 75's and 150's.

Product Identification Mark: ALKA-MINTS embossed on each tablet.

Shown in Product Identification Guide, page 514

ALKA–SELTZER® Effervescent Antacid & Pain Reliever With Specially Buffered Aspirin

Active Ingredients: Each tablet contains: aspirin 325 mg., heat treated sodium bicarbonate 1916 mg., citric acid 1000 mg. ALKA-SELTZER® in water contains principally the antacid sodium citrate and the analgesic sodium acetylsalicylate. Buffered pH is between 6 and 7.

Inactive Ingredients: None.

Indications: ALKA-SELTZER® Effervescent Antacid & Pain Reliever is an analgesic and an antacid and is indicated for relief of sour stomach, acid indigestion or heartburn with headache or body aches and pains. Also for fast relief of upset stomach with headache from over-indulgence in food and drink—especially recommended for taking before bed and again on arising. Effective for pain relief alone: headache or body and muscular aches and pains.

Actions: When the ALKA-SELTZER® Effervescent Antacid & Pain Reliever tablet is dissolved in water, the acetylsalicylate ion differs from acetylsalicylic acid chemically, physically and pharmacologically. Being fat insoluble, it is not absorbed by the gastric mucosal cells. Studies and observations in animals and man including radiochrome determinations of fecal blood loss, measurement of ion fluxes and direct visualization with gastrocamera, have shown that, as contrasted with acetylsalicylic acid, the acetylsalicylate ion delivered in the solution does not alter gastric mucosal permeability to permit back-diffusion of hydrogen ion, and gastric damage and acute gastric mucosal lesions are therefore not seen after administration of the product. ALKA-SELTZER® Effervescent Antacid & Pain Reliever has the capacity to neutralize gastric hydrochloric acid quickly and effectively. In-vitro, 154 ml. of 0.1 N hydrochloric acid are required to decrease the pH of one tablet of ALKA-SELTZER® Effervescent Antacid & Pain Reliever in solution to 4.0. Measured against the in vitro standard established by the Food and Drug Administration one tablet neutralizes 17.2 mEq of acid. In vivo, the antacid activity of two ALKA-SELTZER® Antacid & Pain Reliever tablets is comparable to that of 10 ml. of milk of magnesia. ALKA-SELTZER® Effervescent Antacid & Pain Reliever is able to resist pH changes caused by the continuing secretion of acid in the normal individual and to maintain an elevated pH until emptying occurs.

ALKA-SELTZER® Effervescent Antacid & Pain Reliever provides highly water soluble acetylsalicylate ions which are fat insoluble. Acetylsalicylate ions are not absorbed from the stomach. They empty from the stomach and thereby become available for absorption from the duodenum. Thus, fast drug absorption and high plasma acetylsalicylate levels are achieved. Plasma levels of salicylate following the administration of ALKA-SELTZER® Effervescent Antacid & Pain Reliever solution (acetylsalicylate ion equivalent to 648 mg. acetylsalicylic acid) can reach 29 mg./liter in 10 minutes and rise to peak levels as high as 55 mg./liter within 30 minutes.

Warnings: Children and teenagers should not use this medicine for chicken pox or flu symptoms before a doctor is consulted about Reye syndrome, a rare

Continued on next page

This product information was effective as of November 1, 1994. Current information may be obtained directly from Miles Inc., by writing to P.O. Box 340 Elkhart, IN 46515.

Miles—Cont.

but serious illness reported to be associated with aspirin. As with any drug, if you are pregnant or nursing a baby, seek the advice of a health professional before using this product. IT IS ESPECIALLY IMPORTANT NOT TO USE ASPIRIN DURING THE LAST 3 MONTHS OF PREGNANCY UNLESS SPECIFICALLY DIRECTED TO DO SO BY A DOCTOR BECAUSE IT MAY CAUSE PROBLEMS IN THE UNBORN CHILD OR COMPLICATIONS DURING DELIVERY. Except under the advice and supervision of a physician, do not take more than, Adults: 8 tablets in a 24 hour period. (60 years of age or older: 4 tablets in a 24 hour period), or use the maximum dosage for more than 10 days. Do not use if you are allergic to aspirin or have asthma, if you have bleeding problems, or if you are on a sodium restricted diet. Each tablet contains 567 mg. of sodium. If ringing in the ears or a loss of hearing occurs, consult a doctor before taking any more of this product.

Do not take this product for pain for more than 10 days unless directed by a doctor. If pain persists or gets worse, if new symptoms occur, or if redness or swelling is present, consult a doctor because these could be signs of a serious condition.

Keep this and all drugs out of the reach of children.

Drug Interaction Precaution: Do not take this product if you are taking a prescription drug for anticoagulation (thinning the blood), diabetes, gout or arthritis unless directed by a doctor. Antacids may interact with certain prescription drugs. If you are presently taking a prescription drug, do not take this product without checking with your doctor or other health professional.

Dosage and Administration:
ALKA-SELTZER® must be dissolved in water before taking.
Adults: 2 tablets every 4 hours.
CAUTION: If symptoms persist or recur frequently, or if you are under treatment for ulcer, consult your physician.

Professional Labeling:

ASPIRIN FOR MYOCARDIAL INFARCTION

Indication: The Aspirin contained in ALKA-SELTZER® is indicated to reduce the risk of death and/or non-fatal myocardial infarction in patients with a previous infarction or unstable angina pectoris.

Clinical Trials: The indication is supported by the results of six, large, randomized multicenter, placebo-controlled studies[1–7] involving 10,816, predominantly male, post-myocardial infarction (MI) patients and one randomized placebo-controlled study of 1,266 men with unstable angina. Therapy with aspirin was begun at intervals after the onset of acute MI varying from less than 3 days to more than 5 years and continued for periods of from less than one year to four years. In the unstable angina study, treatment was started within 1 month after the onset of unstable angina and continued for 12 weeks and complicating conditions such as congestive heart failure were not included in the study.

Aspirin therapy in MI patients was associated with about a 20 percent reduction in the risk of subsequent death and/or non-fatal reinfarction, a median absolute decrease of 3 percent from the 12 to 22 percent event rates in the placebo groups. In aspirin-treated unstable angina patients the reduction in risk was about 50 percent, a reduction in event rate of 5 percent from the 10 percent rate in the placebo group over the 12 weeks of the study.

Daily dosage of aspirin in the post-myocardial infarction studies was 300 mg in one study and 900 to 1500 mg in five studies. A dose of 325 mg was used in the study of unstable angina.

Adverse Reactions: Gastrointestinal Reactions: Symptoms and signs of gastrointestinal irritation were not significantly increased in subjects treated for unstable angina with buffered aspirin in solution (ALKA-SELTZER®). Doses of 1000 mg per day of aspirin tablets caused gastrointestinal symptoms and bleeding that in some cases were clinically significant. In the largest post-infarction study (the Aspirin Myocardial Infarction Study (AMIS) with 4,500 people), the percentage incidences of gastrointestinal symptoms for the aspirin (1000 mg of a standard, solid-tablet formulation) and placebo-treated subjects, respectively, were: stomach pain (14.5%; 4.4%); heartburn (11.9%; 4.8%); nausea and/or vomiting (7.6%; 2.1%); hospitalization for gastrointestinal disorder (4.9%; 3.5%). In the AMIS and other trials, aspirin treated patients had increased rates of gross gastrointestinal bleeding. As with all aspirin products ALKA-SELTZER is contraindicated in patients with aspirin sensitivity, with asthma, or with coagulation disease.

Cardiovascular and Biochemical: In the AMIS trial, the dosage of 1000 mg per day of aspirin was associated with small increases in systolic blood pressure (BP) (average 1.5 to 2.1 mm) and diastolic BP (0.5 to 0.6 mm), depending upon whether maximal or last available readings were used. Blood urea nitrogen and uric acid levels were also increased, but by less than 1.0 mg%. Subjects with marked hypertension or renal insufficiency had been excluded from the trial so that the clinical importance of these observations for such subjects or for any subjects treated over more prolonged periods is not known. It is recommended that patients placed on long-term aspirin treatment, even at doses of 300 mg per day, be seen at regular intervals to assess changes in these measurements.

Sodium in Buffered Aspirin for Solution Formulations: One tablet daily of buffered aspirin in solution adds 567 mg of sodium to that in the diet and may not be tolerated by patients with active sodium-retaining states such as congestive heart or renal failure. This amount of sodium adds about 30 percent to the 70 to 90 meq intake suggested as appropriate for dietary treatment of essential hypertension in the 1984 Report of the Joint National Committee on Detection, Evaluation, and Treatment of High Blood Pressure.[8]

Dosage and Administration: Although most of the studies used dosages exceeding 300 mg, daily, two trials used only 300 mg and pharmacologic data indicate that this dose inhibits platelet function fully. Therefore, 300 mg or a conventional 325 mg aspirin dose daily is a reasonable, routine dose that would minimize gastrointestinal adverse reactions. This use of aspirin applies to both solid, oral dosage forms (buffered and plain aspirin) and buffered aspirin in solution.

References:
(1) Elwood, P. C., et al., A Randomized Controlled Trial of Acetysalicylic Acid in the Secondary Prevention of Mortality from Myocardial Infarction," *British Medical Journal* 1:436–440, 1974.
(2) The Coronary Drug Project Research Group, "Aspirin in Coronary Heart Disease," *Journal of Chronic Diseases,* 29:625–642, 1976.
(3) Breddin K., et al., "Secondary Prevention of Myocardial Infarction: A Comparison of Acetylsalicylic Acid, Phenprocoumon or Placebo," *International Congress Series* 470:263–268, 1979.
(4) Aspirin Myocardial Infarction Study Research Group, "A Randomized, Controlled Trial of Aspirin in Persons Recovered from Myocardial Infarction," *Journal American Medical Association* 245:661–669, 1980.
(5) Elwood, P. C., and P. M. Sweetnam, "Aspirin and Secondary Mortality after Myocardial Infarction," *Lancet* pp. 1313–1315, December 22–29, 1979.
(6) The Persantine-Aspirin Reinfarction Study Research Group, "Persantine and Aspirin in Coronary Heart Disease," *Circulation,* 62: 449–460, 1980.
(7) Lewis, H. D., et al., "Protective Effects of Aspirin Against Acute Myocardial Infarction and Death in Men with Unstable Angina, Results of a Veterans Administration Cooperative Study," *New England Journal of Medicine* 309:396–403, 1983.

(8) "1984 Report of the Joint National Committee on Detection, Evaluation, Treatment of High Blood Pressure," U.S. Department of Health and Human Services and United States Public Health Service, National Institutes of Health.

How Supplied: Tablets: foil sealed; box of 12 in 6 foil twin packs; box of 24 in 12 foil twin packs; box of 36 tablets in 18 foil twin packs; 100 tablets in 50 foil twin packs; carton of 72 tablets in 36 foil twin packs. Product Identification Mark: "ALKA-SELTZER" embossed on each tablet.
Shown in Product Identification Guide, page 514

ALKA–SELTZER® Extra Strength Antacid & Pain Reliever

Active Ingredients: Each tablet contains: Aspirin 500mg, heat treated sodium bicarbonate 1985mg, citric acid 1000mg. Alka-Seltzer in water contains principally the antacid sodium citrate and the analgesic sodium acetylsalicylate.

Inactive Ingredient: Flavors

Indications: For fast relief of acid indigestion, sour stomach or heartburn with headache or body aches and pains. Also, for fast relief of upset stomach with headache from overindulgence in food and drink—especially recommended for taking before bed and again on arising. Effective for pain relief alone: headache or body and muscular aches and pains.

Warnings: Children and teenagers should not use this medicine for chicken pox or flu symptoms before a doctor is consulted about Reye syndrome, a rare but serious illness reported to be associated with aspirin. As with any drug, if you are pregnant or nursing a baby, seek the advice of a health professional before using this product. IT IS ESPECIALLY IMPORTANT NOT TO USE ASPIRIN DURING THE LAST 3 MONTHS OF PREGNANCY UNLESS SPECIFICALLY DIRECTED TO DO SO BY A DOCTOR BECAUSE IT MAY CAUSE PROBLEMS IN THE UNBORN CHILD OR COMPLICATIONS DURING DELIVERY. Except under the advice and supervision of a physician, do not take more than, Adults: 7 tablets in a 24-hour period (60 years of age or older, 4 tablets in a 24-hour period), or use the daily maximum dosage for more than 10 days. Do not use if you are allergic to aspirin or have asthma, if you have bleeding problems, or if you are on a sodium restricted diet. Each tablet contains 588mg of sodium. If ringing in the ears or a loss of

hearing occurs, consult a doctor before taking any more of this product.
Do not take this product for pain for more than 10 days unless directed by a doctor. If pain persists or gets worse, if new symptoms occur, or if redness or swelling is present, consult a doctor because these could be signs of a serious condition. Keep this and all drugs out of the reach of children.

Drug Interaction Precaution: Do not take this product if you are taking a prescription drug for anticoagulation (thinning the blood), diabetes, gout, or arthritis unless directed by a doctor. Antacids may interact with certain prescription drugs. If you are presently taking a prescription drug, do not take this product without checking with your doctor or other health professional.

Dosage and Administration: Extra Strength Alka-Seltzer must be dissolved in water before taking. Adults: 2 tablets every 6 hours. Caution: If symptoms persist, or recur frequently, or if you are under treatment for ulcer, consult your physician.

How Supplied: Foil sealed effervescent tablets in cartons of 12's in 6 foil twin packs; 24's in 12 foil twin packs.
Shown in Product Identification Guide, page 514

ALKA–SELTZER® GOLD Effervescent Antacid

Active Ingredients: Each tablet contains heat treated sodium bicarbonate 958 mg, citric acid 832 mg, potassium bicarbonate 312 mg. ALKA-SELTZER® Effervescent Antacid in water contains principally the antacids sodium citrate and potassium citrate.

Inactive Ingredient: A tableting aid. Does not contain aspirin.

Indications: ALKA-SELTZER® Effervescent Antacid is indicated for relief of acid indigestion, sour stomach or heartburn.

Actions: The ALKA-SELTZER® Effervescent Antacid solution provides quick and effective neutralization of gastric acid. Measured by the in vitro standard established by the Food and Drug Administration, one tablet will neutralize 10.6 mEq of acid.

Warnings: Except under the advice and supervision of a physician, do not take more than: Adults: 8 tablets in a 24-hour period (60 years of age or older: 7 tablets in a 24-hour period), Children: 4 tablets

in a 24-hour period; or use the maximum dosage of this product for more than 2 weeks.
Do not use this product if you are on a sodium restricted diet. Each tablet contains 311 mg of sodium.
Keep this and all drugs out of the reach of children. As with any drug, if you are pregnant or nursing a baby, seek the advice of a health professional before using this product.

Drug Interaction Precaution: Antacids may interact with certain prescription drugs. If you are presently taking a prescription drug, do not take this product without checking with your doctor or other health professional.

Dosage and Administration: Adults: Take 2 tablets fully dissolved in water every 4 hours. Children: ½ the adult dosage or as directed by a doctor.

How Supplied: Boxes of 20 tablets in 10 foil twin packs; 36 tablets in 18 foil twin packs.
Shown in Product Identification Guide, page 514

Lemon Lime ALKA-SELTZER® Effervescent Antacid & Pain Reliever

Active Ingredients: Each tablet contains: Aspirin 325 mg, heat treated sodium bicarbonate 1700 mg, citric acid 1000 mg. Alka-Seltzer in water contains principally the antacid sodium citrate and the analgesic sodium acetylsalicylate.

Inactive Ingredients: Aspartame, Flavor, Tableting Aids.

Indications: For fast relief of ACID INDIGESTION, SOUR STOMACH or HEARTBURN with HEADACHE, or BODY ACHES AND PAINS. Also for fast relief of UPSET STOMACH with HEADACHE from overindulgence in food and drink—especially recommended for taking before bed and again on arising. EFFECTIVE FOR PAIN RELIEF ALONE: HEADACHE or BODY and MUSCULAR ACHES and PAINS.

Warnings: Children and teenagers should not use this medicine for chicken pox or flu symptoms before a doctor is consulted about Reye syndrome, a rare but serious illness reported to be associated with aspirin.

Continued on next page

This product information was effective as of November 1, 1994. Current information may be obtained directly from Miles Inc., by writing to P.O. Box 340 Elkhart, IN 46515.

Miles—Cont.

As with any drug, if you are pregnant or nursing a baby, seek the advice of a health professional before using this product. IT IS ESPECIALLY IMPORTANT NOT TO USE ASPIRIN DURING THE LAST 3 MONTHS OF PREGNANCY UNLESS SPECIFICALLY DIRECTED TO DO SO BY A DOCTOR BECAUSE IT MAY CAUSE PROBLEMS IN THE UNBORN CHILD OR COMPLICATIONS DURING DELIVERY.

Except under the advice and supervision of a doctor: Do not take more than, ADULTS: 8 tablets in a 24-hour period, (60 years of age or older: 4 tablets in a 24-hour period), or use the daily maximum dosage for more than 10 days. Do not take this product if you are allergic to aspirin or have asthma, if you have bleeding problems, or if you are on a sodium restricted diet. Each tablet contains 506 mg of sodium. If ringing in the ears or a loss of hearing occurs, consult a doctor before taking any more of this product.

Do not take this product for pain for more than 10 days unless directed by a doctor. If pain persists or gets worse, if new symptoms occur, or if redness or swelling is present, consult a doctor because these could be signs of a serious condition.

Keep this and all drugs out of the reach of children.

Phenylketonurics: Contains Phenylalanine 9 mg per tablet.

Drug Interaction Precaution: Do not take this product if you are taking a prescription drug for anticoagulation (thinning the blood), diabetes, gout, or arthritis unless directed by a doctor. Antacids may interact with certain prescription drugs. If you are presently taking a prescription drug, do not take this product without checking with your doctor or other health professional.

Directions: Alka-Seltzer must be dissolved in water before taking. ADULTS: 2 tablets every 4 hours. CAUTION: If symptoms persist or recur frequently or if you are under treatment for ulcer, consult your physician.

Professional Labeling:

ASPIRIN FOR MYOCARDIAL INFARCTION

Indication: The Aspirin contained in Alka-Seltzer is indicated to reduce the risk of death and/or non-fatal myocardial infarction in patients with a previous infarction or unstable angina pectoris.

Clinical Trials: The indication is supported by the results of six, large, randomized multicenter, placebo-controlled studies[1-7] involving 10,816, predominantly male, post-myocardial infarction (MI) patients and one randomized placebo-controlled study of 1,266 men with unstable angina. Therapy with aspirin was begun at intervals after the onset of

acute MI varying from less than 3 days to more than 5 years and continued for periods of from less than one year to four years. In the unstable angina study, treatment was started within 1 month after the onset of unstable angina and continued for 12 weeks and complicating conditions such as congestive heart failure were not included in the study.

Aspirin therapy in MI patients was associated with about a 20 percent reduction in the risk of subsequent death and/or non-fatal reinfarction, a median absolute decrease of 3 percent from the 12 to 22 percent event rates in the placebo groups. In aspirin-treated unstable angina patients the reduction in risk was about 50 percent, a reduction in event rate of 5 percent from the 10 percent rate in the placebo group over the 12 weeks of the study.

Daily dosage of aspirin in the post-myocardial infarction studies was 300 mg in one study and 900 to 1500 mg in five studies. A dose of 325 mg was used in the study of unstable angina.

Adverse Reactions: Gastrointestinal Reactions: Symptoms and signs of gastrointestinal irritation were not significantly increased in subjects treated for unstable angina with buffered aspirin in solution (ALKA-SELZER®). Doses of 1000 mg per day of aspirin tablets caused gastrointestinal symptoms and bleeding that in some cases were clinically significant. In the largest post-infarction study (the Aspirin Myocardial Infarction Study (AMIS) with 4,500 people), the percentage incidences of gastrointestinal symptoms for the aspirin (1000 mg of a standard, solid-tablet formulation) and placebo-treated subjects, respectively, were: stomach pain (14.5%; 4.4%); heartburn (11.9%; 4.8%); nausea and/or vomiting (7.6%; 2.1%); hospitalization for gastrointestinal disorder (4.9%; 3.5%). In the AMIS and other trials, aspirin treated patients had increased rates of gross gastrointestinal bleeding. As with all aspirin products Alka-Seltzer is contraindicated in patients with aspirin sensitivity, with asthma, or with coagulation disease.

Cardiovascular and Biochemical: In the AMIS trial, the dosage of 1000 mg per day of aspirin was associated with small increases in systolic blood pressure (BP) (average 1.5 to 2.1 mm) and diastolic BP (0.5 to 0.6 mm), depending upon whether maximal or last available readings were used. Blood urea nitrogen and uric acid levels were also increased, but by less than 1.0 mg%. Subjects with marked hypertension or renal insufficiency had been excluded from the trial so that the clinical importance of these observations for such subjects or for any subjects treated over more prolonged periods is not known. It is recommended that patients placed on long-term aspirin treatment, even at doses of 300 mg per day, be seen at regular intervals to assess changes in these measurements.

Sodium in Buffered Aspirin for Solution Formulations: One tablet daily of flavored buffered aspirin in solution adds 506 mg of sodium to that in the diet and may not be tolerated by patients with active sodium-retaining states such as congestive heart or renal failure. This amount of sodium adds about 30 percent to the 70 to 90 meq intake suggested as appropriate for dietary treatment of essential hypertension in the 1984 Report of the Joint National Committee on Detection, Evaluation, and Treatment of High Blood Pressure.[8]

Dosage and Administration: Although most of the studies used dosages exceeding 300 mg, daily, two trials used only 300 mg and pharmacologic data indicate that this dose inhibits platelet function fully. Therefore, 300 mg or a conventional 325 mg aspirin dose daily is a reasonable, routine dose that would minimize gastrointestinal adverse reactions. This use of aspirin applies to both solid, oral dosage forms (buffered and plain aspirin) and buffered aspirin in solution.

References:
(1) Elwood, P. C., et al., A Randomized Controlled Trial of Acetysalicylic Acid in the Secondary Prevention of Mortality from Myocardial Infarction," *British Medical Journal* 1:436–440, 1974.
(2) The Coronary Drug Project Research Group, "Aspirin in Coronary Heart Disease," *Journal of Chronic Diseases,* 29:625–642, 1976.
(3) Breddin K., et al., "Secondary Prevention of Myocardial Infarction: A Comparison of Acetylsalicylic Acid, Phenprocoumon or Placebo," *International Congress Series* 470:263–268, 1979.
(4) Aspirin Myocardial Infarction Study Research Group, "A Randomized, Controlled Trial of Aspirin in Persons Recovered from Myocardial Infarction," *Journal American Medical Association* 245:661–669, 1980.
(5) Elwood, P. C., and P. M. Sweetnam, "Aspirin and Secondary Mortality after Myocardial Infarction," *Lancet* pp. 1313–1315, December 22–29, 1979.
(6) The Persantine-Aspirin Reinfarction Study Research Group, "Persantine and Aspirin in Coronary Heart Disease," *Circulation,* 62: 449–460, 1980.
(7) Lewis, H. D., et al., "Protective Effects of Aspirin Against Acute Myocardial Infarction and Death in Men with Unstable Angina, Results of a Veterans Administration Cooperative Study," *New England Journal of Medicine* 309:396–403, 1983.
(8) "1984 Report of the Joint National Committee on Detection, Evaluation, Treatment of High Blood Pressure," U.S. Department of Health and Human Services and United States Public Health Service, National Institutes of Health.

How Supplied: Foil sealed effervescent tablets in cartons of 12's in 6 foil twin packs; 24's in 12 foil twin packs; 36's in 18 foil twin packs.

Shown in Product Identification Guide, page 514

ALKA-SELTZER PLUS®
COLD & COUGH MEDICINE
LIQUI-GELS®

Directions For Use: ADULTS: Swallow 2 softgels with water. CHILDREN (6–12 years): Swallow 1 softgel with water. CHILDREN (under 6 years): Consult a doctor. Repeat every 4 hours, not to exceed 4 doses per day, or as directed by a doctor.

Indications: Provides temporary relief of these major symptoms of colds and flu with cough: coughing, runny nose, nasal and sinus congestion, headache, body aches and pains, sneezing, fever, and scratchy sore throat.

EACH Softgel CONTAINS THESE ACTIVE INGREDIENTS:	FOR THE TEMPORARY RELIEF OF THESE COLD AND FLU WITH COUGH SYMPTOMS
Cough Suppressant Dextromethorphan Hydrobromide 10 mg	Temporarily reduces the impulse to cough and controls the cough reflex that causes coughing.
Antihistamine Chlorpheniramine Maleate 2 mg	To help relieve the runny nose and sneezing that accompany colds and flu.
Nasal Decongestant Pseudoephedrine HCl 30 mg	To help restore free breathing shrink swollen nasal tissue and relieve sinus congestion due to head colds or flu.
Analgesic Acetaminophen 250 mg	Relieves headache scratchy sore throat, general body aches and the feverish feeling of a cold or flu.

Inactive Ingredients: Artificial Colors, Gelatin, Glycerin, Polyethylene Glycol, Povidone, Propylene Glycol, Purified Water, Sorbitol, Titanium Dioxide.

Warnings: Do not exceed recommended dosage because at higher doses nervousness, dizziness or sleeplessness may occur. Do not take this product for more than 7 days or for fever for more than 3 days unless directed by a doctor. If symptoms do not improve or are accompanied by fever, consult a doctor. A persistent cough may be a sign of a serious condition. If cough persists for more than 1 week, tends to recur or is accompanied by fever, rash or persistent headache, consult a doctor. Do not take this product

for persistent or chronic cough such as occurs with smoking, asthma, emphysema or if cough is accompanied by excessive phlegm (mucus) unless directed by a doctor. If sore throat is severe, persists for more than 2 days, is accompanied by or followed by fever, headache, nausea or vomiting, consult a doctor promptly. May cause excitability especially in children. Do not take this product, unless directed by a doctor, if you have a breathing problem such as emphysema or chronic bronchitis, or glaucoma, difficulty in urination due to enlargement of the prostate gland or heart disease, high blood pressure, diabetes, or thyroid disease. May cause marked drowsiness; alcohol, sedatives and tranquilizers may increase drowsiness effect. Avoid alcoholic beverages while taking this product. Do not take this product if you are taking sedatives or tranquilizers without first consulting your doctor. Use caution when driving a motor vehicle or operating machinery. As with any drug, if you are pregnant or nursing a baby seek the advice of a health professional before using this product. Keep this and all medication out of the reach of children. In case of accidental overdose, contact a physician or Poison Control Center immediately. Prompt medical attention is critical for adults as well as children even if you do not notice any signs or symptoms.

Drug Interaction Precaution: Do not use this product if you are taking a prescription drug for high blood pressure without first consulting your doctor or if you are now taking a prescription monoamine oxidase inhibitor (MAOI) (certain drugs for depression, psychiatric or emotional conditions, or Parkinson's disease), or for 2 weeks after stopping the MAOI drug. If you are uncertain whether your prescription drug contains an MAOI, consult a health professional before taking this product.

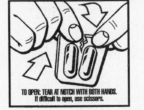

TO OPEN: TEAR AT NOTCH WITH BOTH HANDS. If difficult to open, use scissors.

How Supplied: Cartons of 12 and 20 softgels.
Distributed by Miles Inc., Elkhart, IN 46515 USA

Shown in Product Identification Guide, page 514

ALKA-SELTZER PLUS®
Cold Medicine

Active Ingredients:
Each dry ALKA-SELTZER PLUS® Cold Tablet contains the following active ingredients: Phenylpropanolamine bitartrate 24.08 mg, chlorpheniramine maleate 2 mg, aspirin 325 mg. The product is dissolved in water prior to ingestion and

the aspirin is converted into its soluble ionic form, sodium acetylsalicylate.

Inactive Ingredients: Citric acid, flavors, sodium bicarbonate.

Indications: Provides temporary relief of these major cold and flu symptoms: nasal and sinus congestion, runny nose, sneezing, headache, scratchy sore throat, fever, body aches and pains.

Warnings: Children and teenagers should not use this medicine for chicken pox or flu symptoms before a doctor is consulted about Reye syndrome, a rare but serious illness reported to be associated with aspirin. If sore throat is severe, persists for more than 2 days, is accompanied by high fever, headache, nausea or vomiting, consult a physician promptly. As with any drug, if you are pregnant or nursing a baby, seek the advice of a health professional before using this product. **IT IS ESPECIALLY IMPORTANT NOT TO USE ASPIRIN DURING THE LAST 3 MONTHS OF PREGNANCY UNLESS SPECIFICALLY DIRECTED TO DO SO BY A DOCTOR BECAUSE IT MAY CAUSE PROBLEMS IN THE UNBORN CHILD OR COMPLICATIONS DURING DELIVERY.**
Do not exceed recommended dosage because at higher doses nervousness, dizziness or sleeplessness may occur. May cause excitability, especially in children. Do not take this product unless directed by a doctor if you are allergic to aspirin, have a breathing problem such as emphysema or chronic bronchitis, asthma, glaucoma, difficulty in urination due to enlargement of the prostate gland, heart disease, high blood pressure, diabetes, thyroid disease, bleeding problems or on a sodium restricted diet. Each tablet contains 506 mg of sodium.
May cause drowsiness; alcohol, sedatives and tranquilizers may increase drowsiness effect. Avoid alcoholic beverages while taking this product. Do not take this product if you are taking sedatives or tranquilizers without first consulting your doctor. Use caution when driving a motor vehicle or operating machinery. Do not take this product for more than 7 days. If symptoms do not improve or are accompanied by fever or if fever persists for more than 3 days, consult a doctor. Keep this and all drugs out of the reach of children.

Drug Interaction Precaution: Do not take this product if you are presently taking a prescription drug for anticoagulation (thinning the bood), diabetes, gout, arthritis, high blood pressure or are presently taking a prescription monoamine oxidase inhibitor (MAOI) (certain drugs for depression, psychiatric or emotional conditions, or Parkinson's disease), or for

Continued on next page

This product information was effective as of November 1, 1994. Current information may be obtained directly from Miles Inc., by writing to P.O. Box 340 Elkhart, IN 46515.

Miles—Cont.

2 weeks after stopping the MAOI drug. If you are uncertain whether your prescription drug contains an MAOI, consult a health professional before taking this product.

Dosage and Administration:
ALKA-SELTZER PLUS® is taken in solution; 2 tablets dissolved in approximately 4 ounces of water. Adults: two tablets every 4 hours up to 8 tablets in 24 hours.

How Supplied: Tablets: carton of 12 tablets in 6 foil twin packs; 20 tablets in 10 foil twin packs; carton of 36 tablets in 18 foil twin packs; carton of 48 tablets in 24 foil twin packs.

Product Identification Mark:
"Alka-Seltzer Plus" embossed on each tablet.

Shown in Product Identification Guide, page 514

ALKA-SELTZER PLUS®
COLD MEDICINE
LIQUI-GELS®

Directions For Use: ADULTS: Swallow 2 softgels with water. CHILDREN (6–12 years): Swallow 1 softgel with water. CHILDREN (under 6 years): Consult a doctor. Repeat every 4 hours, not to exceed 4 doses per day, or as directed by a doctor.

Indications: Provides temporary relief of these major symptoms of colds and flu: runny nose, nasal and sinus congestion, headache, body aches and pains, sneezing, fever and scratchy sore throat.

EACH Softgel CONTAINS THESE ACTIVE INGREDIENTS:	FOR THE TEMPORARY RELIEF OF THESE COLD AND FLU SYMPTOMS
Antihistamine Chlorpheniramine Maleate 2 mg	To help relieve the runny nose and sneezing that accompany cold and flu.
Nasal Decongestant Pseudoephedrine HCl 30 mg	To help restore free breathing, shrink swollen nasal tissue and relieve sinus congestion due to head colds or flu.
Analgesic Acetaminophen 250 mg	Relieves headache scratchy sore throat, general body aches and the the feverish feeling of a cold or flu.

Inactive Ingredients: Artificial Colors, Gelatin, Glycerin, Polyethylene Glycol, Povidone, Propylene Glycol, Purified Water, Sorbitol, Titanium Dioxide.
Warnings: Do not exceed recommended dosage because at higher doses nervousness, dizziness or sleeplessness may occur. Do not take this product for more than 7 days or for fever for more than 3 days unless directed by a doctor. If symptoms do not improve or are accompanied by fever, consult a doctor. If sore throat is severe, persists for more than 2 days, is accompanied by or followed by fever, headache, rash, nausea or vomiting, consult a doctor promptly. May cause excitability especially in children. Do not take this product, unless directed by a doctor, if you have a breathing problem such as emphysema or chronic bronchitis, or glaucoma, difficulty in urination due to enlargement of the prostate gland or heart disease, high blood pressure, diabetes or thyroid disease. May cause drowsiness; alcohol, sedatives and tranquilizers may increase drowsiness effect. Avoid alcoholic beverages while taking this product. Do not take this product if you are taking sedatives or tranquilizers without first consulting your doctor. Use caution when driving a motor vehicle or operating machinery. As with any drug, if you are pregnant or nursing a baby, seek the advice of a health professional before using this product. Keep this and all medication out of the reach of children. In case of accidental overdose, contact a physician or Poison Control Center immediately. Prompt medical attention is critical for adults as well as children even if you do not notice any signs or symptoms.

Drug Interaction Precaution: Do not use this product if you are taking a prescription drug for high blood pressure without first consulting your doctor or if you are now taking a prescription monoamine oxidase inhibitor (MAOI) certain drugs for depression, psychiatric or emotional conditions, or Parkinson's disease), or for 2 weeks after stopping the MAOI drug. If you are uncertain whether your prescription drug contains an MAOI, consult a health professional before taking this product.

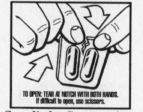

TO OPEN: TEAR AT NOTCH WITH BOTH HANDS. If difficult to open, use scissors.

How Supplied: Cartons of 12 and 20 softgels.
Distributed by Miles Inc., Elkhart, IN 46515 USA

Shown in Product Identification Guide, page 514

ALKA-SELTZER PLUS®
NIGHT-TIME COLD MEDICINE
LIQUI-GELS®

Directions For Use: ADULTS: Swallow 2 softgels with water, once daily, at bedtime. Not recommended for children.
Indications: Provides temporary relief of these major symptoms of colds and flu with cough: coughing, runny nose, nasal and sinus congestion, headache, body aches and pains, sneezing, fever, and scratchy sore throat.

EACH Softgel CONTAINS THESE ACTIVE INGREDIENTS:	FOR THE TEMPORARY RELIEF OF THESE COLD AND FLU SYMPTOMS
Cough Suppressant Dextromethorphan Hydrobromide 10 mg	Temporarily reduces the impulse to cough and controls the cough reflex that causes coughing.
Antihistamine Doxylamine Succinate 6.25 mg	To help relieve the runny nose and sneezing that accompany colds and flu.
Nasal Decongestant Pseudoephedrine HCl 30 mg	To help restore free breathing, shrink swollen nasal tissue, and relieve sinus congestion due to head colds or flu.
Analgesic Acetaminophen 250 mg	Relieves headache, scratchy sore throat, general body aches and the feverish feeling of a cold or flu.

Inactive Ingredients: Artificial Colors, Gelatin, Glycerin, Polyethylene Glycol, Povidone, Propylene Glycol, Purified Water, Sorbitol, Titanium Dioxide. Contains No Alcohol.

Warnings: Do not exceed recommended dosage because at higher doses nervousness, dizziness or sleeplessness may occur. Do not take this product for more than 7 days or for fever for more than 3 days unless directed by a doctor. If symptoms do not improve or are accompanied by fever, consult a doctor. A persistent cough may be a sign of a serious condition. If cough persists for more than 1 week, tends to recur or is accompanied by fever, rash or persistent headache, consult a doctor. Do not take this product for persistent or chronic cough such as occurs with smoking, asthma, emphysema or if cough is accompanied by excessive phlegm (mucus) unless directed by a doctor. If sore throat is severe, persists for more than 2 days, is accompanied by or followed by fever, headache, nausea or vomiting, consult a doctor promptly. May cause excitability especially in children. Do not take this product, unless directed by a doctor, if you have a breathing problem such as emphysema or chronic bronchitis, or glaucoma, difficulty in urination due to enlargement of the prostate gland or heart disease, high blood pressure, diabetes, or thyroid disease. May cause marked drowsiness; alcohol, sedatives and tranquilizers may increase drowsiness effect. Avoid alcoholic beverages while taking this product. Do not take this product if you are taking sedatives or tranquilizers without first consulting your doctor. Use caution when driving a motor vehicle or operating machinery. As with any drug, if you are pregnant or nursing a baby, seek the advice of a health professional before using this product. Keep this and all medication out of the reach of children. In case of accidental overdose, contact a physician or Poison Control Center immediately. Prompt medical attention is critical for adults as well as children even if you do not notice any signs or symptoms.

Drug Interaction Precaution: Do not use this product if you are taking a prescription drug for high blood pressure without first consulting your doctor or if you are now taking prescription monoamine oxidase inhibitor (MAOI) (certain drugs for depression, psychiatric or emotion conditions, or Parkinson's disease), or for 2 weeks after stopping the MAOI drug. If you are uncertain whether your prescription drug contains an MAOI, consult a health professional before taking this product.

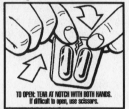

TO OPEN: TEAR AT NOTCH WITH BOTH HANDS.
If difficult to open, use scissors.

How Supplied: Cartons of 12 and 20 softgels.
Distributed by Miles Inc., Elkhart, IN 46515 USA
Shown in Product Identification Guide, page 515

ALKA–SELTZER PLUS®
Night-Time Cold Medicine

Active Ingredients: Each tablet contains aspirin 500 mg, doxylamine succinate 6.25 mg, phenylpropanolamine bitartrate 20 mg, dextromethorphan hydrobromide 15 mg. In water the aspirin is converted into its soluble ionic form, sodium acetylsalicylate.

Inactive Ingredients: Aspartame, citric acid, flavors, sodium bicarbonate, tableting aid.

Indications: For temporary relief of these major cold and flu symptoms: coughing, nasal and sinus congestion, body aches and pains, runny nose, headache, sneezing, fever, scratchy sore throat so you can get the rest you need.

Warning: Children and teenagers should not use this medicine for chicken pox or flu symptoms before a doctor is consulted about Reye syndrome, a rare but serious illness reported to be associated with aspirin. If sore throat is severe, persists for more than 2 days, is accompanied by high fever, headache, nausea or vomiting, consult a physician promptly. As with any drug, if you are pregnant or

nursing a baby, seek the advice of a health professional before using this product. **IT IS ESPECIALLY IMPORTANT NOT TO USE ASPIRIN DURING THE LAST 3 MONTHS OF PREGNANCY UNLESS SPECIFICALLY DIRECTED TO DO SO BY A DOCTOR BECAUSE IT MAY CAUSE PROBLEMS IN THE UNBORN CHILD OR COMPLICATIONS DURING DELIVERY.**
Do not exceed recommended dosage because at higher doses nervousness, dizziness or sleeplessness may occur. May cause excitability, especially in children. Do not take this product unless directed by a doctor if you are allergic to aspirin, have a breathing problem such as emphysema or chronic bronchitis, asthma, glaucoma, difficulty in urination due to enlargement of the prostate gland, heart disease, high blood pressure, diabetes, thyroid disease, bleeding problems or on a sodium restricted diet. Each tablet contains 506 mg of sodium.
May cause marked drowsiness; alcohol, sedatives and tranquilizers may increase drowsiness effect. Avoid alcoholic beverages while taking this product. Do not take this product if you are taking sedatives or tranquilizers without first consulting your doctor. Use caution when driving a motor vehicle or operating machinery. Do not take this product for persistent or chronic cough such as occurs with smoking, asthma, emphysema, or if cough is accompanied by excessive phlegm (mucus), unless directed by a doctor. A persistent cough may be a sign of a serious condition. If cough persists for more than 1 week, tends to recur or is accompanied by fever, rash, or persistent headache, consult a doctor. Do not take this product for more than 7 days. If symptoms do not improve or are accompanied by fever or if fever persists for more than 3 days, consult a doctor. Keep this and all drugs out of the reach of children.

Phenylketonurics: Contains Phenylalanine 16.2 mg per tablet.

Drug Interaction Precaution: Do not take this product if you are presently taking a prescription drug for anticoagulation (thinning the blood), diabetes, gout, arthritis, high blood pressure or are presently taking a monoamine oxidase inhibitor (MAOI) (certain drugs for depression, psychiatric or emotional conditions, or Parkinson's disease), or for 2 weeks after stopping the MAOI drug. If you are uncertain whether your prescription drug contains an MAOI, consult a health professional before taking this product.

Dosage and Administration: Adults: Take 2 tablets fully dissolved in 4 ounces of water (use more or less water to taste). Additional fluid intake is encouraged for cold sufferers. Repeat every 4 hours, not to exceed 8 tablets in any 24-hour period.

How Supplied: Tablets: carton of 12 tablets in 6 foil twin packs; carton of 20

tablets in 10 foil twin packs; carton of 36 tablets in 18 foil twin packs.

Product Identification Mark: "A/S PLUS NIGHT-TIME" etched on each tablet
Shown in Product Identification Guide, page 514

ALKA–SELTZER PLUS®
Sinus Medicine

Active Ingredients: Phenylpropanolamine bitartrate 24.08 mg, brompheniramine maleate 2 mg, aspirin 500 mg. In water the aspirin is converted into its soluble ionic form, sodium acetylsalicylate.

Inactive Ingredients: Aspartame, citric acid, flavors, heat-treated sodium bicarbonate, tableting aids

Indications: For the temporary relief of these major sinusitis, allergic rhinitis or hay fever symptoms: nasal congestion sinus pain and pressure, runny nose, headache, itchy, watery eyes and sneezing.

Warnings: Children and teenagers should not use this medicine for chicken pox or flu symptoms before a doctor is consulted about Reye syndrome, a rare but serious illness reported to be associated with aspirin. As with any drug, if you are pregnant or nursing a baby, seek the advice of a health professional before using this product. **IT IS ESPECIALLY IMPORTANT NOT TO USE ASPIRIN DURING THE LAST 3 MONTHS OF PREGNANCY UNLESS SPECIFICALLY DIRECTED TO DO SO BY A DOCTOR BECAUSE IT MAY CAUSE PROBLEMS IN THE UNBORN CHILD OR COMPLICATIONS DURING DELIVERY.**
Do not exceed recommended dosage because at higher doses nervousness, dizziness or sleeplessness may occur. May cause excitability, especially in children. Do not take this product unless directed by a doctor if you are allergic to aspirin, have a breathing problem such as emphysema or chronic bronchitis, asthma, glaucoma, difficulty in urination due to enlargement of the prostate gland, heart disease, high blood pressure, diabetes, thyroid disease, bleeding problems or on a sodium restricted diet. Each tablet contains 506 mg of sodium.
May cause drowsiness; alcohol, sedatives and tranquilizers may increase the drowsiness effect. Avoid alcoholic beverages while taking this product. Do not take this product if you are taking sedatives or tranquilizers without first consulting your doctor. Use caution when driving a motor vehicle or operating machinery. Do not take this product for more than 7

Continued on next page

This product information was effective as of November 1, 1994. Current information may be obtained directly from Miles Inc., by writing to P.O. Box 340 Elkhart, IN 46515.

Miles—Cont.

days. If symptoms do not improve or are accompanied by fever or if fever persists for more than 3 days, consult a doctor. Keep this and all drugs out of the reach of children.

Phenylketonurics: Contains Phenylalanine 8.98 mg per tablet.

Drug Interaction Precaution: Do not take this product if you are presently taking a prescription drug for anticoagulation (thinning of the blood), diabetes, gout, arthritis, high blood pressure or are presently taking a monoamine oxidase inhibitor (MAOI) (certain drugs for depression, psychiatric or emotional conditions, or Parkinson's disease), or for 2 weeks after stopping the MAOI drug. If you are uncertain whether your prescription drug contains an MAOI, consult a health professional before taking this product.

Directions: Adults: Take 2 tablets dissolved in approximately 4 ounces (½ glass) of water every 4 hours. Do not exceed 8 tablets in any 24-hour period.

How Supplied: Boxes of 20 tablets in 10 foil twin packs.

Product Identification Mark: "AS + Sinus" embossed on each tablet.
Shown in Product Identification Guide, page 515

ALKA-SELTZER PLUS® COLD & COUGH MEDICINE

Active Ingredients: Each ALKA-SELTZER PLUS® COLD AND COUGH tablet contains the following active ingredients: Aspirin 325 mg, Chlorpheniramine Maleate 2 mg, Phenylpropanolamine Bitartrate 20 mg, Dextromethorphan Hydrobromide 10 mg. In water the aspirin is converted into its soluble ionic form, sodium acetylsalicylate.

Inactive Ingredients: Aspartame, Citric Acid, Flavor, Sodium Bicarbonate, Tableting Aids.

Indications: Provides temporary relief of these major symptoms of colds and flu with cough: nasal and sinus congestion, body aches and pains, runny nose, coughing, headache, scratchy sore throat, sneezing, fever.

Warning: Children and teenagers should not use this medicine for chicken pox or flu symptoms before a doctor is consulted about Reye syndrome, a rare but serious illness reported to be associated with aspirin. If sore throat is severe, persists for more than 2 days, is accompanied by high fever, headache, nausea or vomiting, consult a physician promptly. As with any drug, if you are pregnant or nursing a baby, seek the advice of a health professional before using this product. **IT IS ESPECIALLY IMPORTANT NOT TO USE ASPIRIN DURING THE LAST 3 MONTHS OF PREGNANCY UNLESS SPECIFICALLY DI-**

RECTED TO DO SO BY A DOCTOR BECAUSE IT MAY CAUSE PROBLEMS IN THE UNBORN CHILD OR COMPLICATIONS DURING DELIVERY.

Do not exceed recommended dosage because at higher doses nervousness, dizziness or sleeplessness may occur. May cause excitability, especially in children. Do not take this product unless directed by a doctor if you are allergic to aspirin, have a breathing problem such as emphysema or chronic bronchitis, asthma, glaucoma, difficulty in urination due to enlargement of the prostate gland, heart disease, high blood pressure, diabetes, thyroid disease, bleeding problems or on a sodium restricted diet. Each tablet contains 507 mg of sodium.

May cause marked drowsiness; alcohol, sedatives and tranquilizers may increase drowsiness effect. Avoid alcoholic beverages while taking this product. Do not take this product if you are taking sedatives or tranquilizers without first consulting your doctor. Use caution when driving a motor vehicle or operating machinery. Do not take this product for persistent or chronic cough such as occurs with smoking, asthma, emphysema, or if cough is accompanied by excessive phlegm (mucus) unless directed by a doctor. A persistent cough may be a sign of a serious condition. If cough persists for more than 1 week, tends to recur or is accompanied by fever, rash, or persistent headache, consult a doctor. Do not take this product for more than 7 days. If symptoms do not improve or are accompanied by fever or if fever persists for more than 3 days, consult a doctor. Keep this and all drugs out of the reach of children.

Phenylketonurics: Contains Phenylalanine 11.2 mg per tablet.

Drug Interaction Precaution: Do not take this product if you are presently taking a prescription drug for anticoagulation (thinning the blood), diabetes, gout, arthritis, high blood pressure or are presently taking a monoamine oxidase inhibitor (MAOI) (certain drugs for depression, psychiatric or emotional conditions, or Parkinson's disease), or for 2 weeks after stopping the MAOI drug. If you are uncertain whether your prescription drug contains an MAOI, consult a health professional before taking this product.

Dosage and Administration: ALKA-SELTZER PLUS® COLD & COUGH MEDICINE is taken in solution; approximately 4 ounces of water. Additional fluid intake is encouraged for cold sufferers. Adults: 2 tablets every 4 hours up to 8 tablets in 24 hours.

How Supplied: Tablets: carton of 36 tablets in 18 foil twin packs; carton of 20 tablets in 10 foil twin packs; carton of 12 tablets in 6 foil packs.

Product Identification Mark: "AS + Cold Cough" embossed on each tablet.
Shown in Product Identification Guide, page 514

BACTINE® Antiseptic · Anesthetic First Aid Liquid

Active Ingredients: Benzalkonium Chloride 0.13% w/w, Lidocaine HCl 2.5% w/w.

Inactive Ingredients: Edetate Disodium, Fragrances, Octoxynol 9, Propylene Glycol, Purified Water.

Indications: First aid to help prevent bacterial contamination or skin infection and for the temporary relief of pain and itching in minor cuts, scrapes and burns.

Warnings: FOR EXTERNAL USE ONLY. Do not use in the eyes or apply over large areas of the body. In case of deep or puncture wounds, animal bites, or serious burns, consult a doctor. Stop use and consult a doctor if the condition persists or gets worse. Do not use longer than 1 week unless directed by a doctor. Do not use in large quantities, particularly over raw surfaces or blistered areas. Keep this and all drugs out of the reach of children. In case of accidental ingestion, seek professional assistance or contact a Poison Control Center immediately.

Directions: For adults and children 2 years of age and older. Clean the affected area. Apply a small amount of this product on the area 1 to 3 times daily. May be covered with a sterile bandage. If bandaged, let dry first.

How Supplied: 2 oz., 4 oz. and 16 oz. liquid, and 3.5 oz. pump spray.
Shown in Product Identification Guide, page 515

BACTINE® First Aid Antibiotic Plus Anesthetic Ointment

Active Ingredients: Each gram contains Polymyxin B Sulfate 10,000 units; Bacitracin Zinc 500 units; Neomycin Sulfate 5 mg (equivalent to 3.5 mg Neomycin base); Lidocaine 40 mg (pain reliever).

Inactive Ingredient: White Petrolatum.

Indications: First aid to help prevent infection, guard against bacterial contamination, relieve pain and itching in minor cuts, scrapes and burns.

Warning: For external use only. Do not use in the eyes or apply over large areas of the body. In case of deep or puncture wounds, animal bites or serious burns, consult a doctor. Stop use and consult a doctor if the condition persists or gets worse. Do not use longer than 1 week unless directed by a doctor. Keep this and all medicines out of children's reach. In case of accidental ingestion, seek professional assistance or contact a Poison Control Center immediately.

Directions: Clean the affected area. Apply a small amount of the product (an amount equal to the surface area of the tip of a finger) one to three times daily. May be covered with a sterile bandage.

How Supplied: ½ oz. tube.
Shown in Product Identification Guide, page 515

BACTINE® 1.0% Hydrocortisone Anti-Itch Cream

Active Ingredient: Hydrocortisone 1.0%.

Inactive Ingredients: Aluminum Sulfate, Beeswax, Calcium Acetate, Cetearyl Alcohol, Dextrin, Glycerin, Hydrocortisone Alcohol, Light Mineral Oil, Methylparaben, Purified Water, Sodium Lauryl Sulfate, White Petrolatum.

Indications: For the temporary relief of itching associated with minor skin irritations, inflammation and rashes.

Warnings: For external use only. Avoid contact with the eyes. If condition worsens or if symptoms persist for more than seven days or clear up and occur again within a few days, stop use of this product and do not begin use of any other hydrocortisone product unless you have consulted a physician. Do not use for the treatment of diaper rash. Consult a physician.
Keep this and all drugs out of the reach of children. In case of accidental ingestion, seek professional assistance or contact a Poison Control Center immediately.

Directions: For Adults and Children 2 years of age and older. Apply to affected area not more than 3 or 4 times daily. Children under 2 years of age: Do not use, consult a physician.

How Supplied: 1 oz. tube.
Shown in Product Identification Guide, page 515

ASPIRIN REGIMEN BAYER®
Aspirin
Delayed Release Enteric Aspirin
Regular Strength 325 mg Caplets and
Adult Low Strength 81 mg Tablets

Composition: Active Ingredient: ASPIRIN REGIMEN BAYER® is an enteric-coated aspirin available in 325 mg caplet and 81 mg tablet forms. The enteric coating prevents disintegration in the stomach and promotes dissolution in the duodenum, where there is a more neutral to alkaline environment. This action aids in protecting the stomach against injuries that may occur as a result of ingesting non-enteric coated aspirin.

Safety: The safety of enteric-coated aspirin has been demonstrated in a number of endoscopic studies comparing enteric-coated aspirin and plain aspirin, as well as buffered aspirin and "arthritis strength" preparations. In these studies, endoscopies were performed in healthy volunteers before and after either 2-day or 14-day administration of aspirin doses of 3,900 or 4,000 mg per day. Compared to all the other preparations, the enteric-coated aspirin produced signficantly less damage to the gastric mucosa. There was also statistically less duodenal damage when compared with the plain, i.e., non-enteric-coated aspirin.

Bioavailability: The bioavailability of aspirin from **ASPIRIN REGIMEN BAYER®** has been confirmed. In single-dose studies[1] in which plasma acetylsalicylic acid and salicylic acid levels were measured, maximum concentrations were achieved at approximately 5 hours postdosing. **ASPIRIN REGIMEN BAYER®,** when compared with plain aspirin, achieves maximum plasma salicylate levels not significantly different from plain, i.e., non-enteric-coated, aspirin. Dissolution of the enteric coating occurs at a neutral to basic pH and is therefore dependent on gastric emptying into the duodenum. With continued dosing, appropriate therapeutic plasma levels are maintained.

Regular Strength 325mg—D&C Yellow #10, FD&C Yellow #6, Hydroxypropyl Methylcellulose, Methacrylic Acid Copolymer, Starch, Titanium Dioxide, Triacetin.

Adult Low Strength 81mg—Croscarmellose Sodium, D&C Yellow #10, FD&C Yellow #6, Hydroxypropyl Methylcellulose, Iron Oxides, Lactose, Methacrylic Acid, Microcrystalline Cellulose, Polysorbate 80, Sodium Lauryl Sulfate, Starch, Titanium Dioxide, Triacetin.

Indications: ASPIRIN REGIMEN BAYER®is an anti-inflammatory, analgesic, and antiplatelet agent indicated for the relief of painful discomfort and muscular aches and pains associated with conditions requiring long-term aspirin therapy, e.g., arthritis or rheumatism, and for situations where compliance with aspirin usage may be hindered by gastrointestinal side effects of non-enteric-coated or buffered aspirin. For additional **Anti-inflammatory, Antiarthritic,** and **Antiplatelet** indications, see the **PROFESSIONAL LABELING** section.

Directions: The following dosages are provided as appropriate for self-medication:
For analgesic indications the maximum adult nonprescription dosage of aspirin is 4,000 mg per day in divided doses, i.e., two 325 mg caplets or eight 81 mg tablets every 4 hours or three 325 mg caplets or twelve 81 mg tablets every 6 hours. Under a physician's recommendation, the dosage or frequency may be modified as appropriate for the clinical situation.

Consumer Warnings: Children and teenagers should not use this medicine for chicken pox or flu symptoms before a doctor is consulted about Reye Syndrome, a rare but serious illness reported to be associated with aspirin. Do not take for pain for more than 10 days or for fever for more than 3 days unless directed by a doctor. If pain or fever persists or gets worse, if new symptoms occur, or if redness or swelling is present, consult a doctor because these could be signs of a serious condition. Do not take this product if you are allergic to aspirin, have asthma, have stomach problems (such as heartburn, upset stomach or stomach pain) that persist or recur, or have gastric ulcers or bleeding problems unless directed by a doctor. If ringing in the ears or loss of hearing occurs, consult a doctor before taking any more of this product. Keep this and all drugs out of the reach of children. In case of accidental overdose, seek professional assistance or contact a poison control center immediately. As with any drug, if you are pregnant or nursing a baby, seek the advice of a health professional before using this product. IT IS ESPECIALLY IMPORTANT NOT TO USE ASPIRIN DURING THE LAST 3 MONTHS OF PREGNANCY UNLESS SPECIFICALLY DIRECTED TO DO SO BY A DOCTOR BECAUSE IT MAY CAUSE PROBLEMS IN THE UNBORN CHILD OR COMPLICATIONS DURING DELIVERY.

Drug Interaction Precaution: Do not take this product if you are taking a prescription drug for anticoagulation (thinning the blood), diabetes, gout, or arthritis unless directed by a doctor.

Professional Labeling:

Antiarthritic and Anti-inflammatory Effect

Indications: For conditions requiring chronic or long-term aspirin therapy for pain and/or inflammation, e.g., rheumatoid arthritis, juvenile rheumatoid arthritis, systemic lupus erythematosus, osteoarthritis (degenerative joint disease), ankylosing spondylitis, psoriatic arthritis, Reiter's syndrome, and fibrositis.

Antiplatelet Effect
Aspirin for Myocardial Infarction

Indication: Aspirin is indicated to reduce the risk of death and/or nonfatal myocardial infarction in patients with a previous infarction or unstable angina pectoris.

Clinical Trials: The indication is supported by the results of six large, randomized, multicenter, placebo-controlled studies involving 10,816 predominantly male, post-myocardial infarction (MI) patients and one randomized placebo-controlled study of 1,266 men with unstable angina.[2,8] Therapy wih aspirin was begun at intervals after the onset of acute MI varying from less than 3 days to more than 5 years and continued for periods of from less than 1 year to 4 years. In the unstable angina study, treatment was started within 1 month after onset of unstable angina and continued for 12

Continued on next page

This product information was effective as of November 1, 1994. Current information may be obtained directly from Miles Inc., by writing to P.O. Box 340 Elkhart, IN 46515.

Miles—Cont.

weeks, and patients with complicating conditions, such as congestive heart failure, were not included in the study. Aspirin therapy in MI patients was associated with about a 20 percent reduction in the risk of subsequent death and/or nonfatal reinfarction, a median absolute decrease of 3 percent from the 12 to 22 percent event rates in the placebo groups. In aspirin-treated unstable angina patients, the reduction in risk was about 50 percent, a reduction in the event rate of 5 percent from the 10 percent rate in the placebo group over the 12 weeks of the study.

Daily dosage of aspirin in the post-myocardial infarction studies was 300 mg in one study and 900 to 1,500 mg in five studies. A dose of 325 mg was used in the study of unstable angina.

Adverse Reactions: Gastrointestinal Reactions: Doses of 1,000 mg per day of aspirin caused gastrointestinal symptoms and bleeding that in some cases were clinically significant. In the largest post-infarction study (the Aspirin Myocardial Infarction Study [AMIS] with 4,500 people), the percentage incidence of gastrointestinal symptoms for the aspirin- (1,000 mg of a standard, solid tablet formulation) and placebo-treated subjects, respectively, were: stomach pain (14.5 percent, 4.4 percent); heartburn (11.9 percent, 4.8 percent), nausea and/or vomiting (7.6 percent, 2.1 percent); hospitalization for gastrointestinal disorder (4.8 percent, 3.5 percent). In the AMIS and other trials, aspirin-treated patients had increased rates of gross gastrointestinal bleeding. Symptoms and signs of gastrointestinal irritation were not significantly increased in subjects treated for unstable angina with buffered aspirin in solution.

Cardiovascular and Biochemical: In the AMIS trial the dosage of 1,000 mg per day of aspirin was associated with small increases in systolic blood pressure (BP) (average 1.5 to 2.1 mm) and diastolic BP (0.5 to 2.1 mm), depending upon whether maximal or last available readings were used. Blood urea nitrogen and uric acid levels were also increased, but by less than 1.0 mg%. Subjects with marked hypertension or renal insufficiency had been excluded from trial so that the clinical importance of these observations for such subjects or for any subject treated over more prolonged periods is not known. It is recommended that patients placed on long-term aspirin treatment, even at doses of 300 mg per day, be seen at regular intervals to assess changes in these measurements.

Dosage and Administration: Although most of the studies used dosages exceeding 300 mg, two trials used only 300 mg and pharmacological data indicate that this dose inhibits platelet function fully. Therefore, 300 mg or a conventional 325 mg aspirin dose is a reasonable, routine dose that would minimize gastrointestinal adverse reactions. This use of aspirin applies to both solid oral dosage forms (buffered and plain aspirin) and buffered aspirin in solution.

Aspirin for Transient Ischemic Attacks

Indications: For reducing the risk of recurrent Transient Ischemic Attacks (TIAs) or storke in men who have transient ischemia of the brain due to fibrin emboli. There is inadequate evidence that aspirin or buffered aspirin is effective in reducing TIAs in women at the recommended dosage. There is no evidence that aspirin or buffered aspirin is of benefit in the treatment of completed strokes in men or women.

Clinical Trials: The indication is supported by the result of a Canadian study[9] in which 585 patients with threatened stroke followed in a randomized clinical trial for an average of 28 months to determine whether aspirin or sulfinpyrazone, singly or in combination, was superior to placebo in preventing transient ischemic attacks, stroke, or death. The study showed that although sulfinpyrazone had no statistically significant effect, aspirin reduced the risk of continuing transient ischemic attacks, stroke or death by 19 percent and reduced the risk of stroke or death by 31 percent. Another aspirin study trial carried out in the United States with 178 patients showed a statiscally significant number of "favorable outcomes" including reduced transient ischemic attacks, stroke, and death.[10]

Precautions: Patients presenting with signs and symptoms of a TIA should have a complete medical and neurological evaluation. Consideration should be given to other disorders that resemble TIAs. Attention should be given to risk factors; it is important to evaluate and treat, if appropriate, other diseases associated with TIAs and stroke, such as hypertension and diabetes.

Other Precautions: Concurrent administration of absorbable antacids at therapeutic doses may increase the clearance of salicylates in some individuals. The concurrent administration of nonabsorbable antacids may alter the rate of absorption of acetylsalicylic acid, resulting in a decreased acetylsalicylic acid/salicylate ratio in plasma. The clinical significance of these decreases in available aspirin is unknown.

Dosage and Administration: Adult oral dosage for men is 1,300 mg a day, in divided doses of 650 mg twice a day or 325 mg four times daily.

Occasional reports have documented individuals with impaired gastric emptying in whom there may be retention of one or more enteric-coated tablets over time. This phenomenon may occur as a result of outlet obstruction from ulcer disease alone or combined with hypotonic gastric peristalsis. Because of the integrity of the enteric coating in an acidic environment, these tablets may accumulate and form a bezoar in the stomach. Individuals with this condition may present with complaints of early satiety or of vague upper abdominal distress. Diagnosis may be made by endoscopy or by abdominal films, which show opacities suggestive of a mass of small tablets.[11] Management may vary according to the condition of the patient. Options include gastrotomy and alternating slightly basic and neutral lavage.[12] While there have been no clinical reports, it has been suggested that such individuals may also be treated with parenteral cimetidine (to reduce acid secretion) and then given sips of slightly basic liquids to effect gradual dissolution of the enteric coating. Progress may be followed with plasma salicylate levels or via recognition of tinnitus by the patient. **It should be kept in mind that individuals with a history of partial or complete gastrectomy may produce reduced amounts of acid and therefore have less acidic gastric pH. Under these circumstances, the benefits offered by the acid-resistant enteric coating may not exist.**

References: 1. Data on file, Sterling Health. 2. Elwood PC, et al: A randomized controlled trial of acetylsalicylic acid in the secondary preventive of mortality from myocardial infarction. *Br Med J* 1974;1:436–440. 3. The Coronary Drug Project Research Group: Aspirin in coronary heart disease. *J Chronic Dis* 1976;29:625–642. 4. Breddin K, et al: Secondary prevention of myocardial infarction: A comparison of acetylsalicylic acid, phenprocoumon or placebo. *Homeostasis* 1979;470:263–268. 5. Aspirin Myocardial Infarction Study Research Group: A randomized, controlled trial of aspirin in persons recovered from myocardial infarction. *JAMA* 1980;245:661–669. 6. Elwood PC, Sweetnam PM: Aspirin and secondary mortality after myocardial infarction. *Lancet*, December 22–29, 1979, pp 1313–1315. 7. The Persantine-Aspirin Reinfarction Study Research Group: Persantine and aspirin in coronary heart disease. *Circulation* 1980;62:449–460. 8. Lewis HD, et al: Proctective effects of aspirin against acute myocardial infarction and death in men with unstable angina: Results of a Veterans Administration Cooperative Study. *N Engl J Med* 1983;309:396–403. 9. The Canadian Cooperative Study Group: A randomized trial of aspirin and sulfinpyrazone in threatened stroke. *N Eng J Med* 1978;299:53–59. 10. Fields WS, et al: Controlled trial of aspirin in cerebral ischemia. *Stroke* 1977;8:301–316. 11. Bogacz K, Caldron P: Enteric-coated aspirin bezoar: Elevation of serum salicylate level by barium study. *Am J Med* 1987;83:783–786. 12. Baum J: Enteric-coated aspirin and the problem of gastric retention. *J Rheumatol* 1984;11:250–251.

How Supplied: ASPIRIN REGIMEN BAYER—Regular strength 325 mg caplets in bottles of 100 with child-resistant safety closure.

ASPIRIN REGIMEN BAYER—Adult Low Strenth 81 mg tablets in bottles of 120 with child-resistant safety closure.

REV. 11/94

Shown in Product Identification Guide, page 515

Extra Strength BAYER® Aspirin Arthritis Pain Regimen Formula
[aspirin, 500 mg]

EXTRA STRENGTH BAYER®
ASPIRIN
ARTHRITIS PAIN REGIMEN
FORMULA

Enteric Coated Caplets

- Specifically designed for people on a regimen of aspirin, or as directed by your doctor.
- Contains the strongest dose of pain reliever you can buy.
- Safety coated to help protect your stomach.
- Pure BAYER® Aspirin inside.
- Caffeine free and very low sodium.
- Easy-to-swallow caplet shape.

The enteric coating on BAYER® Aspirin Arthritis Pain Regimen Formula is designed to allow the caplet to pass through the stomach to the intestine before it dissolves, providing protection against stomach upset.

Indications: For the temporary relief of minor aches and pains of arthritis or as recommended by your doctor.
For rheumatoid arthritis, juvenile rheumatoid arthritis, systemic lupus erythematosus, osteoarthritis (degenerative joint disease), ankylosing spondylitis, psoriatic arthritis, Reiter's syndrome, and fibrositis.
Because of its delayed action, BAYER® Aspirin Arthritis Pain Regimen Formula will not provide fast relief of headaches, fever or other symptoms needing immediate relief.

Direction: Adults and Children 12 years and over, take 2 caplets with water every 6 hours, as needed, up to a maximum of 8 caplets per 24 hours. Ask your doctor about recommended dosages for other indications.

Warnings: Children and teenagers should not use this medicine for chicken pox or flu symptoms before a doctor is consulted about Reye Syndrome, a rare but serious illness reported to be associated with aspirin. Do not take for pain for more than 10 days or for fever for more than 3 days unless directed by a doctor. If pain or fever persists or gets worse, if new symptoms occur or if redness or swelling is present, consult a doctor because these could be signs of a serious condition. Do not take this product if you are allergic to aspirin, have asthma, have stomach problems (such as heartburn, upset stomach or stomach pain) that persist or recur, gastric ulcers or bleeding problems unless directed by a doctor. If ringing in the ears or loss of hearing occurs, consult a doctor before taking any more of this product. Keep this and all drugs out of the reach

of children. In case of accidental overdose, seek professional assistance or contact a poison control center immediately. As with any drug, if you are pregnant or nursing a baby, seek the advice of a health professional before using this product. IT IS ESPECIALLY IMPORTANT NOT TO USE ASPIRIN DURING THE LAST 3 MONTHS OF PREGNANCY UNLESS SPECIFICALLY DIRECTED TO DO SO BY A DOCTOR BECAUSE IT MAY CAUSE PROBLEMS IN THE UNBORN CHILD OR COMPLICATIONS DURING DELIVERY.

Drug Interaction Precaution: Do not take this product if you are taking a prescription drug for anticoagulation (thinning the blood), diabetes, gout or arthritis unless directed by a doctor.

Active Ingredient: 500 mg Aspirin per caplet.

Inactive Ingredients: D&C Yellow #10 FD&C Yellow #6. Hydroxypropyl Methylcellulose, Iron Oxide, Methacrylic Acid Copolymer, Starch, Titanium Dioxide, Triacetin.
Store at room temperature.

How Supplied: Extra Strength BAYER® Aspirin Arthritis Pain Regimen Formula is supplied in bottles of 50 caplets with a child-resistant safety closure.
Your questions and comments are important to us. Please call 1-800-331-4536 weekdays 9:00–5:00 (Eastern Time).
Store at room temperature.
The Bayer Company,
Sterling Health,
Div. of Sterling Winthrop Inc.,
New York, NY 10016
Shown in Product Identification Guide, page 515

BAYER® Children's Chewable Aspirin
Aspirin (Acetylsalicylic Acid)

Active Ingredients: Bayer Children's Chewable Aspirin—Aspirin 1¼ grains per orange flavored chewable tablet. Also available in cherry flavor.

Inactive Ingredients: Orange Flavored: Dextrose Excipient, FD&C Yellow #6, Flavor, Saccharin Sodium, Starch. Cherry Flavored: D&C Red #27, Dextrose Excipient, FD&C Red #40, Flavor, Saccharin Sodium, Starch.

Indications: For the temporary relief of minor aches, pains and headaches, and to reduce fever associated with colds, sore throats and teething.

Directions: The following dosages are those provided in the packaging, as appropriate for self-medication.
Children's Dose: To be administered only under adult supervision.

Age (Years)	Weight (lb)	Dosage
2 to under 4	32 to 35	2 tablets
4 to under 6	36 to 45	3 tablets
6 to under 9	46 to 65	4 tablets
9 to under 11	66 to 76	4–5 tablets
11 to under 12	77 to 83	4–6 tablets
Adults and Children 12 yrs and over		5–8 tablets

Indicated dosage may be repeated every four hours, while symptoms persist, up to a maximum of five doses per 24 hours or as directed by a doctor. For larger or more frequent doses or for children under 2, consult your doctor before taking.
Ways to Administer: CHEW, then follow with a half a glass of water, milk or fruit juice.
SWALLOW WHOLE with a half a glass of water, milk or fruit juice.
DISSOLVE ON TONGUE, followed with a half a glass of water, milk or fruit juice.
DISSOLVE TABLET in a little water, milk or fruit juice and drink the solution.
CRUSH in a teaspoonful of water—followed with a half a glass of water.

Warnings: Children and teenagers should not use this medicine for chicken pox or flu symptoms before a doctor is consulted about Reye syndrome, a rare but serious illness reported to be associated with aspirin. Do not take this product for pain for more than 10 days (for adults) or 5 days (for children), and do not take for fever for more than 3 days unless directed by a doctor. If pain or fever persists or gets worse, if new symptoms occur, or if redness or swelling is present, consult a doctor because these could be signs of a serious condition. Do not give this product to children for the pain of arthritis unless directed by a doctor. If sore throat is severe, persists for more than 2 days, is accompanied or followed by fever, headache, rash, nausea, or vomiting, consult a doctor promptly. Do not take this product for at least 7 days after tonsillectomy or oral surgery unless directed by a doctor. Do not take this product if you are allergic to aspirin, have asthma, have stomach problems (such as heartburn, upset stomach or stomach pain) that persist or recur or have gastric ulcers or bleeding problems unless directed by a doctor. If ringing in the ears or loss of hearing occurs, consult a doctor before taking any more of this product.
KEEP THIS AND ALL DRUGS OUT OF THE REACH OF CHILDREN. IN CASE OF ACCIDENTAL OVERDOSE, SEEK PROFESSIONAL ASSISTANCE OR CONTACT A POISON CONTROL CENTER IMMEDIATELY. AS WITH ANY DRUG, IF YOU ARE PREGNANT OR NURSING A BABY, SEEK THE ADVICE OF A HEALTH PROFESSIONAL

Continued on next page

This product information was effective as of November 1, 1994. Current information may be obtained directly from Miles Inc., by writing to P.O. Box 340 Elkhart, IN 46515.

Miles—Cont.

BEFORE USING THIS PRODUCT. IT IS ESPECIALLY IMPORTANT NOT TO USE ASPIRIN DURING THE LAST 3 MONTHS OF PREGNANCY UNLESS SPECIFICALLY DIRECTED TO DO SO BY A DOCTOR BECAUSE IT MAY CAUSE PROBLEMS IN THE UNBORN CHILD OR COMPLICATIONS DURING DELIVERY.

Drug Interaction Precaution: Do not take this product if taking a prescription drug for anticoagulation (thinning the blood), diabetes, gout or arthritis unless directed by a doctor.

How Supplied: Bayer Children's Chewable Aspirin 81 mg (1¼ grains) is available in orange and cherry flavors in bottles of 36 tablets with child-resistant safety closure.
Store at room temperature.

*Shown in Product Identification
Guide, page 515*

**Extended-Release
BAYER® 8-Hour Aspirin**
Aspirin (acetylsalicylic acid)

Active Ingredients: Each oblong white scored caplet contains 650 mg (10-grains) of aspirin in microencapsulated form.

Inactive Ingredients: Guar Gum, Microcrystalline Cellulose, Starch and other ingredients.

Indications: Extended-Release BAYER 8-Hour Aspirin is indicated for the temporary relief of nagging, recurring pain of backache, bursitis, minor pain and stiffness of arthritis and rheumatism, sprains, headaches, sinusitis pain, and painful discomfort and fever due to colds and flu.

Directions: Two Extended-Release BAYER 8-Hour Aspirin caplets every 8 hours provide effective long-lasting pain relief. This two-caplet 1300 mg or (20-grain) dose of extended-release aspirin promptly produces salicylate blood levels greater than those achieved by a 650 mg (10-grain) dose of regular aspirin, and in the second 4-hour period produces a salicylate blood level curve which approximates that of two successive 650 mg (10-grain) doses of regular aspirin at 4-hour intervals. The 650 mg (10-grain) scored Extended-Release BAYER 8-Hour Aspirin caplets permit administration of aspirin in multiples of 325 mg (5-grains) allowing individualization of dosage to meet the specific needs of the patient. For the convenience of patients on a regular aspirin dosage schedule, two 650 mg (10-grain) Extended-Release BAYER 8-Hour Aspirin caplets may be administered with water every 8 hours. Whenever necessary, two caplets 1300 mg or (20 grains) should be given before retiring to provide effective analgesic and anti-inflammatory action—for relief of pain throughout the night and lessening of stiffness upon arising. Do not exceed 6 caplets in 24 hours. Extended-Release BAYER 8-Hour Aspirin has been made

in a special caplet to permit easy swallowing. However, for patients who do have difficulty, Extended-Release BAYER 8-Hour Aspirin caplets may be gently crumbled in the mouth and swallowed with water without loss of timed-release effect. There is no bitter "aspirin" taste. For children under 12, consult physician.

Warnings: Children and teenagers should not use this medicine for chicken pox or flu symptoms before a doctor is consulted about Reye syndrome, a rare but serious illness reported to be associated with aspirin. Do not take for pain for more than 10 days or for fever for more than 3 days unless directed by a doctor. If pain or fever persists or gets worse, if new symptoms occur, or if redness or swelling is present consult a doctor because these could be signs of a serious condition. Do not take this product if you are allergic to aspirin, have asthma, stomach problems that persist or recur, gastric ulcers or bleeding problems unless directed by a doctor. If ringing in the ears or loss of hearing occurs, consult a doctor before taking any more of this product. Keep this and all drugs out of the reach of children. In case of accidental overdose, seek professional assistance or contact a poison control center immediately. As with any drug, if you are pregnant or nursing a baby, seek the advice of a health professional before using this product. IT IS ESPECIALLY IMPORTANT NOT TO USE ASPIRIN DURING THE LAST 3 MONTHS OF PREGNANCY UNLESS SPECIFICALLY DIRECTED TO DO SO BY A DOCTOR BECAUSE IT MAY CAUSE PROBLEMS IN THE UNBORN CHILD OR COMPLICATIONS DURING DELIVERY.

Drug Interaction Precaution: Do not take this product if you are taking a prescription drug for anticoagulation (thinning of the blood), diabetes, gout, or arthritis unless directed by a doctor.

How Supplied: Extended-Release Bayer 8-Hour Aspirin 650 mg (10 grains) is supplied in bottles of 50 caplets with a child-resistant safety closure.

*Shown in Product Identification
Guide, page 515*

Extra Strength BAYER® Aspirin
Aspirin (Acetylsalicylic Acid)
Caplets and Tablets

Active Ingredients: Extra Strength Bayer Aspirin—Aspirin 500 mg (7.7 grains) contains a thin, inert, Hydroxypropyl Methylcellulose coating for easier swallowing. This is not an enteric coating and does not alter the onset of action of Bayer Aspirin.

Inactive Ingredients: Starch and Triacetin.

Indications: Analgesic, antipyretic, anti-inflammatory. For relief of head-

ache; painful discomfort and fever of colds; muscular aches and pains; temporary relief of minor pains of arthritis; toothache, and pain following dental procedures; menstrual pain.

Directions: The following dosages are those provided on the packaging, as appropriate for self- medication. Larger or more frequent dosage may be necessary as appropriate for the condition or needs of the patient. The hydroxypropyl methylcellulose coating makes Extra Strength Bayer Aspirin particularly appropriate for those who have difficulty in swallowing uncoated tablets/caplets.
Usual Adult Dose: One or two tablets/caplets with water. May be repeated every four hours as necessary up to 8 caplets/tablets a day. Do not give to children under 12 unless directed by a doctor.

Warnings: Children and teenagers should not use this medicine for chicken pox or flu symptoms before a doctor is consulted about Reye syndrome, a rare but serious illness reported to be associated with aspirin. Do not take this product for pain for more than 10 days or for fever for more than 3 days unless directed by a doctor. If pain or fever persists or gets worse, if new symptoms occur, or if redness or swelling is present consult a doctor because these could be signs of a serious condition. Do not take this product if you are allergic to aspirin, have asthma, stomach problems that persist or recur, gastric ulcers or bleeding problems unless directed by a doctor. If ringing in the ears or loss of hearing occurs, consult a doctor before taking any more of this product. Keep this and all drugs out of the reach of children. In case of accidental overdose, seek professional assistance or contact a poison control center immediately. As with any drug, if you are pregnant or nursing a baby, seek the advice of a health professional before using this product. IT IS ESPECIALLY IMPORTANT NOT TO USE ASPIRIN DURING THE LAST 3 MONTHS OF PREGNANCY UNLESS SPECIFICALLY DIRECTED TO DO SO BY A DOCTOR BECAUSE IT MAY CAUSE PROBLEMS IN THE UNBORN CHILD OR COMPLICATIONS DURING DELIVERY.

Drug Interaction Precaution: Do not take this product if you are taking a prescription drug for anticoagulation (thinning the blood), diabetes, gout, or arthritis unless directed by a doctor.

How Supplied: Extra Strength Bayer Aspirin 500 mg (7.7 grains) is available in bottles of 24, 50 and 100 caplets, and bottles of 50 tablets.
Child-resistant safety closures on 50s bottles of caplets and tablets, 24s bottles of caplets. Bottle of 100s caplets available without safety closure for households without young children.

*Shown in Product Identification
Guide, page 515*

Extra Strength BAYER® PLUS
Buffered Aspirin

Active Ingredients: Each Extra Strength Bayer Plus contains Aspirin (500 mg), in a buffered base of Calcium Carbonate.

Inactive Ingredients: Colloidal Silicon Dioxide, D&C Red #7 Lake, FD&C Blue #2 Lake, FD&C Red #40 Lake, Hydroxypropyl Methylcellulose, Microcrystalline Cellulose, Propylene Glycol, Sodium Starch Glycolate, Starch, Titanium Dioxide, Zinc Stearate.

Indications: Analgesic, antipyretic, anti-inflammatory. For the temporary relief of headache; painful discomfort and fever of colds; muscular aches and pains; temporary relief of minor pains of arthritis; toothache, and pain following dental procedures; menstrual pain.

Directions: The following dosages are those provided in the packaging, as appropriate for self-medication. Larger or more frequent dosage may be necessary as appropriate to the condition or needs of the patient. The addition of buffering agents makes Extra Strength Bayer® Plus particularly appropriate for those who must take frequent doses of aspirin. The hydroxypropyl methylcellulose coating benefits aspirin users who have difficulty in swallowing uncoated caplets. *Usual Adult Dose:* Adults and Children 12 years & over; One or two caplets with water. May be repeated every 4 to 6 hours as necessary up to 8 caplets a day, or as directed by a doctor. Do not give to children under 12 unless directed by a doctor.

Warnings: Children and teenagers should not use this medicine for chicken pox or flu symptoms before a doctor is consulted about Reye syndrome, a rare but serious illness reported to be associated with aspirin. Do not take this product for pain for more than 10 days or for fever for more than 3 days unless directed by a doctor. If pain or fever persists or gets worse, if new symptoms occur, or if redness or swelling is present consult a doctor because these could be signs of a serious condition. Do not take this product if you are allergic to aspirin, have asthma, stomach problems that persist or recur, gastric ulcers or bleeding problems unless directed by a doctor. If ringing in the ears or loss of hearing occurs, consult a doctor before taking any more of this product. Keep this and all drugs out of the reach of children. In case of accidental overdose, seek professional assistance or contact a poison control center immediately. As with any drug, if you are pregnant or nursing a baby, seek the advice of a health professional before using this product. **IT IS ESPECIALLY IMPORTANT NOT TO USE ASPIRIN DURING THE LAST 3 MONTHS OF PREGNANCY UNLESS SPECIFICALLY DIRECTED TO DO SO BY A DOCTOR BECAUSE IT MAY CAUSE PROB-**

LEMS IN THE UNBORN CHILD OR COMPLICATIONS DURING DELIVERY.

Drug Interaction Precaution: Do not take this product if you are taking a prescription drug for anticoagulation (thinning the blood), diabetes, gout, or arthritis unless directed by a doctor.

How Supplied: Extra Strength Bayer® Plus Aspirin (500 mg) is available in bottles of 50 caplets. Child resistant closure on 50s caplets.
Shown in Product Identification Guide, page 515

Extra Strength BAYER® PM Aspirin
[aspirin/diphenhydramine HCl]
EXTRA STRENGTH BAYER® PM ASPIRIN PLUS SLEEP AID
The Only Night Time Aspirin

Indications: For the temporary relief of occasional headaches and minor aches and pains with accompanying sleeplessness.

Directions: Adults and Children 12 years of age and over, take 2 caplets with water at bedtime, if needed, or as directed by a doctor.

Warnings: Do not give to children under 12 years of age. **Children and teenagers should not use this medicine for chicken pox or flu symptoms before a doctor is consulted about Reye Syndrome, a rare but serious illness reported to be associated with aspirin.** Do not take this product for pain for more than 10 days or for fever for more than 3 days unless directed by a doctor. If pain or fever persists or gets worse, if new symptoms occur, or if redness or swelling is present, consult a doctor because these could be signs of a serious condition. Do not take this product if you are allergic to aspirin or if you have asthma unless directed by a doctor. If ringing in the ears or a loss of hearing occurs, consult a doctor before taking any more of this product. Do not take this product if you have stomach problems (such as heartburn, upset stomach, or stomach pain) that persist or recur, or if you have ulcers or bleeding problems, unless directed by a doctor. If sleeplessness persists continuously for more than 2 weeks, consult your doctor. Insomnia may be a symptom of serious underlying medical illness. Do not take this product, unless directed by a doctor, if you have a breathing problem such as emphysema or chronic bronchitis, or if you have glaucoma or difficulty in urination due to enlargement of the prostate gland. Avoid alcoholic beverages while taking this product. Do not take this product if you are taking sedatives or tranquilizers, without first consulting your doctor. Keep this and all drugs out of the reach of children. In case of accidental overdose, seek professional assistance or contact a poison control center immediately. As with any drug, if you are pregnant or

nursing a baby, seek the advice of a health professional before using this product. IT IS ESPECIALLY IMPORTANT NOT TO USE ASPIRIN DURING THE LAST 3 MONTHS OF PREGNANCY UNLESS SPECIFICALLY DIRECTED TO DO SO BY A DOCTOR BECAUSE IT MAY CAUSE PROBLEMS IN THE UNBORN CHILD OR COMPLICATIONS DURING DELIVERY.

Drug Interaction Precaution: Do not take this product if you are taking a prescription drug for anticoagulation (thinning the blood), diabetes, gout, or arthritis unless directed by a doctor.

Active Ingredients: 500 mg Aspirin, 25 mg Diphenhydramine Hydrochloride per caplet.

Inactive Ingredients: Colloidal Silicon Dioxide, Dibasic Calcium Phosphate, Dibutyl Sebacate, Ethylcellulose, FD&C Blue #1 Lake, FD&C Blue #2 Lake, Hydroxypropyl Methylcellulose, Microcrystalline Cellulose, Oleic Acid, Propylene Glycol, Starch, Titanium Dioxide, Zinc Stearate.
Store at room temperature.

How Supplied: Extra Strength BAYER® PM Aspirin is supplied in bottles of 24 caplets with a child-resistant safety closure.
Your questions and comments are important to us. Please call 1-800-331-4536 weekdays 9:00–5:00 (Eastern Time).
The Bayer Company, Sterling Health, Div. of Sterling Winthrop Inc., New York, NY 10016
Shown in Product Identification Guide, page 515

Genuine BAYER® Aspirin
Aspirin (Acetylsalicylic Acid)
Tablets and Caplets

Active Ingredients: Each Genuine Bayer Aspirin contains aspirin 325 mg (5 grains) in a thin, inert, hydroxypropyl methylcellulose coating for easier swallowing. This is not an enteric coating and does not alter the onset of action of Genuine Bayer Aspirin.

Inactive Ingredients: Starch and Triacetin.

Indications: Analgesic, antipyretic, anti-inflammatory. For the temporary relief of headache; painful discomfort and fever of colds; muscular aches and pains; temporary relief of minor pains of arthritis; toothache, and pain following dental procedures; menstrual pain.

Directions: The following dosages are those provided in the packaging, as ap-

Continued on next page

This product information was effective as of November 1, 1994. Current information may be obtained directly from Miles Inc., by writing to P.O. Box 340 Elkhart, IN 46515.

Miles—Cont.

propriate for self-medication. Larger or more frequent dosage may be necessary as appropriate to the condition or needs of the patient. The hydroxypropyl methylcellulose coating makes Genuine Bayer Aspirin particularly appropriate for those who have difficulty in swallowing uncoated tablets and caplets.

Usual Adult Dose: Adults and Children 12 years and over One or two tablets/caplets with water. May be repeated every four hours as necessary up to 12 tablets/caplets a day or as directed by a doctor. Do not give to children under 12 unless directed by a doctor.

Warnings: Children and teenagers should not use this medicine for chicken pox or flu symptoms before a doctor is consulted about Reye syndrome, a rare but serious illness reported to be associated with aspirin. Do not take this product for pain for more than 10 days or for fever for more than 3 days unless directed by a doctor. If pain or fever persists or gets worse, if new symptoms occur, or if redness or swelling is present consult a doctor because these could be signs of a serious condition. Do not take this product if you are allergic to aspirin, have asthma, stomach problems that persist or recur, gastric ulcers or bleeding problems unless directed by a doctor. If ringing in the ears or loss of hearing occurs, consult a doctor before taking any more of this product. Keep this and all drugs out of the reach of children. In case of accidental overdose, seek professional assistance or contact a poison control center immediately. As with any drug, if you are pregnant or nursing a baby, seek the advice of a health professional before using this product. **IT IS ESPECIALLY IMPORTANT NOT TO USE ASPIRIN DURING THE LAST 3 MONTHS OF PREGNANCY UNLESS SPECIFICALLY DIRECTED TO DO SO BY A DOCTOR BECAUSE IT MAY CAUSE PROBLEMS IN THE UNBORN CHILD OR COMPLICATIONS DURING DELIVERY.**

Drug Interaction Precaution: Do not take this product if you are taking a prescription drug for anticoagulation (thinning the blood), diabetes, gout, or arthritis unless directed by doctor.

Professional Labeling:
ANTIARTHRITIC EFFECT
Indication: Conditions requiring chronic or long-term aspirin therapy for pain and/or inflammation, e.g., rheumatoid arthritis, juvenile rheumatoid arthritis, systemic lupus erythematosus, osteoarthritis (degenerative joint disease), ankylosing spondylitis, psoriatic arthritis, Reiter's syndrome, and fibrositis.

ANTIPLATELET EFFECT
In MI Prophylaxis:
Indication: Aspirin is indicated to reduce the risk of death and/or nonfatal myocardial infarction in patients with a previous infarction or unstable angina pectoris.

Clinical Trials: The indication is supported by the results of six large randomized, multicenter, placebo-controlled studies[1-7] involving 10,816 predominantly male post-myocardial infarction (MI) patients and one randomized placebo-controlled study of 1,266 men with unstable angina. Therapy with aspirin was begun at intervals after the onset of acute MI varying from less than three days to more than five years and continuing for periods of from less than one year to four years. In the unstable angina study, treatment was started within one month after the onset of unstable angina and continued for 12 weeks, and complicating conditions, such as congestive heart failure, were not included in the study.

Aspirin therapy in MI patients was associated with about a 20% reduction in the risk of subsequent death and/or nonfatal reinfarction, a median absolute decrease of 3% from the 12% to 22% event rates in the placebo groups. In the aspirin-treated unstable angina patients, the reduction in risk was about 50%, a reduction in the event rate of 5% from the 10% rate in the placebo group over the 12 weeks of study.

Daily dosage of aspirin in the post-myocardial infarction studies was 300 mg in one study and 900–1,500 mg in five studies. A dose of 325 mg was used in the study of unstable angina.

Adverse Reactions: Gastrointestinal reactions: Doses of 1,000 mg per day of aspirin caused gastrointestinal symptoms and bleeding that, in some cases, were clinically significant. In the largest postinfarction study (the Aspirin Myocardial Infarction Study [AMIS] with 4,500 people), the percentage of incidences of gastrointestinal symptoms for the aspirin (1,000 mg of a standard, solid-tablet formulation) and placebo-treated subjects, respectively, were stomach pain (14.5%, 4.4%), heartburn (11.9%, 4.8%), nausea and/or vomiting (7.6%, 2.1%), hospitalization for GI disorder (4.9%, 3.5%). In the AMIS and other trials, aspirin-treated patients had increased rates of gross gastrointestinal bleeding. Symptoms and signs of gastrointestinal irritation were not significantly increased in subjects treated for unstable angina with buffered aspirin in solution.

Cardiovascular and Biochemical: In the AMIS trial, the dosage of 1,000 mg per day of aspirin was associated with small increases in systolic blood pressure (BP) (average 1.5 to 2.1 mm) and diastolic BP (0.5 to 0.6 mm), depending upon whether maximal or last available readings were used. Blood urea nitrogen and uric acid levels were also increased but by less than 1.0 mg percent.

Subjects with marked hypertension or renal insufficiency had been excluded from the trial so that the clinical importance of these observations for such subjects or for any subjects treated over more prolonged periods is not known. It is recommended that patients placed on long-term aspirin treatment, even at doses of 300 mg per day, be seen at regular intervals to assess changes in these measurements.

Dosage and Administration: Although most of the studies used dosages exceeding 300 mg, two trials used only 300 mg daily and pharmacologic data indicate that this dose inhibits platelet function fully. Therefore, 300 mg or a conventional 325 mg aspirin dose daily is a reasonable routine dose that would minimize gastrointestinal adverse reactions. This use of aspirin applies to both solid oral dosage forms (buffered and plain aspirin) and buffered aspirin in solution.

In Transient Ischemic Attacks:
Indication: Aspririn is indicated for reducing the risk of recurrent transient ischemic attacks (TIAs) or stroke in men who have transient ischemia of the brain due to fibrin emboli. There is no evidence that aspirin is effective in reducing TIAs in women, or is of benefit in the treatment of completed strokes in men or women.

Clinical Trials: The indication is supported by the results of a Canadian study[8] in which 585 patients with threatened stroke were followed in a randomized clinical trial for an average of 28 months to determine whether aspirin or sulfinpyrazone, singly or in combination, was superior to placebo in preventing transient ischemic attacks, stroke, or death. The study showed that, although sulfinpyrazone had no statistically significant effect, aspirin reduced the risk of continuing transient ischemic attacks, stroke, or death by 19 percent and reduced the risk of stroke or death by 31 percent. Another aspirin study carried out in the United States with 178 patients showed a statistically significant number of "favorable outcomes," including reduced transient ischemic attacks, stroke, and death.[9]

Precautions: Patients presenting with signs and/or symptoms of TIAs should have a complete medical and neurologic evaluation. Consideration should be given to other disorders which may resemble TIAs. It is important to evaluate and treat, if appropriate, diseases associated with TIAs and stroke, such as hypertension and diabetes.

Concurrent administration of absorbable antacids at therapeutic doses may increase the clearance of salicylates in some individuals. The concurrent administration of nonabsorbable antacids may alter the rate of absorption of aspirin, thereby resulting in a decreased acetylsalicylic acid/salicylate ratio in plasma. The clinical significance of these decreases in available aspirin is unknown. Aspirin at dosages of 1,000 milligrams per day has been associated with small increases in blood pressure, blood urea nitrogen, and serum uric acid levels. It is recommended that patients placed on long-term aspirin treatment be seen at regular intervals to assess changes in these measurements.

Adverse Reactions: At dosages of 1,000 milligrams or higher of aspirin per day, gastrointestinal side effects include stomach pain, heartburn, nausea and/or vomiting, as well as increased rates of gross gastrointestinal bleeding.

Dosage and Administration: Adult oral dosage for men is 1,300 milligrams a day, in divided doses of 650 milligrams twice a day or 325 milligrams four times a day.

References: 1. Elwood PC, et al: A randomized controlled trial of acetylsalicylic acid in the secondary prevention of mortality from myocardial infarction. *Br Med J* 1974;1:436–440. 2. The Coronary Drug Project Research Group: Aspirin in coronary heart disease. *J Chronic Dis* 1976;29:625–642. 3. Breddin K, et al: Secondary prevention of myocardial infarction: A comparison of acetylsalicylic acid, phenprocoumon or placebo. *Homeostasis* 1979;470:263–268. 4. Aspirin Myocardial Infarction Study Research Group: A randomized, controlled trial of aspirin in persons recovered from myocardial infarction. *JAMA* 1980;245:661–669. 5. Elwood PC, Sweetnam PM: Aspirin and secondary mortality after myocardial infarction. *Lancet,* December 22–29, 1979, pp 1313–1315. 6. The Persantine-Aspirin Reinfarction Study Research Group: Persantine and aspirin in coronary heart disease. *Circulation* 1980;62:449–460. 7. Lewis, HD, et al: Protective effects of aspirin against acute myocardial infarction and death in men with unstable angina: Results of a Veterans Administration Cooperative Study. *N Engl J Med* 1983;309:396–403. 8. The Canadian Cooperative Study Group: A randomized trial of aspirin and sulfinpyrazone in threatened stroke. *N Engl J Med* 1978;299:53–59. 9. Fields WS, et al: Controlled trial of aspirin in cerebral ischemia. *Stroke* 1977;8:301–316.

How Supplied:
Genuine Bayer Aspirin 325 mg (5 grains) is supplied in packs of 12 tablets, bottles of 24, 50, 100, 200, 300, and 365 tablets, and bottles of 50 and 100 caplets. Child-resistant safety closures on 12s, 24s, 50s, 200s, 300s, 365s tablets and 50s caplets. Bottles of 100s tablets and caplets available without safety closure for households without small children.
Shown in Product Identification Guide, page 515

BAYER® SELECT™
IBUPROFEN
Pain Relief Formula
Pain Reliever/Fever Reducer

Warning: ASPIRIN SENSITIVE PATIENTS. Do not take this product if you have had a severe allergic reaction to aspirin, e.g.-asthma, swelling, shock or hives, because even though this product contains no aspirin or salicylates, cross-reactions may occur in patients allergic to aspirin.

Active Ingredient: 200 mg Ibuprofen USP per caplet

Inactive Ingredients: Colloidal Silicon Dioxide, Dibasic Calcium Phosphate, Hydroxypropyl Methylcellulose, Magnesium Stearate, Microcrystalline Cellulose, Polyethylene Glycol, Polysorbate 80, Sodium Lauryl Sulfate, Sodium Starch Glycolate, Stearic Acid, Titanium Dioxide.

Indications: For the temporary relief of minor aches and pains associated with the common cold, headache, toothache, muscular aches, backache, for the minor pain of arthritis, for the pain of menstrual cramps and for reduction of fever.

Directions: ADULTS: Take 1 caplet every 4 to 6 hours while symptoms persist. If pain or fever does not respond to 1 caplet, 2 caplets may be used but do not exceed 6 caplets in 24 hours, unless directed by a doctor. The smallest effective dose should be used. Take with food or milk if occasional and mild heartburn, upset stomach, or stomach pain occurs with use. Consult a doctor if these symptoms are more than mild or if they persist. CHILDREN: Do not give this product to children under 12 except under the advice and supervision of a doctor.

Warnings: Do not take for pain for more than 10 days or for fever for more than 3 days unless directed by a doctor. If pain or fever persists or gets worse, if new symptoms occur, or if the painful area is red or swollen, consult a doctor. These could be signs of a serious illness. If you are under a doctor's care for any serious condition, consult a doctor before taking this product. As with aspirin and acetaminophen, if you have any condition which requires you to take prescription drugs or if you have had any problems or serious side effects from taking any non-prescription pain reliever, do not take this product without first discussing it with your doctor. If you experience any symptoms which are unusual or seem unrelated to the condition for which you took ibuprofen, consult a doctor before taking any more of it. Although ibuprofen is indicated for the same conditions as aspirin and acetaminophen, it should not be taken with them except under a doctor's direction. Do not combine this product with any other ibuprofen containing product. As with any drug if you are pregnant or nursing a baby, seek the advice of a health professional before using this product. IT IS ESPECIALLY IMPORTANT NOT TO USE IBUPROFEN DURING THE LAST 3 MONTHS OF PREGNANCY UNLESS SPECIFICALLY DIRECTED TO DO SO BY A DOCTOR BECAUSE IT MAY CAUSE PROBLEMS IN THE UNBORN CHILD OR COMPLICATIONS DURING DELIVERY. Keep this and all drugs out of the reach of children. In case of accidental overdose, seek professional assistance or contact a poison control center immediately.

How Supplied: BAYER® SELECT™ IBUPROFEN Pain Relief Formula is available in 36 count bottles.
Shown in Product Identification Guide, page 516

BAYER® SELECT™
Maximum Strength
Backache Pain Relief Formula
Magnesium Salicylate
Aspirin-Free

Active Ingredient: 580 mg Magnesium Salicylate Tetrahydrate per caplet.

Inactive Ingredients: D&C Red #7 Lake, D&C Yellow #10 Lake, FD&C Blue #2 Lake, FD&C Red #40 Lake, FD&C Yellow #6 Lake Hydroxypropyl Methylcellulose, Microcrystalline Cellulose, Polyethylene Glycol, Polysorbate 80, Sodium Lauryl Sulfate, Sodium Starch Glycolate, Starch, Titanium Dioxide. May also contain Magnesium Stearate, Povidone. Sodium Stearyl Fumarate, Stearic Acid.

Indications: BAYER® SELECT™ BACKACHE Pain Relief Formula contains a specially chosen safe ingredient in a maximum strength dosage form for strong, fast, temporary relief of minor aches and pains associated with BACK-ACHES.

Directions: Adults: Take 2 caplets every 6 hours as needed, not to exceed 8 caplets per 24 hours. Children under 12 years of age: Consult your doctor.

Warnings: Children and teenagers should not use this medicine for chicken pox or flu symptoms before a doctor is consulted about Reye Syndrome, a rare but serious illness reported to be associated with aspirin. Do not take this product for pain for more than 10 days or for fever for more than 3 days unless directed by a doctor. If pain or fever persists or gets worse, if new symptoms occur, or if redness or swelling is present, consult a doctor because these could be signs of a serious condition. Do not take this product if you are allergic to salicylates (including aspirin) unless directed by a doctor. If ringing in the ears or a loss of hearing occurs, consult a doctor before taking any more of this product. Do not take this product if you have stomach problems (such as heartburn, upset stomach or stomach pain) that persist or recur, or if you have ulcers or bleeding problems, unless directed by a doctor. Keep this and all drugs out of the reach of children. As with any drug, if you are pregnant or nursing a baby, seek the advice of a health professional before using this

Continued on next page

This product information was effective as of November 1, 1994. Current information may be obtained directly from Miles Inc., by writing to P.O. Box 340 Elkhart, IN 46515.

Miles—Cont.

product. In case of accidental overdose, seek professional assistance or contact a poison control center immediately.

Drug Interaction Precaution: Do not take this product if you are taking a prescription drug for anticoagulation (thinning the blood), diabetes, gout, or arthritis unless directed by a doctor.
Store at room temperature.

How Supplied: BAYER® SELECT™ Maximum Strength BACKACHE Pain Relief is available in 24 and 50 count bottles.
Shown in Product Identification Guide, page 515

BAYER® SELECT™
Maximum Strength HEADACHE
Pain Relief Formula
Aspirin-Free

Active Ingredients: Acetaminophen 500 mg and Caffeine 65 mg per caplet.

Inactive Ingredients: Croscarmellose Sodium, FD&C Blue #2, Hydroxypropyl Methylcellulose, Magnesium Stearate, Microcrystalline Cellulose, Polyethylene Glycol, Potassium Sorbate, Starch, Titanium Dioxide, Xanthan Gum.

Indications: BAYER® SELECT™ HEADACHE Pain Relief Formula contains a specially chosen combination of safe, aspirin-free ingredients in a maximum dosage form for strong, fast, temporary relief of HEADACHES.

Directions: Adults: Take 2 caplets with water every 4–6 hours, as needed, up to a maximum of 8 caplets per 24 hours. **Children under 12 years of age:** Consult a doctor.

Warnings: Do not give to children 3 years of age or take for more than 10 days unless directed by a doctor. Do not take this product for pain for more than 10 days or for fever for more than 3 days unless directed by a doctor. If pain or fever persists or gets worse, if new symptoms occur, or if redness or swelling is present, consult a doctor because these could be signs of a serious condition. The recommended dose of this product contains about as much caffeine as a cup of coffee. Limit the use of caffeine-containing medications, foods, or beverages while taking this product because too much caffeine may cause nervousness, irritability, sleeplessness, and occasionally, rapid heartbeat. Keep this and all drugs out of the reach of children. In case of accidental overdose, seek professional assistance or contact a poison control center immediately. Prompt medical attention is critical for adults as well as for children even if you do not notice any signs or symptoms. As with any drug, if you are pregnant or nursing a baby, seek the advice of a health professional before using this product.

How Supplied: BAYER® SELECT™ Maximum Strength HEADACHE Pain Relief Formula is available in 36 count bottles.
Shown in Product Identification Guide, page 515

BAYER® SELECT™
Maximum Strength MENSTRUAL
Multi-Symptom Formula
Aspirin-Free

Active Ingredients: Acetaminophen 500 mg and Pamabrom 25 mg per caplet.

Inactive Ingredients: Croscarmellose Sodium, D&C Red #27, Hydroxypropyl Methylcellulose, Iron Oxide, Magnesium Stearate, Microcrystalline Cellulose, Polyethylene Glycol, Polysorbate 80, Starch, Titanium Dioxide.

Indications: BAYER® SELECT™ MENSTRUAL Multi-Symptom Formula contains a specially chosen combination of safe, aspirin-free, caffeine-free ingredients that is not found in any ordinary pain reliever to provide temporary relief of the following symptoms associated with PREMENSTRUAL and MENSTRUAL pain and discomfort:
- Cramps
- Bloating
- Backache
- Water-weight gain
- Headache
- Muscular aches and pains

Directions: Adults: Take 2 caplets with water every 4–6 hours, as needed, up to a maximum of 8 caplets per 24 hours. **Children under 12 years of age:** Consult a doctor.

Warnings: Do not take this product for pain for more than 10 days or for fever for more than 3 days unless directed by a doctor. If pain or fever persists or gets worse, if new symptoms occur, or if redness or swelling is present, consult a doctor because these could be signs of a serious condition. Do not give to children under 3 years of age or take for more than 10 days unless directed by a doctor. Keep this and all drugs out of the reach of children. As with any drug, if you are pregnant or nursing a baby, seek the advice of a health professional before using this product. In case of accidental overdose, seek professional assistance or contact a poison control center immediately. Prompt medical attention is critical for adults as well as for children even if you do not notice any signs or symptoms.

How Supplied: BAYER® SELECT™ Maximum Strength MENSTRUAL Multi-Symptom Formula is available in 24 and 50 count bottles.
Shown in Product Identification Guide, page 516

BAYER® SELECT™
Maximum Strength
NIGHT TIME PAIN RELIEF
Analgesic/Sleep Aid Formula for Pain with Sleeplessness
Aspirin-Free

Active Ingredients: Acetaminophen 500 mg and Diphenhydramine HCl 25 mg per caplet.

Inactive Ingredients: FD&C Blue #1 and #2, Hydroxypropyl Methylcellulose, Polyethylene Glycol, Polysorbate 80, Potassium Sorbate, Povidone, Starch, Stearic Acid, Talc, Titanium Dioxide.

Indications: BAYER® SELECT™ NIGHT TIME PAIN RELIEF Formula contains a specially chosen combination of safe, aspirin-free, caffeine-free ingredients in a maximum dosage form to provide temporary relief of minor aches and NIGHT TIME PAIN while helping you fall asleep safely and gently.

Directions: Adults: Take 2 caplets at bedtime if needed or as directed by a doctor. Do not exceed recommended dosage.

Warnings: Do not give to children under 12 years of age. Do not take this product for pain for more than 10 days or for fever for more than 3 days unless directed by a doctor. If pain or fever persists or gets worse, if new symptoms occur, or if redness or swelling is present, consult a doctor because these could be signs of a serious condition. If sleeplessness persists continuously for more than 2 weeks, consult your doctor. Insomnia may be a symptom of serious underlying medical illness. Do not take this product, unless directed by a doctor, if you have a breathing problem such as emphysema or chronic bronchitis, or if you have glaucoma or difficulty in urination due to enlargement of the prostate gland. Avoid alcoholic beverages while taking this product. Do not take this product if you are taking sedatives or tranquilizers, without first consulting your doctor. Keep this and all drugs out of the reach of children. As with any drug, if you are pregnant or nursing a baby, seek the advice of a health professional before using this product. In case of accidental overdose, seek professional assistance or contact a poison control center immediately. Prompt medical attention is critical for adults as well as for children even if you do not notice any signs or symptoms.

How Supplied: BAYER® SELECT™ Maximum Strength NIGHT TIME PAIN RELIEF FORMULA is available in 24 and 50 count bottles.
Shown in Product Identification Guide, page 516

BAYER® SELECT™
Maximum Strength
SINUS PAIN RELIEF
Analgesic/Decongestant Formula
Aspirin-Free

Active Ingredients: Acetaminophen 500 mg and Pseudoephedrine HCl 30 mg per caplet.

Inactive Ingredients: Colloidal Silicon Dioxide, D&C Yellow #10, FD&C Blue #1, FD&C Yellow #6, Hydroxypropyl Methylcellulose, Iron Oxide, Magnesium Stearate, Microcrystalline Cellulose, Polyethylene Glycol, Polysorbate 80, Povidone, Starch, Titanium Dioxide.

Indications: BAYER® SELECT™ SINUS PAIN RELIEF Formula contains a specially chosen combination of safe, aspirin-free, caffeine-free ingredients in a maximum dosage to provide temporary relief of the following SINUS symptoms without making you drowsy:
● Sinus headache pain and pressure
● Swollen nasal passages
● Nasal congestion due to the common cold, hay fever, other respiratory allergies or associated with sinusitis.

Directions: Adults: Take 2 caplets with water every 4-6 hours, up to a maximum of 8 caplets per 24 hours. **Children under 12 years of age:** Consult your doctor.

Warnings: Do not exceed recommended dosage. If nervousness, dizziness, or sleeplessness occur, discontinue use and consults a doctor. Do not take this product for pain for more than 10 days or for fever for more than 3 days unless directed by a doctor. If symptoms do not improve within 7 days or are accompained by a fever, consult a doctor. If pain or fever persists or gets worse, if new symptoms occur, or if redness or swelling is present, consult a doctor because these could be signs of a serious condition. Do not take this product if you have heart disease, high blood pressure, thyroid disease, diabetes, or difficulty in urination due to enlargement of the prostate gland unless directed by a doctor. Do not give to children under 3 years of age or use for more than 10 days unless directed by a doctor. Keep this and all drugs out of the reach of children. As with any drug, if you are pregnant or nursing a baby, seek the advice of a health professional before using this product. In case of accidental overdose, seek professional assistance or contact a poison control center immediately. Prompt medical attention is critical for adults as well as for children even if you do not notice any signs or symptoms.

Drug Interaction Precaution: Do not use this product if you are now taking a prescription monoamine oxidase inhibitor (MAOI) (certain drugs for depression, psychiatric or emotional conditions, or Parkinson's disease), or for 2 weeks after stopping the MAOI drug. If you are uncertain whether your prescription drug contains an MAOI, consult a health professional before taking this product.

How Supplied: BAYER® SELECT™ Maximum Strength SINUS PAIN RELIEF FORMULA is available in 24 and 50 count bottles.
Shown in Product Identification Guide, page 516

BRONKAID® CAPLETS
BRONCHODILATOR AND
EXPECTORANT

Active Ingredients: Ephedrine Sulfate 25 mg and Guaifenesin 400 mg per caplet.

Inactive Ingredients: Croscarmellose Sodium, Hydroxypropyl Methylcellulose, Magnesium Stearate, Magnesium Trisilicate, Microcrystalline Cellulose, Polyethylene Glycol, Povidone, and Starch.

Indications: For the temporary relief of shortness of breath, tightness in chest, wheezing and cough associated with bronchial asthma. Helps loosen phlegm (mucus) and thin bronchial secretions to rid the bronchial passageways of bothersome mucus and drain bronchial tubes.

Directions: Adults and Children 12 years and over: 1 caplet every 4 hours, not to exceed 6 caplets in 24 hours, or as directed by a doctor. Do not exceed recommended dose unless directed by a doctor. **Children under 12 years of age:** Consult a doctor.

Warnings: Do not use this product unless a diagnosis of asthma has been made by a doctor. Do not use this product if you have heart disease, high blood pressure, thyroid disease, diabetes, or difficulty in urination due to enlargement of the prostate gland unless directed by a doctor. Do not use this product if you have ever been hospitalized for asthma or if you are taking any prescription drug for asthma unless directed by a doctor. **Do not continue to use this product, but seek medical assistance immediately if symptoms are not relieved within 1 hour or become worse.** Some users of this product may experience nervousness, tremor, sleeplessness, nausea, and loss of appetite. If these symptoms persist or become worse, consult a doctor. Do not take this product for persistent or chronic cough such as occurs with smoking, asthma, chronic bronchitis, or emphysema, or where cough is accompanied by excessive phlegm (mucus) unless directed by a doctor. A persistent cough may be a sign of a serious condition. If cough persists for more than 1 week, tends to recur, or is accompanied by a fever, rash, or persistent headache, consult a doctor. Keep this and all drugs out of the reach of children. In case of accidental overdose, seek professional assistance or contact a poison control center immediately. As with any drug, if you are pregnant or nursing a baby, seek the advice of a health professional before using this medication.

Drug Interaction Precaution: Do not take this product if you are presently taking a prescription drug for high blood pressure or depression, including those containing a Monoamine Oxidase Inhibitor (MAOI), without first consulting your doctor.

How Supplied: Boxes of 24 and 60.
Shown in Product Identification Guide, page 516

BRONKAID® MIST
EPINEPHRINE INHALATION
AEROSOL
BRONCHODILATOR
FOR ORAL INHALATION ONLY

Active Ingredient: Epinephrine USP 0.5% (w/w), (as nitrate and hydrochloride salts). Each spray delivers 0.25 mg epinephrine.

Inactive Ingredients: Alcohol 33% (w/w), Ascorbic acid, Dichlorodifluoromethane, Dichlorotetrafluoroethane, Purified water. Contains no sulfites.

Indications: For temporary relief of shortness of breath, tightness of chest and wheezing due to bronchial asthma.

Directions: Adults and children 4 years of age and older: Start with one inhalation, then wait at least one (1) minute. If symptoms are not relieved, use once more. Do not use again for at least 3 hours. The use of this product by children should be supervised by an adult. **Children under 4 years of age:** Consult a doctor. Each spray delivers 0.25 mg epinephrine.
1. Remove cap and mouthpiece from bottle.
2. Remove cap from mouthpiece and check to see that mouthpiece opening is clean and free from foreign objects.
3. Turn mouthpiece sideways and fit metal stem of nebulizer into hole in flattened end of mouthpiece.
4. Exhale, as completely as possible. Now, hold bottle **upside down** between thumb and forefinger and close lips loosely around end of mouthpiece.
5. Inhale deeply while pressing down firmly on bottle, once only.
6. Remove mouthpiece and hold your breath a moment to allow for maximum absorption of medication. Then exhale slowly through nearly closed lips.
7. After use, remove mouthpiece from bottle and replace cap. When possible, rinse mouthpiece with tap water immediately after use. Soap and water will not hurt it. A clean mouthpiece always works better. Slide mouthpiece over bottle for protection.

Warning: Contains CFC-12, and CFC-114, substances which harm public

Continued on next page

This product information was effective as of November 1, 1994. Current information may be obtained directly from Miles Inc., by writing to P.O. Box 340 Elkhart, IN 46515.

Miles—Cont.

health and environment by destroying ozone in the upper atmosphere.

Warnings: FOR ORAL INHALATION ONLY. Avoid spraying in eyes. Do not use this product unless a diagnosis of asthma has been made by a doctor. Do not use this product if you have heart disease, high blood pressure, thyroid disease, diabetes, or difficulty in urination due to enlargement of the prostate gland unless directed by a doctor. Do not use this product if you have ever been hospitalized for asthma or if you are taking any prescription drug for asthma. **Do not use this product more frequently or at higher doses than recommended, unless directed by a doctor.** Excessive use may cause nervousness and rapid heart beat, and possibly, adverse effects on the heart. **Do not continue to use this product, but seek medical assistance immediately if symptoms are not relieved within 20 minutes or become worse.** As with any drug, if you are pregnant or nursing a baby, seek the advice of a health professional before using this medication. Keep this and all drugs out of the reach of children. In case of accidental overdose, seek professional assistance or contact a poison control center immediately. DRUG INTERACTION PRECAUTION: Do not use this product if you are presently taking a prescription drug for high blood pressure or depression, including those containing a monoamine oxidase inhibitor (MAOI), without first consulting your doctor.

Storage and Handling: Store at controlled room temperature 59°F–86°F (15°C–30°C). Contents under pressure. Do not puncture or incinerate. Using or storing near open flame or heating above 120°F may cause bursting.

How Supplied: Bottles of ½ fl oz (15 mL) with actuator. Also available–refills (no mouthpiece) in ½ fl oz (15 mL).
Shown in Product Identification Guide, page 516

BRONKAID® MIST SUSPENSION EPINEPHRINE BITARTRATE INHALATION AEROSOL BRONCHODILATOR FOR ORAL INHALATION ONLY

Active Ingredient: Epinephrine Bitartrate 7.0 mg per ml. Each spray delivers 0.3 mg epinephrine bitartrate equivalent to 0.16 mg epinephrine base. Contains 200 metered inhalations per canister.

Inactive Ingredients: Cetylpyridinium Chloride, dichlorodifluoromethane, dichlorotetrafluoroethane, sorbitan trioleate, trichloromonofluoromethane. Contains no sulfites.

Indications: For temporary relief of shortness of breath, tightness of chest and wheezing due to bronchial asthma.

Directions: Adults and children 4 years of age and older: Start with one inhalation, then wait one (1) minute. If symptoms are not relieved, use once more. Do not use again for at least 3 hours. The use of this product by children should be supervised by an adult.

Children under 4 years of age: Consult a doctor. Each spray delivers 0.3 mg epinephrine bitartrate equivalent to 0.16 mg epinephrine base.

1. **SHAKE WELL.** Remove dust cap and inspect to see that nozzle is clean and free from foreign objects.
2. Hold inhaler with nozzle down while using.
3. Exhale, as completely as possible. Purse the lips as in saying the letter "O" and hold the nozzle up to the lips, keeping the tongue flat. As you start to take a deep breath, squeeze the nozzle and can together, releasing one full application. Complete taking deep breath, drawing medication into your lungs.
4. Hold breath for as long as comfortable. This distributes the medication in the lungs. Then exhale slowly keeping the lips nearly closed.
5. Replace dust cap after each use.
6. Rinse nozzle daily with soap and warm water after removing from vial. Dry with clean cloth.

Warning: Contains CFC-11, CFC-12 and CFC-114, substances which harm public health and environment by destroying ozone in the upper atmosphere.

Warnings: FOR ORAL INHALATION ONLY. Avoid spraying in eyes. Do not use this product unless a diagnosis of asthma has been made by a doctor. Do not use this product if you have heart disease, high blood pressure, thyroid disease, diabetes, or difficulty in urination due to enlargement of the prostate gland. Do not use this product if you have ever been hospitalized for asthma or if you are taking any prescription drug for asthma. **Do not use this product more frequently or at higher doses than recommended, unless directed by a doctor.** Excessive use may cause nervousness and rapid heart beat, and possibly, adverse effects on the heart. **Do not continue to use this product, but seek medical assistance immediately if symptoms are not relieved within 20 minutes or become worse.** As with any drug, if you are pregnant or nursing a baby, seek the advice of a health professional before using this medication. Keep this and all drugs out of the reach of children. In case of accidental overdose, seek professional assistance or contact a poison control center immediately.

Drug Interaction Precaution: Do not use this product if you are presently taking a prescription drug for high blood pressure or depression, including those containing a monoamine oxidase inhibitor (MAOI), without first consulting your doctor.

Storage and Handling: Store at controlled room temperature 59°F–86°F (15°C–30°C). Contents under pressure. Do not puncture or incinerate. Using or storing near open flame or heating above 120°F may cause bursting.

How Supplied: ⅓ fl. oz. (10cc) pocket size inhaler, with actuator.
Shown in Product Identification Guide, page 516

BUGS BUNNY™ Children's Chewable Vitamins Plus Iron (Sugar Free)
FLINTSTONES® Children's Chewable Vitamins
FLINTSTONES® Children's Chewable Vitamins Plus Iron

Vitamin Ingredients: Each multivitamin supplement with iron contains the ingredients listed in the chart below: [See table at top of next page.] FLINTSTONES® Children's Chewable Vitamins provide the same quantities of vitamins, but do not provide iron.

Indication: Dietary supplementation.

Dosage and Administration: One chewable tablet daily. For adults and children two years and older; tablet must be chewed.

Warning For Bugs Bunny Only: Phenylketonurics: Contains Phenylalanine.

Precaution:
IRON SUPPLEMENTS ONLY.
Close tightly and keep out of reach of children. Contains iron, which can be harmful or fatal to children in large doses. In case of accidental overdose, seek professional assistance or contact a Poison Control Center immediately.

How Supplied: Flintstones are supplied in bottles of 60 and 100, Bugs Bunny in bottles of 60 with child-resistant caps.
Shown in Product Identification Guide, page 516

CAMPHO-PHENIQUE® ANTISEPTIC GEL
[kam'fo-finēk]
First Aid Antiseptic/Pain Reliever

Active Ingredient: Camphorated Phenol (Camphor 10.8% and Phenol 4.7% in light mineral oil).

Inactive Ingredients: Colloidal Silicon Dioxide, Eucalyptus Oil, Glycerin, Light Mineral Oil.

Indications: For the temporary relief of pain and itching associated with minor burns, sunburn, minor cuts, scrapes, insect bites or minor skin irritation. Protects against the risk of infection in minor cuts, scrapes and burns.

Directions: Clean the affected area. Apply with cotton 1 to 3 times daily.

Warnings: **For External Use Only.** Do not use in or near the eyes or apply over

BUGS BUNNY™ Children's Chewable Vitamins Plus Iron (Sugar Free)
FLINTSTONES® Children's Chewable Vitamins Plus Iron

Amount per Tablet	%Daily Value for Children 2–4 Years of Age	% Daily Value for Adults and Children 4 or More Years of Age
Vitamin A 2500 I.U. 50% as Beta Carotene	100%	50%
Vitamin C 60 mg	150%	100%
Vitamin D 400 I.U.	100%	100%
Vitamin E 15 I.U.	150%	50%
Thiamin 1.05 mg	150%	70%
Riboflavin 1.2 mg	150%	70%
Niacin 13.5 mg	150%	67%
Vitamin B$_6$ 1.05 mg	150%	52%
Folate 300 mcg	150%	75%
Vitamin B$_{12}$ 4.5 mcg.	150%	75%
Iron (Elemental) 15 mg	150%	83%

large areas of the body. If product gets into the eyes, flush thoroughly with water and obtain medical attention. In case of deep or puncture wounds, animal bites, or serious burns, consult a doctor. Stop use and consult a doctor if condition worsens or if symptoms persist for more than 7 days or clear up and occur again within a few days. Do not use longer than 1 week unless directed by a doctor. Do not bandage. Keep this and all drugs out of the reach of children. In case of accidental ingestion seek professional assistance or contact a poison control center immediately.
DO NOT INDUCE VOMITING before contacting a doctor or poison control center.

How Supplied: 0.5 oz (14g) Tube.
Shown in Product Identification Guide, page 516

CAMPHO-PHENIQUE®
[kam 'fo-finēk]
COLD SORE GEL

Active Ingredient: Camphorated Phenol (Camphor 10.8% and Phenol 4.7% in a light mineral oil).

Inactive Ingredients: Colloidal Silicon Dioxide, Eucalyptus Oil, Glycerin, Light Mineral Oil.

Indications: For the temporary relief of pain and discomfort associated with cold sores/fever blisters.

Directions: Clean the affected area. Apply directly to cold sore or fever blister 1 to 3 times daily.

Warnings: For External Use Only. Do not use in or near the eyes or apply over large areas of the body. If product gets into the eyes, flush thoroughly with water and obtain medical attention. Stop use and consult a doctor if condition worsens or if symptoms persist for more than 7 days or clear up and occur again within a few days. Do not use longer than 1 week unless directed by a doctor. Do not bandage. Keep this and all drugs out of the reach of children. In case of accidental ingestion seek professional assistance or contact a poison control center immediately. DO NOT INDUCE VOMITING before contacting a doctor or poison control center.

How Supplied: 0.23 oz (6.5 g) Tube
Shown in Product Identification Guide, page 516

CAMPHO-PHENIQUE®
[kam 'fo-finēk]
Pain Relieving Antiseptic Liquid

Active Ingredient: Camphorated Phenol (Camphor 10.8% and Phenol 4.7% in light mineral oil).

Inactive Ingredients: Eucalyptus Oil, Light Mineral Oil.

Indications: For the temporary relief of pain and itching associated with minor burns, sunburn, minor cuts, scrapes, insect bites or minor skin irritation. Protects against the risk of infection in minor cuts, scrapes and burns.

Directions: Clean the affected area. Apply with cotton 1 to 3 times daily.

Warnings: For External Use Only. Do not use in or near the eyes or apply over large areas of the body. If product gets into the eyes, flush thoroughly with water and obtain medical attention. In case of deep or puncture wounds, animal bites, or serious burns, consult a doctor. Stop use and consult a doctor if condition worsens or if symptoms persist for more than 7 days or clear up and occur again within a few days. Do not use longer than 1 week unless directed by a doctor. Do not bandage. Keep this and all drugs out of the reach of children. In case of accidental ingestion seek professional assistance or contact a poison control center immediately. DO NOT INDUCE VOMITING before contacting a doctor or a poison control center.

How Supplied: Bottles of 0.75 fl oz (22 ml) and 1.5 fl oz (45 ml).
Shown in Product Identification Guide, page 516

CAMPHO-PHENIQUE®
[kam 'fo-finēk]
First Aid Antibiotic plus Pain Reliever Maximum Strength

Active Ingredients: Each gram contains: Bacitracin Zinc 500 units, Neomycin Sulfate 5 mg (equiv. to 3.5 mg Neomycin Base), Polymyxin B Sulfate 10,000 units, Lidocaine HCl 40 mg (Pain Reliever).

Inactive Ingredient: White Petrolatum

Indications: First aid antibiotic ointment both for temporary relief of pain and to help prevent infection of minor cuts, scrapes and burns.

Directions: Clean the affected area. Apply a small amount (an amount equal to the surface area of the tip of a finger) on the area 1 to 3 times daily. Do not apply more than 3 times daily. May be covered with a sterile bandage. Children under 2 years of age: consult a doctor.

Warnings: For External Use Only. Do not use in or near the eyes or apply over large areas of the body. In case of deep or puncture wounds, animal bites, or serious burns, consult a doctor. Stop use and consult a doctor if the condition worsens or if symptoms persist for more than 7 days or clear up and occur again within a few days. Do not use longer than 1 week unless directed by a doctor. Do not use in large quantities, particularly over raw surfaces or blistered areas. Keep this and all drugs out of the reach of children. In case of accidental ingestion seek professional assistance or contact a poison control center immediately.

Continued on next page

This product information was effective as of November 1, 1994. Current information may be obtained directly from Miles Inc., by writing to P.O. Box 340 Elkhart, IN 46515.

Miles—Cont.

Store at 15°–30°C (59°–86°F).

How Supplied: 0.50 oz (14 g) Tube
Shown in Product Identification Guide, page 516

DAIRY EASE® Tablets/Caplets
Natural Lactase Enzyme Supplement

Ingredients: Each Tablet/Caplet contains 3000 FCC Lactase units (derived from Aspergillus Oryzae). Other ingredients are: (Tablets) Dibasic Calcium Phosphate, Mannitol, Colloidal Silicon Dioxide, Magnesium Stearate. (Caplets): Colloidal Silicon Dioxide, Dibasic Calcium Phosphate, Magnesium Stearate, Microcrystalline Cellulose, Pregelatinized Starch.

Indications: Lactase insufficiency, suspected from gastrointestinal disturbances after consumption of milk or milk-containing products (i.e., Gas, Bloating, Flatulence, Cramps and Diarrhea) or identified by a lactose intolerance test.

Action: Lactase enzyme converts, by hydrolysis, the lactose into its simple sugar components: glucose and galactose.

Product Uses: Dairy Ease is a natural lactase enzyme which supplements the natural level of lactase in the body and helps make lactose more easily digestible. The most common products where lactose can be found are milk, cheese, ice cream & chocolate and it is also found in some vitamins and medications. Dairy Ease can be used with all foods which contain lactose such as pizza, hot dogs, pancakes, creamed salad dressings and soups, instant cocoa mix, puddings and other foods where milk, milk solids, whey, whey protein concentrate, casein or cheese are listed on the ingredient panel.

Dosage: Recommended dosage is 2–3 chewable tablets/swallowable caplets along with or immediately following dairy food consumption. However, since natural lactase levels vary, actual dosage may differ from person to person.

Drug Interactions: None. Dairy Ease tablets and caplets are classified as food products.

Warnings: Do not use if you have had an allergic reaction to products containing lactase enzyme. If symptoms persist consult a doctor about a possible food allergy or other digestive disorder.

Precautions: Diabetics should be aware that the milk sugar will now be metabolically available and must be taken into account (17.5 gm glucose and 17.5 gm galactose per quart at 70% hydrolysis). No reports received of any diabetics' reactions. Galactosemics may not have milk in any form, lactase enzyme modified or not.

Note: Possible adverse reactions are mainly gastrointestinal in nature, sometimes mimicking the symptoms of lactose intolerance and sometimes involving vomiting. Skin rashes possibly due to allergic reactions have been reported. Persons sensitive to penicillin and other molds may be particularly susceptible. Discontinue use of tablets/caplets immediately and consult a physician.

How Supplied: Dairy Ease Chewable Tablets are available in 36, 60 and 100 counts. Dairy Ease Swallowable Caplets are available in a 40 count bottle.
Shown in Product Identification Guide, page 516

DAIRY EASE® Drops
Natural Lactase Enzyme

Ingredients: Water, Glycerol, Lactase Enzyme (derived from Kluyveromyces Lactis). One ml contains no less than 5400 Neutral Lactase units.

Indications: Lactase insufficiency, suspected from gastrointestinal disturbances after consumption of milk or milk-containing products (i.e., Gas, Bloating, Flatulence, Cramps and Diarrhea) or identified by a lactose tolerance test.

Product Uses: Dairy Ease drops are a natural lactase enzyme in liquid form which when added to milk, make it more easily digestible. Dairy Ease drops can be used in any kind of milk including: whole, 1%, 2%, nonfat, canned, powdered and chocolate. Also, cream, baby formulas containing milk and high protein diet formulas. The treated milk can be used for cooking, on cereal or directly from the carton.

Action: Lactase enzyme converts, by hydrolysis, the lactose into its simple sugar components: glucose and galactose.

Dosage: Add Dairy Ease drops to a quart of milk, shake gently and refrigerate for 24 hours. Five drops will remove 70% of the lactose, 10 drops, 90% and 15 drops, 97+%. Since the degree of natural lactase levels varies, each person may have to adjust the number of drops that work best.

Drug Interactions: None known. Dairy Ease drops are classified as a food product.

Warnings: Do not use if you have had an allergic reaction to products containing lactase enzyme. If symptoms persist consult a doctor about a possible food allergy or other digestive disorder.

Precautions: Diabetics should be aware that the milk sugar will now be metabolically available and must be taken into account (17.5 gm glucose and 17.5 gm galactose per quart at 70% hydrolysis). No reports received of any diabetics' reactions. Galactosemics may not have milk in any form, lactase enzyme modified or not.

How Supplied: Dairy Ease drops are available in a 7ml bottle which will treat up to 32 quarts of milk.
Shown in Product Identification Guide, page 516

DAIRY EASE® Real Milk
Lactose Reduced Milk

Dairy Ease is also available in Real Milk which is 70% lactose reduced and contains vitamins A & D. A one quart size in three varieties is available: Nonfat, 1% lowfat, and 2% lowfat. Dairy Ease Real Milk can be used for cooking, on cereal or directly from the carton.

DOMEBORO® Astringent Solution
Powder Packets

Active Ingredients: Each powder packet, when dissolved in water and ready to use, provides the active ingredient aluminum acetate resulting from the reaction of calcium acetate 938 mg, and aluminum sulfate 1191 mg. The resulting astringent solution is buffered to an acid pH.

Inactive Ingredient: Dextrin

Indications: For temporary relief of minor skin irritations due to poison ivy, poison oak, poison sumac, insect bites, athlete's foot or rashes caused by soaps, detergents, cosmetics or jewelry.

Actions: DOMEBORO provides soothing, effective relief of minor skin irritations. For over 50 years, doctors have been recommending DOMEBORO ASTRINGENT SOLUTION to help relieve minor skin irritations.

Warnings: If condition worsens or symptoms persist for more than 7 days, discontinue use of the product and consult a doctor. For external use only. Avoid contact with the eyes. Do not cover compress or wet dressing with plastic to prevent evaporation. Keep this and all drugs out of the reach of children. In case of accidental ingestion, seek professional assistance or contact a Poison Control Center immediately.

Directions: One packet dissolved in 16 ounces of water makes a modified Burow's Solution approximately equivalent to a 1:40 dilution; two packets, a 1:20 dilution; and four packets, a 1:10 dilution. Dissolve one or two packets in water and stir the solution until fully dissolved. Do not strain or filter the solution. Can be used as a compress, wet dressing or as a soak. AS A COMPRESS OR WET DRESSING: Saturate a clean, soft, white cloth (such as a diaper or torn sheet) in the solution; gently squeeze and apply loosely to the affected area. Saturate the cloth in the solution every 15 to 30 minutes and apply to the affected area. Discard solution after each use. Repeat as often as necessary. AS A SOAK: Soak affected area in the solution for 15 to 30 minutes. Discard solution after each use. Repeat 3 times a day.

How Supplied: Boxes of 12 or 100 powder packets.

Shown in Product Identification Guide, page 516

DOMEBORO® Astringent Solution Effervescent Tablets

Active Ingredients: Each effervescent tablet, when dissolved in water and ready to use, provides the active ingredient aluminum acetate resulting from the reaction of calcium acetate 604 mg, and aluminum sulfate 878 mg. The resulting astringent solution is buffered to an acid pH.

Inactive Ingredients: Dextrin, Polyethylene Glycol, Sodium Bicarbonate

Indications: For temporary relief of minor skin irritations due to poison ivy, poison oak, poison sumac, insect bites, athlete's foot or rashes caused by soaps, detergents, cosmetics or jewelry.

Actions: DOMEBORO provides soothing, effective relief of minor skin irritations. For over 50 years doctors have been recommending DOMEBORO ASTRINGENT SOLUTION to help relieve minor skin irritations.

Warnings: If condition worsens or symptoms persist for more than 7 days, discontinue use of the product and consult a doctor. For external use only. Avoid contact with the eyes. Do not cover compress or wet dressing with plastic to prevent evaporation. Keep this and all drugs out of the reach of children. In case of accidental ingestion, seek professional assistance or contact a Poison Control Center immediately.

Directions: One tablet dissolved in 12 ounces of water makes a modified Burow's Solution approximately equivalent to a 1:40 dilution; two tablets, a 1:20 dilution; and four tablets, a 1:10 dilution. Dissolve one or two tablets in water and stir the solution until fully dissolved. Do not strain or filter the solution. Can be used as a compress, wet dressing or as a soak. AS A COMPRESS OR WET DRESSING: Saturate a clean, soft, white cloth (such as a diaper or torn sheet) in the solution; gently squeeze and apply loosely to the affected area. Saturate the cloth in the solution every 15 to 30 minutes and apply to the affected area. Discard solution after each use. Repeat as often as necessary. AS A SOAK: Soak affected area in the solution for 15 to 30 minutes. Discard solution after each use. Repeat 3 times a day.

How Supplied: Boxes of 12 or 100 effervescent tablets.

Shown in Product Identification Guide, page 516

FERGON® Iron Supplement Tablets
[fur-gone]
brand of ferrous gluconate

Ingredients: Each tablet contains 320 mg (5 grains) Ferrous Gluconate equal to approximately 36 mg elemental iron. Also contains: Dextrose, D&C Yellow #10 Lake, FD&C Blue #1 Lake, Hydroxypropyl Methylcellulose, Magnesium Stearate, Polyethylene Glycol, Polysorbate 80, Starch, Talc, Titanium Dioxide.

Action and Uses: For use as a dietary iron supplement.

Directions: Adults: One tablet daily as a Dietary Supplement.

Warnings: CLOSE TIGHTLY AND KEEP OUT OF THE REACH OF CHILDREN. CONTAINS IRON, WHICH CAN BE HARMFUL OR FATAL TO CHILDREN IN LARGE DOSES. IN CASE OF ACCIDENTAL OVERDOSE, SEEK PROFESSIONAL ASSISTANCE OR CONTACT A POISON CONTROL CENTER IMMEDIATELY. If you are pregnant or nursing a baby, seek the advice of a health professional before using this product. AVOID EXCESSIVE HEAT

How Supplied: FERGON Tablets of 320 mg (5 grains) bottle of 100.

Nutrition Facts: Serving Size 1 Tablet Servings Per Container 100

Amount per tablet	% Daily Value
Iron 36 mg	200%

Shown in Product Identification Guide, page 516

FLINTSTONES® COMPLETE
With Iron, Calcium & Minerals Children's Chewable Vitamins

BUGS BUNNY™ COMPLETE
Children's Chewable Vitamins + Minerals With Iron and Calcium (Sugar Free)

Ingredients: Each supplement provides the ingredients listed in the chart below:
[See table at bottom of next page.]

Indication: Dietary Supplementation.

Dosage and Administration: 2–4 years of age: Chew one-half tablet daily. Over 4 years of age: Chew one tablet daily.

Warning for Bugs Bunny only: Phenylketonurics: Contains Phenylalanine.

Precaution: Close tightly and keep out of reach of children. Contains iron, which can be harmful or fatal to children in large doses. In case of accidental overdose, seek professional assistance or contact a Poison Control Center immediately.

How Supplied: Bottles of 60's with child-resistant caps.

Shown in Product Identification Guide, page 516

FLINTSTONES® PLUS CALCIUM
with Beta Carotene
Children's Chewable Vitamins

Ingredients: Calcium Carbonate, Sorbitol, Starch, Sodium Ascorbate, Gelatin, Stearic Acid, Magnesium Stearate, Natural and Artificial Flavors. Vitamin E Acetate, Artificial Colors (including Yellow 6), Silica, Glycerides of Stearic and Palmitic Acids, Malic Acid, Aspartame* (a sweetener), Pyridoxine Hydrochloride, Riboflavin, Thiamine Mononitrate, Vitamin A Acetate, Beta Carotene, Monoammonium Glycyrrhizinate, Folic Acid, Vitamin D, Vitamin B12.

* Phenylketonurics: Contains Phenylalanine

CHEW ONE TABLET DAILY

One Tablet Daily Provides: Vitamins	Quantity Per Tablet	Percent U.S. RDA For Children 2 to 4 Years of Age	For Adults and Children Over 4 Years of Age
Vitamin A (as Acetate and Beta Carotene)	2500 I.U.	100	50
Vitamin D	400 I.U.	100	100
Vitamin E	15 I.U.	150	50
Vitamin C	60 mg	150	100
Folic Acid	0.3 mg	150	75
Thiamine	1.05 mg	150	70
Riboflavin	1.20 mg	150	70
Niacin	13.50 mg	150	67
Vitamin B-6	1.05 mg	150	52
Vitamin B-12	4.5 mcg	150	75

Minerals	Quantity	Percent U.S. RDA	
Calcium	200 mg	25	20

FOR ADULTS AND CHILDREN 2 YEARS AND OLDER; TABLET MUST BE CHEWED

KEEP OUT OF REACH OF CHILDREN.

Do not use this product if safety seal bearing Miles logo under cap is torn or missing.
Child Resistant Cap

How Supplied: Bottle of 60 Tablets

Shown in Product Identification Guide, page 516

Continued on next page

This product information was effective as of November 1, 1994. Current information may be obtained directly from Miles Inc., by writing to P.O. Box 340 Elkhart, IN 46515.

Miles—Cont.

FLINTSTONES® Plus Extra C
Children's Chewable Vitamins
BUGS BUNNY™ With Extra C
Children's Chewable Vitamins
(Sugar Free)

Vitamin Ingredients: Each multivitamin supplement contains the ingredients listed in the chart below:
[See table at top of next page.]

Indication: Dietary supplementation.

Dosage and Administration: One tablet daily for adults and children two years and older; tablet must be chewed.

Warning For Bugs Bunny Only: Phenylketonurics: Contains Phenylalanine.

How Supplied: Flintstones in bottles of 60's & 100's, Bugs Bunny in bottles of 60 with child-resistant caps.
Shown in Product Identification
Guide, page 516

FLINTSTONES® COMPLETE
Children's Chewable Vitamins
BUGS BUNNY™ COMPLETE
Children's Chewable
Vitamins + Minerals
(Sugar Free)
Amount per Tablet

	% Daily Value for Children 2–4 Years of Age	% Daily Value for Adults and Children 4 or More Years of Age
Vitamin A 5000 I.U. 50% as Beta Carotene	100%	100%
Vitamin C 60 mg	75%	100%
Vitamin D 400 I.U.	50%	100%
Vitamin E 30 I.U.	150%	100%
Thiamin 1.5 mg	107%	100%
Riboflavin 1.7 mg	106%	100%
Niacin 20 mg	111%	100%
Vitamin B$_6$ 2 mg	143%	100%
Folate 400 mcg	100%	100%
Vitamin B$_{12}$ 6 mcg	100%	100%
Biotin 40 mcg	13%	13%
Pantothenic Acid 10mg	100%	100%
Calcium 100 mg	6%	10%
Iron (Elemental) 18 mg	90%	100%
Phosphorus 100 mg	6%	10%
Iodine 150 mcg	107%	100%
Magnesium 20 mg	5%	5%
Zinc 15 mg	94%	100%
Copper 2 mg	100%	100%

Teen
Multi-Symptom Formula
MIDOL®
Menstrual Formula

Active Ingredients: Each caplet contains Acetaminophen 400 mg and Pamabrom 25 mg.

Inactive Ingredients: Croscarmellose Sodium, Hydroxpropyl Methylcellulose, Magnesium Stearate, Microcrystaline Cellulose, Pregelatinized Starch and Triacetin.

Indications: Relieves cramps, bloating, water-weight gain, headaches, backaches and muscular aches and pains.
● Provides effective relief of painful menstrual symptoms so you can get on with your life.
● Contains a special combination of safe, aspirin-free, caffeine-free ingredients which is not found in any ordinary pain reliever.
● Non-drowsy formula won't slow you down!

Directions: Adults and children 12 years and over: Take 2 caplets with water. Repeat every 4–6 hours, as needed, up to a maximum of 8 caplets per day. Under age 12: Consult your doctor.

Warnings: Do not use for more than 10 days unless directed by a doctor. If pain persists for more than 10 days, consult a doctor immediately. Keep this and all drugs out of reach of children. In case of accidental overdose, immediate medical attention is essential for adults as well as for children even if you do not notice any signs or symptoms. As with any drug, if you are pregnant or nursing a baby, seek the advice of a health professional before using this product.

How Supplied: White capsule-shaped caplets available in packages of 2 blisters of 8 caplets each and bottles of 32 caplets. Child-resistant safety closure on bottles of 32 caplets.
Shown in Product Identification
Guide, page 517

Maximum Strength
Multi-Symptom Formula
MIDOL®
Menstrual Formula

Active Ingredients: Each caplet or gelcap contains Acetaminophen 500 mg, Caffeine 60 mg and Pyrilamine Maleate 15 mg.

Inactive Ingredients: Caplets—Croscarmellose Sodium, Hydroxypropyl Methylcellulose, Magnesium Stearate, Microcrystalline Cellulose, Pregelatinized Starch and Triacetin.
Gelcaps—Croscarmellose Sodium, D&C Red #33 Lake, EDTA Sodium, FD&C Blue #1 Lake, Gelatin, Glycerin, Hydroxypropyl Methylcellulose, Iron Oxide, Magnesium Stearate, Microcrystalline Cellulose, Starch, Stearic Acid, Titanium Dioxide, Triacetin.

Indications: Relieves all of these physical menstrual symptoms: cramps, bloating, water-weight gain, headaches, backaches, muscular aches and fatigue.
● Provides maximum strength relief of painful physical symptoms suffered during your menstrual cycle.
● Contains a combination of maximum strength, aspirin-free ingredients which is not found in any ordinary pain reliever.

Directions: Adults and children 12 years and over: Take 2 caplets with water. Repeat every 4–6 hours, as needed, up to a maximum of 8 caplets per day. Under age 12: Consult your doctor.

Warnings: Do not use for more than 10 days unless directed by a doctor. If pain persists for more than 10 days, consult a doctor immediately. May cause drowsiness; alcohol, sedatives or tranquilizers may increase drowsiness. Avoid alcoholic beverages while taking this product. Do not take this product if you are taking sedatives or tranquilizers without first consulting your doctor. Use caution

BUGS BUNNY™ With Extra C
  Children's Chewable Vitamins
  (Sugar Free)
FLINTSTONES® Plus Extra C
  Children's Chewable Vitamins

Amount per Tablet	% Daily Value for Children 2–4 Years of Age	% Daily Value for Adults and Children 4 or More Years of Age
Vitamin A 2500 I.U. 50% as Beta Carotene	100%	50%
Vitamin C 60 mg	150%	100%
Vitamin D 400 I.U.	100%	100%
Vitamin E 15 I.U.	150%	50%
Thiamin 1.05 mg	150%	70%
Riboflavin 1.2 mg	150%	70%
Niacin 13.5 mg	150%	67%
Vitamin B_6 1.05 mg	150%	52%
Folate 300 mcg	150%	75%
Vitamin B_{12} 4.5 mcg	150%	75%
Iron (Elemental) 15 mg	150%	83%

when driving or operating machinery. May cause excitability, especially in children. The recommended dose of this product contains about as much caffeine as a cup of coffee. Limit the use of caffeine-containing medications, foods, or beverages while taking this product because too much caffeine may cause nervousness, irritability, sleeplessness, and occasionally, rapid heartbeat. Do not take this product, unless diected by a doctor, if you have a breathing problem such as emphysema or chronic bronchitis or if you have glaucoma or difficulty in urination due to enlargement of the prostate gland. Keep this and all drugs out of reach of children. In case of accidental overdose, immediate medical attention is essential for adults as well as for children even if you do not notice any signs or symptoms. As with any drug, if you are pregnant or nursing a baby, seek the advice of a health professional before using this product.

How Supplied: Caplets—White capsule-shaped caplets available in bottles of 8 and 32 caplets, and packages of 2 blisters of 8 caplets each. Child-resistant safety closures on bottles of 8 and 32 caplets.
Gelcaps—Dark/light blue capsule-shaped gelcaps available in bottles of 24 gelcaps and packages of 2 blisters of 6 gelcaps each. Child-resistant safety closure on bottle of 24 gelcaps.

Shown in Product Identification Guide, page 517

PMS
Multi-Symptom Formula
MIDOL®
Physical Symptom Relief

Active Ingredients: Each caplet or gelcap contains Acetaminophen 500 mg, Pamabrom 25 mg and Pyrilamine Maleate 15 mg.

Inactive Ingredients: Caplets—Croscarmellose Sodium, D&C Red #30, D&C Yellow #10, Hydroxypropyl Methylcellulose, Magnesium Stearate, Microcrystalline Cellulose, Pregelatinized Starch and Triacetin.
Gelcaps—Croscarmellose Sodium, D&C Red #27 Lake, EDTA Disodium, FD&C Blue #1, FD&C Red #40 Lake, Gelatin, Glycerin, Hydroxypropyl Methylcellulose, Iron Oxide, Magnesium Stearate, Microcrystalline Cellulose, Starch, Stearic Acid, Titanium Dioxide, Triacetin.

Indications: Contains maximum strength medication for all these premenstrual symptoms: bloating, water-weight gain, cramps, headaches and backaches.
● Provides maximum strength relief of the physical symptoms of Premenstrual Syndrome so you can feel like yourself again.
● Contains a combination of aspirin-free ingredients which is not found in any ordinary pain reliever: a diuretic to alleviate water retention and an analgesic for pain.

Directions: Adults and children 12 years and over: Take 2 caplets with water. Repeat every 4–6 hours, as needed, up to a maximum of 8 caplets per day. Under age 12: Consult your doctor.

Warnings: Do not use for more than 10 days unless directed by doctor. If pain persists for more than 10 days, consult a doctor immediately. May cause drowsiness; alcohol, sedatives and tranquilizers may increase drowsiness. Avoid alcoholic beverages while taking this product. Do not take this product if you are taking sedatives or tranquilizers without first consulting your doctor. Use caution when driving or operating machinery. May cause excitability especially in children. Do not take this product, unless directed by a doctor, if you have a breathing problem such as emphysema or chronic bronchitis or if you have glaucoma or difficulty in urination due to enlargement of the prostate gland. Keep this and all drugs out of the reach of children. In case of accidental overdose, immediate medical attention is essential for adults as well as for children even if you do not notice any signs or symptoms. As with any drug, if you are pregnant or nursing a baby, seek the advice of a health professional before using this product.

How Supplied: Caplets—White capsule-shaped caplets available in packages of 2 blisters of 8 caplets each and bottles of 32 caplets. Child-resistant safety closure on bottles of 32 caplets. Gelcaps—Dark/light pink capsule-shaped gelcaps available in bottles of 24 gelcaps and packages of 2 blisters of 6 gelcaps each. Child-resistant safety closure on bottle of 24 gelcaps.

Shown in Product Identification Guide, page 517

MILES® Nervine
Nighttime Sleep–Aid

Active Ingredient: Each caplet contains diphenhydramine HCl 25 mg.

Inactive Ingredients: Calcium Phosphate Dibasic, Calcium Sulfate, Carboxymethylcellulose Sodium, Corn Starch, Magnesium Stearate, Microcrystalline Cellulose.

Indications: Miles® Nervine helps you fall asleep and relieves occasional sleeplessness.

Warnings: Do not give to children under 12 years of age. Avoid alcoholic beverages while taking this product. Do not take this product if you are taking sedatives or tranquilizers without first consulting your doctor. If sleeplessness persists continuously for more than 2 weeks, consult your doctor. Insomnia may be a symptom of serious underlying medical

Continued on next page

This product information was effective as of November 1, 1994. Current information may be obtained directly from Miles Inc., by writing to P.O. Box 340 Elkhart, IN 46515.

Miles—Cont.

illness. Do not take this product if you have a breathing problem such as emphysema or chronic bronchitis or if you have glaucoma or difficulty in urination due to enlargement of the prostate gland unless directed by a doctor. As with any drug, if you are pregnant or nursing a baby, seek the advice of a health professional before using this product. Keep this and all drugs out of the reach of children. In case of accidental overdose, seek professional assistance or contact a poison control center immediately.

Dosage and Administration: Adults & children 12 years of age and over, 2 caplets at bedtime if needed or as directed by a doctor.

How Supplied: Blister pack 12's, bottle of 30's with a child-resistant cap.

Shown in Product Identification Guide, page 517

MYCELEX® OTC CREAM ANTIFUNGAL

Active Ingredient: Clotrimazole 1%

Inactive Ingredients: Benzyl alcohol (1%) as a preservative, cetostearyl alcohol, cetyl esters wax, octyldodecanol, polysorbate 60, purified water, sorbitan monostearate.
Store between 2°–30°C (36°–86°F).

Indications: Cures athlete's foot (tinea pedis), jock itch (tinea cruris), and ringworm (tinea corporis). For effective relief of the itching, cracking, burning and discomfort which can accompany these conditions.

Warnings: For external use only. Do not use on children under 2 years of age except under the advice and supervision of a doctor. If irritation occurs or if there is no improvement within 4 weeks (for athlete's foot or ringworm) or within 2 weeks (for jock itch) discontinue use and consult a doctor or pharmacist. Keep this and all drugs out of the reach of children. In case of accidental ingestion seek professional assistance or contact a Poison Control Center immediately. Use only as directed.

Directions: Cleanse skin with soap and water and dry thoroughly. Apply a thin layer and gently massage over affected area morning and evening or as directed by a doctor. For athlete's foot, pay special attention to the spaces between the toes. It is also helpful to wear well-fitting, ventilated shoes and to change shoes and socks at least once daily. Best results in athlete's foot and ringworm are usually obtained with 4 weeks' use of this product and in jock itch with 2 weeks' use. If satisfactory results have not occurred within these times, consult a doctor or pharmacist. Children under 12 years of age should be supervised in the use of this product. This product is not effective on the scalp or nails.

FOR BEST RESULTS, FOLLOW DIRECTIONS AND CONTINUE TREATMENT FOR LENGTH OF TIME INDICATED.

How Supplied: Cream Tube 15 g (½ oz.)

Shown in Product Identification Guide, page 517

MYCELEX® OTC SOLUTION ANTIFUNGAL

Active Ingredient: Clotrimazole 1%

Inactive Ingredient: Polyethylene glycol 400.
Store between 2°–30°C (36°–86°F).

Indications: Cures athlete's foot (tinea pedis), jock itch (tinea cruris), and ringworm (tinea corporis). For effective relief of the itching, cracking, burning and discomfort which can accompany these conditions.

Warnings: For external use only. Do not use on children under 2 years of age except under the advice and supervision of a doctor. If irritation occurs or if there is no improvement within 4 weeks (for athlete's foot or ringworm) or within 2 weeks (for jock itch) discontinue use and consult a doctor or pharmacist. Keep this and all drugs out of the reach of children. In case of accidental ingestion seek professional assistance or contact a Poison Control Center immediately. Use only as directed.

Directions: Cleanse skin with soap and water and dry thoroughly. Apply a thin layer and gently massage over affected area morning and evening or as directed by a doctor. For athlete's foot, pay special attention to the spaces between the toes. It is also helpful to wear well-fitting, ventilated shoes and to change shoes and socks at least once daily. Best results in athlete's foot and ringworm are usually obtained with 4 weeks' use of this product and in jock itch with 2 weeks' use. If satisfactory results have not occurred within these times, consult a doctor or pharmacist. Children under 12 years of age should be supervised in the use of this product. This product is not effective on the scalp or nails.

FOR BEST RESULTS, FOLLOW DIRECTIONS AND CONTINUE TREATMENT FOR LENGTH OF TIME INDICATED.

How Supplied: Solution Bottle 10 mL (⅓ fluid ounce)

MYCELEX-7® VAGINAL CREAM ANTIFUNGAL

Active Ingredient: Clotrimazole 1%

Inactive Ingredients: Benzyl alcohol, cetostearyl alcohol, cetyl esters wax, octyldodecanol, polysorbate 60, purified water, sorbitan monostearate

Indications: For treatment of vaginal yeast (Candida) infection.

Actions: Cures most vaginal yeast infections. MYCELEX®-7 Antifungal Vaginal Cream can kill the yeast that may cause vaginal infection. It is greaseless and does not stain clothes.

Precautions: IF THIS IS THE **FIRST** TIME YOU HAVE HAD VAGINAL ITCH AND DISCOMFORT, CONSULT YOUR DOCTOR. IF YOU HAVE HAD A DOCTOR DIAGNOSE A VAGINAL YEAST INFECTION BEFORE AND HAVE THE SAME SYMPTOMS NOW, USE THIS CREAM AS DIRECTED FOR 7 CONSECUTIVE DAYS.

**WARNING: DO NOT USE IF YOU HAVE ABDOMINAL PAIN, FEVER, OR FOUL-SMELLING DISCHARGE. CONTACT YOUR DOCTOR IMMEDIATELY.
IF YOU DO NOT IMPROVE IN 3 DAYS OR IF YOU DO NOT GET WELL IN 7 DAYS, YOU MAY HAVE A CONDITION OTHER THAN A YEAST INFECTION. CONSULT YOUR DOCTOR.** If your symptoms return within two months or if you have infections that do not clear up easily with proper treatment, consult your doctor. You could be pregnant or there could be a serious underlying medical cause for your infections, including diabetes or a damaged immune system (including damage from infection with HIV-the virus that causes AIDS). (PLEASE READ PATIENT PACKAGE PAMPHLET.)
Do not use during pregnancy except under the advice and supervision of a doctor. Do not use tampons while using this medication. Keep this and all drugs out of the reach of children. In case of accidental ingestion, seek professional assistance or contact a Poison Control Center immediately. NOT FOR USE IN CHILDREN LESS THAN 12 YEARS OF AGE.

Dosage and Administration: Before using, read the enclosed pamphlet.
Directions: Fill the applicator and insert one applicatorful of cream into the vagina, preferably at bedtime. Repeat this procedure daily for 7 consecutive days.

How Supplied: 1.5 oz. (45 g) tube and applicator. (7-Day Therapy)

Shown in Product Identification Guide, page 517

MYCELEX-7 VAGINAL ANTIFUNGAL CREAM WITH 7 DISPOSABLE APPLICATORS

Description: MYCELEX®-7 Antifungal Vaginal Cream can kill the yeast that may cause vaginal infection. It is greaseless and does not stain clothes.

Indications: For treatment of vaginal yeast (Candida) infection.
IF THIS IS THE **FIRST** TIME YOU HAVE HAD VAGINAL ITCH AND DISCOMFORT, CONSULT YOUR DOC-

TOR. IF YOU HAVE HAD A DOCTOR DIAGNOSE A VAGINAL YEAST INFECTION BEFORE AND HAVE THE SAME SYMPTOMS NOW, USE THIS CREAM AS DIRECTED FOR 7 CONSECUTIVE DAYS.
WARNING: DO NOT USE IF YOU HAVE ABDOMINAL PAIN, FEVER, OR FOUL-SMELLING DISCHARGE. CONTACT YOUR DOCTOR IMMEDIATELY.
Before using, read the enclosed pamphlet.
Directions: Fill the applicator and insert one applicatorful of cream into the vagina, preferably at bedtime. Dispose of each applicator after use. Do not flush in toilet. Repeat this procedure daily with a new applicator for 7 consecutive days.
WARNING: IF YOU DO NOT IMPROVE IN 3 DAYS OR IF YOU DO NOT GET WELL IN 7 DAYS, YOU MAY HAVE A CONDITION OTHER THAN A YEAST INFECTION. CONSULT YOUR DOCTOR. If your symptoms return within two months or if you have infections that do not clear up easily with proper treatment, consult your doctor. You could be pregnant or there could be a serious underlying medical cause for your infections, including diabetes or a damaged immune system (including damage from infection with HIV— the virus that causes AIDS). (PLEASE READ PATIENT PACKAGE PAMPHLET.)
Do not use during pregnancy except under the advice and supervision of a doctor. Do not use tampons while using this medication. Keep this and all drugs out of the reach of children.
In case of accidental ingestion, seek professional assistance or contact a Poison Control Center immediately. **NOT FOR USE IN CHILDREN LESS THAN 12 YEARS OF AGE.**
If you have any questions about MYCELEX®-7 or vaginal yeast infection, contact your physician.
Store at room temperature between 2° **and 30°C (36° and 86°F).**
See end panel of carton and tube crimp for lot number and expiration date.
Active Ingredient: Clotrimazole 1%.
Inactive Ingredients: Benzyl alcohol, cetostearyl alcohol, cetyl esters wax, octyldodecanol, polysorbate 60, purified water, sorbitan monostearate.
How Supplied: One 45g (1.5 oz.) tube of vaginal cream and 7 applicators (7 day therapy)
Consumer Questions or Comments Call 1-800-800-4793
8:30–5:00 EST M–F
Shown in Product Identification Guide, page 517

MYCELEX-7®
VAGINAL INSERTS ANTIFUNGAL

Active Ingredient: Each insert contains 100 mg clotrimazole.
Inactive Ingredients: Corn starch, lactose, magnesium stearate, povidone.

Indications: For treatment of vaginal yeast (Candida) infection.

Actions: Cures most vaginal yeast infections. MYCELEX-7 Antifungal Vaginal Inserts can kill the yeast that may cause vaginal infection. They do not stain clothes.

Precautions: IF THIS IS THE **FIRST** TIME YOU HAVE HAD VAGINAL ITCH AND DISCOMFORT, CONSULT YOUR DOCTOR. IF YOU HAVE HAD A DOCTOR DIAGNOSE A VAGINAL YEAST INFECTION BEFORE AND HAVE THE SAME SYMPTOMS NOW, USE THESE INSERTS AS DIRECTED FOR 7 CONSECUTIVE DAYS.

WARNING: DO NOT USE IF YOU HAVE ABDOMINAL PAIN, FEVER, OR FOUL-SMELLING DISCHARGE. CONTACT YOUR DOCTOR IMMEDIATELY.

IF YOU DO NOT IMPROVE IN 3 DAYS OR IF YOU DO NOT GET WELL IN 7 DAYS, YOU MAY HAVE A CONDITION OTHER THAN A YEAST INFECTION. CONSULT YOUR DOCTOR. If your symptoms return within two months or if you have infections that do not clear up easily with proper treatment, consult your doctor. You could be pregnant or there could be a serious underlying medical cause for your infections, including diabetes or a damaged immune system (including damage from infection with HIV-the virus that causes AIDS). (PLEASE READ PATIENT PACKAGE PAMPHLET) Do not use during pregnancy except under the advice and supervision of a doctor. Do not use tampons while using this medication. Keep this and all drugs out of the reach of children. In case of accidental ingestion, seek professional assistance or contact a Poison Control Center immediately. **NOT FOR USE IN CHILDREN LESS THAN 12 YEARS OF AGE.**

Dosage and Administration: Before using, read the enclosed pamphlet.
Directions: Unwrap one insert, place it in the applicator, and use the applicator to place the insert into the vagina, preferably at bedtime. Repeat this procedure daily for 7 consecutive days.

How Supplied: 7 vaginal inserts and applicator. (7-Day Therapy)

MYCELEX-7 Combination-Pack
VAGINAL INSERTS &
EXTERNAL VULVAR CREAM

- **Cures Most Vaginal Yeast Infections**
- **Relieves Associated External Vulvar Itching and Irritation**

MYCELEX®-7 Antifungal Vaginal Inserts and External Vulvar Cream can kill the yeast that may cause vaginal infection. They do not stain clothes.

Indications: For treatment of vaginal yeast *(Candida)* infection and the relief of external vulvar itching and irritation associated with vaginal yeast infection.
IF THIS IS THE **FIRST** TIME YOU HAVE HAD VAGINAL OR VULVAR ITCH AND DISCOMFORT, CONSULT YOUR DOCTOR. IF YOU HAVE HAD A DOCTOR DIAGNOSE A VAGINAL YEAST INFECTION BEFORE AND HAVE THE SAME SYMPTOMS NOW, USE THESE INSERTS AND CREAM AS DIRECTED.
WARNING: DO NOT USE IF YOU HAVE ABDOMINAL PAIN, FEVER, OR FOUL-SMELLING DISCHARGE. CONTACT YOUR DOCTOR IMMEDIATELY.
Before using, read the enclosed pamphlet.

Directions:
Inserts: Unwrap one insert, place it in the applicator, and use the applicator to place the insert into the vagina, preferably at bedtime. Repeat this procedure daily for 7 consecutive days to treat vaginal *(Candida)* yeast infection.

Cream: Squeeze a small amount of cream onto your finger and gently spread the cream onto the irritated area of the vulva. Use once or twice daily for up to 7 days as needed to relieve external vulvar itching. THE CREAM SHOULD NOT BE USED FOR VULVAR ITCHING DUE TO CAUSES OTHER THAN A YEAST INFECTION.
WARNING: IF YOU DO NOT IMPROVE IN 3 DAYS OR IF YOU DO NOT GET WELL IN 7 DAYS, YOU MAY HAVE A CONDITION OTHER THAN A YEAST INFECTION. CONSULT YOUR DOCTOR. If your symptoms return within two months or if you have infections that do not clear up easily with proper treatment, consult your doctor. You could be pregnant or there could be a serious underlying medical cause for your infections, including diabetes or a damaged immune system (including damage from infection with HIV— the virus that causes AIDS). (PLEASE READ ENCLOSED PATIENT PACKAGE PAMPHLET.)
Do not use during pregnancy except under the advice and supervision of a doctor.
Do not use tampons while using this medication.
Keep this and all drugs out of the reach of children. In case of accidental ingestion, seek professional assistance or contact a Poison Control Center immediately.

Continued on next page

This product information was effective as of November 1, 1994. Current information may be obtained directly from Miles Inc., by writing to P.O. Box 340 Elkhart, IN 46515.

Miles—Cont.

NOT FOR USE IN CHILDREN LESS THAN 12 YEARS OF AGE.
If you have any questions about MYCE-LEX®-7 Combination-Pack or vaginal yeast infection, contact your physician.

Active Ingredient:
Inserts: Each insert contains 100 mg clotrimazole
Cream: Clotrimazole 1%

Inactive Ingredients:
Inserts: Corn starch, lactose, magnesium stearate, povidone
Cream: Benzyl alcohol, cetostearyl alcohol, cetyl esters wax, octyldodecanol, polysorbate 60, purified water, sorbitan monostearate

How Supplied: 7 vaginal inserts and applicator (7-day therapy) and one 7g. (.25 oz.) tube of external vulvar cream.
Store at room temperature between 2° and 30°C (36° and 86°F).
See end panel of carton, foil wrappers and tube crimp for lot number and expiration date.
Consumer Questions or Comments call
1-800-800-4793
8:30–5:00 EST M-F
Shown in Product Identification Guide, page 517

NaSal™ Moisturizer AF
Saline (buffered)
0.65% Sodium chloride
Nasal Spray and Drops

Description: The nasal spray and nose drops contain Sodium Chloride 0.65%. Also contains: Benzalkonium Chloride and Thimerosal 0.001% as preservative, Mono- and Dibasic Sodium Phosphates as buffers, Purified Water.
Contains No Alcohol.

Actions: Immediate relief for dry nose. Formulated to match the pH of normal nasal secretions to help prevent stinging or burning.

Indications: Provides gentle relief for dry, irritated nasal passages due to colds, low humidity, air travel, allergies, minor nose bleeds, overuse of decongestant sprays/drops and other nasal irritations. As an ideal moisturizer, it can be used with cold, allergy, and sinus medications.

Warnings: The use of this dispenser by more than one person may spread infection. Keep out of the reach of children.

Dosage and Administration: Spray: Spray twice in each nostril as often as needed or as directed by doctor.
Drops: For infants, children and adults, 2 to 6 drops in each nostril as often as needed or as directed by doctor.

How Supplied: Nasal Spray—plastic squeeze bottles of 30 mL (1 fl. oz.).
Nose Drops—MonoDrop® bottles of 15 mL (½ fl. oz.).
Shown in Product Identification Guide, page 517

NEO-SYNEPHRINE®
Pediatric Formula, Mild Formula, Regular Strength, and Extra Strength.
phenylephrine hydrochloride

Description: This line of Nasal Sprays, Drops and Spray Pumps contains Phenylephrine Hydrochloride in strengths ranging from 0.125% (drops only) to 1%. Also contains: Benzalkonium Chloride and Thimerosal 0.001% as preservatives, Citric Acid, Purified Water, Sodium Chloride, Sodium Citrate.

Action: Rapid-acting nasal decongestant.

Directions: For a 0.125% solution: Children 2 to under 6 years of age (with adult supervision): 2 or 3 drops or sprays in each nostril not more often than every 4 hours. **Use only recommended amount.** Children under 2 years of age: consult a doctor.
For a 0.25% solution (Mild):
Adults and children 6 to under 12 years of age (with adult supervision): 2 or 3 drops or sprays in each nostril not more often than every 4 hours. Children under 6 years of age: consult a doctor.
For a 0.5% solution (Regular):
Adults and children 12 years of age and over: 2 or 3 drops or sprays in each nostril not more often than every 4 hours. Do not give to children under 12 years of age unless directed by a doctor.
For a 1% solution (Extra):
Adults and children 12 years of age and over: 2 or 3 drops or sprays in each nostril not more often than every 4 hours. Do not give to children under 12 years of age unless directed by a doctor.

Indications: For temporary relief of nasal congestion due to common cold, hay fever, sinusitis, or other upper respiratory allergies.

Warnings: For adults:
Do not exceed recommended dosage. This product may cause temporary discomfort such as burning, stinging, sneezing, or an increase in nasal discharge. The use of this container by more than one person may spread infection. Do not use this product for more than 3 days. Use only as directed. Frequent or prolonged use may cause nasal congestion to recur or worsen. If symptoms persist, consult a doctor. Do not use this product if you have heart disease, high blood pressure, thyroid disease, diabetes, or difficulty in urination due to enlargement of the prostate gland unless directed by a doctor.
For children under 12 years of age:
Do not exceed recommended dosage. This product may cause temporary discomfort such as burning, stinging, sneezing, or an increase in nasal discharge. The use if this container by more than one person may spread infection. Do not use this product for more than 3 days. Use only as directed. Frequent or prolonged use may cause nasal congestion to recur or worsen. If symptoms persist, consult a doctor. Do not use this product

---

in a child who has heart disease, high blood pressure, thyroid disease, or diabetes unless directed by a doctor.
Prolonged exposure to air or strong light will cause oxidation and some loss of potency. Do not use if brown in color or contains a precipitate.
Keep these and all drugs out of the reach of children. In case of accidental ingestion seek professional assistance or contact a poison control center immediately.

How Supplied: Pediatric Formula (0.125%) in 15 mL drops. Mild Formula (0.25%) in 15 mL drops and spray. Regular Strength (0.5%) in 15 mL drops and spray. Extra Strength (1.0%) in 15 mL drops and spray.
Shown in Product Identification Guide, page 517

NEO-SYNEPHRINE®
Maximum Strength 12 Hour and Maximum Strength 12 Hour Extra Moisturizing
oxymetazoline hydrochloride
Nasal Spray 0.05%

Description: *Maximum Strength 12 Hour Nasal Spray* and *Nasal Spray Pump* contain: Oxymetazoline Hydrochloride 0.05%. Also contain: Benzalkonium Chloride and Phenylmercuric Acetate 0.002% as preservatives, Glycine, Purified Water, Sorbitol, may also contain Sodium Chloride.
Maximum Strength 12 Hour Extra-Moisturizing Nasal Spray contains: Oxymethazoline Hydrochloride 0.05%. Also contains: Benzalkonium Chloride and Phenylmercuric Acetate 0.002% as preservatives, Glycerin, Glycine, Purified Water, Sorbitol, and may also contain Sodium Chloride.

Action: 12 HOUR Nasal Decongestant.

Indications: Provides temporary relief, for up to 12 HOURS, of nasal congestion due to colds, hay fever, sinusitis, or other upper respiratory allergies. NEO-SYNEPHRINE MAXIMUM STRENGTH 12-HOUR Nasal Spray and Pump contain oxymetazoline which provides the longest-lasting relief of nasal congestion available. Neo-Synephrine Maximum Strength 12-hour Extra Moisturizing Nasal Spray soothes and moisturizes dry nasal passages as it goes to the core of your congestion.

Warnings: Do not exceed recommended dosage. This product may cause temporary discomfort such as burning, stinging, sneezing, or an increase in nasal discharge. The use of this container by more than one person may spread infection. Do not use this product for more than 3 days. Use only as directed. Frequent or prolonged use may cause nasal congestion to recur or worsen. If symptoms persist, consult a doctor. Do not use this product if you have heart disease, high blood pressure, thyroid disease, diabetes, or difficulty in urination due to enlargement of the prostate gland unless directed by a doctor.

Keep this and all drugs out of the reach of children. In case of accidental ingestion, seek professional assistance or contact a poison control center immediately. As with any drug, if you are pregnant or nursing a baby, seek the advice of a health professional before using this product.

Directions: Adults and children 6 to under 12 years of age (with adult supervision): 2 or 3 drops or sprays in each nostril not more often than every 10 to 12 hours. Do not exceed 2 doses in any 24-hour period. Children 6 years of age: consult a doctor.

How Supplied: *Nasal Spray Maximum Strength* — plastic squeeze bottles of 15 ml (½ fl. oz.); *Nasal Spray Pump* —15 ml bottle (½ fl. oz.). Maximum Strength 12 Hour Extra Moisturizing Nasal Spray — 15 ml (½ fl. oz)
Shown in Product Identification Guide, page 517

NTZ®
Long Acting
Oxymetazoline hydrochloride
Nasal Spray 0.05%
Nose Drops 0.05%

Description: Both the nasal spray and nose drops contain Oxymetazoline Hydrochloride 0.05%. Also contain: Benzalkonium Chloride and Phenylmercuric Acetate 0.002% as preservatives, Glycine, Purified Water, Sorbitol, and may also contain Sodium Chloride.

Actions: 12 Hour Nasal Decongestant.

Indications: Provides temporary relief, for up to 12 hours, of nasal congestion due to colds, hay fever, sinusitis, or other upper respiratory allergies. Oxymetazoline hydrochloride provides the longest-lasting relief of nasal congestion available. It decongests nasal passages up to 12 hours, reduces swelling of nasal passages, and temporarily restores freer breathing through the nose.

Warnings: Do not exceed recommended dosage. This product may cause temporary discomfort such as burning, stinging, sneezing, or an increase in nasal discharge. The use of this container by more than one person may spread infection. Do not use this product for more than 3 days. Use only as directed. Frequent or prolonged use may cause nasal congestion to recur or worsen. If symptoms persist, consult a doctor. Do not use this product if you have heart disease, high blood pressure, thyroid disease, diabetes, or difficulty in urination due to enlargement of the prostate gland unless directed by a doctor. Keep these and all drugs out of the reach of children. In case of accidental ingestion seek professional assistance or contact a poison control center immediately.

Directions: Adults and children 6 to under 12 years of age (with adult supervision): 2 or 3 drops or sprays in each nostril not more often than every 10 to 12

hours. Do not exceed 2 doses in any 24-hour period. Children under 6 years of age: consult a doctor.

How Supplied: *Nasal Spray* —plastic squeeze bottles of 15 ml (½ fl. oz.). *Nose Drops* —bottles of 15 ml (½ fl. oz.) with dropper.

ONE-A-DAY® 55 PLUS

Description: *ONE-A-DAY 55 Plus is specially formulated for mature adults with more Vitamin C, B-1, B-2, B-6, and E. ONE-A-DAY continues to apply the latest and best nutritional knowledge to help keep nutrition understandable and help protect your health. Trust ONE-A-DAY to be your partner in nutrition.*

MULTIVITAMIN/MULTIMINERAL SUPPLEMENT

Directions For Use: Adults take one tablet daily with food.
[See table above.]

Nutrient Information: Vitamin A is essential for the normal function of vision. **Niacin** plays a role in synthesis of DNA. **Vitamin D** helps properly utilize calcium and phosphorus necessary for strong bones and teeth. **Folic Acid** is essential to the formation of red blood cells. **Biotin** is essential in the metabolism of fat, sugar and some amino acids. **Pantothenic Acid** is essential for the metabolism of fat and sugar.

Ingredients: Calcium Carbonate, Magnesium Hydroxide, Ascorbic Acid, Potassium Chloride, Cellulose, Gelatin, Vitamin E Acetate, Zinc Sulfate, Acacia, Hydroxypropyl Methylcellulose, Modified Cellulose Gum, Calcium Pantothenate, Niacinamide, Citric Acid, Magnesium Stearate, Hydroxypropyl Cellulose, Selenium Yeast, Povidone, Artificial Colors (including Yellow 6), Pyridoxine Hydrochloride, Manganese Sulfate, Starch, Thiamine Mononitrate, Cupric Sulfate, Chromium Yeast, Molybdenum Yeast, Riboflavin, Dicalcium Phosphate, Dextrose, Vitamin A Acetate, Beta Carotene, Folic Acid, Potassium Iodide, Lecithin, Sodium, Haxametaphosphate, Vitamin K, Biotin, Vitamin B-12, Vitamin D.

VITAMINS	QUANTITY	% U.S. RDA	MINERALS	QUANTITY	% U.S. RDA
Vitamin A (as Acetate) and Beta Carotene	6000 I.U.	120	Calcium (elemental)	220 mg	22
Vitamin C	120 mg	200	Iodine	150 mcg	100
Thiamine (B-1)	4.5 mg	300	Magnesium	100 mg	25
Riboflavin (B-2)	3.4 mg	200	Copper	2 mg	100
Niacin	20 mg	100	Zinc	15 mg	100
Vitamin D	400 I.U.	100	Chromium	10 mcg	*
Vitamin E	60 I.U.	200	Selenium	10 mcg	*
Vitamin B-6	6 mg	300	Molybdenum	10 mcg	*
Folic Acid	0.4 mg	100	Manganese	2.5 mg	*
Vitamin B-12	25 mcg	417	Potassium	37.5 mg	*
Biotin	30 mg	10	Chloride	34 mg	*
Pantothenic Acid	20 mg	200			
Vitamin K	25 mcg	*			

*No U.S. RDA established.

How Supplied: Bottles of 50's and 80's with child-resistant caps.
Shown in Product Identification Guide, page 517

ONE-A-DAY® Essential Vitamins
11 Essential Vitamins

Ingredients: Calcium Carbonate, Ascorbic Acid, Gelatin, Vitamin E Acetate, Starch, Niacinamide, Calcium Pantothenate, Calcium Silicate, Hydroxypropyl Methylcellulose, Artificial Color, Hydroxypropylcellulose, Vitamin A Acetate, Pyridoxine Hydrochloride, Riboflavin, Thiamine Mononitrate, Magnesium Stearate, Folic Acid, Beta Carotene, Sodium Hexametaphosphate, Vitamin D, Vitamin B-12, Lecithin.

Vitamins	Quantity	U.S. RDA
Vitamin A (as Acetate and Beta Carotene)	5000 I.U.	100
Vitamin C	60 mg	100
Thiamine (B₁)	1.5 mg	100
Riboflavin (B₂)	1.7 mg	100
Niacin	20 mg	100
Vitamin D	400 I.U.	100
Vitamin E	30 I.U.	100
Vitamin B₆	2 mg	100
Folic Acid	0.4 mg	100
Vitamin B₁₂	6 mcg	100
Pantothenic Acid	10 mg	100

Indication: Dietary supplementation.

Dosage and Administration: Adults take one tablet daily.

How Supplied: Bottles of 75's and 130's with child-resistant caps.
Shown in Product Identification Guide, page 517

Continued on next page

This product information was effective as of November 1, 1994. Current information may be obtained directly from Miles Inc., by writing to P.O. Box 340 Elkhart, IN 46515.

Miles—Cont.

ONE-A-DAY® EXTRAS ANTIOXIDANT

Ingredients: Ascorbic Acid, Vitamin E Acetate, Gelatin, Glycerin, Soybean Oil, Selenium Yeast, Lecithin, Zinc Oxide, Vegetable Oil (Partially Hydrogenated Cottonseed and Soybean Oils), Yellow Wax (Beeswax, Yellow) Manganese Sulfate, Beta Carotene, Cupric Oxide, Titanium Dioxide, Artificial Colors including FD&C Yellow #5 (Tartrazine). **EXTRAS** individual supplements can be taken alone or with your everyday multivitamin.

Directions for Use: Adults take one softgel capsule daily. To preserve quality and freshness, keep bottle tightly closed.

VITAMINS	QUANTITY	% US RDA
Vitamin E	200 I.U.	667
Vitamin C	250 mg	417
Vitamin A	5000 I.U.	100
(as Beta Carotene)		

MINERALS	QUANTITY	% US RDA
Zinc	7.5 mg	50
Copper	1.0 mg	50
Selenium	15.0 mcg	*
Manganese	1.5 mg	*

*No. U.S. RDA established

Indications: ONE-A-DAY EXTRAS ANTIOXIDANT is specially formulated to create a *high potency* **antioxidant supplement that meets a wide range of dietary needs. Antioxidants** may neutralize the effects of free radicals (oxidants) which many scientists believe can be a cause of cell damage.
ONE-A-DAY EXTRAS ANTIOXIDANT formula combines the antioxidant nutrients with the essential trace minerals necessary for antioxidant enzyme activity.
Easy to swallow softgel capsule.
CHILD RESISTANT CAP
Do not use this product if safety seal bearing Miles logo under cap is torn or missing.

How Supplied: Bottle of 50 softgels.
Shown in Product Identification Guide, page 517

ONE-A-DAY® EXTRAS GARLIC

Ingredients: Garlic Oil Macerate, Gelatin, Glycerin, Sorbitol, Xylose.
EXTRAS individual supplements can be taken alone or with your everyday multivitamin.

Directions For Use: Adults take one softgel capsule daily. Do not chew. Swallow whole to ensure maximum strength and breath freshness. To preserve quality and freshness, keep bottle tightly closed.

KEEP OUT OF REACH OF CHILDREN

Indications: ONE-A-DAY EXTRAS GARLIC contains 600 mg of concentrated garlic which is equivalent to one garlic clove. Provides the benefits of fresh garlic in one softgel capsule. Easy to swallow high potency softgel capsule.
CHILD RESISTANT CAP
Do not use this product if safety seal bearing Miles logo under cap is torn or missing.

How Supplied: Bottles of 45 softgels
Shown in Product Identification Guide, page 518

ONE-A-DAY® EXTRAS VITAMIN C

Ingredients: Ascorbic Acid, Starch, Cellulose, Stearic Acid, Crospovidone, Lactose, Magnesium Stearate.
EXTRAS individual supplements can be taken alone or with your everyday multivitamin.

Directions for Use:
Adults take one tablet daily.

VITAMINS	QUANTITY	% U.S. RDA
Vitamin C	500 mg	833

KEEP OUT OF REACH OF CHILDREN

Indications: ONE-A-DAY EXTRAS VITAMIN C is formulated to give you 500 mg of Vitamin C. Contains high potency level of Vitamin C in one tablet. Vitamin C is an antioxidant nutrient which may neutralize the effects of free radicals (oxidants) which many scientists believe can be a cause of cell damage.
CHILD RESISTANT CAP
Do not use this product if safety seal bearing Miles logo under cap is torn or missing.

How Supplied: Bottle of 100 Tablets
Shown in Product Identification Guide, page 518

ONE-A-DAY® EXTRAS VITAMIN E

Ingredients: Vitamin E Acetate, Gelatin, Glycerin.
EXTRAS individual supplements can be taken alone or with your everyday multivitamin.

Directions for Use:
Adults take one softgel capsule daily. To preserve quality and freshness, keep bottle tightly closed.

VITAMIN	QUANTITY	% U.S. RDA
Vitamin E	400 I.U.	1,333

KEEP OUT OF REACH OF CHILDREN

Indications: ONE-A-DAY EXTRAS VITAMIN E is formulated to give you 400 I.U. of Vitamin E. High potency level of Vitamin E in one easy to swallow softgel capsule. Vitamin E is an antioxidant nutrient which may neutralize the effects of free radicals (oxidants) which many scientists believe can be a cause of cell damage.
CHILD RESISTANT CAP
Do not use this product if safety seal bearing Miles logo under cap is torn or missing.

How Supplied: Bottle of 60 Softgels.
Shown in Product Identification Guide, page 518

ONE-A-DAY® Maximum Multivitamin/Multimineral Supplement for Adults

Ingredients: Dicalcium Phosphate, Magnesium Hydroxide, Cellulose, Potassium Chloride, Ascorbic Acid, Gelatin, Ferrous Fumarate, Zinc Sulfate, Modified Cellulose Gum, Vitamin E Acetate, Citric Acid, Niacinamide, Hydroxypropyl Methylcellulose, Magnesium Stearate, Calcium Pantothenate, Selenium Yeast, Artifical Color, Polyvinylpyrrolidone, Hydroxypropylcellulose, Manganese Sulfate, Silica, Copper Sulfate, Chromium Yeast, Molybdenum Yeast, Pyridoxine Hydrochloride, Riboflavin, Thiamine Mononitrate, Beta Carotene, Vitamin A Acetate, Folic Acid, Potassium Iodide, Sodium Hexametaphosphate, Biotin, Vitamin D, Vitamin B-12, Lecithin.
One tablet daily of ONE-A-DAY® Maximum provides:

Vitamins	Quantity	% of U.S. RDA
Vitamin A (as Acetate and Beta Carotene)	5000 I.U.	100
Vitamin C	60 mg	100
Thiamine (B1)	1.5 mg	100
Riboflavin (B2)	1.7 mg	100
Niacin	20 mg	100
Vitamin D	400 I.U.	100
Vitamin E	30 I.U.	100
Vitamin B6	2 mg	100
Folic Acid	0.4 mg	100
Vitamin B12	6 mcg	100
Biotin	30 mcg	10
Pantothenic Acid	10 mg	100

Minerals	Quantity	% of U.S. RDA
Iron (Elemental)	18 mg	100
Calcium (Elemental)	130 mg	13
Phosphorus	100 mg	10
Iodine	150 mcg	100
Magnesium	100 mg	25
Copper	2 mg	100
Zinc	15 mg	100
Chromium	10 mcg	*
Selenium	10 mcg	*
Molybdenum	10 mcg	*
Manganese	2.5 mg	*
Potassium	37.5 mg	*
Chloride	34 mg	*

*No U.S. RDA established

Indication: Dietary supplementation.

Dosage and Administration: Adults take one tablet daily with food.

Precaution: Contains iron, which can be harmful in large doses. Close tightly and keep out of reach of children. In case of overdose, contact a physician or Poison Control Center immediately.

How Supplied: Bottles of 60 and 100 with child-resistant caps.

Shown in Product Identification Guide, page 517

ONE-A-DAY® MEN'S MULTIVITAMIN SUPPLEMENT

Ingredients: Ascorbic Acid, Calcium Carbonate, Gelatin, Vitamin E Acetate, Starch, Niacinamide, Cellulose, Calcium Silicate, Calcium Pantothenate, Hydroxypropyl Methylcellulose, Artificial Color (FD&C Yellow #6), Hydroxypropylcellulose, Magnesium Stearate, Pyridoxine Hydrochloride, Riboflavin, Thiamine Mononitrate, Vitamin A Acetate, Beta Carotene, Folic Acid, Sodium Hexametaphosphate, Vitamin D, Vitamin B-12, Lecithin.

Directions for Use: Adults take one tablet daily.

Vitamins	Quantity	% U.S. RDA
Vitamin A (as Acetate and Beta Carotene)	5000 I.U.	100
Vitamin C	200 mg	333
Thiamine (B-1)	2.25 mg	150
Riboflavin (B-2)	2.55 mg	150
Niacin	20 mg	100
Vitamin D	400 I.U.	100
Vitamin E	45 I.U.	150
Vitamin B-6	3 mg	150
Folic Acid	0.4 mg	100
Vitamin B-12	9 mcg	150
Pantothenic Acid	10 mg	100

KEEP OUT OF REACH OF CHILDREN

Indications: Dietary Supplementation.
CHILD RESISTANT CAP
Do not use this product if safety seal bearing Miles logo under cap is torn or missing.

How Supplied: Bottles of 60's & 100's with child-resistant caps.

Shown in Product Identification Guide, page 517

ONE-A-DAY® WOMEN'S
**Multivitamin/Mineral Supplement
A formula which gives
you 11 essential vitamins plus
extra iron, and calcium & zinc.**

Ingredients: Calcium Carbonate, Acacia, Ferrous Fumarate, Ascorbic Acid, Gelatin, Vitamin E Acetate, Microcrystalline Cellulose, Hydroxypropyl Methylcellulose, Modified Cellulose Gum, Niacinamide, Zinc Oxide, Magnesium Stearate, Calcium Pantothenate, Artificial Colors including FD&C Yellow #5 (Tartrazine) and #6, Hydroxypropylcellulose, Starch, Pyridoxine Hydrochloride, Riboflavin, Thiamine Mononitrate,

Beta Carotene, Vitamin A Acetate, Folic Acid, Sodium Hexametaphosphate, Lecithin, Vitamin D, Vitamin B-12.

Vitamins	Quantity	% of U.S. RDA
Vitamin A (as Acetate and Beta Carotene)	5000 I.U.	100
Vitamin C	60 mg	100
Thiamine (B₁)	1.5 mg	100
Riboflavin (B₂)	1.7 mg	100
Niacin	20 mg	100
Vitamin D	400 I.U.	100
Vitamin E	30 I.U.	100
Vitamin B₆	2 mg	100
Folic Acid	0.4 mg	100
Vitamin B₁₂	6 mcg	100
Pantothenic Acid	10 mg	100

Minerals	Quantity	% of U.S. RDA
Iron (Elemental)	27 mg	150
Calcium (Elemental)	450 mg	45
Zinc	15 mg	100

Indication: Dietary supplementation.

Dosage and Administration: Adults take one tablet daily with food.

Precaution: Contains iron, which can be harmful in large doses. Close tightly and keep out of reach of children. In case of overdose, contact a physician or Poison Control Center immediately.

How Supplied: Bottles of 60 and 100 with child-resistant caps.

Shown in Product Identification Guide, page 517

PHILLIPS'® GELCAPS
Laxative plus Stool Softener

Active Ingredients: A combination of phenolphthalein (90 mg) and docusate sodium (83 mg) per gelcap.

Inactive Ingredients: FD&C Blue # 2, gelatin, glycerin, PEG 400 and 3350, propylene glycol, sorbitol, and titanium dioxide.

Indications: For relief of occasional constipation (irregularity). This product generally produces bowel movement in 6 to 12 hours.

Action: Phenolphthalein is a stimulant laxative which increases the peristaltic activity of the intestine. Docusate sodium is a stool softener which allows easier passage of the stool.

Directions: Adults and children 12 and over take one (1) or two (2) gelcaps daily with a full glass (8 oz) of liquid, or as directed by a doctor. For children under 12, consult your doctor.

Drug Interaction Precaution: Do not take this product if you are presently taking mineral oil, unless directed by a doctor.

Warnings: Do not take any laxative if abdominal pain, nausea or vomiting are present unless directed by a doctor. If you

have noticed a sudden change in bowel habits persisting for over 2 weeks, consult a doctor before using a laxative. Laxative products should not be used for a period longer than 1 week, unless directed by a doctor. Rectal bleeding or failure to have a bowel movement after use of a laxative may indicate a serious condition. Discontinue use and consult your doctor. If skin rash appears, do not use this product or any other preparation containing phenolphthalein. Keep this and all drugs out of the reach of children. In case of accidental overdose, seek professional assistance or contact a poison control center immediately. As with any drug, if you are pregnant or nursing a baby, seek the advice of a health professional before using this product.

How Supplied: Blister packs of 30 and 60 gelcaps.

Shown in Product Identification Guide, page 518

PHILLIPS'® MILK OF MAGNESIA
Laxative/Antacid

Active Ingredients: A suspension of magnesium hydroxide in purified water meeting all USP specifications. Phillips' Milk of Magnesia contains 400 mg per teaspoon (5 mL) of magnesium hydroxide.

Inactive Ingredients: Original—Purified water. Mint—Flavor, Mineral Oil, Purified water, Saccharin Sodium. Cherry—Carboxymethylcellulose Sodium, Citric Acid, D&C Red #28, Flavor, Glycerine, Microcrystalline Cellulose, Propylene Glycol, Purified water, Sorbitol, Sugar, Xantham Gum.

Indications: For relief of occasional constipation (irregularity), relief of acid indigestion, sour stomach and heartburn. The laxative dosage generally produces bowel movement in ½ to 6 hours.

Action at Laxative Dosage: Phillips' Milk of Magnesia is a mild saline laxative which acts by drawing water into the gut, increasing intraluminal pressure, and increasing intestinal motility.

Action at Antacid Dosage: Phillips' Milk of Magnesia is an effective acid neutralizer.

Directions: As a laxative, adults and children 12 years and older, 2–4 tbsp followed by a full glass (8 oz) of liquid; children 6–11 years, 1–2 tbsp followed by a full glass (8 oz) of liquid; children 2–5 years, 1–3 tsp followed by a full glass (8 oz) of liquid. Children under 2, consult a doctor.

Continued on next page

This product information was effective as of November 1, 1994. Current information may be obtained directly from Miles Inc., by writing to P.O. Box 340 Elkhart, IN 46515.

Miles—Cont.

As an antacid, adults & children 12 & older, 1–3 tsp with a little water, up to four times a day, or as directed by a doctor.

Drug Interaction Precaution: Antacids may interact with certain prescription drugs. If you are presently taking a prescription drug do not take this product without checking with your doctor or other health professional.

Laxative Warnings: Do not take any laxative if abdominal pain, nausea, vomiting or kidney disease are present unless directed by a doctor. If you have noticed a sudden change in bowel habits persisting for over 2 weeks, consult a doctor before using a laxative. Laxative products should not be used for a period longer than 1 week, unless directed by a doctor. Rectal bleeding or failure to have a bowel movement after use of a laxative may indicate a serious condition. Discontinue use and consult your doctor. Phillips® Milk of Magnesia is a saline laxative.

Antacid Warnings: Do not take more than the maximum recommended daily dosage in a 24-hour period (see Directions), or use the maximum dosage of this product for more than two weeks, or use this product if you have kidney disease, except under the advice and supervision of a doctor. May have laxative effect.

General Warnings: As with any drug, if you are pregnant or nursing a baby, seek the advice of a health professional before using this product. Keep this and all drugs out of reach of children. In case of accidental overdose, seek professional assistance or contact a poison control center immediately.

How Supplied: Phillips' Milk of Magnesia is available in original, mint and cherry flavor in 4, 12 and 26 fl oz bottles. Also available in tablet form and concentrated liquid form.
Shown in Product Identification Guide, page 518

STRI-DEX®
[*Strī-dex*]
ANTIBACTERIAL CLEANSING BAR
ANTIBACTERIAL FACE WASH

Active Ingredient: Triclosan 1%.

Inactive Ingredients: Stri-Dex® Bar: Sodium Tallowate, Sodium Cocoate and/ or Sodium Palm Kernelate, Water, Glycerin, Sucrose, Potassium Cyclocarboxypropyloleate, Bentonite, Cetyl Acetate, Acetylated Lanolin Alcohol, Pentasodium Pentanate, Tetrasodium Etidronate, D&C Yellow #10, D&C Orange #4. Stri-Dex® Face Wash: Citric Acid, Cocamidopropyl Betaine, DMDM Hydantoin, Glycerin, PEG-120, Methyl-Glucose Dioleate, PEG-8, Sodium Laureth Sulfate, Tetrasodium EDTA, Water

Indications:
Stri-Dex® Bar: Antibacterial Soap.
Stri-Dex® Face Wash: Antibacterial Face Wash.

Directions: Use Stri-Dex® Antibacterial cleansers in place of ordinary soap. For best results use three times daily. Wet face and neck. Put soap or facewash into hands and work up an abundant lather with warm water and massage into the skin. Rinse thoroughly and pat dry with a towel. Gentle enough to use daily. Cleansers can be used for facial cleansing as well as in the bath. After deep cleaning the skin with Stri-Dex® Antibacterial Cleansing Bar or Antibacterial Face Wash, continue on acne treatment program with Stri-Dex® Medicated Acne Pads or Sti-Dex® Clear Gel Acne Medication.

Warnings: Do not use on infants under 6 months of age. For external use only. Do not get into eyes. Keep this and all drugs out of the reach of children. In case of accidental ingestion, seek professional assistance or contact a poison control center immediately.

How Supplied: Stri-Dex® Antibacterial Cleansing Bar is available in a 3.5 ounce package (single bar) Stri-Dex® Antibacterial Face Wash is available in an 8 oz. pump bottle.
Shown in Product Indentification Guide, page 518

STRI-DEX®
[*Strī-dex*]
CLEAR GEL ACNE MEDICATION

Active Ingredient: Salicylic Acid 2.0%.

Inactive Ingredients: Carbomer 940, Citric Acid, DMDM Hydantoin, Glycerin, Phenoxyethanol, Polyglycerylmethacrylate, Propylene Glycol, Purified Water, SD Alcohol 9.3% (w/w), Tetrasodium EDTA, Triethanolamine.

Indications: For the treatment of acne. Reduces the number of blackheads and allows the skin to heal. Helps prevent new acne pimples from forming.

Directions: Clean the skin thoroughly before use. Apply a thin layer to acne pimple areas of face, neck and body 1 to 3 times daily. Because excessive drying of the skin may occur, start with one application daily, then gradually increase to two or three times daily if needed or as directed by a doctor. If bothersome dryness or peeling occurs, reduce application to once a day or every other day.

Warnings: FOR EXTERNAL USE ONLY. Using other topical acne medications at the same time or immediately following use of this product may increase dryness or irritation of the skin. If this occurs, only one medication should be used unless directed by a doctor. Persons who are sensitive to or have a known allergy to salicylic acid should not use this medication. If excessive itching,

dryness, redness or swelling occurs, discontinue use. If these symptoms persist, consult a doctor promptly. Keep away from eyes, lips and other mucous membranes. Keep this and all drugs out of the reach of children. In case of accidental ingestion, seek professional assistance or contact a poison control center immediately.

How Supplied: 1oz Tube.
Shown in Product Identification Guide, page 518

STRI-DEX® PADS
Regular Strength
STRI-DEX® PADS
Maximum Strength
STRI-DEX® PADS
Sensitive Skin
STRI-DEX® SUPER SCRUB PADS
Oil Fighting Formula
STRI-DEX® DUAL TEXTURED PADS
Maximum Strength

Active Ingredients:
Stri-Dex® Regular Strength: Salicylic Acid 0.5%.
Stri-Dex® Maximum Strength: Salicylic Acid 2.0%.
Stri-Dex® Sensitive Skin: Salicylic Acid 0.5%.
Stri-Dex® Super Scrub: Salicylic Acid 2.0%.
Stri-Dex® Dual Textured Maximum Strength: Salicylic Acid 2.0%.

Inactive Ingredients:
Stri-Dex® Regular Strength: Citric Acid, Fragrance Menthol, Purified Water, SD Alcohol 28%, Simethicone Emulsion, Sodium Carbonate, Sodium Dodecylbenzenesulfonate, Sodium Xylenesulfonate.
Stri-Dex® Maximum Strength: Purified Water, SD Alcohol 44%, Ammonium Xylenesulfonate, Sodium Dodecylbenzenesulfonate, Citric Acid, Sodium Carbonate, Fragrance, Menthol, Simethicone Emulsion.
Stri-Dex® Sensitive Skin: Aloe Vera Gel, Citric Acid, Fragrance, Menthol, Purified Water, SD Alcohol 28%, Simethicone Emulsion, Sodium Carbonate, Sodium Dodecylbenzenesulfonate, Sodium Xylenesulfonate.
Stri-Dex® Super Scrub: Ammonium Xylenesulfonate, Citric Acid, Fragrance, Menthol, Purified Water, SD Alcohol 54%, Simethicone Emulsion, Sodium Carbonate, Sodium Dodecylbenzenesulfonate, Sodium Lauroyl Sarcosinate,
Stri-Dex® Dual Textured Maximum Strength: Ammonium Xylenesulfonate, Citric Acid, Fragrance, Menthol, Purified Water, SD Alcohol 44%, Simethicone Emulsion, Sodium Carbonate, Sodium Dodecylbenzenesulfonate.

Indications: Stri-Dex® Pads for the treatment of acne. Reduces the number of acne pimples and blackheads, and allows the skin to heal. Helps prevent new acne pimples from forming.

Directions:
Stri-Dex® Pads. Cleanse the skin thoroughly before using all varieties of Stri-Dex medicated pads. Use the pad to open pores and loosen the oil and dirt that can clog them. Then wipe away oil and dirt and leave behind a tough pimple fighting medicine that will treat pimples and help prevent new ones from forming. Use the pad to wipe the entire affected area one to three times daily. Because excessive drying of the skin may occur, start with one application daily, then gradually increase to two or three times daily if needed or as directed by a doctor.

Warnings: FOR EXTERNAL USE ONLY: Using other topical acne medications at the same time or immediately following use of this product may increase dryness or irritation of the skin. If this occurs, only one medication should be used unless directed by a doctor. Persons with very sensitive skin or known allergy to salicylic acid should not use this medication. If irritation or excessive dryness and/or peeling occurs, reduce frequency of use or dosage. If excessive itching, dryness, redness, or swelling occurs, discontinue use. If these symptoms persist, consult a physician promptly. Keep away from eyes, lips, and other mucous membranes. Keep this and all drugs out of reach of children. In the case of accidental ingestion, seek professional assistance or contact a Poison control center immediately.

How Supplied:
Stri-Dex Regular Strength is available in a package of 55 pads.
Stri-Dex Maximum Strength is available in a package of 55 and 90 pads.
Stri-Dex Sensitive Skin is available in a package of 55 pads.
Stri-Dex Super Scrub is available in a package of 55 pads.
Stri-Dex Dual Textured Maximum Strength is available in a package of 32 pads.
Shown in Product Identification Guide, page 518

VANQUISH® Analgesic Caplets

Active Ingredients: Each caplet contains aspirin 227 mg, acetaminophen 194 mg, caffeine 33 mg, dried aluminum hydroxide gel 25 mg, magnesium hydroxide 50 mg in a thin, inert hydroxypropyl methylcellulose coating for easier swallowing.

Inactive Ingredients: Microcrystalline Cellulose, Polyethylene Glycol, Polysorbate 80, Silicon Dioxide, Starch, Titanium Dioxide, Zinc Stearate.

Indications: A buffered analgesic, antipyretic for relief of headache; muscular aches and pains; neuralgia and neuritic pain; toothache; pain following dental procedures; for painful discomforts and fever of colds; functional menstrual pain, headache and pain due to cramps; temporary relief from minor pains of arthritis, rheumatism, bursitis, lumbago, sciatica.

Directions: Adults and children 12 years and over: Two caplets with water. May be repeated every four hours if necessary up to 12 caplets per day. Larger or more frequent doses may be prescribed by doctor if necessary.

Warnings: Children and teenagers should not use this medicine for chicken pox or flu symptoms before a doctor is consulted about Reye syndrome, a rare but serious illness reported to be associated with aspirin. Do not take this product for pain for more than 10 days or for fever for more than 3 days unless directed by a doctor. If pain or fever persists or gets worse, if new symptoms occur, or if redness or swelling is present consult a doctor immediately. Do not take this product if you are allergic to aspirin, have asthma, stomach problems that persist or recur, gastric ulcers or bleeding problems unless directed by a doctor. If ringing in the ears or loss of hearing occurs, consult a doctor before taking any more of this product. Keep this and all drugs out of the reach of children. In case of accidental overdose, immediate medical attention is essential for adults as well as for children even if you do not notice any sign or symptoms. As with any drug, if you are pregnant or nursing a baby, seek the advice of a health professional before using this product. **IT IS ESPECIALLY IMPORTANT NOT TO USE ASPIRIN DURING THE LAST 3 MONTHS OF PREGNANCY UNLESS SPECIFICALLY DIRECTED TO DO SO BY A DOCTOR BECAUSE IT MAY CAUSE PROBLEMS IN THE UNBORN CHILD OR COMPLICATIONS DURING DELIVERY.**

Drug Interaction Precaution: Do not take this product if you are taking a prescription drug for anticoagulation (thinning of the blood), diabetes, gout, or arthritis unless directed by a doctor.

How Supplied:
White, capsule-shaped caplets in bottles of 30, 60 and 100 caplets. Child-resistant safety closures on bottles of 30 and 60 caplets. Bottle of 100 caplets available without safety closure for households without young children.
Shown in Product Identification Guide, page 518

IF YOU SUSPECT AN INTERACTION...
The 1,400-page
*PDR Guide to Drug Interactions •
Side Effects • Indications*
can help.
Use the order form
in the front of this book.

Miles Inc.
Diagnostics Division
511 BENEDICT AVENUE
TARRYTOWN, NY 10591

GLUCOMETER ELITE®
Diabetes Care System

With the GLUCOMETER ELITE Diabetes Care System, there are no buttons to push, no test strips to wipe or blot, and no test pad to cover. Even the right amount of blood is measured automatically. Its unique, state-of-the-art design provides more ease of use and less chance for operator error. For consistent, accurate results. From a smaller sample than any other blood glucose meter.
Simply insert the GLUCOMETER ELITE Test Strip to activate the meter.

1 Peel back the foil surrounding a GLUCOMETER ELITE Test Strip and insert the strip in the GLUCOMETER ELITE Meter.

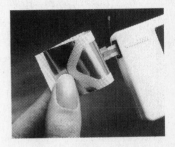

No buttons, no bother. Meter turns on automatically when test strip is inserted
Just touch the tip of test strip to apply the blood sample. The correct amount of blood is automatically drawn into a sample chamber within the test strip, and timing is started.

2 Stick your finger with the GLUCOLET® Automatic Lancing Device. Touch the tip of the GLUCOMETER ELITE Test Strip to the drop of blood.

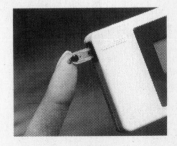

The right amount of blood is automatically drawn into the test strip to help ensure testing accuracy. No wiping or blotting is required. The GLUCOMETER ELITE Meter uses less blood than other meters.

Continued on next page

Miles—Cont.

Read the results in 60 seconds. Remove the test strip to turn off the meter (automatic shutoff occurs in 3 minutes if the strip is left inserted).

3 Read your blood glucose result.

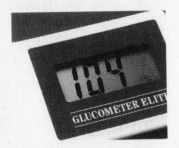

Results appear in the display in 60 seconds. With less to do, there is less chance for mistakes and greater confidence in test results. The GLUCOMETER ELITE... making accuracy effortless.

The GLUCOMETER ELITE System comes with everything you need to start blood glucose testing:

- GLUCOMETER ELITE Blood Glucose Meter
- GLUCOMETER ELITE Test Strips
- GLUCOMETER ELITE Normal Control
- GLUCOMETER ELITE Check Strip
- GLUCOLET® Lancing Device
- CLINILOG® Record Diary
- GLUCOMETER ELITE User Guide
- Instructional Videotape

GLUCOMETER ELITE PRECISION PATIENT STUDY*

Control	No. of Tests	Mean (mg/dL)	Overall S.D. (mg/dL)	Overall C.V. (%)
Normal	456	92.0	5.08	5.5
High	465	282.6	12.78	4.5

- Soft Leather Carrying Case
- Hard Sided Carrying Case

A significant advance in testing technology.

[See figure at bottom of page]

- Unique test strip design with capillary gap action eliminates the drawbacks of traditional reagent strips.
- There's no need to keep the strip level or to wipe or blot it.
- The sealed sample chamber prevents contamination and eliminates regular cleanings.
- Automatic sampling eliminates the need for obtaining a hanging drop of blood or precisely covering the reagent area.
- Blood is touched to the tip, not the top, of the test strip.
- Capillary gap action draws just 3 μL of blood into the test chamber.
- Advanced testing technology senses the correct amount and starts the test.

An impressive benchmark for accuracy and precision.

- Extensive testing documents excellent correlation with laboratory methods for accuracy.*
- Reliable precision shown in test after test.*
- Wide testing range produces reliable results from 40 to 500 mg/dL.

- Acceptable results obtained for hematocrits from 20% to 60%.

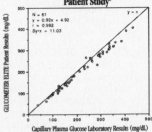

GLUCOMETER ELITE Accuracy Patient Study*

N = 61
y = 0.92x + 4.92
r = 0.992
Sy·x = 11.03

[See table above.]

An exceptional edge in patient preference.

- Three out of four patients in a recent survey gave the GLUCOMETER ELITE System an overall rating of "excellent" or "very good."*
- Features like ease of use, small size, and large display also were consistently rated "excellent" or "very good."*
- Recommend the GLUCOMETER ELITE System for frequent testers or for anyone who demands the maximum in simplicity and accuracy.

[See figure at top of next page]

A significant advance in testing technology.

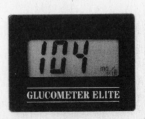

Capillary Gap

Conductive Bars

Test Chamber

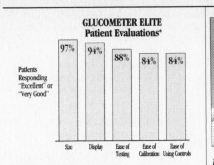

GLUCOMETER ELITE
Patient Evaluations*

Patients Responding "Excellent" or "Very Good"

Size	Display	Ease of Testing	Ease of Calibration	Ease of Using Controls
97%	94%	88%	84%	84%

* Data on file, Miles Inc.

PRODUCT GUIDE	PRODUCT CODE
GLUCOMETER ELITE Diabetes Care System	3901
GLUCOMETER ELITE Test Strips 25s	3911
GLUCOMETER ELITE Normal Control	3926
GLUCOMETER ELITE High Control	3927
Ames GLUCO System Lancet 100s	5509G

MILES
Diagnostics Division
Miles Inc.
Tarrytown, NY 10591

GLUCOMETER ENCORE™
Diabetes Care System

Indications: The GLUCOMETER EN-CORE™ Diabetes Care System lets your patients enjoy easy blood glucose testing and convenience at an affordable price. Yet they still receive the exceptional performance they need for tighter diabetes control and better long-term diabetes care. Fast operation, a no-wipe procedure, and accurate test results make the GLUCOMETER ENCORE System ideal for patients who need economy plus ease of use.
Fast, straightforward operation.

Directions:

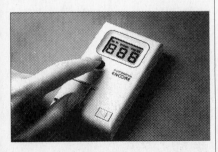

Press and release button to activate the meter.

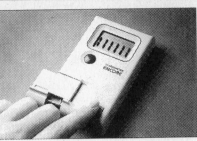

Press slide release to open test slide.

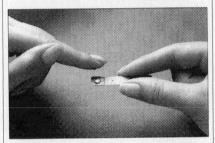

Apply blood to test strip. No need to wipe or blot.

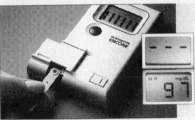

Insert test strip. Timing begins automatically and results appear within 15 to 60 seconds.

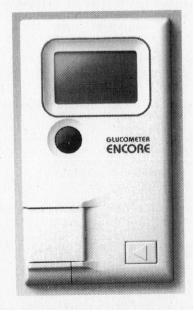

Virtually technique independent.
- No wiping, blotting or timing for quick, simple blood glucose testing.
- Automatic test activation and easy, one-step programming.

- Specially designed test strip for easy handling and sample application.
- 10-test memory for easy tracking of test results.
- Test average for estimating blood glucose levels over time.

Convenience and economy combined.
- Small, compact size ideal for pocket or purse.
- Large, easy-to-read display.
- Foil-wrapped test strips.
- Batteries guaranteed for up to 15,000 tests or 5 years.
- Fully backed by Miles Inc., Diagnostics Division toll-free service and customer support.

Accurate and reliable results.
- Hexokinase chemistry method, referenced to plasma or serum glucose, allows direct comparisons with laboratory results.
- Wide testing range provides reliable results from 10 to 600 mg/dL.
- Accurate results obtained for hematocrits from 20% to 60%.
- Reliable precision shown across multiple tests and blood glucose ranges.

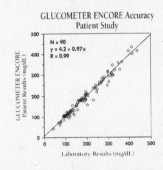

GLUCOMETER ENCORE Accuracy
Patient Study

N = 90
y = 4.2 + 0.97x
R = 0.99

GLUCOMETER ENCORE Patient Results (mg/dL)

Laboratory Results (mg/dL)

The GLUCOMETER ENCORE System comes with everything your patients need to start enjoying the benefits of easy, economical blood glucose testing.
MILES
Diagnostics Division
Miles Inc.
Tarrytown, NY 10591

Muro Pharmaceutical, Inc.
890 EAST STREET
TEWKSBURY, MA 01876-1496

BROMFED® SYRUP
Antihistamine-Nasal Decongestant
ORANGE-LEMON FLAVOR

Each 5 mL (1 teaspoonful) contains: 2 mg brompheniramine maleate and 30 mg pseudoephedrine hydrochloride; also contains citric acid, FD & C Yellow #6, flavor, glycerin, methyl paraben, sodium benzoate, sodium citrate, sodium saccharin, sorbitol, sucrose, purified water.

Indications: For temporary relief of nasal congestion, sneezing, itchy and watery eyes and running nose due to

Continued on next page

Muro—Cont.

common cold, hay fever or other upper respiratory allergies.

Directions: Adults and children 12 years of age and over: 2 teaspoonfuls every 4–6 hours. Children 6 to 12 years of age: 1 teaspoonful every 4–6 hours. Do not exceed 4 doses in 24 hours. Children under 6 years of age, consult a physician.

Warnings: If symptoms do not improve within seven days or are accompanied by high fever, consult a physician before continuing use. May cause drowsiness. May cause excitability especially in children. DO NOT exceed recommended daily dosage because at higher doses nervousness, dizziness, or sleeplessness may occur. **Except under the advice and supervision of a physician:** DO NOT give this product to children under six years. DO NOT take this product if you have asthma, glaucoma, difficulty in urination due to enlargement of the prostate gland, high blood pressure, heart disease, diabetes, or thyroid disease. As with any drug, if you are pregnant or nursing a baby, seek the advice of a health professional before using this product.

Caution: Avoid operating a motor vehicle or heavy machinery and alcoholic beverages while taking this product. Keep this and all drugs out of the reach of children.

Drug Interaction Precaution: Do not take this product if you are presently taking a prescription antihypertensive or antidepressant drug containing a monoamine oxidase inhibitor except under the advice and supervision of a physician.

Overdosage: In case of accidental overdose, seek professional assistance or contact a Poison Control Center immediately.

Store at controlled room temperature, between 15° and 30°C (59° and 86°F). Dispense in tight, light resistant, child resistant containers as defined in USP.

How Supplied: NDC 0451-4201-16, for 16 fl. oz. (480 mL), NDC 0451-4201-04, for 4 fl. oz. (120 mL).

GUAIFED® SYRUP
Expectorant/Nasal Decongestant

A red colored, berry citrus flavored syrup.
Each 5mL (teaspoonful) contains:
Pseudoephedrine HCl, USP   30mg
Guaifenesin, USP   200mg
CONTAINS NO ANTIHISTAMINE which may cause drowsiness or excessive drying.

Guaifed® Syrup also contains inactive ingredients:
Benzoic Acid, Berry Citrus Flavor, Citric Acid, FD&C Red #40, Glycerin, Menthol, Polyethylene Glycol, Povidone, Purified Water, Saccharin Sodium, Sodium Citrate, Sorbitol, Vanillin.

Directions: Guaifed® Syrup—Adults and children 12 years of age and over: Two teaspoonfuls every 4–6 hours, not to exceed eight teaspoonfuls in 24 hours. Children 6 to under 12 years of age: One teaspoonful every 4–6 hours, not to exceed four teaspoonfuls in 24 hours. Children 2 to under 6 years of age: ½ teaspoonful every 4–6 hours, not to exceed two teaspoonfuls in 24 hours. Children under 2 years of age: consult a physician.

How Supplied: Guaifed® Syrup is a red colored, berry citrus flavored syrup supplied in 473 mL bottles (NDC #0451-2601-16) and 118 mL bottles (NDC #0451-2601-04).

Store at controlled room temperature between 15°C and 30°C (59°F and 86°F). Dispense in Child Resistant, tight and light resistant containers.

GUAITAB® TABLETS
Expectorant/Nasal Decongestant

A purple layered tablet
Each tablet contains:
Pseudoephedrine HCl   60mg
Guaifenesin   400mg

GUAITAB® TABLET also contains inactive ingredients: colloidal silicon dioxide, lactose, magnesium stearate, microcrystalline cellulose, pharmaceutical glaze, sodium starch glycolate, starch, talc, FD&C Blue #2, D&C Red #27.

Indications: For the temporary relief of nasal congestion associated with the common cold, sinusitis, hay fever or other upper respiratory allergies. Also helps loosen phlegm (mucus) and thin bronchial secretions to rid the bronchial passageways of bothersome mucus, drain bronchial tubes, and make coughs more productive.

Warnings: Do not exceed recommended dosage because at higher doses nervousness, dizziness or sleeplessness may occur. Do not use if you have high blood pressure, heart disease, diabetes, thyroid disease or a persistent chronic cough, except under the advice and supervision of a physician. Do not take this product for persistent or chronic cough such as occurs with smoking, asthma, chronic bronchitis, or emphysema, or where cough is accompanied by excessive phlegm (mucus) unless directed by a doctor. A persistent cough may be a sign of a serious condition. If cough persists for more than 1 week, tends to recur, or is accompanied by a fever, rash or persistent headache, consult a doctor.

Contraindications: Hypersensitivity to guaifenesin or sympathomimetic amines; marked hypertension, hyperthyroidism; or in patients receiving monoamine oxidase (MAO) inhibitors.

Adverse Reactions: Possible side effects include nausea, vomiting, nervousness, restlessness, rash (including urticaria), headache, or dry mouth.

Drug Interaction Precautions: Do not take this medication if you are presently taking a prescription antihypertensive or antidepressant drug containing a monoamine oxidase inhibitor except under the advice and supervision of a physician.

Geriatrics: Pseudoephedrine should be used with caution in the elderly because they may be more sensitive to the effect of the sympathomimetics.

Note: As with any drug, if you are pregnant or nursing a baby, seek the advice of a health professional before using this product.

In the case of accidental overdose, seek professional assistance or contact a Poison Control Center immediately.

Guaifenesin has been shown to produce a color interference with certain clinical laboratory determinations of 5-hydroxyindoleacetic acid (5-HIAA) and vanillylmandelic acid (VMA).

Directions: Guaitab® Tablets — Adults and Children 12 years of age and over: One Tablet every 4–6 hours, not to exceed four tablets in 24 hours. Children 6 to under 12 years of age: ½ the adult dosage (break tablet in half): ½ tablet every 4–6 hours, not to exceed two tablets in 24 hours.

How Supplied: Guaitab® Tablet is a purple layered Tablet in bottles of 100's. Each scored Tablet is coded "60/400" on one side and "Muro" on the other side. NDC 0451-4600-50.

Store at controlled room temperature between 15°C and 30°C (59°F and 86°F). Dispense in Child Resistant, tight and light resistant containers.

SALINEX® NASAL MIST AND DROPS
Buffered Isotonic Saline Solutions

Ingredients: Sodium Chloride 0.4%. Also contains edetate disodium, hydroxypropyl methylcellulose, sodium phosphate, polyethylene glycol, propylene glycol and purified water. Preservative used is benzalkonium chloride 0.01%.

Indications: A nasal moisturizer formulated to be physiologically compatible with nasal membranes, providing soothing relief for clogged nasal passages without stinging or burning. Salinex restores moisture to relieve dry, inflamed nasal membranes due to low humidity, colds, allergies and overuse of nasal decongestants.

Directions: Spray: Squeeze twice in each nostril as needed. Drops: Two drops in each nostril as needed or as directed by physician.

How Supplied: SPRAY: 50 ml plastic spray bottle. NDC 0451-4500-50. DROPS: 15 ml plastic dropper bottle. NDC 0451-4500-85.

Nature's Bounty, Inc.
90 ORVILLE DRIVE
BOHEMIA, NY 11716

ENER–B®
Vitamin B-12 Nasal Gel
Dietary Supplement

Description: ENER-B™ is the first intra-nasal application for Vitamin B-12.

Each delivery supplies 400 mcg. of Vitamin B-12. This method of delivery provides the highest Vitamin B-12 blood levels that can be obtained without a prescription. Clinical tests show that ENER-B produced 8.4 to 10 times more Vitamin B-12 in the blood than tablets.

Measured Vitamin B-12 Increase In Blood Levels

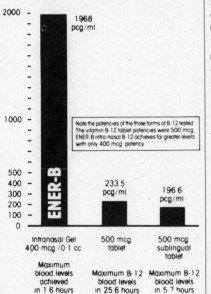

Clinical Tests results are available by writing Nature's Bounty.

Potency and Administration: Each nasal applicator delivers $\frac{1}{10}$ cc of gel into the nose which adheres to the mucous membranes providing 400 mcg. of Vitamin B-12. Odorless and non-irritating to the nose.

Directions: As a dietary supplement, one unit every two to three days.

How Supplied: Packages of 12 unit doses. Supplies 400 mcg. of B-12 each.
Shown in Product Identification Guide, page 518

Niché Pharmaceuticals, Inc.
**200 N. OAK STREET
P O BOX 449
ROANOKE, TX 76262**

MAGTAB® SR
[măg-tăb]
**(Magnesium L-lactate dihydrate)
Sustained-release Magnesium
Supplement**

Description: MagTab® SR is a sustained release oral magnesium supplement. Each pale yellow caplet contains 7mEq (84 Mg) magnesium as magnesium L-lactate dihydrate (835 Mg in a sustained release wax matrix formulation).

Indications/Uses: As a dietary supplement, MagTab® SR is indicated for patients with, or at risk for, magnesium deficiency. Hypomagnesemia and/or magnesium deficiency can result from inadequate nutritional intake or absorption, alcoholism, or magnesium depleting drugs such as diuretics.

Warnings/Side Effects: Patients with renal disease should not take magnesium supplements without the advice and direct supervision of a physician. Excessive dosage of magnesium can cause loose stools or diarrhea.

Dosage/How Supplied: As a dietary supplement, take 1 or 2 caplets b.i.d. or as directed by a physician. MagTab® SR is available for oral administration as uncoated yellow caplets, in bottles of 60 and 100.
U.S. Patent Number: 5,002,774

Ohm Laboratories, Inc.
**P. O. BOX 279
FRANKLIN PARK, NJ 08823**

CRAMP END
**Ibuprofen Tablets, USP, 200 mg
Menstrual Pain & Cramp Reliever**

WARNING: ASPIRIN-SENSITIVE PATIENTS: Do not take this product if you have had a severe allergic reaction to aspirin, e.g., asthma, swelling, shock or hives, because even though this product contains no aspirin or salicylates, cross-reactions may occur in patients allergic to aspirin.

Indications: For the temporary relief of painful menstrual cramps (Dysmenorrhea); also headaches, backaches and muscular aches and pains associated with Premenstrual Syndrome.

Directions: Adults: Take 1 tablet every 4 to 6 hours at the onset of menstrual symptoms and while pain persists. If pain does not respond to 1 tablet, 2 tablets may be used but do not exceed 6 tablets in 24 hours, unless directed by a doctor. The smallest effective dose should be used. Take with food or milk if occasional and mild heartburn, upset stomach, or stomach pain occurs with use. Consult a doctor if these symptoms are more than mild or if they persist.
Children: Do not give this product to children under 12 except under the advice and supervision of a doctor.

Warnings: Do not take for pain for more than 10 days unless directed by a doctor. If pain persists or gets worse, or if new symptoms occur, consult a doctor. These could be signs of serious illness. If you are under a doctor's care for any serious condition, consult a doctor before taking this product. As with aspirin and acetaminophen, if you have any condition which requires you to take prescription drugs or if you have had any problems or serious side effects from taking any non-prescription pain reliever, do not take this product without first discussing it with your doctor. If you experience any symptoms which are unusual or seem unrelated to the condition for which you took ibuprofen, consult a doctor before taking any more of it. Although ibuprofen is indicated for the same conditions as aspirin and acetaminophen, it should not be taken with them except under a doctor's direction. Do not combine this product with any other ibuprofen-containing product. As with any drug, if you are pregnant or nursing a baby, seek the advice of a health professional before using this product. **IT IS ESPECIALLY IMPORTANT NOT TO USE IBUPROFEN DURING THE LAST 3 MONTHS OF PREGNANCY UNLESS SPECIFICALLY DIRECTED TO DO SO BY A DOCTOR BECAUSE IT MAY CAUSE PROBLEMS IN THE UNBORN CHILD OR COMPLICATIONS DURING DELIVERY.** Keep this and all drugs out of the reach of children. In case of accidental overdose, seek professional assistance or contact a poison control center immediately.

How Supplied: Coated tablets in blister packs of 12's
Store at room temperature; avoid excessive heat 40°C (104°F).

Active Ingredient: Each tablet contains Ibuprofen 200 mg.
Manufactured by OHM LABORATORIES, INC, Franklin Park, NJ 08823
Shown in Product Identification Guide, page 518

IBUPROHM®
**Ibuprofen Tablets, USP
Ibuprofen Caplets, USP**

Active Ingredient: Each tablet contains Ibuprofen USP, 200 mg.

Warning: ASPIRIN SENSITIVE PATIENTS: Do not take this product if you have had a severe allergic reaction to aspirin, e.g., asthma, swelling, shock or hives, because even though this product contains no aspirin or salicylates, cross-reactions may occur in patients allergic to aspirin.

Indications: For the temporary relief of minor aches and pains associated with the common cold, headache, toothache, muscular aches, backache, for the minor pain of arthritis, for the pain of menstrual cramps, and for reduction of fever.

Directions: Adults: Take 1 tablet every 4 to 6 hours while symptoms persist. If pain or fever does not respond to 1 tablet, 2 tablets may be used but do not exceed 6 tablets in 24 hours, unless directed by a doctor. The smallest effective dose should be used. Take with food or milk if occasional and mild heartburn, upset stomach, or stomach pain occurs with use. Consult a doctor if these symptoms are more than mild or if they persist.
Children: Do not give this product to children under 12 except under the advice and supervision of a doctor.

Warnings: Do not take for pain for more than 10 days or for fever for more than 3 days unless directed by a doctor. If

Continued on next page

Ohm—Cont.

pain or fever persists or gets worse, if new symptoms occur, or if the painful area is red or swollen, consult a doctor. These could be signs of serious illness. If you are under a doctor's care for any serious condition, consult a doctor before taking this product. As with aspirin and acetaminophen, if you have any condition which requires you to take prescription drugs or if you have had any problems or serious side effects from taking any nonprescription pain reliever, do not take this product without first discussing it with your doctor. If you experience any symptoms which are unusual or seem unrelated to the condition for which you took ibuprofen, consult a doctor before taking any more of it. Although ibuprofen is indicated for the same conditions as aspirin and acetaminophen, it should not be taken with them except under a doctor's direction. Do not combine the product with any other ibuprofen-containing product. As with any drug, if you are pregnant or nursing a baby, seek the advice of a health professional before using this product. IT IS ESPECIALLY IMPORTANT NOT TO USE IBUPROFEN DURING THE LAST 3 MONTHS OF PREGNANCY UNLESS SPECIFICALLY DIRECTED TO DO SO BY A DOCTOR BECAUSE IT MAY CAUSE PROBLEMS IN THE UNBORN CHILD OR COMPLICATIONS DURING DELIVERY. Keep this and all drugs out of the reach of children. In case of accidental overdose, seek professional assistance or contact a poison control center immediately.

How Supplied: Coated tablets in bottles of 24, 50, 100, 165, 250, 500 and 1000. Coated caplets in bottles of 24, 50, 100 and 250.

Storage: Store at room temperature; avoid excessive heat 40° (104°F).

Shown in Product Identification Guide, page 518

LOPERAMIDE HYDROCHLORIDE CAPLETS*

2 mg (Nonprescription Formula)
(Antidiarrheal)

Loperamide Hydrochloride Caplet relieves diarrhea for both adults and children 6 years of age and older, in many cases with just one dose. Each caplet contains loperamide hydrochloride, previously available only in a prescription product. This ingredient has been prescribed for millions of people, and has proven to be an exceptionally safe and effective antidiarrheal medication. Loperamide HCl caplets are small and easy to swallow.

Indication: Loperamide hydrochloride controls the symptoms of diarrhea.

Directions: Drink plenty of clear fluids to help prevent dehydration, which may accompany diarrhea.

Dosage and Administration:
[See table below.]

Warnings: DO NOT USE FOR MORE THAN TWO DAYS UNLESS DIRECTED BY A PHYSICIAN. Do not use if diarrhea is accompanied by high fever (greater than 101°F), or if blood is present in the stool, or if you have had a rash or other allergic reaction to loperamide HCl. If you are taking antibiotics or have a history of liver disease, consult a physican before using this product. As with any drug, if you are pregnant or nursing a baby, seek the advice of a health professional before using this product. Keep this and all drugs out of the reach of children. In case of accidental overdose, seek professional assistance or contact a poison control center immediately.

Active Ingredient: Loperamide HCl 2 mg per caplet.

Inactive Ingredients: Croscarmellose sodium, Crospovidone, Hydrogenated vegetable oil, lactose, magnesium stearate, powdered cellulose, pregelatinized starch, FD&C Blue #1 and D&C Yellow #10.
See side panel for expiration date. Store at room temperature 15°–25°C (59°–77°F).

How Supplied: Green scored caplet with "122" engraved on the other side. The caplets in 6's, 10's, 12's, and 20's blister packaging which is tamper resistant and child resistant.
* Each Caplet (capsule-shaped tablet) contains 2 mg of Loperamide Hydrochloride.

Shown in Product Identification Guide, page 518

Adults and Children 12 Years of Age and Older	Take 2 caplets after the first loose bowel movement and 1 caplet after each subsequent loose bowel movement but no more than 4 caplets a day for no more than two days.
Children 9–11 Years (60–95 lbs)	Take 1 caplet after the first loose bowel movement and ½ caplet after each subsequent loose bowel movement but no more than 3 caplets a day for no more than two days.
Children 6–8 Years (48–59 lbs)	Take 1 caplet after the first loose bowel movement and ½ caplet after each subsequent loose bowel movement but no more than 2 caplets a day for no more than two days.
Under 6 years old (up to 47 lbs):	**Consult a physician. Not intended for children under 6 years old.**

Ortho Pharmaceutical Corporation
Advanced Care Products
RARITAN, NJ 08869

CONCEPTROL®
Contraceptive Gel
Single use applicators

How to use
CONCEPTROL Gel
Single Use Applicators:

Please read the following instructions carefully before use.

1. Twist off cap.

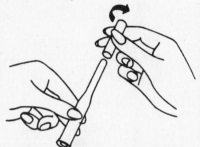

2. Put open end of cap over rubber stopper.

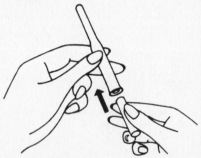

3. Hold finger over cap and gently insert small end of applicator well into vagina. Hold applicator in place and push cap all the way into applicator to deposit gel. Remove the applicator and discard it in a waste container.

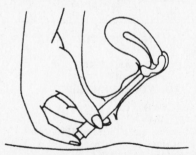

Insertion of the applicator is easier when lying on back with knees bent.
For maximum protection, CONCEPTROL should be applied not more than an hour before intercourse.

Action: Spermicidal

Indication: Contraception

Warning: Keep out of reach of children.

IMPORTANT: EACH APPLICATOR IS INDIVIDUALLY WRAPPED. IF AN APPLICATOR IS UNWRAPPED OR THE WRAPPER IS TORN, <u>DO NOT USE</u> AND RETURN ENTIRE CONTENTS TO PLACE OF PURCHASE.

Precautions: When a pregnancy is medically contraindicated, the contraceptive program should be prescribed by your physician.
CONCEPTROL provides a high degree of contraceptive protection. No product, however, can provide an absolute guarantee against becoming pregnant.

Adverse Reactions: The following side effects have been reported: occasional burning and/or irritation of the vagina or penis. If this occurs, discontinue use and consult your physician.

Dosage and Administration: CONCEPTROL should be inserted prior to each intercourse. One applicatorful of CONCEPTROL inserted just before intercourse is adequate for one time only. An additional applicatorful is required each time intercourse is repeated. For maximum protection, CONCEPTROL should be applied not more than one hour before intercourse.
Douching is not recommended after using CONCEPTROL. However, if desired for cleansing purposes, wait at least six hours following last intercourse to allow for full spermicidal activity of CONCEPTROL.
Refer to directions and diagram for detailed instructions.
Always keep an extra package of CONCEPTROL Single Use Contraceptives on hand. Every package of CONCEPTROL is dated to ensure freshness.

Storage: Store at room temperature; avoid exposure to extremes of heat or cold.
In case of accidental ingestion, call a Poison Control Center, Emergency Medical Facility, or a doctor.
If vaginal irritation occurs, and continues, contact your physician.

631-09-571-2
Shown in Product Identification Guide, page 518

CONCEPTROL®
Contraceptive Inserts

Description: CONCEPTROL Contraceptive Inserts are an effective and convenient method of vaginal contraception when used as directed. CONCEPTROL may be used with a condom or alone. Please read the following instructions carefully before use.

Instructions for use alone or with a condom

1. Tear off a single insert from the strip and separate tabs of the protective wrap with your thumb. With thumb and forefinger of each hand, grasp the tabs and pull downward (see illustration). CONCEPTROL is now ready for insertion.

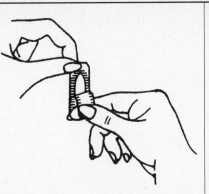

2. At least 10 minutes prior to intercourse, insert one CONCEPTROL Contraceptive Insert with the index finger as far as possible into the vagina. The best protection will occur when CONCEPTROL is placed deep into the vagina near the cervix. (Refer to Dosage and Administration section.)

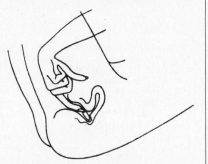

IMPORTANT: WAIT AT LEAST 10 MINUTES after insertion to assure proper dispersion which is necessary for contraceptive protection.

Action: Spermicidal

Warning: Keep out of reach of children.
IMPORTANT: EACH INSERT IS INDIVIDUALLY WRAPPED. IF AN INSERT IS UNWRAPPED OR THERE IS AN OPENING IN THE WRAPPER. <u>DO NOT USE</u> AND RETURN ENTIRE CONTENTS TO PLACE OF PURCHASE.

Precautions: When pregnancy is medically contraindicated, your contraceptive program should be recommended by a physician.
CONCEPTROL is an effective method of contraception. No product, however, can provide an absolute guarantee against becoming pregnant.

Adverse Reactions: Occasional burning or irritation of the vagina or penis have been reported. If this occurs, discontinue use and consult your physician.

Dosage and Administration: CONCEPTROL should be inserted into the vagina at least 10 minutes prior to male penetration to insure proper dispersion. CONCEPTROL provides protection from 10 minutes to 1 hour <u>after product insertion.</u> Insert a new CONCEPTROL Con-

traceptive Insert each time intercourse is repeated.
Douching after use of CONCEPTROL is not recommended; however, should you desire to do so, wait at least six hours after intercourse to avoid interfering with contraceptive protection.
Always keep an extra package of CONCEPTROL on hand. Each CONCEPTROL package is dated to ensure freshness.

Storage Instructions: Store at room temperature. Avoid excessive heat (over 86°F or 30°C).

How Supplied: 150 mg nonoxyhol-9 per insert.

634-09-580-4

Advanced Care Products
Ortho Pharmaceutical Corp.
Raritan, NJ 08869
Shown in Product Identification Guide, page 518

DELFEN®
Contraceptive Foam

Description: USED BY MILLIONS OF WOMEN IN THE UNITED STATES FOR OVER A PERIOD OF TEN YEARS DELFEN Foam provides effective contraceptive protection when used alone. If used together with another contraceptive method, there will probably be better protection against pregnancy.
DELFEN FOAM STARTS WORKING IMMEDIATELY
For maximum protection, DELFEN should be applied just before intercourse, preferably not more than an hour before. There is no waiting with DELFEN. It starts working immediately. DELFEN blankets the vaginal folds with a protective shield that fits natural contours, forming a barrier between the sperm and the egg.
KILLS SPERM ON CONTACT
DELFEN has sufficient potency that only one applicatorful before intercourse is necessary for protection. **An additional applicatorful is required each time intercourse is repeated.**
GENTLE TO DELICATE TISSUES
DELFEN is a vaginal foam made to approximate the natural condition of a normal healthy vagina. It is well-tolerated by most women and can be used as often as desired over a long period of time without irritation. However, burning and/or irritation of the vagina or penis have been reported. **In such cases, the medication should be discontinued and your physician consulted.**
STABLE
DELFEN is unaffected in all but extreme (above 120°F) fluctuations in temperature or humidity. It cannot melt and its ingredients will not break down or separate in hot weather.

Continued on next page

Ortho—Cont.

Directions for use:

Indications: Contraception

Action: Spermicidal

Precautions: When pregnancy is medically contraindicated, your physician should be consulted for a contraceptive program.

Side Effects: Should sensitivity to the ingredients or irritation of the vagina or penis develop, discontinue use and consult your physician.

IMPORTANT: THIS AEROSOL CONTAINER IS TAMPER RESISTANT BY DESIGN

Warning: Contents under pressure. Do not puncture or incinerate container. Do not expose to heat or store at temperature above 120°F. **Keep Out of Reach of Children.**

Dosage and Administration: One applicatorful of DELFEN Contraceptive Foam should be inserted prior to each intercourse. You may have intercourse any time up to one hour after you have inserted the foam. If you repeat intercourse, insert another applicator of DELFEN Foam.

DELFEN CONTRACEPTIVE FOAM IS EASY TO USE
Just these simple steps:

1. Shake the can before each use.
2. Remove the cap after shaking the can.
3. Place can upright on a level surface.
4. Place applicator on top of can. Press applicator down *very gently* to fill. Fill the bottom of ribbed section on the applicator. (See illustration A.)

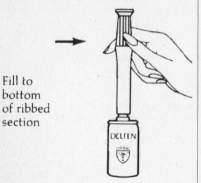

Fill to bottom of ribbed section

DELFEN
ORTHO

5. Remove applicator from can to stop flow of foam.
6. Hold the filled applicator by the barrel and gently insert well into the vagina. This can be done most easily while lying on your back with knees bent. Hold applicator in place and push plunger to deposit foam near the cervix. (See illustration B.) With the plunger still depressed, remove applicator. That's all. DELFEN Contraceptive Foam is effective immediately.

[See illustration on top of next column.]

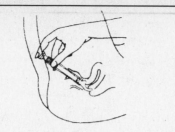

(Correct method of inserting DELFEN Contraceptive Foam.)

7. **Cleaning and storage:** After each use, clean excess foam from top of can. Replace cap. Store at room temperature not over 120°F. Wash the applicator with mild soap and warm water. Do not boil. Rinse thoroughly. The applicator may be pulled apart for easy cleaning. (See illustration C.) To reassemble, gently push plunger back into barrel as far as it will go.

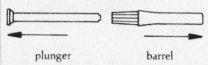

plunger   barrel

8. **When to replace the can:** The can is almost empty when the applicator fills more slowly than normal and a sputtering sound can be heard. **Always keep and extra can available.**
9. **Douching** is not recommended after using DELFEN Foam. However, if desired for cleansing purposes, wait at least six hours following last intercourse to allow for the full spermicidal activity of DELFEN Foam.

Although DELFEN Contraceptive Foam provides a high degree of contraceptive protection, it cannot provide an absolute guarantee against becoming pregnant.

Shown in Product Identification Guide, page 518

GYNOL II®
Original Formula
CONTRACEPTIVE JELLY
AND THE DIAPHRAGM

Description: 97% Effective in Preventing Pregnancy.
In a closely controlled study involving more than 200 women, the majority of whom completed 12 months or more of continuous use, the combination of GYNOL II Contraceptive Jelly and the diaphragm was found to be 97% effective when used according to directions. This effective protection results from the barrier effect of the diaphragm and from GYNOL II Contraceptive Jelly. The GYNOL II spermicidal formula encourages use with each and every act of intercourse because it is unscented, stainless, colorless, and greaseless.
The effectiveness of the GYNOL II diaphragm contraceptive method is dependent upon highly motivated use—use with every act of intercourse in accordance with directions. In fact, the effectiveness of the GYNOL II diaphragm

method was only 90% in the above-mentioned study when those are included who failed to use GYNOL II and the diaphragm in accordance with directions.

Directions For Use:
PREPARING THE DIAPHRAGM
Before handling the diaphragm, it is recommended that you wash your hands with soap and water. Prior to inserting your diaphragm, put an applicatorful (about a teaspoonful) of GYNOL II into the cup of the dome and spread a small amount around the edge with your fingertip. Then insert.

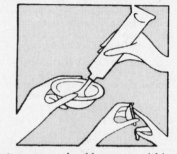

Intercourse should occur within six hours after the diaphragm and GYNOL II have been inserted. An additional application of GYNOL II must be applied prior to each act of intercourse. DO NOT REMOVE THE DIAPHRAGM—simply add more GYNOL II with the applicator, being careful not to dislodge the diaphragm.

1. Remove cap from tube and attach applicator to tube by turning applicator clockwise.

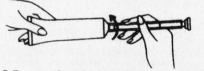

2. Squeeze the tube from the bottom, forcing the contents into the barrel until the plunger is pushed out as far as it will go and the barrel is completely filled.

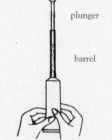

plunger

barrel

3. Always roll the tube from the bottom. After each use replace cap and roll tube as shown. Avoid storing in a cold place.

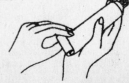

4.After detaching from the tube, hold the filled applicator by the barrel and gently insert the barrel well into the vagina. Press the plunger; then, with the plunger still depressed remove the applicator holding it by the barrel. Insertion of the applicator is accomplished more easily when lying on your back with the knees bent. Note diagram.

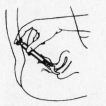

IMPORTANT:—For contraceptive effectiveness, the diaphragm should remain in place for six hours after intercourse and should be removed as soon as possible thereafter. Continuous wearing of the diaphragm for more than 24 hours is not recommended. Retention of the diaphragm for prolonged periods may encourage growth of certain bacteria in the vaginal tract. It has been suggested that under certain as yet unestablished conditions overgrowth of these bacteria may lead to symptoms of toxic shock syndrome (TSS). For further information, consult your physician. Women with a known or suspected history of TSS should not use the diaphragm. **This method of contraception must be used each and every time intercourse takes place, regardless of the time of month.**

Douching is not recommended after using GYNOL II. However, if desired for cleansing purposes, wait at least six hours following last intercourse to allow for the full spermicidal activity of GYNOL II.

AFTER EACH USE
Wash the applicator with mold soap and warm water. Do not boil. Rinse thoroughly. The applicator may be pulled apart for easy cleaning to reassemble gently push plunger back as far as it will go.

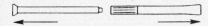

Precaution: If you have been advised against pregnancy for medical reasons, your birth control method should be thoroughly discussed with your physician so that both you and your physician are satisfied that the method you have selected is right for you.

Adverse Reactions: Occasional burning and/or irritation of the vagina or penis have been reported. If this occurs, discontinue use and consult your physician.

Warning: Keep out of reach of children.
IMPORTANT UNSCREW THE CAP. THE TUBE OPENING IS SEALED. DO NOT USE IF SEAL IS PUNCTURED OR NOT VISIBLE AND RETURN PRODUCT TO PLACE OF PURCHASE. TO PUNCTURE THE SEAL REVERSE THE CAP AND PLACE THE PUNCTURE-TOP ONTO THE TUBE. PUSH DOWN FIRMLY UNTIL SEAL IS OPEN. TO CLOSE, SCREW THE CAP BACK ONTO THE TUBE.

Remember, no method of birth control can absolutely guarantee against pregnancy. For maximum protection, all methods-including these-must be used according to directions.

Every package of GYNOL II is dated to ensure freshness.

634-09-130-1

Advanced Care Products
Ortho Pharmaceutical Corp.
Raritan, NJ 08869
Shown in Product Identification Guide, page 519

GYNOL II®
Extra Strength
CONTRACEPTIVE JELLY

Efficacy: In a closely controlled study involving more than 200 women using nonoxynol-9 2% jelly (GYNOL II) and a diaphragm, the effectiveness was found to be 97% when used according to directions. GYNOL II Extra Strength contains 3% nonoxynol-9 and is, therefore, at least as effective as GYNOL II when used with a diaphragm.

The effectiveness of the GYNOL II Extra Strength/diaphragm contraceptive method is dependent upon highly motivated use—use with every act of intercourse in accordance with directions. In fact, the effectiveness of the method was only 90% in the above-mentioned study when users are included who failed to use GYNOL II and the diaphragm in accordance with directions.

GYNOL II Extra Strength can also be used to provide extra protection when used with a condom. It also effectively aids in the prevention of pregnancy when used by itself; however, use with a diaphragm may provide extra protection.

Action: Spermicidal

Indication: Contraception

Directions for Use With the Diaphragm: Before handling the diaphragm, it is recommended that you wash your hands with soap and water. Prior to inserting your diaphragm, put an applicatorful (about a teaspoonful) of GYNOL II Extra Strength into the cup of the dome and spread a small amount around the edge with your fingertip. Then insert. Intercourse should occur within six hours after the diaphragm with GYNOL II Extra Strength has been inserted. An additional application of GYNOL II Extra Strength must be applied prior to each act of intercourse. DO NOT REMOVE THE DIAPHRAGM —simply add more jelly with the applicator being careful not to dislodge the diaphragm.

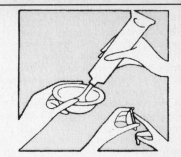

1.Remove cap from tube and attach applicator to tube by turning applicator clockwise.

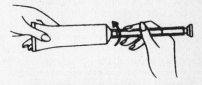

2.Squeeze the tube from the bottom, forcing the contents into the barrel until the plunger is pushed out as far as it will go and the barrel is completely filled.

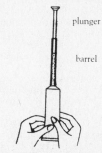

plunger

barrel

3.Always roll the tube from the bottom. After each use, replace cap and roll tube as shown. Avoid storing in a cold place.

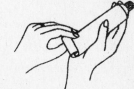

4.After detaching from the tube, hold the filled applicator by the barrel and gently insert the barrel well into the vagina. Press the plunger; then, with the plunger still depressed, remove the applicator, holding it by the barrel. Insertion of the applicator is accomplished more easily when lying on your back with the knees bent. Note diagram.

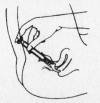

Continued on next page

Ortho—Cont.

IMPORTANT—An association has been reported between diaphragm use and toxic shock syndrome (TSS), a serious condition which can be fatal. For contraceptive effectiveness, the diaphragm should remain in place for six hours after intercourse and should be removed as soon as possible thereafter. Continuous wearing of a contraceptive diaphragm for more than twenty-four hours is not recommended. Retention of the diaphragm for any period of time may encourage the growth of certain bacteria in the vaginal tract. It has been suggested that under certain as yet unestablished conditions overgrowth of these bacteria may lead to symptoms of TSS. For further information, please contact your physician. Women with a known or suspected history of TSS should not use the diaphragm. **This method of contraception must be used each and every time intercourse takes place, regardless of the time of month.**

Directions For Use With A Condom Or As A Use Alone Product: Insert an applicatorful of GYNOL II Extra Strength into the vagina as shown in the illustration. Intercourse should occur within 1 hour after GYNOL II Extra Strength has been inserted. An additional application must be used prior to each additional act of intercourse. This method of contraception must be used each and every time intercourse takes place, regardless of the time of the month.

After Each Use: Wash the applicator with mild soap and warm water. Do not boil. Rinse thoroughly. The applicator may be pulled apart for easy cleaning. To reassemble, gently push plunger back into barrel as far as it will go.

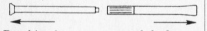

Douching is not recommended after using GYNOL II Extra Strength. However, if desired for cleansing purposes, wait at least six hours following your last intercourse to allow for the full spermicidal activity of GYNOL II Extra Strength.

Precaution: If you have been advised against pregnancy for medical reasons, your birth control method should be thoroughly discussed with your physician so that both you and your physician are satisfied that the method you have selected is right for you.

Adverse Reactions: Burning and/or irritation of the vagina or penis may be experienced. If this occurs, discontinue use and consult your physician.

Warning: Keep out of reach of children.

TAMPER-RESISTANT FEATURE: THE TUBE OPENING IS COVERED WITH A SEAL EMBOSSED WITH THIS DESIGN: . UNSCREW THE CAP. DO NOT USE IF SEAL IS PUNCTURED OR EMBOSSED DESIGN IS NOT VISIBLE AND RETURN PRODUCT TO PLACE OF PURCHASE.

TO PUNCTURE THE SEAL, REVERSE THE CAP AND PLACE THE PUNCTURE-TOP ONTO THE TUBE. PUSH DOWN FIRMLY UNTIL SEAL IS OPEN. TO CLOSE, SCREW THE CAP BACK ONTO THE TUBE.

Because of the higher concentration of the spermicide nonoxynol-9 in GYNOL II Extra Strength (150 mg nonoxynol-9 per applicatorful), vaginal or penile burning or irritation may occur. If this occurs, diaphragm users may wish to try GYNOL II Original Formula (100 mg nonoxynol-9 per applicatorful). Non-diaphragm users may wish to try CONCEPTROL® Contraceptive Gel (100 mg nonoxynol-9 per applicatorful). If the burning or irritation continues, discontinue use and consult your physician. Remember, no method of birth control can absolutely guarantee against pregnancy. For maximum protection, all methods—including these—must be used according to directions.

Every package of GYNOL II Extra Strength is dated to ensure freshness.

Shown in Product Identification Guide, page 519

ORTHO-GYNOL®
Contraceptive Jelly
For Use With Diaphragm

Directions For Use
PREPARING THE DIAPHRAGM
Before handling the diaphragm, it is recommended that you wash your hands with soap and water. Prior to inserting your diaphragm, put an applicatorful (about a teaspoonful) of ORTHO-GYNOL into the cup of the dome and spread a small amount around the edge with your fingertip. Then insert.

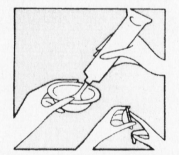

Intercourse should occur within six hours after the diaphragm and ORTHO-GYNOL have been inserted. An additional application of ORTHO-GYNOL must be applied prior to each act of intercourse. DO NOT REMOVE THE DIAPHRAGM—simply add more ORTHO-GYNOL with the applicator, being careful not to dislodge the diaphragm.

1. Remove cap from tube and attach applicator to tube by turning applicator clockwise.

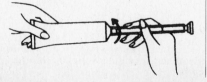

2. Squeeze the tube from the bottom, forcing the contents into the barrel until the plunger is pushed out as far as it will go and the barrel is completely filled.

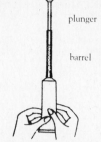

plunger

barrel

3. Always roll the tube from the bottom. After each use, replace cap and roll tube as shown. Avoid storing in a cold place.

4. After detaching from the tube, hold the filled applicator by the barrel and gently insert the barrel well into the vagina. Press the plunger; then, with the plunger still depressed, remove the applicator, holding it by the barrel. Insertion of the applicator is accomplished more easily when lying on your back with the knees bent. Note diagram

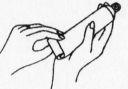

IMPORTANT—An association has been reported between diaphragm use and toxic shock syndrome (TSS), a serious condition which can be fatal. For contraceptive effectiveness, the diaphragm should remain in place for six hours after intercourse and should be removed as soon as possible thereafter. Continuous wearing of a contraceptive diaphragm for more than twenty-four hours is not recommended. Retention of the diaphragm for any period of time may encourage the growth of certain bacteria in the vaginal tract. It has been suggested that under certain as yet unestablished conditions overgrowth of these bacteria may lead to symptoms of TSS. For further information please contact your physician. Women with a known or suspected history of TSS should not use the diaphragm. **This method of contraception must be used each and every time intercourse takes place, regardless of the time of month.**

Douching is not recommended after using ORTHO-GYNOL. However, if desired for cleansing purposes, wait at least six hours following last intercourse to allow for the full spermicidal activity of ORTHO-GYNOL.

AFTER EACH USE
Wash the applicator with mild soap and warm water. Do not boil. Rinse thoroughly. The applicator may be pulled apart for easy cleaning. To reassemble, gently push plunger back into barrel as far as it will go.

Precaution: If you have been advised against pregnancy for medical reasons, your birth control method should be thoroughly discussed with your physician so that both you and your physician are satisfied that the method you have selected is right for you.

Adverse Reactions: Occasional burning and/or irritation of the vagina or penis have been reported. If this occurs, discontinue use and consult your physician.

Warning: Keep out of reach of children.
Important: UNSCREW THE CAP. THE TUBE OPENING IS SEALED. DO NOT USE IF SEAL IS PUNCTURED OR NOT VISIBLE AND RETURN PRODUCT TO PLACE OF PURCHASE.
TO PUNCTURE THE SEAL, REVERSE THE CAP AND PLACE THE PUNCTURE-TOP ONTO THE TUBE. PUSH DOWN FIRMLY UNTIL SEAL IS OPEN. TO CLOSE, SCREW THE CAP BACK ONTO THE TUBE.
Remember, no method of birth control can absolutely guarantee against pregnancy. For maximum protection, all methods—including these—must be used according to directions.
Every package of ORTHO-GYNOL is dated to ensure freshness.
Shown in Product Identification Guide, page 519

P & S Laboratories
**210 WEST 131st STREET
LOS ANGELES, CA 90061**

See Standard Homeopathic Company.

UNKNOWN DRUG?
Consult the
Product Identification Guide
(Gray Pages)
for full-color photos of
leading over-the-counter
medications

The Parthenon Co., Inc.
**3311 W. 2400 SOUTH
SALT LAKE CITY, UTAH 84119**

DEVROM® CHEWABLE TABLETS

Description: DEVROM® is a safe and effective internal (oral) deodorant. Each tablet contains 200 mg of Bismuth Subgallate powder.

Indications: DEVROM® is indicated for the control of odors from ileostomies, colostomies and fecal incontinence.

Dosage: Take one or two tablets of **DEVROM®** three times a day with meals or as directed by physician. Chew or swallow whole if desired.

Note: The beneficial ingredient in **DEVROM®** may coat the tongue which may also darken in color. This condition is harmless and temporary. Darkening of the stool is also possible and equally harmless.

Warning: This product cannot be expected to be effective in the reduction of odor due to faulty personal hygiene.
KEEP THIS BOTTLE AND ALL MEDICATION OUT OF THE REACH OF CHILDREN.

Inactive Ingredients: Mannitol, U.S.P., Lactose, N.F., Corn Starch, N.F., Confectioner's Sugar, N.F., Acacia Powder, N.F., Purified Water, U.S.P., Magnesium Stearate, N.F.
NO PHYSICIAN'S PRESCRIPTION IS NECESSARY

How Supplied: DEVROM® is supplied in bottles of 100 tablets.
DO NOT USE IF PRINTED OUTER SAFETY SEAL OR PRINTED INNER SAFETY SEAL IS BROKEN.
THE PARTHENON CO., INC./
3311 W. 2400 So./
Salt Lake City, Utah 84119

Pfizer Consumer Health Care Division
**Division of Pfizer Inc.
100 JEFFERSON ROAD
PARSIPPANY, NJ 07054**

BENGAY® External Analgesic Products

Description: BENGAY products contain menthol in an alcohol base gel, combinations of methyl salicylate and menthol in cream and ointment bases, as well as a combination of methyl salicylate, menthol and camphor in a non-greasy cream base; all suitable for topical application.
In addition to the Original Formula Pain Relieving Ointment (methyl salicylate, 18.3%; menthol, 16%), BENGAY is offered as BENGAY Greaseless Pain Relieving Cream (methyl salicylate, 15%; menthol, 10%), an Arthritis Formula NonGreasy Pain Relieving Cream (methyl salicylate, 30%; menthol, 8%), an Ultra Strength NonGreasy Pain Re-

lieving Cream (methyl salicylate 30%; menthol 10%; camphor 4%), and Vanishing Scent NonGreasy Pain Relieving Gel (3% menthol).

Action and Uses: Methyl salicylate, menthol and camphor are external analgesics which stimulate sensory receptors of warmth and/or cold. This produces a counter-irritant response which provides temporary relief of minor aches and pains of muscles and joints associated with simple backache, arthritis, strains, bruises and sprains.
Several double-blind clinical studies of BENGAY products containing menthol-methyl salicylate have shown the effectiveness of this combination in counteracting minor pain of skeletal muscle stress and arthritis.
Three studies involving a total of 102 normal subjects in which muscle soreness was experimentally induced showed statistically significant beneficial results from use of the active product vs. placebo for lowered Muscle Action Potential (spasms), greater rise in threshold of muscular pain and greater reduction in perceived muscular pain.
Six clinical studies of a total of 207 subjects suffering from minor pain due to osteoarthritis and rheumatoid arthritis showed the active product to give statistically significant beneficial results vs. placebo for greater relief of perceived pain, increased range of motion of the affected joints and increased digital dexterity. In two studies designed to measure the effect of topically applied BENGAY vs. Placebo on muscular endurance, discomfort, onset of exercise pain and fatigue, 30 subjects performed a submaximal three-hour run and another 30 subjects performed a maximal treadmill run. BENGAY was found to significantly decrease the discomfort during the submaximal and maximal runs, and increase the time before onset of fatigue during the maximal run.
Applied before workouts, BENGAY relaxes tight muscles and increases circulation to make exercising more comfortable, longer.
To help reduce muscle ache and soreness after exercise, BENGAY can be applied and allowed to work before taking a shower.

Directions: Apply generously and gently massage into painful area until BENGAY disappears. Repeat 3 to 4 times daily.

Warning: For external use only. Do not use with a heating pad. Keep away from children to avoid accidental poisoning. Do not bandage tightly. Do not swallow. If swallowed, induce vomiting and call a physician. Keep away from eyes, mucous membranes, broken or irritated skin. If skin redness or irritation develops, pain lasts for more than 10 days, or with arthritis—like conditions in children under 12, do not use and call a physician.

Continued on next page

Pfizer Consumer—Cont.

BONINE®   OTC
(Meclizine hydrochloride)
Chewable Tablets

Action: BONINE (meclizine) is an H_1 histamine receptor blocker of the piperazine side chain group. It exhibits its action by an effect on the Central Nervous System (CNS), possibly by its ability to block muscarinic receptors in the brain.

Indications: BONINE is effective in the management of nausea, vomiting and dizziness associated with motion sickness.

Contraindications: Do not take this product, unless directed by a doctor, if you have a breathing problem such as emphysema or chronic bronchitis, or if you have glaucoma or difficulty in urination due to enlargement of the prostate gland.

Warnings: May cause drowsiness; alcohol, sedatives and tranquilizers may increase the drowsiness effect. Avoid alcoholic beverages while taking this product. Do not take this product if you are taking sedatives or tranquilizers without first consulting your doctor. Do not drive or operate dangerous machinery while taking this medication.
Usage in Children:
Clinical studies establishing safety and effectiveness in children have not been done; therefore, usage is not recommended in children under 12 years of age.
Usage in Pregnancy:
As with any drug, if you are pregnant or nursing a baby, seek advice of a health care professional before taking this product.

Adverse Reactions: Drowsiness, dry mouth, and on rare occasions, blurred vision have been reported.

Dosage and Administration: For motion sickness, take one or two tablets of Bonine once daily, one hour before travel starts, for up to 24 hours of protection against motion sickness. The tablet can be chewed with or without water or swallowed whole with water. Thereafter, the dose may be repeated every 24 hours for the duration of the travel.

How Supplied: BONINE (meclizine HCl) is available in convenient packets of 8 chewable tablets of 25 mg. meclizine HCl.

Inactive Ingredients: FD&C Red #40, Lactose, Magnesium Stearate, Purified Siliceous Earth, Raspberry Flavor, Saccharin Sodium, Starch, Talc.

DESITIN CORNSTARCH BABY POWDER
(with Zinc Oxide)

Description: Desitin Cornstarch Baby Powder combines zinc oxide (10%) with topical starch (cornstarch) for topical application. Also contains: fragrance and tribasic calcium phosphate.

Actions and Uses: Desitin Cornstarch Baby Powder with zinc oxide and topical starch (cornstarch) is designed to protect from wetness, help prevent and treat diaper rash, and other minor skin irritations. It offers all the benefits of a talc-free, absorbent cornstarch powder, but with the addition of zinc oxide, the same protective ingredient found in Desitin Ointment. Cornstarch also prevents friction. Zinc oxide provides an additional physical barrier by forming a protective coating over the skin or mucous membranes which serves to reduce further effects of irritants on affected areas.

Directions: Prevention: Change wet and soiled diapers promptly, cleanse the diaper area, and allow to dry.
Apply powder close to the body away from child's face. Carefully shake the powder into the diaper or into the hand and apply to diaper area. Apply liberally as often as necessary with each diaper change, especially at bedtime, or anytime when exposure to wet diapers may be prolonged.

Treatment: Use liberally in all body creases, and whenever chafing, prickly heat or other minor skin irritations occur.

Warning: For external use only. Do not use on broken skin. Avoid contact with eyes. Keep powder away from child's face to avoid inhalation. If diaper rash worsens or does not improve within 7 days, consult a doctor.

How Supplied: Desitin Cornstarch Baby Powder with Zinc Oxide is available in 1 ounce (28g), and 14 ounce (397g) containers with sifter-top caps.
Shown in Product Identification Guide, page 519

DAILY CARE™ from DESITIN®
Diaper Rash Prevention Ointment
Skin Protectant (10% Zinc Oxide)

Description: Daily Care from DESITIN contains Zinc Oxide (10%) in a petrolatum base suitable for topical application. Also contains: cyclomethicone, dimethicone, fragrance, methylparaben, mineral oil, mineral wax, propylparaben, sodium borate, sorbitan sesquioleate, white wax and purified water.

Actions and Uses: Daily Care helps treat and prevent diaper rash. It helps seal out irritating wetness that can cause diaper rash by creating a protective wetness barrier at every diaper change. Daily Care has a pleasant formula that's easy to apply, easy to clean up and has a fresh scent.

Directions: Prevention—To help prevent diaper rash, change wet and soiled diaper promptly, cleanse the diaper area and allow to dry. Apply Daily Care ointment liberally as often as necessary with each diaper change—especially at bedtime or anytime when exposure to a wet diaper may be prolonged.

Treatment—At the first sign of redness or minor skin irritation, apply Daily Care liberally over the affected area and repeat as necessary. After the rash has cleared, continue to use Daily Care at every diaper change to help protect skin from future diaper rash.

Warnings: For external use only. Avoid contact with eyes. If condition worsens or does not improve within 7 days, consult your doctor. Keep out of reach of children. In case of accidental ingestion, seek professional assistance or contact a Poison Control Center immediately. Store between 2 and 30°C (36 and 86°F).

How Supplied: Daily Care Ointment is available in 2 oz. (57g) and 4 oz. (113g) tubes.
Shown in Product Identification Guide, page 519

DESITIN® OINTMENT

Description: Desitin Ointment combines Zinc Oxide (40%) with Cod Liver Oil in a petrolatum-lanolin base suitable for topical application. Also contains: BHA, fragrances, methylparaben, talc and water.

Actions and Uses: Desitin Ointment is designed to provide relief of diaper rash, superficial wounds and burns, and other minor skin irritations. It helps prevent incidents of diaper rash, protects against urine and other irritants, and soothes chafed skin.
Relief and protection is afforded by Zinc Oxide and Cod Liver Oil. These ingredients together with the petrolatum-lanolin base provide a physical barrier by forming a protective coating over skin or mucous membranes which serves to reduce further effects of irritants on the affected area and relieves burning, pain or itch produced by them.
Several studies have shown the effectiveness of Desitin Ointment in the relief and prevention of diaper rash.
Two clinical studies involving 90 infants demonstrated the effectiveness of Desitin Ointment in curing diaper rash. The diaper rash area was treated with Desitin Ointment at each diaper change for a period of 24 hours, while the untreated site served as controls. A significant reduction was noted in the severity and area of diaper dermatitis on the treated area.
Ninety-seven (97) babies participated in a 12-week study to show that Desitin Ointment helps prevent diaper rash. Approximately half of the infants (49) were treated with Desitin Ointment on a regular daily basis. The other half (48) received the ointment as necessary to treat any diaper rash which occurred. The incidence as well as the severity of diaper rash was significantly less among the babies using the ointment on a regular daily basis.

In a comparative study of the efficacy of Desitin Ointment vs. a baby powder, forty-five (45) babies were observed for a total of eight (8) weeks. Results support the conclusion that Desitin Ointment is a better prophylactic against diaper rash than the baby powder.

In another study, Desitin was found to be dramatically more effective in reducing the severity of medically diagnosed diaper rash than a commercially available diaper rash product in which only anhydrous lanolin and petrolatum were listed as ingredients. Fifty (50) infants participated in the study, half of whom were treated with Desitin and half with the other product. In the group (25) treated with Desitin, seventeen (17) infants showed significant improvement within 10 hours which increased to twenty-three improved infants within 24 hours. Of the group (25) treated with the other product, only three showed improvement at ten hours with a total of four improved within twenty-four hours. These results are statistically valid to conclude that Desitin Ointment reduces severity of diaper rash within ten hours.

Several other studies show that Desitin Ointment helps relieve other skin disorders, such as contact dermatitis.

Directions: Prevention: To prevent diaper rash, apply Desitin Ointment to the diaper area—especially at bedtime when exposure to wet diapers may be prolonged.

Treatment: If diaper rash is present, or at the first sign of redness, minor skin irritation or chafing, simply apply Desitin Ointment three or four times daily as needed. In superficial noninfected surface wounds and minor burns, apply a thin layer of Desitin Ointment, using a gauze dressing, if necessary. For external use only.

How Supplied: Desitin Ointment is available in 1 ounce (28g), 2 ounce (57g), and 4 ounce (114g) tubes, and 9 ounce (255g) and 1 lb. (454g) jars.

Shown in Product Identification Guide, page 519

RHEABAN® Maximum Strength FAST ACTING CAPLETS
[rē'ăban]
(attapulgite)

Description: Maximum Strength Rheaban is an anti-diarrheal medication containing activated attapulgite and is offered in caplets form.
Each white Rheaban caplets contains 750 mg. of colloidal activated attapulgite. Rheaban provides the maximum level of medication when taken as directed. Rheaban contains no narcotics, opiates or other habit-forming drugs.

Actions and Uses: Rheaban is indicated for relief of diarrhea and the cramps and pains associated with it. Attapulgite, which has been activated by thermal treatment, is a highly sorptive substance which absorbs nutrients and digestive enzymes as well as noxious gases, irritants, toxins and some bacteria and viruses that are common causes of diarrhea.

In clinical studies to show the effectiveness in relieving diarrhea and its symptoms, 100 subjects suffering from acute gastroenteritis with diarrhea participated in a double-blind comparison of Rheaban to a placebo. Patients treated with the attapulgite product showed significantly improved relief of diarrhea and its symptoms vs. the placebo.

Dosage and Administration:
CAPLETS
Adults—2 caplets after initial bowel movement, 2 caplets after each subsequent bowel movement. For a maximum of 12 caplets in 24 hours.
Children 6 to 12 years—1 caplet after initial bowel movement, 1 caplet after each subsequent bowel movement. For a maximum of 6 caplets in 24 hours, or as directed by a physician.

Warnings: Do not exceed 12 caplets in 24 hours. Swallow caplets with water, do not chew. Do not use for more than two days, or in the presence of high fever. Caplets should not be used for infants or children under 6 years of age unless directed by physician. If diarrhea persists consult a physician.

How Supplied:
Caplets—Boxes of 12 caplets.

Inactive Ingredients: Carnauba Wax, Croscarmellose Sodium, D&C Yellow No. 10 Aluminum Lake, FD&C Blue No. 1 Aluminum Lake, Hydroxypropyl Cellulose, Hydroxypropyl Methylcellulose, Methylparaben, Pectin, Pharmaceutical Glaze, Propylene Glycol, Propylparaben, Sucrose, Talc Titanium Dioxide, Zinc Stearate.

RID® Spray   OTC
Lice Control Spray

PRODUCT OVERVIEW

Key Facts: Rid Lice Control Spray is a pediculicide spray for controlling lice and louse eggs on inanimate objects, to help prevent reinfestation. It contains a highly active synthetic pyrethroid that kills lice and their eggs on inanimate objects.

Major Uses: Rid Lice Control Spray effectively kills lice and louse eggs on garments, bedding, furniture and other inanimate objects that cannot be either laundered or dry cleaned.

Safety Information: Rid Lice Control Spray is intended for use on inanimate objects only; it is not for use on humans or animals. It is harmful if swallowed. It should not be sprayed in the eyes or on the skin and should not be inhaled. The product should be used only in well ventilated areas; room(s) should be vacated after treatment and ventilated before reoccupying.

PRESCRIBING INFORMATION

RID® Spray
Lice Control Spray

THIS PRODUCT IS NOT FOR USE ON HUMANS OR ANIMALS

Active Ingredient:

Permethrin*	0.5%
Inert Ingredients	99.5%
	100.00%

*(3-phenoxyphenol)methyl $\pm$ cis/trans 3-(2,2-dichloroethenyl) 2,2-dimethylcyclopropane-carboxylate, cis/trans ratio: Minimum 35% ($\pm$ cis) and maximum 65% ($\pm$ trans).

Actions: A highly active synthetic pyrethroid for the control of lice and louse eggs on garments, bedding, furniture and other inanimate objects.

Warnings: Avoid contamination of feed and foodstuffs. Remove pets and birds and cover fish aquaria before space spraying on surface applications. HARMFUL IF SWALLOWED. This product is not for use on humans or animals. If lice infestations should occur on humans, consult either your physician or pharmacist for a product for use on humans.

Physical and Chemical Hazards: Contents under pressure. Do not use or store near heat or open flame. Do not puncture or incinerate container. Exposure to temperatures above 130° F may cause bursting. Store in cool, dry area. Do not store below 32° F.
CAUTION: Avoid spraying in eyes. Avoid breathing spray mist. Use only in well ventilated areas. Avoid contact with skin. In case of contact wash immediately with soap and water. Vacate room after treatment and ventilate before reoccupying.
Statement of Practical Treatment:
If inhaled: Remove affected person to fresh air. Apply artifical respiration if indicated.
If in eyes: Flush with plenty of water. Contact physician if irritation persists.
If on skin: Wash affected areas immediately with soap and water.

Direction for Use: It is a violation of Federal law to use this product in a manner inconsistent with its labeling.
Shake well before using.
To kill lice and louse eggs: Spray in an inconspicuous area to test for possible staining or discoloration. Inspect again after drying, then proceed to spray entire area to be treated. Hold container upright with nozzle away from you. Depress valve and spray from a distance of 8 to 10 inches.
Spray each square foot for 3 seconds. Spray only those garments, parts of bedding, including mattresses and furniture that cannot be either laundered or dry cleaned.
Allow all sprayed articles to dry thoroughly before use.

Continued on next page

Pfizer Consumer—Cont.

Buyer assumes all risks of use, storage or handling of this material not in strict accordance with directions given herewith.

DISPOSAL OF CONTAINER
Wrap container in several layers of newspaper and dispose of in trash. Do not incinerate or puncture.

How Supplied: 5 ounce aerosol can. Also available in combination with RID® Lice Killing Shampoo as the RID® Lice Elimination Kit.

RID®
Lice Killing Shampoo

PRODUCT OVERVIEW

Key Facts: The Rid® Lice Killing Shampoo contains a liquid pediculicide effective against head, body, and pubic (crab) lice and their eggs. The active ingredients in Rid® are pyrethrum extract and piperonyl butoxide, technical which attack the louse's nervous system. Piperonyl butoxide is a synergist. The pyrethrum extract in Rid® rinses out completely after treatment, and is poorly absorbed through the skin. Each Rid® Lice Killing Shampoo package also contains a patented nit (egg) removal comb with an exclusive handle design that provides gentle combing action to remove the nits (eggs).

Major Uses: Rid® has proved to be clinically effective in treating infestations of head lice and their eggs. It is also effective in the treatment of infestations of body lice, pubic (crab) lice and their eggs.

Safety Information: Rid® should be used with caution by ragweed sensitized persons. It is intended for external use on humans only and is harmful if swallowed. It should not be inhaled or allowed to come in contact with the eyes or mucous membranes. Contamination of feed or foodstuffs should be avoided.

PRESCRIBING INFORMATION
RID®
Lice Killing Shampoo

Description: Rid® contains a liquid pediculicide whose active ingredients are pyrethrum extract 0.33% and piperonyl butoxide, technical 4.00%, equivalent to min. 3.2% (butylcarbityl) (6-propylpiperonyl) ether and 0.8% related compounds. Inert ingredients (95.67%) are: C13–C14 isoparaffin, fragrance, isopropyl alcohol, PEG-25 hydrogenated castor oil, water, xanthan gum.

Actions: Rid® kills head lice (Pediculus humanus capitis), body lice (Pediculus humanus humanus), and pubic (crab) lice (Phthirus pubis), and their eggs. The pyrethrum extract acts as a contact poison and affects the parasite's nervous system, resulting in paralysis and death. The efficacy of the pyrethrum extract is enhanced by a synergist, piperonyl butoxide. The pyrethrum extract rinses out completely after treatment and is not designed to leave long-acting residues. In addition, pyrethrum extract is poorly absorbed through the skin. Of the relatively minor amounts that are absorbed, they are rapidly metabolized to water-soluble compounds and eliminated from the body without ill effects.

Indications: For the treatment of head, pubic (crab), and body lice.

Warnings: Use with caution on persons allergic to ragweed. For external use only. Do not use near the eyes or permit contact with mucous membranes, such as inside the nose, mouth, or vagina, as irritation may occur. Keep out of eyes when rinsing hair. Adults and children: Close eyes tightly and do not open eyes until product is rinsed out. Also, protect children's eyes with washcloth, towel, or other suitable material, or by a similar method. If product gets into the eyes, immediately flush with water. If skin irritation or infection is present or develops, discontinue use and consult a doctor. Consult a doctor if infestation of eyebrows or eyelashes occurs.

Storage and Disposal: Do not store below 32°F (0°C) or above 120°F. Do not reuse empty container. Wrap in several layers of newspaper and discard in trash.

Dosage and Administration: Apply to affected area until all hair is thoroughly wet with product. Allow product to remain on area for 10 minutes but not longer. Add sufficient warm water to form a lather and shampoo as usual. Rinse thoroughly. A fine tooth comb or special lice/nit removing comb may be used to help remove dead lice or their eggs (nits) from hair. A second treatment must be done in 7 to 10 days to kill any newly hatched lice. Since there is no immunity from lice, personal cleanliness and the avoidance of infested persons and their bedding and clothes will aid in preventing infestation. These additional steps are important in order to minimize the chance of possible reinfestation.
- Inspect all family members daily for at least two weeks, and if they become infested, treat with Rid®.
- Wash all personal clothing, nightwear and bedding of any infested person in hot water, at least 130°F, or by dry cleaning.
- Soak all personal articles such as combs, brushes, etc. in Rid® solution or hot, soapy water (at least 130°F) for ten minutes.
- Tell children not to use any borrowed combs or brushes, nor to wear anyone else's clothes.

LICE WHICH INFEST HUMANS

Head Lice: Head lice live on the scalp and lay small white eggs (nits) on the hair shaft close to the scalp. The nits are most easily found on the nape of the neck or behind the ears. All personal headgear, scarfs, coats, and bed linen should be disinfected by machine washing in hot water and drying, using the hot cycle of a dryer for at least 20 minutes. Personal articles of clothing or bedding that cannot be washed may be dry-cleaned, sealed in a plastic bag for a period of about 2 weeks, or sprayed with a product specifically designed for this purpose. Personal combs and brushes may be disinfected by soaking in hot water (above 130°F) for 5 to 10 minutes. Thorough vacuuming of rooms inhabited by infected patients is recommended.

Pubic (Crab) Lice: Pubic lice may be transmitted by sexual contact; therefore, sexual partners should be treated simultaneously to avoid reinfestation. The lice are very small and look almost like brown or gray dots on the skin. Pubic lice usually cause intense itching and lay small white eggs (nits) on the hair shaft generally close to the skin surface. In hairy individuals, pubic lice may be present on the short hairs of the thighs and trunk, underarms, and occasionally on the beard and mustache. Underwear should be disinfected by machine washing in hot water, then drying, using the hot cycle for at least 20 minutes.

Body Lice: Body lice and their eggs are generally found in the seams of clothing, particularly in the waistline and armpit area. They move to the skin to feed, then return to the seams of the clothing where they lay their eggs. Clothing worn and not laundered before treatment should be disinfected by the same procedure as described for head lice, except that sealing clothing in a plastic bag is not recommended because the nits (eggs) from these lice can remain dormant for a period of up to 30 days.

How Supplied: In 2, 4 and 8 fl. oz. plastic bottles. Exclusive nit (egg) removal comb that removes all nits (eggs) and patient instruction booklet (English and Spanish) are included in each package of Rid®. Also available in combination with Rid® Lice Control Spray as the Rid® Lice Elimination Kit.

MAXIMUM STRENGTH   OTC
UNISOM SLEEPGELS
Nighttime Sleep Aid

Description: Maximum Strength Unisom SleepGels are liquid-filled, blue soft gelatin capsules.

Active Ingredient: Diphenhydramine Hydrochloride 50 mg.

Inactive Ingredients: FD&C Blue No. 1, Gelatin, Glycerin, Pharmaceutical Glaze, Polyethylene Glycol, Propylene Glycol, Purified Water, Sorbitol, Titanium Dioxide.

Indications: Helps to reduce difficulty falling asleep.

Action: Diphenhydramine Hydrochloride is an ethanolamine antihistamine with anticholinergic and sedative effects.

Administration and Dosage: Adults and children 12 years of age and over: Oral dosage is one softgel (50 mg.) at bedtime if needed, or as directed by a doctor.

Warnings: Do not take this product, unless directed by a doctor, if you have a breathing problem such as emphysema or chronic bronchitis, or if you have glaucoma or difficulty in urination due to enlargement of the prostate gland. Do not take this product if pregnant or nursing a baby.

- Do not give to children under 12 years of age.
- If sleeplessness persists continuously for more than two weeks, consult your doctor. Insomnia may be a symptom of serious underlying medical illness.
- Avoid alcoholic beverages while taking this product. Do not take this product if you are taking sedatives or tranquilizers, without first consulting your doctor.
- Keep this and all drugs out of the reach of children.
- In case of accidental overdose, seek professional assistance or contact a Poison Control Center immediately.

Drug Interaction: Monoamine oxidase (MAO) inhibitors prolong and intensify the anticholinergic effects of antihistamines. The CNS depressant effect is heightened by alcohol and other CNS depressant drugs.

Symptoms of Oral Overdosage: Antihistamine overdosage reactions may vary from central nervous system depression to stimulation. Stimulation is particularly likely in children. Atropine-like signs and symptoms, such as dry mouth, fixed and dilated pupils, flushing, and gastrointestinal symptoms, may also occur.

Attention: Use only if softgel blister seals are unbroken.

How Supplied: Boxes of 16 liquid filled softgels in child resistant blisters and boxes of 8 with non-child resistant packaging. Also in a 32 count child resistant bottle.
Store between 15° and 30°C (59° and 86°F)

UNISOM®   OTC
[yu 'na-som]
**Nighttime Sleep Aid
(doxylamine succinate)**

PRODUCT OVERVIEW

Key Facts: Unisom is an ethanolamine antihistamine (doxylamine) which characteristically shows a high incidence of sedation. It produces a reduced latency to end of wakefulness and early onset of sleep.

Major Uses: Unisom has been shown to be clinically effective as a sleep aid when 1 tablet is given 30 minutes before retiring.

Safety Information: Unisom is contraindicated in pregnancy and nursing mothers. It is also contraindicated in patients with asthma, glaucoma, and enlargement of the prostate. Caution should be used if taken when alcohol is being consumed. Caution is also indicated when taken concurrently with other medications due to the anticholinergic properties of antihistamines.

PRESCRIBING INFORMATION

UNISOM®   OTC
[yu 'na-som]
**Nighttime Sleep Aid
(doxylamine succinate)**

Description: Pale blue oval scored tablets containing 25 mg. of doxylamine succinate, 2-[α-(2-dimethylaminoethoxy)α-methylbenzyl]pyridine succinate.

Action and Uses: Doxylamine succinate is an antihistamine of the ethanolamine class, which characteristically shows a high incidence of sedation. In a comparative clinical study of over 20 antihistamines on more than 3000 subjects, doxylamine succinate 25 mg. was one of the three most sedating antihistamines, producing a significantly reduced latency to end of wakefulness and comparing favorably with established hypnotic drugs such as secobarbital and pentobarbital in sedation activity. It was chosen as the antihistamine, based on dosage, causing the earliest onset of sleep. In another clinical study, doxylamine succinate 25 mg. scored better than secobarbital 100 mg. as a nighttime hypnotic. Two additional, identical clinical studies, involving a total of 121 subjects demonstrated that doxylamine succinate 25 mg. reduced the sleep latency period by a third, compared to placebo. Duration of sleep was 26.6% longer with doxylamine succinate, and the quality of sleep was rated higher with the drug than with placebo. An EEG study on 6 subjects confirmed the results of these studies. In yet another study, no statistically significant difference was found between doxylamine succinate and flurazepam in the average time required for 200 patients with mild to moderate insomnia to fall asleep over 5 nights following a nightly dose of doxylamine succinate 25 mg. or flurazepam 30 mg., nor was any statistically significant difference found in the total time the 200 patients slept. Patients on doxylamine succinate awoke an average of 1.2 times per night while those on flurazepam awoke an average of 0.9 times per night. In either case the patients awoke rested the following morning. On a rating scale of 1 to 5, doxylamine succinate was given a 3.0, flurazepam a 3.4 by patients rating the degree of restfulness provided by their medication (5 represents "very well rested"). Although statistically significant, the difference between doxylamine succinate 25 mg. and flurazepam 30 mg. in the number of awakenings and degree of restfulness is clinically insignificant.

Administration and Dosage: One tablet 30 minutes before retiring. Not for children under 12 years of age.

Side Effects: Occasional anticholinergic effects may be seen.

Precautions: Unisom® should be taken only at bedtime.

Contraindications: Do not take this product, unless directed by a doctor, if you have a breathing problem such as emphysema or chronic bronchitis, or if you have glaucoma or difficulty in urination due to enlargement of the prostate gland. This product should not be taken by pregnant women or those who are nursing a baby.

Warnings: Should be taken with caution if alcohol is being consumed. Product should not be taken if patient is concurrently on any other drug, without prior consultation with physician. Should not be taken for longer than two weeks unless approved by physician.

How Supplied: Boxes of 8, 16, 32 or 48 tablets.

Inactive Ingredients: Dibasic Calcium Phosphate, FD&C Blue #1 Aluminum Lake, Magnesium Stearate, Microcrystalline Cellulose, Sodium Starch Glycolate.

UNISOM® WITH PAIN   OTC
RELIEF®
[yu 'na-som]
Nighttime Sleep Aid and Pain Reliever

PRODUCT OVERVIEW

Key Facts: Unisom With Pain Relief (diphenhydramine sleep aid/acetaminophen pain relief formula) is a product with a dual antihistamine sleep aid/analgesic action to utilize the sedative effects of an antihistamine and relieve mild to moderate pain that may disturb normal sleep patterns. If patients have difficulty in falling asleep but are not experiencing pain at the same time, regular Unisom Sleep Aid which contains doxylamine succinate or Maximum Strength Unisom Sleepgels which contains diphenhydramine is indicated.

Major Uses: One Unisom With Pain Relief is indicated 30 minutes before retiring to help reduce difficulty in falling asleep while relieving accompanying minor aches and pains, such as headache, muscle aches or menstrual discomfort.

Safety Information: Do not take this product, unless directed by a doctor, if you have a breathing problem such as emphysema or chronic bronchitis, or if you have glaucoma or difficulty in urination due to enlargement of the prostate gland. Unisom With Pain Relief is contraindicated in pregnancy or in nursing mothers. Excessive dosing may lead to liver damage. Product is intended for patients 12 years and older. Alcoholic beverages should be avoided while taking this product. This product should not be

Continued on next page

Pfizer Consumer—Cont.

taken without first consulting a physician if sedatives or tranquilizers are being taken.

PRESCRIBING INFORMATION
UNISOM WITH PAIN RELIEF®
[yu 'na-som]
Nighttime Sleep Aid and Pain Reliever

Description: Unisom With Pain Relief® is a pale blue, capsule-shaped, coated tablet.

Active Ingredients: 650 mg. acetaminophen and 50 mg. diphenhydramine HCl per tablet.

Indications: Unisom With Pain Relief (diphenhydramine sleep aid formula) is indicated to help reduce difficulty in falling asleep while relieving accompanying minor aches and pains such as headache, muscle ache or menstrual discomfort. If there is difficulty in falling asleep, but pain is not being experienced at the same time, regular Unisom sleep aid is indicated which contains doxylamine succinate as its active ingredient.

Administration and Dosage: One tablet at bedtime if needed, or as directed by a physician.

Contraindications: Do not take this product, unless directed by a doctor, if you have a breathing problem such as emphysema or chronic bronchitis, or if you have glaucoma or difficulty in urination due to enlargement of the prostate gland. Do not take this product if pregnant or nursing a baby.
Do not take this product for treatment of arthritis except under the advice and supervision of a physican.

Warnings: Do not exceed recommended dosage because severe liver damage may occur. If symptoms persist continuously for more than ten days, consult your physician. Insomnia may be a symptom of serious underlying medical illness. Avoid alcoholic beverages while taking this product. Do not take this product if you are taking sedatives or tranquilizers, without first consulting your doctor. For adults only. Do not give to children under 12 years of age. Keep this and all medications out of reach of children. IN CASE OF ACCIDENTAL OVERDOSE SEEK PROFESSIONAL ADVICE OR CONTACT A POISON CONTROL CENTER IMMEDIATELY.

Caution: This product contains an antihistamine and will cause drowsiness. It should be used only at bedtime.

Drug Interaction: Monoamine oxidase (MAO) inhibitors prolong and intensify the anticholinergic effects of antihistamines. The CNS depressant effect is heightened by alcohol and other CNS depressant drugs.

Attention: Use only if tablet blister seals are unbroken. Child resistant packaging.

How Supplied: Boxes of 8 and 16 tablets in child resistant blisters.

Inactive Ingredients: Crospovidone, FD&C Blue #1 Aluminum Lake, FD&C Blue #2 Aluminum Lake, Hydroxypropyl Methylcellulose, Magnesium Stearate, Polyethylene Glycol, Polysorbate 80, Povidone, Pregelatinized Starch, Stearic Acid, Titanium Dioxide.

VISINE L. R.™ EYE DROPS
(oxymetazoline hydrochloride)

Description: Visine L. R. is a sterile, isotonic, buffered ophthalmic solution containing oxymetazoline hydrochloride 0.025%, boric acid, sodium borate, sodium chloride and water. It is preserved with benzalkonium chloride 0.01% and edetate disodium 0.1%.
Visine L. R. is produced by a process that assures sterility.

Indications: Visine L. R. is a decongestant ophthalmic solution designed for the relief of redness of the eye due to minor eye irritations. Visine L. R. is specially formulated to relieve redness of the eye in minutes with effective relief that lasts up to 6 hours.

Directions: *Adults and children 6 years of age and older*—Place 1 or 2 drops in the affected eye(s). This may be repeated as needed every 6 hours or as directed by a physician.

Warning: If you experience eye pain, changes in vision, continued redness or irritation of the eye, or if the condition worsens or persists for more than 72 hours, discontinue use and consult a physician. If you have glaucoma, do not use this product except under the advice and supervision of a physician. As with any medication, if you are pregnant seek the advice of a physician before using this product. Overuse of this product may produce increased redness of the eye. If solution changes color or becomes cloudy, do not use. To avoid contamination of this product, do not touch tip of container to any surface. Replace cap after using. Remove contact lenses before using this product.

Parents: Before using with children under 6 years of age, consult your physician. Keep this and all medications out of the reach of children. In case of accidental ingestion, seek professional assistance or contact a poison control center immediately.

Caution: Should not be used if Visine-imprinted neckband on bottle is broken or missing.

Storage: Store between 2° and 30°C (36° and 86°F).

How Supplied: In 0.5 fl. oz. and 1 fl. oz. plastic dispenser bottle.
Shown in Product Identification Guide, page 519

VISINE MAXIMUM STRENGTH ALLERGY RELIEF®
Astringent/Redness Reliever Eye Drops

Description: Visine with allergy relief is a sterile, isotonic, buffered ophthalmic solution containing tetrahydrozoline hydrochloride 0.05%, zinc sulfate 0.25%, boric acid, sodium chloride, sodium citrate and purified water. It is preserved with benzalkonium chloride 0.01% and edetate disodium 0.1%. Visine with allergy relief is an ophthalmic solution combining the effects of the vasoconstrictor tetrahydrozoline hydrochloride with the astringent effects of zinc sulfate. The vasoconstrictor provides symptomatic relief of conjunctival edema and hyperemia secondary to minor irritation due to conditions such as dust and airborne pollutants as well as so-called nonspecific or catarrhal conjunctivitis, while zinc sulfate provides relief from burning and itching, symptoms often associated with hay fever, allergies, etc. Beneficial effects include amelioration of burning, irritation, pruritis, and removal of mucus from the eye. Relief is afforded by both ingredients, tetrahydrozoline hydrochloride and zinc sulfate.
Tetrahydrozoline hydrochloride is a sympathomimetic agent, which brings about decongestion by vasoconstriction. Reddened eyes are rapidly whitened by this effective vasoconstrictor, which limits the local vascular response by constricting the small blood vessels. The onset of vasoconstriction becomes apparent within minutes. Zinc sulfate is an ocular astringent which, by precipitating protein, helps to clear mucus from the outer surface of the eye.
The effectiveness of Visine with allergy relief in relieving conjunctival hyperemia and associated symptoms induced by allergies has been clinically demonstrated. In one double-blind study allergy sufferers experienced acute episodes of minor eye irritation. Visine with allergy relief produced statistically significant beneficial results versus a placebo of normal saline solution in relieving irritation of bulbar conjunctiva, irritation of palpebral conjunctiva, and mucous build-up. Treatment with Visine with allergy relief containing zinc sulfate also significantly improved burning and itching symptoms.

Indications: For temporary relief of discomfort and redness due to minor eye irritations.

Directions: Instill 1 to 2 drops in the affected eye(s) up to 4 times daily.

Warning: To avoid contamination, do not touch tip of container to any surface. Replace cap after using. If you experience eye pain, changes in vision, continued redness or irritation of the eye, or if the condition worsens or persists for more than 72 hours, discontinue use and consult a doctor. If you have glaucoma, do not use this product except under the advice and supervision of a doctor. Overuse of this product may produce in-

creased redness of the eye. If solution changes color or becomes cloudy, do not use. Remove contact lenses before using.
Parents: Before using with children under 6 years of age, consult your physician. Keep this and all other drugs out of the reach of children. In case of accidental ingestion, seek professional assistance or contact a poison control center immediately.

How Supplied: In 0.5 fl. oz. and 1.0 fl. oz. plastic dispenser bottle.
Shown in Product Identification Guide, page 519

VISINE MOISTURIZING
Redness Reliever/Lubricant Eye Drops

Description: Visine Moisturizing is a sterile, isotonic, buffered ophthalmic solution containing tetrahydrozoline hydrochloride 0.05%, polyethylene glycol 400 1.0%, boric acid, sodium borate, sodium chloride and water. It is preserved with benzalkonium chloride 0.013% and edetate disodium 0.1%.

Visine Moisturizing is an ophthalmic solution combining the effects of the decongestant tetrahydrozoline hydrochloride with the demulcent effects of polyethylene glycol. It provides symptomatic relief of conjunctival edema and hyperemia secondary to ocular allergies, minor irritations and so-called nonspecific or catarrhal conjunctivitis. Tetrahydrozoline hydrochloride is a sympathomimetic agent, which brings about decongestion by vasoconstriction. Reddened eyes are rapidly whitened by this effective vasoconstrictor, which limits the local vascular response by constricting the small blood vessels. The onset of vasoconstriction becomes apparent within minutes. Additional effects include amelioration of burning, irritation, pruritus, soreness, and excessive lacrimation. Relief is afforded by polyethylene glycol.

Polyethylene glycol is an ophthalmic demulcent which has been shown to be effective for the temporary relief of discomfort of minor irritations of the eye due to exposure to wind or sun. It is effective as a protectant and lubricant against further irritation or to relieve dryness of the eye.

The effectiveness of tetrahydrozoline hydrochloride in relieving conjunctival hyperemia and associated symptoms has been demonstrated by numerous clinicals, including several double-blind studies, involving more than 2000 subjects suffering from acute or chronic hyperemia induced by a variety of conditions. Visine Moisturizing is a product that combines the redness relieving effects of a vasoconstrictor and the soothing moisturizing and protective effects of a demulcent.

Indications: Relieves redness of the eye due to minor eye irritations. For use as a protectant against further irritation or to relieve dryness.

Directions: Instill 1 to 2 drops in the affected eye(s) up to 4 times daily.
Warning: To avoid contamination, do not touch tip of container to any surface. Replace cap after using. If you experience eye pain, changes in vision, continued redness or irritation of the eye, or if the condition worsens or persists for more than 72 hours, discontinue use and consult a doctor. If you have glaucoma, do not use this product except under the advice and supervision of a doctor. Overuse of this product may produce increased redness of the eye. If solution changes color or becomes cloudy, do not use. Remove contact lenses before using.
Parents: Before using with children under 6 years of age, consult your physician. Keep this and all other drugs out of the reach of children. In case of accidental ingestion, seek professional assistance or contact a poison control center immediately.

How Supplied: In 0.5 fl. oz. and 1.0 fl. oz. plastic dispenser bottle.
Shown in Product Identification Guide, page 519

VISINE® ORIGINAL
Tetrahydrozoline Hydrochloride Redness Reliever Eye Drops

Description: Visine is a sterile, isotonic, buffered ophthalmic solution containing tetrahydrozoline hydrochloride 0.05%, boric acid, sodium borate, sodium chloride and water. It is preserved with benzalkonium chloride 0.01% and edetate disodium 0.1%. Visine is a decongestant ophthalmic solution designed to provide symptomatic relief of conjunctival edema and hyperemia secondary to minor irritations, due to conditions such as smoke, dust, other airborne pollutants, swimming etc. and so-called nonspecific or catarrhal conjunctivitis. Relief is afforded by tetrahydrozoline hydrochloride, a sympathomimetic agent, which brings about decongestion by vasoconstriction. Reddened eyes are rapidly whitened by this effective vasoconstrictor, which limits the local vascular response by constricting the small blood vessels. The onset of vasoconstriction becomes apparent within minutes.

The effectiveness of Visine in relieving conjunctival hyperemia has been demonstrated by numerous clinicals, including several double-blind studies, involving more than 2,000 subjects suffering from acute or chronic hyperemia induced by a variety of conditions. Visine was found to be efficacious in providing relief from conjunctival hyperemia.

Indications: Relieves redness of the eye due to minor eye irritations.

Directions: Instill 1 to 2 drops in the affected eye(s) up to four times daily.

Warning: To avoid contamination, do not touch tip of container to any surface. Replace cap after using. If you experience eye pain, changes in vision, continued redness or irritation of the eye, or if the condition worsens or persists for

more than 72 hours, discontinue use and consult a doctor. If you have glaucoma, do not use this product except under the advice and supervision of a doctor. Overuse of this product may produce increased redness of the eye. If solution changes color or becomes cloudy, do not use. Remove contact lenses before using.
Parents: Before using with children under 6 years of age, consult your physician. Keep this and all other drugs out of the reach of children. In case of accidental ingestion, seek professional assistance or contact a poison control center immediately.

How Supplied: In 0.5 fl. oz., 0.75 fl. oz., and 1.0 fl. oz. plastic dispenser bottle and 0.5 fl. oz. plastic bottle with dropper.
Shown in Product Identification Guide, page 519

WART–OFF®
Liquid

Active Ingredient: Salicylic Acid 17% w/w.

Inactive Ingredients: Alcohol, 26.35% w/w, Flexible Collodion, Propylene Glycol Dipelargonate.

Indications: For the removal of common warts and plantar warts on the bottom of the foot. The common wart is easily recognized by the rough "cauliflower-like" appearance of the surface. The plantar wart is recognized by its location only on the bottom of the foot, its tenderness, and the interruption of the footprint pattern.

Warnings: For external use only. Keep this and all medications out of the reach of children to avoid accidental poisoning. In case of accidental ingestion, contact a physician or a Poison Control Center immediately. Do not use this product on irritated skin, on any area that is infected or reddened, if you are a diabetic, or if you have poor blood circulation. Do not use on moles, birthmarks, warts with hair growing from them, genital warts, or warts on the face or mucous membranes. If product gets into the eye, flush with water for 15 minutes. Avoid inhaling vapors. If discomfort persists, see your doctor.
Extremely Flammable—Keep away from fire or flame. Cap bottle tightly and store at room temperature away from heat (59°–86°F).

Instructions For Use: Read warnings and enclosed instructional brochure. Wash affected area. Dry area thoroughly. Using the special pinpoint applicator, apply one drop at a time to sufficiently cover each wart. Apply Wart-Off to warts only—not to surrounding skin. Let dry. Repeat this procedure once or twice daily as needed (until wart is removed) for up to 12 weeks. Replace cap tightly to prevent evaporation.

How Supplied: 0.45 fluid ounce bottle with special pinpoint plastic applicator and instructional brochure.

Pharmavite Corp.
15451 SAN FERNANDO
MISSION BLVD.
MISSION HILLS, CA 91345

NATURE MADE® ANTIOXIDANT FORMULA
(Vitamins C, E, & Beta Carotene)

Description: Nature Made® Antioxidant Formula contains high levels of Vitamin C, Vitamin E and Beta Carotene which are "free radical fighters". This product meets USP standards for purity, potency and disintegration. Like all Nature Made products, this product is manufactured to contain no artificial colors, no artificial flavors, no preservatives, no chemical solvents, no yeast, no sugar, no sodium and no starch.

Nutrition Facts
Serving Size 1 softgel

Amount Per Softgel	%Daily Value
Vitamin A 10,000 I.U.	200%
100% as Beta Carotene	
Vitamin C 250 mg	417%
Vitamin E 200 I.U.	667%

Active Ingredients: Ascorbic Acid, dl-Alpha Tocopheryl Acetate and Beta Carotene.

Inactive Ingredients: Cottonseed Oil, Gelatin, Glycerin, Water, Partially Hydrogenated Cottonseed and Soybean Oils.

Indications: Supplementation to diet as only one in ten Americans consume the recommended 5 servings of fruits and vegetables daily. Antioxidant vitamins (Vitamin C, Vitamin E and Beta Carotene) may help protect cells against the damaging effects of free radicals. Free radicals are highly reactive oxygen molecules created by environmental factors such as ultraviolet light, pollution, X-rays and alcohol, as well as by normal body processes.

Recommended Intake: Take one softgel daily, with a meal. Nature Made Antioxidant Formula can be taken by itself or with a multiple vitamin.

Warnings: Keep out of the reach of children.

How Supplied: Softgels, bottle of 60. Store at room temperature.

Shown in Product Identification Guide, page 519

NATURE MADE®
ESSENTIAL BALANCE®
Complete High Potency Multivitamin-Multimineral Formula

Description: Nature Made® Essential Balance® offers a complete and more natural multivitamin/multimineral with higher levels of antioxidant vitamins C and Natural E than the leading multivitamin brand. This product meets USP standards for purity, potency and dissolution. Like all Nature Made products, this product is manufactured to contain no artificial colors, no artificial flavors, no preservatives, no yeast and no gluten.

Each tablet contains: For adults percentage of U.S. Recommended Daily Allowance (U.S.RDA):
[See table below.]

Inactive Ingredients: Cellulose, Glycerides of Fatty Acids, Croscarmellose Sodium, Stearic Acid, Hydroxypropyl Methylcellulose, Magnesium Stearate, Corn Starch, Polyethylene Glycol, Carnauba Wax.

Recommended Intake: Take one tablet daily, with a meal.

Warnings: Keep out of the reach of children.

How Supplied: Oval shaped scored tablet, bottles of 100 plus 30. Store at room temperature.

Shown in Product Identification Guide, page 519

Suggested use: As a dietary supplement, take one tablet daily.

Each Essential Balance tablet contains:	Quantity	% DAILY VALUE
Vitamin A (As Acetate and Beta Carotene)	5000 I.U.	100
Vitamin E (From d-Alpha Tocopheryl Succinate)	**40 I.U.**	**133**
Vitamin C (With Rose Hips)	**120 mg**	**200**
Folic Acid	400 mcg	100
Vitamin B1 (As Thiamine Mononitrate)	1.5 mg	100
Vitamin B2 (Riboflavin)	1.7 mg	100
Niacin (From Niacinamide Ascorbate)	20 mg	100
Vitamin B6 (From Pyridoxine Hydrochloride)	2 mg	100
Vitamin B12 (Cyanocobalamin)	6 mcg	100
Vitamin D	400 I.U.	100
Biotin	30 mcg	10
Pantothenic Acid (From d-Calcium Pantothenate)	10 mg	100
Vitamin K (As Phylloquinone)	25 mcg	*
Calcium (From Dibasic Calcium Phosphate)	100 mg	10
Phosphorus (From Dibasic Calcium Phosphate)	77 mg	8
Iodine (From Kelp and Potassium Iodide)	150 mcg	100
Iron (From Ferrous Fumarate)	18 mg	100
Magnesium (From Magnesium Oxide)	100 mg	25
Copper (From Cupric Oxide)	2 mg	100
Zinc (From Zinc Oxide)	15 mg	100
Manganese (From Manganese Sulfate)	2.5 mg	*
Potassium (From Potassium Chloride)	40 mg	1
Chloride (From Potassium Chloride)	36.3 mg	*
Chromium (From Chromium Chloride)	25 mcg	*
Molybdenum (From Sodium Molybdate)	25 mcg	*
Selenium (From Sodium Selenate)	25 mcg	*
Nickel (From Nickelous Sulfate)	5 mcg	*
Tin (From Stannous Chloride)	10 mcg	*
Silicon (From Sodium Metasilicate & Silicon Dioxide)	2 mg	*
Vanadium (From Sodium Metavanadate)	10 mcg	*
Boron (As Borates)	150 mcg	*

In a base containing Rose Hips-50 mg, Lemon Bioflavonoid Complex-2.5 mg, Rutin-2.5 mg, Hesperidin Complex-2.5 mg.

* DAILY VALUE NOT ESTABLISHED.

PolyMedica Pharmaceuticals (U.S.A.), Inc.
11 STATE STREET
WOBURN, MA 01801

ALCONEFRIN®
Phenylephrine hydrochloride
Nasal Decongestant

How Supplied:
Drops 1 oz., 0.16%, 0.25%, 0.50%
Spray 1 oz., 0.25%

AZO-STANDARD™
Phenazopyridine hydrochloride
Urinary Tract Analgesic Tablets

Description: Each tablet contains phenazopyridine hydrochloride 95mg.

Indication: An analgesic for use as an aid for the prompt temporary relief of minor pain, urgency, frequency and burning of urination.

Directions: Adults: 2 tablets 3 times a day after meals. Use is only recommended for up to 2 days. For children under 12, consult a physician.

Warnings: Do not administer to children under 12 unless directed by a physician. Individuals with any hepatic or renal trouble should not use this product unless directed by a physician. Do not use for more than two days without consulting a physician. If you are pregnant or nursing a baby, seek the advice of a physician before using this product. Keep out of the reach of children. If symptoms persist, consult a physician.
Store at room temperature.

How Supplied: Cartons of 30 tablets.

NEOPAP®
Acetaminophen, 125mg
Analgesic

How Supplied: Pediatric Suppositories, 12's

EDUCATIONAL MATERIAL

An educational brochure is available
Title: "What Every Woman Needs to Know about Urinary Discomfort"
Subject: Urinary discomfort
Description: Educational brochure discussing the causes, symptoms, and possible prevention of urinary discomfort
Size: Height = 8.5 inches, Length = 3.5 inches, 6 panels
Quantity Available: 25 brochures per store; includes one counter top holder
Available to: physicians, pharmacists, consumers
Brochures carry no charge (from requests sent to our office)
No samples available

Premier, Inc.
GREENWICH OFFICE PARK ONE
GREENWICH, CT 06831

EXACT™
[Ex-áct]
Benzoyl Peroxide Acne Medication
Vanishing and Tinted Creams

Vanishing Cream Active Ingredient:
Benzoyl Peroxide 5.0% in a colorless, odorless, and greaseless cream base containing water, acrylates copolymer, glycerin, sorbitol, cetyl alcohol, glyceryl dilaurate, stearyl alcohol, sodium lauryl sulfate, magnesium aluminum silicate, sodium citrate, silica, citric acid, methylparaben, xanthan gum and propylparaben.
Tinted Cream Active Ingredient:
Benzoyl Peroxide 5.0% in a flesh-toned, odorless, and greaseless cream base containing water, acrylates copolymer, glycerin, titanium dioxide, sorbitol, cetyl alcohol, glyceryl dilaurate, stearyl alcohol, sodium lauryl sulfate, magnesium aluminum silicate, sodium citrate, silica, iron oxides, citric acid, methylparaben, xanthan gum and propylparaben.

Indications: For the topical treatment of acne vulgaris.

Actions: Exact Vanishing and Tinted Creams contain 5% benzoyl peroxide. Each product clears existing pimples and helps prevent new pimples from forming.

Additional Benefits: Exact utilizes a patented Microsponge® system to provide prolonged release of benzoyl peroxide to the skin. This special Microsponge formula was designed for low irritancy and to provide 50% higher oil absorbancy than other benzoyl peroxide medications. Exact Tinted Cream is flesh-toned to hide acne pimples while it treats them.

Warning: For external use only. Using other topical acne medications at the same time or immediately following use of this product may increase dryness or irritation of the skin. If this occurs, only one medication should be used unless directed by a doctor. Do not use this medication if you have very sensitive skin or if you are sensitive to benzoyl peroxide. This product may cause irritation, characterized by redness, burning, itching, peeling, or possibly swelling. Mild irritation may be reduced by using the product less frequently or in a lower concentration. If irritation becomes severe, discontinue use; if irritation still continues, consult a doctor. Keep away from eyes, lips, and mouth. This product may bleach hair or dyed fabrics. Store at room temperature. Keep away from flame, fire and heat.
KEEP THIS AND ALL DRUGS OUT OF REACH OF CHILDREN.
In case of accidental ingestion, seek professional assistance or contact a Poison Control Center immediately.

Symptoms and Treatment of Ingestion: These symptoms are based upon medical judgement, not on actual experience. Theoretically, ingestion of very large amounts may cause nausea, vomiting, abdominal discomfort and diarrhea. Treatment is symptomatic, with bed rest and observation.

Directions for Use: Cleanse the skin thoroughly before applying medication. Cover the entire affected area with a thin layer one to three times daily. Because excessive drying of the skin may occur, start with one application daily, then gradually increase to two or three times daily if needed or as directed by a doctor. If bothersome dryness or peeling occurs, reduce application to once a day or every other day.

How Supplied: .65 oz. (18 g) plastic squeeze tubes.

Procter & Gamble
P. O. BOX 5516
CINCINNATI, OH 45201

ALEVE®   OTC
[ə lēv']
Naproxen Sodium Tablets, USP
Pain Reliever/Fever Reducer

Allergy Warning: Do not take this product if you have had either hives or a severe allergic reaction after taking any pain reliever. Even though this product may not contain the same ingredient, ALEVE could cause similar reactions in patients allergic to other pain relieving drugs.

Alcohol Warning: If you generally consume 3 or more alcohol-containing drinks per day, you should consult your physician for advice on when and how you should take ALEVE and other pain relievers.

Active Ingredient: Each [tablet] [caplet] contains naproxen sodium 220 mg (naproxen 200 mg and sodium 20 mg).

Inactive Ingredients: Magnesium Stearate, Microcrystalline Cellulose, Povidone, Talc, Opadry YS-1-4215.

Indications: For the temporary relief of minor aches and pains associated with the common cold, headache, toothache, muscular aches, backache, for the minor pain of arthritis, for the pain of menstrual cramps and for the reduction of fever.

Dosage and Administration:
Adults: Take one [tablet] [caplet] every 8 to 12 hours while symptoms persist. With experience, some people may find that an initial dose of two [tablets] [caplets] followed by one [tablet] [caplet] 12 hours later, if necessary, will give better relief. *Do not exceed three [tablets] [caplets] in 24 hours unless directed to do so by a doctor.* The smallest effective dose should be used. A full glass of water or other liquid is recommended with each dose.
Adults over age 65: Do not take more than one [tablet] [caplet] every 12 hours, unless directed to do so by a doctor.
Children under age 12: Do not give this product to children under 12, except under the advice and supervision of a doctor.

General Warnings: Do not take ALEVE for more than 10 days for pain, or for more than 3 days for fever, unless directed by a doctor.
Consult a doctor if:
*your pain or fever persists or gets worse
*the painful area is red or swollen
*you take any other drugs on a regular basis
*you have had serious side effects from any pain reliever
*you have any new or unusual symptoms
*more than mild heartburn, upset stomach, or stomach pain occurs with use of

Continued on next page

Procter & Gamble—Cont.

this product or if even mild symptoms persist

Although naproxen sodium is indicated for the same conditions as aspirin, ibuprofen and acetaminophen, it should not be taken with them or other naproxen-containing products except under a doctor's direction. As with any drug, if you are pregnant or nursing a baby, seek the advice of a health professional before using this product. IT IS ESPECIALLY IMPORTANT NOT TO USE NAPROXEN SODIUM DURING THE LAST 3 MONTHS OF PREGNANCY UNLESS SPECIFICALLY DIRECTED TO DO SO BY A DOCTOR BECAUSE IT MAY CAUSE PROBLEMS IN THE UNBORN CHILD OR COMPLICATIONS DURING DELIVERY.
KEEP THIS AND ALL DRUGS OUT OF THE REACH OF CHILDREN. In case of accidental overdose, seek professional assistance or contact a poison control center immediately.
If you have questions, comments or problems, call 1-800-395-0689 to report them.

How Supplied: Light blue round tablets or oval-shaped caplets debossed with "ALEVE". Child-resistant "Safety SquEASE" bottles of 24, 50, and 100 tablets or caplets, with fold-out back label on the 24 and 50 count bottles containing important information.

Storage: Store at room temperature (typically 59–85F° or 15–30°C). Avoid excessive heat (104°F or 40°C).

CREST® Sensitivity Protection Toothpaste for sensitive teeth and cavity prevention

Active Ingredients: Potassium Nitrate (5%), Sodium Fluoride (0.15% w/v fluoride ion).

Actions: Builds protection against sensitive tooth pain. Contains **Fluoride** for cavity prevention. Gentle on tooth enamel, leaves teeth feeling clean.
WHAT ARE SENSITIVE TEETH?
If you experience flashes of tooth pain or discomfort from cold or hot foods and drinks, or even when you touch your teeth with your toothbrush, you may suffer from **Dentinal Hypersensitivity** (or "sensitive teeth.") **Hypersensitivity** can occur when dentin, which surrounds the pulp cavity and tooth nerve, is not protected. Dentin can become exposed when gums recede and the protective layer covering the root surface is worn away, leaving dentin exposed. Crest Sensitivity Protection helps relieve the pain of sensitive teeth by soothing the nerves in your teeth when the dentin is exposed.
This product has been given the Seal of Acceptance from the ADA Council on Dental Therapeutics.

Uses: When used regularly, builds increasing protection against painful sensitivity of the teeth to cold, heat, acids,

sweets, or contact, and aids in the prevention of cavities.

Directions: Adults and children 12 years of age and older: Apply at least a 1-inch strip of the product onto a soft bristle toothbrush. Brush teeth thoroughly for at least 1 minute twice a day (morning and evening) or as recommended by a dentist or physician. Make sure to brush all sensitive areas of the teeth. Do not swallow. Children under 12 years of age: ask a dentist or physician.

Warnings: Sensitive teeth may indicate a serious problem that may need prompt care by a dentist. See your dentist if the problem persists or worsens. Do not use this product longer than four weeks unless recommended by a dentist or physician. **Keep this and all drugs out of the reach of children.**

Inactive Ingredients: Water, Hydrated Silica, Glycerin, Sorbitol, Trisodium Phosphate, Sodium Lauryl Sulfate, Cellulose Gum, Xanthan Gum, Flavor, Sodium Saccharin, Titanium Dioxide.

How Supplied: 6.2 OZ (175g), 2.5 OZ (70g) and 1.0 OZ (28g) tubes in cartons.

HEAD & SHOULDERS® INTENSIVE TREATMENT DANDRUFF SHAMPOO

Head & Shoulders Intensive Treatment Dandruff Shampoo offers effective control of persistent dandruff, and beautiful hair from a pleasant-to-use formula. Double-blind and expert-graded testing have proven that Intensive Treatment Dandruff Shampoo reduces persistent dandruff. It is also gentle enough to use every day for clean, manageable hair.

Active Ingredient: 1% selenium sulfide suspended in a mild surfactant base. Shampoo also includes mild conditioning agents.

Indications: For effective control of seborrheic dermatitis and dandruff of the scalp.

Actions: Selenium sulfide is substantive to the scalp and remains after rinsing. Its mechanism is believed to be antiproliferative, and to also control the microorganisms associated with persistent dandruff flaking and itching.

WARNINGS: For external use only. Avoid contact with eyes—if this happens, rinse thoroughly with water. If scalp condition worsens, or does not improve, consult a doctor. Keep out of reach of children.

Caution: If used on light, gray, or chemically treated hair, rinse **VIGOROUSLY** for 5 minutes.

Dosage and Administration: For best results in controlling persistent dandruff, Head & Shoulders Intensive Treatment Dandruff Shampoo should be used regularly. It is gentle enough to use for every shampoo.

Composition: Lotion—Intensive Treatment Regular Formula: Ingredients: Selenium sulfide in a shampoo base of water, ammonium laureth sulfate, ammonium lauryl sulfate, cocamide MEA, glycol distearate, ammonium xylenesulfonate, dimethicone, fragrance, tricetylmonium chloride, cetyl alcohol, DMDM hydantoin, sodium chloride, stearyl alcohol, hydroxypropyl methylcellulose, FD&C Red no. 4.
Lotion—Intensive Treatment 2-in-1 (Persistent Dandruff Shampoo plus Conditioner in One) Formula: Selenium sulfide in a shampoo base of water, ammonium laureth sulfate, ammonium lauryl sulfate, cocamide MEA, glycol distearate, dimethicone, ammonium xylenesulfonate, fragrance, tricetylmonium chloride, cetyl alcohol, DMDM hydantoin, sodium chloride, stearyl alcohol, hydroxypropyl methylcellulose, FD&C Red no. 4.

How Supplied: Intensive Treatment Regular Lotion is available in 7.0 and 11.0 fl. oz. unbreakable plastic bottles. Intensive Treatment 2-in-1 is available in 6.0 and 8.9 fl. oz. unbreakable plastic bottles.

METAMUCIL®
[met 'uh-mū 'sil]
(psyllium hydrophilic mucilloid)

Description: Metamucil is a bulk-forming natural therapeutic fiber for restoring and maintaining regularity as recommended by a physician. It contains hydrophilic mucilloid, a highly efficient dietary fiber derived from the husk of the psyllium seed (*Plantago ovata*). Metamucil contains no chemical stimulants and does not disrupt normal bowel function. Each dose contains approximately 3.4 grams of psyllium hydrophilic mucilloid. Inactive ingredients, sodium, potassium, calories, carbohydrate, fat and phenylalanine content are shown in Table 1 for all forms and flavors. NutraSweet®* brand sweetener (aspartame) is used in flavored sugar-free Metamucil powdered products. Phenylketonurics should be aware that phenylalanine is present in Metamucil products that contain Nutrasweet. Metamucil Sugar-Free Regular Flavor contains no sugar and no artificial sweeteners.
Metamucil in powdered forms is gluten-free. Wafers contain gluten: Apple Crisp contains 0.7 g/dose, Cinnamon Spice contains 0.5 g/dose.

Actions: The active ingredient in Metamucil is psyllium, a natural fiber which promotes elimination due to its bulking effect in the colon. This bulking effect is due to both the water-holding capacity of undigested fiber and the increased bacterial mass following partial fiber digestion. These actions result in enlargement of the lumen of the colon, and softer stool, thereby decreasing intraluminal pressure and straining, and speeding colonic transit in constipated patients.

TABLE 1

Forms/ Flavors	Inactive Ingredients	Sodium mg/ Dose	Potassium mg/ Dose	Calories per Dose	Carbo- hy- drate g/ Dose	Fat g/ Dose	Phenyl- alanine mg/Dose	Dosage 1–3 Times Daily. Each Dose Contains 3.4 g Psyllium Hydrophilic Mucilloid	How Supplied
Smooth Texture Orange Flavor **METAMUCIL** Powder	Citric acid, D&C Yellow No. 10, FD&C Yellow No. 6, Flavoring, Sucrose	<5	30	35	12	—	—	1 rounded tablespoonful 12 g	Canisters: 13, 20.3, and 30.4 ozs. (Doses: 30, 48 and 72); Cartons: 30 single-dose packets (OTC)
Smooth Texture Sugar-Free Orange Flavor **METAMUCIL** Powder	Aspartame, Citric acid, D&C Yellow No. 10, FD&C Yellow No. 6, Flavoring, Maltodextrin	<5	30	10	5	—	25	1 rounded teaspoonful 5.8 g	Canisters: 10, 15 and 23.3 ozs. (Doses: 48, 72 and 114); Cartons: 30 single-dose packets (OTC), 100 single-dose packets (Institutional)
Smooth Texture Citrus Flavor **METAMUCIL** Powder	Citric acid, D&C Yellow No. 10, FD&C Yellow No. 6, Flavoring, Sucrose	<5	40	35	12	—	—	1 rounded tablespoonful 12 g	Canisters: 13, 20.3 and 30.4 ozs. (Doses: 30, 48 and 72); Cartons: 30 single-dose packets (OTC) 100 single-dose packets (Institutional)
Smooth Texture Sugar-Free Citrus Flavor **METAMUCIL** Powder	Aspartame, Citric acid, D&C Yellow No. 10, FD&C Yellow No. 6, Flavoring, Maltodextrin	<5	30	10	5	—	25	1 rounded teaspoonful 5.8 g	Canisters: 10, 15 and 23.3 ozs. (Doses: 48, 72 and 114); Cartons: 30 single-dose packets (OTC)
Smooth Texture Sugar-Free Regular Flavor **METAMUCIL** Powder	Citric acid (less than 1%), Magnesium sulfate**, Maltodextrin	<5	30	10	5	—	—	1 rounded teaspoonful 5.8 g	Canisters: 10, 15 and 23.3 ozs. (Doses: 48, 72 and 114)
Regular Flavor **METAMUCIL** Powder	Dextrose	<5	30	14	6	—	—	1 rounded teaspoonful 7 g	Canisters: 13, 19, and 29 ozs. (Doses: 48, 72 and 114)
Orange Flavor **METAMUCIL** Powder	Citric acid, FD&C Yellow No. 6, Flavoring, Sucrose	<5	35	30	10	—	—	1 rounded tablespoonful 11 g	Canisters: 13, 19 and 29 ozs. (Doses: 30, 48 and 72)
Sugar-Free Lemon-Lime Flavor **METAMUCIL** Effervescent Powder	Aspartame, Calcium carbonate, Citric acid, Flavoring, Potassium bicarbonate, Silicon dioxide, Sodium bicarbonate	10	280	6	4	—	30	1 packet 5.4 g	Cartons: 30 single-dose packets (OTC), 100 single-dose packets (Institutional)
Sugar-Free Orange-Flavor **METAMUCIL** Effervescent Powder	Aspartame, Citric acid, FD&C Yellow No. 6, Flavoring, Potassium bicarbonate, Silicon dioxide, Sodium bicarbonate	5	280	6	4	—	28	1 packet 5.2 g	Cartons: 30 single-dose packets (OTC)

Continued on next page

Procter & Gamble—Cont.

TABLE 1 (continued)

Forms/ Flavors	Inactive Ingredients	Sodium mg/ Dose	Potassium mg/ Dose	Calories per Dose	Carbohydrate g/ Dose	Fat g/ Dose	Phenylalanine mg/Dose	Dosage 1–3 Times Daily. Each Dose Contains 3.4 g Psyllium Hydrophilic Mucilloid	How Supplied
Apple Crisp **METAMUCIL** Wafers	Ascorbic acid, Brown sugar, Cinnamon, Corn oil, Flavors, Fructose, Lecithin, Modified food starch, Molasses, Oat hull fiber, Sodium bicarbonate, Sucrose, Water, Wheat flour	20	50	100	19	5	—	2 wafers 25 g	Cartons: 12 doses; 24 doses
Cinnamon Spice **METAMUCIL** Wafers	Ascorbic acid, Cinnamon, Corn oil, Flavors, Fructose, Lecithin, Modified food starch, Molasses, Nutmeg, Oat hull fiber, Oats, Sodium bicarbonate, Sucrose, Water Wheat flour	15	45	100	18	5	—	2 wafers 25 g	Cartons: 12 doses; 24 doses

*NutraSweet® is a registered trademark of the NutraSweet Company.
**Metamucil Sugar-Free Regular Flavor contains 26 mg of magnesium per dose.

Indications: Metamucil is indicated in the management of chronic constipation, in irritable bowel syndrome, as adjunctive therapy in the constipation of diverticular disease, in the bowel management of patients with hemorrhoids, for constipation associated with convalescence and senility and for occasional constipation during pregnancy when under the care of a physician. Pregnancy: Category B.

Contraindications: Intestinal obstruction, fecal impaction. Known allergy to any component.

Warnings: Patients are advised they should not use the product without consulting a doctor when abdominal pain, nausea, or vomiting are present or if they have noticed a sudden change in bowel habits that persists over a period of 2 weeks, or rectal bleeding. Patients are advised to consult a physician if constipation persists for longer than one week, as this may be a sign of a serious medical condition. **PATIENTS ARE CAUTIONED THAT TAKING THIS PRODUCT WITHOUT ADEQUATE FLUID MAY CAUSE IT TO SWELL AND BLOCK THE THROAT OR ESOPHAGUS AND MAY CAUSE CHOKING. THEY SHOULD NOT TAKE THE PRODUCT IF THEY HAVE DIFFICULTY IN SWALLOWING. IF THEY EXPERIENCE CHEST PAIN, VOMITING, OR DIFFICULTY IN SWALLOWING OR BREATHING AFTER TAKING THIS PRODUCT, THEY ARE ADVISED TO SEEK IMMEDIATE MEDICAL ATTENTION.** Psyllium products may cause allergic reaction in people sensitive to inhaled or ingested psyllium. Keep this and all medications out of the reach of children.

Precaution: *Notice to Health Care Professionals:* To minimize the potential for allergic reaction, health care professionals who frequently dispense powdered psyllium products should avoid inhaling airborne dust while dispensing these products. *Handling and Dispensing:* To minimize generating airborne dust, spoon product from the canister into a glass according to label directions.

Dosage and Administration: The usual adult dosage is 1 rounded teaspoonful or 1 rounded tablespoonful depending on product form. Generally the sugar-free products are dosed by the teaspoonful, sucrose-containing products by the tablespoonful. Some forms are available in packets. The appropriate dose should be mixed with 8 oz. of liquid (e.g. cool water, fruit juice, milk) following the labeled instructions. Metamucil wafers should be consumed with 8 oz. of liquid. **THE PRODUCT (CHILD OR ADULT DOSE) SHOULD BE TAKEN WITH AT LEAST 8 OZ (A FULL GLASS) OF WATER OR OTHER FLUID. TAKING THIS PRODUCT WITHOUT ENOUGH LIQUID MAY CAUSE CHOKING (SEE WARNINGS).** Metamucil can be taken orally one to three times a day, depending on the need and response. It may require continued use for 2 to 3 days to provide optimal benefit. For children (6 to 12 years old), use ½ the adult dose in/with 8 oz. of liquid, 1 to 3 times daily.

New Users: (Label statement) Your doctor can recommend the right dosage of Metamucil to best meet your needs. In general, start by taking one dose each day. Gradually increase to three doses per day, if needed or recommended by your doctor. If minor gas or bloating occurs when you increase doses, try slightly reducing the amount you are taking.

How Supplied: Powder: canisters (OTC) and cartons of single-dose packets (OTC and Institutional). Wafers: cartons of single-dose packets (OTC). (See Table 1).
[See table on preceding page and above.]

OIL OF OLAY®—Daily UV Protectant SPF 15 Beauty Fluid—Original & Fragrance Free Versions (Olay Co., Inc.)

Oil of Olay Daily UV Protectant Beauty Fluid is a light, greaseless lotion that is specially formulated to provide effective moisturization and SPF 15 protection with minimal migration to reduce the likelihood of eye sting. Oil of Olay Daily UV Protectant is PABA free. It is non-comedogenic and is suitable for daily use under facial make-up.

Active Ingredients: Octyl Methoxycinnamate, Phenylbenzimidazole Sulfonic Acid

Inactive Ingredients: Water, Isohexadecane, Butylene Glycol, Triethanolamine, Glycerin, Stearic Acid, Cetyl Alcohol, Cetyl Palmitate, DEA-Cetyl Phosphate, Aluminum Starch Octenylsuccinate, Titanium Dioxide, Imidazolidinyl Urea, Methylparaben, Propylparaben, Carbomer, Acrylates/C10–30 Alkyl Acrylate Crosspolymer, PEG-10 Soya Sterol, Disodium EDTA, Castor Oil, Fragrance, FD&C Red No. 4, FD&C Yellow No. 5.
Available in both lightly scented original version and a 100% color free and fragrance free version.

Indications: Filters out the sun's harmful rays to help prevent skin damage. Provides SPF 15 protection in a light, greaseless moisturizer. Regular use over the years may reduce the chance of skin damage, some types of skin cancer, and other harmful effects due to the sun.

Directions: Adults and children 6 months of age and over: Apply liberally as often as necessary. Children under 6 months of age: Consult a doctor.

WARNINGS: For external use only, not to be swallowed. Avoid contact with the eyes. If contact occurs, rinse eyes thoroughly with water. Discontinue use if signs of irritation or rash appear. If irritation or rash persists, consult a doctor. **KEEP OUT OF REACH OF CHILDREN.**

How Supplied: Available in 3.5 fl. oz. and 5.25 fl. oz. plastic bottles.

PEPTO-BISMOL® ORIGINAL LIQUID AND ORIGINAL AND CHERRY TABLETS AND CAPLETS

For diarrhea, heartburn, indigestion, upset stomach and nausea.

Multi-symptom Pepto-Bismol contains bismuth subsalicylate and is the only leading OTC stomach remedy clinically proven effective for both upper and lower GI symptoms. Pepto-Bismol is in more households than any other stomach remedy, making it a convenient recommendation with a name your patients will know. It has been clinically-proven in double-blind placebo-controlled trials for relief of upset stomach symptoms and diarrhea.

Description: Each tablespoon (15 ml) of Pepto-Bismol Liquid contains 262 mg bismuth subsalicylate. Each tablespoonful of liquid contains a total of 130 mg salicylate. Pepto-Bismol liquid contains no sugar and is very low in sodium (less than 3 mg/tablespoonful). Inactive ingredients: benzoic acid, D&C Red No. 22, D&C Red No. 28, flavor, magnesium aluminum silicate, methylcellulose, saccharin sodium, salicylic acid, sodium salicylate, sorbic acid and water.
Each Pepto-Bismol Tablet contains 262 mg bismuth subsalicylate. Each tablet contains a total of 102 mg salicylate (99 mg salicylate for Cherry). Pepto-Bismol tablets contain no sugar and are very low in sodium (less than 2 mg/tablet). Inactive ingredients include: adipic acid (in Cherry only), calcium carbonate, D&C Red No. 27, FD&C Red No. 40 (in Cherry only), flavors, magnesium stearate, mannitol, povidone, saccharin sodium and talc.
Caplets: Each caplet contains 262 mg bismuth subsalicylate. Each caplet contains a total of 99 mg salicylate. Caplets contain no sugar and are low in sodium (less

than 2 mg/caplet). Inactive ingredients include: calcium carbonate, mannitol, sodium starch glycolate, povidone, magnesium stearate, D&C Red No. 27, silicon dioxide, and polysorbate 80.

Indications: Pepto-Bismol controls diarrhea within 24 hours, relieving associated abdominal cramps; soothes heartburn and indigestion without constipating; and relieves nausea and upset stomach.

Actions: For upset stomach symptoms (i.e. heartburn, indigestion, nausea and fullness caused by over-indulgence), the active ingredient is believed to work via a topical effect on the stomach mucosa. For diarrhea, it is believed to work by several mechanisms in the gastrointestinal tract, including: 1) normalizing fluid movement via an antisecretory mechanism and 2) binding bacterial toxins and antimicrobial activity.

Warnings: Children and teenagers who have or are recovering from chicken pox or flu should not use this medicine to treat nausea or vomiting. If nausea or vomiting is present, patients are advised to consult a doctor because this could be an early sign of Reye's syndrome, a rare but serious illness.
This product contains salicylates. If taken with aspirin and ringing in the ears occurs, discontinue use. This product does not contain aspirin, but should not be administered to those patients who have a known allergy to aspirin or salicylates. Caution is advised in the administration to patients taking medication for anticoagulation, diabetes and gout.
If diarrhea is accompanied by a high fever or continues more than 2 days, patients are advised to consult a physician. As with any drug, caution is advised in the administration to pregnant or nursing women.
Note: This medication may cause a temporary and harmless darkening of the tongue and/or stool. Stool darkening should not be confused with melena.

Overdosage: In case of overdose, patients are advised to contact a physician or Poison Control Center. Emesis induced by ipecac syrup is indicated in large ingestions provided ipecac can be administered within one hour of ingestion. Activated charcoal may be administered after gastric emptying. Patients should be evaluated for signs and symptoms of salicylate toxicity.

Dosage and Administration:
Liquid: Shake well before using.
  Adults—2 tablespoonsful (1 dose cup)
  Children (according to age)—

9–12 yrs.	1 tablespoonful (½ dose cup)
6–9 yrs.	2 teaspoonsful (⅓ dose cup)
3–6 yrs.	1 teaspoonful (⅙ dose cup)

Repeat dosage every ½ to 1 hour, if needed, to a maximum of 8 doses in a 24-hour period. Drink plenty of clear fluids

to help prevent dehydration which may accompany diarrhea.
For children under 3 years of age, consult physician.

Tablets:
  Adults—Two tablets
  Children (according to age)—

9–12 yrs.	1 tablet
6–9 yrs.	⅔ tablet
3–6 yrs.	⅓ tablet

Chew or dissolve in mouth. Repeat every ½ to 1 hour as needed, to a maximum of 8 doses in a 24-hour period. Drink plenty of clear fluids to help prevent dehydration, which may accompany diarrhea.
Caplets:
  Adults—Two caplets
  Children (according to age)—

9–12 yrs.	1 tablet
6–9 yrs.	⅔ tablet
3–6 yrs.	⅓ tablet

Swallow caplet(s) with water, do not chew. Repeat every ½ to 1 hour as needed, to a maximum of 8 doses in a 24-hour period. Drink plenty of clear fluids to help prevent dehydration, which may accompany diarrhea.

How Supplied: Pepto-Bismol Liquid is available in: 4, 8, 12, and 16 fl. oz. bottles. Pepto-Bismol Tablets are pink, round, chewable tablets imprinted with "Pepto-Bismol" on one side. Tablets are available in: boxes of 30 and 48 and roll pack of 12 (cherry only). Caplets are available in: bottles of 24 and 40.

PEPTO-BISMOL®MAXIMUM STRENGTH LIQUID

For diarrhea, heartburn, indigestion, upset stomach and nausea.

Multi-symptom Pepto-Bismol contains bismuth subsalicylate and is the only leading OTC stomach remedy clinically proven effective for both upper and lower GI symptoms. Pepto-Bismol is in more households than any other stomach remedy, making it a convenient recommendation with a name your patients will know. It has been clinically-proven in double-blind placebo-controlled trials for relief of upset stomach symptoms and diarrhea.

Description: Each tablespoonful (15ml) of Maximum Strength Pepto-Bismol Liquid contains 525 mg bismuth subsalicylate (236 mg salicylate). Maximum Strength Pepto-Bismol Liquid contains no sugar and is low in sodium (less than 3 mg/tablespoonful). Inactive ingredients include: benzoic acid, D&C Red No. 22, D&C Red No. 28, flavor, magnesium aluminum silicate, methylcellulose, saccharin sodium, salicylic acid, sodium salicylate, sorbic acid, and water.

Indications: Maximum Strength Pepto-Bismol controls diarrhea within 24

Continued on next page

Procter & Gamble—Cont.

hours, relieving associated abdominal cramps; soothes heartburn and indigestion without constipating; and relieves nausea and upset stomach.

Actions: For upset stomach symptoms (i.e. heartburn, indigestion, nausea and fullness caused by over-indulgence), the active ingredient is believed to work via a topical effect on the stomach mucosa. For diarrhea, it is believed to work by several mechanisms in the gastro-intestinal tract, including: 1) by normalizing fluid movement via an antisecretory mechanism and 2) by binding bacterial toxins and antimicrobial activity.

Warnings: Children and teenagers who have or are recovering from chicken pox or flu should NOT use this medicine to treat nausea or vomiting. If nausea or vomiting is present, patients are advised to consult a doctor because this could be an early sign of Reye Syndrome, a rare but serious illness.
This product contains salicylates. If taken with aspirin and ringing in the ears occurs, discontinue use. This product does not contain aspirin, but should not be administered to those patients who have a known allergy to aspirin or salicylates. Caution is advised in the administration to patients taking medication for anticoagulation, diabetes and gout.
If diarrhea is accompanied by a high fever or continues more than 2 days, patients are advised to consult a physician. As with any drug, caution is advised in the administration to pregnant or nursing women.

Note: This medication may cause a temporary and harmless darkening of the tongue and/or stool. Stool darkening should not be confused with melena.

Overdosage: In case of overdose, patients are advised to contact a physician or Poison Control Center. Emesis induced by ipecac syrup is indicated in large ingestions provided ipecac can be administered within one hour of ingestion. Activated charcoal should be administered after gastric emptying. Patients should be evaluated for signs and symptoms of salicylate toxicity.

Dosage and Administration: Shake well before using.

Adults—2 tablespoonfuls (1 dose cup)
Children (according to age)—

9–12 yrs.	1 tablespoonful (½ dose cup)	
6–9 yrs.	2 teaspoonfuls (⅓ dose cup)	
3–6 yrs.	1 teaspoonful (⅙ dose cup)	

Repeat dosage every hour, if needed, to a maximum of 4 doses in a 24-hour period. Drink plenty of clear fluids to help prevent dehydration, which may accompany diarrhea.

How Supplied: Maximum Strength Pepto-Bismol is available in:

4 fl. oz. bottle
8 fl. oz. bottle
12 fl. oz. bottle

PEPTO DIARRHEA CONTROL®
Loperamide Hydrochloride Oral Solution & Caplets

Description: Each 5 ml (teaspoon) of Pepto Diarrhea Control liquid contains Loperamide Hydrochloride 1 mg. Pepto Diarrhea Control is a non-chalky, cherry flavored, clear liquid. Each caplet of Pepto Diarrhea Control contains 2 mg of Loperamide Hydrochloride and is scored and colored white.

Actions: Pepto Diarrhea Control contains a clinically proven antidiarrheal medication, Loperamide Hydrochloride, that works in many cases with just one dose. Loperamide Hydrochloride acts by slowing intestinal motility and by affecting water and electrolyte movement through the bowel.

Indication: Pepto Diarrhea Control controls the symptoms of diarrhea.

Directions: A dose cup is provided to accurately measure liquid doses as noted below. Drink plenty of clear fluids to help prevent dehydration, which may accompany diarrhea.

Usual Dosage: Adults and children 12 years of age and older: Take four teaspoonfuls or two caplets after first loose bowel movement followed by two teaspoonfuls or one caplet after each subsequent loose bowel movement but not more than eight teaspoonfuls or four caplets a day for no more than two days. Children 9–11 years old (60–95 lbs.): Two teaspoonfuls or one caplet after first loose bowel movement, followed by one teaspoonful or one-half caplet after each subsequent loose bowel movement. Do not exceed six teaspoonfuls or three caplets a day for no more than two days. Children 6–8 years old (48–59 lbs.): Two teaspoonfuls or one caplet after first loose bowel movement, followed by one teaspoonful or one-half caplet after each subsequent loose bowel movement. Do not exceed four teaspoonfuls or two caplets a day for no more than two days. Professional Dosage Schedule for children 2–5 years old (24–47 lbs.): One teaspoon after first loose bowel movement, followed by one after each subsequent loose bowel movement. Do not exceed three teaspoonfuls a day.

Warnings: DO NOT USE FOR MORE THAN TWO DAYS UNLESS DIRECTED BY A PHYSICIAN. Do not use if diarrhea is accompanied by high fever (greater than 101°F), or if blood is present in the stool, or if you have had a rash or other allergic reaction to Loperamide Hydrochloride. If you are taking antibiotics or have a history of liver disease, consult a physician before using this product. As with any drug, if you are pregnant or nursing a baby, seek the ad-

vice of a health professional before using this product. Keep this and all drugs out of the reach of children. In case of accidental overdose, seek professional assistance or contact a poison control center immediately. Store at room temperature.

Overdosage: Overdosage of Loperamide Hydrochloride in man may result in constipation, CNS depression and nausea. A slurry of activated charcoal administered promptly after ingestion of Loperamide Hydrochloride can reduce the amount of drug which is absorbed. If vomiting occurs spontaneously upon ingestion, a slurry of 100 grams of activated charcoal should be administered orally as soon as fluids can be retained. If vomiting has not occurred, and CNS depression is evident, gastric lavage should be performed followed by administration of 100 gms of the activated charcoal slurry through the gastric tube. In the event of overdosage, patients should be monitored for signs of CNS depression for at least 24 hours. Children may be more sensitive to central nervous system effects than adults. If CNS depression is observed, naloxone may be administered. If responsive to naloxone, vital signs must be monitored carefully for recurrence of symptoms of drug overdose for at least 24 hours after the last dose of naloxone.

Inactive Ingredients: Liquid: Alcohol (5.25%), citric acid, flavors, glycerin, methylparaben, propylparaben and purified water.
Caplets: Corn starch, lactose, magnesium stearate, microcrystalline cellulose.

How Supplied: Cherry flavored liquid (clear) 2 fl. oz. and 4 fl. oz. tamper resistant bottles with child resistant safety caps and special dosage cups. White scored caplets in 6's, 12's and 18's blister packaging which is tamper resistant and child resistant.

PERCOGESIC®
[pĕr′kō-jē′zĭk]
Analgesic Tablets
Pain Reliever/Fever Reducer

Active Ingredients: Each tablet contains:
Acetaminophen .... 325 mg
Phenyltoloxamine citrate .... 30 mg

Inactive Ingredients: Cellulose, FD&C Yellow No. 6, Flavor, Hydroxypropyl Methylcellulose, Magnesium Stearate, Polyethylene Glycol, Povidone, Silica Gel, Starch, Stearic Acid, Sucrose.

Indications: For temporary relief of minor aches and pains associated with headaches, muscular aches, backaches, premenstrual and menstrual periods, colds, the flu, toothaches, as well as for minor pain from arthritis, and to reduce fever.

Dosage and Administration: Adults (12 years and over)—1 or 2 tablets every four hours. Maximum daily dose—8 tablets.

Children (6 to under 12 years)—1 tablet every 4 hours. Maximum daily dose—4 tablets.

Children under 6 years of age: consult a doctor.

Warnings: Do not take this product for pain for more than 10 days (adults) or 5 days (children), and do not take for fever for more than 3 days unless directed by a doctor. If pain or fever persists or worsens, new symptoms occur or redness or swelling is present, consult a doctor as these could be signs of a serious condition. Do not give to children for arthritis pain unless directed by a doctor. May cause excitability especially in children. Do not take this product if you have asthma, glaucoma, emphysema, chronic pulmonary disease, shortness of breath, or difficulty in breathing unless directed by a doctor. May cause drowsiness; alcohol, sedatives, and tranquilizers may increase the drowsiness effect. Avoid alcoholic beverages while taking this product. Do not take this product if you are taking sedatives or tranquilizers without first consulting your doctor. Use caution when driving a motor vehicle or operating machinery. **KEEP THIS AND ALL DRUGS OUT OF THE REACH OF CHILDREN.** In case of accidental overdose, seek professional assistance or contact a poison control center immediately. Prompt medical attention is critical for adults as well as for children even if you do not notice any signs or symptoms. As with any drug, if you are pregnant or nursing a baby, seek the advice of a health professional before using this product.

How Supplied: Light orange tablets engraved with "Percogesic". Child-resistant bottles of 24 and 90 tablets, and non-child-resistant bottles of 50 tablets.

VICKS® 44 DRY HACKING COUGH
Dextromethorphan HBr/ Cough Suppressant

Active Ingredient per 2 tsp. (10 mL): Dextromethorphan Hydrobromide 30 mg

Inactive Ingredients: Alcohol 10%, Caramel, Carboxymethylcellulose Sodium, Citric Acid, FD&C Red No. 40, Flavor, Invert Sugar, Propylene Glycol, Purified Water, Sodium Citrate.

Indications: VICKS® 44 provides temporary relief of coughs due to minor throat and bronchial irritation associated with a cold.

Actions: VICKS® 44 is a cough suppressant.

Directions:
Adults and Children 12 years of age and over: 2 teaspoons

Children under 12 years of age: consult a doctor.

Repeat every 6–8 hours. No more than 4 doses per day or as directed by doctor.

WARNINGS: A persistent cough may be a sign of a serious condition. If cough persists for more than 1 week, tends to recur, or is accompanied by fever, rash, or persistent headache, consult a doctor. Do not take this product for persistent or chronic cough such as occurs with smoking, asthma, emphysema, or if cough is accompanied by excessive phlegm (mucus) unless directed by a doctor. *Drug Interaction Precaution:* Do not use this product if you are now taking a prescription monoamine oxidase inhibitor (MAOI) (certain drugs for depression, psychiatric or emotional conditions, or Parkinson's disease), or for two weeks after stopping the MAOI drug. If you are uncertain whether your prescription drug contains an MAOI, consult a health professional before taking this product. **Keep this and all drugs out of the reach of children.** In case of accidental overdose, seek professional assistance or contact a poison control center immediately. As with any drug, if you are pregnant or nursing a baby, seek the advice of a health professional before using this product.

How Supplied: Available in 4 FL. OZ. (118 mL) squeeze bottles with Vicks® AccuTip® Dispenser for accurate, easy dosing.

VICKS® 44D DRY HACKING COUGH & HEAD CONGESTION
Cough Suppressant/ Nasal Decongestant

Active Ingredients per 3 tsp. (15 mL): Dextromethorphan Hydrobromide 30 mg, Pseudoephedrine Hydrochloride 60 mg.

Inactive Ingredients: Alcohol 10%, Citric Acid, FD&C Red No. 40, Flavor, Glycerin, Propylene Glycol, Purified Water, Saccharin Sodium, Sodium Citrate, Sucrose.

Indications: VICKS® 44D provides temporary relief of coughs and nasal congestion due to a common cold.

Actions: VICKS® 44D is a cough suppressant and a nasal decongestant.

Dosage Directions: Adults and children 12 years of age and older: 3 teaspoons

Children under 12 years of age: consult a doctor.

Repeat every 6 hours. No more than 4 doses per day or as directed by a doctor.

WARNINGS: A persistent cough may be a sign of a serious condition. If cough persists for more than 1 week, tends to recur, or is accompanied by fever, rash, or persistent headache, consult a doctor. Do not take this product for persistent or chronic cough such as occurs with smoking, asthma, emphysema, or if cough is accompanied by excessive phlegm (mucus) unless directed by a doctor. Do not

exceed recommended dosage because at higher doses nervousness, dizziness, or sleeplessness may occur. Do not take this product for more than 7 days. If symptoms do not improve or are accompanied by fever, consult a doctor. Do not take this product if you have heart disease, high blood pressure, thyroid disease, diabetes, or difficulty in urination due to enlargement of the prostate gland unless directed by a doctor. *Drug Interaction Precaution:* Do not use this product if you are now taking a prescription monoamine oxidase inhibitor (MAOI) (certain drugs for depression, psychiatric or emotional conditions, or Parkinson's disease), or for two weeks after stopping the MAOI drug. If you are uncertain whether your prescription drug contains an MAOI, consult a health professional before taking this product. **Keep this and all drugs out of the reach of children.** In case of accidental overdose, seek professional assistance or contact a poison control center immediately. As with any drug, if you are pregnant or nursing a baby, seek the advice of a health professional before using this product.

How Supplied: Available in 4 FL. OZ. (118 mL) and 8 FL. OZ. (236 mL) squeeze bottles with Vicks® AccuTip® Dispenser for accurate, easy dosing.

VICKS® 44 LIQUICAPS® COUGH, COLD & FLU RELIEF
Cough Suppressant ● Nasal Decongestant ● Antihistamine ● Pain Reliever/Fever Reducer

Active Ingredient (per softgel): Dextromethorphan Hydrobromide 10 mg, Pseudoephedrine Hydrochloride 30 mg, Chlorpheniramine Maleate 2 mg, Acetaminophen 250 mg.

Inactive Ingredients: D&C Red No. 33 Lake, FD&C Blue No. 1 Lake, Gelatin, Glycerin, Polyethylene Glycol, Povidone, Propylene Glycol, Purified Water, Edible Ink.

Indications: Vicks® 44 LiquiCaps® Cough, Cold & Flu Relief provides temporary relief of coughing, nasal congestion, runny nose and sneezing due to a cold. Also for temporary relief of headache, fever, muscular aches and sore throat pain due to a cold or flu.

Directions: Adults and Children 12 years and older: Swallow 2 softgels with water.
Children (6 to under 12 years): Swallow 1 softgel with water. Do not chew. Repeat every 4 hours not to exceed 4 doses per day. Not recommended for children under 6 years.

WARNINGS: Do not take this product for persistent or chronic cough such as occurs with smoking, asthma, emphysema, or if cough is accompanied by excessive phlegm (mucus) unless directed

Continued on next page

Procter & Gamble—Cont.

by a doctor. Do not exceed recommended dosage because at higher doses nervousness, dizziness, or sleeplessness may occur. Do not take this product if you have heart disease, high blood pressure, thyroid disorder, diabetes, glaucoma, or difficulty in urination due to enlargement of the prostate gland unless directed by a doctor. *Drug Interaction Precaution:* Do not use this product if you are now taking a prescription monoamine oxidase inhibitor (MAOI) (certin drugs for depression, psychiatric or emotional conditions, or Parkinson's disease), or for take two weeks after stopping the MAOI drug. If you are uncertain whether your prescription drug contains an MAOI, consult a health professional before taking this product. May cause excitability especially in children. Do not take this product, unless directed by a doctor, if you have a breathing problem such as emphysema or chronic bronchitis. May cause marked drowsiness; alcohol, sedatives and tranquilizers may increase the drowsiness effect. Avoid alcoholic beverages while taking this product. Do not take this product if you are taking sedatives or tranquilizers, without first consulting your doctor. Use caution when driving a motor vehicle or operating machinery. Do not take this product for more than 7 days (for adults) or 5 days (for children). A persistent cough may be a sign of a serious condition. If cough persists for more than 7 days, tends to recur, or is accompanied by rash, or persistent headache, fever that lasts for more than three days or if new symptoms occur, consult a doctor. If sore throat is severe, persists for more than 2 days, is accompanied or followed by fever, headache, rash, nausea, or vomiting, consult a doctor promptly. **Keep this and all drugs out of the reach of children.** In case of accidental overdose, seek professional assistance or contact a poison control center immediately. Prompt medical attention is critical for adults as well as for children even if you do not notice any signs or symptoms. As with any drug, if you are pregnant or nursing a baby, seek the advice of a health professional before using this product.

How Supplied: Available in 12-count child-resistant blister packages. Each blue liquicap is imprinted: "44".

VICKS® 44
LIQUICAPS®NON-DROWSY COUGH & COLD RELIEF
Cough Suppressant/ Nasal Decongestant

Active Ingredient (per softgel): Dextromethorphan Hydrobromide 30 mg, Pseudoephedrine Hydrochloride 60 mg.

Inactive Ingredients: D&C Red No. 33, FD&C Blue No. 1, FD&C Red No. 40, Gelatin, Glycerin, Polyethylene Glycol, Povidone, Purified Water, Sorbitol, Edible Ink.

Indications: VICKS® 44 LiquiCaps® Non-Drowsy Cough & Cold Relief provides for the temporary relief of coughs and nasal congestion due to the common cold.

Directions: Adults and children 12 years of age and over: Swallow 1 softgel with water. Do not chew. Repeat every 6 hours, not to exceed 4 softgels per day. Not recommended for children under 12.

WARNINGS: A persistent cough may be a sign of a serious condition. If cough persists for more than 1 week, tends to recur, or is accompanied by fever, rash, or persistent or chronic headache, consult a doctor. Do not take this product for persistent or chronic cough such as occurs with smoking, asthma, emphysema, or if cough is accompanied by excessive phlegm (mucus) unless directed by a doctor. Do not exceed recommended dosage because at higher doses nervousness, dizziness, or sleeplessness may occur. Do not take this product for more than 7 days. If symptoms do not improve or are accompanied by fever, consult a doctor. Do not take this product if you have heart disease, high blood pressures, thyroid disease, diabetes, or difficulty; in urination due to enlargement of the prostate gland. *Drug Interaction Precaution:* Do not use this product if you are now taking a prescription monoamine oxidase inhibitor (MAOI) (certain drugs for depression, psychiatric or emotional conditions, or Parkinson's disease), or for 2 weeks after stopping the MAOI drug. If you are uncertain whether your prescription drug contains an MAOI, consult a health professional before taking this product. **Keep this and all drugs out of the reach of children.** In case of accidental overdose, seek professional assistance or contact a poison control center immediately. As with any drug, if you are pregnant or nursing a baby, seek the advice of a health professional before using this product.

How Supplied: Available in 10 count blister packages. Each red softgel is imprinted "44".

VICKS® 44E
Chest Cough & Chest Congestion
Cough Suppressant/Expectorant

Active Ingredients: per 3 teaspoons (15 mL): Dextromethorphan Hydrobromide 20 mg, Guaifenesin 200 mg

Inactive Ingredients: Alcohol 10%, Citric Acid, FD&C Blue No. 1, FD&C Red No. 40, Flavor, Glycerin, Propylene Glycol, Purified Water, Saccharin Sodium, Sodium Citrate, Sucrose.

Indications: VICKS® 44E provides temporary relief of coughs due to the common cold and helps loosen phlegm to rid the bronchial passageways of bothersome mucus.

Actions: VICKS® 44E is a cough suppressant and expectorant.

Directions: Adults and Children 12 years of age and over: 3 teaspoons Children under 12 years of age: consult a doctor.
Repeat every 4 hours. No more than 6 doses per day, or as directed by a doctor.

WARNINGS: A persistent cough may be a sign of a serious condition. If cough persists for more than 1 week, tends to recur, or is accompanied by fever, rash, or persistent headache, consult a doctor. Do not take this product for persistent or chronic cough such as occurs with smoking, asthma, chronic bronchitis, or emphysema, or if cough is accompanied by excessive phlegm (mucus) unless directed by a doctor. *Drug Interaction Precaution:* Do not use this product if you are now taking a prescription monoamine oxidase inhibitor (MAOI) (certain drugs for depression, psychiatric or emotional conditions, or Parkinson's disease), or for two weeks after stopping the MAOI drug. If you are uncertain whether your prescription drug contains an MAOI, consult a health professional before taking this product. **Keep this and all drugs out of the reach of children.** In case of accidental overdose, seek professional assistance or contact a poison control center immediately. As with any drug, if you are pregnant or nursing a baby, seek the advice of a health professional before using this product.

How Supplied: Available in 4 FL. OZ. (118 mL) and 8 FL. OZ. (236 mL) squeeze bottles with Vicks AccuTip® Dispenser for accurate, easy dosing.

VICKS® 44M
COUGH, COLD & FLU RELIEF
Cough Suppressant/Nasal Decongestant/Antihistamine/ Pain Reliever–Fever Reducer

Active Ingredients: per 4 tsp. (20 mL): Dextromethorphan Hydrobromide 30 mg, Pseudoephedrine Hydrochloride 60 mg, Chlorpheniramine Maleate 4 mg, Acetaminophen 650 mg

Inactive Ingredients: Alcohol 10%, Citric Acid, FD&C Blue No. 1, FD&C Red No. 40, Flavor, Glycerin, Purified Water, Saccharin Sodium, Sodium Benzoate, Sodium Citrate, Sorbitol, and Sucrose.

Indications: VICKS® 44M provides temporary relief of coughing, nasal congestion, runny nose, and sneezing due to a cold. Also for temporary relief of headache, fever, muscular aches and sore throat due to a cold or flu.

Actions: VICKS® 44M is a cough suppressant, nasal decongestant, antihistamine and analgesic.

Directions: Adults and children 12 years of age and older:
fill cup to top line or 4 teaspoons

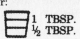
1 TBSP.
½ TBSP.

Repeat every 6 hours. No more than 4 doses per day or as directed by a doctor. Children under 12 years of age: consult a doctor.

WARNINGS: Do not take this product for persistent or chronic cough such as occurs with smoking, asthma, or emphysema, or if cough is accompanied by excessive phlegm (mucus) unless directed by a doctor. Do not exceed recommended dosage because at higher doses nervousness, dizziness, or sleeplessness may occur. Do not take this product if you have heart disease, high blood pressure, thyroid disease, diabetes, glaucoma, or difficulty in urination due to enlargement of the prostate gland unless directed by a doctor. *Drug Interaction Precaution:* Do not use this product if you are now taking a prescription monoamine oxidase inhibitor (MAOI) (certain drugs for depression, psychiatric or emotional conditions, or Parkinson's disease), or for two weeks after stopping the MAOI drug. If you are uncertain whether your prescription drug contains an MAOI, consult a health professional before taking this product. May cause excitability especially in children. Do not take this product, unless directed by a doctor, if you have a breathing problem such as emphysema or chronic bronchitis. May cause marked drowsiness; alcohol, sedatives, and tranquilizers may increase the drowsiness effect. Avoid alcoholic beverages while taking this product. Do not take this product if you are taking sedatives or tranquilizers, without first consulting your doctor. Use caution when driving a motor vehicle or operating machinery. Do not take this product for more than 7 days. A persistent cough may be a sign of a serious condition. If cough persists for more than 7 days, tends to recur, or is accompanied by rash, persistent headache, fever that lasts for more than 3 days, or if new symptoms occur, consult a doctor. If symptoms do not improve or are accompanied by fever that lasts for more than 3 days, or if new symptoms occur, consult a doctor. If sore throat is severe, persists for more than 2 days, is accompanied or followed by fever, headache, rash, nausea or vomiting, consult a doctor. **Keep this and all drugs out of the reach of children.** In case of accidental overdose, seek professional assistance or contact a poison control center immediately. Prompt medical attention is critical for adults as well as for children, even if you do not notice any signs or symptoms. As with any drug, if you are pregnant or nursing a baby, seek the advice of a health professional before using this product.

How Supplied: Available in 4 FL. OZ. (118 mL) and 8 FL. OZ. (236 mL) squeeze bottles with Vicks® AccuTip® Dis-

penser for accurate, easy dosing. A calibrated dose cup accompanies each bottle.

**CHILDREN'S VICKS®
CHLORASEPTIC®
SORE THROAT LOZENGES
Benzocaine/Oral Anesthetic
(Grape Flavor)**

Active Ingredient: Benzocaine 5 mg per lozenge.

Inactive Ingredients: Corn syrup, FD&C Blue No. 1, FD&C Red No. 40, flavor, and sucrose.

Indications: For temporary relief of occasional minor mouth irritation and pain, sore mouth and sore throat. Also for pain associated with canker sores.

Directions: Adults and children 2 years of age and older: Allow 1 lozenge to dissolve slowly in mouth. May be repeated every 2 hours as needed or as directed by a physician or dentist. Children under 2 years of age: Consult a physician or a dentist.

WARNINGS: If sore throat is severe, or is accompanied by difficulty in breathing, or persists for more than two days, do not use, and consult a doctor promptly. If sore throat is accompanied or followed by fever, headache, rash, swelling, nausea, or vomiting, consult a doctor promptly. If sore mouth symptoms do not improve in 7 days, or if irritation, pain, or redness persists or worsens, see your doctor promptly. Do not use this product if you have a history of allergy to local anesthetics such as procaine, butacaine, benzocaine, or other "caine" anesthetics. **Keep this and all drugs out of the reach of children.** In case of accidental overdose seek professional assistance or contact a poison control center immediately. As with any drug, if you are pregnant or nursing a baby, seek the advice of a health professional before using this product.

How Supplied: Cartons of 18. Each purple lozenge is debosed with "CC".

**CHILDREN'S VICKS®
CHLORASEPTIC®
SORE THROAT SPRAY
Phenol/Oral
Anesthetic/Antiseptic**

Children's Chloraseptic® is specially formulated with a reduced concentration of phenol, the active ingredient in Chloraseptic®, to provide fast, effective relief in a great-tasting grape flavor your child will like.

Active Ingredient: Phenol 0.5%

Inactive Ingredients: FD&C Blue No. 1, FD&C Red No. 40, flavor, glycerin, purified water, saccharin sodium, and sorbitol.

Indications: For temporary relief of occasional minor sore throat pain and sore mouth. Also, for temporary relief of pain due to canker sores, minor irritation or injury of the mouth and gums, minor dental procedures, or orthodontic appliances.

Directions—Children 2 Years of Age and Older: Spray 5 times directly into throat or affected area and swallow. Repeat every two hours or as directed by a physician or dentist. Children under 12 years of age should be supervised in product use.

Children Under 2 Years of Age: Consult a physician or dentist.

WARNINGS: If sore throat is severe, or is accompanied by difficulty in breathing, or persists for more than 2 days, do not use, and consult a doctor promptly. If sore throat is accompanied or followed by fever, headache, rash, swelling, nausea or vomiting, consult a doctor promptly. If sore mouth symptoms do not improve in 7 days, or if irritation, pain, or redness persists or worsens, see your doctor promptly. **Keep this and all drugs out of the reach of children.** In case of accidental overdose, seek professional assistance or contact a poison control center immediately. As with any drug, if you are pregnant or nursing a baby, seek the advice of a health professional before using this product.

How Supplied: Available in 6 FL. OZ. (177 mL) plastic bottles with sprayer.

**CHILDREN'S VICKS® DAYQUIL®
ALLERGY RELIEF
Antihistamine/Nasal Decongestant**

Children's Vicks® DayQuil® Allergy Relief was specially formulated with two effective ingredients to relieve allergy symptoms and head colds without coughs.

Active Ingredients per ½ FL. OZ., Dose (1 TBSP): Chlorpheniramine Maleate 2 mg, Pseudoephedrine HCl 30 mg.

Inactive Ingredients: Citric Acid, FD&C Blue No. 1, FD&C Red No. 40, Flavor, Methylparaben, Potassium Sorbate, Propylene Glycol, Purified Water, Sodium Citrate, Sorbitol and Sucrose.

Indications: For temporary relief of nasal and sinus congestion, sneezing, runny nose, and itchy, watery eyes due to hay fever or other upper respiratory allergies.

Directions: Take as directed. Use medicine cup provided. A total of 4 doses may be given per day, each 6 hours apart, or use as directed by a doctor.

Continued on next page

Procter & Gamble—Cont.

Age	Weight	Dose
Under 6 yrs	Under 48 lbs.	Consult physician*
6–11 yrs	48–95 lbs.	1 TABLESPOON (TBSP.)
12 yrs and older	96 lbs. and over	2 TABLESPOONS (TBSP.)

*Professional Labeling:** Children under 6 years of age: Use only as directed by a physician. Suggested doses for children under 6 years of age:

Age	Weight	Dose
*6–11 mo.	17–21 lbs.	1 teaspoon (tsp.) (5 mL)
*12–23 mo.	22–27 lbs.	1¼ teaspoon (tsp.) (6.25 mL)
2–5 yrs.	28–47 lbs.	½ TABLE-SPOON (TBSP.) (7.5 mL)

Repeat every 6 hours, not to exceed 4 doses in 24 hours, or as directed by doctor.
*Based on extrapolation from studies on the safety and efficacy of active ingredients conducted among older children and adults. Use caution in treating children under 2 years of age who were born prematurely.

WARNINGS: Do not exceed recommended dosage, because at higher doses nervousness, dizziness or sleeplessness may occur. Do not take this product for more than 7 days. If symptoms do not improve or are accompanied by fever, consult a doctor. Do not take this product if you have heart disease, high blood pressure, thyroid disease, diabetes, glaucoma, or difficulty in urination due to enlargement of the prostate gland unless directed by a doctor. *Drug Interaction Precaution:* Do not use this product if you are now taking a prescription monoamine oxidase inhibitor (MAOI) (certain drugs for depression, psychiatric or emotional conditions, or Parkinson's disease), or for two weeks after stopping the MAOI drug. If you are uncertain whether your prescription drug contains an MAOI, consult a health professional before taking this product. May cause excitability especially in children. Do not take this product, unless directed by a doctor, if you have a breathing problem such as emphysema or chronic bronchitis. May cause drowsiness; alcohol, sedatives, and tranquilizers may increase the drowsiness effect. Avoid alcoholic beverages while taking this product. Do not take this product if you are taking sedatives or tranquilizers, without first consulting your doctor. Use caution when driving a motor vehicle or operating machinery. **Keep this and all drugs out of the reach of children.** In case of acci-

dental overdose, seek professional assistance or contact a poison control center immediately. As with any drug, if you are pregnant or nursing a baby, seek the advice of a health professional before using this product.

How Supplied: Available in 4 FL. OZ. (118 mL) plastic bottles with child-resistant, tamper-evident cap and a calibrated medicine cup.

CHILDREN'S VICKS® NYQUIL® COLD/COUGH RELIEF
Antihistamine/Nasal Decongestant/Cough Suppressant

Children's NyQuil® was specially formulated with three effective ingredients to relieve nighttime cough, nasal congestion, and runny nose so children can rest. Children's NyQuil® is alcohol free and analgesic free and has a pleasant cherry flavor.

Active Ingredients: Per 1 TBSP.: Chlorpheniramine Maleate 2 mg, Pseudoephedrine HCl 30 mg, Dextromethorphan Hydrobromide 15 mg.

Inactive Ingredients: Citric Acid, FD&C Red No. 40, Flavor, Potassium Sorbate, Propylene Glycol, Purified Water, Sodium Citrate, Sucrose.

Indications: For temporary relief of nasal congestion, runny nose, sneezing, and coughing due to a cold, so your child can rest.

Directions: Take at bedtime as directed. Use medicine cup provided. If cold symptoms keep your child at home, 4 doses may be given per day, each 6 hours apart, or use as directed by a doctor.

| | 1 TBSP. |
| | ½ TBSP. |

Age	Weight	Dose
Under 6 yrs	Under 48 lbs.	Consult physician*
6–11 yrs	48–95 lbs.	1 TABLESPOON (TBSP.)
12 yrs and older	96 lbs. and over	2 TABLESPOONS (TBSP.)

*Professional Labeling:** Children under 6 years of age: Use only as directed by a physician. Suggested doses for children under 6 years of age:

Age	Weight	Dose
*6–11 mo.	17–21 lbs.	1 teaspoon (tsp.) (5 mL)
*12–23 mo.	22–27 lbs.	1¼ teaspoon (tsp.) (6.25 mL)
2–5 yrs.	28–47 lbs.	½ TABLE-SPOON (TBSP.) (7.5 mL)

Repeat every 6 hours, not to exceed 4 doses in 24 hours, or as directed by doctor.

* Based on extrapolation from studies on the safety and efficacy of active ingredients conducted among older children and adults. Use caution in treating children under 2 years of age who were born prematurely.

WARNINGS: Do not exceed recommended dosage because at higher doses nervousness, dizziness, or sleeplessness may occur. Do not take this product for more than 7 days. If symptoms do not improve or are accompanied by fever, consult a doctor. Do not take this product if you have heart disease, high blood pressure, thyroid disease, diabetes, glaucoma, or difficulty in urination due to enlargement of the prostate gland unless directed by a doctor. *Drug Interaction Precaution:* Do not use this product if you are now taking a prescription monoamine oxidase inhibitor (MAOI) (certain drugs for depression, psychiatric or emotional conditions, or Parkinson's disease), or for two weeks after stopping the MAOI drug. If you are uncertain whether your prescription drug contains an MAOI, consult a health professional before taking this product. May cause excitability especially in children. Do not take this product, unless directed by a doctor, if you have a breathing problem such as emphysema or chronic bronchitis. May cause marked drowsiness; alcohol, sedatives, and tranquilizers may increase the drowsiness effect. Avoid alcoholic beverages while taking this product. Do not take this product if you are taking sedatives or tranquilizers, without first consulting your doctor. Use caution when driving a motor vehicle or operating machinery. A persistent cough may be a sign of a serious condition. If cough persists for more than 1 week, tends to recur, or is accompanied by fever, rash, or persistent headache, consult a doctor. Do not take this product for persistent or chronic cough such as occurs with smoking, asthma, emphysema, or if cough is accompanied by excessive phlegm (mucus) unless directed by a doctor.

Keep this and all drugs out of the reach of children. In case of accidental overdose, seek professional assistance or contact a poison control center immediately. As with any drug, if you are pregnant or nursing a baby, seek the advice of a health professional before using this product.

How Supplied: Available in 4 FL. OZ. (118 mL) bottles with child-resistant, tamper-evident cap and a calibrated medicine cup.

VICKS® CHLORASEPTIC® COUGH & THROAT DROPS
Menthol Cough Suppressant/Oral Anesthetic

Flavors: Available in Menthol, Cherry, and Honey Lemon flavors.

Active Ingredients: Menthol Flavor: Menthol 8.4 mg, Cherry and Honey Lemon: Menthol 10 mg.

Inactive Ingredients: Menthol Flavor: Corn Syrup, FD&C Blue No. 1, Flavor, Sucrose. Cherry Flavor: Corn Syrup, FD&C Blue No. 2, FD&C Red No. 40, Flavor, Sucrose. Honey Lemon: Citric Acid, Corn Syrup, D&C Yellow No. 10, FD&C Yellow No. 6, Flavor, Sucrose.

Indications: Temporarily relieves sore throat and coughs due to colds or inhaled irritants.

Directions: Adults and children 5 to 12 years: Allow drop to dissolve slowly in mouth. **Cough:** may be repeated every hour as needed or as directed by a doctor. **Sore Throat:** may be repeated every 2 hours as needed or as directed by a doctor.
Children under 5 years of age: consult a doctor.

WARNINGS: A persistent cough may be a sign of a serious condition. If cough persists for more than 1 week, tends to recur, or is accompanied by fever, rash, or persistent headache, consult a doctor. Do not take this product for persistent or chronic cough such as occurs with smoking, asthma, emphysema, or if cough is accompanied by excessive phlegm (mucus), unless directed by a doctor. If sore throat is severe, or is accompanied by difficulty in breathing, or persists for more than 2 days, do not use, and consult a doctor promptly. If sore throat is accompanied or followed by fever, headache, rash, swelling, nausea, or vomiting, consult a doctor promptly. **Keep this and all drugs out of the reach of children.** As with any drug, if you are pregnant or nursing a baby, seek the advice of a health professional before using this product.

How Supplied: Vicks® Chloraseptic® Cough & Throat Drops are available in single sticks of 9 drops each and bags of 25 drops. Each drop is debossed with "V".

VICKS® CHLORASEPTIC® SORE THROAT LOZENGES
Menthol, Cherry, and Cool Mint Flavor
Menthol/Benzocaine
Oral Anesthetic

Active Ingredients: Benzocaine 6 mg, Menthol 10 mg.

Inactive Ingredients: Menthol Lozenges: Corn syrup, D&C Yellow No. 10, FD&C Blue No. 1, FD&C Yellow No. 6, flavor and sucrose. Cherry Lozenges: Corn syrup, FD&C Blue No. 1, FD&C Red No. 40, flavor and sucrose. Cool Mint Lozenges: Corn syrup, FD&C Blue No. 1, flavor and sucrose.

Indications: For temporary relief of occasional minor mouth pain and irritation, sore mouth and sore throat. Also, for pain associated with canker sores.

Directions: Adults and children 2 years of age and older: Allow 1 lozenge to dissolve slowly in mouth. May be repeated every 2 hours as needed or as directed by a physician or dentist. Children under 2 years of age: Consult a physician or a dentist.

WARNINGS: If sore throat is severe, or is accompanied by difficulty in breathing, or persists for more than 2 days, do not use, and consult a doctor promptly. If sore throat is accompanied or followed by fever, headache, rash, swelling, nausea, or vomiting, consult a doctor promptly. If sore mouth symptoms do not improve in 7 days, see your doctor promptly. Do not use this product if you have a history of allergy to local anesthetics such as procaine, butacaine, or other "caine" anesthetics. **Keep this and all drugs out of the reach of children.** In case of accidental overdose seek professional assistance or contact a poison control center immediately. As with any drug if you are pregnant or nursing a baby, seek the advice of a health professional before using this product.

How Supplied: Available in Menthol, Cherry, and Cool Mint lozenges in packages of 18. Each green or red lozenge is debossed with "VC".

VICKS® CHLORASEPTIC® SORE THROAT SPRAY GARGLE & MOUTH RINSE
Phenol/oral anesthetic/antiseptic
Menthol, Cherry and Cool Mint Flavors

Active Ingredient: Gargle and Spray— Phenol 1.4%.

Inactive Ingredients: Original Menthol Liquid: D&C Green No. 5, D&C Yellow No. 10, FD&C Green No. 3, flavor, glycerin, purified water, saccharin sodium. Cherry Liquid: FD&C Red No. 40, flavor, glycerin, purified water, saccharin sodium. Cool Mint Liquid: FD&C Blue No. 1, flavor, glycerin, purified water, saccharin sodium.

Indications: For temporary relief of occasional minor sore throat pain and sore mouth. Also for the temporary relief of pain due to canker sores, minor irritation or injury of the mouth and gums, minor dental procedures, dentures or orthodontic appliances.

Administration and Dosage: Chloraseptic Spray (Pump): **Spray 5 times** directly into throat or affected area and swallow. Children 2–12 years of age, spray 3 times and swallow. Repeat every 2 hours or as directed by a physician or dentist. Children under 12 years of age should be supervised in product use. Children under 2 years: consult a physician or dentist.
Chloraseptic Gargle: Adults and children 12 years of age and older: Gargle or swish around the mouth for at least 15 seconds and then spit out. Use every 2 hours or as directed by a physician or dentist. Children 6 to under 12 years: Gargle or swish around in mouth 2 teaspoonsful for at least 15 seconds and then spit out. Use every 2 hours or as directed by a physician or dentist. Children under 12 years should be supervised in product use. Children under 6 years: Consult a physician or dentist.

WARNINGS: If sore throat is severe, or is accompanied by difficulty in breathing, or persists for more than 2 days, do not use, and consult a doctor promptly. If sore throat is accompanied or followed by fever, headache, rash, swelling, nausea, or vomiting, consult a doctor promptly. If sore mouth symptoms do not improve in 7 days, or if irritation, pain, or redness persists or worsens, consult your doctor promptly. **Keep this and all drugs out of the reach of children.** In case of accidental overdose, seek professional assistance or contact a poison control center immediately. As with any drug, if you are pregnant or nursing a baby, seek the advice of a health professional before using this product.

How Supplied: Available in Original Menthol, Cherry, and Cool Mint flavors in 6 FL. OZ. (177 mL) plastic bottles with sprayer. Menthol Flavor is also available in 12 FL. OZ. (355 mL) gargle.

VICKS® COUGH DROPS
Menthol Cough Suppressant/Oral Anesthetic

Flavors: Available in two popular flavors: Menthol and Cherry.

Active Ingredient: Menthol.

Inactive Ingredients: Menthol Flavor: Benzyl Alcohol, Camphor, Caramel, Corn Syrup, Eucalyptus Oil, Flavor, Sucrose, Tolu Balsam, Thymol. Cherry Flavor: Citric Acid, Corn Syrup, FD&C Blue No. 1, FD&C Red No. 40, Flavor, Sucrose.

Indications: Temporarily relieves sore throat and coughs due to colds or inhaled irritants.

Directions: Adults and children 3 to 12 years: [Menthol] Allow drop to dissolve slowly in mouth. [Cherry] Allow 2 drops to dissolve slowly in mouth. **Cough:** may be repeated every hour as needed or as directed by a doctor. **Sore Throat:** may be repeated every 2 hours —as needed or as directed by a doctor. **Children under 3 years of age:** consult a doctor.

Continued on next page

Procter & Gamble—Cont.

WARNINGS: A persistent cough may be a sign of a serious condition. If cough persists for more than 1 week, tends to recur, or is accompanied by fever, rash, or persistent headache, consult a doctor. Do not take this product for persistent or chronic cough such as occurs with smoking, asthma, emphysema, or if cough is accompanied by excessive phlegm (mucus), unless directed by a doctor. If sore throat is severe, or is accompanied by difficulty in breathing, or persists for more than 2 days, do not use, and consult a doctor promptly. If sore throat is accompanied or followed by fever, headache, rash, swelling, nausea, or vomiting, consult a doctor promptly. **Keep this and all drugs out of the reach of children.** As with any drug, if you are pregnant or nursing a baby, seek the advice of a health professional before using this product.

How Supplied: Vicks® Chloraseptic® Cough & Throat Drops are available in boxes of 14 drops each and bags of 30 drops. Each red or green drop is debossed with "V".

**EXTRA STRENGTH VICKS®
COUGH DROPS
Menthol Cough Suppressant/Oral Anesthetic**

Flavors: Available in Cherry, Menthol, Honey Lemon and Peppermint flavors.

Active Ingredient: Menthol Flavor: Menthol 8.4 mg. Cherry: Menthol 10 mg, Honey Lemon: Menthol 10 mg, Peppermint: Menthol 10 mg.

Inactive Ingredients:
Menthol Flavor: Corn Syrup, FD&C Blue No. 1, Flavor, Sucrose, Cherry Flavor: Corn Syrup, FD&C Blue No. 2, FD&C Red No. 40, Flavor, Sucrose Honey Lemon: Citric Acid, Corn Syrup, D&C Yellow No. 10, FD&C Yellow No. 6, Flavor, Sucrose, Peppermint: Corn Syrup, Flavor, Peppermint Oil, Sucrose.

Indications: Temporarily relieves sore throat and coughs due to colds or inhaled irritants.

Directions: **Adults and children 3 to 12 years:** Allow drop to dissolve slowly in mouth. **Cough:** may be repeated every hour as needed or as directed by a doctor. **Sore Throat:** may be repeated every 2 hours as needed or as directed by a doctor. **Children under 3 years of age:** consult a doctor.

WARNINGS: A persistent cough may be a sign of a serious condition. If cough persists for more than 1 week, tends to recur, or is accompanied by fever, rash, or persistent headache, consult a doctor. Do not take this product for persistent or chronic cough such as occurs with smok-ing, asthma, emphysema, or if cough is accompanied by excessive phlegm (mucus), unless directed by a doctor. If sore throat is severe, or is accompanied by difficulty in breathing, or persists for more than 2 days, do not use, and consult a doctor promptly. If sore throat is accompanied or followed by fever, headache, rash, swelling, nausea, or vomiting, consult a doctor promptly. **Keep this and all drugs out of the reach of children.** As with any drug, if you are pregnant or nursing a baby, seek the advice of a health professional before using this product.

How Supplied: Extra Strength Vicks Cough Drops are available in single sticks of 9 drops each and bags of 30 drops.

**VICKS® DAYQUIL® ALLERGY RELIEF 4 HOUR TABLETS
Nasal Decongestant/Antihistamine**

Active Ingredients: Each Extended Release Tablet Contains:
75 mg Phenylpropanolamine Hydrochloride, 12 mg Brompheniramine Maleate.

Inactive Ingredients: D&C Blue No. 1 Aluminum Lake, Magnesium Stearate, Microcrystalline Cellulose, Starch.

Indications: For the temporary relief of nasal congestion due to the common cold, hay fever or other upper respiratory allergies or associated with sinusitis; temporarily relieves runny nose, sneezing, and itchy and watering eyes as may occur in allergic rhinitis (such as hay fever). Temporarily restores freer breathing through the nose.

Directions: Adults and children 12 years of age and older: one tablet every 4 hours. Do not exceed 1 tablet every 4 hours or 6 tablets in a 24-hour period. Children under 12 years of age: consult a doctor.

WARNINGS: Do not exceed recommended dosage because at higher doses nervousness, dizziness, or sleeplessness may occur. Do not take this product for more than 7 days. If symptoms do not improve or are accompanied by fever, consult a doctor. Do not take this product if you have heart disease, high blood pressure, thyroid disease, diabetes, glaucoma, or difficulty in urination due to enlargement of the prostate gland unless directed by a doctor. *Drug Interaction Precaution:* Do not take this product if you are presently taking a prescription drug for high blood pressure or depression without first consulting your doctor. May cause excitability especially in children. Do not take this product, unless directed by a doctor, if you have a breathing problem such as emphysema or chronic bronchitis. May cause drowsiness: alcohol, sedatives and tranquilizers may increase the drowsiness effect. Avoid alcoholic beverages while taking this product. Do not take this product if you are taking sedatives or tranquilizers

without first consulting your doctor. Use caution when driving a motor vehicle or operating machinery. **Keep this and all drugs out of the reach of children.** In case of accidental overdose, seek professional assistance or contact a poison control center immediately. As with any drug, if you are pregnant or nursing a baby, seek the advice of a health professional before using this product.

How Supplied: Available in 12 and 24 count blister packages. Each blue tablet is imprinted with the letter A inside the Vicks® shield .

**VICKS® DAYQUIL® ALLERGY RELIEF 12 HOUR EXTENDED RELEASE TABLETS
Nasal Decongestant/Antihistamine**

Active Ingredients: Each Extended Release Tablet Contains:
75 mg Phenylpropanolamine Hydrochloride, 12 mg Brompheniramine Maleate

Inactive Ingredients: Dimethyl Polysiloxane Oil, FD&C Blue No. 1 Aluminum Lake, Hydroxypropyl Methylcellulose, Lactose, Magnesium Stearate, Polyethylene Glycol. Talc, Titanium Dioxide.

Indications: For the temporary relief of nasal congestion due to the common cold, hay fever or other upper respiratory allergies, or associated with sinusitis; temporarily relieves runny nose, sneezing, and itchy and watery eyes as may occur in allergic rhinitis (such as hay fever). Temporarily restores freer breathing through the nose.

Action: Nasal Decongestant and Antihistamine. The anytime stuffy nose, sneezing, runny nose, itchy, watery eyes, so you can face your allergy season medicine.™

Directions: Adults and children 12 years of age and older: One tablet every 12 hours. DO NOT EXCEED 1 TABLET EVERY 12 HOURS, OR 2 TABLETS IN A 24-HOUR PERIOD. Children under 12 years of age: consult a doctor.

Warnings: This product may cause excitability, especially in children. Do not take this product if you have heart disease, high blood pressure, thyroid disease, diabetes, glaucoma, or difficulty in urination due to enlargement of the prostate gland, except under the advice and supervision of a doctor. Do not take this product, unless directed by a doctor, if you have a breathing problem such as emphysema or chronic bronchitis. Do not give this product to children under 12 years, except under the advice and supervision of a doctor. May cause drowsiness. Do not exceed recommended dosage because at higher doses nervousness, dizziness, or sleeplessness may occur. If symptoms do not improve within 7 days or are accompanied by fever, consult a doctor before continuing use. Do not take if hypersensitive to any of the ingredients. As with any drug, if you are pregnant or nursing a baby, seek the advice of a health professional before using this product. **CAUTION:** Avoid driving a motor vehicle or operating machinery and avoid alcoholic beverages while taking this product. **DRUG INTERACTION PRECAUTION:** Do not take this product if you are presently taking a prescription antihypertensive or antidepressant drug containing a monoamine oxidase inhibitor, except under the advice and supervision of a doctor. KEEP THIS AND ALL DRUGS OUT OF THE REACH OF CHILDREN. IN CASE OF ACCIDENTAL OVERDOSE, SEEK PROFESSIONAL ASSISTANCE OR CONTACT A POISON CONTROL CENTER IMMEDIATELY.

How Supplied: Available in 12 and 24 count blister packages. Each blue tablet is imprinted with the letter A inside the Vicks shield.

VICKS® DAYQUIL® LIQUID
VICKS® DAYQUIL® LIQUICAPS®
Multi-Symptom Cold/Flu Relief
Nasal Decongestant/Expectorant/
Pain Reliever/Cough
Suppressant/Fever Reducer

Active Ingredients: LIQUID—per fluid ounce (2 TBSP.) or LIQUICAPS—per two softgels, contains: Pseudoephedrine Hydrochloride 60 mg, Guaifenesin 200 mg, Acetaminophen 650 mg (Liquid) or 500 mg (softgels), Dextromethorphan Hydrobromide 20 mg.

Inactive Ingredients: Liquid: Citric Acid, FD&C Yellow No. 6, Flavor, Glycerin, Polyethylene Glycol, Propylene Glycol, Purified Water, Saccharin Sodium, Sodium Citrate, Sucrose. Softgels: FD&C Red No. 40, FD&C Yellow No. 6, Gelatin, Glycerin, Polyethylene Glycol, Povidone, Propylene Glycol, Purified Water. May contain Sorbitol.

Indications: For the temporary relief of minor aches, pains, headache, muscular aches, sore throat pain, and fever associated with a cold or flu. Temporarily relieves nasal congestion and coughing due to a cold. Helps loosen phlegm (mucus) and thin secretions to drain bronchial tubes and make coughs more productive.

Directions: Take as directed.
Adults 12 years and over: 1 FL. OZ. in medicine cup (2 Tablespoons-TBSP), or swallow 2 softgels with water.
Children 6 to under
12 years of age: ½ FL. OZ. in medicine cup (1 Tablespoon-TBSP), or swallow 1 softgel with water.
Children under 6 years of age: Consult a doctor.
Repeat every 4 hours, not to exceed 4 doses per day, or as directed by a doctor.

Warnings: Do not exceed recommended dosage because at higher doses nervousness, dizziness, or sleeplessness may occur. Do not take this product if you have heart disease, high blood pressure, thyroid disease, diabetes, or difficulty in urination due to enlargement of the prostate gland unless directed by a doctor. *Drug Interaction Precaution:* Do not take this product if you are now taking a prescription monoamine oxidase inhibitor (MAOI) (certain drugs for depression, psychiatric or emotional conditions, or Parkinson's disease), or for two weeks after stopping the MAOI drug. If you are uncertain whether your prescription drug contains an MAOI, consult a health professional before taking this product. Do not take this product for persistent or chronic cough such as occurs with smoking, asthma, chronic bronchitis, emphysema, or if cough is accompanied by excessive phlegm (mucus) unless directed by a doctor. Do not take this product for more than 7 days (for adults) or 5 days (for children). A persistent cough may be a sign of serious condition. If cough persists for more than 7 days, tends to recur, or is accompanied by rash, or persistent headache, consult a doctor. If symptoms do not improve or are accompanied by fever that lasts for more than 3 days, or if new symptoms occur, consult a doctor. If sore throat is severe, persists for more than 2 days, is accompanied or followed by fever, headache, rash, nausea, or vomiting, consult a doctor promptly. **Keep this and all drugs out of the reach of children.** In case of accidental overdose, seek professional assistance or contact a poison control center immediately. Prompt medical attention is critical for adults as well as for children even if you do not notice any signs or symptoms. As with any drug, if you are pregnant or nursing a baby, seek the advice of a health professional before using this product.

How Supplied: Available in: **LIQUID** 6 FL. OZ. (177 mL) plastic bottles with child-resistant, tamper-evident cap and a calibrated medicine cup.
LIQUICAP: in 12-count child-resistant packages and 20-count non child-resistant packages. Each softgel is imprinted: "DayQuil."

VICKS® DAYQUIL® SINUS
PRESSURE & CONGESTION RELIEF
Nasal Decongestant/Expectorant

Active Ingredients: (per caplet) contains Guaifenesin 200 mg, Phenylpropanolamine Hydrochloride 25 mg.

Inactive Ingredients: Colloidal Silicone Dioxide, Crospovidone, FD&C Yellow No. 6 Aluminum Lake, Hydroxypropyl Methylcellulose, Microcrystalline Cellulose, Polyethylene Glycol, Polysorbate 80, Povidone, Stearic Acid, Titanium Dioxide.

Indications: For the temporary relief of nasal/sinus congestion and pressure associated with sinusitis, hay fever, upper respiratory allergies or the common cold. Also helps loosen phlegm and thin bronchial secretions to relieve chest congestion.

Directions: Take as directed.
Adults 12 years and older: 1 FL. OZ. in medicine cup (2 Tablespoons-TBSP), or swallow 2 softgels with water.
Children 6 to under
12 years of age: ½ FL. OZ. in medicine cup (1 Tablespoon-TBSP), or swallow 1 softgel with water.
Children under 6 years of age: Consult a doctor. Repeat every 4 hours, not to exceed 4 doses per day, or as directed by a doctor.

WARNINGS: Do not exceed recommended dosage because at higher doses nervousness, dizziness, or sleeplessness may occur. Do not take this product if you have heart disease, high blood pressure, thyroid disease, diabetes, or difficulty in urination due to enlargement of the prostate gland unless directed by a doctor. *Drug Interaction Precaution:* Do not use this product if you are now taking a prescription monoamine oxidase inhibitor (MAOI) (certain drugs for depression, psychiatric or emotional conditions, or Parkinson's disease), or for two weeks after stopping the MAOI drug. If you are uncertain whether your prescription drug contains an MAOI, consult a health professional before taking this product. Do not take this product for persistent or chronic cough such as occurs with smoking, asthma, chronic bronchitis, emphysema, or if cough is accompanied by excessive phlegm (mucus) unless directed by a doctor. Do not take this product for more than 7 days (for adults) or 5 days (for children). A persistent cough may be a sign of serious condition. If cough persists for more than 7 days, tends to recur, or is accompanied by rash, or persistent headache, consult a doctor. If symptoms do not improve or are accompanied by fever that lasts for more than 3 days, or if new symptoms occur, consult a doctor. If sore throat is severe, persists for more than 2 days, is accompanied or followed by fever, headache, rash, nausea, or vomiting, consult a doctor promptly. **Keep this and all drugs out of the reach of children.** In case of accidental overdose, seek professional assistance or contact a poison control center immediately. Prompt medical attention is critical for adults as well as for children even if you do not notice any signs or symptoms. As with any drug, if you are pregnant or nursing a baby, seek the advice of a health professional before using this product.

How Supplied: Available in:
LIQUID: 6 FL. OZ. (177 mL) plastic bottles with child-resistant, tamper-evident cap and a calibrated medicine cup.
LIQUICAP: in 12-count child-resistant packages and 20-count non child-resistant packages. Each softget is imprinted: "DayQuil."

Continued on next page

Procter & Gamble—Cont.

VICKS® DAYQUIL® SINUS
**Pressure & PAIN Relief
WITH IBUPROFEN*
IBUPROFEN/PSEUDOEPHEDRINE
HCL
Pain Reliever/Fever Reducer/
Nasal Decongestant
*NEW FORMULA—SEE NEW
WARNINGS**

Warning: ASPIRIN SENSITIVE PATIENTS. Do not take this product if you have had a severe reaction to aspirin (e.g., asthma, swelling, shock or hives) because even though this product contains no aspirin or salicylates, cross-reactions may occur in patients allergic to aspirin.

Indications: For temporary relief of symptoms associated with the common cold, sinusitis or flu including nasal congestion, headache, fever, body aches, and pains.

Directions: Adults: Take 1 caplet every 4 to 6 hours while symptoms persist. If symptoms do not respond to 1 caplet, 2 caplets may be used but do not exceed 6 caplets in 24 hours, unless directed by a doctor. The smallest effective dose should be used. Take with food or milk if occasional and mild heartburn, upset stomach, or stomach pain occurs with use. Consult a doctor if these symptoms are more than mild or they persist. Children: Do not give this product to children under 12 years of age except under the advice and supervision of a doctor.

WARNINGS: Do not take for colds for more than 7 days or for fever for more than 3 days unless directed by a doctor. If the cold or fever persists or gets worse or if new symptoms occur, consult a doctor. These could be signs of serious illness. As with aspirin and acetaminophen, if you have any condition which requires you to take prescription drugs or if you have had problems or serious side effects from taking any non-prescription pain reliever, do not take this product without first discussing it with your doctor. IF YOU EXPERIENCE ANY SYMPTOMS WHICH ARE UNUSUAL OR SEEM UNRELATED TO THE CONDITION FOR WHICH YOU TOOK THIS PRODUCT, CONSULT A DOCTOR BEFORE TAKING ANY MORE OF IT. If you are under a doctor's care for any serious condition, consult a doctor before taking this product. Do not exceed recommended dosage because at higher doses nervousness, dizziness or sleeplessness may occur. Do not take this product if you have high blood pressure, heart disease, diabetes, thyroid disease or difficulty in urination due to enlargement of the prostate gland, except under the advice and supervision of a doctor. Drug Interaction Precaution: Do not take this product if you are presently taking a prescription drug for high blood pressure or depression without first consulting your doctor. Do not combine this product with other non-prescription pain relievers. Do not combine this product with any other ibuprofen-containing product. As with any drug, if you are pregnant or nursing a baby, seek the advice of a health professional before using this product. IT IS ESPECIALLY IMPORTANT NOT TO USE THIS PRODUCT DURING THE LAST 3 MONTHS OF PREGNANCY UNLESS SPECIFICALLY DIRECTED TO DO SO BY A DOCTOR BECAUSE IT MAY CAUSE PROBLEMS IN THE UNBORN CHILD OR COMPLICATIONS DURING DELIVERY. Keep this and all drugs out of reach of children. In case of accidental overdose, seek professional assistance or contact a poison control center immediately.

Active Ingredients: each caplet contains Ibuprofen 200 mg, Pseudoephedrine Hydrochloride 30 mg.

Inactive Ingredients: Carnuba or Equivalent Wax, Croscarmellose Sodium, Iron Oxide, Methylparaben, Microcrystalline Cellulose, Propylparaben, Silicon Dioxide, Sodium Benzoate, Sodium Lauryl Sulfate, Starch, Stearic Acid, Sucrose, Titanium Dioxide.

How Supplied: Available in 20 count blister package and 40 count bottle. Each white caplet is imprinted: "DAYQUIL®

VICKS® NYQUIL®
**HOT THERAPY™
ADULT NIGHTTIME COLD/FLU
HOT LIQUID MEDICINE
Honey Lemon Hot Liquid Drink
Antihistamine/Cough Suppressant/
Pain Reliever/Nasal Decongestant/
Fever Reducer**

Active Ingredients: (per packet) Doxylamine Succinate 12.5 mg, Dextromethorphan Hydrobromide 30 mg, Acetaminophen 1000 mg, Pseudoephedrine Hydrobromide 30 mg.

Inactive Ingredients: Citric Acid, Flavor, and Sucrose.

Indications: For the temporary relief of minor aches, pains, headache, muscular aches, sore throat pain, and fever associated with a cold or flu. Temporarily relieves nasal congestion, cough due to minor throat and bronchial irritations, runny nose and sneezing associated with the common cold.

Actions: The nighttime sniffling, sneezing, coughing, aching, stuffy head, fever, so you can rest HOT LIQUID medicine.™

Directions: Adults and Children 12 years and over: Take one dose at bedtime. **DISSOLVE ONE PACKET IN 6 OZ. CUP OF HOT WATER. SIP WHILE HOT.** If your cold or flu symptoms keep you confined to bed or at home, a total of 4 doses may be taken per day, each 6 hours apart, or as directed by a doctor. **MICROWAVE HEATING INSTRUCTIONS:** Add contents of packet and 6 ounces of cool water to a microwave-safe cup and stir briskly. Microwave on high 1½ minutes or until hot. **DO NOT BOIL.** Sweeten to taste if desired.

WARNINGS: Do not exceed recommended dosage because at higher doses nervousness, dizziness, or sleeplessness may occur. Do not take this product if you have heart disease, high blood pressure, thyroid disease, diabetes, glaucoma, or difficulty in urination due to enlargement of the prostate gland unless directed by a doctor. Drug Interaction Precaution: Do not use this product if you are now taking a prescription monoamine oxidase inhibitor (MAOI) (certain drugs for depression, psychiatric or emotional conditions, or Parkinson's disease), or for two weeks after stopping the MAOI drug. If you are uncertain whether your prescription drug contains an MAOI, consult a health professional before taking this product. Do not take this product for persistent or chronic cough such as occurs with smoking, asthma, emphysema, or if cough is accompanied by excessive phlegm (mucus) unless directed by a doctor. May cause excitability especially in children. Do not take this product, unless directed by a doctor, if you have a breathing problem such as emphysema or chronic bronchitis. May cause marked drowsiness; alcohol, sedatives and tranquilizers may increase the drowsiness effect. Avoid alcoholic beverages while taking this product. Do not take this product if you are taking sedatives or tranquilizers without first consulting your doctor. Use caution when driving a motor vehicle or operating machinery. Do not take this product for more than 7 days. A persistent cough may be a sign of a serious condition. If cough persists for more than 7 days, tends to recur, or is accompanied by rash, or persistent headache, consult a doctor. If symptoms do not improve or are accompanied by fever that lasts for more than 3 days, or if new symptoms occur, consult a doctor. If sore throat is severe, persists for more than 2 days, is accompanied or followed by fever, headache, rash, nausea or vomiting, consult a doctor promptly. **Keep this and all drugs out of the reach of children.** In case of accidental overdose, seek professional assistance or contact a poison control center immediately. Prompt medical attention is critical for adults as well as for children even if you do not notice any signs or symptoms. As with any drug, if you are pregnant or nursing a baby, seek the advice of a health professional before using this product.

How Supplied: Available in child-resistant packages of 6 and 10 individual dose pouches.

VICKS® NYQUIL® LIQUICAPS®
VICKS® NYQUIL® LIQUID
(Original and Cherry)
Multi-Symptom Cold/Flu Relief/
Antihistamine/Cough
Suppressant/Pain Reliever/
Nasal Decongestant/
Fever Reducer

Active Ingredients (per softgel): Doxylamine Succinate 6.25 mg, Dextromethorphan HBr 10 mg, Acetaminophen 250 mg, Pseudoephedrine HCl 30 mg. **(per fluid oz) (2 TBSP):** Doxylamine succinate 12.5 mg, Dextromethorphan HBr 30 mg, Acetaminophen 1000 mg, Pseudoephedrine HCl 60 mg.

Inactive Ingredients: (per softgel): D&C Yellow No. 10, FD&C Blue No. 1, Gelatin, Glycerin, Polyethylene Glycol, Povidone, Propylene Glycol and Purified Water. May contain Edible Ink. Contains no alcohol. **(Liquid):** Alcohol 10%, Citric Acid, Flavor, Glycerin, Polyethylene Glycol, Propylene Glycol, Purified Water, Saccharin Sodium, Sodium Citrate, Sucrose.
Original flavor also has D&C Yellow No. 10, FD&C Green No. 3, FD&C Yellow No. 6.
Cherry flavor also has FD&C Blue No. 1, FD&C Red No. 40.

Indications: For the temporary relief of minor aches, pains, headache, muscular aches, sore throat pain, and fever associated with a cold or flu. Temporarily relieves nasal congestion, cough due to minor throat and bronchial irritations, runny nose and sneezing associated with the common cold.

Actions: The nighttime sniffling, sneezing, coughing, aching, stuffy head, fever, so you can rest medicine.®

Directions: **(LiquiCaps®)** ADULTS (12 years and older): Swallow two softgels. If your cold or flu symptoms keep you confined to bed or at home a total of 4 doses may be taken per day, each 4 hours apart, or as directed by a doctor.
(Liquid) Take one fluid ounce (2 tablespoons) at bedtime in medicine cup provided. If your cold or flu symptoms keep you confined to bed or at home, a total of 4 doses may be taken per day, each 6 hours apart, or as directed by a doctor. **NOT RECOMMENDED FOR CHILDREN.**

WARNINGS: Do not exceed recommended dosage because at higher doses nervousness, dizziness or sleeplessness may occur. Do not take this product if you have heart disease, high blood pressure, thyroid disease, diabetes, glaucoma, or difficulty in urination due to enlargement of the prostate gland unless directed by a doctor. *Drug Interaction Precaution:* Do not use this product if you are now taking a prescription monoamine oxidase inhibitor (MAOI) (certain drugs for depression, psychiatric or emotional conditions, or Parkinson's disease), or for two weeks after stopping the MAOI drug. If you are uncertain whether your prescription drug contains an MAOI, consult a health professional before taking this product. Do not take this product for persistent or chronic cough such as occurs with smoking, asthma, emphysema, or if cough is accompanied by excessive phlegm (mucus) unless directed by a doctor. May cause excitability especially in children. Do not take this product, unless directed by a doctor, if you have a breathing problem such as emphysema or chronic bronchitis. May cause marked drowsiness; alcohol, sedatives, and tranquilizers may increase the drowsiness effect. Avoid alcoholic beverages while taking this product. Do not take this product if you are taking sedatives or tranquilizers, without first consulting your doctor. Use caution when driving a motor vehicle or operating machinery. Do not take this product for more than 7 days. A persistent cough may be a sign of a serious condition. If cough persists for more than 7 days, tends to recur, or is accompanied by rash, or persistent headache, consult a doctor. If symptoms do not improve or are accompanied by fever that lasts for more than 3 days, or if new symptoms occur, consult a doctor. If sore throat is severe, persists for more than 2 days, is accompanied or followed by fever, headache, rash, nausea, or vomiting, consult a doctor promptly. **Keep this and all drugs out of the reach of children.** In case of accidental overdose, seek professional assistance or contact a poison control center immediately. Prompt medical attention is critical for adults as well as for children even if you do not notice any signs or symptoms. As with any drug, if you are pregnant or nursing a baby, seek the advice of a health professional before using this product.

How Supplied: (LiquiCaps®) Available in 12-count child-resistant blister packages and 20-count non-child resistant blister packages. Each softgel is imprinted: "NyQuil".
(Liquid) Available in 6, 10, and 14 fl. oz (177, 295, and 414 mL, respectively) plastic bottles with child-resistant, tamper-evident cap and calibrated medicine cup.

PEDIATRIC VICKS®
44d DRY HACKING
COUGH & HEAD CONGESTION

Active Ingredients: Per 1 tablespoon (TBSP.) (15 mL): Dextromethorphan Hydrobromide 15 mg, Pseudoephedrine Hydrochloride 30 mg.

CONTAINS NO ALCOHOL

Inactive Ingredients: Carboxymethylcellulose Sodium, Cellulose, Citric Acid, FD&C Red No. 40, Flavor, Glycerin, Polysorbate 80, Potassium Sorbate, Propylene Glycol, Purified Water, Sodium Citrate, Sorbitol, Sucrose.

Indications: For temporary relief of coughs and nasal congestion due to the common cold.

Actions: PEDIATRIC VICKS® 44d is an alcohol-free cough suppressant and nasal decongestant.

Administration and Dosage:
Directions: SHAKE WELL BEFORE USING
Squeeze bottle to accurately dispense medicine into dosage cup provided. 1 TBSP. ½ TBSP.

Dosage:

Age	Weight	Dose
Under 2 yrs	Under 28 lbs.	Consult physician*
2–5 yrs	28–47 lbs.	Fill cup to ½ TABLESPOON (TBSP.)
6–11 yrs	48–95 lbs.	Fill cup to 1 TABLESPOON (TBSP.)
12 yrs. and older	96 lbs. and over	2 TABLESPOONS (TBSP.) or Try one of the Adult Formula 44® Medicines

Repeat every 6 hours, no more than 4 doses in 24 hours, or as directed by a doctor.

***Professional Dosage:**
Physicians: Suggested doses for children under 2 years of age.

Age	Weight	Dose
* 6–11 mo.	17–21 lbs.	1 teaspoon (tsp.) (5 mL)
*12–23 mo.	22–27 lbs.	1¼ teaspoon (tsp.) (6.25 mL)

Repeat every 6 hours. No more than 4 doses in 24 hours, or as directed by doctor.
*Based on extrapolation from studies on the safety and efficacy of active ingredients conducted among older children and adults. Use caution in treating children under 2 years who were born prematurely.

WARNINGS: A persistent cough may be a sign of a serious condition. If cough persists for more than 1 week, tends to recur, or is accompanied by fever, rash, or persistent headache, consult a doctor. Do not take this product for persistent or chronic cough such as occurs with smoking, asthma, emphysema, or if cough is accompanied by excessive phlegm (mucus) unless directed by a doctor. Do not exceed recommended dosage because at higher doses nervousness, dizziness, or sleeplessness may occur. Do not take this product for more than 7 days. If symptoms do not improve or are accompanied

Continued on next page

Procter & Gamble—Cont.

by fever, consult a doctor. Do not take this product if you have heart disease, high blood pressure, thyroid disease, diabetes, or difficulty in urination due to enlargement of the prostate gland unless directed by a doctor. *Drug Interaction Precaution:* Do not use this product if you are now taking a prescription monoamine oxidase inhibitor (MAOI) (certain drugs for depression, psychiatric or emotional conditions, or Parkinson's disease), or for two weeks after stopping the MAOI drug. If you are uncertain whether your prescription drug contains an MAOI, consult a health professional before taking this product. **Keep this and all drugs out of the reach of children.** In case of accidental overdose, seek professional assistance or contact a poison control center immediately. As with any drug, if you are pregnant or nursing a baby, seek the advice of a health professional before using this product.

How Supplied: 4 FL. OZ. (118 mL) squeeze bottle with Vicks® AccuTip® Dispenser for accurate, easy dosing. A calibrated dose cup accompanies each bottle.

PEDIATRIC VICKS® 44e
Chest Cough & Chest Congestion

Active Ingredients per 1 tablespoon (TBSP.) (15 mL):
Dextromethorphan Hydrobromide 10 mg, Guaifenesin 100 mg.

CONTAINS NO ALCOHOL

Inactive Ingredients: Carboxymethylcellulose Sodium, Cellulose, Citric Acid, FD&C Red No. 40, Flavor, Glycerin, Polysorbate 80, Potassium Sorbate, Propylene Glycol, Purified Water, Sodium Citrate, Sorbitol, Sucrose.

Indications: Provides temporary relief of coughs due to a common cold and helps loosen phlegm to rid the bronchial passageways of bothersome mucus.

Actions: PEDIATRIC VICKS® 44e is an alcohol-free cough suppressant and expectorant.

**Administration and Dosage:
Directions: (SHAKE WELL BEFORE USING)**

Squeeze bottle to accurately dispense medicine into dosage cup provided. 1 TBSP. ½ TBSP.

Dosage:

Age	Weight	Dose
Under 2 yrs	Under 28 lbs.	Consult physician*
2–5 yrs	28–47 lbs.	Fill cup to ½ TABLESPOON (TBSP.)
6–11 yrs	48–95 lbs.	Fill cup to 1 TABLESPOON (TBSP.)
12 yrs and older	96 lbs. and over	2 TABLESPOONS (TBSP.) or Try one of the Adult Formula 44® Medicines

Repeat every 4 hours. No more than 6 doses in 24 hours, or as directed by a doctor.

*Professional Dosage:

Physicians: Suggested doses for children under 2 years of age.

Age	Weight	Dose
* 6–11 mo.	17–21 lbs.	1 teaspoon (tsp.) (5 mL)
*12–23 mo.	22–27 lbs.	1¼ teaspoon (tsp.) (6.25 mL)

Repeat every 4 hours. No more than 6 doses in 24 hours, or as directed by doctor.

* Based on extrapolation from studies on the safety and efficacy of active ingredients conducted among older children and adults. Use caution in treating children under 2 years who were born prematurely.

WARNINGS: A persistent cough may be a sign of a serious condition. If cough persists for more than 1 week, tends to recur, or is accompanied by fever, rash, or persistent headache, consult a doctor. Do not take this product for persistent or chronic cough such as occurs with smoking, asthma, chronic bronchitis, emphysema, or if cough is accompanied by excessive phlegm (mucus) unless directed by a doctor. *Drug Interaction Precaution:* Do not use this product if you are now taking a prescription monoamine oxidase inhibitor (MAOI) (certain drugs for depression, psychiatric or emotional conditions, or Parkinson's disease), or for two weeks after stopping the MAOI drug. If you are uncertain whether your prescription drug contains an MAOI, consult a health profesional before taking this product. **Keep this and all drugs out of the reach of children.** In case of accidental overdose, seek professional assistance or contact a poison control center immediately. As with any drug, if you are pregnant or nursing a baby, seek the advice of a health professional before using this product.

How Supplied: 4 FL. OZ. (118 mL) squeeze bottle with Vicks® AccuTip® Dispenser for accurate, easy dosing. A calibrated dose cup accompanies each bottle.

PEDIATRIC VICKS® 44m
COUGH & COLD RELIEF
Cough Suppressant/Nasal Decongestant/Antihistamine

Active Ingredients Per 1 tablespoon (TBSP.) (15 mL): Dextromethorphan Hydrobromide 15 mg, Pseudoephedrine Hydrochloride 30 mg, Chlorpheniramine Maleate 2 mg

CONTAINS NO ALCOHOL

Inactive Ingredients: Carboxymethylcellulose Sodium, Cellulose, Citric Acid, FD&C Red No. 40, Flavor, Glycerin, Polysorbate 80, Potassium Sorbate, Propylene Glycol, Purified Water, Sodium Citrate, Sorbitol, Sucrose.

Indications: For the temporary relief of coughs, nasal congestion, runny nose and sneezing due to the common cold.

Actions: PEDIATRIC VICKS® 44m is an alcohol-free cough suppressant, nasal decongestant and antihistamine.

**Administration and Dosage:
Directions: SHAKE WELL BEFORE USING**

Squeeze bottle to accurately dispense medicine into dosage cup provided. 1 TBSP. ½ TBSP.

Dosage:

Age	Weight	Dose
Under 6 yrs	Under 48 lbs.	Consult Physician*
6–11 yrs	48–95 lbs.	Fill cup to 1 TABLESPOON (TBSP.)
12 yrs and older	96 lbs. and over	2 TABLESPOONS (TBSP.) or try one of the Adult Formula 44 Medicines

Repeat every 6 hours. No more than 4 doses in 24 hours, or as directed by a doctor.

Professional Dosage:

*Physicians: Suggested doses for children under 6 years of age.

Age	Weight	Dose
* 6–11 mo.	17–21 lbs.	1 teaspoon (tsp.) (5 mL)
*12–23 mo.	22–27 lbs.	1¼ teaspoon (tsp.) (6.25 mL)
2–5 yrs.	28–47 lbs.	½ TABLESPOON (TBSP.) (7.5 mL)

Repeat every 6 hours, no more than 4 doses in 24 hours, or as directed by doctor.

*Based on extrapolation from studies on the safety and efficacy of active ingredients conducted among older children and adults. Use caution in treating children under 2 years of age who were born prematurely.

WARNINGS: A persistent cough may be a sign of a serious condition. If cough persists for more than 1 week, tends to recur, or is accompanied by fever, rash, or persistent headache, consult a doctor. Do not take this product for persistent or chronic cough such as occurs with smoking, asthma, emphysema, or if cough is accompanied by excessive phlegm (mucus) unless directed by a doctor. Do not exceed recommended dosage because at higher doses nervousness, dizziness, or sleeplessness may occur. Do not take this product for more than 7 days. If symptoms do not improve or are accompanied by fever, consult a doctor. Do not take this product if you have heart disease, high blood pressure, thyroid disease, diabetes, glaucoma, or difficulty in urination due to enlargement of the prostate gland unless directed by a doctor. *Drug Interaction Precaution:* Do not use this product if you are now taking a prescription monoamine oxidase inhibitor (MAOI) (certain drugs for depression, psychiatric or emotional conditions, or Parkinson's disease), or for two weeks after stopping the MAOI drug. If you are uncertain whether your prescription drug contains an MAOI, consult a health professional before taking this product. May cause excitability especially in children. Do not take this product, unless directed by a doctor, if you have a breathing problem such as emphysema or chronic bronchitis. May cause marked drowsiness; alcohol, sedatives, and tranquilizers may increase the drowsiness effect. Avoid alcoholic beverages while taking this product. Do not take this product if you are taking sedatives or tranquilizers, without first consulting your doctor. Use caution when driving a motor vehicle or operating machinery. **Keep this and all drugs out of the reach of children.** In case of accidental overdose, seek professional assistance or contact a poison control center immediately. As with any drug, if you are pregnant or nursing a baby, seek the advice of a health professional before using this product.

How Supplied: 4 FL OZ (118 mL) squeeze bottle with Vicks® AccuTip® Dispenser for accurate easy dosing. A calibrated dose cup accompanies each bottle.

VICKS® SINEX® NASAL SPRAY
[sī′něx]
Nasal Decongestant Spray and Ultra Fine Mist

Active Ingredient: Phenylephrine Hydrochloride 0.5%.

Inactive Ingredients: Aromatic Vapors (Camphor, Eucalyptol, Menthol), Citric Acid, Purified Water, Tyloxapol. Preservatives: Benzalkonium Chloride, Chlorhexidine Gluconate, Disodium EDTA.

Indications: For temporary relief of sinus/nasal congestion due to colds, hay fever, upper respiratory allergies or sinusitis.

Dosage and Administration: Keep head and dispenser upright. May be used every 4 hours as needed.
Ultra Fine Mist: Remove protective cap. Before using for the first time, prime the pump by firmly depressing its rim several times. Hold container with thumb at base and nozzle between first and second fingers. Without tilting your head, insert nozzle into nostril. Fully depress rim with a firm even stroke and inhale deeply. Adults and Children—age 12 and over: 2 or 3 sprays in each nostril not more often than every 4 hours. Do not give to children under 12 years of age unless directed by a doctor.
Squeeze Bottle: Adults and Children— age 12 and over: 2 or 3 sprays in each nostril not more often than every 4 hours. Do not give to children under 12 years of age unless directed by a doctor.

WARNINGS: Do not exceed recommended dosage because burning, stinging, sneezing, or increase of nasal discharge may occur. The use of this container by more than one person may spread infection. Do not use this product for more than 3 days. If symptoms persist, consult a doctor. Do not use this product if you have heart disease, high blood pressure, thyroid disease, diabetes, or difficulty in urination due to enlargement of the prostate gland unless directed by a doctor. **Keep this and all drugs out of the reach of children.** In case of accidental ingestion, seek professional assistance or contact a poison control center immediately.

How Supplied: Available in ½ FL. OZ. (14 mL) plastic squeeze bottle and ½ FL. OZ. (14 mL) measured dose Ultra Fine mist pump.

VICKS® SINEX®
[sī′něx]
12-HOUR Nasal Decongestant Spray and Ultra Fine Mist

Active Ingredient: Oxymetazoline Hydrochloride 0.05%.

Inactive Ingredients: Aromatic Vapors (Camphor, Eucalyptol, Menthol), Potassium Phosphate, Purified Water, Sodium Chloride, Sodium Phosphate, Tyloxapol. Preservatives: Benzalkonium Chloride, Chlorhexidine Gluconate, Disodium EDTA.

Indications: For temporary relief of nasal congestion due to colds, hay fever, upper respiratory allergies or sinusitis.

Dosage and Administration: Keep head and dispenser upright. May be used twice daily (morning and evening) or as directed by a physician.

Ultra Fine Mist: Remove protective cap. Before using for the first time, prime the pump by firmly depressing its rim several times. Hold container with thumb at base and nozzle between first and second fingers. Without tilting head, insert nozzle into nostril. Fully depress rim with a firm even stroke and inhale deeply.
Adults and children 6 years of age and over (with adult supervision): 2 or 3 sprays in each nostril not more often than every 10 to 12 hours. Do not exceed 2 applications in any 24-hour period. Children under 6 years of age: consult a doctor.
Squeeze Bottle: Adults and children 6 years of age and over (with adult supervision): 2 or 3 sprays in each nostril not more often than every 10 to 12 hours. Do not exceed 2 applications in any 24-hour period. Children under 6 years of age: consult a doctor.

WARNINGS: Do not exceed recommended dosage because burning, stinging, sneezing or increase of nasal discharge may occur. The use of this container by more than one person may spread infection. Do not use this product for more than 3 days. If symptoms persist, consult a doctor. Do not use this product if you have heart disease, high blood pressure, thyroid disease, diabetes, or difficulty in urination due to enlargement of the prostate gland unless directed by a doctor. **Keep this and all drugs out of the reach of children.** In case of accidental ingestion, seek professional assistance or contact a poison control center immediately.

How Supplied: Available in ½ FL. OZ. (14 mL) plastic squeeze bottle and ½ FL. OZ. (14 mL) measured-dose Ultra Fine mist pump.

VICKS® VAPOR INHALER
l-Desoxyephedrine/Nasal Decongestant

Active Ingredient per inhaler: *l*-Desoxyephedrine 50 mg.

Inactive Ingredients: Special Vicks Vapors (bornyl acetate, camphor, lavender oil, menthol).

Indications: For the temporary relief of nasal congestion due to the common cold, hay fever, upper respiratory allergies or sinusitis.

Directions: Adults: 2 inhalations in each nostril not more often than every 2 hours. **Children 6 to under 12 years of age** (with adult supervision): 1 inhalation in each nostril not more often than every 2 hours. Children under 6 years of age: consult a doctor.

WARNINGS: Do not exceed recommended dosage because burning, stinging, sneezing, or increase of nasal dis-

Continued on next page

Procter & Gamble—Cont.

charge may occur. The use of this container by more than one person may spread infection. Do not use this product for more than 7 days. If symptoms persist, consult a doctor. **Keep this and all drugs out of the reach of children.** In case of accidental ingestion, seek professional assistance or contact a poison control center immediately.

VICKS® VAPOR INHALER is effective for a minimum of 3 months after first use. Keep tightly closed.

How Supplied: Available as a cylindrical plastic nasal inhaler.
Net weight: 0.007 OZ (198 mg).

VICKS® VAPORUB®
VICKS® VAPORUB® CREAM
[vā'pō-rub]
Nasal Decongestant/Cough Suppressant/Topical Analgesic

Active Ingredients: Camphor (5.2% cream) 4.8% oint.), Menthol (2.8% cream) 2.6% oint.), Eucalyptus Oil 1.2%.

USE on Chest & Throat: For temporary relief of nasal congestion and coughs associated with a cold.

Active Ingredients: Camphor (5.2% cream) 4.8% oint.), Menthol (2.8% cream) 2.6% oint.).

USE: For temporary relief of minor aches and pains of muscles.

Directions: Adults and children 2 years of age and over:
Chest & Throat: rub on a thick layer. [If desired, cover with a dry, soft cloth, but keep clothing loose to let vapors rise to the nose and mouth. (oint.)]
Rub on sore area.
Repeat up to three times daily or as directed by a doctor.
Children under two years of age: consult a doctor.
Do not heat. Never expose VapoRub® to flame, microwave, or place in any container in which you are heating water. [Such improper use may cause the mixture to splatter. (oint.)]

WARNINGS: For external use only. Do not take by mouth or place in nostrils. A persistent cough may be a sign of a serious condition. If cough persists for more than 1 week, recur, or are accompanied by fever, rash, or persistent headache, discontinue using this product and consult a doctor. Do not apply to wounds or damaged skin. **Keep this and all drugs out of the reach of children.** In case of accidental ingestion, seek professional assistance or contact a poison control center immediately.

Inactive Ingredients: (ointment) Cedarleaf Oil, Mineral Oil, Nutmeg Oil, Petrolatum, Spirits of Turpentine, Thymol. **(cream)** Carbomer, Cedarleaf Oil, Cetyl Alcohol, Cetyl Palmitate, Cyclomethicone and Dimethicone Copolyol, Dimethicone, EDTA, Glycerin, Imidazolidinyl Urea, Isopropyl Palmitate, Methylparaben, Nutmeg Oil, PEG-100, Stearate, Propylparaben, Purified Water, Sodium Hydroxide, Spirits of Turpentine, Stearic Acid, Stearyl Alcohol, Thymol, Titanium Dioxide.

How Supplied: (ointment) Available in 1.5 OZ. (42.5 g), 3.0 OZ. (85 g) and 6.0 OZ. (1700 g) plastic jars. **(cream)** 2.0 oz. (56.7 g) tube.

VICKS® VAPOSTEAM®
[vā'pō "stēm]
Liquid Medication for Hot Steam Vaporizers.
Nasal Decongestant/Cough Suppressant

Active Ingredients: Camphor 6.2%, Menthol 3.2%, Eucalyptus Oil 1.5%.

Inactive Ingredients: Alcohol 74%, Cedarleaf Oil, Nutmeg Oil, Poloxamer 124, Polyoxyethylene Dodecanol, Silicone.

Indications: For temporary relief of nasal congestion due to colds, hay fever or other upper respiratory allergies. Temporarily relieves cough occurring with a cold.

Actions: VAPOSTEAM increases the action of steam to relieve cold symptoms in the following ways: relieves coughs of colds, eases nasal congestion, and moistens dry, irritated breathing passages.

Directions:
Adults and children 2 years of age and older: Use VAPOSTEAM only in hot/warm steam vaporizers, as described below. Follow directions for use carefully. Breathe in medicated vapors. May be repeated up to 3 times daily or as directed by a doctor.
Children under 2 years of age: consult a doctor.
In Hot/Warm Steam Vaporizers: VAPOSTEAM is formulated to be added directly to the water in your hot/warm steam vaporizer. Add one tablespoon of VAPOSTEAM with each quart of water added to the vaporizer. Do not direct steam from vaporizer close to face. For best performance, vaporizer should be thoroughly cleaned after each use according to manufacturer's instructions. To promote steaming, follow directions of vaporizer manufacturer.
Never expose VAPOSTEAM to flame, microwave, or place in any container in which you are heating water except for a hot-warm steam vaporizer. Never use VAPOSTEAM in any bowl or washbasin with hot water. Improper use may cause the mixture to splatter and cause burns.

Warnings: For hot/warm steam vaporizers only. Do not use in cold steam vaporizers or humidifiers. **Not to be taken by mouth.** A persistent cough may be a sign of a serious condition. If cough persists for more than one week, tends to recur or is accompanied by fever, rash, or persistent headache, consult a doctor. Do not use this product for persistent or chronic cough such as occurs with smoking, asthma, emphysema, or if cough is accompanied by excessive phlegm (mucus) unless directed by a doctor. **Keep this and all drugs out of the reach of children.**

Accidental Ingestion: In case of accidental ingestion, seek professional assistance or contact a poison control center immediately.

How Supplied: Available in 4 FL. OZ. (118 mL) and 8 FL. OZ. (236 mL) bottles.

Quintex Pharmaceuticals, Ltd.
ONE EXECUTIVE DRIVE
FORT LEE, NJ 07024

ALCOMED® 2-60 TABLETS
Antihistamine—Nasal Decongestant
Dexbrompheniramine Maleate 2 mg and Pseudoephedrine HCl 60 mg

How Supplied: Blister Packs of 24

EXPRESSIN® 400 CAPLETS
Expectorant—Nasal Decongestant
Guaifenesin 400 mg and Pseudoephedrine HCl 60 mg

How Supplied: Blister Packs of 20

ISOHIST® 2.0 TABLETS
Antihistamine
Dexbrompheniramine Maleate 2 mg

How Supplied: Blister Packs of 24

PEDIAPRESSIN® DROPS
Pediatric Cough and Cold Drops
Pseudoephedrine HCl 15 mg
Guaifenesin 50 mg
Dextromethorphan HBr 5 mg

How Supplied: 1 Oz. with Dropper

RESTYN® 76 CAPLETS
Sleep Aid
Diphenhydramine Citrate 76 mg

How Supplied: Blister Packs of 21

SUPRESSIN® DM CAPLETS
Cough Suppressant—Expectorant
Dextromethorphan HBr 15 mg and Guaifenesin 200 mg

How Supplied: Blister Packs of 20

Reed & Carnrick
Division of Block Drug Company, Inc.
257 CORNELISON AVENUE
JERSEY CITY, NJ 07302

PHAZYME® and PHAZYME®-95
[*fay-zime*]
Tablets

Description: Contains simethicone, an antiflatulent to alleviate or relieve the symptoms of gas. It has no known side effects or drug interactions.

Actions: Simethicone minimizes gas formation and relieves gas entrapment in both the stomach and the lower G.I. tract. This action combats the distress due to gastrointestinal gas.

Indication: To alleviate or relieve the symptoms of gas. May also be used for postoperative gas pain.

Warnings: Keep this and all drugs out of the reach of children. If condition persists, consult your physician.

Store at controlled room temperature 59°–86°F (15°–30°C).

PHAZYME®

Active Ingredient: Each tablet contains simethicone 60 mg.

Inactive Ingredients: Acacia, calcium sulfate, carnauba wax, crospovidone, D&C red No. 7 calcium lake, FD&C blue No. 1 aluminum lake, gelatin, lactose, methylparaben, microcrystalline cellulose, polyoxyl-40 stearate, povidone, pregelatinized starch, propylparaben, rice starch, sodium benzoate, sucrose, talc, titanium dioxide, white wax.

Dosage: One tablet four times a day after meals and at bedtime. Do not exceed 8 tablets a day unless directed by a physician.

How Supplied: Pink coated tablet imprinted "Phazyme" in bottles of 100.

PHAZYME® 95

Active Ingredient: Each tablet contains simethicone 95 mg.

Inactive Ingredients: Acacia, carnauba wax, compressible sugar, crosscarmellose sodium, FD&C red No. 40 aluminum lake, FD&C yellow No. 6 aluminum lake, hydroxypropyl methylcellulose, microcrystalline cellulose, polyoxyl 40 stearate, povidone, sodium benzoate, sucrose, talc, titanium dioxide, white wax.

Dosage: One tablet four times a day after meals and at bedtime. Do not exceed 5 tablets per day unless directed by a physician.

How Supplied: Red coated tablet imprinted "Phazyme 95" in 10 pack, 30 pack and bottles of 50's and 100's.

PHAZYME® DROPS
[*fay-zime*]

Description: Contains simethicone, an antiflatulent to alleviate or relieve the symptoms of gas. It has no known side effects or drug interactions.

Active Ingredients: Each 0.6 mL contains simethicone, 40 mg.
Inactive Ingredients: Carbomer 934 P, citric acid, flavor (natural orange), hydroxypropyl methylcellulose, PEG-8 stearate, potassium sorbate, sodium citrate, sodium saccharin, water.

Actions: Simethicone minimizes gas formation and relieves gas entrapment in both the stomach and the lower G.I. tract. This action combats the distress due to gastrointestinal gas.

Indication: To alleviate or relieve the symptoms of gas. May also be used for postoperative gas pain or endoscopic examination.

Warnings: Keep this and all drugs out of the reach of children. If condition persists, consult your physician.

Store at controlled room temperature 59°–86°F (15°–30°C).

Dosage/Administration: Shake well before using.
Infants (under 2 years):
0.3 ml four times daily after meals and at bedtime or as directed by a physician. Can also be mixed with liquids for easier administration.
Children (2 to 12 years):
0.6 ml four times daily after meals and at bedtime or as directed by a physician.
Adults: 1.2 ml (take two 0.6 ml doses) four times daily after meals and at bedtime. Do not take more than six times per day unless directed by a physician.

How Supplied: Dropper bottles of 15 mL (0.5 fl oz) and 30 mL (1 fl oz).
Shown in Product Identification Guide, page 519

Maximum Strength
PHAZYME®-125 Chewable Tablets
[*fayzime*]

Description: Phazyme Chewables contain the highest dose of simethicone available in a single clean, fresh mint tasting chewable tablet. It has no known side effects or drug interactions.

Active Ingredient: Each tablet contains simethicone 125 mg.

Inactive Ingredients: Citric acid, D&C Yellow #10, dextrates, FD&C Blue #1, peppermint flavor, sorbitol, starch, sucrose, talc, tribasic calcium phosphate.

Actions: Simethicone minimizes gas formation and relieves gas entrapment in both the stomach and the lower G.I. tract. This action combats the distress due to gastrointestinal gas.

Indication: To alleviate or relieve the symptoms of gas. May also be used for postoperative gas pain.

Warnings: Keep this and all drugs out of the reach of children. If condition persists, consult your physician.

Store at controlled room temperature 59°–89°F (15°–30°C).

Dosage: One tablet, chewed thoroughly, four times a day after meals and at bedtime. Do not exceed 4 chewable tablets per day unless directed by a physician.

How Supplied: White, bevel-edged tablets with green speckles and imprinted with "Phazyme 125" in 10 pack, 30 pack and 50 pack.

Maximum Strength
PHAZYME®-125 Softgel Capsules
[*fayzime*]

Description: A red softgel containing the highest dose of simethicone available in a single capsule. It has no known side effects or drug interactions.
Active Ingredient: Each capsule contains simethicone, 125 mg.
Inactive Ingredients: FD&C red No. 40, gelatin, glycerin, hydrogenated soybean oil, lecithin, methylparaben, polysorbate 80, propylparaben, soybean oil, titanium dioxide, vegetable shortening, yellow wax.

Actions: Simethicone minimizes gas formation and relieves gas entrapment in both the stomach and the lower G.I. tract. This action combats the distress due to gastrointestinal gas.

Indication: To alleviate or relieve the symptoms of gas. May also be used for postoperative gas pain.

Warnings: Keep this and all drugs out of the reach of children. If condition persists, consult your physician.

Store at controlled room temperature 59°–86°F (15°–30°C).

Dosage: One softgel capsule four times a day after meals and at bedtime. Do not exceed 4 softgel capsules per day unless directed by a physician.

How Supplied: Red softgel capsule imprinted Phazyme 125 in 10 pack, 30 pack and 50 count bottle.

**IF YOU SUSPECT
AN INTERACTION...**
The 1,400-page
*PDR Guide to Drug Interactions •
Side Effects • Indications*
can help.
Use the order form
in the front of this book.

Requa, Inc.
BOX 4008
1 SENECA PLACE
GREENWICH, CT 06830

CHARCOAID
Poison Adsorbent, liquid has sweet, pleasant taste and feel.

Active Ingredient: Activated vegetable charcoal U.S.P., 30 g per bottle, suspended in 70% sorbitol solution U.S.P., 110 g.

Indication: For the emergency treatment of acute ingested poison.

Action: Adsorbent

Warnings: Before using call a poison control center, emergency room, or a physician for advice. If the patient has been given Ipecac Syrup, do not give activated charcoal until after patient has vomited. Do not use in a semi-conscious or unconscious person.

Precaution: May cause laxation. Careful attention to fluids and electrolytes is important, especially with young children. Not recommended for multiple dose therapy.

Dosage and Administration: Adults: Shake well and drink entire contents (add water if too sweet). To insure a full dose, rinse bottle with water and drink. For children, refer to Poison Control Center.

Professional Labeling: Some dilution may be necessary for administration via lavage tube. Add a small amount of water to bottle and shake.

How Supplied: 5 fl. oz. unit dose bottle, 30 g activated charcoal U.S.P., suspended in 70% sorbitol solution U.S.P., 110 g.
U.S. Patent #4,122,169

CharcoAid 2000
Emergency Poison Adsorbent with super activated charcoal.

Active Ingredient: Super Activated Charcoal U.S.P., 50g

Indication: For the emergency treatment of acute ingested poison.

Action: Adsorbent

Warnings: See Charcoaid

Dosage and Administration: Shake bottle vigorously for at least 15 seconds. Drink entire contents, or for children use as directed by a health professional.

How Supplied: 240 ml bottle contains 50g charcoal in water suspension

Richardson-Vicks Inc.
(See Procter & Gamble.)

Roberts Pharmaceutical Corporation
4 INDUSTRIAL WAY WEST
EATONTOWN, NJ 07724

CHERACOL® Nasal Spray Pump
Cherry Scented

Description: CHERACOL® NASAL SPRAY PUMP is a cherry scented long acting topical nasal decongestant. One application lasts up to 12 hours.

Indications: For the temporary relief of nasal congestion associated with colds ("flu"), hay fever, and sinusitis.

Active Ingredients: Oxymetazoline hydrochloride USP 0.05% (0.5 mg/ml).

Inactive Ingredients: Benzalkonium chloride, glycine, sodium hydroxide, phenylmercuric acetate (0.02 mg/ml), sorbitol, artificial cherry flavor, and purified water.

Dosage and Administration: CHERACOL Nasal Spray has a long duration of action lasting up to 12 hours with each topical application. One application mornings and at bedtime is usually sufficient for round-the-clock action. For adults and children 6 years of age and over: Two or three sprays in each nostril twice daily—morning and bedtime. Remove protective cap. Hold bottle with thumb at base and nozzle between first and second fingers. With head upright, insert metered pump spray nozzle in nostril. Depress pump 2 or 3 times all the way down with a firm even stroke and sniff deeply. Repeat in other nostril. Do not tilt head backward while spraying. Wipe tip clean after each use. Before using the first time, remove the protective cap from the tip and prime the metered pump by depressing pump firmly several times.

Warning: Do not give this product to children under 6 years of age except under the advice and supervision of a physician. Do not exceed recommended dosage because burning, stinging, sneezing, or increase in nasal discharge may occur. The use of this container by more than one person may spread infection. Do not use this product for more than 3 days. If symptoms persist, consult a doctor. Do not use this product if you have heart disease, high blood pressure, thyroid disease, diabetes, or difficulty in urination due to enlargement of the prostate gland unless directed by a doctor. Do not give this product to children who have heart disease, high blood pressure, thyroid disease, or diabetes, unless directed by a doctor. As with any drug, if you are pregnant or nursing a baby seek the advice of a health professional before using this product. The use of this dispenser by more than one person may spread infection. Store at room temperature. Keep this and all medicines out of children's reach.

Overdose: In case of accidental overdose contact a physician or regional poison control center immediately.

How Supplied: Available in 1 fluid ounce bottles fitted with a metered pump (NDC 54092-880-30).
Manufactured for:
Roberts Laboratories Inc.,
a subsidiary of
ROBERTS PHARMACEUTICAL CORPORATION
Eatontown, NJ 07724 USA

CHERACOL® SINUS
12 Hour Formula

Description: Cheracol® SINUS sustained-action tablets combine a nasal decongestant with an antihistamine in a special continuous-acting timed-release tablet to provide temporary relief of nasal congestion due to the common cold, and associated with sinusitis. Also alleviates running nose and sneezing due to hay fever.

Each Cheracol® SINUS Sustained-Action Tablet Contains: 6 mg of dexbrompheniramine maleate and 120 mg of pseudoephedrine sulfate. Half of the medication is released after the tablet is swallowed and the remaining amount of medication is sustained-release, providing continuous long-lasting relief for 12 hours.

Indications: For temporary relief of nasal congestion due to the common cold, hay fever, or other upper respiratory allergies, and associated with sinusitis. Helps decongest sinus openings, sinus passages. Reduces swelling of nasal passages; shrinks swollen membranes; and temporarily restores freer breathing through the nose. Alleviates running nose, sneezing, itching of the nose or throat, and itchy and watery eyes as may occur in allergic rhinitis (such as hay fever).

Directions: Adults and Children 12 Years and Over—one tablet every 12 hours. Do not exceed two tablets in 24 hours.

Warnings: If symptoms do not improve within 7 days or are accompanied by high fever, consult a physician before continuing use. May cause drowsiness; alcohol may increase the drowsiness effect. Avoid alcoholic beverages while taking this product. Use caution when driving a motor vehicle or operating machinery. May cause excitability especially in children. Do not exceed recommended dosage, because at higher doses nervousness, dizziness, or sleeplessness may occur. Do not give this product to children under 12 years, except under the advice and supervision of a physician. Do not take this product if you have emphysema, chronic pulmonary disease, shortness of breath, and difficulty in breathing, asthma, glaucoma, difficulty in urination due to enlargement of the prostate gland, high blood pressure, heart disease, diabetes, or thyroid disease except under the advice and supervision of a physician. As with any drug, if you are pregnant or nursing a baby, seek the advice of a health professional before using this product. Keep this and all drugs out of the reach of children. In case of accidental overdose, seek professional assistance or contact a Poison Control Center immediately.

Drug Interaction Precaution: Do not take this product if you are presently taking a prescription drug for high blood pressure or depression, without first consulting your doctor.

Active Ingredients: Dexbrompheniramine Meleate 6 mg, Pseudoephedrine Sulfate 120 mg.

Also Contains: Acacia, Calcium Carbonate, Carnauba Wax, Confectioner's Sugar, D&C Yellow #10, FD&C Blue #1, FD&C Yellow #6, Gelatin, Hydrogenated Castor Oil, Magnesium Stearate, Methylparaben, Povidone, Propylparaben, Shellac, Sodium Benzoate, Sucrose, Talc, Titanium Dioxide.
Use by expiration date printed on package.
Store between 2° and 30°C (36° and 86°F). Protect from excessive moisture.

How Supplied: 10 sustained-action release tablets. NDC 54092-045-10
Manufactured for:
Roberts Laboratories Inc.,
a subsidiary of
ROBERTS   PHARMACEUTICAL CORPORATION
Eatontown, NJ 07724, USA

CHERACOL® Sore Throat Spray
Anesthetic/Antiseptic Liquid

Description: A pleasant tasting cherry flavored liquid spray with anesthetic and antiseptic properties.

Indications: For the temporary relief of occasional minor sore throat pain and irritation. Also for temporary relief of pain associated with sore mouth, canker sores, tonsillitis, pharyngitis and throat infections.

Active Ingredients: Phenol 1.4%.

Inactive Ingredients: Alcohol 12.5%, citric acid, FD&C Red No. 40, flavor, glycerin, propylene glycol, sodium citrate, sodium saccharin, sorbitol and purified water.

Directions For Use: Mouthwash and gargle: Irritated throat: Spray 5 times (children 3–12 years of age, 3 times) and swallow. May be used as a gargle. Repeat every 2 hours or as directed by physician or dentist. Children under 12 years of age should be supervised in the use of this product.

Warning: If sore throat is severe, persists for more than 2 days, is accompanied or followed by fever, headache, rash, nausea or vomiting, consult a doctor promptly. If sore throat or mouth symptoms do not improve in 7 days, see your doctor or dentist promptly. As with any drug, if you are pregnant or nursing a baby, seek the advice of a health professional before using this product. Do not administer to children under 3 years unless directed by a physician or dentist. Keep this and all medicines out of the reach of children.

Overdose: In case of accidental overdose contact a physician or a poison control center immediately.

How Supplied: Available in 6 fluid ounce spray pump bottle (NDC 54092-340-06).
Manufactured for:
Roberts Laboratories Inc.,
a subsidiary of
ROBERTS PHARMACEUTICAL CORPORATION
Eatontown, NJ 07724 USA

CHERACOL–D® Cough Formula
Maximum Strength Cough Formula

Description: CHERACOL-D® is a non-narcotic cough formula which combines two important medicines in one safe, fast-acting pleasant tasting liquid:
● The highest level of cough suppressant available without prescription.
● A clinically proven expectorant to help loosen phlegm and drain bronchial tubes.

Indications: CHERACOL-D® cough formula helps quiet dry, hacking coughs, and helps loosen phlegm and mucus. Recommended for adults and children 2 years of age and older.

Active Ingredients: Each teaspoonful (5 ml) contains dextromethorphan hydrobromide, 10 mg; guaifenesin, 100 mg; alcohol, 4.75%. Also contains benzoic acid, FD&C Red #40, flavors, fragrances, fructose, glycerin, propylene glycol, sodium chloride, sucrose, and purified water.

Dosage—Adults and children 12 years of age and over: Oral dosage is 2 teaspoonfuls every 4 hours, not to exceed 12 teaspoonfuls in 24 hours, or as directed by a doctor. **Children 6 to under 12 years of age:** Oral dosage is 1 teaspoonful every 4 hours, not to exceed 6 teaspoonfuls in 24 hours, or as directed by a doctor. **Children 2 to under 6 years of age:** Oral dosage is ½ teaspoonful every 4 hours, not to exceed 3 teaspoonfuls in 24 hours, or as directed by a doctor. **Children under 2 years of age:** Consult a doctor.

Warnings: Keep this and all drugs out of the reach of children. Do not give this product to children under 2 years of age except under the advice and supervision of a physician. Do not use this product for persistent or chronic cough such as oc-

curs with smoking, asthma, or emphysema or where cough is accompanied by excessive secretions except under the advice and supervision of a physician. As with any drug, if you are pregnant or nursing a baby, seek the advice of a health professional before using this product.

Caution: A persistent cough may be a sign of a serious condition. If cough persists for more than 1 week, tends to recur or is accompanied by high fever, rash or persistent headache, consult a physician.

Overdose: In case of accidental overdose contact a physician or a poison control center immediately.

How Supplied: Available in 2 oz bottle (NDC 54092-400-60), 4 oz bottle (NDC 54092-400-04), and 6 oz bottle (NDC 54092-400-06).
Manufactured for:
Roberts Laboratories Inc.,
a subsidiary of
ROBERTS PHARMACEUTICAL CORPORATION
Eatontown, NJ 07724 USA
Shown in Product Identification Guide, page 519

CHERACOL PLUS® Cough Syrup
Multisymptom cough/cold formula

Description: CHERACOL PLUS® Cough Syrup is a pleasant tasting 3-ingredient non-narcotic liquid formulation.

Indications: Cheracol Plus syrup is an effective 3-ingredient, maximum strength formula for the temporary relief of head cold symptoms and cough (without narcotic side effects).

Active Ingredients: Each tablespoonful (15ml) contains phenylpropanolamine HCl, 25 mg; dextromethorphan hydrobromide, 20 mg; chlorpheniramine maleate, 4 mg; and alcohol, 8%.

Inactive Ingredients: Flavors, glycerin, methylparaben, propylene glycol, propylparaben, FD&C Red No. 40, sodium chloride, sorbitol solution, and purified water.

Dosage and Administration: Adults and children over 12 years of age: 1 tablespoonful (15ml) every 4 hours or as directed by a physician. Do not take more than 6 tablespoonfuls in a 24 hour period. Do not administer to children under 12 years of age.

Uses: Cheracol Plus® multisymptom head cold/cough formula provides cough suppressant and decongestant activity and controls runny nose associated with the common cold ("flu").

Warnings: Do not take this product for persistent or chronic cough such as occurs with smoking, asthma, or emphysema or where cough is accompanied by excessive secretions or if you have high blood pressure, heart or thyroid disease,

Continued on next page

Roberts—Cont.

diabetes, asthma, glaucoma, or difficulty in urination due to enlargement of the prostate gland except under the advice and supervision of a physician. If symptoms do not improve within 7 days or are accompanied by high fever, consult a physician before continuing use. May cause excitability, especially in children. Do not give this product to children under 12 years except under the advice and supervision of a physician. May cause marked drowsiness. Avoid alcoholic beverages, driving a motor vehicle or operating heavy machinery while taking this product. As with any drug, if you are pregnant or nursing a baby consult a health professional before using this product. Keep out of the reach of children.

Drug Interaction Precaution: Do not use this product if you are now taking a prescription monoamine oxidase inhibitor (MAOI) (certain drugs for depression, psychiatric or emotional conditions, or Parkinson's disease), or for 2 weeks after stopping the MAOI drug. If you are uncertain whether your prescription drug contains an MAOI, consult a health professional before taking this product.

Overdose: In case of accidental overdose contact a physician or a poison control center immediately.

How Supplied: Available in 4 oz bottle (NDC 54092-401-04), 6 oz bottle (54092-401-06).
Manufactured for:
Roberts Laboratories Inc.,
a subsidiary of
ROBERTS PHARMACEUTICAL CORPORATION
Eatontown, NJ 07724 USA

CITROCARBONATE® Antacid

Active Ingredients: When dissolved, each 4.1 grams (1 teaspoonful) contains approximately: sodium bicarbonate, 0.78 gram and sodium citrate anhydrous, 1.82 grams. **As derived from (per teaspoonful):** sodium bicarbonate, 2.34 gram; citric acid anhydrous, 1.19 gram; sodium citrate hydrous, 254 mg; calcium lactate pentahydrate, 151 mg; sodium chloride, 79 mg; monobasic sodium phosphate anhydrous, 44 mg; magnesium sulfate dried, 42 mg. Each 4.1 grams (teaspoonful) contains 30.46 mEq (700.6 mg) of sodium.

Indications: For the relief of heartburn, acid indigestion, and sour stomach; and upset stomach associated with these symptoms.

Dosage and Administration: Adults: 1 to 2 teaspoonfuls (not to exceed 5 level teaspoonfuls per day) in a glass of cold water after meals. Persons 60 years or older: $\frac{1}{2}$ to 1 teaspoonful after meals. Children 6 to 12 years: $\frac{1}{4}$ to $\frac{1}{2}$ teaspoonful. For children under 6 years: Consult physician.

Warnings: Do not use this product if you are on a restricted sodium diet, or take more than the above recommended dosage in a 24-hour period, or use the maximum dosage of this product for more than 2 weeks, except under the advice and supervision of a physician. Keep this and all drugs out of the reach of children.

How Supplied: Available in 5 oz (NDC 54092-900-05) and 10 oz (NDC 54092-900-10) bottles.
Manufactured for:
Roberts Laboratories Inc.,
a subsidiary of
ROBERTS PHARMACEUTICAL CORPORATION
Eatontown, NJ 07724 USA

CLOCREAM®
Skin Protectant Cream

Description: CLOCREAM® skin protectant cream contains Vitamins A and D in a greaseless vanishing cream base that leaves no residue. Also contains cetyl palmitate, cholecalciferol, cottonseed oil, glycerin, glyceryl monostearate, fragrance, methylparaben, mineral oil, potassium stearate, propylparaben, sodium citrate, Vitamin A palmitate and purified oil. Each ounce of CLOCREAM® contains Vitamins A and D equivalent to 1 ounce of cod liver oil.

Indications: CLOCREAM® is indicated for the temporary relief of chapped skin, diaper rash, wind burn, sunburn and minor non-infected skin irritations. CLOCREAM® promotes epithelization.

Uses: CLOCREAM® may be particularly useful for health care personnel or others who frequently wash their hands and for general patient care to reduce dermal excoriation and breakdown from prolonged bed rest, bedwetting and abrasions. The vanishing action of CLOCREAM® skin protectant cream makes it cosmetically acceptable when the skin treated is on an exposed part of the body such as the hands or arms.

Warnings: CLOCREAM® skin protectant cream is for external use only. Avoid contact with the eyes. If condition worsens or if symptoms persist for more than 7 days, discontinue use of this product and consult a physician. Keep this and all medications out of the reach of children. In case of accidental ingestion seek professional assistance or contact a poison control center immediately.

Dosage and Administration: Gently massage or apply liberally to unbroken skin or abraded skin where promotion of epitheliazation is desired. Use as often as desired.

How Supplied: Available in 1 ounce tubes (NDC 54092-300-30).
Manufactured for:
Roberts Laboratories Inc.,
a subsidiary of

ROBERTS PHARMACEUTICAL CORPORATION
Eatontown, NJ 07724 USA

COLACE®
[kōlās]
docusate sodium,
capsules • syrup • liquid (drops)

Description: Colace® (docusate sodium) is a stool softener.
Colace® Capsules, 50 mg, contain the following inactive ingredients: citric acid, D&C Red No. 33, FD&C Red No. 40, nonporcine gelatin, edible ink, polyethylene glycol, propylene glycol, and purified water.
Colace® Capsules, 100 mg, contain the following inactive ingredients: citric acid, D&C Red No. 33, FD&C Red No. 40, FD&C Yellow No. 6, nonporcine gelatin, edible ink, polyethylene glycol, propylene glycol, titanium dioxide, and purified water.
Colace® Liquid, 1%, contains the following inactive ingredients: citric acid, D&C Red No. 33, methylparaben, poloxamer, polyethylene glycol, propylene glycol, propylparaben, sodium citrate, vanillin, and purified water.
Colace® Syrup, 20 mg/5 mL, contains the following inactive ingredients: alcohol (not more than 1%), citric acid, D&C Red No. 33, FD&C Red No. 40, flavor (natural), menthol, methylparaben, peppermint oil, poloxamer, polyethylene glycol, propylparaben, sodium citrate, sucrose, and purified water.

Actions and Uses: Colace®, a surface-active agent, helps to keep stools soft for easy, natural passage and is not a laxative, thus, not habit forming. Useful in constipation due to hard stools, in painful anorectal conditions, in cardiac and other conditions in which maximum ease of passage is desirable to avoid difficult or painful defecation, and when peristaltic stimulants are contraindicated. *Note:* When peristaltic stimulation is needed due to inadequate bowel motility, see Peri-Colace® (laxative and stool softener).

Contraindications: There are no known contraindications to Colace®.

Warning: As with any drug, pregnant or nursing women should seek the advice of a health professional before using this product.

Side Effects: The incidence of side effects—none of a serious nature—is exceedingly small. Bitter taste, throat irritation, and nausea (primarily associated with the use of the syrup and liquid) are the main side effects reported. Rash has occurred.

Administration and Dosage: *Orally*—Suggested daily Dosage: *Adults and older children:* 50 to 200 mg *Children 6 to 12:* 40 to 120 mg *Children 3 to 6:* 20 to 60 mg. *Infants and children under 3:* 10 to 40 mg. The higher doses are recommended for initial therapy. Dosage should be adjusted to individual response. The effect on stools is usually apparent 1 to 3 days after the first dose. Colace® liquid or syrup must be given in a 6 oz. to 8 oz. glass of milk or fruit juice or in infant's formula to prevent throat irritation. In *enemas*—Add 50 to 100 mg Colace® 5 to 10 mL Colace® liquid) to a retention or flushing enema.

How Supplied: Colace® capsules, 50 mg
    NDC 54092-052-30 Bottles of 30
    NDC 54092-052-60 Bottles of 60
    NDC 54092-052-52 Cartons of 100
       single unit packs
Colace® capsules, 100 mg
    NDC 54092-053-30 Bottles of 30
    NDC 54092-053-60 Bottles of 60
    NDC 54092-053-02 Bottles of 250
    NDC 54092-053-10 Bottles of 1000
    NDC 54092-053-52 Cartons of 100
       single unit packs
Note: Colace® capsules should be stored at controlled room temperature (59°–86°F or 15°–30°C)
Colace® liquid, 1% solution; 10 mg/mL (with calibrated dropper)
    NDC 54092-414-16 Bottles of 16 fl oz
    NDC 54092-414-30 Bottles of 30 mL
Colace® syrup, 20 mg/5-mL teaspoon; contains not more than 1% alcohol
    NDC 54092-415-08 Bottles of 8 fl oz
    NDC 54092-415-16 Bottles of 16 fl oz
Manufactured for:
Roberts Laboratories Inc.,
a subsidiary of
ROBERTS PHARMACEUTICAL CORPORATION
Eatontown, NJ 07724 USA
Shown in Product Identification Guide, page 519

HALTRAN® Tablets
Ibuprofen/Analgesic
MENSTRUAL CRAMP RELIEVER
WARNING: ASPIRIN SENSITIVE PATIENTS. Do not take this product if you have had a severe allergic reaction to aspirin, eg—asthma, swelling, shock or hives, because even though this product contains no aspirin or salicylates cross-reactions may occur in patients allergic to aspirin.

Indications: For the pain of menstrual cramps and also the temporary relief of minor aches and pains associated with the common cold, headache, toothache, muscular aches, backache, for the minor pain of arthritis and for reduction of fever.

Directions: *Adults:* Take 1 tablet every 4 to 6 hours while symptoms persist. If pain or fever does not respond to 1 tablet, 2 tablets may be used, but do not exceed 6 tablets in 24 hours, unless directed by a doctor. The smallest effective dose should be used. Take with food or milk if occasional and mild heartburn, upset stomach, or stomach pain occurs with use. Consult a doctor if these symptoms are more than mild or if they persist. *Children:* Do not give this product to children under 12 except under the advice and supervision of a doctor.

Warnings: Do not take for pain for more than 10 days or for fever for more than 3 days unless directed by a doctor. If pain or fever persists or gets worse, if new symptoms occur, or if the painful area is red or swollen, consult a doctor. These could be signs of serious illness. If you are under a doctor's care for any serious condition, consult a doctor before taking this product. As with aspirin and acetaminophen, if you have any condition which requires you to take prescription drugs or if you have had any problems or serious side effects from taking any non-prescription pain reliever, do not take HALTRAN® Tablets (ibuprofen) without first discussing it with your doctor. If you experience any symptoms which are unusual or seem unrelated to the condition for which you took ibuprofen, consult a doctor before taking any more of it. Although ibuprofen is indicated for the same conditions as aspirin and acetaminophen, it should not be taken with them except under a doctor's direction. Before using any drug, including HALTRAN®, you should seek the advice of a health professional if you are pregnant or nursing a baby. IT IS ESPECIALLY IMPORTANT NOT TO USE IBUPROFEN DURING THE LAST 3 MONTHS OF PREGNANCY UNLESS SPECIFICALLY DIRECTED TO DO SO BY A DOCTOR BECAUSE IT MAY CAUSE PROBLEMS IN THE UNBORN CHILD OR COMPLICATIONS DURING DELIVERY. Keep this and all drugs out of the reach of children. In case of accidental overdose, seek professional assistance or contact a poison control center immediately.

Active Ingredient: Each tablet contains ibuprofen USP 200 mg.

Other Ingredients: Carnauba wax, cornstarch, hydroxypropyl methylcellulose, propylene glycol, silicon dioxide, pregelatinized starch, stearic acid, and titanium dioxide.
Store at room temperature. Avoid excessive heat 40°C (104°F).

How Supplied: Available in bottles of 30 (NDC 54092-020-30).
Manufactured for:
Roberts Laboratories Inc.,
a subsidiary of
ROBERTS PHARMACEUTICAL CORPORATION
Eatontown, NJ 07724 USA
Shown in Product Identification Guide, page 519

PERI-COLACE® capsules • syrup
(casanthranol and docusate sodium)

Description: Peri-Colace® is a combination of the mild stimulant laxative casanthranol, and the stool-softener Colace® (docusate sodium). Each capsule contains 30 mg of casanthranol and 100 mg of Colace®; the syrup contains 30 mg of casanthranol and 60 mg of Colace® per 15-mL tablespoon (10 mg of casan-

thranol and 20 mg of Colace® per 5-mL teaspoon) and 10% alcohol.
Peri-Colace® Capsules contain the following inactive ingredients: D&C Red No. 33, FD&C Red No. 40, non-porcine gelatin, edible ink, polyethylene glycol, propylene glycol, titanium dioxide, and purified water.
Peri-Colace® Syrup contains the following inactive ingredients: alcohol (10% v/v), citric acid, flavors, methyl salicylate, methylparaben, poloxamer, polyethylene glycol, propylparaben, sodium citrate, sorbitol solution, sucrose, and purified water.

Action and Uses: Peri-Colace® provides gentle peristaltic stimulation and helps to keep stools soft for easier passage. Bowel movement is induced gently—usually overnight or in 8 to 12 hours. Nausea, griping, abnormally loose stools, and constipation rebound are minimized. Useful in management of chronic or temporary constipation.
Note: To prevent hard stools when laxative stimulation is not needed or undesirable, see Colace® (stool softener).

Warnings: Do not use when abdominal pain, nausea, or vomiting is present. Frequent or prolonged use of this preparation may result in dependence on laxatives.
As with any drug, pregnant or nursing women should seek the advice of a health professional before using this product.

Side Effects: The incidence of side effects—none of a serious nature—is exceedingly small. Nausea, abdominal cramping or discomfort, diarrhea, and rash are the main side effects reported.

Administration and Dosage:
Adults—1 or 2 capsules, or 1 or 2 tablespoons syrup at bedtime, or as indicated. In severe cases, dosage may be increased to 2 capsules or 2 tablespoons twice daily, or 3 capsules at bedtime. *Children*—1 to 3 teaspoons of syrup at bedtime, or as indicated. Peri-Colace® syrup must be given in a 6 oz. to 8 oz. glass of milk or fruit juice or in infant's formula to prevent throat irritation.

Overdosage: In addition to symptomatic treatment, gastric lavage, if timely, is recommended in cases of large overdosage.

How Supplied: Peri-Colace® ® Capsules
    NDC 54092-054-30 Bottles of 30
    NDC 54092-054-60 Bottles of 60
    NDC 54092-054-02 Bottles of 250
    NDC 54092-054-10 Bottles of 1000
    NDC 54092-054-52 Cartons of 100 single unit packs
Note: Peri-Colace® capsules should be stored at controlled room temperatures (59°–86°F or 15°–30°C).
Peri-Colace® ® Syrup
    NDC 54092-418-08 Bottles of 8 fl oz
    NDC 54092-418-16 Bottles of 16 fl oz
Manufactured for:
Roberts Laboratories Inc.,

Continued on next page

Roberts—Cont.

a subsidiary of
**ROBERTS PHARMACEUTICAL
CORPORATION**
Eatontown, NJ 07724 USA
*Shown in Product Identification
Guide, page 519*

**PYRROXATE® Caplets
Extra Strength Decongestant/
Antihistamine/
Analgesic Caplets**

Description: *Pyrroxate®* provides single-caplet, multisymptom relief for colds, allergies, nasal/sinus congestion, runny nose, sneezing, and watery eyes. Because it contains the non-aspirin analgesic **acetaminophen,** *Pyrroxate®* gives temporary relief of occasional minor aches, pains, headache, and helps in the reduction of fever. *Pyrroxate®* is caffeine and aspirin-free.

Active Ingredients: Each *Pyrroxate®* Caplet contains: chlorpheniramine maleate, 4 mg; phenylpropanolamine HCl, 25 mg; acetaminophen, 650 mg.

Inactive Ingredients: Cellulose, sodium croscarmellose, silicon dioxide, stearic acid, magnesium stearate, hydroxpropyl methylcellulose, yellow No. 10 lake, yellow No. 6 lake, titanium dioxide, polyethylene glycol.

Indications: *Pyrroxate®* Caplets are for the temporary relief of runny nose, sneezing, itching of the nose or throat; for the temporary relief of nasal congestion due to the common cold, allergies (hay fever), sinus congestion and for the temporary relief of occasional minor aches, pains, headache, and for the reduction of fever.

Actions: Chlorpheniramine maleate is an antihistamine effective in controlling runny nose, sneezing, watery eyes, and itching of the nose and throat. Phenylpropanolamine HCl is an oral nasal decongestant effective in relieving nasal/sinus congestion due to the common cold or allergies (hay fever). Acetaminophen is a clinically effective analgesic and antipyretic without aspirin side effects.

Warnings: Do not take this product for more than 7 days. If symptoms persist, do not improve, or new ones occur, or if fever persists for more than 3 days, discontinue use and consult your physician. Do not take this product if you have asthma, glaucoma, difficulty in urination due to the enlargement of the prostate gland, high blood pressure, diabetes, thyroid disease, or if you are presently taking a prescription antihypertensive or antidepressant drug containing a monamine oxidase inhibitor, except under the advice and supervision of a physician. As with any drug, if you are pregnant or nursing a baby, seek the advice of a health professional before using this product. Do not exceed recommended dosage because severe liver damage may occur and at higher doses, nervousness, dizziness or sleeplessness may occur. Do not take other medications containing acetaminophen simultaneously, to avoid the risk of overdosage. Do not take this product for the treatment of arthritis except under the advice and supervision of a physician.

Cautions: Avoid alcoholic beverages, driving a motor vehicle, or operating heavy machinery while taking this product. This product may cause drowsiness or excitability, especially in children. Keep this and all drugs out of the reach of children. In case of accidental overdose, seek professional assistance or contact a poison control center immediately.

Dosage and Administration: Take 1 caplet every 4 hours or as directed by a physician. Do not take more than 6 caplets in a 24-hour period. Do not administer to children under 12 years of age.

How Supplied: Yellow caplets available in bottles of 24 (NDC 54092-041-24) and 500 (NDC 54092-041-05).
Manufactured for:
Roberts Laboratories Inc.,
a subsidiary of
**ROBERTS PHARMACEUTICAL
CORPORATION**
Eatontown, NJ 07724 USA
*Shown in Product Identification
Guide, page 519*

**SIGTAB® Tablets
High Potency Vitamin Supplement**

Each Tablet Contains:		% U.S. RDA*
Vitamin A	5000 IU	100
Vitamin D	400 IU	100
Vitamin E	15 IU	50
Vitamin C	333 mg	555
Folic Acid	0.4 mg	100
Thiamine	10.3 mg	687
Riboflavin	10 mg	588
Niacin	100 mg	500
Vitamin B₆	6 mg	300
Vitamin B₁₂	18 mcg	300
Pantothenic Acid	20 mg	200

*Percentage of U.S. Recommended Daily Allowance.

Recommended Dosage: For adults, 1 tablet daily

Ingredient List: Sucrose, sodium ascorbate (Vit. C), Calcium Sulfate, Niacinamide, Vitamin E Acetate, Calcium Pantothenate, Vitamin A Acetate, Thiamine Mononitrate (B-1), Riboflavin (B-2), Gelatin, Pyridoxine HCl (B-6), Povidone, Lacca, Magnesium Stearate, Silica, Artificial Color, Sodium Benzoate, Folic Acid, Polyethylene Glycol, Cholecalciferol (Vit. D), Carnauba Wax, Cyanocobalamin (B-12), Medical Antifoam, Sesame Seed Oil and Titanium Dioxide.

How Supplied: Available in bottles of 90 (NDC 54092-033-90) and 500 (NDC 54092-033-05).

Warning: Keep out of the reach of children.

Manufactured for:
Roberts Laboratories Inc.,
a subsidiary of
**ROBERTS PHARMACEUTICAL
CORPORATION**
Eatontown, NJ 07724 USA

SIGTAB®-M Tablets
[See table at top of next page.]

How Supplied: Bottle of 100 tablets.
NDC 54092-038-01
Recommended dosage for adults: 1 tablet daily.

Warning: Keep out of the reach of children.
**Keep container tightly closed. Store at room temperature.
Do not use if seal under cap is broken.**
Manufactured for:
Roberts Laboratories Inc.,
a subsidiary of
**ROBERTS PHARMACEUTICAL
CORPORATION**
Eatontown, NJ 07724, USA
*Shown in Product Identification
Guide, page 519*

**ZYMACAP® Capsules
High Potency Vitamin Supplement**

Description: Dietary multivitamin supplement providing 150% of the RDA for Vitamin B and Vitamin C plus 100% of the RDA for Vitamins A and D.

Each Capsule Contains:		% US RDA*
Vitamin A	5,000 IU	100
Vitamin D	400 IU	100
Vitamin E	15 IU	50
Vitamin C	90 mg	150
Folic Acid	400 mcg	100
Thiamine	2.25 mg	150
Riboflavin	2.6 mg	150
Niacin	30 mg	150
Vitamin B-6	3 mg	150
Vitamin B-12	9 mcg	150
Pantothenic Acid	15 mg	150

*Percentage of U.S. recommended daily allowance.

Recommended Dosage: 1 Capsule daily.

Ingredient List: Soybean oil, ascorbic acid (Vitamin C), gelatin, glycerin, niacinamide, calcium pantothenate, Vitamin E acetate, lecithin, pyridoxine hydrochloride (Vitamin B-6), yellow wax, thiamine mononitrate (Vitamin B-1), riboflavin (Vitamin B-2), Vitamin A palmitate, FD&C Red No. 40, folic acid, titanium dioxide, ethyl vanillin, vanilla enhancer, cholecalciferol (Vitamin D), cyanocobalamin (Vitamin B-12).

How Supplied: Available in bottles of 90 capsules (NDC 54092-030-90).
Manufactured for:
Roberts Laboratories Inc.,
a subsidiary of
**ROBERTS PHARMACEUTICAL
CORPORATION**
Eatontown, NJ 07724 USA

SIGTAB®-M Tablets
Each Tablet Contains:

Active Ingredients:

		% U.S. RDA*
Vitamin A (From Vit. A & Beta Carotene)	6000 Intl. Units	120
Vitamin D3	400 Intl. Units	100
Vitamin E (DL-Alpha Tocopherol Acetate)	45 Intl. Units	150
Vitamin C (Ascorbic Acid)	100 mg	166
Niacinamide	25 mg	125
Thiamine Mononitrate	5 mg	333
Riboflavin	5 mg	294
Pyridoxine (Pyridoxine HCl)	3 mg	150
Folic Acid	400 mcg	100
Pantothenic Acid (D-Calcium Pant.)	15 mcg	150
Vitamin B12	18 mcg	300
Vitamin K1	25 mcg	8
Biotin	45 mcg	15
Calcium	200 mg	20
Phosphorus (Dicalcium Phosphate)	150 mg	15
Iron (Ferrous Fumarate)	18 mg	100
Magnesium (Magnesium Oxide)	100 mg	25
Copper (Copper Oxide)	2 mg	100
Zinc (Zinc Oxide)	15 mg	100
Iodine (Potassium Iodide)	150 mcg	100
Manganese (Manganese Sulfate)	5 mg	**
Potassium (Potassium Chloride)	40 mg	**
Chloride	36.3 mg	**
Selenium (Sodium Selenate)	25 mcg	**
Molybdenum (Sodium Molybdate)	25 mcg	**
Chromium (Chromium Chloride)	25 mcg	**
Nickel	5 mcg	**
Tin	10 mcg	**
Vanadium	10 mcg	**
Silicon	2 mcg	**
Boron	150 mcg	**

Inactive Ingredients:
Microcrystalline Cellulose NF, Stearic Acid NF, Croscarmellose Sodium NF, Magnesium Stearate NF, Hydroxypropyl Methylcellulose NF, Propylene Glycol, USP, FD&C Yellow #6
 *Percentage of U.S. Recommended Daily Allowances
 **These beneficial minerals are in addition to the Recommended Daily Allowances of the vitamins.

A. H. Robins Consumer Products
**American Home Products Corporation
FIVE GIRALDA FARMS
MADISON, NJ 07940-0871**

DIMETAPP® Cold & Allergy
[di 'mĕ-tap]
Chewable Tablets

Description: Each chewable tablet contains:
Brompheniramine Maleate, USP ... 1 mg
Phenylpropanolamine Hydrochloride, USP ... 6.25 mg

Inactive Ingredients: Aspartame, Citric Acid, Crospovidone, D&C Red 30 Aluminum Lake, D&C Red 7 Calcium Lake, FD&C Blue 1 Aluminum Lake, Flavor, Glycine, Magnesium Stearate, Mannitol, Microcrystalline Cellulose, Pregelatinized Starch, Silicon Dioxide, Sorbitol, Stearic Acid.

Indications: For temporary relief of nasal congestion due to the common cold, hay fever, or other upper respiratory allergies or associated with sinusitis. Temporarily relieves runny nose, sneezing, and itchy, watery eyes due to allergic rhinitis (hay fever). Temporarily restores freer breathing through the nose.

Warnings: Do not to give this product to children who have a breathing problem such as chronic bronchitis, glaucoma, high blood pressure, heart disease, diabetes, or thyroid disease, without first consulting the child's physician. This product may cause drowsiness: sedatives and tranquilizers may increase the drowsiness effect. Do not give this product to children who are taking sedatives or tranquilizers without first consulting the child's physician. May cause excitability, especially in children.
Do not exceed the recommended dosage, because at higher doses, nervousness, dizziness, or sleeplessness may occur. Do not give this product to children for more than 7 days. If symptoms do not improve, or are accompanied by a fever, consult a physician. Do not give this product to children if they are hypersensitive to any of the ingredients. As with any drug, if you are pregnant or nursing a baby, seek the advice of a health professional before using this product.

Drug Interaction Precaution: Do not use this product if you are now taking a prescription monoamine oxidase inhibitor (MAOI) (certain drugs for depression, psychiatric or emotional conditions, or Parkinson's disease) or for 2 weeks after stopping the MAOI drug. If you are uncertain whether your prescription drug contains an MAOI, consult a health professional before taking this product.
KEEP THIS AND ALL DRUGS OUT OF THE REACH OF CHILDREN. IN CASE OF ACCIDENTAL OVERDOSE, SEEK PROFESSIONAL ASSISTANCE OR CONTACT A POISON CONTROL CENTER IMMEDIATELY.
Phenylketonurics are advised that this product contains 8 mg of phenylalanine per tablet.

Directions: Children 6 to under 12 years of age: 2 chewable tablets every 4 hours. Children under 6: Consult a physician. DO NOT EXCEED 6 DOSES IN A 24-HOUR PERIOD.

Professional Labeling: The suggested dosage for children age 2 to under 6 years, only when the child is under the care of a physician, is 1 tablet every 4 hours, not to exceed 6 doses in a 24-hour period.

How Supplied: Purple tablet scored on one side and engraved with AHR 2290 on the other in bottles of 24 tablets (NDC 0031–2290–54).
Store at Controlled Room Temperature, Between 15°C and 30°C (59°F and 86°F).

DIMETAPP® Elixir
[dī ' mĕ-tap]

Description: Each 5 mL (1 teaspoonful) contains:
Brompheniramine Maleate, USP ... 2 mg
Phenylpropanolamine Hydrochloride, USP ... 12.5 mg

Inactive Ingredients: Citric Acid, FD&C Blue 1, FD&C Red 40, Flavors, Glycerin, Saccharin Sodium, Sodium Benzoate, Sorbitol, Water.

Indications: For temporary relief of nasal congestion due to the common cold, hay fever or other upper respiratory allergies or associated with sinusitis. Temporarily relieves runny nose, sneezing, itching of the nose or throat, and itchy and watery eyes due to allergic rhinitis (hay fever). Temporarily restores freer breathing through the nose.

Warnings: Do not take this product if you have a breathing problem such as emphysema or chronic bronchitis, high

Continued on next page

Prescribing information on A. H. Robins products listed here is based on official labeling in effect November 1, 1994, with Indications, Contraindications, Warnings, Precautions, Adverse Reactions, and Dosage stated in full.

A. H. Robins—Cont.

blood pressure, heart disease, diabetes, thyroid disease, glaucoma, or difficulty in urination due to enlargement of the prostate gland, unless directed by a physician. May cause drowsiness; alcohol, sedatives and tranquilizers may increase the drowsiness effect. Avoid alcoholic beverages while taking this product. Do not take this product if you are taking sedatives or tranquilizers without first consulting your physician. Use caution when driving a motor vehicle or operating machinery. May cause excitability, especially in children.

Do not exceed the recommended dosage because at higher doses, nervousness, dizziness or sleeplessness may occur. Do not take this product for more than 7 days. If symptoms do not improve, or are accompanied by fever, consult a physician.

Do not take this product if you are hypersensitive to any of the ingredients. As with any drug, if you are pregnant or nursing a baby, seek the advice of a health professional before using this product.

KEEP THIS AND ALL DRUGS OUT OF THE REACH OF CHILDREN. IN CASE OF ACCIDENTAL OVERDOSE, SEEK PROFESSIONAL ASSISTANCE OR CONTACT A POISON CONTROL CENTER IMMEDIATELY.

Drug Interaction Precaution: Do not use this product if you are now taking a prescription monoamine oxidase inhibitor (MAOI) (certain drugs for depression, psychiatric or emotional conditions, or Parkinson's disease) or for 2 weeks after stopping the MAOI drug. If you are uncertain whether your prescription drug contains an MAOI, consult a health professional before taking this product.

Directions: Adults and children 12 years of age and over: 2 teaspoonfuls every 4 hours; children 6 to under 12 years: 1 teaspoonful every 4 hours; DO NOT EXCEED 6 DOSES IN A 24-HOUR PERIOD. Children under 6 years: consult a physician.

Professional Labeling: The suggested dosage for children age 2 to under 6 years, only when the child is under the care of a physician, is ½ teaspoonful every 4 hours, not to exceed 6 doses in a 24-hour period. The dosage for children under 2 years should be determined by the physician on the basis of the patient's weight, physical condition, or other appropriate consideration. Dimetapp Elixir is contraindicated in neonates (children under the age of one month).

How Supplied: Purple, grape-flavored liquid in bottles of 4 fl. oz. (NDC 0031-2230-12), 8 fl. oz. (NDC 0031-2230-18), 12 fl. oz. (NDC 0031-2230-22), pints (NDC 0031-2230-25), and gallons (NDC 0031-2230-29).

Store at Controlled Room Temperature, between 20°C and 25°C (68°F and 77°F). Not a USP elixir.

Shown in Product Identification Guide, page 520

DIMETAPP® DM ELIXIR
[dī'mĕ-tap]

Description: Each 5 mL (1 teaspoonful) contains:
Brompheniramine
  Maleate, USP .... 2 mg
Phenylpropanolamine
  Hydrochloride, USP .... 12.5 mg
Dextromethorphan
  Hydrobromide, USP .... 10.0 mg

Inactive Ingredients: Citric Acid, FD&C Blue 1, FD&C Red 40, Flavors, Glycerin, Propylene Glycol, Saccharin Sodium, Sodium Benzoate, Sorbitol, Water.

Indications: Temporarily relieves cough due to minor throat and bronchial irritation as may occur with a cold. For temporary relief of nasal congestion due to the common cold, hay fever or other upper respiratory allergies or associated with sinusitis. Temporarily relieves runny nose, sneezing, itching of the nose or throat and itchy and watery eyes due to allergic rhinitis (hay fever). Temporarily restores freer breathing through the nose.

Warnings: Do not take this product if you have a breathing problem such as emphysema or chronic bronchitis or persistent or chronic cough such as occurs with smoking or asthma, or cough that is accompanied by excessive phlegm (mucus) unless directed by a physician. Likewise, if you have high blood pressure, heart disease, diabetes, thyroid disease, glaucoma, or difficulty in urination due to enlargement of the prostate gland, do not take this product unless directed by a physician.

May cause marked drowsiness; alcohol, sedatives and tranquilizers may increase the drowsiness effect. Avoid alcoholic beverages while taking this product. Do not take this product if you are taking sedatives or tranquilizers without first consulting your physician. Use caution when driving a motor vehicle or operating machinery. May cause excitability, especially in children.

Do not exceed the recommended dosage because at higher doses, nervousness, dizziness or sleeplessness may occur. Do not take the product for more than 7 days. A persistent cough may be a sign of a serious condition. If cough or other symptoms persist for more than one week without improvement, tend to recur, or are accompanied by fever, rash or persistent headache, consult a physician. Do not take this product if you are hypersensitive to any of the ingredients. As with any drug, if you are pregnant or nursing a baby, seek the advice of a health professional before using this product.

KEEP THIS AND ALL DRUGS OUT OF THE REACH OF CHILDREN. IN CASE OF ACCIDENTAL OVERDOSE, SEEK PROFESSIONAL ASSISTANCE OR CONTACT A POISON CONTROL CENTER IMMEDIATELY.

Drug Interaction Precaution: Do not use this product if you are now taking a prescription monoamine oxidase inhibitor (MAOI) (certain drugs for depression, psychiatric or emotional conditions, or Parkinson's disease) or for 2 weeks after stopping the MAOI drug. If you are uncertain whether your prescription drug contains an MAOI, consult a health professional before taking this product.

Directions: Adults and children 12 years of age and over: Two teaspoonfuls every 4 hours; children 6 to under 12 years: one teaspoonful every 4 hours. DO NOT EXCEED 6 DOSES IN A 24-HOUR PERIOD. Children under 6 years: consult a physician.

Professional Labeling: The suggested dosage for children age 2 to under 6 years, only when the child is under the care of a physician, is ½ teaspoonful every 4 hours, not to exceed 6 doses in a 24-hour period. The dosage for children under 2 years should be determined by the physician on the basis of the patient's weight, physical condition, or other appropriate consideration. Dimetapp DM Elixir is contraindicated in neonates (children under the age of one month).

How Supplied: Red, grape-flavored liquid in bottles of 4 fl. oz. (NDC 0031-2240-12), 8 fl. oz. (NDC 0031-2240-18), and 12 fl. oz. (NDC 0031-2240-22). Store at Controlled Room Temperature, Between 20°C and 25°C (68°F and 77°F) Not a USP elixir.

DIMETAPP® Extentabs®
[dī' mĕ-tap]

Description: Each **Dimetapp Extentabs®** Tablet contains:
Brompheniramine Maleate,
  USP .... 12 mg
Phenylpropanolamine
  Hydrochloride, USP .... 75 mg

Inactive Ingredients: Acacia, Acetylated Monoglycerides, Calcium Sulfate, Carnauba Wax, Castor Wax or Oil, Citric Acid, Edible Inks, FD&C Blue 1, FD&C Blue 2 Aluminum Lake, Gelatin, Magnesium Stearate, Magnesium Trisilicate, Pharmaceutical Glaze, Polysorbates, Povidone, Silicon Dioxide, Stearyl Alcohol, Sucrose, Titanium Dioxide, Wheat Flour, White Wax. May contain FD&C Red 40 and FD&C Yellow 6 Aluminum Lakes.

Indications: For temporary relief of nasal congestion due to the common cold, hay fever or other upper respiratory allergies or associated with sinusitis; temporarily relieves runny nose, sneezing, and itchy and watery eyes due to allergic rhinitis (hay fever). Temporarily restores freer breathing through the nose.

Warnings: Do not take this product, unless directed by a physician, if you have a breathing problem such as emphysema or chronic bronchitis, or if you have high blood pressure, heart disease, diabetes, thyroid disease, glaucoma, or difficulty in urination due to enlargement of the prostate gland.

This product may cause drowsiness; alcohol, sedatives and tranquilizers may increase the drowsiness effect. Avoid alcoholic beverages while taking this product. Do not take this product if you are taking sedatives or tranquilizers without first consulting your physician. Use caution when driving a motor vehicle or operating machinery. May cause excitability, especially in children.

Do not exceed the recommended dosage because at higher doses nervousness, dizziness or sleeplessness may occur. Do not take this product for more than 7 days. If symptoms do not improve, or are accompanied by fever, consult a physician.

Do not give this product to children under 12 years, except under the advice and supervision of a physician. Do not take this product if you are hypersensitive to any of the ingredients. As with any drug, if you are pregnant or nursing a baby, seek the advice of a health professional before using this product.

KEEP THIS AND ALL DRUGS OUT OF THE REACH OF CHILDREN. IN CASE OF ACCIDENTAL OVERDOSE, SEEK PROFESSIONAL ASSISTANCE OR CONTACT A POISON CONTROL CENTER IMMEDIATELY.

Drug Interaction Precaution: Concomitant administration of phenylpropanolamine with other sympathomimetic agents may produce additive effects and increased toxicity; with monoamine oxidase inhibitors (MAOIs) may produce a hypertensive crisis; with certain antihypertensive agents may diminish their antihypertensive effect.

Directions: Adults and children 12 years of age and over: one tablet every 12 hours. DO NOT EXCEED 1 TABLET EVERY 12 HOURS OR 2 TABLETS IN A 24-HOUR PERIOD.

How Supplied: Pale blue sugar-coated tablets monogrammed DIMETAPP AHR in bottles of 100 (NDC 0031-2277-63), 500 (NDC 0031-2277-70); Dis-Co® Unit Dose Packs of 100 (NDC 0031-2277-64); and consumer packages of 12 tablets (NDC 0031-2277-46), 24 tablets (NDC 0031-2277-54) and 48 tablets (NDC 0031-2277-59) (individually packaged).

Store at Controlled Room Temperature, between 15°C and 30°C (59°F and 86°F).

Dimetapp Extentabs® Tablets are the A. H. Robins Company's uniquely constructed extended action tablets.

Shown in Product Identification Guide, page 520

DIMETAPP® Sinus Caplets*
[di'mĕ-tap]
*Oval-Shaped tablets

Description: Each Dimetapp Caplet contains:

Ibuprofen .... 200 mg
Pseudoephedrine Hydro-
chloride .... 30 mg

Inactive Ingredients: Carnauba or Equivalent Wax, Croscarmellose Sodium, Iron Oxide, Methylparaben, Microcrystalline Cellulose, Propylparaben, Silicon Dioxide, Sodium Benzoate, Sodium Lauryl Sulfate, Starch, Stearic Acid, Sucrose, Titanium Dioxide.

Indications: For temporary relief of symptoms associated with the common cold, sinusitis or flu, including nasal congestion, headache, fever, body aches, and pains.

Warnings: ASPIRIN SENSITIVE PATIENTS. Do not take this product if you have had a severe allergic reaction to aspirin, e.g. - asthma, swelling, shock, or hives because, even though this product contains no aspirin or salicylates, cross-reactions may occur in patients allergic to aspirin.

Do not take for colds for more than 7 days or for fever for more than 3 days unless directed by a doctor. If the cold or fever persists or gets worse or if new symptoms occur, consult a doctor. These could be signs of serious illness. As with aspirin and acetaminophen, if you have any condition which requires you to take prescription drugs or if you have had any problems or serious side effects from taking any non-prescription pain reliever, do not take this product without first discussing it with your doctor. IF YOU EXPERIENCE ANY SYMPTOMS WHICH ARE UNUSUAL OR SEEM UNRELATED TO THE CONDITION FOR WHICH YOU TOOK THIS PRODUCT, CONSULT A DOCTOR BEFORE TAKING ANY MORE OF IT. If you are under a doctor's care for any serious condition, consult a doctor before taking this product. Do not exceed the recommended dosage because at higher doses nervousness, dizziness or sleeplessness may occur. Do not take this product if you have high blood pressure, heart disease, diabetes, thyroid disease or difficulty in urination due to enlargement of the prostate gland, except under the advice and supervision of a doctor. As with any drug, if you are pregnant or nursing a baby, seek the advice of a health professional before using this product. Women are warned that IT IS ESPECIALLY IMPORTANT NOT TO USE THIS PRODUCT DURING THE LAST 3 MONTHS OF PREGNANCY UNLESS SPECIFICALLY DIRECTED TO DO SO BY A DOCTOR BECAUSE IT MAY CAUSE PROBLEMS IN THE UNBORN CHILD OR COMPLICATIONS DURING DELIVERY. Keep this and all drugs out of the reach of children. In case of accidental overdose, seek professional assistance or contact a poison control center immediately.

Drug Interaction Precaution: Do not take this product if you are presently taking a prescription drug for high blood pressure or depression without first consulting your doctor. Do not combine this product with other non-prescription pain relievers. Do not combine this product with any other ibuprofen-containing product.

Directions: Adults: 1 caplet every 4 to 6 hours while symptoms persist. If symptoms do not respond to 1 caplet, 2 caplets may be used but do not exceed 6 caplets in 24 hours, unless directed by a doctor. The smallest effective dose should be used. Take with food or milk if occasional and mild heartburn, upset stomach, or stomach pain occurs with use. Consult a doctor if these symptoms are more than mild or if they persist. Children: Do not give this product to children under 12 years of age except under the advice and supervision of a doctor.

How Supplied: White coated caplet monogrammed DIMETAPP SINUS in packages of 20 tablets (NDC 0031–2260–52), and bottles of 40 tablets (NDC 0031–2260–56).

Store at room temperture; avoid excessive heat (40°C, 104°F).

DIMETAPP® Tablets and Liqui-Gels®
[dī' mĕ-tap]

Description: Each **Dimetapp** Tablet or Liquigel® contains:
Brompheniramine
Maleate, USP .... 4 mg
Phenylpropanolamine
Hydrochloride, USP .... 25 mg

Inactive Ingredients: Tablets: Corn Starch, FD&C Blue 1 Aluminum Lake, Magnesium Stearate, Microcrystalline Cellulose. Liqui-Gels: D&C Red 33, FD&C Blue 1, Gelatin, Glycerin, Mannitol, Pharmaceutical Glaze, Polyethylene Glycol, Povidone, Propylene Glycol, Sorbitan, Sorbitol, Titanium Dioxide, Water.

Indications: For temporary relief of nasal congestion due to the common cold, hay fever or other upper respiratory allergies or associated with sinusitis; temporarily relieves runny nose, sneezing, and itchy and watery eyes due to allergic rhinitis (hay fever). Temporarily restores freer breathing through the nose.

Warnings: Do not take take this product, unless directed by a physician, if you have a breathing problem such as emphysema or chronic bronchitis, or if you have high blood pressure, heart disease, diabetes, thyroid disease, glaucoma, or difficulty in urination due to enlargement of the prostate gland. This product may cause drowsiness; alcohol, sedatives and tranquilizers may increase the drow-

Continued on next page

Prescribing information on A. H. Robins products listed here is based on official labeling in effect November 1, 1994, with Indications, Contraindications, Warnings, Precautions, Adverse Reactions, and Dosage stated in full.

A. H. Robins—Cont.

siness effect. Avoid alcoholic beverages while taking this product. Do not take this product if you are taking sedatives or tranquilizers without first consulting your physician. Use caution when driving a motor vehicle or operating machinery. May cause excitability, especially in children. Do not exceed the recommended dosage because at higher doses, nervousness, dizziness or sleeplessness may occur. Do not take this product for more than 7 days. If symptoms do not improve, or are accompanied by fever, consult a physician.

Do not take this product if you are hypersensitive to any of the ingredients. As with any drug, if you are pregnant or nursing a baby, seek the advice of a health professional before using this product.

KEEP THIS AND ALL DRUGS OUT OF THE REACH OF CHILDREN. IN CASE OF ACCIDENTAL OVERDOSE, SEEK PROFESSIONAL ASSISTANCE OR CONTACT A POISON CONTROL CENTER IMMEDIATELY.

Drug Interaction Precaution: Do not use this product if you are now taking a prescription monoamine oxidase inhibitor (MAOI) (certain drugs for depression, psychiatric or emotional conditions, or Parkinson's disease) or for 2 weeks after stopping the MAOI drug. If you are uncertain whether your prescription drug contains an MAOI, consult a health professional before taking this product.

Directions: Tablets: Adults and children 12 years of age and over: one tablet every 4 hours. Children 6 to under 12 years: one-half tablet every 4 hours. DO NOT EXCEED 6 DOSES IN A 24-HOUR PERIOD. Children under 6 years: Use only as directed by a physician. Liqui-Gels: Adults and children 12 years of age and over: one Liquigel every 4 hours. Children under 12 years: consult a physician. DO NOT EXCEED 6 LIQUI-GELS IN A 24-HOUR PERIOD.

How Supplied: Tablets: Blue, scored compressed tablets engraved AHR and 2254 in consumer packages of 24 (NDC 0031-2254-54) (individually packaged). Liqui-Gels: Purple Liquigel imprinted AHR and 2255 in consumer packages of 12 (NDC 0031-2255-46) and 24 (NDC 0031-2255-54) (individually packaged). Tablets and Liqui-Gels: Store at Controlled Room Temperature, between 15°C and 30°C (59°F and 86°F).

Liqui-Gels and Liquigel are registered trademarks of R.P. Scherer International Corporation.

ROBITUSSIN® COLD & COUGH LIQUI-GELS®

[ro "bĭ-tuss 'ĭn]

Description: Each Softgel contains:

Guaifenesin, USP .... 200 mg
Pseudoephedrine Hydrochloride,
  USP .... 30 mg

Dextromethorphan Hydrobromide,
  USP .... 10 mg

Inactive Ingredients: FD&C Blue 1, FD&C Red 40, Gelatin, Glycerin, Mannitol, Pharmaceutical Glaze, Polyethylene Glycol, Povidone, Propylene Glycol, Sorbitan, Sorbitol, Titanium Dioxide, Water.

Indications: Temporarily relieves coughs due to minor throat and bronchial irritation and nasal congestion due to the common cold, hay fever or other upper respiratory allergies, associated with sinusitis. Helps loosen phlegm (mucus) and thin bronchial secretions to make coughs more productive.

Warnings: Do not take this product for persistent or chronic cough such as occurs with smoking, asthma, chronic bronchitis, emphysema, or if cough is accompanied by excessive phlegm (mucus), unless directed by a physician. Likewise, if you have heart disease, high blood pressure, thyroid disease, diabetes, or difficulty in urination due to enlargement of the prostate gland, do not take this product unless directed by a physician.

Do not exceed the recommended dosage because at higher doses, nervousness, dizziness or sleeplessness may occur. Do not take this product for more than 7 days. A persistent cough may be a sign of a serious condition. If cough or other symptoms persist for more than one week without improvement, tend to recur, or are accompanied by fever, rash, or persistent headache, consult a physician. Do not take this product if you are hypersensitive to any of the ingredients. As with any drug, if you are pregnant or nursing a baby, seek the advice of a health professional before using this product.

KEEP THIS AND ALL DRUGS OUT OF THE REACH OF CHILDREN. IN CASE OF ACCIDENTAL OVERDOSE, SEEK PROFESSIONAL ASSISTANCE OR CONTACT A POISON CONTROL CENTER IMMEDIATELY.

Drug Interaction Precaution: Do not use this product if you are now taking a prescription monoamine oxidase inhibitor (MAOI) (certain drugs for depression, psychiatric or emotional conditions, or Parkinson's disease) or for 2 weeks after stopping the MAOI drug. If you are uncertain whether your prescription drug contains an MAOI, consult a health professional before taking this product.

Directions: Follow dosage below: DO NOT EXCEED 4 DOSES IN A 24-HOUR PERIOD. Adults and children 12 years of age and over: swallow two Softgels every 4 hours. Children 6 to under 12 years: swallow one Softgel every 4 hours. Children under 6–consult your doctor.

How Supplied: Red Liquigel imprinted AHR and 8600 in consumer packages of 12 (NDC 0031-8600-46) and 20 (NDC 0031-8600-52) (individually packaged).

Store at controlled room temperature, between 20°C and 25°C (68°F and 77°F) Liqui-Gels and Liquigel are registered trademarks of R.P. Scherer International Corporation.

Note: Guaifenesin had been shown to produce a color interference with certain clinical laboratory determinations of 5-hydroxyindoleacetic acid (5-HIAA) and vanillylmandelic acid (VMA).

ROBITUSSIN® SEVERE CONGESTION LIQUI-GELS®

[ro "bĭ-tuss 'ĭn]

Description: Each Robitussin Severe Congestion Liquigel® contains:

Guaifenesin, USP .... 200 mg
Pseudoephedrine Hydrochloride,
  USP .... 30 mg

Inactive Ingredients: FD&C Green 3, Gelatin, Glycerin, Mannitol, Pharmaceutical Glaze, Polyethylene Glycol, Povidone, Propylene Glycol, Sorbitan, Sorbitol, Titanium Dioxide, Water.

Indications: For the temporary relief of nasal congestion due to the common cold, hay fever or other upper respiratory allergies, or associated with sinusitis. Helps loosen phlegm (mucus) and thin bronchial secretions to make coughs more productive.

Warnings: Do not take this product for persistent or chronic cough such as occurs with smoking, asthma, chronic bronchitis, emphysema, or if cough is accompanied by excessive phlegm (mucus). Likewise, if you have heart disease, high blood pressure, thyroid disease, diabetes, or difficulty in urination due to enlargement of the prostate gland, do not take this product unless directed by a physician.

Do not exceed the recommended dosage because at higher doses, nervousness, dizziness or sleeplessness may occur. Do not take this product for more than 7 days. A persistent cough may be a sign of a serious condition. If cough or other symptoms persist for more than one week without improvement, tend to recur, or are accompanied by fever, rash, or persistent headache, consult a physician. Do not take this product if you are hypersensitive to any of the ingredients. As with any drug, if you are pregnant or nursing a baby, seek the advice of a health professional before using this product.

KEEP THIS AND ALL DRUGS OUT OF THE REACH OF CHILDREN. IN CASE OF ACCIDENTAL OVERDOSE, SEEK PROFESSIONAL ASSISTANCE OR CONTACT A POISON CONTROL CENTER IMMEDIATELY.

Drug Interaction Precaution: Do not use this product if you are now taking a prescription monoamine oxidase inhibitor (MAOI) (certain drugs for depression, psychiatric or emotional conditions, or Parkinson's disease) or for 2 weeks after stopping the MAOI drug. If you are uncertain whether your prescription drug contains an MAOI, consult a health professional before taking this product.

Directions: Follow dosage below: DO NOT EXCEED 4 DOSES IN A 24-HOUR PERIOD. Adults and children 12 years of age and over: swallow two Softgels every 4 hours. Children 6 to under 12 years: swallow one Softgel every 4 hours. Children under 6, consult a physician.

How Supplied: Aqua Liquigel imprinted AHR and 8501 in consumer packages of 12 (NDC 0031-8601-46) and 20 (NDC 0031-8601-52) (individually packaged).
Store at controlled room temperature, between 20°C and 25°C (68°F and 77°F).
Liqui-Gels and Liquigel are registered trademarks of R.P. Scherer International Corporation.
Note: Guaifenesin has been shown to produce a color interference with certain clinical laboratory determinations of 5-hydroxyindoleacetic acid (5-HIAA) and vanillylmandelic acid (VMA).

Shown in Product Identification Guide, page 520

ROBITUSSIN®
[ro"bĭ-tuss'ĭn]
(Guaifenesin Syrup, USP)

Active Ingredients: Each teaspoonful (5 mL) contains:
Guaifenesin, USP .... 100 mg

Inactive Ingredients: Caramel, Citric Acid, FD&C Red 40, Flavors, Glucose, Glycerin, High Fructose Corn Syrup, Saccharin Sodium, Sodium Benzoate, Water.

Indications: Helps loosen phlegm (mucus) and thin bronchial secretions to make coughs more productive.

Professional Labeling: Helps loosen phlegm and thin bronchial secretions in patients with stable chronic bronchitis.

Warnings: Do not take this product for persistent or chronic cough such as occurs with smoking, asthma, chronic bronchitis, emphysema, or where cough is accompanied by excessive phlegm (mucus) unless directed by a physician.
A persistent cough may be a sign of a serious condition. If cough persists for more than one week, tends to recur, or is accompanied by fever, rash, or persistent headache, consult a physician.
Do not take this product if you are hypersensitive to any of the ingredients. As with any drug, if you are pregnant or nursing a baby, seek the advice of a health professional before using this product.
KEEP THIS AND ALL DRUGS OUT OF THE REACH OF CHILDREN. IN CASE OF ACCIDENTAL OVERDOSE, SEEK PROFESSIONAL ASSISTANCE OR CONTACT A POISON CONTROL CENTER IMMEDIATELY.

Directions: Follow dosage below. Dosage cup provided. Do Not Exceed Recommended Dosage. Adults and children 12 years and over: 2–4 teaspoonfuls every 4 hours; children 6 years to under 12 years: 1–2 teaspoonfuls every 4 hours. Children 2 years to under 6 years: ½–1 teaspoonful every 4 hours. Children under 2 years—consult your doctor.

How Supplied: Robitussin (wine-colored) in bottles of 4 fl. oz. (NDC 0031-8624-12), 8 fl. oz. (NDC 0031-8624-18), pint (NDC 0031-8624-25).
Robitussin also available in 1 fl. oz. bottles (4 × 25's) (NDC 0031-8624-02).
Store at controlled room temperature, between 20°C and 25°C (68°F and 77°F).
Note: Guaifenesin has been shown to produce a color interference with certain clinical laboratory determinations of 5-hydroxyindoleacetic acid (5-HIAA) and vanillylmandelic acid (VMA).

ROBITUSSIN®-CF
[ro"bĭ-tuss'ĭn]

Active Ingredients: Each teaspoonful (5 mL) contains:
Guaifenesin, USP .... 100 mg
Phenylpropanolamine
   Hydrochloride, USP .... 12.5 mg
Dextromethorphan
   Hydrobromide, USP .... 10 mg

Inactive Ingredients: Citric Acid, FD&C Red 40, Flavors, Glycerin, Propylene Glycol, Saccharin Sodium, Sodium Benzoate, Sorbitol, Water.

Indications: Temporarily relieves coughs due to minor throat and bronchial irritation and nasal congestion as may occur with a cold. Helps loosen phlegm (mucus) and thin bronchial secretions to make coughs more productive.

Warnings: Do not take this product for persistent or chronic cough such as occurs with smoking, asthma, chronic bronchitis, emphysema, or if cough is accompanied by excessive phlegm (mucus) unless directed by a physician. Likewise, if you have heart disease, high blood pressure, thyroid disease, diabetes, or difficulty in urination due to enlargement of the prostate gland, do not take this product unless directed by a physician.
Do not exceed the recommended dosage because at higher doses, nervousness, dizziness or sleeplessness may occur. Do not take this product for more than 7 days. A persistent cough may be a sign of a serious condition. If cough or other symptoms persist for more than one week without improvement, tend to recur, or are accompanied by fever, rash, or persistent headache, consult a physician.
Do not take this product if you are hypersensitive to any of the ingredients. As with any drug, if you are pregnant or nursing a baby, seek the advice of a health professional before using this product.
KEEP THIS AND ALL DRUGS OUT OF THE REACH OF CHILDREN. IN CASE OF ACCIDENTAL OVERDOSE, SEEK PROFESSIONAL ASSISTANCE OR

CONTACT A POISON CONTROL CENTER IMMEDIATELY.

Drug Interaction Precautions: Do not use this product if you are now taking a prescription monoamine oxidase inhibitor (MAOI) (certain drugs for depression, psychiatric or emotional conditions, or Parkinson's disease) or for 2 weeks after stopping the MAOI drug. If you are uncertain whether your prescription drug contains an MAOI, consult a health professional before taking this product.

Directions: Follow dosage below: Dosage cup provided. DO NOT EXCEED 6 DOSES IN A 24-HOUR PERIOD. Adults and children 12 years and over: 2 teaspoonfuls every 4 hours; children 6 years to under 12 years, 1 teaspoonful every 4 hours; children 2 years to under 6 years, ½ teaspoonful every 4 hours; children under 2 years—consult your doctor.

How Supplied: Robitussin-CF (red-colored) in bottles of 4 fl. oz. (NDC 0031-8677-12), 8 fl. oz. (NDC 0031-8677-18), and 12 fl. oz. (NDC 0031-8677-22).
Store at Controlled Room Temperature, between 20°C and 25°C (68°F and 77°F).
Note: Guaifenesin has been shown to produce a color interference with certain clinical laboratory determinations of 5-hydroxyindoleacetic acid (5-HIAA) and vanillylmandelic acid (VMA).

ROBITUSSIN®-DM
[ro"bĭ-tuss'ĭn]

Active Ingredients: Each teaspoonful (5 mL) contains:
Guaifenesin, USP .... 100 mg
Dextromethorphan Hydrobromide,
   USP .... 10 mg

Inactive Ingredients: Citric Acid, FD&C Red 40, Flavors, Glucose, Glycerin, High Fructose Corn Syrup, Saccharin Sodium, Sodium Benzoate, Water.

Indications: Temporarily relieves cough due to minor throat and bronchial irritation as may occur with a cold and helps loosen phlegm (mucus) and thin bronchial secretions to make coughs more productive.

Warnings: Do not take this product for persistent or chronic cough such as occurs with smoking, asthma, chronic bronchitis, emphysema, or if cough is accompanied by excessive phlegm (mucus) unless directed by a physician.
A persistent cough may be a sign of a serious condition. If cough persists for more than one week, tends to recur, or is

Continued on next page

Prescribing information on A. H. Robins products listed here is based on official labeling in effect November 1, 1994, with Indications, Contraindications, Warnings, Precautions, Adverse Reactions, and Dosage stated in full.

A. H. Robins—Cont.

accompanied by a fever, rash, or persistent headache, consult a physician.

Do not take this product if you are hypersensitive to any of the ingredients. As with any drug, if you are pregnant or nursing a baby, seek the advice of a health professional before using this product.

KEEP THIS AND ALL DRUGS OUT OF THE REACH OF CHILDREN. IN CASE OF ACCIDENTAL OVERDOSE, SEEK PROFESSIONAL ASSISTANCE OR CONTACT A POISON CONTROL CENTER IMMEDIATELY.

Drug Interaction Precaution: Do not use this product if you are now taking a prescription monoamine oxidase inhibitor (MAOI) (certain drugs for depression, psychiatric or emotional conditions, or Parkinson's disease) or for 2 weeks after stopping the MAOI drug. If you are uncertain whether your prescription drug contains an MAOI, consult a health professional before taking this product.

Directions: Follow dosage below or use as directed by a doctor. Dosage cup provided. DO NOT EXCEED 6 DOSES IN A 24-HOUR PERIOD. Adults and children 12 years and over: 2 teaspoonfuls every 4 hours; children 6 years to under 12 years, 1 teaspoonful every 4 hours; children 2 years to under 6 years, ½ teaspoonful every 4 hours; children under 2 years—consult your doctor.

How Supplied: Robitussin-DM (cherry-colored) in bottles of 4 fl. oz. (NDC 0031-8685-12), 8 fl. oz. (NDC 0031-8685-18), 12 fl. oz. (NDC 0031-8685-22), pint (NDC 0031-8685-25) and single doses: 6 premeasured doses—⅓ fl. oz. each (NDC 0031-8685-06).

Store at Controlled Room Temperature, between 20°C and 25°C (68°F and 77°F).

Note: Guaifenesin has been shown to produce a color interference with certain clinical laboratory determinations of 5-hydroxyindoleacetic acid (5-HIAA) and vanillylmandelic acid (VMA).

Shown in Product Identification Guide, page 520

ROBITUSSIN®-PE
[ro "bĭ-tuss 'ĭn]

Active Ingredients: Each teaspoonful (5 mL) contains:
Guaifenesin, USP .... 100 mg
Pseudoephedrine Hydrochloride, USP .... 30 mg

Inactive Ingredients: Citric Acid, FD&C Red 40, Flavors, Glucose, Glycerin, High Fructose Corn Syrup, Maltol, Propylene Glycol, Saccharin Sodium, Sodium Benzoate, Water.

Indications: Temporarily relieves nasal congestion as may occur with a cold. Helps loosen phlegm (mucus) and thin bronchial secretions to make coughs more productive.

Warnings: Do not take this product for persistent or chronic cough such as occurs with smoking, asthma, chronic bronchitis, emphysema, or if cough is accompanied by excessive phlegm (mucus) unless directed by a physician. Likewise, if you have heart disease, high blood pressure, thyroid disease, diabetes, or difficulty in urination due to enlargement of the prostate gland, do not take this product unless directed by a physician.

Do not exceed the recommended dosage because at higher doses, nervousness, dizziness or sleeplessness may occur. Do not take this product for more than 7 days. A persistent cough may be a sign of a serious condition. If cough or other symptoms persist for more than one week without improvement, tend to recur, or are accompanied by fever, rash, or persistent headache, consult a physician.

Do not take this product if you are hypersensitive to any of the ingredients. As with any drug, if you are pregnant or nursing a baby, seek the advice of a health professional before using this product.

KEEP THIS AND ALL DRUGS OUT OF THE REACH OF CHILDREN. IN CASE OF ACCIDENTAL OVERDOSE, SEEK PROFESSIONAL ASSISTANCE OR CONTACT A POISON CONTROL CENTER IMMEDIATELY.

Drug Interaction Precautions: Do not use this product if you are now taking a prescription monoamine oxidase inhibitor (MAOI) (certain drugs for depression, psychiatric or emotional conditions, or Parkinson's disease) or for 2 weeks after stopping the MAOI drug. If you are uncertain whether your prescription drug contains an MAOI, consult a health professional before taking this product.

Directions: Follow dosage below. Dosage cup provided. DO NOT EXCEED 4 DOSES IN A 24-HOUR PERIOD. Adults and children 12 years and over: 2 teaspoonfuls every 4 hours; children 6 years to under 12 years, 1 teaspoonful every 4 hours; children 2 years to under 6 years, ½ teaspoonful every 4 hours; children under 2 years—consult your doctor.

How Supplied: Robitussin-PE (orange-red) in bottles of 4 fl. oz. (NDC 0031-8695-12), and 8 fl. oz. (NDC 0031-8695-18).

Store at Controlled Room Temperature, Between 20°C and 25°C (68°F and 77°F).

Note: Guaifenesin has been shown to produce a color interference with certain clinical laboratory determinations of 5-hydroxyindoleacetic acid (5-HIAA) and vanillylmandelic acid (VMA).

ROBITUSSIN® MAXIMUM STRENGTH COUGH SUPPRESSANT
[ro "bĭ-tuss 'ĭn]

Description: Each 5 mL (1 teaspoonful) contains:

Dextromethorphan
Hydrobromide, USP .... 15 mg

Inactive Ingredients: Alcohol 1.4%, Citric Acid, FD&C Red 40, Flavors, Glycerin, Glucose, High Fructose Corn Syrup, Saccharin Sodium, Sodium Benzoate, Water.

Indications: Temporarily relieves coughs due to minor throat and bronchial irritation as may occur with a cold.

Warnings: Do not take this product for persistent or chronic cough such as occurs with smoking, asthma, emphysema, or if cough is accompanied by excessive phlegm (mucus) unless directed by a physician.

A persistent cough may be a sign of a serious condition. If cough persists for more than one week, tends to recur, or is accompanied by fever, rash, or persistent headache, consult a physician.

Do not take this product if you are hypersensitive to any of the ingredients. As with any drug, if you are pregnant or nursing a baby seek, the advice of a health professional before using this product.

KEEP THIS AND ALL DRUGS OUT OF THE REACH OF CHILDREN. IN CASE OF ACCIDENTAL OVERDOSE, SEEK PROFESSIONAL ASSISTANCE OR CONTACT A POISON CONTROL CENTER IMMEDIATELY.

Drug Interaction Precaution: Do not use this product if you are now taking a prescription monoamine oxidase inhibitor (MAOI) (certain drugs for depression, psychiatric or emotional conditions, or Parkinson's disease) or for 2 weeks after stopping the MAOI drug. If you are uncertain whether your prescription drug contains an MAOI, consult a health professional before taking this product.

Directions: Follow dosage recommendations below or use as directed by a doctor. Repeat every 6–8 hours as needed. DO NOT EXCEED 4 DOSES IN A 24-HOUR PERIOD. Adults and children 12 years and over: 2 teaspoonfuls every 6–8 hours, in medicine cup. Children under 12 years: consult your doctor.

Professional Labeling: Children 6 years to under 12 years, 1 teaspoonful every 6–8 hours; children 2 years to under 6 years, ½ teaspoonful every 6–8 hours. Do not exceed 4 doses in a 24-hour period.

How Supplied: Robitussin Maximum Strength (dark red-colored) in bottles of 4 fl. oz. (NDC 0031-8670-12) and 8 fl. oz. (NDC 0031-8670-18).

Store at Controlled Room Temperature, between 20°C and 25°C (68°F and 77°F).

ROBITUSSIN® MAXIMUM STRENGTH COUGH & COLD
[ro "bĭ-tuss 'ĭn]

Description: Each teaspoonful (5 mL) contains:

Dextromethorphan Hydrobomide,
USP .... 15 mg
Pseudoephedrine Hydrochloride,
USP .... 30 mg

Inactive Ingredients: Alcohol 1.4%, Citric Acid, FD&C Red 40, Flavors, Glycerin, Glucose, High Fructose Corn Syrup, Saccharin Sodium, Sodium Benzoate, Water.

Indications: Temporarily relieves coughs due to minor throat and bronchial irritation and nasal congestion as may occur with a cold.

Warnings: Do not take this product for persistent or chronic cough such as occurs with smoking, asthma, emphysema, or if cough is accompanied by excessive phlegm (mucus) unless directed by a physician. Likewise, if you have heart disease, high blood pressure, thyroid disease, diabetes, or difficulty in urination due to enlargement of the prostate gland, do not take this product unless directed by a physician.
Do not exceed the recommended dosage because at higher doses nervousness, dizziness or sleeplessness may occur. Do not take this product for more than 7 days. A persistent cough may be a sign of a serious condition. If cough or other symptoms persist for more than one week without improvement, tend to recur, or are accompanied by fever, rash, or persistent headache, consult a physician.
Do not take this product if you are hypersensitive to any of the ingredients. As with any drug, if you are pregnant or nursing a baby, seek the advice of a health professional before using this product.
KEEP THIS AND ALL DRUGS OUT OF THE REACH OF CHILDREN. IN CASE OF ACCIDENTAL OVERDOSE, SEEK PROFESSIONAL ASSISTANCE OR CONTACT A POISON CONTROL CENTER IMMEDIATELY.

Drug Interaction Precaution: Do not use this product if you are now taking a prescription monoamine oxidase inhibitor (MAOI) (certain drugs for depression, psychiatric or emotional conditions, or Parkinson's disease) or for 2 weeks after stopping the MAOI drug. If you are uncertain whether your prescription drug contains an MAOI, consult a health professional before taking this product.

Directions: Follow dosage recommendations below or use as directed by a doctor. Repeat every 6 hours as needed. DO NOT EXCEED 4 DOSES IN A 24-HOUR PEROID. Adults and children 12 years and over: 2 teaspoonfuls every 6 hours in medicine cup. Children under 12 years: consult your doctor.

How Supplied: Red syrup in bottles of 4 fl. oz. (NDC 0031-8671-12) and 8 fl. oz. (NDC-0031-8671-18).
Store at Controlled Room Temperature, Between 20°C and 25°C (68°F and 77°F).

Age	Weight	Dose
Under 2 yrs.	Under 24 lbs.	Consult doctor
2 to under 6 yrs.	24–47 lbs.	1 Teaspoonful
6 to under 12 yrs.	48–95 lbs.	2 Teaspoonfuls
12 yrs. and older	96 lbs. and over	4 Teaspoonfuls

ROBITUSSIN® PEDIATRIC COUGH & COLD FORMULA
[ro "bĭ-tuss 'ĭn]

Description: Each 5 mL (1 teaspoonful) contains:
Dextromethorphan
  Hydrobromide, USP .... 7.5 mg
Pseudoephedrine
  Hydrochloride .... 15 mg

Inactive Ingredients: Citric Acid, FD&C Red 40, Flavors, Glycerin, Propylene Glycol, Saccharin Sodium, Sodium Benzoate, Sorbitol, Water.

Indications: Temporarily relieves cough due to minor throat and bronchial irritation and nasal congestion as may occur with a cold.

Warnings: Do not take this product for persistent chronic cough such as occurs with smoking, asthma, or emphysema, or if cough is accompanied by excessive phlegm (mucus) unless directed by a physician. Likewise if you have heart disease, high blood pressure, thyroid disease, diabetes, or difficulty in urination due to enlargement of the prostate gland, do not take this product unless directed by a physician.
Do not exceed the recommended dosage because at higher doses, nervousness, dizziness or sleeplessness may occur. Do not take this product for more than 7 days. A persistent cough may be a sign of a serious condition. If cough or other symptoms persist for more than one week without improvement, tend to recur, or are accompanied by fever, rash, or persistent headache, consult a physician.
Do not take this product if you are hypersensitive to any of the ingredients. As with any drug, if you are pregnant or nursing a baby, seek the advice of a health professional before using this product.
KEEP THIS AND ALL DRUGS OUT OF THE REACH OF CHILDREN. IN CASE OF ACCIDENTAL OVERDOSE, SEEK PROFESSIONAL ASSISTANCE OR CONTACT A POISON CONTROL CENTER IMMEDIATELY.

Drug Interaction Precautions: Do not use this product if you are now taking a prescription monoamine oxidase inhibitor (MAOI) (certain drugs for depression, psychiatric or emotional conditions, or Parkinson's disease) or for 2 weeks after stopping the MAOI drug. If you are uncertain whether your prescription drug contains an MAOI, consult a health professional before taking this product.

Directions: Follow dosage recommendations below or use as directed by a physician. Repeat every 6 hours. DO NOT EXCEED 4 DOSES IN A 24-HOUR PERIOD. Dosage: choose by weight, if known; if weight is not known, choose by age.
[See table above.]

How Supplied: Robitussin Pediatric Cough & Cold formula (bright red) in bottles of 4 fl. oz. (NDC 0031-8609-12) and 8 fl. oz. (NDC 0031-8609-18).
Store at Controlled Room Temperature, Between 20°C and 25°C (68°F and 77°F).

ROBITUSSIN® PEDIATRIC COUGH SUPPRESSANT
[ro "bĭ-tuss 'ĭn]

Description: Each 5 mL (1 teaspoonful) contains:
Dextromethorphan
  Hydrobromide, USP .... 7.5 mg

Inactive Ingredients: Citric Acid, FD&C Red 40, Flavors, Glycerin, Propylene Glycol, Saccharin Sodium, Sodium Benzoate, Sorbitol, Water.

Indications: Temporarily relieves coughs due to minor throat and bronchial irritation as may occur with a cold.

Warnings: Do not take this product for persistent or chronic cough such as occurs with smoking, asthma, or emphysema, or if cough is accompanied by excessive phlegm (mucus) unless directed by a physician.
A persistent cough may be a sign of a serious condition. If cough persists for more than one week, tends to recur, or is accompanied by fever, rash, or persistent headache, consult a physician.
Do not take this product if you are hypersensitive to any of the ingredients. As with any drug, if you are pregnant or nursing a baby, seek the advice of a health professional before using this product.
KEEP THIS AND ALL DRUGS OUT OF THE REACH OF CHILDREN. IN CASE OF ACCIDENTAL OVERDOSE, SEEK PROFESSIONAL ASSISTANCE OR CONTACT A POISON CONTROL CENTER IMMEDIATELY.

Drug Interaction Precaution: Do not use this product if you are now taking a prescription monoamine oxidase inhibitor (MAOI) (certain drugs for depression, psychiatric or emotional conditions, or Parkinson's disease) or for 2 weeks after stopping the MAOI drug. If you are un-

Continued on next page

Prescribing information on A. H. Robins products listed here is based on official labeling in effect November 1, 1994, with Indications, Contraindications, Warnings, Precautions, Adverse Reactions, and Dosage stated in full.

A. H. Robins—Cont.

Age	Weight	Dose
Under 2 yrs.	Under 24 lbs.	Consult doctor
2 to under 6 yrs.	24–47 lbs.	1 Teaspoonful
6 to under 12 yrs.	48–95 lbs.	2 Teaspoonfuls
12 yrs. and older	96 lbs. and over	4 Teaspoonfuls

certain whether your prescription drug contains an MAOI, consult a health professional before taking this product.

Directions: Follow dosage recommendations below or use as directed by a physician. Repeat every 6–8 hours. DO NOT EXCEED 4 DOSES IN A 24 HOUR PERIOD. Dosage: choose by weight, if known; if weight is not known, choose by age.
[See table above.]

How Supplied: Robitussin Pediatric (cherry-colored) in bottles of 4 fl. oz. (NDC 0031-8610-12) and 8 fl. oz. (NDC 0031-8610-18).
Store at Controlled Room Temperature, Between 20°C and 25°C (68°F and 77°F).

Ross Products Division
Abbott Laboratories
COLUMBUS, OHIO 43215-1724
PEDIATRIC NUTRITIONAL PRODUCTS

Alimentum® Protein Hydrolysate Formula With Iron

Isomil® Soy Formula With Iron

Isomil® DF Soy Formula For Diarrhea

Isomil® SF Sucrose-Free Soy Formula With Iron

PediaSure® Complete Liquid Nutrition

PediaSure® With Fiber Complete Liquid Nutrition

RCF® Ross Carbohydrate Free Low-Iron Soy Formula Base

Similac® Low-Iron Infant Formula

Similac® NeoCare™ Premature Infant Formula With Iron

Similac® PM 60/40 Low-Iron Infant Formula

Similac® Special Care® With Iron 24 Premature Infant Formula

Similac® Toddler's Best™ Milk-Based Nutritional Beverage

Similac® With Iron Infant Formula

For most current information, refer to product labels.

CLEAR EYES®
[klēr īz]
Lubricant Eye Redness Reliever Eye Drops

Description: Clear Eyes is a sterile, isotonic buffered solution containing the active ingredients naphazoline hydrochloride (0.012%) and glycerin (0.2%). It also contains boric acid, purified water and sodium borate. Edetate disodium and benzalkonium chloride are added as preservatives. Clear Eyes is a lubricating, decongestant ophthalmic solution specially designed for temporary relief of redness and drying due to minor eye irritation caused by dust, smoke, smog, sun glare, wearing contact lenses or swimming. Clear Eyes contains laboratory-tested and scientifically blended ingredients, including an effective vasoconstrictor which narrows swollen blood vessels and rapidly whitens reddened eyes in a formulation which also contains a lubricant and produces a refreshing, soothing effect. Clear Eyes is a sterile, isotonic solution compatible with the natural fluids of the eye.

Indications: For the temporary relief of redness due to minor eye irritation AND for protection against further irritation or dryness of the eye.

Warnings: To avoid contamination, do not touch tip of container to any surface. Replace cap after using. If you experience eye pain, changes in vision, continued redness or irritation of the eye, or if the condition worsens or persists for more than 72 hours, discontinue use and consult a doctor. If you have glaucoma, do not use this product except under the advice and supervision of a doctor. Overuse of this product may produce increased redness of the eye. If solution changes color or becomes cloudy, do not use. Keep this and all drugs out of the reach of children. In case of accidental ingestion, seek professional assistance or contact a Poison Control Center immediately.

Directions: Instill 1 or 2 drops in the affected eye(s), up to four times daily.

How Supplied: In 0.5-fl-oz (15 mL) and 1.0-fl-oz (30 mL) plastic dropper bottles. (FAN 3178)

CLEAR EYES® ACR
[klēr īz]
Astringent/Lubricant Redness Reliever Eye Drops

Description: Clear Eyes ACR is a sterile, isotonic buffered solution containing the active ingredients naphazoline hydrochloride (0.012%), zinc sulfate (0.25%) and glycerin (0.2%). It also contains boric acid, purified water, sodium chloride and sodium citrate. Edetate disodium and benzalkonium chloride are added as preservatives. Clear Eyes ACR is a triple-action formula that: (1) has an extra ingredient to clear away mucus buildup and relieve itching associated with exposure to airborne allergens, (2) immediately removes redness and (3) moisturizes irritated eyes. Clear Eyes ACR contains laboratory-tested and scientifically blended ingredients, including an effective vasoconstrictor which narrows swollen blood vessels and rapidly whitens reddened eyes in a formulation which also contains a lubricant and produces a refreshing, soothing effect. Clear Eyes ACR also contains an ocular astringent (zinc sulfate) that precipitates the sticky mucus buildup on the eye often associated with exposure to airborne allergens, and this helps clear the mucus from the outer surface of the eye. Clear Eyes ACR is a sterile, isotonic solution compatible with the natural fluids of the eye.

Indications: For the temporary relief of redness due to minor eye irritation AND for protection against further irritation or dryness of the eye.

Warnings: To avoid contamination, do not touch tip of container to any surface. Replace cap after using. If you experience eye pain, changes in vision, continued redness or irritation of the eye, or if the condition worsens or persists for more than 72 hours, discontinue use and consult a doctor. If you have glaucoma, do not use this product except under the advice and supervision of a doctor. Overuse of this product may produce increased redness of the eye. If solution changes color or becomes cloudy, do not use. Keep this and all drugs out of the reach of children. In case of accidental ingestion, seek professional assistance or contact a Poison Control Center immediately.

Directions: Instill 1 or 2 drops in the affected eye(s), up to four times daily.

How Supplied: In 0.5-fl-oz (15 mL) and 1.0-fl-oz (30 mL) plastic dropper bottles. (FAN 3178)

EAR DROPS BY MURINE®
[myūr'ēn]
See Murine Ear Wax Removal System/Murine Ear Drops.

MURINE® EAR WAX REMOVAL SYSTEM/MURINE® EAR DROPS
[myūr'ēn]
Carbamide Peroxide
Ear Wax Removal Aid

Description: MURINE EAR DROPS contains the active ingredient carbamide peroxide, 6.5%. It also contains alcohol (6.3%), anhydrous glycerin, polysorbate 20 and other ingredients in a buffered vehicle. The MURINE EAR WAX REMOVAL SYSTEM includes a 1.0-fl-oz soft bulb ear syringe. This system is a complete, medically approved system to safely remove ear wax. Application of carbamide peroxide drops followed by warm-water irrigation is an effective, medically recommended way to help loosen excessive and/or hardened ear wax.

Actions: The carbamide peroxide formula in MURINE EAR DROPS is an aid in the removal of wax from the ear canal. Anhydrous glycerin penetrates and softens wax while the release of oxygen from carbamide peroxide provides a mechanical action resulting in the loosening of the softened wax accumulation. It is usually necessary to remove the loosened wax by gently flushing the ear with warm water, using the soft bulb ear syringe provided.

Indications: The MURINE EAR WAX REMOVAL SYSTEM is indicated for occasional use as an aid to soften, loosen and remove excessive ear wax.

Warnings: DO NOT USE if you have ear drainage or discharge, ear pain, irritation or rash in the ear or are dizzy: Consult a doctor. DO NOT USE if you have an injury or perforation (hole) of the eardrum or after ear surgery, unless directed by a doctor.
DO NOT USE for more than 4 days; if excessive ear wax remains after use of this product, consult a doctor. Avoid contact with the eyes. If accidental contact with eyes occurs, flush eyes with water and consult a doctor. KEEP THIS AND ALL MEDICINES OUT OF THE REACH OF CHILDREN. In case of accidental ingestion, seek professional assistance or contact a Poison Control Center immediately.

Directions: FOR USE IN THE EAR ONLY. Adults and children over 12 years of age: Tilt head sideways and place 5 to 10 drops in ear. Tip of applicator should not enter ear canal. Keep drops in ear for several minutes by keeping head tilted or placing cotton in the ear. Use twice daily for up to 4 days if needed, or as directed by a doctor. Any wax remaining after treatment may be removed by gently flushing the ear with warm water, using a soft bulb ear syringe. Children under 12 years: Consult a doctor.

Note: When the ear canal is irrigated, the tip of the ear syringe should not obstruct the flow of water leaving the ear canal.

How Supplied: The MURINE EAR WAX REMOVAL SYSTEM contains 0.5-fl-oz (15 mL) drops and a 1.0-fl-oz (30 mL) soft bulb ear syringe.
Also available in 0.5-fl-oz (15 mL) drops only, MURINE EAR DROPS.
(FAN 3178)

MURINE®
[*myūr'ēn*]
Lubricant Eye Drops

Description: Murine eye lubricant is a sterile, buffered solution containing the active ingredients 0.5% polyvinyl alcohol and 0.6% povidone. Also contains benzalkonium chloride, dextrose, disodium edetate, potassium chloride, puri-

fied water, sodium bicarbonate, sodium chloride, sodium citrate and sodium phosphate (mono- and dibasic). Murine is a sterile, hypotonic solution formulated to more closely match the natural tear fluid of the eye for gentle, soothing relief from minor eye irritation while moisturizing and relieving dryness. Use as desired to temporarily relieve minor eye irritation, dryness and burning.

Indications: For the temporary relief or prevention of further discomfort due to minor eye irritations and symptoms related to dry eyes.

Warnings: To avoid contamination, do not touch tip of container to any surface. Replace cap after using. If you experience eye pain, changes in vision, continued redness or irritation of the eye, or if the condition worsens or persists for more than 72 hours, discontinue use and consult a doctor. If solution changes color or becomes cloudy, do not use. Keep this and all drugs out of the reach of children. In case of accidental ingestion, seek professional assistance or contact a Poison Control Center immediately.

Directions: Instill 1 or 2 drops in the affected eye(s) as needed.

How Supplied: In 0.5-fl-oz (15 mL) and 1.0-fl-oz (30 mL) plastic dropper bottles. (FAN 3178)

MURINE® PLUS
[*myūr'ēn*]
Lubricant Redness Reliever Eye Drops

Description: Murine Plus is a sterile, non-staining, buffered solution containing the active ingredients 0.5% polyvinyl alcohol, 0.6% povidone and 0.05% tetrahydrozoline hydrochloride. Also contains benzalkonium chloride, dextrose, disodium edetate, potassium chloride, purified water, sodium bicarbonate, sodium chloride, sodium citrate and sodium phosphate (mono- and dibasic). Murine Plus is a sterile, hypotonic, ophthalmic solution formulated to more closely match the natural fluid of the eye. It contains demulcents for gentle, soothing relief from minor eye irritation as well as the sympathomimetic agent, tetrahydrozoline hydrochloride, which produces local vasoconstriction in the eye. Thus, the drug effectively narrows swollen blood vessels locally and provides symptomatic relief of edema and hyperemia of conjunctival tissues due to eye allergies, minor local irritations and conjunctivitis. Use up to four times daily, to remove redness due to minor eye irritation. The effect of Murine Plus is prompt (apparent within minutes).

Indications: For the temporary relief or prevention of further discomfort due to minor eye irritations and symptoms related to dry eyes PLUS removal of redness.

Warnings: To avoid contamination, do not touch tip of container to any surface.

Replace cap after using. If you experience eye pain, changes in vision, continued redness or irritation of the eye, or if the condition worsens or persists for more than 72 hours, discontinue use and consult a doctor. If you have glaucoma, do not use this product except under the advice and supervision of a doctor. Overuse of this product may produce increased redness of the eye. If solution changes color or becomes cloudy, do not use. Keep this and all drugs out of the reach of children. In case of accidental ingestion, seek professional assistance or contact a Poison Control Center immediately.

Directions: Instill 1 or 2 drops in the affected eye(s), **up to four times daily.**

How Supplied: In 0.5-fl-oz (15 mL) and 1.0-fl-oz (30 mL) plastic dropper bottles. (FAN 3178)

PEDIALYTE®
[*pē'dē-ah-līt"*]
Oral Electrolyte Maintenance Solution

Usage: To quickly restore fluids and minerals lost in diarrhea and vomiting; for maintenance of water and electrolytes following corrective parenteral therapy for severe diarrhea.

Features:
- Ready To Use—no mixing or dilution necessary.
- Balanced electrolytes to replace stool losses and provide maintenance requirements.
- Provides glucose to promote sodium and water absorption.
- Unflavored form available for younger infants; Bubble Gum and Fruit-flavored forms available to enhance compliance in older infants and children.
- Plastic liter bottles are resealable and easy to pour.
- Widely available in grocery, drug and convenience stores.

Availability:
1 quart 1.8 fl oz (1 liter) plastic bottles; 8 per case; Unflavored, No. 336; Fruit-flavored, No. 365; Bubble Gum-flavored, No. 51752.
8-fl-oz (237 mL) bottles; 4 six-packs per case; Unflavored, No. 160. For hospital use, Pedialyte is available in the Ross Hospital Formula System.

Dosage: See Administration Guide to restore fluids and minerals lost in diarrhea and vomiting (Pedialyte Unflavored, Bubble Gum-flavored or Fruit-flavored) and management of mild to moderate dehydration secondary to mod-

Continued on next page

Ross—Cont.

erate to severe diarrhea (Rehydralyte® Oral Electrolyte Rehydration Solution). Pedialyte (Unflavored, Bubble Gum-flavored or Fruit-flavored) or Rehydralyte should be offered frequently in amounts tolerated. Total daily intake should be adjusted to meet individual needs, based on thirst and response to therapy. The following suggested intakes for maintenance are based on water requirements for ordinary energy expenditure.[1] For dehydrated children, the suggested intakes are for replacement and for maintenance, based on a fluid deficit of 5% or 10% of body weight (including maintenance requirement). The fluid deficit

should be replaced as quickly as possible, usually in the first 4 to 6 hours. [See table below.]

Reference:
1. Extrapolated from Barness L: Nutrition and nutritional disorders, in Behrman RE, Kliegman RM, Nelson WE, Vaughan VC III: *Nelson Textbook of Pediatrics*, ed 14. Philadelphia: WB Saunders Co, 1992, pp 105-107.

Composition: Unflavored Pedialyte (Bubble Gum-flavored and Fruit-flavored Pedialyte have similar composition and nutrient value. For specific information, see product label.)

Ingredients: (Pareve, Ⓤ) Water, dextrose, potassium citrate, sodium chloride and sodium citrate.

Provides:	Per 8 Fl Oz	Per Liter	Per 32 Fl Oz
Sodium (mEq)	10.6	45	42.4
Potassium (mEq)	4.7	20	18.8
Chloride (mEq)	8.3	35	33.2
Citrate (mEq)	7.1	30	28.4
Dextrose (g)	5.9	25	23.6
Calories	24	100	96

(FAN 3106-01)

Shown in Product Identification Guide, page 520

PEDIASURE® And PEDIASURE® WITH FIBER
[pē'dē-ah-shur"]
Complete Liquid Nutrition
For Children 1 to 10 years old.

Usage: As a liquid food providing complete, balanced nutrition for children 1 to

---

Pedialyte, Rehydralyte Administration Guide*

For Infants and Young Children

Age	2 Weeks	3	6 Months	9	1	1½	2	2½ Years	3	3½	4	5	6
Approximate Weight†													
(lb)	7	13	17	20	23	25	28	30	32	35	38	41	46
(kg)	3.2	6.0	7.8	9.2	10.2	11.4	12.6	13.6	14.6	16.0	17.0	18.7	20.7
PEDIALYTE UNFLAVORED, BUBBLE GUM-FLAVORED or FRUIT-FLAVORED fl oz/day for maintenance**	13 to 16	28 to 32	34 to 40	38 to 44	41 to 46	45 to 50	48 to 53	51 to 56	54 to 58	56 to 60	57 to 62	59 to 66	62 to 69
REHYDRALYTE fl oz/day for Replacement for 5% Dehydration (including maintenance)**	18 to 21	38 to 42	47 to 53	53 to 59	58 to 63	64 to 69	69 to 74	74 to 79	78 to 82	83 to 87	85 to 90	90 to 97	96 to 104
REHYDRALYTE fl oz/day for Replacement for 10% Dehydration (including maintenance)**	23 to 26	48 to 52	60 to 66	68 to 74	75 to 80	83 to 88	90 to 95	97 to 102	102 to 106	110 to 114	113 to 118	121 to 128	131 to 138

* Administration Guide does not apply to infants less than 1 week of age.

**Fluid intakes do not take into account ongoing stool losses. Fluid loss in the stool should be replaced by consumption of an extra amount of Pedialyte or Rehydralyte equal to stool losses, in addition to the amounts indicated in this Administration Guide.

† Weight based on the 50th percentile of weight for age of the National Center for Health Statistics (NCHS) reference growth data. Hamill PVV, Drizd TA, Johnson CL, et al: Physical growth: National Center for Health Statistics percentiles. *Am J Clin Nutr* 1979; 32:607-629.

10 years of age. May be used for total nutritional support or as a nutritional supplement with and between meals.

Features: PediaSure and PediaSure With Fiber

- Doctor recommended and hospital used
- Nutrition to help recover from illness
- For unpredictable/"picky" eaters
- Ideal for busy, active lifestyles
- A dietary source of fiber (PediaSure With Fiber only)
- Lactose free, * easily digested
- Convenient, ready to drink, great tasting

*Not for patients with galactosemia.

PediaSure and PediaSure With Fiber contain 100% or more of the NAS-NRC Recommended Dietary Allowances (RDA) for protein, vitamins and minerals in 1000 mL (approx. 34 fl oz) for children 1 to 6 years of age and in 1300 mL (approx. 44 fl oz) for children 7 to 10 years of age.

Availability: Ready To Use 8-fl-oz (237 mL) cans in 6-packs; 24 cans per case. PediaSure: Vanilla, No. 373; Chocolate, No. 51812; Strawberry, No. 51810; Banana Cream, No. 51808. PediaSure With Fiber: Vanilla, No. 50652.

Directions for Use: Shake very well. Delicious chilled. Do not add water. Suggest 1 to 3 cans per day for supplemental use. Once opened, cover, refrigerate and use within 48 hours. Consult your health care professional regarding your child's specific needs. Not intended for infants under 1 year of age unless specified by a physician.

Ingredients† PediaSure and PediaSure With Fiber (Vanilla flavor): Ⓤ-D Water, hydrolyzed cornstarch, sugar (sucrose), sodium caseinate, high-oleic safflower oil, soy oil, fractionated coconut oil (medium-chain triglycerides), whey protein concentrate, soy fiber (PediaSure With Fiber only), calcium phosphate tribasic, natural and artificial flavor, potassium citrate, magnesium chloride, potassium phosphate dibasic, potassium chloride, soy lecithin, mono- and diglycerides, choline chloride, carrageenan, ascorbic acid, m-inositol, taurine, ferrous sulfate, zinc sulfate, niacinamide, alpha-tocopheryl acetate, L-carnitine, calcium pantothenate, manganese sulfate, thiamine chloride hydrochloride, pyridoxine hydrochloride, riboflavin, cupric sulfate, vitamin A palmitate, folic acid, biotin, potassium iodide, sodium selenite, sodium molybdate, phylloquinone, vitamin D_3 and cyanocobalamin.
Nutrients (grams/8 fl oz): Protein, 7.1; Fat, 11.8; Carbohydrate, 26 (26.9‡, PediaSure With Fiber); L-Carnitine, 0.004; Taurine, 0.017; Water, 200. Calories per mL, 1.0; Calories per fl oz, 29.6.

† For Vanilla product; minor differences exist in other PediaSure flavors. For specific information, see product labels.

‡ Includes soy fiber (a source of dietary fiber that provides 3.4 Calories and 1.2 g of total dietary fibers).
(FAN 3139-02) (PediaSure)
(FAN 3139-01) (PediaSure With Fiber)
Shown in Product Identification Guide, page 520

REHYDRALYTE®
[rē-hī´drə-līt″]
Oral Electrolyte Rehydration Solution

Usage: To restore fluids and minerals lost during moderate to severe diarrhea.
Features:
- Ready To Use—no mixing or dilution necessary.
- Safe, economical alternative to IV therapy.
- 75 mEq of sodium per liter for effective replacement of fluid deficits.
- 2½% glucose solution to promote sodium and water absorption and provide energy.
- Available in pharmacies.

Availability: 8-fl-oz (237 mL) bottles; 4 six-packs per case; No. 162.

Dosage: (See Administration Guide under Pedialyte®.)

Ingredients: (Pareve, Ⓤ) Water, dextrose, sodium chloride, potassium citrate and sodium citrate.

Provides:	Per 8 Fl Oz	Per Liter
Sodium (mEq)	17.7	75
Potassium (mEq)	4.7	20
Chloride (mEq)	15.4	65
Citrate (mEq)	7.1	30
Dextrose (g)	5.9	25
Calories	24	100

(FAN 3106-01)

SELSUN BLUE®
[sel´sun blü]
Dandruff Shampoo
(selenium sulfide lotion, 1%)

Description: Selsun Blue is a non-prescription anti-dandruff shampoo containing the active ingredient selenium sulfide, 1%, in a freshly scented, pH-balanced formula to leave hair clean and manageable. Available in Regular, Extra Conditioning and Medicated Treatment formulas.

Inactive Ingredients:
Regular hair formula —Ammonium laureth sulfate, ammonium lauryl sulfate, citric acid, cocamide DEA, cocamidopropyl betaine, DMDM hydantoin, FD&C blue No. 1, fragrance, hydroxypropyl methylcellulose, magnesium aluminum silicate, purified water, sodium chloride and titanium dioxide.
Extra Conditioning formula — Aloe, ammonium laureth sulfate, ammonium lauryl sulfate, citric acid, cocamide DEA, di (hydrogenated) tallow phthalic acid amide, dimethicone, DMDM hydantoin, FD&C blue No. 1, fragrance, hydroxypropyl methylcellulose, purified

water, sodium citrate, sodium isostearoyl lactylate and titanium dioxide.
Medicated Treatment formula — Ammonium laureth sulfate, ammonium lauryl sulfate, citric acid, cocamide DEA, cocamidopropyl betaine, DMDM hydantoin, D&C red No. 33, FD&C blue No. 1, fragrance, hydroxypropyl methylcellulose, magnesium aluminum silicate, menthol, purified water, sodium chloride and TEA-lauryl sulfate.
Clinical testing has shown Selsun Blue to be as safe and effective as other leading shampoos in helping control dandruff symptoms with regular use. May be used on color-treated or permed hair, if used as directed.

Directions: Shake well. Shampoo and rinse thoroughly. For best results, use regularly, at least twice a week or as directed by a doctor.

Warnings: For external use only. Avoid contact with the eyes. If contact occurs, rinse eyes thoroughly with water. If condition worsens or does not improve after regular use of this product as directed, consult a doctor. Keep this and all drugs out of the reach of children. In case of accidental ingestion, seek professional assistance or contact a Poison Control Center immediately.

How Supplied: 4 (118 mL), 7 (207 mL) and 11 (325 mL) fl oz plastic bottles. (FAN 3178)

SELSUN GOLD FOR WOMEN®
[sel´sun gōld]
Dandruff Shampoo
(selenium sulfide lotion, 1%)

Description: Selsun Gold for Women is a non-prescription anti-dandruff shampoo containing the active ingredient selenium sulfide, 1%. This formula allows you to shampoo, condition and control dandruff flaking and itching with one shampoo. This formula contains patented ingredients to leave hair soft, shiny and manageable. You won't need a separate conditioner to have beautiful hair. May be used on color-treated or permed hair, if used as directed.

Inactive Ingredients: Ammonium lauryl sulfate, ammonium laureth sulfate, citric acid, cocamide DEA, di (hydrogenated) tallow phthalic acid amide, dimethicone, DMDM hydantoin, hydroxypropyl methylcellulose, purified water, sodium citrate and fragrance.

Directions: Shake well. Shampoo and rinse thoroughly. For best results, use regularly, at least twice a week or as directed by a doctor.

Continued on next page

If desired, additional information on any Ross product will be provided upon request to Ross Products Division, Abbott Laboratories, Columbus, Ohio 432 15-1724.

Ross—Cont.

Warnings: For external use only. Avoid contact with the eyes. If contact occurs, rinse eyes thoroughly with water. If condition worsens or does not improve after regular use of this product as directed, consult a doctor. Keep this and all drugs out of the reach of children. In case of accidental ingestion, seek professional assistance or contact a Poison Control Center immediately.

How Supplied: 4 (118 mL), 7 (207 mL) and 11 (325 mL) fl oz plastic bottles. (FAN 3178)

SIMILAC® Toddler's Best™
[sim 'e-lak täd 'lərs best]
Milk-Based Nutritional Beverage For Toddlers Over 12 Months Old.

Usage: As an iron-fortified, milk-based alternative to cow's milk or juice for children over 12 months of age.

Features:
- Caloric density: 20 Cal/fl oz
- 2.9 mg of iron per 8 fl oz to help avoid iron deficiency
- Iron content per 8 fl oz is 30% of the Daily Value (DV)
- Contains 40% of the DV for vitamin C per 8 fl oz (6 times the amount in whole cow's milk)
- Contains 50% of the DV for vitamin E per 8 fl oz (17 times the amount in whole cow's milk)
- Higher in many essential nutrients than whole cow's milk

Availability: Ready To Use 8-fl-oz (237 mL) drink box; 27 8-fl-oz drink boxes per case (9 units of 3 drink boxes); Vanilla, No. 52154; Chocolate, No. 52152; Berry, No. 52156.

Directions for Use: Shake well before using. Serve one 8-fl-oz drink box as an alternative to cow's milk or fruit juice with or between regular meals. Delicious at room temperature or chilled. Once opened, refrigerate unused portion and use within 24 hours.

Composition: Ready To Use Vanilla (Chocolate and Berry flavors have similar composition and nutrient values. For specific information, see product labels.)

Ingredients: Ⓤ-D Water, nonfat milk, sugar (sucrose), lactose, high-oleic safflower oil, coconut oil, soy oil, natural and artificial flavor, calcium carbonate, soy lecithin, ascorbic acid, choline chloride, ferrous sulfate, taurine, m-inositol, alpha-tocopheryl acetate, zinc sulfate, niacinamide, calcium pantothenate, vitamin A palmitate, cupric sulfate, thiamine chloride hydrochloride, riboflavin, pyridoxine hydrochloride, folic acid, manganese sulfate, phylloquinone, biotin, sodium selenite, vitamin D_3 and cyanocobalamin.
[See table below.]
(FAN 3148-01)
Shown in Product Identification Guide, page 520

TRONOLANE®
[tron 'ə-lān]
Anesthetic Cream for Hemorrhoids

Description: The active ingredient in Tronolane cream is the topical anesthetic agent, pramoxine hydrochloride, 1% (chemically unrelated to the benzoate esters of the "caine" type), which is chemically designated as a 4-n-butoxyphenyl gammamor-pholinopropyl-ether hydrochloride. Also contains the following inactive ingredients: A nongreasy cream base containing beeswax, cetyl alcohol, cetyl esters wax, glycerin, methylparaben, propylparaben, sodium lauryl sulfate and zinc oxide.
Tronolane cream contains a rapidly acting topical anesthetic producing analgesia that lasts up to 5 hours. Because the drug is chemically unrelated to other anesthetics, cross-sensitization is unlikely. Patients who are already sensitized to the "caine" anesthetics can generally use Tronolane cream.
The emollient/emulsion base of Tronolane cream provides soothing lubrication. Tronolane cream is in a nondrying base that is nongreasy and nonstaining to undergarments.

Indications: Tronolane cream is indicated for the temporary relief of pain, itching, burning and soreness associated with hemorrhoids.

Warnings: If condition worsens or does not improve within 7 days, consult a doctor. Do not exceed the recommended

daily dosage, unless directed by a doctor. In case of bleeding, consult a doctor promptly. Do not put this product into the rectum by using fingers or any mechanical device or applicator. Certain persons can develop allergic reactions to ingredients in this product. If the symptom being treated does not subside, or if redness, irritation, swelling, pain or other symptoms develop or increase, discontinue use and consult a doctor. As with any drug, if you are pregnant or nursing a baby, seek the advice of a health care professional before using this product. Keep this and all drugs out of the reach of children. In case of accidental ingestion, seek professional assistance or contact a Poison Control Center.

Dosage and Administration (Directions): Adults—When practical, cleanse the affected area with mild soap and warm water and rinse thoroughly or cleanse by patting or blotting with an appropriate cleansing pad. Gently dry by patting or blotting with toilet tissue or a soft cloth before application of this product. Apply externally to the affected area up to five times daily. Children under 12 years of age—Consult a doctor.

How Supplied: Tronolane cream is available in 1-oz (28g) and 2-oz (57g) tubes.
(FAN 2393)

TRONOLANE®
[tron 'ə-lān]
Hemorrhoidal Suppositories

Description: The active ingredients in Tronolane suppositories are zinc oxide, 5%, and hard fat, 95%. Zinc oxide (an astringent) and hard fat (a skin protectant) afford temporary relief of hemorrhoidal itching and burning and protect irritated hemorrhoidal areas.

Indications: Tronolane suppositories are indicated for the temporary relief of the itching, burning and irritation associated with hemorrhoids.

Warnings: If condition worsens or does not improve within 7 days, consult a doctor. Do not exceed the recommended daily dosage, unless directed by a doctor. In case of bleeding, consult a doctor promptly. As with any drug, if you are pregnant or nursing a baby, seek the ad-

Similac® Toddler's Best™ Compared With Whole Cow's Milk: Selected Nutrients

Nutrient	NLEA* Labeling Daily Values (DV)	Similac Toddler's Best		Whole Cow's Milk	
	Children <4 years of age	8 fl oz	% DV	8 fl oz	% DV
Protein, g	16	5.6	35	8.0	50
Fat, g	NA	7.5	NA	8.2	NA
Carbohydrate, g	NA	17.6	NA	11.5	NA
Iron, mg	10	2.9	30	0.12	2
Vitamin E, IU	10	4.8	50	0.28	2
Vitamin C, mg	40	15.2	40	2.24	6

*Nutrition Labeling and Education Act, 1990
NA Not applicable

vice of a health care professional before using this product. **Do not store above 86°F.** Keep this and all drugs out of the reach of children. In case of accidental ingestion, seek professional assistance or contact a Poison Control Center immediately.

Dosage and Administration (Directions): Adults—When practical, cleanse the affected area with mild soap and warm water and rinse thoroughly or cleanse by patting or blotting with an appropriate cleansing pad. Gently dry by patting or blotting with toilet tissue or a soft cloth before application of this product. Remove foil wrapper before inserting into the rectum. Use up to six times daily or after each bowel movement. Children under 12 years of age—Consult a doctor.

How Supplied: Tronolane suppositories are available in 10- and 20-count boxes.
(FAN 2393)

Sandoz Pharmaceuticals Corporation/ Consumer Division
59 ROUTE 10 EAST HANOVER, NJ 07936

ACID MANTLE® CREME
[ă'sĭd-mănt'l]
Acid pH

Description: Restores and maintains protective acidity of the skin. Provides relief of mildly irritated skin due to exposure to soaps, detergents, chemicals and alkalis. Aids in the treatment of diaper rash; bath dermatitis; winter eczema and dry, rough, scaly skin of varied causes.

Ingredients: Water, cetostearyl alcohol, white petrolatum, glycerin, synthetic beeswax, light mineral oil, sodium lauryl sulfate, aluminum sulfate, calcium acetate, methylparaben, white potato dextrin.

Caution: For external use only. Avoid contact with the eyes.

Directions: Apply several times daily, especially after wet work.

How Supplied: 1 oz. tubes; 4 oz. and 1 lb. jars.

BiCOZENE® Creme External Analgesic
[bĭ-cō-zēn]

Active Ingredients: Benzocaine 6%, resorcinol 1.67% in a specially prepared cream base.

Inactive Ingredients: Castor Oil, Chlorothymol, Ethanolamine Stearates, Glycerin, Glyceryl Borate, Glyceryl Stearates, Parachlorometaxylenol, Polysorbate 80, Sodium Stearate, Triglycerol Diisostearate, Perfume.

Indications: For the temporary relief of pain and itching associated with minor burns, sunburn, minor cuts, scrapes, insect bites or minor skin irritations.

Actions: Benzocaine is a topical anesthetic and resorcinol is a topical antipruritic, at the concentrations used in BiCozene Creme. Both exert their actions by depressing cutaneous sensory receptors.

Warnings: Do not apply over large areas of the body. Caution: Use only as directed. Keep away from the eyes. Not for prolonged use. If the symptoms persist for more than seven days or clear up and reoccur within a few days, or if a rash or irritation develops, discontinue use and consult a physician. For external use only. **KEEP THIS AND ALL DRUGS OUT OF THE REACH OF CHILDREN.** In case of accidental ingestion, seek professional assistance or contact a Poison Control Center immediately.

Drug Interaction Precautions: No known drug interaction.

Dosage and Administration: Adults and children 2 years of age and older: apply to affected area not more than 3 to 4 times daily. Children under 2 years of age: consult a physician. Apply liberally to affected area as needed, several times a day.

How Supplied: BiCozene Creme is available in 1-ounce tubes.
Shown in Product Identification Guide, page 520

CAMA® ARTHRITIS PAIN RELIEVER
[kă'măh]

Description: Each CAMA Inlay-Tab contains: aspirin USP, 500 mg (7.7 grains); magnesium oxide, USP, 150 mg; dried aluminum hydroxide gel, USP, equivalent to 125 mg aluminum hydroxide. Other ingredients: colloidal silicon dioxide, croscarmellose sodium, hydrogenated vegetable oil, methylcellulose, methylparaben, microcrystalline cellulose, polyethylene glycol, povidone, pregelatinized starch, starch, Yellow 6, Yellow 10.

Indications: For the temporary relief of minor arthritic pain.

Warnings: Children and teenagers who have or are recovering from chicken pox, flu symptoms, or flu should NOT use this product. If nausea, vomiting or fever occur, consult a doctor because these symptoms could be an early sign of Reye Syndrome, a rare but serious illness. If redness or swelling is present, consult a doctor because these could be signs of a serious condition. Do not take this drug if you have asthma unless directed by a doctor. Do not take this product if you have stomach problems (such as heartburn, upset stomach, or stomach pain) that persist or recur, or if you have ulcers or bleeding problems, unless directed by

a doctor. Do not take this product for more than 10 days or for fever for more than 3 days unless directed by a doctor. If pain persists or gets worse, if new symptoms occur, or if redness or swelling is present, consult a doctor because these could be signs of a serious condition. As with any drug, if you are pregnant or nursing a baby, seek the advice of a health professional before using this product. **IT IS ESPECIALLY IMPORTANT NOT TO USE ASPIRIN DURING THE LAST 3 MONTHS OF PREGNANCY UNLESS SPECIFICALLY DIRECTED TO DO SO BY A DOCTOR BECAUSE IT MAY CAUSE PROBLEMS IN THE UNBORN CHILD OR COMPLICATIONS DURING DELIVERY.** Stop taking this product if ringing in the ears, loss of hearing, or dizziness occur. Do not take this product if you are presently taking a prescription drug for anticoagulation (thinning the blood), diabetes, arthritis, gout or if you have an aspirin allergy unless directed by a doctor. **Keep this and all medicines out of the reach of children. In case of accidental overdose, contact a physician immediately.**

Directions For Use: Adults: 2 tablets with a full glass of water every 6 hours. Not to exceed 8 tablets in 24 hours unless directed by a physician. Do not use in children under 12 years of age except under the advice and supervision of a physician.

How Supplied: CAMA Arthritis Pain Reliever Tablets (white with salmon inlay), imprinted "Cama 500" on one side, "Dorsey" on the other, in bottles of 100.

DORCOL® CHILDREN'S COUGH SYRUP
[door'call]

Description: Each teaspoonful (5 ml) of DORCOL Children's Cough Syrup contains pseudoephedrine hydrochloride 15 mg, guaifenesin 50 mg, dextromethorphan hydrobromide 5 mg. Other ingredients: benzoic acid, Blue 1, edetate disodium, flavors, glycerin, propylene glycol, purified water, Red 40, sodium hydroxide, sucrose, tartaric acid.

Indications: Temporarily relieves your child's cough due to minor throat and bronchial irritation as may occur with the common cold. Helps loosen phlegm (mucus) and thin bronchial secretions to rid the bronchial passageways of bothersome mucus. Helps drain bronchial tubes and makes coughs more productive. Temporarily relieves nasal stuffiness due to the common cold, hay fever or upper respiratory allergies, and promotes nasal and/or sinus drainage.

Warnings: Keep this and all drugs out of the reach of children. In case of accidental overdose, seek professional assistance or contact a Poison Control Center immediately.

Continued on next page

Sandoz—Cont.

Do not exceed recommended dosage because at higher doses nervousness, dizziness, or sleeplessness may occur. Do not give your child this product for more than 7 days. If symptoms persist, are accompanied by fever, rash or persistent headache, or if cough recurs, consult a doctor. A persistent cough may be a sign of a serious condition. Do not give this product: 1) if cough is accompanied by excessive phlegm (mucus), 2) for persistent or chronic cough such as occurs with asthma, or 3) if your child has heart disease, high blood pressure, thyroid disease, or diabetes.

Drug Interactions Precaution: Do not give this product to a child who is taking a prescription monoamine oxidase inhibitor (MAOI) (certain drugs for depression, psychiatric or emotional conditions) or for 2 weeks after stopping the MAOI drug. If you are uncertain whether your prescription drug contains an MAOI, consult a health professional before giving this product.

Directions For Use: Children under 2 years—consult physician.
By age:
Children 2 to under 6 years: 1 teaspoonful every 4 hours.
Children 6 to under 12 years: 2 teaspoonfuls every 4 hours.
By weight:
Children 25 to 45 pounds: 1 teaspoonful every 4 hours.
Children 46 to 85 pounds: 2 teaspoonfuls every 4 hours.
Unless directed by a physician, do not exceed 4 doses in 24 hours.

Professional Labeling: The suggested dosage for pediatric patients is:

3–12 months	3 drops/Kg of body weight every 4 hours
12–24 months	7 drops (0.2 ml)/Kg of body weight every 4 hours

Maximum 4 doses in 24 hours.

How Supplied: DORCOL Children's Cough Syrup (grape colored), in 4 fl oz and 8 fl oz plastic bottles with tamper-evident band around child-resistant cap.

Shown in Product Identification Guide, page 520

EX–LAX® Chocolated Laxative Tablets

Active Ingredient: Yellow phenolphthalein, 90 mg. phenolphthalein per tablet.

Inactive Ingredients: Cocoa, Confectioner's Sugar, Hydrogenated Palm Kernel Oil, Lecithin, Nonfat Dry Milk, Vanillin.

Indication: For relief of occasional constipation (irregularity).

Caution: Do not take any laxative when abdominal pain, nausea, or vomiting are present. Frequent or prolonged use of this or any other laxative may result in dependence on laxatives. If skin rash appears, do not use this or any other preparation containing phenolphthalein.

Warnings: Keep this and all drugs out of the reach of children. In case of accidental overdose, seek professional assistance or contact a poison control center immediately. As with any drug, if you are pregnant or nursing a baby, seek the advice of a health care professional before using this product.

Dosage and Administration: Adults and children 12 years old and over: Chew 1 to 2 tablets, preferably at bedtime. Children over 6 years: Chew ½ tablet.

How Supplied: Available in boxes of 6, 18, 48, and 72 chewable chocolate-flavored tablets.

Shown in Product Identification Guide, page 520

EX–LAX® Laxative Pills

Regular Strength Ex-Lax®
Laxative Pills
Extra Gentle Ex-Lax® Laxative Pills
Maximum Relief Formula Ex-Lax®
Laxative Pills
Ex-Lax® Gentle Nature® Laxative Pills

Active Ingredients: Regular Strength Ex-Lax Laxative Pills—Yellow phenolphthalein, 90 mg. phenolphthalein per pill. **Extra Gentle Ex-Lax Laxative Pills**—Docusate sodium, 75 mg. and yellow phenolphthalein, 65 mg. per pill. **Maximum Relief Formula Ex-Lax Laxative Pills**—Yellow phenolphthalein, 135 mg. phenolphthalein per pill. **Ex-Lax Gentle Nature Laxative Pills**—Sennosides, 20 mg. per pill.

Inactive Ingredients: Regular Strength Ex-Lax Laxative Pills—Acacia, Alginic Acid, Carnauba Wax, Colloidal Silicon Dioxide, Dibasic Calcium Phosphate, Iron Oxides, Magnesium Stearate, Microcrystalline Cellulose, Sodium Benzoate, Sodium Lauryl Sulfate, Starch, Stearic Acid, Sucrose, Talc, Titanium Dioxide. **Extra Gentle Ex-Lax Laxative Pills**—Acacia, Croscarmellose Sodium, Dibasic Calcium Phosphate, Colloidal Silicon Dioxide, Magnesium Stearate, Microcrystalline Cellulose, Red 7, Stearic Acid, Sucrose, Talc, Titanium Dioxide. **Maximum Relief Formula Ex-Lax Laxative Pills**—Acacia, Alginic Acid, Blue No. 1, Carnauba Wax, Colloidal Silicon Dioxide, Dibasic Calcium Phosphate, Magnesium Stearate, Microcrystalline Cellulose, Povidone, Sodium Benzoate, Sodium Lauryl Sulfate, Starch, Stearic Acid, Sucrose, Talc, Titanium Dioxide. **Ex-Lax Gentle Nature Laxative Pills**—Alginic Acid, Colloidal Silicon Dioxide, Dibasic Calcium Phosphate, Magnesium Stearate, Microcrystalline Cellulose, Pregelatinized Starch, Sodium Lauryl Sulfate, Stearic Acid.

Indication: For relief of occasional constipation (irregularity).

Caution: Do not take any laxative when abdominal pain, nausea, or vomiting are present. Frequent or prolonged use of this or any other laxative may result in dependence on laxatives. If skin rash appears, do not use this or any other preparation containing phenolphthalein.

Warnings: Keep this and all drugs out of the reach of children. In case of accidental overdose, seek professional assistance or contact a Poison Control Center immediately. As with any drug, if you are pregnant or nursing a baby, seek the advice of a health care professional before using this product.

Dosage and Administration: Regular Strength Ex-Lax Laxative Pills, Extra Gentle Ex-Lax Laxative Pills, and Ex-Lax Gentle Nature Laxative Pills—Adults and children 12 years old and over: Take 1 to 2 pills with a glass of water, preferably at bedtime. Consult with a physician for children under 12 years of age. **Maximum Relief Formula Ex-Lax Laxative Pills**—Adults and children over 12 years of age, take 1 to 2 pills with a glass of water, preferably at bedtime. Consult with a physician for children under 12 years of age.

How Supplied: Regular Strength Ex-Lax Laxative Pills—Available in boxes of 8, 30, and 60 pills. **Extra Gentle Ex-Lax Laxative Pills and Maximum Relief Formula Ex-Lax Laxative Pills**—Available in boxes of 24 pills. **Ex-Lax Gentle Nature Laxative Pills**—Available in boxes of 16 pills.

Shown in Product Identification Guide, page 520

GAS–X® AND
EXTRA STRENGTH GAS-X®
Antiflatulent, Anti-Gas Tablets

Active Ingredients: GAS-X®—Each tablet contains 80 mg. simethicone. EXTRA STRENGTH GAS-X®—Each tablet contains 125 mg. simethicone.

Inactive Ingredients: calcium phosphates dibasic and tribasic, calcium silicate, colloidal silicon dioxide, compressible sugar, microcrystalline cellulose and talc. GAS-X cherry creme flavored tablets also contain Red 30. Extra Strength GAS-X peppermint creme and Extra Strength GAS-X cherry creme flavored tablets also contain Red 30 and Yellow 10.

Indications: For relief of the pain and pressure symptoms of excess gas in the digestive tract, which is often accompanied by complaints of bloating, distention, fullness, pressure, pain, cramps or excess anal flatus.

Actions: GAS-X acts in the stomach and intestines to disperse and reduce the formation of mucus-trapped gas bubbles. The GAS-X defoaming action reduces the surface tension of gas bubbles so that they are more easily eliminated.

Warning: Keep this and all medicines out of the reach of children.

Drug Interaction Precautions: No known drug interaction.

Dosage and Administration: Adults: Chew thoroughly and swallow one or two tablets as needed after meals and at bedtime. Do not exceed six GAS-X tablets or four EXTRA STRENGTH GAS-X tablets in 24 hours, except under the advice and supervision of a physician.

Professional Labeling: GAS-X may be used in the alleviation of postoperative gas pain, and for use in endoscopic examination.

How Supplied: GAS-X is available in peppermint creme and cherry creme flavored, chewable, scored tablets in boxes of 36 tablets and 12 tablets.
EXTRA STRENGTH GAS-X is available in peppermint creme and cherry creme flavored, chewable, scored tablets in boxes of 18 tablets and 48 tablets.
Shown in Product Identification Guide, page 520

TAVIST-1® TABLETS

Description: Each tablet contains: clemastine fumarate, USP, 1.34 mg (equivalent to 1 mg clemastine). Other ingredients: lactose, povidone, starch, stearic acid, and talc.

Indications: Temporarily reduces runny nose and relieves sneezing, itching of the nose or throat, and itchy, watery eyes due to hay fever or other upper respiratory allergies.

Warnings: May cause drowsiness; alcohol, sedatives, and tranquilizers may increase the drowsiness effect. Do not take this product if you are taking sedatives or tranquilizers without first consulting your doctor. Use caution when driving a motor vehicle or operating machinery. May cause excitability especially in children. Do not take this product if you have glaucoma, a breathing problem such as emphysema or chronic bronchitis, or difficulty in urination due to enlargement of the prostate gland unless directed by a doctor. As with any drug, if you are pregnant or nursing a baby, seek the advice of a health professional before using this product. Keep this and all drugs out of reach of children. In case of accidental overdose, seek professional assistance or contact a Poison Control Center immediately.

Directions: Adults and children 12 years of age and over: Take one tablet every 12 hours, not to exceed 2 tablets in 24 hours, or as directed by a doctor. Children under 12 years: Consult a doctor.

How Supplied: Tavist-1 tablets (white) imprinted "Tavist-1" on both sides in blister packs of 8, 16, and 32.

Shown in Product Identification Guide, page 520

TAVIST-D® TABLETS

Description: Each tablet contains: clemastine fumarate, USP, 1.34 mg (equivalent to 1 mg clemastine) immediate release and 75 mg phenylpropanolamine hydrochloride, USP, extended release. Other ingredients: Colloidal silicon dioxide, dibasic calcium phosphate, lactose, magnesium stearate, methylcellulose, polyethylene glycol, povidone, starch, synthetic polymers, titanium dioxide and Yellow 10.

Indications: For the temporary relief of nasal congestion associated with upper respiratory allergies or sinusitis when accompanied by other symptoms of hay fever or allergies, including runny nose, sneezing, itchy nose or throat or itchy, watery eyes.

Warnings: May cause drowsiness; alcohol, sedatives, and tranquilizers may increase the drowsiness effect. Avoid alcoholic beverages while taking this product. Do not take this product if you are taking sedatives or tranquilizers without first consulting your doctor. Use caution when driving a motor vehicle or operating machinery. May cause excitability especially in children. **Do not exceed recommended dosage because at higher doses nervousness, dizziness, or sleeplessness may occur.** Do not take this product for more than 7 days. If symptoms do not improve or are accompanied by fever, consult a doctor. Do not take this product if you have diabetes, glaucoma, heart disease, high blood pressure, thyroid disease, a breathing problem such as emphysema or chronic bronchitis, or difficulty in urination due to enlargement of the prostate gland unless directed by a doctor. As with any drug, if you are pregnant or nursing a baby, seek the advice of a health professional before using this product. Keep this and all drugs out of reach of children. In case of accidental overdose, seek professional assistance or contact a Poison Control Center immediately.

Drug Interaction Precaution: Do not take this product if you are presently taking a decongestant or prescription drug for high blood pressure or depression, without first consulting your doctor.

Directions: Adults and children 12 years of age and over: Take one tablet swallowed whole every 12 hours, not to exceed 2 tablets in 24 hours, or as directed by a doctor. Children under 12 years: Consult a doctor.

How Supplied: Tavist-D tablets (white) imprinted "Tavist-D" on both sides, in blister packs of 8, 16, and 32; and Bottles of 50

Shown in Product Identification Guide, page 521

THERAFLU®
Flu and Cold Medicine
Flu, Cold & Cough Medicine

Description: Each packet of TheraFlu Flu and Cold Medicine contains: acetaminophen 650 mg, pseudoephedrine hydrochloride 60 mg, and chlorpheniramine maleate 4 mg. Each packet of TheraFlu Flu, Cold & Cough Medicine also contains dextromethorphan hydrobromide 20 mg. Other ingredients: ascorbic acid (vitamin C), citric acid, natural lemon flavors, pregelatinized starch, silicon dioxide, sodium citrate, sucrose, titanium dioxide, tribasic calcium phosphate, Yellow 6, and Yellow 10.

Indications: Provides temporary relief of the symptoms associated with flu, common cold and other upper respiratory infections including: headache, body aches, fever, minor sore throat pain, nasal and sinus congestion, runny nose and sneezing. TheraFlu Flu, Cold & Cough Medicine also suppresses coughs due to minor throat and bronchial irritation.

Warnings: Keep this and all drugs out of the reach of children. In case of accidental overdose, contact a doctor or a Poison Control Center immediately. Prompt medical attention is critical for adults as well as children even if you do not notice any signs or symptoms.
Do not take this product for more than 7 days. Do not exceed recommended dosage because at higher doses nervousness, dizziness, or sleeplessness may occur. May cause excitability, especially in children. Unless directed by a doctor, do not take this product if you have heart disease, high blood pressure, thyroid disease, diabetes, glaucoma, a breathing problem such as emphysema or chronic bronchitis, or difficulty in urination due to enlargement of the prostate gland.
Unless directed by a doctor, do not take this product for fever for more than 3 days. If pain or fever persists or gets worse, if new symptoms occur, or if redness or swelling is present, consult a doctor because these could be signs of a serious condition. If sore throat is severe, persists for more than 2 days, is accompanied or followed by fever, headache, rash, nausea, or vomiting, consult a doctor promptly.
May cause marked drowsiness. Alcohol, sedatives, and tranquilizers may increase the drowsiness effect. Avoid alcoholic beverages while taking this product. Do not take this product if you are taking sedatives or tranquilizers without first consulting your doctor. Use caution when driving a motor vehicle or operating machinery.
Do not take the Flu, Cold & Cough formula for persistent or chronic cough such as occurs with smoking, asthma, or emphysema, or if cough is accompanied by excessive phlegm (mucus) unless directed by a doctor. A persistent cough may be a sign of a serious condition. If cough persists for more than 1 week,

Continued on next page

Sandoz—Cont.

tends to recur, or is accompanied by a fever, rash, or persistent headache, consult a doctor.

As with any drug, if you are pregnant or nursing a baby, seek the advice of a health professional before using this product.

Drug Interaction Precaution: Do not take this product if you are now taking a prescription monoamine oxidase inhibitor (MAOI) (certain drugs for depression, psychiatric or emotional conditions, or Parkinson's disease) or for 2 weeks after stopping the MAOI drug. If you are uncertain whether your prescription drug contains an MAOI, consult a health professional before taking this product.

Directions: Adults and children 12 years and over—dissolve one packet in 6 oz. cup of hot water. Sip while hot. Microwave Heating Instructions: Add contents of packet and 6 oz. of cool water to a microwave-safe cup and stir briskly. Microwave on high 1½ minutes or until hot. Do not boil water or overheat and remember to stir liquid between reheatings. Sweeten to taste if desired. May repeat every 4 hours, but not to exceed 4 doses in 24 hours.

How Supplied: TheraFlu Flu and Cold Medicine powder in foil packets, 6 or 12 packets per carton. TheraFlu Flu, Cold & Cough Medicine powder in foil packets, 6 or 12 packets per carton.
Shown in Product Identification Guide, page 521

THERAFLU®
MAXIMUM STRENGTH NIGHTTIME
Flu, Cold & Cough Medicine

Description: Each packet of TheraFlu Maximum Strength Nighttime Flu, Cold & Cough Medicine contains: acetaminophen 1000 mg, dextromethorphan HBr 30 mg, pseudoephedrine HCl 60 mg, and chlorpheniramine maleate 4 mg. Other ingredients: ascorbic acid (Vitamin C), citric acid, natural lemon flavors, maltol, pregelatinized starch, silicon dioxide, sodium citrate, sucrose, titanium dioxide, tribasic calcium phosphate, Yellow 6 and Yellow 10.

Indications: Provides temporary relief of the symptoms associated with flu, common cold and other upper respiratory infections including: headache, body aches, fever, minor sore throat pain, nasal and sinus congestion, runny nose, sneezing, watery and itchy eyes. TheraFlu Maximum Strength Flu, Cold, & Cough Medicine also suppresses coughs due to minor throat and bronchial irritation.

Warnings: Keep this and all drugs out of the reach of children. In case of accidental overdose, contact a doctor or a Poison Control Center immediately. Prompt medical attention is critical for adults as well as children even if you do not notice any signs or symptoms.

Do not take this product for more than 7 days. Do not exceed recommended dosage because at higher doses nervousness, dizziness, or sleeplessness may occur. May cause excitability, especially in children. Unless directed by a doctor, do not take this product if you have heart disease, high blood pressure, thyroid disease, diabetes, glaucoma, a breathing problem such as emphysema or chronic bronchitis, or difficulty in urination due to enlargement of the prostate gland.

A persistent cough may be a sign of a serious condition. If cough persists for more than one week, tends to recur, or is accompanied by a fever, rash, or persistent headache, consult a doctor. Do not take this product for persistent or chronic cough such as occurs with smoking, asthma, or emphysema, or if cough is accompanied by excessive phlegm (mucus) unless directed by a doctor.

Unless directed by a doctor, do not take this product for fever for more than 3 days. If pain or fever persists or gets worse, if new symptoms occur, or if redness or swelling is present, consult a doctor because these could be signs of a serious condition. If sore throat is severe, persists for more than 2 days, is accompanied or followed by fever, headache, rash, nausea, or vomiting, consult a doctor promptly.

May cause marked drowsiness. Alcohol, sedatives, and tranquilizers may increase the drowsiness effect. Avoid alcoholic beverages while taking this product. Do not take this product if you are taking sedatives or tranquilizers without first consulting your doctor. Use caution when driving a motor vehicle or operating machinery.

As with any drug, if you are pregnant or nursing a baby, seek the advice of a health professional before using this product.

Drug Interaction Precaution: Do not take this product if you are now taking a prescription monoamine oxidase inhibitor (MAOI) (certain drugs for depression, psychiatric or emotional conditions, or Parkinson's disease) or for 2 weeks after stopping the MAOI drug. If you are uncertain whether your prescription drug contains an MAOI, consult a health professional before taking this product.

Directions: Adults and children 12 years and over: Dissolve one packet in 6 oz. cup of hot water. Sip while hot. Microwave Heating Instructions: Add contents of packet and 6 oz. of cool water to a microwave-safe cup and stir briskly. Microwave on high 1½ minutes or until water is hot. Do not boil water or overheat and remember to stir liquid between reheatings. Sweeten to taste if desired. May repeat every 6 hours, but not to exceed 4 doses in 24 hours.

How Supplied: TheraFlu Maximum Strength Nighttime Flu, Cold, & Cough Medicine powder in foil packets, 6 or 12 packets per carton.
Shown in Product Identification Guide, page 521

THERAFLU®
MAXIMUM STRENGTH
NON-DROWSY FORMULA
Flu, Cold & Cough Medicine

Description: Each packet of TheraFlu Maximum Strength Non-Drowsy Formula contains: acetaminophen 1000 mg, dextromethorphan 30 mg, pseudoephedrine HCl 60 mg. Other Ingredients: ascorbic acid (Vitamin C), citric acid, natural lemon flavors, maltol, pregelatinized starch, silicon dioxide, sodium citrate, sucrose, titanium dioxide, tribasic calcium phosphate, Yellow 6 and Yellow 10.

Indications: Provides temporary relief of the symptoms associated with flu, common cold, and other upper respiratory infections including: headache, body aches, fever, minor sore throat pain, nasal and sinus congestion, runny nose, sneezing, watery and itchy eyes. TheraFlu Maximum Strength Non-Drowsy Formula also suppresses coughs due to minor throat and bronchial irritation.

Warnings: Keep this and all drugs out of the reach of children. In case of accidental overdose, seek professional assistance or contact a Poison Control Center immediately. Prompt medical attention is critical for adults as well as children even if you do not notice any signs or symptoms.

Do not take this product for more than 7 days. Do not exceed recommended dosage because at higher doses nervousness, dizziness, or sleeplessness may occur. Unless directed by a doctor, do not take this product if you have heart disease, high blood pressure, thyroid disease, diabetes, or difficulty in urination due to enlargement of the prostate gland.

A persistent cough may be the sign of a serious condition. If cough persists for more than 1 week, tends to recur, or is accompanied by a fever, rash, or persistent headache, consult a doctor. Do not take this product for persistent or chronic cough such as occurs with smoking, asthma, or emphysema, or if cough is accompanied by excessive phlegm (mucus) unless directed by a doctor.

Unless directed by a doctor, do not take this product for fever for more than 3 days. If pain or fever persists or gets worse, if new symptoms occur, or if redness or swelling is present, consult a doctor, because these could be signs of a serious condition. If sore throat is severe, persists for more than 2 days, is accompanied or followed by fever, headache, rash, nausea, or vomiting, consult a doctor promptly.

As with any drug, if you are pregnant or nursing a baby, seek the advice of a health professional before using this product.

Drug Interaction Precaution: Do not take this product if you are now taking a prescription monoamine oxidase inhibitor (MAOI) (certain drugs for depression, psychiatric or emotional conditions, or Parkinson's disease) or for 2 weeks after stopping the MAOI drug. If you are uncertain whether your prescription drug contains an MAOI, consult a health professional before taking this product.

Directions: Adults and children 12 years and over: Dissolve one packet in 6 oz. cup of hot water; sip while hot. Microwave Heating Instructions: Add contents of packet and 6 oz. of cool water to a microwave-safe cup and stir briskly. Microwave on high 1 1/2 minutes or until hot. Do not boil or overheat, and remember to stir liquid between reheatings. Sweeten to taste if desired. May repeat every 6 hours, but not to exceed 4 doses in 24 hours.

Shown in Product Identification Guide, page 521

THERAFLU® MAXIMUM STRENGTH NON-DROWSY FORMULA CAPLETS

Description: Each TheraFlu Maximum Strength Non-Drowsy caplet contains: Acetaminophen 500 mg, dextromethorphan HBr 15 mg, and pseudoephedrine HCl 30 mg. Other ingredients: colloidal silicon dioxide, croscarmellose sodium, gelatin, hydroxypropyl cellulose, hydroxpropyl methylcellulose, lactose, magnesium stearate, methylparaben, polydextrose, polyethylene glycol, pregelatinized starch, Red 40, titanium dioxide, triacetin, Yellow 6, Yellow 10.

Indications: Provides temporary relief of the symptoms associated with flu, common cold, and other upper respiratory infections including: headache, body aches, fever, minor sore throat pain, nasal and sinus congestion, runny nose, sneezing, watery and itchy eyes. TheraFlu Maximum Strength Non-Drowsy Formula Caplets also suppress coughs due to minor throat and bronchial irritation.

Warnings: Keep this and all drugs out of the reach of children. In case of accidental overdose, contact a doctor or Poison Control Center immediately. Prompt medical attention is critical even if you do not notice any signs or symptoms. Unless directed by a doctor, do not take this product: 1) if cough is accompanied by excessive phlegm (mucus), 2) for persistent or chronic cough such as occurs with smoking, asthma or emphysema, or 3) if you have heart disease, high blood pressure, thyroid disease, diabetes or difficulty in urination due to enlargement of the prostate gland. Do not exceed dosage because at higher doses nervousness, dizziness, or sleeplessness may occur. Do not take for more than 7 days. If symptoms persist or new ones occur, or if fever persists for more than 3 days, or recurs, consult a doctor. A persistent cough may be a sign of a serious condition. If cough persists for more than 1 week, tends to recur, or is accompanied by fever, rash, or persistent headache, consult a doctor. If

sore throat is severe, persists for more than 2 days, is accompanied or followed by fever, headache, rash, nausea, or vomiting, consult a doctor promptly. As with any drug, if you are pregnant or nursing a baby, seek the advice of a health professional before using this product.

Drug Interaction Precaution: Do not take this product if you are now taking a prescription monoamine oxidase inhibitor (MAOI) (certain drugs for depression, psychiatric or emotional conditions, or Parkinson's disease) or for 2 weeks after stopping the MAOI drug. If you are uncertain whether your prescription drug contains an MAOI, consult a health professional before taking this product.

Directions: Adults and children 12 and over: Two caplets every 6 hours, not to exceed eight caplets in 24 hours.

How Supplied: TheraFlu Maximum Strength Non-Drowsy Formula gelatin film coated caplets (yellow) in blister packs of 12 and 24.

Shown in Product Identification Guide, page 521

TRIAMINIC® ALLERGY TABLETS
[*trī″ah-mĭn′ĭc*]

Description: Each tablet contains: phenylpropanolamine hydrochloride 25 mg and chlorpheniramine maleate 4 mg. Other ingredients: calcium stearate, calcium sulfate, colloidal silicon dioxide, methylcellulose, methylparaben, microcrystalline cellulose, polyethylene glycol, povidone, pregelatinized starch, titanium dioxide, Yellow 10.

Indications: For the temporary relief of runny nose, nasal congestion, sneezing, itching of the eyes, nose or throat and watery eyes as may occur in hay fever or other upper respiratory allergies (allergic rhinitis).

Warnings: Do not take this product if you have high blood pressure, heart disease, diabetes, thyroid disease, glaucoma, a breathing problem such as emphysema or chronic bronchitis, or difficulty in urination due to enlargement of the prostate gland unless directed by a doctor. Do not exceed the recommended dosage because at higher doses nervousness, dizziness or sleeplessness may occur, or take for more than 7 days. This preparation may cause drowsiness; alcohol, sedatives and tranquilizers may increase the drowsiness effect; avoid alcoholic beverages; do not operate machinery or drive a motor vehicle while taking this product; this preparation may cause excitability, especially in children. If symptoms do not improve within seven days or are accompanied by high fever, consult a doctor. As with any drug, if you are pregnant or nursing a baby, seek the advice of a health professional before using this product. Keep this and all drugs out of the reach of children. In case of accidental overdose, seek professional assistance or contact a Poison Control Center immediately.

Drug Interaction Precaution: Do not take this product if you are now taking a prescription monoamine oxidase inhibitor (MAOI) (certain drugs for depression, psychiatric or emotional conditions, or Parkinson's disease) or for 2 weeks after stopping the MAOI drug. If you are uncertain whether your prescription drug contains an MAOI, consult a health professional before taking this product.

Directions: Adults and children over 12 years of age—1 tablet every 4 hours. Children 6 to under 12 years, ½ tablet every 4 hours. Unless directed by physician, do not exceed 6 doses in 24 hours or give to children under 6 years.

How Supplied: Triaminic Allergy Tablets (yellow), scored, in blister packs of 24.

TRIAMINIC® AM COUGH AND DECONGESTANT FORMULA

Description: Each teaspoonful (5 ml) of TRIAMINIC AM COUGH AND DECONGESTANT FORMULA contains: Dextromethorphan hydrobromide, USP 7.5 mg, and pseudoephedrine hydrochloride, USP 15 mg. in a palatable, orange flavored, dye-free, non-drowsy, alcohol-free liquid. Other ingredients: Benzoic acid, citric acid, dibasic sodium phosphate, edetate disodium, flavors, propylene glycol, purified water, sorbitol, sucrose.

Indications: Temporarily quiets coughs due to minor throat and bronchial irritations and relieves stuffy noses.

Warnings: Keep this and all drugs out of the reach of children. In case of accidental overdose, seek professional assistance or contact a Poison Control Center immediately.
Do not exceed recommended dosage because at higher doses nervousness, dizziness, or sleeplessness may occur. Do not take this product for more than 7 days. If symptoms do not improve or are accompanied by fever, consult a doctor. Do not take this product if you have heart disease, high blood pressure, thyroid disease, diabetes or difficulty in urination due to enlargement of the prostate gland, unless directed by a doctor.
A persistent cough may be a sign of a serious condition. If cough persists for more than 1 week, tends to recur, or is accompanied by fever, rash or persistent headache, consult a doctor. Do not take this product for persistent or chronic cough such as occurs with smoking, asthma, or emphysema or if cough is accompanied by excessive phlegm (mucus) unless directed by doctor.
As with any drug, if you are pregnant or nursing a baby, seek the advice of a health professional before using this product.

Drug Interaction Precaution: Do not take this product if you are now taking a

Continued on next page

Sandoz—Cont.

prescription monoamine oxidase inhibitor (MAOI) (certain drugs for depression, psychiatric or emotional conditions, or Parkinson's disease) or for 2 weeks after stopping the MAOI drug. If you are uncertain whether your prescription drug contains an MAOI, consult a health professional before taking this product.

Dosage and Administration: Adults and children 12 and over 96+ lbs)—4 teaspoons every 6 hours. Children 6 to under 12 years (48–95 lbs)—2 teaspoons every 6 hours. Children 2 to under 6 years (24–47 lbs)—1 teaspoon every 6 hours. Unless directed by physician, do not exceed 4 doses in 24 hours or give to children under 2 years of age. For convenience, a True-Dose® dosage cup is provided with each 4 fl. oz. and 8 fl. oz. bottle.

Professional Labeling: The suggested dosage for pediatric patients is:

3–12 months	1.25 ml (¼ tsp)
(12–17 lbs)	every 6 hours
12–24 months	2.5 ml (½ tsp)
(18–23 lbs)	every 6 hours

How Supplied: TRIAMINIC AM COUGH AND DECONGESTANT FORMULA (clear liquid) in 4 fl. oz. and 8 fl. oz. plastic bottles with tamper-evident band around child-resistant cap. Orange flavored. Alcohol-free. Dye-free. Non-drowsy.

Shown in Product Identification Guide, page 521

TRIAMINIC® AM DECONGESTANT FORMULA

Description: Each teaspoonful (5 ml) of TRIAMINIC AM DECONGESTANT FORMULA contains: Pseudoephedrine hydrochloride, USP 15 mg. in a palatable, orange flavored, dye-free, non-drowsy, alcohol-free liquid. Other ingredients: Benzoic acid, edetate disodium, flavors, purified water, sodium hydroxide, sorbitol, sucrose

Indications: For temporary relief of nasal congestion due to the common cold, hay fever or upper respiratory allergies or associated with sinusitis. Reduces swelling of nasal passages; shrinks swollen membranes.

Warnings: Keep this and all drugs out of the reach of children. In case of accidental overdose, seek professional assistance or contact a Poison Control Center immediately.
Do not exceed recommended dosage because at higher doses nervousness, dizziness, or sleeplessness may occur. Do not take this product for more than 7 days. If symptoms do not improve or are accompanied by fever, consult a doctor. Do not take this product if you have heart disease, high blood pressure, thyroid disease, diabetes or difficulty in urination due to enlargement of the prostate gland, unless directed by a doctor.

As with any drug, if you are pregnant or nursing a baby, seek the advice of a health professional before using this product.

Drug Interaction Precaution: Do not take this product if you are now taking a prescription monoamine oxidase inhibitor (MAOI) (certain drugs for depression, psychiatric or emotional conditions, or Parkinson's disease) or for 2 weeks after stopping the MAOI drug. If you are uncertain whether your prescription drug contains an MAOI, consult a health professional before taking this product.

Dosage and Administration: Adults and children 12 and over (96+ lbs)—4 teaspoons every 4–6 hours. Children 6 to under 12 years (48–95 lbs)—2 teaspoons every 4–6 hours. Children 2 to under 6 years (24–47 lbs)—1 teaspoon every 4–6 hours. Unless directed by physician, do not exceed 4 doses in 24 hours or give to children under 2 years of age. For convenience, a True-Dose® dosage cup is provided with each 4 fl. oz. and 8 fl. oz. bottle.

Professional Labeling: The suggested dosage for pediatric patients is:

3–12 months	1.25 ml (¼ tsp)
(12–17 lbs)	every 6 hours
12–24 months	2.5 ml (½ tsp)
(18–23 lbs)	every 6 hours

How Supplied: TRIAMINIC AM DECONGESTANT FORMULA (clear liquid) in 4 fl oz and 8 fl oz plastic bottles with tamper-evident band around child-resistant cap. Orange flavored. Alcohol-free. Dye-free. Non-drowsy.

Shown in Product Identification Guide, page 521

TRIAMINIC® COLD TABLETS
[trī"ah-mĭn'ĭc]

Description: Each tablet contains: phenylpropanolamine hydrochloride 12.5 mg and chlorpheniramine maleate 2 mg. Other ingredients: calcium stearate, colloidal silicon dioxide, flavor, lactose, methylcellulose, methylparaben, microcrystalline cellulose, polyethylene glycol, povidone, pregelatinized starch, Red 40, saccharin sodium, titanium dioxide, Yellow 6.

Indications: For the temporary relief of nasal congestion due to the common cold, hay fever or other upper respiratory allergies and symptoms associated with sinusitis. Helps decongest sinus openings, sinus passages, promotes nasal and/or sinus drainage, temporarily restores freer breathing through the nose. For temporary relief of runny nose, sneezing, itching of the nose or throat and itchy and watery eyes as may occur in allergic rhinitis (such as hay fever).

Warnings: Do not take this product if you have high blood pressure, heart disease, diabetes, thyroid disease, glaucoma, a breathing problem such as emphysema or chronic bronchitis, or difficulty in urination due to enlargement of

the prostate gland unless directed by a doctor. Do not exceed the recommended dosage because at higher doses nervousness, dizziness or sleeplessness may occur. Do not take for more than 7 days. This preparation may cause drowsiness; alcohol, sedatives and tranquilizers may increase the drowsiness effect; avoid alcoholic beverages; do not operate machinery or drive a motor vehicle while taking this product; this preparation may cause excitability, especially in children. If symptoms do not improve within seven days or are accompanied by high fever, consult a doctor. As with any drug, if you are pregnant or nursing a baby, seek the advice of a health professional before using this product. Keep this and all drugs out of the reach of children. In case of accidental overdose, seek professional assistance or contact a Poison Control Center immediately.

Drug Interaction Precaution: Do not take this product if you are now taking a prescription monoamine oxidase inhibitor (MAOI) (certain drugs for depression, psychiatric or emotional conditions, or Parkinson's disease) or for 2 weeks after stopping the MAOI drug. If you are uncertain whether your prescription drug contains an MAOI, consult a health professional before taking this product.

Directions: Adults and children 12 years of age and older: 2 tablets every 4 hours. Children 6 to under 12 years, 1 tablet every 4 hours. Unless directed by physician, do not exceed 6 doses in 24 hours or give to children under 6 years.

How Supplied: Triaminic Cold Tablets (orange) imprinted "DORSEY" on one side, "TRIAMINIC" on the other, in blister packs of 24.

Shown in Product Identification Guide, page 521

TRIAMINIC® EXPECTORANT
[trī"ah-mĭn'ĭc]

Description: Each teaspoonful (5 ml) of TRIAMINIC Expectorant contains: phenylpropanolamine hydrochloride 6.25 mg and guaifenesin 50 mg in a palatable, citrus-flavored alcohol-free liquid. Other ingredients: benzoic acid, edetate disodium, flavors, glycerin, polyethylene glycol, propylene glycol, purified water, sorbitol, sucrose, Yellow 6, Yellow 10.

Indications: Relieves chest congestion by loosening phlegm to help clear bronchial passageways. Temporarily relieves stuffy nose.

Warnings: Keep this and all drugs out of the reach of children. In case of accidental overdose, seek professional assistance or contact a Poison Control Center immediately.
Do not exceed recommended dosage because at higher doses nervousness, dizziness, or sleeplessness may occur. Do not take for more than 7 days. If symptoms persist, are accompanied by fever, rash or persistent headache, or if cough recurs,

consult a doctor. A persistent cough may be a sign of a serious condition. Do not take this product: 1) if cough is accompanied by excessive phlegm (sputum), 2) for persistent or chronic cough such as occurs with smoking, asthma, chronic bronchitis or emphysema, or 3) if you have heart disease, high blood pressure, thyroid disease, diabetes, difficulty in urination due to enlargement of the prostate gland, or if you are presently taking another product containing phenylpropanolamine.

As with any drug, if you are pregnant or nursing a baby, seek the advice of a health professional before using this product.

Drug Interaction Precaution: Do not take this product if you are now taking a prescription monoamine oxidase inhibitor (MAOI) (certain drugs for depression, psychiatric or emotional conditions, or Parkinson's disease) or for 2 weeks after stopping the MAOI drug. If you are uncertain whether your prescription drug contains an MAOI, consult a health professional before taking this product.

Dosage and Administration: Adults and children 12 and over (96+ lbs)—4 teaspoons every 4 hours. Children 6 to under 12 years (48–95 lbs)—2 teaspoons every 4 hours. Children 2 to under 6 years (24–47 lbs)—1 teaspoon every 4 hours. Unless directed by physician, do not exceed 6 doses in 24 hours or give to children under 2 years of age. For convenience, a True-Dose® dosage cup is provided with each 4 fl. oz. and 8 fl. oz. bottle.

Professional Labeling: The suggested dosage for pediatric patients is:

3–12 months	1.25 ml (¼ tsp)
(12–17 lbs)	every 4 hours
12–24 months	2.5 ml (½ tsp)
(18–23 lbs)	every 4 hours

How Supplied: TRIAMINIC Expectorant (yellow), in 4 fl oz and 8 fl oz plastic bottles with tamper-evident band around child-resistant cap. Citrus flavored, Alcohol free.

Shown in Product Identification Guide, page 521

TRIAMINIC® NITE LIGHT®
Nighttime Cough and Cold Medicine for Children
[tri″ah-min′ic]

Description: Each teaspoonful (5 ml) of Triaminic® Nite Light® contains: Pseudoephedrine hydrochloride 15 mg, chlorpheniramine maleate 1 mg, dextromethorphan hydrobromide 7.5 mg in a palatable, grape-flavored, alcohol-free liquid. Other ingredients: benzoic acid, Blue 1, citric acid, flavors, propylene glycol, purified water, Red 33, dibasic sodium phosphate, sorbitol, sucrose.

Indications: Temporarily relieves cold symptoms, including coughs due to minor throat and bronchial irritation, runny nose, stuffy nose, sneezing, itching nose or throat and itchy, watery eyes.

Warnings: Keep this and all drugs out of the reach of children. In case of accidental overdose, seek professional assistance or contact a Poison Control Center immediately.

Do not exceed recommended dosage because at higher doses nervousness, dizziness, or sleeplessness may occur. Do not take for more than 7 days. If symptoms persist, are accompanied by fever, rash or persistent headache, or if cough recurs, consult a doctor. A persistent cough may be a sign of a serious condition. Do not take this product: 1) if cough is accompanied by excessive phlegm (sputum), 2) for persistent or chronic cough such as occurs with smoking, asthma or emphysema, or 3) if you have heart disease, high blood pressure, thyroid disease, diabetes, glaucoma, a breathing problem such as emphysema or chronic bronchitis, or difficulty in urination due to enlargement of the prostate gland, or 4) if you are taking sedatives or tranquilizers, unless directed by a doctor. May cause excitability, especially in children. May cause drowsiness. Alcohol, sedatives or tranquilizers may increase drowsiness. Avoid driving or operating machinery while taking this product.

As with any drug, if you are pregnant or nursing a baby, seek the advice of a health professional before using this product.

Drug Interaction Precaution: Do not take this product if you are now taking a prescription monoamine oxidase inhibitor (MAOI) (certain drugs for depression, psychiatric or emotional conditions, or Parkinson's disease) or for 2 weeks after stopping the MAOI drug. If you are uncertain whether your prescription drug contains an MAOI, consult a health professional before taking this product.

Dosage and Administration: Adults and children 12 and over (96+ lbs.)—4 teaspoons every 6 hours. Children 6 to under 12 years (48–95 lbs.)—2 teaspoons every 6 hours. Unless directed by physician, do not exceed 4 doses in 24 hours or give to children under 6 years of age. For convenience, a True-Dose® dosage cup is provided with each 4 fl. oz. and 8 fl. oz. bottle.

Professional Labeling: The suggested dosage for pediatric patients is:

3 to under 12 months (12–17 lbs.)	¼ teaspoon or 1.25 ml
12 months to under 2 years (18–23 lbs.)	½ teaspoon or 2.5 ml
2 to under 6 years	1 teaspoon or 5 ml

How Supplied: Triaminic® Nite Light® Nighttime Cough and Cold Medicine for Children (purple), in 4 fl. oz. and 8 fl. oz. plastic bottles packaged in cartons with tamper-evident band around child-resistant cap. Grape flavored. Alcohol free.

Shown in Product Identification Guide, page 521

TRIAMINIC®
Sore Throat Formula
[tri″ah-min′ic]

Description: Each teaspoonful (5 ml) of Triaminic Sore Throat Formula contains: acetaminophen, USP 160 mg, dextromethorphan hydrobromide, USP 7.5 mg, and pseudoephedrine hydrochloride, USP 15 mg. in a palatable, grape-flavored, alcohol-free liquid. Other ingredients: benzoic acid, Blue 1, dibasic sodium phosphate, edetate disodium, flavors, glycerin, polyethylene glycol, propylene glycol, purified water, Red 33, Red 40, sucrose, tartaric acid.

Indications: Temporarily relieves sore throat pain and other minor aches and pains, quiets coughs due to minor throat and bronchial irritations, relieves stuffy noses, and reduces fever.

Warnings: Keep this and all drugs out of the reach of children. In case of accidental overdose, seek professional assistance or contact a Poison Control Center immediately. Prompt medical attention is critical for adults as well as for children even if you do not notice any signs or symptoms.

Do not exceed recommended dosage because at higher doses nervousness, dizziness, or sleeplessness may occur. Do not take this product for more than 4 days. If symptoms persist or new ones occur, if sore throat is severe or persists for more than 2 days, if fever persists for more than 3 days, if symptoms are accompanied by rash, fever, nausea, vomiting, persistent headache or if cough recurs, consult a doctor. A persistent cough may be the sign of a serious condition. Do not take this product: 1) if cough is accompanied by excessive phlegm (mucus), 2) for persistent or chronic cough such as occurs with smoking, asthma or emphysema, or 3) if you have heart disease, high blood pressure, thyroid disease, diabetes, difficulty in urination due to enlargement of the prostate gland, unless directed by a doctor.

As with any drug, if you are pregnant or nursing a baby, seek advice from a health professional before using this product.

Drug Interaction Precaution: Do not take this product if you are now taking a prescription monoamine oxidase inhibitor (MAOI) (certain drugs for depression, psychiatric or emotional conditions, or Parkinson's disease) or for 2 weeks after stopping the MAOI drug. If you are uncertain whether your prescription drug contains an MAOI, consult a health professional before taking this product.

Dosage and Administration: Adults and children 12 and over (96+lbs)—4 teaspoons every 6 hours. Children 6 to under 12 years (48–95 lbs)—2 teaspoons every 6 hours. Children 2 to under 6 years (24–47 lbs)—1 teaspoon every 6 hours. Unless directed by a physician, do not exceed 4 doses in 24 hours or give to children under 2 years of age. For conve-

Continued on next page

Sandoz—Cont.

nience, a True-Dose® dosage cup is provided with each 4 fl. oz and 8 fl. oz. bottle.

Professional Labeling: The suggested dosage for pediatric patients is:
3–12 months   1.25 ml (¼ tsp)
(12–17 lbs)   every 6 hours
12–24 months 2.5 ml (½ tsp)
(18–23 lbs)   every 6 hours
2–6 years   5 ml (1 tsp)
(24–47 lbs)   every 6 hours

How Supplied: Triaminic Sore Throat Formula (purple), in 4 fl. oz. and 8 fl. oz. plastic bottles with tamper-evident band around child resistant cap. Grape flavored, alcohol-free.
Shown in Product Identification Guide, page 521

TRIAMINIC® SYRUP
[trī"ah-mĭn'ĭc]

Description: Each teaspoonful (5 ml) of TRIAMINIC Syrup contains: phenylpropanolamine hydrochloride 6.25 mg and chlorpheniramine maleate 1 mg in a palatable, orange-flavored, alcohol-free liquid. Other ingredients: benzoic acid, edetate disodium, flavors, purified water, sodium hydroxide, sorbitol, sucrose. Contains FD&C Yellow No. 6 as a color additive.

Indications: Temporarily relieves cold and allergy symptoms, including runny nose, stuffy nose, sneezing, itching nose or throat, and itchy, watery eyes.

Warnings: Keep this and all drugs out of the reach of children. In case of accidental overdose, seek professional assistance or contact a Poison Control Center immediately.
Do not exceed recommended dosage because at higher doses nervousness, dizziness or sleeplessness may occur. Do not take for more than 7 days. If symptoms persist or are accompanied by fever, consult a doctor. Do not take this product: 1) if you have heart disease, high blood pressure, thyroid disease, diabetes, glaucoma, a breathing problem such as emphysema or chronic bronchitis, or difficulty in urination due to enlargement of the prostate gland, 2) if you are taking sedatives or tranquilizers, or 3) if you are presently taking another product containing phenylpropanolamine, unless directed by a doctor. May cause excitability, especially in children. May cause drowsiness. Alcohol, sedatives or tranquilizers may increase drowsiness. Avoid driving or operating machinery while taking this product.
As with any drug, if you are pregnant or nursing a baby, seek the advice of a health professional before using this product.

Drug Interaction Precaution: Do not take this product if you are now taking a prescription monoamine oxidase inhibitor (MAOI) (certain drugs for depression, psychiatric or emotional conditions, or

Parkinson's disease) or for 2 weeks after stopping the MAOI drug. If you are uncertain whether your prescription drug contains an MAOI, consult a health professional before taking this product.

Dosage and Administration: Adults and children 12 and over (96+ lbs)—4 teaspoons every 4 hours. Children 6 to under 12 years (48–95 lbs)—2 teaspoons every 4 hours. Unless directed by physician, do not exceed 6 doses in 24 hours. Consult physician for dosage under 6 years of age. For convenience, a True-Dose® dosage cup is provided with each 4 fl. oz. and 8 fl. oz. bottle.

Professional Labeling: The suggested dosage for pediatric patients is:
3–12 months   1.25 ml (¼ tsp)
(12–17 lbs)   every 4 hours
12–24 months 2.5 ml (½ tsp)
(18–23 lbs)   every 4 hours
2–6 years   5 ml (1 tsp)
(24–47 lbs)   every 4 hours

How Supplied: TRIAMINIC Syrup (orange), in 4 fl oz and 8 fl oz plastic bottles with tamper-evident band around child-resistant cap. Orange flavored. Alcohol-free.
Shown in Product Identification Guide, page 521

TRIAMINIC–DM® SYRUP
[trī"ah-mĭn'ĭc]

Description: Each teaspoonful (5 ml) of TRIAMINIC-DM Syrup contains: phenylpropanolamine hydrochloride 6.25 mg and dextromethorphan hydrobromide 5 mg in a palatable, berry-flavored alcohol-free liquid. Other ingredients: benzoic acid, Blue 1, flavors, propylene glycol, purified water, Red 40, sodium chloride, sorbitol, sucrose.

Indications: Temporarily quiets coughs due to minor throat and bronchial irritation, and relieves stuffy nose. The decongestant and antitussive are provided in an alcohol-free and antihistamine-free formula.

Warnings: Keep this and all drugs out of the reach of children. In case of accidental overdose, seek professional assistance or contact a Poison Control Center immediately.
Do not exceed recommended dosage because at higher doses nervousness, dizziness, or sleeplessness may occur. Do not take for more than 7 days. If symptoms persist, are accompanied by fever, rash or persistent headache or if cough recurs, consult a doctor. A persistent cough may be a sign of a serious condition. Do not take this product: 1) if cough is accompanied by excessive phlegm (sputum), 2) for persistent or chronic cough such as occurs with smoking, asthma or emphysema, 3) if you have heart disease, high blood pressure, thyroid disease, diabetes, difficulty in urination due to enlargement of the prostate gland, or 4) if you are presently taking another product

containing phenylpropanolamine, unless directed by a doctor.
As with any drug, if you are pregnant or nursing a baby, seek the advice of a health professional before using this product.

Drug Interaction Precaution: Do not take this product if you are now taking a prescription monoamine oxidase inhibitor (MAOI) (certain drugs for depression, psychiatric or emotional conditions, or Parkinson's disease) or for 2 weeks after stopping the MAOI drug. If you are uncertain whether your prescription drug contains an MAOI, consult a health professional before taking this product.

Dosage and Administration: Adults and children 12 and over (96+ lbs)—4 teaspoons every 4 hours. Children 6 to under 12 years (48–95 lbs)—2 teaspoons every 4 hours. Children 2 to under 6 years (24–47 lbs) 1 teaspoon every 4 hours. Unless directed by physician, do not exceed 6 doses in 24 hours or give to children under 2 years of age. For convenience, a True-Dose® dosage cup is provided with each 4 fl. oz. and 8 fl. oz. bottle.

Professional Labeling: The suggested dosage for pediatric patients is:
3–12 months   1.25 ml (¼ tsp)
(12–17 lbs)   every 4 hours
12–24 months 2.5 ml (½ tsp)
(18–23 lbs)   every 4 hours

How Supplied: TRIAMINIC-DM Syrup (dark red), in 4 fl oz and 8 fl oz plastic bottles with tamper-evident band around child-resistant cap. Berry flavored. Alcohol-free.
Shown in Product Identification Guide, page 521

TRIAMINIC–12® TABLETS
[trī"ah-mĭn'ĭc]

Description: Each tablet contains: phenylpropanolamine hydrochloride 75 mg and chlorpheniramine maleate 12 mg. Other ingredients: carnauba wax, colloidal silicon dioxide, lactose, methylcellulose, polyethylene glycol, povidone, Red 30, stearic acid, titanium dioxide, Yellow 6. Triaminic-12 Tablets contain the nasal decongestant phenylpropanolamine, and the antihistamine chlorpheniramine, in a formulation providing 12 hours of symptomatic relief.

Indications: For the temporary relief of nasal congestion due to the common cold, hay fever or other upper respiratory allergies and symptoms associated with sinusitis. Helps decongest sinus openings, sinus passages; promotes nasal and/or sinus drainage; temporarily restores freer breathing through the nose. For temporary relief of running nose, sneezing, itching of the nose or throat and itchy and watery eyes as may occur in allergic rhinitis (such as hay fever).

Warnings: Do not give this product to children under 12 years except under the advice and supervision of a physician. Do not take this product if you are taking another medication containing phenyl-propanolamine. Do not take this preparation if you have high blood pressure, heart disease, diabetes, thyroid disease, glaucoma, a breathing problem such as emphysema or chronic bronchitis or difficulty in urination due to enlargement of the prostate gland except under the advice and supervision of a physician. Do not exceed the recommended dosage because at higher doses nervousness, dizziness or sleeplessness may occur. This preparation may cause drowsiness; alcohol, sedatives and tranquilizers may increase the drowsiness effect; this preparation may cause excitability, especially in children. If symptoms do not improve within seven days or are accompanied by high fever, consult a physician before continuing use. As with any drug, if you are pregnant or nursing a baby, seek the advice of a health professional before using this product. Keep this and all drugs out of the reach of children. In case of accidental overdose, seek professional assistance or contact a Poison Control Center immediately.

Caution: Avoid driving a motor vehicle or operating heavy machinery. Avoid alcoholic beverages while taking this product.

Drug Interaction Precaution: Do not take this product if you are now taking a prescription monoamine oxidase inhibitor (MAOI) (certain drugs for depression, psychiatric or emotional conditions, or Parkinson's disease) or for 2 weeks after stopping the MAOI drug. If you are uncertain whether your prescription drug contains an MAOI, consult a health professional before taking this product.

Directions: Adults and children over 12 years of age—1 tablet swallowed whole every 12 hours. Unless directed by physician, do not exceed 2 tablets in 24 hours.

Note: The nonactive portion of the tablet that supplies the active ingredients may occasionally appear in your stool as a soft mass.

How Supplied: Triaminic-12 Tablets (orange) imprinted "DORSEY" on one side, "TRIAMINIC-12" on the other, in blister packs of 10 and 20.
Shown in Product Identification Guide, page 521

TRIAMINICIN® TABLETS
[trī"ah-min'ĭ-sĭn]

Description: Each tablet contains: phenylpropanolamine hydrochloride 25 mg and chlorpheniramine maleate 4 mg and acetaminophen 650 mg. Other ingredients: colloidal silicon dioxide, croscarmellose sodium, hydroxypropyl cellulose, lactose, magnesium stearate, methylcellulose, methylparaben, polyethylene glycol, povidone, pregelatinized starch, Red 40, titanium dioxide, Yellow 10.

Indications: Temporarily relieves runny nose, sneezing, itching of the nose

or throat, and itchy, watery eyes due to hay fever or other upper respiratory allergies (allergic rhinitis). Temporarily relieves nasal congestion due to hay fever or other upper respiratory allergies or symptoms associated with sinusitis. Temporarily relieves nasal congestion, runny nose and sneezing associated with the common cold. For the temporary relief of occasional minor aches, pains, headache and for the reduction of fever associated with the common cold.

Warnings: Do not take this product if you have high blood pressure, heart disease, diabetes, thyroid disease, glaucoma, a breathing problem such as emphysema or chronic bronchitis, or difficulty in urination due to enlargement of the prostate gland unless directed by a doctor. Do not exceed recommended dosage because at higher doses nervousness, dizziness, or sleeplessness may occur. This preparation may cause drowsiness; alcohol, sedatives and tranquilizers may increase the drowsiness effect; avoid alcoholic beverages; do not operate machinery or drive a motor vehicle while taking this product; this preparation may cause excitability, especially in children. Do not take this product for more than 7 days. If symptoms do not improve, new ones occur, or if fever persists for more than 3 days (72 hours) or recurs, consult a doctor. As with any drug, if you are pregnant or nursing a baby, seek the advice of a health professional before using this product. Keep this and all drugs out of the reach of children. In case of accidental overdose, seek professional assistance or contact a Poison Control Center immediately. Prompt medical attention is critical for adults as well as for children even if you do not notice any signs or symptoms.

Drug Interaction Precaution: Do not take this product if you are now taking a prescription monoamine oxidase inhibitor (MAOI) (certain drugs for depression, psychiatric or emotional conditions, or Parkinson's disease) or for 2 weeks after stopping the MAOI drug. If you are uncertain whether your prescription drug contains an MAOI, consult a health professional before taking this product.

Directions: Adults and children 12 years and older: Take 1 tablet every 4 hours. Unless directed by a doctor, do not exceed 6 doses in 24 hours or give to children under 12 years.

How Supplied: TRIAMINICIN Tablets (yellow) imprinted "DORSEY" on one side, "TRIAMINICIN" on the other, in blister packs of 12, 24 and 48, and bottles of 100 tablets.
Shown in Product Identification Guide, page 521

TRIAMINICOL® MULTI-SYMPTOM COLD TABLETS
[trī"ah-min'ĭ-call]

Description: Each tablet contains: phenylpropanolamine hydrochloride

12.5 mg, chlorpheniramine maleate 2 mg and dextromethorphan hydrobromide 10 mg. Other ingredients: calcium stearate, colloidal silicon dioxide, lactose, methylcellulose, methylparaben, microcrystalline cellulose, polyethylene glycol, povidone, pregelatinized starch, Red 40, titanium dioxide.

Indications: For the temporary relief of nasal congestion due to the common cold, hay fever or other upper respiratory allergies and symptoms associated with sinusitis. Helps decongest sinus openings, sinus passages, promotes nasal and/or sinus drainage, temporarily restores freer breathing through the nose. For temporary relief of runny nose, sneezing, itching of the nose or throat and itchy and watery eyes as may occur in allergic rhinitis (such as hay fever). For temporary relief of cough due to minor throat and bronchial irritation as may occur with the common cold or with inhaled irritants.

Warnings: Do not take this product: 1) if cough is accompanied by excessive secretions, 2) for persistent cough such as occurs with smoking, asthma or emphysema, or 3) if you have high blood pressure, heart disease, diabetes, thyroid disease, glaucoma, a breathing problem such as emphysema or chronic bronchitis, or difficulty in urination due to enlargement of the prostate gland unless directed by a doctor. A persistent cough may be a sign of a serious condition. If cough persists for more than one week, tends to recur, or is accompanied by high fever, rash, or persistent headaches, consult a doctor. Do not exceed recommended dosage because at higher doses nervousness, dizziness, or sleeplessness may occur or take for more than 7 days. This preparation may cause drowsiness; alcohol, sedatives, and tranquilizers may increase the drowsiness effect; avoid alcoholic beverages; do not operate machinery or drive a motor vehicle while taking this product; this preparation may cause excitability, especially in children. If symptoms do not improve within seven days or are accompanied by fever, rash or persistant headache or if cough recurs, consult a doctor. As with any drug, if you are pregnant or nursing a baby, seek the advice of a health professional before using this product. Keep this and all drugs out of the reach of children. In case of accidental overdose, seek professional assistance or contact a Poison Control Center immediately.

Drug Interaction Precaution: Do not take this product if you are now taking a prescription monoamine oxidase inhibitor (MAOI) (certain drugs for depression, psychiatric or emotional conditions, or Parkinson's disease) or for 2 weeks after stopping the MAOI drug. If you are uncertain whether your prescription drug contains an MAOI, consult a health professional before taking this product.

Continued on next page

Sandoz—Cont.

Directions: Adults and children 12 years of age and older: 2 tablets every 4 hours. Children 6 to under 12 years, 1 tablet every 4 hours. Unless directed by physician, do not exceed 6 doses in 24 hours or give to children under 6 years.

How Supplied: Triaminicol Tablets (cherry red) imprinted "DORSEY" on one side, "TRIAMINICOL" on the other, in blister packs of 24.

Shown in Product Identification Guide, page 521

TRIAMINICOL® MULTI-SYMPTOM RELIEF
[trī"ah-mĭn'ĭ-call]

Description: Each teaspoonful (5 ml) of TRIAMINICOL Multi-Symptom Relief contains: phenylpropanolamine hydrochloride 6.25 mg, chlorpheniramine maleate 1 mg, dextromethorphan hydrobromide 5 mg in a palatable, cherry flavored alcohol-free liquid. Other ingredients: benzoic acid, flavor, propylene glycol, purified water, Red 40, sodium chloride, sorbitol, sucrose.

Indications: Temporarily relieves cold symptoms, including coughs due to minor throat and bronchial irritation, runny nose, stuffy nose, sneezing, itching nose or throat and itchy, watery eyes.

Warnings: Keep this and all drugs out of the reach of children. In case of accidential overdose, seek professional assistance or contact a Poison Control Center immediately.
Do not exceed recommended dosage because at higher doses nervousness, dizziness, or sleeplessness may occur. Do not take for more than 7 days. If symptoms persist, are accompanied by fever, rash or persistent headache, or if cough recurs, consult a doctor. A persistent cough may be a sign of a serious condition. Do not take this product: 1) if cough is accompanied by excessive phlegm (sputum), 2) for persistent or chronic cough such as occurs with smoking, asthma or emphysema, or 3) if you have heart disease, high blood pressure, thyroid disease, diabetes, glaucoma, a breathing problem such as emphysema or chronic bronchitis, or difficulty in urination due to enlargement of the prostate gland, 4) if you are presently taking another product containing, phenylpropanolamine, or 5) if you are taking sedatives or tranquilizers, unless directed by a doctor. May cause excitability, especially in children. May cause drowsiness. Alcohol, sedatives or tranquilizers may increase drowsiness. Avoid driving or operating machinery while taking this product.
As with any drug, if you are pregnant or nursing a baby, seek the advice of a health professional before using this product.

Drug Interaction Precaution: Do not take this product if you are now taking a prescription monoamine oxidase inhibitor (MAOI) (certain drugs for depression, psychiatric or emotional conditions, or Parkinson's disease) or for 2 weeks after stopping the MAOI drug. If you are uncertain whether your prescription drug contains an MAOI, consult a health professional before taking this product.

Dosage and Administration: Adults and children 12 and over (96+ lbs)— 4 teaspoons every 4 hours. Children 6 to under 12 years (48–95 lbs)—2 teaspoons every 4 hours. Unless directed by physician, do not exceed 6 doses in 24 hours or give to children under 6 years of age. For convenience, a True-Dose® Dosage cup is provided with each 4 fl. oz. and 8 fl. oz. bottle.

Professional Labeling: The suggested dosage for pediatric patients is:

3–12 months	1.25 ml (¼ tsp)
(12–17 lbs)	every 4 hours
12–24 months	2.5 ml (½ tsp)
(18–23 lbs)	every 4 hours
2–6 years	5 ml (1 tsp)
(24–47 lbs)	every 4 hours

How Supplied: TRIAMINICOL Multi-Symptom Relief (red), in 4 fl oz and 8 fl oz plastic bottles with tamper-evident band around child-resistant cap. Cherry flavored. Alcohol-free.

Shown in Product Identification Guide, page 522

URSINUS® INLAY–TABS®
[yur"sĭgn'us]

Description: Each URSINUS Inlay-Tab contains: pseudoephedrine hydrochloride 30 mg and aspirin (USP) 325 mg. Other ingredients: calcium stearate, glycolate, lactose, microcrystalline cellulose, pregelatinized starch, sodium starch, starch, Yellow 6, Yellow 10.

Indications: For the temporary relief of nasal congestion due to the common cold, hay fever or symptoms associated with sinusitis. For the temporary relief of occasional minor aches, pains and headache and for the reduction of fever associated with the common cold.

Warnings: Children and teenagers who have or are recovering from chicken pox, flu symptoms, or flu should NOT use this product. If nausea, vomiting or fever occur, consult a doctor because these symptoms could be an early sign of Reye Syndrome, a rare but serious illness. Unless directed by a doctor: 1) Do not take this product if you are allergic to aspirin or if you have asthma, or if you have stomach distress, ulcers or bleeding problems; 2) Do not take this product if you have heart disease, thyroid disease, or difficulty in urination due to enlargement of the prostate gland, and 3) Do not exceed recommended dosage because at higher doses nervousness, dizziness, or sleeplessness may occur. Do not take this product for more than 7 days. If symptoms do not improve, are accompanied by fever, or new symptoms occur, consult a doctor. Stop taking this product if ringing in the ears or other symptoms occur. As with any drug, if you are pregnant or nursing a baby, seek the advice of a health professional before using this product. IT IS ESPECIALLY IMPORTANT NOT TO USE ASPIRIN DURING THE LAST 3 MONTHS OF PREGNANCY UNLESS SPECIFICALLY DIRECTED TO DO SO BY A DOCTOR BECAUSE IT MAY CAUSE PROBLEMS IN THE UNBORN CHILD OR COMPLICATIONS DURING DELIVERY.
Keep this and all medicines out of the reach of children. In case of accidental overdose, contact a physician immediately.

Drug Interaction Precaution: Do not take this product if you are now taking a prescription monoamine oxidase inhibitor (MAOI) (certain drugs for depression, psychiatric or emotional conditions, or Parkinson's disease) or for 2 weeks after stopping the MAOI drug. If you are uncertain whether your prescription drug contains an MAOI, consult a health professional before taking this product.
Do not take this product is you are presently taking a prescription drug for anticoagulation (thinning the blood), diabetes, arthritis or gout unless directed by a doctor.

Directions for Use: Adults and children 12 years and older: 2 tablets with a full glass of water every 4 hours while symptoms persist or as directed by a physician. Do not take more than 4 doses in 24 hours. For chicken pox or flu see Warnings.

How Supplied: URSINUS INLAY-TABS (white with yellow inlay), in bottles of 24.

Sanofi Winthrop Pharmaceuticals
90 PARK AVENUE
NEW YORK, NY 10016

DRISDOL®
ergocalciferol oral solution, USP in propylene glycol
Vitamin D Supplement

Description: 200 International Units (5 µg) per drop. (Contains 8000 IU ergocalciferol per gram. The dropper supplied delivers 40 drops per mL.)

Indication: For the prevention of vitamin D deficiency in infants, children, and adults.

Warnings: As with any drug, if you are pregnant or nursing a baby, seek the advice of a health professional before using this product. Keep this and all drugs out of the reach of children. In case of accidental overdose, seek professional assistance or contact a poison control center immediately.

Dosage: 2 drops daily. This dose provides the US Recommended Daily Allowance of vitamin D for infants, children, and adults.

How Supplied: Bottles of 2 fl oz (NDC 0024-0391-02)

ZEPHIRAN® CHLORIDE
brand of benzalkonium chloride
ANTISEPTIC
AQUEOUS SOLUTION 1:750
TINTED TINCTURE 1:750
SPRAY–TINTED TINCTURE 1:750

Description: ZEPHIRAN Chloride, brand of benzalkonium chloride, NF, a mixture of alkylbenzyldimethylammonium chlorides, is a cationic quaternary ammonium surface-acting agent. It is very soluble in water, alcohol, and acetone. Aqueous solutions of ZEPHIRAN Chloride are neutral to slightly alkaline, generally colorless, and nonstaining. They have a bitter taste, aromatic odor, and foam when shaken. ZEPHIRAN Chloride Tinted Tincture 1:750 contains alcohol 50 percent and acetone 10 percent by volume. ZEPHIRAN Chloride Spray–Tinted Tincture 1:750 contains alcohol 92 percent. The Tinted Tincture and Spray also contain an orange-red coloring agent.

Clinical Pharmacology: ZEPHIRAN Chloride solutions are rapidly acting anti-infective agents with a moderately long duration of action. They are active against bacteria and some viruses, fungi, and protozoa. Bacterial spores are considered to be resistant. Solutions are bacteriostatic or bactericidal according to their concentration. The exact mechanism of bactericidal action is unknown but is thought to be due to enzyme inactivation. Activity generally increases with increasing temperature and pH. Gram-positive bacteria are more susceptible than gram-negative bacteria (TABLE 1).

TABLE 1
Highest Dilution of ZEPHIRAN Chloride Aqueous Solution Destroying the Organism in 10 but not in 5 Minutes

Organisms	20°C
Streptococcus pyogenes	1:75,000
Staphylococcus aureus	1:52,500
Salmonella typhosa	1:37,500
Escherichia coli	1:10,500

Pseudomonas is the most resistant gram-negative genus. Using the AOAC Use-Dilution Confirmation Method, no growth was obtained when *Staphylococcus aureus, Salmonella choleraesuis,* and *Pseudomonas aeruginosa* (strain PRD-10) were exposed for ten minutes at 20°C to ZEPHIRAN Chloride Aqueous Solution 1:750 and Tinted Tincture 1:750. ZEPHIRAN Chloride Aqueous Solution 1:750 has been shown to retain its bactericidal activity following autoclaving for 30 minutes at 15 lb pressure, freezing, and then thawing.
The tubercle bacillus may be resistant to aqueous ZEPHIRAN Chloride solutions

but is susceptible to the 1:750 tincture (AOAC Method, 10 minutes at 20°C). ZEPHIRAN Chloride solutions also demonstrate deodorant, wetting, detergent, keratolytic, and emulsifying activity.

Indications and Usage: ZEPHIRAN Chloride aqueous solutions in appropriate dilutions (see Recommended Dilutions) are indicated for the antisepsis of skin, mucous membranes, and wounds. They are used for preoperative preparation of the skin, surgeons' hand and arm soaks, treatment of wounds, preservation of ophthalmic solutions, irrigations of the eye, body cavities, bladder, urethra, and vaginal douching.
ZEPHIRAN Chloride Tinted Tincture 1:750 and Spray are indicated for preoperative preparation of the skin and for treatment of minor skin wounds and abrasions.

Contraindication: The use of ZEPHIRAN Chloride solutions in occlusive dressings, casts, and anal or vaginal packs is inadvisable, as they may produce irritation or chemical burns.

Warnings: Sterile Water for Injection, USP, should be used as diluent in preparing diluted aqueous solutions intended for use on deep wounds or for irrigation of body cavities. Otherwise, freshly distilled water should be used. Tap water, containing metallic ions and organic matter, may reduce antibacterial potency. Resin deionized water should not be used since it may contain pathogenic bacteria.
Organic, inorganic, and synthetic materials and surfaces may adsorb sufficient quantities of ZEPHIRAN Chloride to significantly reduce its antibacterial potency in solutions. This has resulted in serious contamination of solutions of ZEPHIRAN Chloride with viable pathogenic bacteria. Solutions should not be stored in bottles stoppered with cork closures, but rather in those equipped with appropriate screw-caps. Cotton, wool, rayon, and other materials should not be stored in ZEPHIRAN Chloride solutions. Gauze sponges and fiber pledgets used to apply solutions of ZEPHIRAN Chloride to the skin should be sterilized and stored in separate containers. Only immediately prior to application should they be immersed in ZEPHIRAN Chloride solutions.
Since ZEPHIRAN Chloride solutions are inactivated by soaps and anionic detergents, thorough rinsing is necessary if these agents are employed prior to their use.
Antiseptics such as ZEPHIRAN Chloride solutions must not be relied upon to achieve complete sterilization, because they do not destroy bacterial spores and certain viruses, including the etiologic agent of infectious hepatitis, and may not destroy *Mycobacterium tuberculosis* and other rare bacterial strains.
ZEPHIRAN Chloride Tinted Tincture 1:750 and Spray contain flammable organic solvents and should not be used near an open flame or cautery.

If solutions stronger than 1:3000 enter the eyes, irrigate immediately and repeatedly with water. Prompt medical attention should then be obtained. Concentrations greater than 1:5000 should not be used on mucous membranes, with the exception of the vaginal mucosa (see Recommended Dilutions).

Precautions: In preoperative antisepsis of the skin, ZEPHIRAN Chloride solutions should not be permitted to remain in prolonged contact with the patient's skin. Avoid pooling of the solution on the operating table.
ZEPHIRAN Chloride solutions that are used on inflamed or irritated tissues must be more dilute than those used on normal tissues (see Recommended Dilutions). ZEPHIRAN Chloride Tinted Tincture 1:750 and Spray, which contain irritating organic solvents, should be kept away from the eyes or other mucous membranes.
Preoperative periorbital skin or head prep should be performed only before the patient, or eye, is anesthetized.

Adverse Reactions: ZEPHIRAN Chloride solutions in normally used concentrations have low systemic and local toxicity and are generally well tolerated, although a rare individual may exhibit hypersensitivity.

Directions for Use:
General: For most surgical applications, the recommended concentration of ZEPHIRAN Chloride Aqueous Solution or ZEPHIRAN Chloride Tinted Tincture is 1:750 (0.13 percent). Liberal use of the solution is recommended to compensate for any adsorption of ZEPHIRAN Chloride by cotton or other materials.
To use ZEPHIRAN Chloride Spray–Tinted Tincture 1:750, remove protective cap, hold in an UPRIGHT position several inches away from the surgical field or injured area, and apply by spraying freely.
Preoperative preparation of skin: ZEPHIRAN Chloride solutions 1:750 are recommended as an antiseptic for use on unbroken skin in the preoperative preparation of the surgical field. Detergents and soaps should be thoroughly rinsed from the skin before applying ZEPHIRAN Chloride solutions. The detergent action of ZEPHIRAN Chloride solutions, particularly when used alternately with alcohol, leaves the skin smooth and clean. When ZEPHIRAN Chloride solutions are applied by friction (using several changes of sponges), dirt, skin fats, desquamating epithelium, and superficial bacteria are effectively removed, thus exposing the underlying

Continued on next page

This product information was effective as of October 31, 1994. Current detailed information may be obtained directly from Sanofi Winthrop Pharmaceuticals by writing to 90 Park Avenue, New York, NY 10016.

Sanofi Winthrop—Cont.

skin to the antiseptic activity of the solutions.

The following procedure has been found satisfactory for preparation of the surgical field. On the day prior to surgery, the operative site is shaved and then scrubbed thoroughly with ZEPHIRAN Chloride Aqueous Solution 1:750. Immediately before surgery, ZEPHIRAN Chloride Tinted Tincture 1:750 or Spray is applied to the site in the usual manner (see Precautions). If the red tinted solution turns yellow during the preparation of patient's skin for surgery, it usually indicates the presence of soap (alkali) residue which is incompatible with ZEPHIRAN solutions. Therefore, rinse thoroughly and reapply the antiseptic. Because ZEPHIRAN Chloride Tinted Tincture 1:750 contains alcohol and acetone, its cleansing action on the skin is particularly effective and it dries more rapidly than the aqueous solution. The Tinted Tincture is recommended when it is desirable to outline the operative site.

Recommended Dilutions: For specific directions, see Tables 2 and 3.

Surgery

Preoperative preparation of skin: Aqueous solution 1:750 and Tinted Tincture 1:750 or Spray

Surgeons' hand and arm soaks: Aqueous solution 1:750

Treatment of minor wounds and lacerations: Tinted Tincture 1:750 or Spray

Irrigation of deep infected wounds: Aqueous solution 1:3000 to 1:20,000

Denuded skin and mucous membranes: Aqueous solution 1:5000 to 1:10,000

Obstetrics and Gynecology

Preoperative preparation of skin: Aqueous solution 1:750 and Tinted Tincture 1:750 or Spray

Vaginal douche and irrigation: Aqueous solution 1:2000 to 1:5000

Postepisiotomy care: Aqueous solution 1:5000 to 1:10,000

Breast and nipple hygiene: Aqueous solution 1:1000 to 1:2000

Urology

Bladder and urethral irrigation: Aqueous solution 1:5000 to 1:20,000

Bladder retention lavage: Aqueous solution 1:20,000 to 1:40,000

Dermatology

Oozing and open infections: Aqueous solution 1:2000 to 1:5000

Wet dressings by irrigation or open dressing (Use in occlusive dressings is inadvisable.): Aqueous solution 1:5000 or less

Ophthalmology

Eye irrigation: Aqueous solution 1:5000 to 1:10,000

Preservation of ophthalmic solutions: Aqueous solution 1:5000 to 1:7500
[See table below.]

TABLE 2
Correct Use of ZEPHIRAN Chloride

ZEPHIRAN Chloride solutions must be prepared, stored, and used correctly to achieve and maintain their antiseptic action. Serious inactivation and contamination of ZEPHIRAN Chloride solutions may occur with misuse.

CORRECT DILUENTS	INCOMPATIBILITIES	PREFERRED FORM
Sterile Water for Injection is recommended for irrigation of body cavities. *Sterile distilled water* is recommended for irrigating traumatized tissue and in the eye. *Freshly distilled water* is recommended for skin antisepsis. *Resin deionized water* should not be used because the deionizing resins can carry pathogens (especially gram-negative bacteria); they also inactivate quaternary ammonium compounds. *Stored water* is not recommended since it may contain many organisms. *Saline* should not be used since it may decrease the antibacterial potency of ZEPHIRAN Chloride solutions.	Anionic detergents and soaps should be thoroughly rinsed from the skin or other areas prior to use of ZEPHIRAN Chloride solutions because they reduce the antibacterial activity of the solutions. Serum and protein material also decrease the activity of ZEPHIRAN Chloride solutions. Corks should not be used to stopper bottles containing ZEPHIRAN Chloride solutions. Fibers or fabrics when stored in ZEPHIRAN Chloride solutions adsorb ZEPHIRAN from the surrounding liquid. Examples are:	ZEPHIRAN Chloride Tinted Tincture 1:750 is recommended for preoperative skin preparation because it contains alcohol and acetone which enhance its cleansing action and promote rapid drying. ZEPHIRAN Chloride Tinted Tincture 1:750, containing acetone, is recommended when it is desirable to outline the operative site. (Aqueous solutions of ZEPHIRAN Chloride used in skin preparation have a tendency to "run off" the skin.) Caution: Because of the flammable organic solvents in ZEPHIRAN Chloride Tinted Tincture 1:750 and Spray, these products should be kept away from open flame or cautery.

Cotton — Gauze sponges
Wool — Rayon
Rubber materials

Applicators or sponges, intended for a skin prep, should be stored separately and dipped in ZEPHIRAN Chloride solutions immediately before use.

Under certain circumstances the following commonly encountered substances are incompatible with ZEPHIRAN Chloride solutions:

Iodine — Aluminum
Silver nitrate — Caramel
Fluorescein — Kaolin
Nitrates — Pine oil
Peroxide — Zinc sulfate
Lanolin — Zinc oxide
Potassium — Yellow oxide
  permanganate — of mercury

TABLE 3
Dilutions of ZEPHIRAN Chloride
Aqueous Solution 1:750

Final Dilution	ZEPHIRAN Chloride Aqueous Solution 1:750 (parts)	Distilled Water (parts)
1:1000	3	1
1:2000	3	5
1:2500	3	7
1:3000	3	9
1:4000	3	13
1:5000	3	17
1:10,000	3	37
1:20,000	3	77
1:40,000	3	157

Accidental Ingestion: If ZEPHIRAN Chloride solution, particularly a concentrated solution, is ingested, marked local irritation of the gastrointestinal tract, manifested by nausea and vomiting, may occur. Signs of systemic toxicity include restlessness, apprehension, weakness, confusion, dyspnea, cyanosis, collapse, convulsions, and coma. Death occurs as a result of paralysis of the respiratory muscles.
Treatment: Immediate administration of several glasses of a mild soap solution, milk, or egg whites beaten in water is recommended. This may be followed by gastric lavage with a mild soap solution. Alcohol should be avoided as it promotes absorption.
To support respiration, the airway should be clear and oxygen should be administered, employing artificial respiration if necessary. If convulsions occur, a short-acting barbiturate may be given parenterally with caution.

How Supplied:
ZEPHIRAN Chloride Aqueous Solution 1:750
 Bottles of 8 fl oz (NDC 0024-2521-04) and 1 gallon (NDC 0024-2521-08)
ZEPHIRAN Chloride Tinted Tincture 1:750 *(flammable)*
 Bottles of 1 gallon (NDC 0024-2523-08)
ZEPHIRAN Chloride Spray–Tinted Tincture 1:750 *(flammable)*
 Bottles of 1 fl oz (NDC 0024-2527-01) and 6 fl oz (NDC 0024-2527-03)
ZSW-3

Scandinavian Natural Health & Beauty Products, Inc. Scandinavian Pharmaceuticals
**13 NORTH SEVENTH STREET
PERKASIE, PA 18944**

SALIX SST Lozenges
Saliva Stimulant

Active Ingredients: sorbitol, malic acid, sodium citrate, dicalcium phosphate, citric acid.

Indications and Usage: SALIX is an aid for mild oral dryness or severe xero-

stomia conditions such as in autoimmune conditions/Sjogren's, post-irradiation or side effect from dozens of medications. Also helpful in oral candidiasis. Helps defend against dental and denture wear, caries, gum disease, halitosis, swallowing difficulties, reduced oral defense.... SALIX helps provide a regulated stimulation to salivary glands with buffering action to protect the teeth and balance the oral ph.
Note: Primary or secondary saliva cells must be functioning to some degree. The acidic content, although quickly buffered, may irritate conditions of active localized oral tissue inflammation.

Dosage: as needed or up to 1 per hour in severe xerostomia conditions.

Schering-Plough HealthCare Products
LIBERTY CORNER, NJ 07938

A AND D® MEDICATED DIAPER RASH OINTMENT

Description: An ointment containing White Petrolatum and Zinc Oxide. Also contains: Benzoic Acid, Benzyl Alcohol, Cholecalciferol, Cod Liver Oil, Cyclomethicone, Glyceryl Monostearate, Light Mineral Oil, Magnesium Aluminum Silicate, Ozokerite, Propylparaben.

Indications: Helps treat and prevent diaper rash. Protects chafed skin due to diaper rash and helps seal out wetness.

Dosage and Administration: Change wet and soiled diapers promptly, cleanse the diaper area and allow to dry. Apply ointment liberally as often as necessary, with each diaper change, especially at bedtime or anytime when exposure to wet diapers is prolonged.
Warning: Keep this and all drugs out of the reach of children. In case of accidental ingestion, seek professional assistance or contact a Poison Control Center immediately.

How Supplied: A and D® Medicated Ointment is available in 1 ½-ounce (42.5g) and 4-ounce (113g) tubes.
Store between 15° and 25°C (59° and 77°F).

Shown in Product Identification Guide, page 522

A and D® Ointment

Description: An ointment containing the emollients, lanolin and petrolatum. Also contains: Cholecalciferol, Fish Liver Oil, Fragrance, Mineral Oil, Paraffin.

Indications: *Diaper rash—*A and D Ointment provides prompt, soothing relief for diaper rash and helps heal baby's tender skin; forms a moisture-proof shield that helps protect against urine and detergent irritants; comforts baby's skin and helps prevent chafing.
*Chafed Skin—*A and D Ointment helps skin retain its vital natural moisture; quickly soothes chafed skin in adults and children and helps prevent abnormal dryness.

*Abrasions and Minor Burns—*A and D Ointment soothes and helps relieve the smarting and pain of abrasions and minor burns, encourages healing and prevents dressings from sticking to the injured area.

Warning: Keep this and all drugs out of the reach of children. In case of accidental ingestion, seek professional assistance or contact a poison control center immediately.

Dosage and Administration: Apply as needed or consult your physician.

How Supplied: A and D Ointment is available in 1½-ounce (42.5 g) and 4-ounce (113 g) tubes and 1-pound (454 g) jars and 2.5 oz. pumps.
Shown in Product Identification Guide, page 522

AFRIN®
[a 'frin]
**Nasal Spray 0.05%
Nasal Spray Pump 0.05%
Sinus Nasal Spray 0.05%
Cherry Scented Nasal Spray 0.05%
Menthol Nasal Spray 0.05%
Extra Moisturizing Nasal
Spray 0.05%
Nose Drops 0.05%**

Description: AFRIN products contain oxymetazoline hydrochloride, the longest acting topical nasal decongestant available.
Each mL of **AFRIN Nasal Spray, Nasal Spray Pump, and Nose Drops** contains Oxymetazoline Hydrochloride, 0.05%. **Also contains:** Benzalkonium Chloride, Edetate Disodium, Polyethlene Glycol 1450, Povidone, Propylene Glycol, Sodium Phosphate Dibasic, Sodium Phosphate Monobasic, Water.
Each mL of **AFRIN Sinus** contains Oxymetazoline Hydrochloride 0.05%. **Also contains:** Benzalkonium Chloride, Benzyl Alcohol, Edetate Disodium, Mentanase-12™ (Camphor, Eucalyptol, Menthol), Polysorbate 80, Propylene Glycol, Sodium Phosphate Dibasic, Sodium Phosphate Monobasic, Water.
AFRIN Extra Moisturizing Nasal Spray is specially formulated to sooth dry, irritated nasal passages.
AFRIN Menthol Nasal Spray contains cooling aromatic vapors of menthol, eucalyptol, camphor and polysorbate in addition to the ingredients of AFRIN Nasal Spray.
AFRIN Cherry Scented Nasal Spray contains artificial cherry flavor in addition to the ingredients in regular AFRIN.

Indications: For the temporary relief of nasal congestion due to a cold, due to hay fever or other upper respiratory allergies, or associated with sinusitis. Reduces swelling of nasal passages; shrinks

Continued on next page

Information on Schering-Plough HealthCare Products appearing on these pages is effective as of November 1994.

Schering-Plough—Cont.

swollen membranes. Temporarily restores freer breathing through the nose.

Actions: The sympathomimetic action of AFRIN products constricts the smaller arterioles of the nasal passages, producing a prolonged, gentle and predictable decongesting effect. In just a few minutes a single dose, as directed, provides prompt, temporary relief of nasal congestion that lasts up to 12 hours. AFRIN products last up to 3 or 4 times longer than most ordinary nasal sprays.

Warnings: Do not exceed recommended dosage. This product may cause temporary discomfort such as burning, stinging, sneezing, or an increase in nasal discharge. Do not use this product for more than 3 days. Use only as directed. Frequent or prolonged use may cause nasal congestion to recur or worsen. If symptoms persist, consult a doctor. The use of this container by more than one person may spread infection. Do not use this product if you have heart disease, high blood pressure, thyroid disease, diabetes, or difficulty in urination due to enlargement of the prostate gland unless directed by a doctor. Do not use this product in a child who has heart disease, high blood pressure, thyroid disease, or diabetes unless directed by a doctor. As with any drug, if you are pregnant or nursing a baby, seek the advice of a health professional before using this product. Keep this and all medicines out of the reach of children. In case of accidental ingestion, seek professional assistance or contact a Poison Control Center immediately.

Directions: Adults and children 6 to under 12 years of age (with adult supervision): 2 or 3 sprays in each nostril not more often than every 10 to 12 hours. Do not exceed 2 doses in any 24-hour period. **Children under 6 years of age:** consult a doctor. To spray, squeeze bottle quickly and firmly. Do not tilt head backward while spraying. Wipe nozzle clean after use.

How Supplied: AFRIN Nasal Spray 0.05%, 15 ml and 30 ml plastic squeeze bottles.
AFRIN Nasal Spray Pump 0.05% (1:2000), 15 ml spray pump bottles.
AFRIN Sinus Nasal Spray 0.05%, 15 ml plastic squeeze bottles.
AFRIN Extra Moisturizing Nasal Spray 0.05%, 15 ml and 30 ml plastic squeeze bottles.
AFRIN Cherry Scented Nasal Spray 0.05% (1:2000), 15 ml plastic squeeze bottle.
AFRIN Menthol Nasal Spray 0.05% (1:2000), 15 ml plastic squeeze bottle.
AFRIN Nose Drops 0.05% (1:2000), 20 ml dropper bottle.
Store all nasal sprays and nose drops between 2° and 30°C (36° and 86°F)
Shown in Product Identification Guide, page 522

AFRIN®
[a 'frin]
Saline Mist

Ingredients: Water, PEG-32, Sodium Chloride, Sodium Benzoate, Benzalkonium Chloride, Disodium EDTA, Benzoic Acid.

Indications: Provides soothing moisture to dry, inflamed nasal membranes due to colds, allergies, low humidity, and other minor nasal irritations. Afrin Saline Mist loosens and thins mucus secretions to aid removal of mucus from nose and sinuses. Afrin Saline Mist can be used as often as needed, and is safe to use with cold, allergy, and sinus medications.

Directions: For infants, children, and adults, 2 to 6 sprays/drops in each nostril as often as needed or as directed by a physician. For a fine mist, keep bottle upright; for nose drops, keep bottle upside down; for a stream, keep bottle horizontal. Wipe nozzle clean after use.

Keep out of the reach of children. If you are pregnant or nursing a baby, seek the advice of a health professional before using this product.
The use of this dispenser by more than one person may spread infection.
CONTAINS NO ALCOHOL

AFTATE® Antifungal
Aerosol Liquid
Aerosol Powder

Active Ingredient: Tolnaftate 1%.
Also Contains:
Aftate Spray Powder for Athlete's Foot—Alcohol 14% w/w, (from SD alcohol 40-2), BHT, isobutane, PPG-12-buteth-16, talc. **Aftate Spray Liquid**—Alcohol 36% w/w, (from SD alcohol 40-2), BHT, isobutane, PPG-12-buteth-16. **Aftate Spray Powder for Jock Itch**—Alcohol 14% w/w, (from SD alcohol 40-2), BHT, isobutane, PPG-12-buteth-16, talc.

Indications: Aftate Spray Powder for Athlete's Foot and Aftate Spray Liquid effectively soothe and relieve symptoms of athlete's foot (tinea pedis), including itching, burning and cracking. Clinically proven to **cure** athlete's foot and when used daily, helps **prevent** it from recurring.
Aftate Spray Powder for Jock Itch effectively soothes and relieves the painful symptoms of Jock Itch (tinea cruris), including itching, chafing and burning rash. Clinically proven to **cure** Jock Itch.

Directions: Wash the affected area and dry thoroughly. Shake can well. Spray a thin layer of the product over the affected area twice daily (morning and night) or as directed by a doctor. Supervise children in the use of this product. For Athlete's Foot: pay special attention to spaces between the toes; wear well-fitting, ventilated shoes and change

shoes and socks at least once daily. Use daily for 4 weeks for Athlete's Foot and for 2 weeks for Jock Itch. If condition persists longer, consult a doctor. This product is not effective on the scalp or nails. To prevent Athlete's Foot, apply once or twice daily (morning and/or night).

Warnings: Do not use on children under 2 years of age unless directed by a doctor. For external use only. If irritation occurs or if there is no improvement within 4 weeks for Athlete's Foot or within 2 weeks for Jock Itch, discontinue use and consult a doctor. Flammable. Do not use while smoking or near heat or flame. Avoid spraying in eyes. Contents under pressure. Do not puncture or incinerate. Do not store at temperature above 120°F. Use only as directed. Intentional misuse by deliberately concentrating and inhaling contents can be harmful or fatal. Keep this and all drugs out of the reach of children. In case of accidental ingestion, seek professional assistance or contact a Poison Control Center Immediately.

How Supplied:
AFTATE for Athlete's Foot
  Aerosol Spray Powder—3.5 oz can
  Aerosol Spray Liquid—4 oz. can
AFTATE for Jock Itch
  Aerosol Spray Powder—3.5 oz. can
  Shown in Product Identification Guide, page 522

CHLOR–TRIMETON®
[klor-tri 'mĕ-ton]
4 Hour Allergy Tablets
8 Hour Allergy Tablets
12 Hour Allergy Tablets

Active Ingredients: Each 4 Hour Allergy Tablet contains: 4 mg chlorpheniramine maleate, USP; also contains: Corn Starch, D&C Yellow No. 10 Aluminum Lake, Lactose, Magnesium Stearate. **Each 8 Hour Allergy Tablet contains:** 8 mg chlorpheniramine maleate; also contains: Acacia, Butylparaben, Calcium Phosphate, Calcium Sulfate, Carnauba Wax, Corn Starch, D&C Yellow No. 10 Aluminum Lake, FD&C Yellow No. 6 Aluminum Lake, FD&C Yellow No. 6, Lactose, Magnesium Stearate, Neutral Soap, Oleic Acid, Potato Starch, Rosin, Sugar, Talc, White Wax, Zein.
Each 12 Hour Allergy Tablet contains: 12 mg chlorpheniramine maleate; also contains: Acacia, Butylparaben, Calcium Phosphate, Calcium Sulfate, Carnauba Wax, Corn Starch, D&C Yellow No. 10 Aluminum Lake, FD&C Blue No. 2 Aluminum Lake, FD&C Yellow No. 6, FD&C Yellow No. 6 Aluminum Lake, Lactose, Magnesium Stearate, Neutral Soap, Oleic Acid, Potato Starch, Rosin, Sugar, Talc, White Wax, Zein.

Indications: For effective relief of sneezing, itchy, watery eyes, itchy throat, and runny nose due to hay fever and other upper respiratory allergies.

Warnings: May cause excitability especially in children. Do not give the 8 Hour or 12 Hour Allergy Tablets to children under 12 years, or 4 Hour Allergy Tablets to children under 6 years except under the advice and supervision of a doctor. Do not take this product, unless directed by a doctor, if you have a breathing problem such as emphysema or chronic bronchitis, or if you have glaucoma, difficulty in urination due to enlargement of the prostate gland. May cause drowsiness; alcohol may increase the drowsiness effect. Avoid alcoholic beverages while taking this product. Do not take this product if you are taking sedatives or tranquilizers, without first consulting your doctor. Use caution when driving a motor vehicle or operating machinery. As with any drug, if you are pregnant or nursing a baby, seek the advice of a health professional before using this product. Keep this and all drugs out of the reach of children. In case of accidental overdose, seek professional assistance or contact a Poison Control Center immediately.

Dosage and Administration: 4 Hour Allergy Tablets—Adults and Children 12 years of age and over: Oral dosage is one tablet (4 mg) every 4 to 6 hours, not to exceed 6 tablets in 24 hours. Children 6 to under 12 years of age: Oral dosage is one half the adult dose (2 mg) (break tablet in half) every 4 to 6 hours, not to exceed 3 whole tablets (12 mg) in 24 hours, or as directed by a doctor. Children under 6 years of age: consult a doctor.
8 Hour Allergy Tablets—Adults and Children 12 years and over—One tablet every 8 to 12 hours. Do not take more than one tablet every 8 hours or 3 tablets in 24 hours.
12 Hour Allergy Tablets—Adults and children 12 years and over—One tablet every 12 hours. Do not exceed 2 tablets in 24 hours.

How Supplied: CHLOR-TRIMETON 4 Hour Allergy Tablets, box of 24, bottles of 100.
CHLOR-TRIMETON 8 Hour Allergy Tablets, boxes of 15, bottles of 100.
CHLOR-TRIMETON 12 Hour Allergy Tablets, boxes of 10 and 24, bottles of 100. Store between 2° and 30°C (36° and 86°F). Protect from excessive moisture.
Shown in Product Identification Guide, page 522

CHLOR–TRIMETON®
[*klortri 'mĕ-ton*]
4 Hour Allergy/Decongestant Tablets
12 Hour Allergy/Decongestant Tablets

Active Ingredients: Each 4 Hour Allergy/Decongestant Tablet contains: 4 mg chlorpheniramine maleate, USP and 60 mg pseudoephedrine sulfate; also contains: Corn Starch, FD&C Blue No. 1, Lactose, Magnesium Stearate, Povidone. **Each 12 Hour Allergy/Decongestant Tablet contains:** 8 mg chlorpheniramine maleate and 120 mg pseudoephedrine sulfate; also contains: Acacia, Butylparaben, Calcium Sulfate, Carnauba Wax, Corn Starch, D&C Yellow No. 10 Aluminum Lake, FD&C Blue No. 1 Aluminum Lake, FD&C Yellow No. 6 Aluminum Lake, Gelatin, Lactose, Magnesium Stearate, Neutral Soap, Oleic Acid, Povidone, Rosin, Sugar, Talc, White Wax, Zein.

Indications: For effective temporary relief of sneezing, itchy, watery eyes, itchy throat, and runny nose due to hay fever and other upper respiratory allergies. Helps decongest sinus openings and sinus passages; relieves sinus pressure. Temporarily restores freer breathing through the nose.

Warnings: May cause excitability, especially in children. Do not exceed recommended dosage because at higher doses nervousness, dizziness, or sleeplessness may occur. Do not take this product for more than 7 days. If symptoms do not improve or are accompanied by fever, consult a doctor. Do not take this product, unless directed by a doctor, if you have a breathing problem such as emphysema or chronic bronchitis, or if you have glaucoma, heart disease, high blood pressure, thyroid disease, diabetes, or difficulty in urination due to enlargement of the prostate gland. May cause drowsiness; alcohol, sedatives, and tranquilizers may increase the drowsiness effect. Avoid alcoholic beverages while taking this product. Do not take this product if you are taking sedatives or tranquilizers without first consulting your doctor. Use caution when driving a motor vehicle or operating machinery. As with any drug, if you are pregnant or nursing a baby, seek the advice of a health professional before using this product. Keep this and all drugs out of the reach of children. In case of accidental overdose, seek professional assistance or contact a Poison Control Center immediately.

Drug Interaction Precaution: Do not use this product if you are taking a prescription drug containing a monoamine oxidase inhibitor (MAOI) (certain drugs for depression or psychiatric or emotional conditions), without first consulting your doctor. If you are uncertain whether your prescription drug contains an MAOI, consult a health professional before taking this product.

Dosage and Administration: 4 Hour Allergy/Decongestant Tablets — ADULTS AND CHILDREN 12 YEARS OF AGE AND OVER: Oral dosage is one tablet every 4 to 6 hours, not to exceed 4 tablets in 24 hours, or as directed by a doctor. CHILDREN 6 TO UNDER 12 YEARS OF AGE: Oral dosage is one half the adult dose (break tablet in half) every 4 to 6 hours, not to exceed 2 whole tablets in 24 hours, or as directed by a doctor. CHILDREN UNDER 6 YEARS OF AGE: Consult a doctor. **12 Hour Allergy/Decongestant Tablets**—ADULTS AND CHILDREN 12 YEARS AND OVER: one tablet every 12 hours. Do not exceed 2 tablets in 24 hours.

How Supplied: CHLOR-TRIMETON 4 Hour Allergy/Decongestant Tablets— boxes of 24. CHLOR-TRIMETON 12 Hour Allergy/Decongestant Tablets boxes of 10.
Store these CHLOR-TRIMETON Products between 2° and 30°C (36° and 86°F); and protect from excessive moisture.
Shown in Product Identification Guide, page 522

CHOOZ® ANTACID GUM

Active Ingredients: 500 mg. of calcium carbonate per tablet.

Inactive Ingredients: Sucrose, gum base, glucose, corn starch, peppermint oil, hydrated silica, gelatin, glycerin, acacia, carnauba wax, beeswax, sodium benzoate.

Indications: For relief from acid indigestion, sour stomach, heartburn, and upset stomach associated with these symptoms. Five tablets provide 100% of the adult U.S. Recommended Daily Allowance for calcium. Chooz Antacid Gum is dietically sodium-free, an important benefit for those watching their sodium and salt consumption.

Warnings: Adults—Do not take more than 14 tablets in a 24-hour period. Do not use the maximum dosage of this product for more than 2 weeks except under the advice and supervision of a physician. Children 6 to 12 years—Do not take more than 8 tablets in a 24-hour period. Keep this and all drugs out of reach of children.

Dosage and Administration: Adults chew 1 to 2 tablets every 2 to 4 hours. Children 6 to 12 years of age chew 1 tablet every 2 to 4 hours. Or take as directed by physician.

How Supplied: Tablets—individually foil-backed safety sealed blister packaging in boxes of 16 tablets.
Shown in Product Identification Guide, page 522

COMPLEX 15®
Therapeutic Moisturizing Lotion
Contains Phospholipids
Formulated For Mild To Severe Dry Skin

Ingredients: Water, Caprylic/Capric Triglyceride, Glycerin, Glyceryl Stearate, Dimethicone, PEG-50 Stearate, Squalane, Cetyl Alcohol, Glycol Stearate, Myristyl Myristate, Stearic Acid, Lecithin, C10–30 Cholesterol/Lanosterol Esters, Diazolidinyl Urea, Carbomer, Magnesium Aluminum Silicate, Sodium Hydroxide, BHT, Tetrasodium EDTA
COMPLEX 15® Therapeutic Moisturizing Lotion is formulated for mild to se-

Continued on next page

Information on Schering-Plough HealthCare Products appearing on these pages is effective as of November 1994.

Schering-Plough—Cont.

vere dry skin with a system modeled from nature. It contains lecithin, a phospholipid water-binding agent found naturally in the skin. Each phospholipid molecule holds 15 molecules of water, restoring the natural moisture balance. COMPLEX 15 Therapeutic Moisturizing Lotion is nongreasy and absorbs quickly into the skin. COMPLEX 15 Therapeutic Moisturizing Lotion is unscented, contains no parabens, lanolin, or mineral oil. COMPLEX 15 Therapeutic Moisturizing Lotion is proven to be hypoallergenic and noncomedogenic.

Directions: Apply to the hands and body as needed, or as directed by a physician. Avoid contact with eyes.

FOR EXTERNAL USE ONLY

How Supplied: COMPLEX 15® Therapeutic Moisturizing Lotion is available in 8 fluid ounce bottles (0085-4115-08).

Shown in Product Identification Guide, page 522

COMPLEX 15®
Therapeutic Moisturizing
Face Cream
Contains Phospholipids

Ingredients: Water, Caprylic/Capric Triglyceride, Glycerin, Squalane, Glyceryl Stearate, Propylene Glycol, PEG-50 Stearate, Cetyl Alcohol, Dimethicone, Glycol Stearate, Myristyl Myristate, Stearic Acid, Carbomer, Magnesium Aluminum Silicate, Diazolidinyl Urea, Lecithin, Sodium Hydroxide, C10–30 Cholesterol/Lanosterol Esters, BHT, Tetrasodium EDTA

COMPLEX 15® Therapeutic Moisturizing Face Cream is formulated for mild to severe dry skin with a system modeled from nature. It contains lecithin, a phospholipid water-binding agent found naturally in the skin. Each phospholipid molecule holds 15 molecules of water, restoring the natural moisture balance. COMPLEX 15 Therapeutic Moisturizing Face Cream is nongreasy and absorbs quickly into the skin. COMPLEX 15 Therapeutic Moisturizing Face Cream is unscented, contains no parabens, lanolin or mineral oil. COMPLEX 15 Therapeutic Moisturizing Face Cream is proven to be hypoallergenic and noncomedogenic.

Directions: Apply to the face as needed or as directed by a physician. Avoid contact with eyes.

FOR EXTERNAL USE ONLY

How Supplied: COMPLEX 15® Moisturizing Face Cream is available in 2.5 oz. tubes (0085-4100-25).

Shown in Product Identification Guide, page 522

CORICIDIN® Tablets
[*kor-a-see'din*]

CORICIDIN 'D'® Decongestant Tablets

Active Ingredients: CORICIDIN Tablets—2 mg chlorpheniramine maleate, 325 mg (5 gr) acetaminophen.
CORICIDIN 'D' Decongestant Tablets—2 mg chlorpheniramine maleate, 12.5 mg phenylpropanolamine hydrochloride, 325 mg (5 gr) acetaminophen.

Inactive Ingredients: CORICIDIN Tablets—Acacia, Butylparaben, Calcium Sulfate, Carnauba Wax, Cellulose, Corn Starch, FD&C Red No. 40 Aluminum Lake, FD&C Yellow No. 6 Aluminum Lake, Lactose, Magnesium Stearate, Povidone, Sugar, Talc, Titanium Dioxide, White Wax.
CORICIDIN 'D' Decongestant Tablets —Acacia, Butylparaben, Calcium Sulfate, Carnauba Wax, Cellulose, Corn Starch, Magnesium Stearate, Povidone, Sugar, Talc, Titanium Dioxide, White Wax.

Indications: CORICIDIN Tablets temporarily relieve minor aches, pains and headache, and reduce the fever associated with colds or flu; temporarily relieve sneezing, runny nose and itchy watery eyes due to hay fever, other upper respiratory allergies or the common cold. **Unlike other cold remedies, CORICIDIN Tablets do not contain a decongestant and therefore are suitable for hypertensive patients.**
CORICIDIN 'D' Tablets temporarily relieve minor aches, pains, and reduce the fever associated with a cold or flu; temporarily relieve sneezing and stuffy/runny nose associated with the common cold; provide temporary relief of sinus headache and pressure and reduce swelling of nasal passages. **CORICIDIN 'D' Tablets do contain a decongestant.**

Warnings: CORICIDIN Tablets—Do not take this product for pain for more than 10 days (adults) or 5 days (children 6 to under 12 years of age) and do not take for fever for more than 3 days unless directed by a doctor. If pain or fever persists or gets worse, if new symptoms occur, or if redness or swelling is present, consult a doctor because these could be signs of a serious condition. May cause excitability especially in children. Do not take this product, unless directed by a doctor, if you have a breathing problem such as emphysema or chronic bronchitis, or if you have glaucoma or difficulty in urination due to enlargement of the prostate gland. May cause drowsiness; alcohol, sedatives, and tranquilizers may increase the drowsiness effect. Avoid alcoholic beverages while taking this product. Do not take this product if you are taking sedatives or tranquilizers without first consulting your doctor. Use caution when driving a motor vehicle or operating machinery. As with any drug if you are pregnant or nursing a baby, seek the advice of a health professional before using this product. Keep this and all drugs

out of the reach of children. In case of accidental overdose, seek professional assistance or contact a Poison Control Center immediately. Prompt medical attention is critical for adults as well as for children even if you do not notice any signs or symptoms.
CORICIDIN 'D' Decongestant Tablets— Do not take this product for pain or congestion for more than 7 days (adults) or 5 days (children 6 to under 12 years of age) and do not take for fever for more than 3 days unless directed by a doctor. If pain or fever persists or gets worse, if new symptoms occur, or if redness or swelling is present, consult a doctor because these could be signs of a serious condition. May cause excitability, especially in children. Do not exceed recommended dosage because at higher doses nervousness, dizziness, or sleeplessness may occur. Do not take this product, unless directed by a doctor if you have a breathing problem such as emphysema or chronic bronchitis, or if you have glaucoma, heart disease, high blood pressure, thyroid disease, diabetes, or difficulty in urination due to enlargement of the prostate gland. May cause drowsiness; alcohol, sedatives, and tranquilizers may increase the drowsiness effect. Avoid alcoholic beverages while taking this product. Do not take this product if you are taking sedatives or tranquilizers without first consulting your doctor. Use caution when driving a motor vehicle or operating machinery. As with any drug, if you are pregnant or nursing a baby, seek the advice of a health professional before using this product. Keep this and all drugs out of the reach of children. In case of accidental overdose, seek professional assistance or contact a Poison Control Center immediately. Prompt medical attention is critical for adults as well as for children even if you do not notice any signs or symptoms.

Drug Interaction Precaution: CORICIDIN 'D' Decongestant Tablets—Do not take this product if you are taking a prescription drug containing a monoamine oxidase inhibitor (MAOI) (certain drugs for depression or psychiatric or emotional conditions), without first consulting your doctor. If you are uncertain whether your prescription drug contains an MAOI, consult a health professional before taking this product. Do not take this product if you are taking an appetite-controlling medication containing phenylpropanolamine without first consulting your doctor.

Dosage and Administration: CORICIDIN Tablets—**Adults and children 12 years of age and over:** oral dosage is 2 tablets every 4 to 6 hours, not to exceed 12 tablets in 24 hours, or as directed by a doctor. **Children 6 to under 12 years of age:** oral dosage is 1 tablet every 4 to 6 hours, not to exceed 5 tablets in 24 hours, or as directed by a doctor. **Children under 6 years of age:** consult a doctor. CORICIDIN 'D' Decongestant Tablets —**Adults and children 12 years of age and over:** oral dosage is 2 tablets every 4 hours not to exceed 12 tablets in 24 hours, or as directed by a doctor. **Children 6 to under 12 years of age:** oral dosage is 1 tablet every 4 hours not to exceed 5 tablets in 24 hours, or as directed by a doctor. **Children under 6 years of age:** consult a doctor.

How Supplied: CORICIDIN Tablets—Bottles of 12, 48, and 100 tablets, blisters of 24.
CORICIDIN 'D' Decongestant Tablets—Bottles of 12, 48, and 100 tablets, blisters of 24.
Store between 2° and 30°C (36° and 86°F).
Shown in Product Identification Guide, page 522

CORRECTOL®
Laxative
Tablets & Caplets

Active Ingredients: Tablets and Caplets—Yellow phenolphthalein, 65 mg. and docusate sodium, 100 mg. per tablet/caplet.

Inactive Ingredients: Butylparaben, calcium gluconate, calcium sulfate, carnauba wax, D&C Red No. 7 calcium lake, gelatin, magnesium stearate, sugar, talc, titanium dioxide, wheat flour, white wax, and other ingredients.

Indications: For relief of occasional constipation or irregularity. CORRECTOL generally produces bowel movement in 6 to 8 hours.

Actions: Yellow phenolphthalein—stimulant laxative; docusate sodium—fecal softener.

Warnings: Not to be taken in case of nausea, vomiting, abdominal pain, or signs of appendicitis. Take only as needed —as frequent or continued use of laxatives may result in dependence on them. If skin rash appears, do not use this or any other preparation containing phenolphthalein. Keep out of children's reach. In case of accidental overdose, seek professional assistance or contact a poison control center immediately.

Dosage and Administration
Dosage: Adults—1 or 2 tablets or caplets daily as needed, at bedtime or on arising. Children over 6 years—1 tablet or caplet daily as needed.

How Supplied: Tablets—Individual foil-backed safety sealed blister packaging in boxes of 15, 30 , 60 and 90 tablets. Caplets—Individual foil-backed safety sealed blister packaging in boxes of 30 and 60 caplets.
Shown in Product Identification Guide, page 523

CORRECTOL® EXTRA GENTLE
Stool Softener

Active Ingredient: Docusate sodium 100 mg. per soft gel.
Also Contains—D&C Red No. 33, FD&C Red No. 40, FD&C Yellow No. 6, gelatin, glycerin, polyethylene glycol 400, propylene glycol, sorbitol.

Indications: For relief of constipation without cramps for sensitive systems. Correctol Extra Gentle will work gradually to return you to regularity in 1 to 3 days.

Warning: Keep out of reach of children. In case of accidental overdose, seek professional assistance or contact a poison control center immediately.

Directions: Adults: For gradual relief of constipation, take 2 soft gels daily, as needed. Children 6–12: Take 1 daily, as needed.

How Supplied: Tablets—individual foil-backed safety sealed blister packaging in boxes of 30 tablets.
Store below 86°F. Protect from freezing.
Shown in Product Identification Guide, page 523

DI–GEL®
Antacid · Anti-Gas
Tablets/Liquid

DI-GEL Tablets: Active Ingredients: (Per Tablet)—Simethicone 20 mg., Calcium Carbonate 280 mg., Magnesium Hydroxide 128 mg. **Inactive Ingredients:** D & C yellow No. 10 aluminum lake, dextrin, FD&C yellow No. 6 aluminum lake, flavor, magnesium stearate, mannitol, povidone, stearic acid, sucrose, talc.
Dietetically sodium free, calcium rich.

DI-GEL Liquid: Active Ingredients—per teaspoonful (5 ml): Simethicone 20 mg., aluminum hydroxide (equivalent to aluminum hydroxide dried gel USP 200 mg.), magnesium hydroxide 200 mg. **Also contains:** Flavor, hydroxypropyl methylcellulose, methylcellulose, methylparaben, propylparaben, sodium saccharin, sorbitol, water.
Dietetically sodium free.

Indications: For fast, temporary relief of acid indigestion, heartburn, sour stomach and accompanying painful gas symptoms.

Actions: The antacid system in DI-GEL relieves and soothes acid indigestion, heartburn and sour stomach. At the same time, the simethicone "defoamers" eliminate gas.
When air becomes entrapped in the stomach, heartburn and acid indigestion can result, along with sensations of fullness, pressure and bloating.

Warnings: Do not take more than 20 teaspoonfuls or 24 tablets in a 24 hour period, or use the maximum dosage of this product for more than 2 weeks, except under the advice and supervision of a physician. If you have kidney disease do not use this product except under the advice and supervision of a physician. Tablets may cause constipation or have a laxative effect. Keep this and all drugs out of the reach of children.

Drug Interaction: (Liquid Only) This product should not be taken if patient is presently taking a prescription antibiotic drug containing any form of tetracycline.

Dosage and Administration: Two teaspoonfuls or tablets every 2 hours, or after or between meals and at bedtime, not to exceed 20 teaspoonfuls or 24 tablets per day, or as directed by a physician.

How Supplied:
DI-GEL Liquid in Mint Flavor - 6 and 12 fl. oz. bottles, safety sealed and Lemon/Orange Flavor - 12 fl. oz. bottles, safety sealed.
DI-GEL Tablets in Mint and Lemon/Orange Flavor - In boxes of 30 and 90 in handy portable safety sealed blister packaging. Also available in Mint 60-tablet bottles.
Shown in Product Identification Guide, page 523

DRIXORAL® COUGH Liquid Caps
Cough Suppressant
Liquid Caps

Description: Each DRIXORAL® COUGH Liquid Cap contains 30 mg Dextromethorphan Hydrobromide. Also contains: FD&C Blue No. 1, FD&C Red No. 40, Gelatin, Glycerin, Polyethylene Glycol 400, Povidone, Propylene Glycol, Sorbitol, Water.

Indications: Temporarily relieves coughs due to minor throat and bronchial irritations as may occur with a cold. Each DRIXORAL® COUGH Liquid Cap contains a maximum strength dose of cough suppressant to control daytime and nighttime coughs without narcotic side effects. Safe for individuals with diabetes.

Warnings: A persistent cough may be a sign of a serious condition. If cough persists for more than 1 week, tends to recur, or is accompanied by fever, rash or persistent headache, consult a doctor. Do not take this product for persistent or chronic cough such as occurs with smoking, asthma, emphysema, or if cough is accompanied by excessive phlegm (mucus) unless directed by a doctor. As with any drug, if you are pregnant or nursing a baby, seek the advice of a health professional before using this product. Keep this and all drugs out of the reach of children. In case of accidental overdose, seek professional assistance or contact a Poison Control Center immediately.

Drug Interaction Precaution: Do not use this product if you are taking a prescription drug containing a monoamine oxidase inhibitor (MAOI) (certain drugs for depression or psychiatric or emotional conditions), without first consulting your doctor. If you are uncertain whether your prescription drug contains

Continued on next page

Information on Schering-Plough HealthCare Products appearing on these pages is effective as of November 1994.

Schering-Plough—Cont.

an MAOI, consult a health professional before taking this product.

Dosage and Administration: Adults: Swallow one liquid cap (30 mg.) with water every 6 to 8 hours, not to exceed 4 liquid caps (120 mg.) in 24 hours, or as directed by a doctor. This product is not for children under 12 years of age.
Store below 86°. Protect from freezing. Protect from excessive moisture.

How Supplied: DRIXORAL® COUGH Caps are available in boxes of 10's and 20's.

Shown in Product Identification Guide, page 523

DRIXORAL® COLD & ALLERGY
[*dricks-or'al*]
Sustained-Action Tablets

Description: EACH DRIXORAL® COLD & ALLERGY SUSTAINED-ACTION TABLET CONTAINS: 120 mg of pseudoephedrine sulfate and 6 mg of dexbrompheniramine maleate. Half of the medication is released after the tablet is swallowed and the remaining amount of medication is released hours later providing continuous long-lasting relief for 12 hours. Also contains: Acacia, Butylparaben, Calcium Sulfate, Carnauba Wax, Corn Starch, D&C Yellow No. 10 Aluminum Lake, FD&C Blue No. 1 Aluminum Lake, FD&C Yellow No. 6 Aluminum Lake, Gelatin, Lactose, Magnesium Stearate, Neutral Soap, Oleic Acid, Povidone, Rosin, Sugar, Talc, White Wax, Zein.

Indications: The decongestant (pseudoephedrine sulfate) temporarily relieves nasal congestion due to the common cold, hay fever or other upper respiratory allergies, and associated with sinusitis. Helps decongest sinus openings and sinus passages. Reduces swelling of nasal passages; shrinks swollen membranes; and temporarily restores freer breathing through the nose. The antihistamine (dexbrompheniramine maleate) alleviates runny nose, sneezing, itching of the nose or throat and itchy and watery eyes as may occur in allergic rhinitis (such as hay fever).

Warnings: If symptoms do not improve within 7 days or are accompanied by fever, consult a physician before continuing use. May cause excitability especially in children. Do not exceed recommended dosage because at higher doses nervousness, dizziness, or sleeplessness may occur. Do not take this product if you have asthma, glaucoma, emphysema, chronic pulmonary disease, shortness of breath, difficulty in breathing, heart disease, high blood pressure, thyroid disease, diabetes, difficulty in urination due to enlargement of the prostate gland or give this product to children under 12 years, unless directed by a physician. May cause drowsiness; alcohol may increase the drowsiness effect. Avoid alcoholic beverages while taking this product. Use

caution when driving a motor vehicle or operating machinery. Keep this and all drugs out of the reach of children. In case of accidental overdose, seek professional assistance or contact a Poison Control Center immediately. As with any drug, if you are pregnant or nursing a baby, seek the advice of a health professional before using this product.

Drug Interaction Precaution: Do not take use this product if you are taking a prescription drug containing monoamine oxidase inhibitor (MAOI) (certain drugs for depression or psychiatric or emotional conditions), without first consulting your doctor. If you are uncertain whether your prescription contains an MAOI, consult a health professional before taking this product.

Dosage and Administration: ADULTS AND CHILDREN 12 YEARS AND OVER—one tablet every 12 hours. Do not exceed two tablets in 24 hours.

How Supplied: DRIXORAL® Cold & Allergy Sustained-Action Tablets, green, sugar-coated tablets branded in black with the product name, boxes of 10, 20, and 40, bottle of 100.
Store between 2° and 25°C (36° and 77°F).
Protect from excessive moisture.
Shown in Product Identification Guide, page 523

DRIXORAL® COUGH & CONGESTION Liquid Caps
Cough Suppressant/Nasal Decongestant
Liquid Caps

Description: Each DRIXORAL® COUGH & CONGESTION Liquid Cap contains 30 mg Dextromethorphan Hydrobromide, and 60 mg Pseudoephedrine Hydrochloride. **Also contains:** D&C Red No. 33 Aluminum Lake, FD&C Blue No. 1 Aluminum Lake, Gelatin, Glycerin, Polyethylene Glycol 400, Povidone, Propylene Glycol, Sorbitol, Water.

Indications: The **cough suppressant** temporarily relieves coughs due to minor throat and bronchial irritations as may occur with a cold. The **decongestant** temporarily relieves nasal congestion due to the common cold.

Warnings: A persistent cough may be a sign of a serious condition. If cough persists for more than 1 week, tends to recur, or is accompanied by fever, rash, or persistent headache, consult a doctor. Do not take this product for persistent or chronic cough such as occurs with smoking, asthma, emphysema, or if cough is accompanied by excessive phlegm (mucus), unless directed by a doctor. Do not exceed recommended dosage because at higher doses nervousness, dizziness, or sleeplessness may occur. Do not take this product for more than 7 days. If symptoms do not improve, or are accompanied by a fever, consult a doctor. Do not take this product if you have heart disease,

high blood pressure, thyroid disease, diabetes, or difficulty in urination due to the enlargement of the prostate gland unless directed by a doctor. As with any drug, if you are pregnant or nursing a baby, seek the advice of a health professional before using this product. Keep this and all drugs out of reach of children. In case of accidental overdose, seek professional assistance or contact a Poison Control Center immediately.

Drug Interaction Precaution: Do not use this product if you are taking a prescription drug containing a monoamine oxidase inhibitor (MAOI) (certain drugs for depression or psychiatric or emotional conditions), without first consulting your doctor. If you are uncertain whether your prescription contains an MAOI consult a health professional before taking this product.

Dosage and Administration: Adults (12 yrs and older): Swallow one liquid cap with water every 6 hours, not to exceed 4 liquid caps in 24 hours, or as directed by a doctor. This product is not for children under 12 years of age.
Store below 86°F. Protect from freezing. Protect from excessive moisture.

How Supplied: DRIXORAL® COUGH & CONGESTION Liquid Caps are available in boxes of 10's.
Shown in Product Identification Guide, page 523

DRIXORAL® COUGH & SORE THROAT Liquid Caps
Cough Suppressant/Pain Reliever-Fever Reducer
Liquid Caps

Description: Each DRIXORAL® COUGH & SORE THROAT Liquid Cap contains 15 mg. Dextromethorphan Hydrobromide, and 325 mg Acetaminophen. **Also contains:** Colloidal Silicon Dioxide, D&C Red No. 33, FD&C Blue No. 1, Gelatin, Glycerin, Polyethylene Glycol 400, Povidone, Propylene Glycol, Sorbitol, Titanium Dioxide.

Indications: The **cough suppressant** temporarily relieves coughs due to minor throat and bronchial irritations as may occur with a cold. The **pain reliever-fever reducer** temporarily relieves minor aches, pains, fever and sore throat. **Safe for individuals with diabetes.**

Warnings: A persistent cough may be a sign of a serious condition. If cough persists for more than 1 week, tends to recur, or is accompanied by fever, rash, or persistent headache, consult a doctor. Do not take this product for persistent or chronic cough such as occurs with smoking, asthma, emphysema, or if cough is accompanied by excessive phlegm (mucus), unless directed by a doctor. Do not take this product for pain for more than 10 days (adults) or 5 days (children 6 to under 12 years of age) or for fever for more than 3 days unless directed by a doctor. If pain or fever persists or gets worse, if new symptoms occur, or if redness or swelling is present, consult a doctor because these could be signs of a serious condition. If sore throat is severe, persists for more than 2 days, is accompanied or followed by fever, headache, rash, nausea, or vomiting, consult a doctor promptly. As with any drug, if you are pregnant or nursing a baby, seek the advice of a health professional before using this product. Keep this and all drugs out of reach of children. In case of accidental overdose, seek professional assistance or contact a Poison Control Center immediately. Prompt medical attention is critical for adults as well as children, even if you do not notice any signs or symptoms.

Drug Interaction Precaution: Do not use this product if you are taking a prescription drug containing a monoamine oxidase inhibitor (MAOI) (certain drugs for depression or psychiatric or emotional conditions), without first consulting your doctor. If you are uncertain whether your prescription contains an MAOI consult a health professional before taking this product.

Dosage and Administration: Adults (12 yrs and older): Swallow two liquid caps with water every 6 to 8 hours, not to exceed 8 liquid caps in 24 hours, or as directed by a doctor. **Children (6 to under 12 yrs old):** Swallow one liquid cap with water every 6 to 8 hours, not to exceed 4 liquid caps in 24 hours or as directed by a doctor.
Store below 86°F. Protect from freezing. Protect from excessive moisture.

How Supplied: DRIXORAL® COUGH & SORE THROAT Liquid Caps are available in boxes of 10's.
Shown in Product Identification Guide, page 523

DRIXORAL® NON-DROWSY FORMULA
[dricks-or 'al]
Long-Acting Nasal Decongestant

DRIXORAL® NON-DROWSY FORMULA Long-Acting Nasal Decongestant Tablets contain 120 mg pseudoephedrine sulfate, a nasal decongestant, in an extended-release tablet providing up to 12 hours of continuous relief ... without drowsiness. Also contains: Acacia, Butylparaben, Calcium Sulfate, Carnauba Wax, Corn Starch, FD&C Blue No. 1 Aluminum Lake, Gelatin, Lactose, Magnesium Stearate, Neutral Soap, Oleic Acid, Povidone, Rosin, Sugar, Talc, White Wax, Zein.

Indications: For temporary relief of nasal congestion due to the common cold, hay fever or other upper respiratory allergies, and nasal congestion associated with sinusitis. Helps decongest sinus openings and sinus passages.

Directions: Adults and Children 12 Years and Over—One tablet every 12 hours. Do not exceed two tablets in 24 hours. DRIXORAL® NON-DROWSY

FORMULA is not recommended for children under 12 years of age.

Warnings: Do not exceed recommended dosage because at higher doses, nervousness, dizziness, or sleeplessness may occur. Do not take this product if you have heart disease, high blood pressure, thyroid disease, diabetes, difficulty in urination due to enlargement of the prostate gland, or give this product to children under 12 years unless directed by a physician. If symptoms do not improve within 7 days or are accompanied by fever, consult your physician before continuing use. Keep this and all drugs out of the reach of children. In case of accidental overdose, seek professional assistance or contact a Poison Control Center immediately. As with any drug, if you are pregnant or nursing a baby, seek the advice of a health professional before using this product.

Drug Interaction Precautions: Do not take this product if you are presently taking a prescription drug for high blood pressure or depression, without first consulting your physician.

How Supplied: DRIXORAL® NON-DROWSY FORMULA Long-Acting Nasal Decongestant Tablets are available in boxes of 10's and 20's.
Store between 2° and 25°C (36° and 77°F).
Protect from excessive moisture.
Shown in Product Identification Guide, page 523

DRIXORAL® COLD & FLU
[dricks-or 'al]
Extended-Release Tablets

Active Ingredients: 500 mg Acetaminophen, 3 mg Dexbrompheniramine Maleate, 60 mg Pseudoephedrine Sulfate.

Also Contains: Calcium Phosphate, Carnauba Wax, D&C Yellow No. 10 Aluminum Lake, FD&C Blue No. 1 Aluminum Lake, FD&C Yellow No. 6 Aluminum Lake, Hydroxypropyl Methylcellulose, Magnesium Stearate, Methylparaben, PEG, Propylparaben, Stearic Acid.
DRIXORAL® COLD & FLU Extended-Release Tablets combine a nasal decongestant and an antihistamine with a nonaspirin analgesic in a special 12-hour continuous-acting timed-release tablet.

Indications: The *decongestant* temporarily relieves nasal congestion due to the common cold, hay fever or other upper respiratory allergies, and associated with sinusitis. Reduces swelling of nasal passages; shrinks swollen membranes; and temporarily restores freer breathing through the nose. Also helps decongest sinus openings, sinus passages. The *nonaspirin analgesic* temporarily relieves minor aches, pains, and headache and reduces fever due to the common cold. The *antihistamine* alleviates running

nose, sneezing, itching of the nose or throat, and itchy and watery eyes as may occur in allergic rhinitis (such as hay fever).

Directions: ADULTS AND CHILDREN 12 YEARS AND OVER—two tablets every 12 hours. Do not exceed four tablets in 24 hours. **CHILDREN UNDER 12 YEARS OF AGE:** consult a doctor.

Warnings: Do not take this product for more than 7 days. If symptoms do not improve, or are accompanied by fever that lasts for more than three days (72 hours) or recurs, or if new symptoms occur, consult a physician before continuing use. If pain or fever persists or gets worse, or if redness or swelling is present, consult a physician because these could be signs of a serious condition. May cause excitability especially in children. Do not exceed recommended dosage because at higher doses nervousness, dizziness, or sleeplessness may occur. Do not take this product if you have asthma, glaucoma, emphysema, chronic pulmonary disease, shortness of breath, difficulty in breathing, heart disease, high blood pressure, thyroid disease, diabetes, difficulty in urination due to enlargement of the prostate gland, or give this product to children under 12 years unless directed by a physician. May cause drowsiness; alcohol, sedatives, and tranquilizers may increase the drowsiness effect. Avoid alcoholic beverages while taking this product. Use caution when driving a motor vehicle or operating machinery. Keep this and all drugs out of the reach of children. In case of accidental overdose, seek professional assistance or contact a Poison Control Center immediately. Prompt medical attention is critical for adults as well as for children even if you do not notice any signs or symptoms. As with any drug, if you are pregnant or nursing a baby, seek the advice of a health professional before using this product.

Drug Interaction Precaution: Do not take this product if you are presently taking a prescription drug for high blood pressure or depression, sedatives or tranquilizers, without first consulting your physician.

How Supplied: DRIXORAL® COLD & FLU Extended-Release Tablets are available in boxes of 12's and 24's.
Store between 2° and 25°C (36° and 77°F).
Protect from excessive moisture.
Shown in Product Identification Guide, page 523

Continued on next page

Information on Schering-Plough HealthCare Products appearing on these pages is effective as of November 1994.

Schering-Plough—Cont.

DRIXORAL® ALLERGY/SINUS
[*dricks-or 'al*]
Nasal decongestant/Pain reliever/
Antihistamine

DRIXORAL® ALLERGY/SINUS Extended-Release Tablets combine a nasal decongestant, a non-aspirin analgesic, and an antihistamine in a 12-hour timed-release tablet.

Indications: The *decongestant* temporarily relieves nasal congestion due to sinusitis, the common cold, and hay fever or other upper respiratory allergies. Helps decongest sinus openings, sinus passages; relieves sinus pressure. Reduces swelling of nasal passages; shrinks swollen membranes; and temporarily restores freer breathing through the nose. The *non-aspirin analgesic* temporarily relieves headaches, and minor aches and pains. The *antihistamine* alleviates runny nose, sneezing, itching of the nose or throat, and itchy and watery eyes as may occur in allergic rhinitis (such as hay fever).

Each DRIXORAL® ALLERGY/SINUS Extended-Release Tablet Contains: 60 mg of pseudoephedrine sulfate, 3 mg of dexbrompheniramine maleate, and 500 mg of acetaminophen. These ingredients are released continuously, providing long-lasting relief for 12 hours. Also contains: Calcium Phosphate, Carnauba Wax, D&C Yellow No. 10 Aluminum Lake, FD&C Yellow No. 6 Aluminum Lake, Hydroxypropyl Methylcellulose, Magnesium Stearate, Methylparaben, PEG, Propylparaben, Stearic Acid.

Directions: ADULTS AND CHILDREN 12 YEARS AND OVER—two tablets every 12 hours. Do not exceed four tablets in 24 hours. CHILDREN UNDER 12 YEARS OF AGE: consult a physician.
Store between 2° and 25°C (36° and 77°F).

Warnings: Do not take this product for more than 7 days. If symptoms do not improve, or are accompanied by fever that lasts for more than three days (72 hours) or recurs, or if new symptoms occur, consult a physician before continuing use. If pain or fever persists or gets worse, or if redness or swelling is present, consult a physician because these could be signs of a serious condition. May cause excitability especially in children. Do not exceed recommended dosage because at higher doses nervousness, dizziness, or sleeplessness may occur. Do not take this product unless directed by a doctor, if you have a breathing problem such as emphysema or chronic bronchitis, or if you have glaucoma, heart disease, high blood pressure, thyroid disease, diabetes or difficulty in urination due to enlargement of the prostate gland or give this product to children under 12 years of age. May cause drowsiness; alcohol, sedatives, and tranquilizers may increase the drowsiness effect. Avoid alcoholic beverages while taking this product. Do not take this product if you are taking sedatives or tranquilizers, without first consulting your doctor. Use caution when driving a motor vehicle or operating machinery. Keep this and all drugs out of the reach of children. In case of accidental overdose, seek professional assistance or contact a Poison Control Center immediately. Prompt medical attention is critical for adults as well as for children even if you do not notice any signs or symptoms. As with any drug, if you are pregnant or nursing a baby, seek the advice of a health care professional before using this product.
Drug Interaction Precaution: Do not use this product if you are taking a prescription drug containing a monoamine oxidase inhibitor (MAOI) (certain drugs for depression or psychiatric or emotional conditions), without first consulting your doctor. If you are uncertain whether your prescription contains an MAOI, consult a health professional before taking this product.

How Supplied: DRIXORAL® ALLERGY/SINUS Extended-Release Tablets are available in boxes of 12's and 24's.
Shown in Product Identification Guide, page 523

DUOFILM® LIQUID
Wart Remover

Active Ingredient: Salicylic Acid 17% (w/w).

Inactive Ingredients: Alcohol 15.8% w/w, castor oil, ether 42.6% w/w, ethyl lactate, and polybutene in flexible collodion.

Indications: For the removal of common and plantar warts. Common warts can be easily recognized by the rough, cauliflower-like appearance of the surface. Plantar warts are found on the bottom of the foot.

Warnings: For external use only. Do not use this product on irritated skin, on any area that is infected or reddened, if you are a diabetic, or if you have poor blood circulation. If discomfort persists, see your doctor. Do not use on moles, birthmarks, warts with hair growing from them, genital warts, or warts on the face or mucous membranes. Keep out of reach of children. If DuoFilm Liquid gets in eyes, flush with water for 15 minutes. Avoid inhaling vapors. DuoFilm Liquid is extremely flammable. Keep away from fire or flame. Cap bottle tightly when not in use. Store at room temperature away from heat.

Directions: Wash affected area. May soak wart in warm water for 5 minutes. Dry area thoroughly.
Apply one thin layer (with brush applicator) at a time to sufficiently cover each wart. Let dry. Repeat this procedure once or twice daily as needed (until wart is removed) for up to 12 weeks.
Note: Adhesive bandage may be used to cover treated area.

How Supplied: DuoFilm Liquid is available in ½ fluid oz. spill-resistant bottles with brush applicator for pinpoint application.
Shown in Product Identification Guide, page 523

DUOFILM® PATCH
Wart Remover

Active Ingredient: Salicylic Acid 40% in a rubber-based vehicle.

Indications: For the concealment and removal of common warts. Common warts can be easily recognized by the rough, cauliflower-like appearance of the surface.

Warnings: For external use only. Do not use this product on irritated skin, on any area that is infected or reddened, if you are a diabetic, or if you have poor blood circulation. If discomfort persists, see your doctor. Do not use on moles, birthmarks, warts with hair growing from them, genital warts, or warts on the face or mucous membranes. Keep out of reach of children.

Directions: Wash affected area. May soak wart in warm water for five minutes. Dry area thoroughly. Apply Medicated Patch (packet A). If necessary, cut patch to fit wart. Repeat procedure every 48 hours as needed (until wart is removed) for up to 12 weeks.
Note: Self-adhesive cover-up patches (packet B) may be used to conceal Medicated Patch and wart.

How Supplied: DuoFilm Patch includes 54 Medicated Patches of varying sizes, with 20 self-adhesive Cover-Up patches for concealment while treatment is ongoing.
Shown in Product Identification Guide, page 523

DUOPLANT® GEL
Plantar Wart Remover

Active Ingredient: Salicylic Acid 17% (w/w).

Inactive Ingredients: Alcohol 57.6% w/w, ether 16.42% w/w, ethyl lactate, hydroxypropyl cellulose, and polybutene in flexible collodion, USP.

Indications: For the removal of plantar and common warts. Plantar warts are found on the bottom of the foot. Common warts can be easily recognized by the rough, cauliflower-like appearance of the surface.

Warnings: For external use only. Do not use this product on irritated skin, on any area that is infected or reddened, if you are a diabetic, or if you have poor blood circulation. If discomfort persists, see your doctor. Do not use on moles, birthmarks, warts with hair growing from them, genital warts, or warts on the face or mucous membranes. Keep out of reach of children. If DuoPlant Gel gets in eyes, flush with water for 15 minutes. Avoid inhaling vapors. DuoPlant Gel is extremely flammable. Keep away from fire or flame. Keep tube tightly capped when not in use. Store at room temperature away from heat.

Directions: Wash affected area. May soak wart in warm water for five minutes. Dry area thoroughly. Apply a thin layer to sufficiently cover each wart. Let dry. Repeat this procedure once or twice daily as needed (until wart is removed) for up to 12 weeks.
Note: Adhesive bandage may be used to cover treated area.

How Supplied: DuoPlant Gel is available in ½ oz. tubes with applicator tip for pinpoint application.

Shown in Product Identification Guide, page 523

DURATION
12 Hour Nasal Spray 0.05%

Description: DURATION products contain oxymetazoline hydrochloride, the longest acting topical nasal decongestant available. Each ml of DURATION Nasal Spray contains Oxymetazoline Hydrochloride, USP 0.5 mg (0.05%). **Also Contains:** Benzalkonium Chloride, Edetate Disodium, Polyethylene Glycol 1450, Povidone, Propylene Glycol, Sodium Phosphate Dibasic, Sodium Phosphate Monobasic, Water.

Indications: For prompt, temporary relief for up to 12 hours of nasal congestion due to colds, hay fever and sinusitis, and other upper respiratory allergies.

Actions: The sympathomimetic action of DURATION products constricts the smaller arterioles of the nasal passages, producing a prolonged, gentle and predictable decongesting effect. In just a few minutes a single dose, as directed, provides prompt, temporary relief of nasal congestion that lasts up to 12 hours. DURATION products last up to 3 times longer than most ordinary nasal sprays.

Warnings: Do not exceed recommended dosage because burning, stinging, sneezing or increase of nasal discharge may occur. The use of this container by more than one person may spread infection. Do not use this product for more than 3 days. If symptoms persist, consult a doctor. Do not use this product if you have heart disease, high blood pressure, thyroid disease, diabetes or difficulty in urination due to enlargement of the prostate gland unless directed by a doctor. As with any drug, if you are pregnant or nursing a baby seek the advice of a health professional before using this product. Keep this and all medicines out of the reach of children. In case of accidental ingestion, seek professional assistance or contact a Poison Control Center immediately.

Directions: Adults and children 6 to under 12 years of age (with adult supervision): 2 or 3 sprays in each nostril not more often than every 10 to 12 hours. Do not exceed 2 applications in any 24-hour period. **Children under 6 years of age:** consult a doctor. To spray squeeze bottle quickly and firmly. Do not tilt head backward while spraying. Wipe nozzle clean after use.

How Supplied: DURATION 12 Hour Nasal Spray 0.05%—½ oz and 1 oz plastic squeeze bottles

Shown in Product Identification Guide, page 523

FEEN-A-MINT®
Laxative Gum/Pills

Active Ingredients: Gum—yellow phenolphthalein 97.2 mg. per tablet. **Pills**—yellow phenolphthalein 65 mg., and docusate sodium 100 mg. per pill.

Inactive Ingredients: Gum—Acacia, butylated hydroxyanisole, carnauba wax, corn starch, gelatin, glucose, glycerin, gum base, peppermint oil, sodium benzoate, sugar, water, white wax.
Pills—Butylparaben, calcium gluconate, calcium sulfate, carnauba wax, gelatin, magnesium stearate, sugar, talc, titanium dioxide, wheat flour, white wax and other ingredients.

Indications: For relief of occasional constipation or irregularity. FEEN-A-MINT generally produces bowel movement in 6 to 8 hours.

Warning: Do not take any laxative in case of nausea, vomiting, or abdominal pain or any signs of appendicitis. Take only as needed as frequent or continued use of laxatives may result in dependence on them. If skin rash appears, do not take this or any other preparation containing phenolphthalein. Keep out of the reach of children. In case of accidental overdose, seek professional assistance or contact a Poison Control Center immediately.

How Supplied: Gum—Individual foil-backed safety sealed blister packaging in boxes of 5 and 16 tablets.
Pills—Safety sealed boxes of 15, 30, and 60 tablets.

Shown in Product Identification Guide, page 523

GYNE-LOTRIMIN®
Clotrimazole
Vaginal Cream
Antifungal

Active Ingredient: Clotrimazole 1%

Inactive Ingredients: Benzyl alcohol, cetearyl alcohol, cetyl esters wax, octyldodecanol, polysorbate 60, purified water, sorbitan monostearate.

Indications: Gyne-Lotrimin® will cure most recurrent vaginal yeast (Candida) infections. Gyne-Lotrimin® usually starts to relieve the itching and other symptoms of vaginal yeast infection within 3 days. If the patient does not improve in 3 days or if the infection isn't gone in 7 days, a condition other than a yeast infection may exist. The patient should discontinue use of the product and consult a doctor. Also, if symptoms recur within a 2-month period, patient should consult a doctor.

Important: In order to kill the yeast completely, GYNE-LOTRIMIN must be used the full seven days, even if symptoms are relieved sooner.

Warnings:
• Do not use if you have abdominal pain, fever, or a foul-smelling vaginal discharge. You may have a condition which is more serious than a yeast infection. Contact your doctor immediately.
• Do not use if this is your first experience with vaginal itch and discomfort. See your doctor.
• If there is no improvement within 3 days, you may have a condition other than a yeast infection. Stop using this product and see your doctor.
• If you may have been exposed to the human immunodeficiency virus (HIV, the virus that causes AIDS) and are now having recurrent vaginal infections, especially infections that don't clear up easily with proper treatment, see your doctor promptly to determine the cause of your symptoms and to receive proper medical care.
• If your symptoms return within two months or if you have infections that do not clear up easily with proper treatment, consult your doctor. You could be pregnant or there could be a serious underlying medical cause for your infections, including diabetes or a damaged immune system (including damage from infection with HIV—the virus that causes AIDS). (PLEASE READ EDUCATIONAL PAMPHLET FOUND INSIDE PACKAGE.)
• Do not use during pregnancy except under the advice and supervision of a doctor.
• This medication is for vaginal use only. It is not for use in the mouth or the eyes. In case of accidental ingestion, seek professional assistance or contact a Poison Control Center immediately.
• Keep this and all drugs out of reach of children. This product is not to be used on children less than 12 years of age.

Directions: Fill the applicator with the cream and then insert one applicatorful of cream into the vagina every day, preferably at bedtime. Repeat this procedure for seven consecutive days. For relief of external vulvar itching, squeeze a small amount of cream onto your finger

Continued on next page

Information on Schering-Plough HealthCare Products appearing on these pages is effective as of November 1994.

Schering-Plough—Cont.

and gently spread the cream onto the irritated area of the vulva. Use once or twice a day for up to 7 days as needed to relieve external vulvar itching. THE CREAM SHOULD NOT BE USED FOR VULVAR ITCHING DUE TO CAUSES OTHER THAN A YEAST INFECTION. *Cream also available with 7 disposable applicators and 7 pre-filled applicators.

GYNE-LOTRIMIN®
Clotrimazole
Vaginal Inserts
Antifungal

Active Ingredient: Each insert contains Clotrimazole 100 mg.

Inactive Ingredients: Corn starch, lactose, magnesium stearate, povidone.

Indications: Gyne-Lotrimin® will cure most vaginal yeast (Candida) infections. Gyne-Lotrimin® usually starts to relieve the itching and other symptoms of vaginal yeast infection within 3 days. If the patient does not improve in 3 days or if the infection isn't gone in 7 days, a condition other than a yeast infection may exist. The patient should discontinue use of the product and consult a doctor. Also, if symptoms recur within a 2-month period, patient should consult a doctor.

Important: In order to kill the yeast completely, GYNE-LOTRIMIN must be used the full seven days, even if symptoms are relieved sooner.

Warnings:
• Do not use if you have abdominal pain, fever, or a foul-smelling vaginal discharge. You may have a condition which is more serious than a yeast infection. Contact your doctor immediately.
• Do not use if this is your first experience with vaginal itch and discomfort. See your doctor.
• If there is no improvement within 3 days, you may have a condition other than a yeast infection. Stop using this product and see your doctor.
• If you may have been exposed to the human immunodeficiency virus (HIV, the virus that causes AIDS) and are now having recurrent vaginal infections, especially infections that don't clear up easily with proper treatment, see your doctor promptly to determine the cause of your symptoms and to receive proper medical care.
• If your symptoms return within two months or if you have infections that do not clear up easily with proper treatment, consult your doctor. You could be pregnant or there could be a serious underlying medical cause for your infections, including diabetes or a damaged immune system (including damage from infection with HIV—the virus that causes AIDS). (PLEASE READ EDUCATIONAL PAMPHLET FOUND INSIDE PACKAGE.)

• Do not use during pregnancy except under the advice and supervision of a doctor.
• This medication is for vaginal use only. It is not to be taken by mouth. In case of accidental ingestion, seek professional assistance or contact a Poison Control Center immediately.
• Keep this and all drugs out of reach of children. This product is not to be used on children less than 12 years of age.

Directions: Using the applicator, place one insert into the vagina, preferably at bedtime. Repeat this procedure for seven consecutive days.
*Inserts also available in a Combination Pack, which includes external vulvar cream for the relief of associated external vulvar itching and irritation.

GYNE-MOISTRIN®
Vaginal Moisturizing Gel

Description: Gyne-Moistrin Vaginal Moisturizing Gel is specially designed to soothe and relieve vaginal dryness associated with menopause. Gyne-Moistrin provides natural feeling moisture and lubrication. It is clear, colorless, odorless and proven to be non-irritating. Gyne-Moistrin is water-based, greaseless and non-staining; and it contains no hormones or medication, so it can be used as often as needed.

Actions: When used as directed, Gyne-Moistrin will relieve vaginal dryness. Gyne-Moistrin forms a non-occlusive layer of moisture over the vaginal epithelium, gradually hydrating a dry irritated area. Gyne-Moistrin can be used as often as needed.
Externally, in the vulvar area, Gyne-Moistrin will also moisturize tissues.

Ingredients: Polyglycerylmethacrylate, water, propylene glycol, methylparaben, propylparaben.

Warnings: Gyne-Moistrin is not a contraceptive. Does not harm condoms.

Directions: Gyne-Moistrin may be applied externally and internally according to personal preference using fingertip application or the reusable applicator.
FOR FINGERTIP APPLICATION: Squeeze out small amount of gel to cover fingertip and apply to the vaginal opening and external area as needed. Actual amount applied may be increased or decreased according to personal preference.
FOR INTERNAL USE: Remove reusable applicator from sealed wrapper. Fill with gel to line on applicator. Gently insert front end well into vagina; push end of applicator to fully release gel; remove applicator. Actual amount used may be increased or decreased according to personal preference. Wash applicator in warm soapy water then thoroughly rinse and dry before and after each use.

Store at room temperature.

How Supplied: Gyne-Moistrin is available in 1.5 oz. and 2.5 oz. tubes.
Shown in Product Identification Guide, page 523

LOTRIMIN® AF ANTIFUNGAL
[lo-tre-min]
Clotrimazole
Cream 1%
Solution 1%
Lotion 1%

Description: Lotrimin® AF Cream 1% is a white fully vanishing homogeneous cream containing 1% clotrimazole. The cream contains no sensitizing parabens and is totally grease free and non-staining.
Lotrimin® AF Solution 1% is a non-aqueous liquid, containing polyethylene glycol.
Lotrimin® AF Lotion 1% is a light penetrating buffered emulsion also containing no common sensitizing agents and is greaseless and nonstaining.

Indications: Lotrimin® AF Cream, Solution and Lotion contain 1% clotrimazole, a synthetic broad-spectrum antifungal agent. Clotrimazole is used for the treatment of dermal infections caused by a variety of pathogenic dermatophytes, yeasts and *Malassezia furfur*. The primary action of clotrimazole is against dividing and growing organisms. Lotrimin® AF was first made available as an over-the-counter drug in 1990 and is indicated for superficial dermatophyte infections: athlete's foot (tinea pedis), jock itch (tinea cruris) and ringworm (tinea corporis). Lotrimin® AF remains on prescription for topical candidiasis due to *Candida albicans* and tinea versicolor due to *Malassezia furfur*.

Directions: Cleanse skin with soap and water and dry thoroughly. Apply a thin layer over affected area morning and evening or as directed by a physician. For athlete's foot, pay special attention to the spaces between the toes. It is also helpful to wear well-fitting, ventilated shoes and to change shoes and socks at least once daily. Best results in athlete's foot and ringworm are usually obtained with 4 weeks use of this product, and in jock itch, with 2 weeks use. If satisfactory results have not occurred within these times, consult a physician or pharmacist. Children under 12 years of age should be supervised in the use of this product. This product is not effective on the scalp or nails.

How Supplied: Lotrimin® AF Antifungal Cream is available in a 0.42 oz. tube (12 grams) and a 0.84 oz. tube (24 grams).
Inactive ingredients include: benzyl alcohol, cetearyl alcohol, cetyl esters wax, octyldodecanol, polysorbate, sorbitan monostearate and water.
Lotrimin® AF Antifungal Solution is available in a 0.33 fl. oz. (10 milliliters) bottle. Inactive ingredients include PEG.
Lotrimin® AF Antifungal Lotion is available in a 0.66 fl. oz. (20 milliliters) bottle. Inactive ingredients include ben-

zyl alcohol, cetearyl alcohol, cetyl esters wax, octyldodecanol, polysorbate, sodium biphosphate, sodium phosphate dibasic, sorbitan monostearate and water.

Storage: Keep Lotrimin® AF products between 2° and 30°C (36° and 86°F).

Shown in Product Identification Guide, page 523

LOTRIMIN® AF ANTIFUNGAL
Miconazole Nitrate 2%
Athlete's Foot Spray Liquid
Athlete's Foot Spray Powder
Athlete's Foot Powder
Jock Itch Spray Powder

Active Ingredients:
SPRAY LIQUID contains Miconazole Nitrate 2%. Also contains: Alcohol SD-40 (17% w/w), Cocamide DEA, Isobutane, Propylene Glycol, Tocopherol (vitamin E).
SPRAY POWDER (Athlete's Foot/Jock Itch) contains Miconazole Nitrate 2%. Also contains: Alcohol SD-40 (10% w/w), Isobutane, Stearalkonium Hectorite, Talc.
POWDER contains Miconazole Nitrate 2%. Also contains: Talc.

Indications: LOTRIMIN AF Athlete's Foot Spray Liquid, Spray Powder and Powder are proven clinically effective in the treatment of athlete's foot (tinea pedis), jock itch (tinea cruris) and ringworm (tinea corporis). For effective relief of the itching, cracking, burning, scaling and discomfort that can accompany these conditions.
LOTRIMIN AF Powder also aids in the drying of naturally moist areas.
LOTRIMIN AF Jock Itch Spray Powder cures jock itch (tinea cruris). For effective relief of the itching, burning, scaling and discomfort associated with jock itch.

Warnings: For Athlete's Foot Spray Powder, Spray Liquid and Jock Itch Spray Powder: Do not use on children under 2 years of age except under the advice and supervision of a doctor. For external use only. If irritation occurs or if there is no improvement within 4 weeks (for athlete's foot or ringworm) or within 2 weeks (for jock itch), discontinue use and consult a doctor or a pharmacist. Avoid spraying in eyes. Contents under pressure. Do not puncture or incinerate. Flammable mixture: do not use or store near heat or open flames. Do not use while smoking. Exposure to temperatures above 120°F may cause bursting. Never throw container into fire or incinerator. Use only as directed. Intentional misuse by deliberately concentrating and inhaling contents may be harmful or fatal. Keep this and all drugs out of the reach of children. In case of accidental ingestion, seek professional assistance or contact a Poison Control Center immediately.
Lotrimin AF Powder: Do not use on children under 2 years of age except under the advice and supervision of a doc-

tor. For external use only. If irritation occurs, or if there is no improvement within 4 weeks (for athlete's foot or ringworm) or within 2 weeks (for jock itch) discontinue use and consult a doctor or pharmacist. Keep this and all drugs out of the reach of children. In case of accidental ingestion, seek professional assistance or contact a Poison Control Center immediately.

Directions: For Athlete's Foot Spray Liquid, Spray Powder and Jock Itch Spray Powder: Cleanse skin with soap and water and dry thoroughly. Shake can well before using. Hold can about six inches from the area to be treated. Apply a thin layer over affected area morning and night or as directed by a doctor. For athlete's foot, pay special attention to spaces between the toes. It is helpful to wear well fitting, ventilated shoes and to change socks and shoes at least once daily. Best results in athlete's foot and ringworm are usually obtained with 4 weeks use of this product and in jock itch with 2 weeks use. If satisfactory results have not occurred within these times, consult a doctor or pharmacist. Children under 12 years of age should be supervised in the use of this product. This product is not effective on the scalp or nails.
Powder: Cleanse skin with soap and water and dry thoroughly. Sprinkle powder liberally over affected area morning and night or as directed by a physician. For athlete's foot, pay special attention to the spaces between the toes. It is also helpful to wear well-fitting, ventilated shoes and to change socks and shoes at least once daily. Best results in athlete's foot and ringworm are usually obtained with 4 weeks use of this product and in jock itch with 2 weeks use. If satisfactory results have not occurred within these times, consult a doctor or pharmacist. Children under 12 years of age should be supervised in the use of this product. This product is not effective on the scalp or nails.
Store between 2° and 30° C (36° and 86°F).

How Supplied: LOTRIMIN AF Athlete's Foot Spray Powder and Jock Itch Spray Powder—3.5 oz. cans. LOTRIMIN AF Spray Liquid—4 oz. can. LOTRIMIN AF POWDER—3 oz. plastic bottle.

Shown in Product Identification Guide, page 523

SHADE® SUNBLOCK GEL SPF 30

Active Ingredients: Ethylhexyl p-methoxycinnamate, homosalate, oxybenzone.

Other Ingredients: SD alcohol 40 (73% V/V), water, PVP/VA copolymer, tetrahydroxypropyl ethylenediamine, acrylates/C10-30 alkyl acrylate crosspolymer, acrylates/octylacrylamide copolymer.

Indications: PABA-FREE Shade SPF 30 Oil-Free Clear Gel is clinically tested to protect your skin from the sun's burning UVA and UVB rays. This clean, clear

gel vanishes quickly without any greasy residue. It leaves your skin feeling fresh and clean while providing 30 times your natural protection against sunburn. This unique formula blocks UVB rays that are primarily responsible for sunburn and long-term skin damage caused by overexposure to the sun. It also protects your skin against the deeper penetrating UVA rays that have been associated with skin damage resulting in premature aging and wrinkling. Regular use of Shade 30 Oil-Free Clear Gel may help prevent skin cancer caused by long-term overexposure to the sun.

Non-greasy/Non-oily: Fresh, clear, lightweight greaseless formula that absorbs quickly—feels cool. Specially formulated for people with normal to oily skin.

Waterproof Maintains its degree of protection (SPF 30) for 80 minutes or more in the water.

Non-acnegenic/Non-comedogenic: Won't clog pores or cause blemishes.

Fragrance-free: Free of fragrances that may irritate those with sensitive skin.

Hypoallergenic: Won't irritate or sting sensitive skin like some protective sunscreens. Gentle enough for children's delicate skin.

Warnings: Flammable, do not use near heat or flame. Avoid contact with eyes, if skin irritation or rash develops discontinue use.

Directions for Use: Smooth evenly and liberally on all exposed areas. To ensure maximum protection, reapply often especially after swimming or excessive perspiration.

How Supplied: 4 oz. plastic bottles.
Shown in Product Identification Guide, page 523

SHADE® SUNBLOCK LOTION SPF 45

Active Ingredients: Ethylhexyl p-methoxycinnamate, octocrylene, oxybenzone, 2-ethylhexyl salicylate.

Other Ingredients: Water, sorbitan isostearate, sorbitol, octadecene/MA copolymer, triethanolamine, stearic acid, benzyl alcohol, barium sulfate, dimethicone, methylparaben, imidazolidinyl urea, phenethyl alcohol, propylparaben, carbomer, disodium EDTA.

Indications: PABA-FREE Shade SPF 45 is clinically tested to protect your skin from the sun's burning UVA and UVB rays. This ultra moisturizing formula keeps your skin feeling soft yet provides 45 times your natural protection against

Continued on next page

Information on Schering-Plough HealthCare Products appearing on these pages is effective as of November 1994.

Schering-Plough—Cont.

sunburn. It blocks UVB rays that are primarily responsible for sunburn and long-term skin damage caused by overexposure to the sun. It also protects your skin against the deeper penetrating UVA rays that have been associated with skin damage resulting in premature aging and wrinkling. Regular use of Shade 45 may help prevent skin cancer caused by long-term overexposure to the sun.

Moisturizing: Rich moisturizing formula helps keep your skin feeling smooth, soft and supple.

Waterproof: Maintains its degree of protection (SPF 45) for 80 minutes or more in the water.

Non-comedogenic: Won't clog pores.

Hypoallergenic: Won't irritate or sting sensitive skin like some protective sunscreens. Gentle enough for children's delicate skin.

Fragrance Free: Free of fragrances that may irritate those with sensitive skin.

Warnings: Avoid contact with eyes. If skin irritation or rash develops, discontinue use.

Directions for Use: Smooth evenly and liberally on all exposed areas. To ensure maximum protection, reapply often especially after swimming or excessive perspiration.

How Supplied: 4 oz. plastic bottles
Shown in Product Identification Guide, page 523

SHADE® UVAGUARD™
SPF 15 Sunscreen Lotion

Active Ingredients: Octyl methoxycinnamate, 7.5%; avobenzone (Parsol® 1789), 3%; oxybenzone, USP, 3%.

Other Ingredients: Benzyl alcohol, carbomer-941, dimethicone, edetate disodium, glyceryl stearate SE, isopropyl myristate, methylparaben, octadecene/MA copolymer, propylparaben, purified water, sorbitan monooleate, sorbitol, stearic acid and trolamine.

Indications: While all sunscreens protect your skin from the sun's burning rays, Shade® UVAGUARD™ sunscreen, with the patented ingredient Parsol®1789, offers extra protection from the UVA rays that may contribute to skin damage and premature aging of the skin. Shade UVAGUARD is clinically tested to provide 15 times your natural sunburn protection (UVB). And the moisturizing formula of Shade UVAGUARD keeps your skin feeling soft and is PABA-free. Regular use of Shade UVAGUARD may help reduce the chance of acute and long-term skin damage associated with exposure to UVA and UVB rays. Overexposure to the sun may lead to premature aging of the skin and skin cancer.

Water-resistant: Maintains its degree of protection (SPF 15) for 40 minutes or more in water.

Fragrance-free: Free of fragrance that may irritate those with sensitive skin.

Moisturizing: Moisturizing formula helps keep your skin feeling smooth and soft.

Non-comedogenic: Won't clog pores.

Warnings: Do not use if sensitive to cinnamates, benzophenones or any other ingredient in this product. Avoid contact with the eyes, if contact occurs, rinse eyes thoroughly with water. For external use only, not to be swallowed. Discontinue use if signs of irritation or rash appear. Keep this and all drugs out of the reach of children. In case of accidental ingestion, seek professional assistance or contact a Poison Control Center immediately.

Directions for Use: Shake well before using. Before sun exposure, apply evenly and liberally on all exposed areas and reapply after 40 minutes in the water or after excessive sweating. There is no recommended dosage for children under six (6) months of age except under the advice and supervision of a physician.

How Supplied: 4 oz. plastic bottles.
Shown in Product Identification Guide, page 523

ST. JOSEPH®
ADULT CHEWABLE ASPIRIN
Low Strength Tablets (81 mg. each)

Active Ingredient: Each St. Joseph Adult Chewable Aspirin Tablet contains 81 mg. aspirin in a chewable, orange flavored form.

Inactive Ingredients: Corn Starch, FD&C Yellow No. 6 Aluminum Lake, Flavor, Hydrogenated Vegetable Oil, Maltodextrin, Mannitol, Saccharin.

Indications: St. Joseph® Adult Chewable Aspirin Tablets provide safe, effective, temporary relief from: Headaches, muscular aches, minor aches and pain associated with overexertion; sprains; menstrual cramps; neuralgia; bursitis; and discomforts of fever due to colds.

Warnings: Children and teenagers should not use this medicine for chicken pox or flu symptoms before a doctor is consulted about Reye Syndrome, a rare but serious illness reported to be associated with aspirin. If symptoms persist, or new ones occur, consult your doctor. NOTE: SEVERE OR PERSISTENT SORE THROAT, HIGH FEVER, HEADACHE, NAUSEA OR VOMITING, MAY BE SERIOUS, DISCONTINUE USE AND CONSULT YOUR DOCTOR IF NOT RELIEVED IN 24 HOURS. Do not take this product for more than five days unless directed by your doctor. Do not exceed recommended dosage. When using St. Joseph Adult Chewable Aspirin,

do not give any other medications containing aspirin unless directed by your doctor. As with any drug, if you are pregnant or nursing a baby, seek the advice of a health professional before using this product. **IT IS ESPECIALLY IMPORTANT NOT TO USE ASPIRIN THE LAST 3 MONTHS OF PREGNANCY UNLESS SPECIFICALLY DIRECTED TO DO SO BY A DOCTOR BECAUSE IT MAY CAUSE PROBLEMS IN THE UNBORN CHILD OR COMPLICATIONS DURING DELIVERY.** Keep this and all drugs out of reach of children. In case of accidental overdose, seek professional assistance or contact a Poison Control Center immediately.

Dosage and Administration: Take from 4 to 8 tablets (325 mg. to 650 mg.) every 4 hours as needed. Do not exceed 48 tablets in 24 hours. For professional dosage see below.

Professional Labeling: Aspirin for Myocardial Infarction.

Indication: Aspirin is indicated to reduce the risk of death and/or nonfatal myocardial infarction in patients with a previous infarction or unstable angina pectoris.

Clinical Trials: The indication is supported by the results of six large randomized, multicenter, placebo-controlled studies[1-7] involving 10,816 predominantly male post–myocardial infarction (MI) patients and one randomized placebo-controlled study of 1,266 men with unstable angina. Therapy with aspirin was begun at intervals after the onset of acute MI varying from less than three days to more than five years and continued for periods of from less than one year to four years. In the unstable angina study, treatment was started within one month after the onset of unstable angina and continued for 12 weeks, and complicating conditions, such as congestive heart failure, were not included in the study. Aspirin therapy in MI patients was associated with about a 20% reduction in the risk of subsequent death and/or nonfatal reinfarction, a median absolute decrease of 3% from the 12% to 22% event rates in the placebo groups. In the aspirin-treated unstable angina patients, the reduction in risk was about 50%, a reduction in the event rate of 5% from the 10% rate in the placebo group over the 12 weeks of study.

Daily dosage of aspirin in the post-myocardial infarction studies was 300 mg in one study and 900–1,500 mg in five studies. A dose of 325 mg was used in the study of unstable angina.

Adverse Reactions: Gastrointestinal Reactions: Doses of 1,000 mg per day of aspirin caused gastrointestinal symptoms and bleeding that, in some cases, were clinically significant. In the largest postinfarction study (the Aspirin Myocardial Infarction Study [AMIS] with 4,500 people), the percentage of incidences of gastrointestinal symptoms for the aspirin (1,000 mg of a standard, solid-tablet formulation) and placebo-treated subjects, respectively, were stomach pain (14.5%, 4.4%), heartburn, (11.9%, 4.8%), nausea and/or vomiting (7.6%, 2.1%), hospitalization for GI disorder (4.9%, 3.5%). In the AMIS and other trials, aspirin-treated patients had increased rates of gross gastrointestinal bleeding. Symptoms and signs of gastrointestinal irritation were not significantly increased in subjects treated for unstable angina with buffered aspirin in solution.

Cardiovascular and Biochemical: In the AMIS trial, the dosage of 1,000 mg per day of aspirin was associated with small increases in systolic blood pressure (BP) (average 1.5 to 2.1 mm) and diastolic BP (0.5 to 0.6 mm), depending upon whether maximal or last available readings were used. Blood urea nitrogen and uric acid levels were also increased, but by less than 1.0 mg percent. Subjects with marked hypertension or renal insufficiency had been excluded from the trial so that the clinical importance of these observations for such subjects or for any subjects treated over more prolonged periods is not known. It is recommended that patients placed on long-term aspirin treatment, even at doses of 300 mg per day, be seen at regular intervals to assess changes in these measurements.

Dosage and Administration: Although most of the studies used dosage exceeding 300 mg, two trials used only 300 mg daily and pharmacologic data indicate that this dose inhibits platelet function fully. Therefore, 300 mg or 325 mg (4 tablets) aspirin dose daily is a reasonable routine dose that would minimize gastrointestinal adverse reactions.

References:
1. Elwood PC, et al: A randomized controlled trial of acetylsalicylic acid in the secondary prevention of mortality from myocardial infarction, *BR Med J.* 1974;1;436–440.
2. The Coronary Drug Project Research Group: Aspirin in coronary heart disease. *J Chronic Dis.* 1976;29:625–642.
3. Breddin K, et al: Secondary prevention of myocardial infarction: a comparison of acetylsalicylic acid, phenprocoumon or placebo. *Homeostasis.* 1979;470:263–268.
4. Aspirin Myocardial Infarction Study Research Group: A randomized, controlled trial of aspirin in persons recovered from myocardial infarction, *JAMA.* 1980;245:661–669.
5. Elwood PC, and Sweetnam, PM: Aspirin and secondary mortality after myocardial infarction. *Lancet.* December 22–29, 1979, pp 1313–1315.
6. The Persantine-Aspirin Reinfarction Study Research Group: Persantine and aspirin in coronary heart disease. *Circulation.* 1980;62:449–460.
7. Lewis HD. et al: Protective effects of aspirin against acute myocardial infarction and death in men with unstable angina: Results of a Veterans Administration Cooperative Study, *N Engl J Med* 1983;309:396–403.

How Supplied: Chewable, orange flavored tablets in plastic bottles of 36 tablets each.
Shown in Product Identification Guide, page 524

TINACTIN® Antifungal
[*tin-ak 'tin*]
Cream 1%
Solution 1%
Powder 1%
Powder (1%) Aerosol
Liquid (1%) Aerosol
Deodorant Powder Aerosol 1%
Jock Itch Cream 1%
Jock Itch Spray Powder 1%

Description: TINACTIN Cream 1% is a white homogeneous, nonaqueous preparation containing the highly active synthetic fungicidal agent, tolnaftate. Each gram contains 10 mg tolnaftate solubilized in BHT, Carbomer, Monoamylamine, PEG-8, Propylene Glycol, and Titanium Dioxide.
TINACTIN Jock Itch Cream 1% is a smooth white homogeneous cream containing the highly active synthetic fungicidal agent, tolnaftate. Each gram contains 10 mg tolnaftate finely dispersed in a water-washable emulsion containing: Cetearyl Alcohol, Ceteareth-30, Chlorocresol, Mineral Oil, Petrolatum, Propylene Glycol, Sodium Phosphate and Water. Phosphoric acid and sodium hydroxide used to adjust pH.
TINACTIN Solution 1% contains in each ml tolnaftate 10 mg, BHT, and PEG. The solution solidifies at low temperatures but liquefies readily when warmed, retaining its potency.
TINACTIN Liquid Aerosol contains 91 mg tolnaftate in a vehicle of Alcohol SD-40-2 (36%), BHT, Isobutane and PPG-12-Buteth-16. The spray deposits solution containing a concentration of 1% tolnaftate.
Each gram of **TINACTIN Powder 1%** contains tolnaftate 10 mg in a vehicle of corn starch and talc.
TINACTIN Powder Aerosol contains 91 mg tolnaftate in a vehicle of Alcohol SD-40-2 (14% w/w), BHT, Isobutane, PPG-12-Buteth-16 and Talc. The spray deposits a white clinging powder containing a concentration of 1% tolnaftate.
TINACTIN Deodorant Powder Aerosol contains tolnaftate in a vehicle of Isobutane, SD Alcohol 40 (14% w/w), Talc, PPG-12-Buteth-16, Starch/Acrylates/Acrylamide Copolymer, Fragrance, BHT. The spray deposits a white clinging powder containing a concentration of 1% tolnaftate.
TINACTIN Jock Itch Spray Powder contains 91 mg tolnaftate in a vehicle of Alcohol SD-40-2 (14% w/w), BHT, Isobutane, PPG-12 Buteth-16, Talc. The spray deposits a white clinging powder containing a concentration of 1% tolnaftate.

Indications: TINACTIN Cream, Solution, Liquid Aerosol, Powder Aerosol, Powder, and Deodorant Powder Aerosol effectively soothe and relieve symptoms of athlete's foot (tinea pedis), including itching, burning and cracking. Clinically proven to **cure** athlete's foot and when used daily, helps **prevent** it from recurring.
TINACTIN Jock Itch Cream, Jock Itch Powder Aerosol effectively soothes and relieves the painful symptoms of Jock Itch (tinea cruris), including itching, chafing and burning rash. Clinically proven to **cure** Jock Itch.

Warnings: TINACTIN Cream, Powder, Solution and TINACTIN Jock Itch Cream: Do not use on children under 2 years of age unless directed by a doctor. For external use only. Avoid contact with the eyes. If irritation occurs or if there is no improvement within 4 weeks for Athlete's Foot or within 2 weeks for Jock Itch, discontinue use and consult a doctor. Keep this and all drugs out of the reach of children. In case of accidental ingestion, seek professional assistance or contact a Poison Control Center Immediately.
TINACTIN Powder Aerosol, Liquid Aerosol, Deodorant Powder Aerosol and TINACTIN Jock Itch Spray Powder: Do not use on children under 2 years of age unless directed by a doctor. For external use only. If irritation occurs or if there is no improvement within 4 weeks for Athlete's Foot or within 2 weeks for Jock Itch, discontinue use and consult a doctor. Flammable. Do not use while smoking or near heat or flame. Avoid spraying in eyes. Contents under pressure. Do not puncture or incinerate. Do not store at temperature above 120°F. Use only as directed. Intentional misuse by deliberately concentrating and inhaling contents can be harmful or fatal. Keep this and all drugs out of the reach of children. In case of accidental ingestion, seek professional assistance or contact a Poison Control Center Immediately.

Directions: TINACTIN Cream, Solution, Powder and TINACTIN Jock Itch Cream: Wash the affected area and dry thoroughly. Apply a thin layer of the product over the affected area twice daily (morning and night) or as directed by a doctor. Supervise children in the use of this product. For Athlete's Foot: pay special attention to spaces between the toes; wear well-fitting, ventilated shoes and change shoes and socks at least once daily. Use daily for 4 weeks for Athlete's Foot and for 2 weeks for Jock Itch. If condition persists longer, consult a doctor. This product is not effective on the scalp or nails. To prevent Athlete's Foot, apply once or twice daily (morning and/or night).

Continued on next page

Information on Schering-Plough HealthCare Products appearing on these pages is effective as of November 1994.

Schering-Plough—Cont.

TINACTIN Powder Aerosol, Deodorant Powder Aerosol, Liquid Aerosol and TINACTIN Jock Itch Spray Powder: Wash the affected area and dry thoroughly. Shake can well. Spray a thin layer of the product over the affected area twice daily (morning and night) or as directed by a doctor. Supervise children in the use of this product. For Athlete's Foot: pay special attention to spaces between the toes; wear well-fitting, ventilated shoes and change shoes and socks at least once daily. Use daily for 4 weeks for Athlete's Foot and for 2 weeks for Jock Itch. If condition persists longer, consult a doctor. This product is not effective on the scalp or nails. To prevent Athlete's Foot, apply once or twice daily (morning and/or night).

How Supplied: TINACTIN Antifungal Cream 1%, 15 g (½ oz) and 30 g (1 oz) collapsible tube with dispensing tip. **TINACTIN Antifungal Solution 1%,** 10 ml (⅓ oz) plastic squeeze bottle. **TINACTIN Antifungal Liquid (1%) Aerosol,** 113 g (4 oz) spray can. **TINACTIN Antifungal Powder 1%,** 45 g (1.5 oz) and 90 g (3.0 oz) plastic containers. **TINACTIN Antifungal Powder (1%) Aerosol,** 100 g (3.5 oz) and 150 g (5.0 oz) spray containers. TINACTIN Antifungal Deodorant Powder Aerosol 100 g (3.5 oz.) spray container. **TINACTIN Antifungal Jock Itch Cream 1%,** 15 g (½ oz) collapsible tube with dispensing tip. **TINACTIN Antifungal Jock Itch Spray Powder (1%),** 100 g (3.5 oz) spray can.
Store TINACTIN products between 36° and 86°F (2° and 30°C).
Shown in Product Identification Guide, page 524

Scot-Tussin Pharmacal Co., Inc.
P.O. BOX 8217
CRANSTON, RI 02920-0217

The following SCOT-TUSSIN® may be taken by individuals with diabetes, heart condition and/or high blood pressure and/or on Sugar restricted diet.

SCOT-TUSSIN SUGAR-FREE DM
Antitussive-Antihistaminic
Dextromethorphan
Chlorpheniramine Maleate

(Dextromethorphan 15 mg/5 ml, chlorpheniramine maleate 2 mg/5 ml).
No alcohol, sorbitol, saccharin, or decongestant.
#036

SCOT-TUSSIN® SUGAR-FREE ALLERGY RELIEF FORMULA
Antihistaminic
Diphenhydramine HCl

(Diphenhydramine HCl 12.5 mg/5 ml). No alcohol, sorbitol, saccharin, dye.
#047-04

SCOT-TUSSIN® SUGAR-FREE COUGH CHASERS Lozenges
Antitussive
Dextromethorphan

No sodium, dye. DM 2.5 mg/lozenge.
#044-20

SCOT-TUSSIN® SUGAR-FREE; ALCOHOL-FREE EXPECTORANT
Guaifenesin

(Guaifenesin 100 mg/5 ml). No alcohol, sorbitol, sodium, dye, saccharin.
#006-04

Smart Pharmaceuticals, Inc./SMARTRX@AOL.COM
214 E. 16TH STREET
VANCOUVER, WA 98663-3409

HEALTHPRIN™ BRAND ASPIRIN
Adult Low Strength 81 mg. tablets and 162.5 mg half-dose tablets and 325 mg full strength tablets.
THIS PRODUCT NOT FOR CHILDREN OR TEENAGERS

Active Ingredient: Acetylsalicylic Acid (Aspirin)

Consumer Information: Healthprin® brand aspirin is available in 81 mg white heart-shaped tablets, 162.5 mg pink, heart-shaped tablets and 325 mg white, heart-shaped tablets. The 325 mg white, heart-shaped tablet will be available the second quarter of '95. All tablets are bisected for easy splitting. Tablets have a heart imprint on both sides except the 325 mg. tablet which has the heart imprint on one side and the word SMART on the other side.

OBSERVE WARNINGS ON BOTTOM OF BOX

Important: See your doctor before taking this product for your heart or for other new uses of aspirin, because serious side effects could occur with self treatment.

Directions: For simple headache relief take 4–8 tablets (325mg–650mg) with a full glass of water every four hours as needed or while symptoms persist. Not to exceed 48 tablets in 24 hours, or as directed by a doctor. Unlike other aspirins, 100% pure Healthprin™ does not contain artificial flavors or colors. Nor will you find saccharin, sugar or sodium. In addition, Healthprin™ has no caffeine or preservatives. The coating on each tablet makes swallowing easy, no aspirin taste in the mouth or throat and offers

protection from moisture and potency loss.

Warnings: Follow the usual directions and standard warnings for aspirin. Observe warnings on package.

How Supplied: Healthprin® brand aspirin is supplied in a 100 tablet count bottle in box and a 500 tablet count stand alone bottle with a retail list price of under 1 cent per dose.

Drug Interaction Precaution: Do not take this product if you are taking a prescription drug for anticoagulation (thinning of the blood), diabetes, gout, or arthritis unless directed by a doctor. Heart shape tablet and imprint, trademarks of Smart Pharmaceuticals.
Shown in Product Identification Guide, page 524

SmithKline Beecham Consumer Healthcare, L.P.
Unit of SmithKline Beecham, Inc.
POST OFFICE BOX 1467
PITTSBURGH, PA 15230

CĒPASTAT®
[sē'pə-stăt]
Sore Throat Lozenges
Cherry Flavor and Extra Strength

Description: Each <u>Cherry Flavor</u> lozenge contains: Phenol 14.5 mg. Also contains: Antifoam Emulsion, D&C Red No. 33, FD&C Yellow No. 6, Flavor, Gum Crystal, Mannitol, Menthol, Saccharin Sodium, and Sorbitol.
Each <u>Extra Strength</u> lozenge contains: Phenol 29 mg. Also contains: Antifoam Emulsion, Caramel, Eucalyptus Oil, Gum Crystal, Mannitol, Menthol, Saccharin Sodium, and Sorbitol.

Actions: Phenol is a recognized topical anesthetic. The sugar-free formula should not promote tooth decay as sugar-based lozenges can.

Indications: For fast, temporary relief of minor sore throat pain.

Warnings: If sore throat is severe, persists for more than 2 days, is accompanied or followed by fever, headache, rash, nausea, or vomiting, consult a physician promptly. If sore mouth symptoms do not improve in 7 days, see your dentist or physician promptly. Keep this and all drugs out of the reach of children. In case of accidental overdose, seek professional assistance or contact a Poison Control Center immediately. As with any drug, if you are pregnant or nursing a baby, seek the advice of a health professional before using this product.
Note to Diabetics: Each lozenge contributes approximately 8 calories from 2 grams of sorbitol.

Dosage and Administration:
<u>Lozenges–Cherry Flavor</u>
Adults and children 12 years of age and older: Allow the lozenge to dissolve

slowly in the mouth. May be repeated every 2 hours, not to exceed 18 lozenges per day, or as directed by a dentist or physician. Children 6 to under 12 years of age: Allow lozenge to dissolve slowly in the mouth. May be repeated every 2 hours, not to exceed 10 lozenges per day, or as directed by a dentist or physician. Children under 6 years of age: Consult a dentist or physician.

Lozenges–Extra Strength

Adults and children 12 years of age and older: Allow the lozenge to dissolve slowly in the mouth. May be repeated every 2 hours, or as directed by a dentist or physician. Children 6 to under 12 years of age: Allow lozenge to dissolve slowly in the mouth. May be repeated every 2 hours, not to exceed 10 lozenges per day, or as directed by a dentist or physician. Children under 6 years of age: Consult a dentist or physician.

How Supplied:

Lozenges–Cherry Flavor

Trade package: Boxes of 18 lozenges as 2 pocket packs of 9 lozenges each.

Lozenges–Extra Strength

Trade package: Boxes of 18 lozenges as 2 pocket packs of 9 lozenges each. Store at room temperature, below 86°F (30°C). Protect contents from humidity.

Shown in Product Identification Guide, page 524

Orange Flavor
CITRUCEL®
[sĭt 'rə-sĕl]
(Methylcellulose)
Bulk-forming Fiber Laxative

Description: Each 19 g adult dose (approximately one heaping measuring tablespoonful) contains Methylcellulose 2 g. Each 9.5 g child's dose (one-half the adult dose) contains Methylcellulose 1 g. Methylcellulose is a nonallergenic fiber. Also contains: Citric Acid, FD&C Yellow No. 6, Orange Flavors (natural and artificial), Potassium Citrate, Riboflavin, Sucrose, and other ingredients. Each adult dose contains approximately 3 mg of sodium, 105 mg of potassium, and contributes 60 calories from Sucrose.

Actions: Promotes elimination by providing additional fiber (bulk) to the diet. This product generally produces bowel movement in 12 to 72 hours.

Indications: For relief of constipation (irregularity). May also be used for relief of constipation associated with other bowel disorders such as irritable bowel syndrome, diverticular disease, and hemorrhoids as well as for bowel management during postpartum, postsurgical, and convalescent periods when recommended by a physician.

Contraindications: Intestinal obstruction, fecal impaction, known hypersensitivity to formula ingredients.

Warnings: Patients should be instructed to consult their physician before using any laxative if they have noticed a sudden change in bowel habits which persists for two weeks. Unless directed by a physician, patients should be advised not to use laxative products when abdominal pain, nausea, or vomiting is present. Patients should also be advised to discontinue use and consult a physician if rectal bleeding or failure to have a bowel movement occurs after use of any laxative product. Unless recommended by a physician, patients should not exceed the recommended maximum daily dose. Patients should not use laxative products for a period longer than one week unless directed by a physician. **TAKING THIS PRODUCT WITHOUT ADEQUATE FLUID MAY CAUSE IT TO SWELL AND BLOCK YOUR THROAT OR ESOPHAGUS AND MAY CAUSE CHOKING. DO NOT TAKE THIS PRODUCT IF YOU HAVE DIFFICULTY IN SWALLOWING. IF YOU EXPERIENCE CHEST PAIN, VOMITING, OR DIFFICULTY IN SWALLOWING OR BREATHING AFTER TAKING THIS PRODUCT, SEEK IMMEDIATE MEDICAL ATTENTION. KEEP THIS AND ALL DRUGS OUT OF THE REACH OF CHILDREN.**

Dosage and Administration: Adult Dose: *one rounded tablespoonful* (19 g) stirred briskly into at least 8 ounces of cold water up to three times daily at the first sign of constipation. Children age 6 to 12 years of age: *one-half the adult dose* stirred briskly into at least 8 ounces of cold water, once daily at the first sign of constipation. The mixture should be administered promptly and drinking another glass of water is highly recommended (see warnings). Children under 6 years of age: *Use only as directed by a physician.* Continued use for 12 to 72 hours may be necessary for full benefit. **TAKE THIS PRODUCT (CHILD OR ADULT DOSE) WITH AT LEAST 8 OZ. (A FULL GLASS) OF WATER OR OTHER FLUID. TAKING THIS PRODUCT WITHOUT ENOUGH LIQUID MAY CAUSE CHOKING. SEE WARNINGS.**

How Supplied: 16 oz. and 30 oz. containers.
Boxes of 20-single-dose packets.
Store below 86°F (30°C). Protect contents from humidity; keep tightly closed.
Shown in Product Identification Guide, page 524

Sugar Free Orange Flavor
CITRUCEL®
[sĭt 'rə-sĕl]
(Methylcellulose)
Bulk-forming Fiber Laxative

Description: Each 10.2 g adult dose (approximately one rounded measuring tablespoonful) contains Methylcellulose 2 g. Each 5.1 g child's dose (one-half the adult dose) contains Methylcellulose 1 g. Methylcellulose is a nonallergenic fiber. Also contains: Aspartame*, Dibasic Calcium Phosphate, FD&C Yellow No. 6, Malic Acid, Maltodextrin, Orange Flavors (natural and artificial), Potassium Citrate and Riboflavin. Each 10.2 g dose contributes 24 calories from Maltodextrin.

Actions: Promotes elimination by providing additional fiber (bulk) to the diet. This product generally produces bowel movement in 12 to 72 hours.

Indications: For relief of constipation (irregularity). May also be used for relief of constipation associated with other bowel disorders such as irritable bowel syndrome, diverticular disease, and hemorrhoids as well as for bowel management during postpartum, postsurgical, and convalescent periods when recommended by a physician.

Contraindications: Intestinal obstruction, fecal impaction, known hypersensitivity to formula ingredients.

Warnings: Patients should be instructed to consult their physician before using any laxative if they have noticed a sudden change in bowel habits which persists for two weeks. Unless directed by a physician, patients should be advised not to use laxative products when abdominal pain, nausea, or vomiting is present. Patients should also be advised to discontinue use and consult a physician if rectal bleeding or failure to have a bowel movement occurs after use of any laxative product. Unless recommended by a physician, patients should not exceed the recommended maximum daily dose. Patients should not use laxative products for a period longer than one week unless directed by a physician. **TAKING THIS PRODUCT WITHOUT ADEQUATE FLUID MAY CAUSE IT TO SWELL AND BLOCK YOUR THROAT OR ESOPHAGUS AND MAY CAUSE CHOKING. DO NOT TAKE THIS PRODUCT IF YOU HAVE DIFFICULTY IN SWALLOWING. IF YOU EXPERIENCE CHEST PAIN, VOMITING, OR DIFFICULTY IN SWALLOWING OR BREATHING AFTER TAKING THIS PRODUCT, SEEK IMMEDIATE MEDICAL ATTENTION. KEEP THIS AND ALL DRUGS OUT OF THE REACH OF CHILDREN.**
Phenylketonurics: CONTAINS PHENYLALANINE 52 mg per adult dose. Individuals with phenylketonuria and other individuals who must restrict their intake of phenylalanine should be warned that each 10.2 g adult dose contains aspartame which provides 52 mg of phenylalanine.

Dosage and Administration: Adult Dose: *one rounded tablespoonful* (10.2 g) stirred briskly into at least 8 ounces of cold water up to three times daily at the first sign of constipation. Children age 6 to 12 years of age: *one-half the adult dose* stirred briskly into at least 8 ounces of cold water, once daily at the first sign of constipation. The mixture should be administered promptly and drinking another glass of water is highly recommended (see warnings). Children under 6 years of age: *Use only as directed by a*

Continued on next page

SmithKline Beecham—Cont.

physician. Continued use for 12 to 72 hours may be necessary for full benefit. **TAKE THIS PRODUCT (CHILD OR ADULT DOSE) WITH AT LEAST 8 OZ. (A FULL GLASS) OF WATER OR OTHER FLUID. TAKING THIS PRODUCT WITHOUT ENOUGH LIQUID MAY CAUSE CHOKING. SEE WARNINGS.**

How Supplied:
8.6 oz and 16.9 oz containers.
Boxes of 20 single-dose packets.
Store below 86°F (30°C). Protect contents from humidity; keep tightly closed.

*NutraSweet and the NutraSweet symbol are trademarks of the NutraSweet Company.

Shown in Product Identification Guide, page 524

CONTAC
Day & Night Allergy/Sinus

Product Information: Contac Day & Night Allergy/Sinus includes 15 day caplets and 5 night caplets in each package to provide:
● 5 days of relief from stuffy nose, sinus pressure and headache pain without drowsiness.
● 5 nights of relief from stuffy, runny nose, sinus pressure, sneezing and headache pain to let your rest.

Day Caplets
Product Benefits: Contac Day Caplets provide an ANALGESIC and a DECONGESTANT.

Indications: Temporarily relieves headache pain and nasal congestion due to hay fever or other upper respiratory allergies or associated with sinusitis. Promotes nasal and/or sinus drainage; temporarily relieves sinus congestion and pressure.

Directions: Adults (12 years and older): Take one White Day Caplet every 6 hours, or as directed by a doctor. DO NOT EXCEED A TOTAL OF 4 CAPLETS (whether all Day or all Night or combination of each) IN 24 HOURS. ALL CAPLETS SHOULD BE TAKEN AT LEAST 6 HOURS APART. Children under 12 years of age: Consult a doctor.

Night Caplets
Product Benefits: Contac Night Caplets provide an ANALGESIC, an ANTIHISTAMINE, and a DECONGESTANT

Indication: Temporarily relieves headache pain and nasal congestion, runny nose, sneezing and itchy, watery eyes due to hay fever or other upper respiratory allergies or associated with sinusitis. Promotes nasal and/or sinus drainage; temporarily relieves sinus congestion and pressure.

Directions: Adults (12 years and older): Take one Green Night Caplet every 6 hours, or as directed by a doctor. DO NOT EXCEED A TOTAL OF 4 CAP-

LETS (whether all Day or all Night or combination of each) IN 24 HOURS. ALL CAPLETS SHOULD BE TAKEN AT LEAST 6 HOURS APART. Children under 12 years of age: Consult a doctor.

Warnings for Day and Night Caplets: Do not take this product for more than 10 days. If symptoms do not improve or are accompanied by fever that lasts for more than 3 days, or if new symptoms occur, consult a doctor. Do not take this product, unless directed by a doctor, if you have a breathing problem such as emphysema or chronic bronchitis, or if you have heart disease, high blood pressure, thyroid disease, diabetes, glaucoma or difficulty in urination due to enlargement of the prostate gland. **Do not exceed recommended dosage.** If nervousness, dizziness, or sleeplessness occur, discontinue use and consult a doctor. **KEEP THIS AND ALL DRUGS OUT OF THE REACH OF CHILDREN.** Prompt medical attention is critical for adults as well as for children even if you do not notice any signs or symptoms. In case of accidental overdose, seek professional assistance or contact a Poison Control Center immediately. As with any drug, if you are pregnant or nursing a baby, seek the advice of a health professional before using this product.

Additional Warnings for Night Caplets: May cause excitability especially in children. May cause marked drowsiness; alcohol, sedatives, and tranquilizers may increase the drowsiness effect. Avoid alcoholic beverages while taking this product. Do not take this product if you are taking sedatives or tranquilizers, without first consulting your doctor. Use caution when driving a motor vehicle or operating machinery.

Drug Interaction Precaution: Do not use this product if you are now taking a prescription monoamine oxidase inhibitor (MAOI) (certain drugs for depression, psychiatric or emotional conditions, or Parkinson's disease), or for 2 weeks after stopping the MAOI drug. If you are uncertain whether your prescription drug contains an MAOI, consult a health professional before taking this product.

Active Ingredients: EACH DAY AND NIGHT CAPLET CONTAINS: Acetaminophen 650 mg, Pseudoephedrine Hydrochloride 60 mg. NIGHT CAPLETS ALSO CONTAIN: Diphenhydramine Hydrochloride 50 mg.

Inactive Ingredients: EACH DAY AND NIGHT CAPLET CONTAINS: Hydroxpropyl Methylcellulose, Magnesium Stearate, Microcrystalline Cellulose, Polyethylene Glycol, Polysorbate 80, Silicon Dioxide, Starch, Stearic Acid, Titanium Dioxide. NIGHT CAPLETS ALSO CONTAIN: D&C Yellow 10, FD&C Blue 1, FD&C Yellow 6.

How Supplied: Consumer package of 5 Night Caplets and 15 Day Caplets (see previous Day Caplet listing).

Note: There are other CONTAC products. Make sure this is the one you are interested in.

Shown in Product Identification Guide, page 524

CONTAC
Day & Night Cold/Flu

Composition:

Product Information: Contac Day & Night Cold/Flu includes 15 day caplets and 5 night caplets in each package to provide:
● 5 days of relief from stuffy nose, coughing and aches and pains without drowsiness
● 5 nights of relief from stuffy runny, nose, sneezing and aches and pains to let you rest.

Day Caplets

Product Benefits: Contac Day Caplets provide an ANALGESIC, a DECONGESTANT, and a COUGH SUPPRESSANT.

Indications: For the temporary relief of headache, minor aches and pains, fever, nasal congestion and coughs due to the common cold or flu.

Directions: Adults (12 years and older): Take one Yellow Day Caplet every 6 hours, or as directed by a doctor. DO NOT EXCEED A TOTAL OF 4 CAPLETS (whether all Day or all Night or combination of each) IN 24 HOURS. ALL CAPLETS SHOULD BE TAKEN AT LEAST 6 HOURS APART. Children under 12 years of age: Consult a doctor.

Night Caplets

Product Benefits: Contac Night Caplets provide an ANALGESIC, an ANTIHISTAMINE, and a DECONGESTANT.

Indications: For the temporary relief of headache minor aches and pains, fever, nasal congestion, runny nose, and sneezing due to the common cold and flu.

Directions: Adults (12 years and older): Take one Blue Night Caplet every 6 hours, or as directed by a doctor. DO NOT EXCEED A TOTAL OF 4 CAPLETS (whether all Day or all Night or combination of each) IN 24 HOURS. ALL CAPLETS SHOULD BE TAKEN AT LEAST 6 HOURS APART. Children under 12 years of age: Consult a doctor.

Warnings for Day and Night Caplets: Do not take this product for more than 10 days. If symptoms do not improve or are accompanied by fever that lasts for more than 3 days, or if new symptoms occur, consult a doctor. Do not take this product, unless directed by a doctor, if you have a breathing problem such as emphysema or chronic bronchitis, or if you have heart disease, high blood pressure, thyroid disease, diabetes, glaucoma or difficulty in urination due to enlargement of the prostate gland. **Do not exceed recommended dosage.** If nervousness, dizziness, or sleeplessness occur, discontinue use and consult a doctor. **KEEP THIS AND ALL DRUGS OUT**

OF THE REACH OF CHILDREN.
Prompt medical attention is critical for adults as well as for children even if you do not notice any signs or symptoms. In case of accidental overdose, seek professional assistance or contact a Poison Control Center immediately. As with any drug, if you are pregnant or nursing a baby, seek the advice of a health professional before using this product.

Additional Warnings for Day Caplets: A persistent cough may be a sign of a serious condition. If cough persists for more than 7 days, tends to recur, or is accompanied by rash, persistent headache, fever that lasts for more than 3 days, or if new symptoms occur, consult a doctor. Do not take this product for persistent or chronic cough such as occurs with smoking, asthma, emphysema, or if cough is accompanied by excessive phlegm (mucus) unless directed by a doctor.

Additional Warnings for Night Caplets: May cause excitability especially in children. May cause marked drowsiness; alcohol, sedatives, and tranquilizers may increase the drowsiness effect. Avoid alcoholic beverages while taking this product. Do not take this product if you are taking sedatives or tranquilizers, without first consulting your doctor. Use caution when driving a motor vehicle or operating machinery.

Drug Interaction Precaution: Do not use this product if you are now taking a prescription monoamine oxidase inhibitor (MAOI) (certain drugs for depression, psychiatric or emotional conditions, or Parkinson's disease), or for 2 weeks after stopping the MAOI drug. If you are uncertain whether your prescription drug contains an MAOI, consult a health professional before taking this product.

Active Ingredients: EACH DAY CAPLET CONTAINS: Acetaminophen 650 mg, Pseudoephedrine Hydrochloride 60 mg. Dextromethorphan Hydrobromide 30 mg. EACH NIGHT CAPLET CONTAINS: Acetaminophen 650 mg, Pseudoephedrine Hydrochloride 60 mg, Diphenhydramine Hydrochloride 50 mg.

Inactive Ingredients: EACH DAY AND NIGHT CAPLET CONTAINS: Hydroxypropyl Methylcellulose, Magnesium Stearate, Microcrystalline Cellulose, Polyethylene Glycol, Polysorbate 80, Silicon Dioxide, Starch, Stearic Acid, Titanium Dioxide. DAY CAPLETS ALSO CONTAIN: D&C Yellow 10, FD&C Yellow 6. NIGHT CAPLETS ALSO CONTAIN: FD&C Blue 1.

How Supplied: Consumer package of 5 Night Caplets and 15 Day Caplets (see previous Day Caplet listing).
Note: There are other CONTAC products. Make sure this is the one you are interested in.
Shown in Product Identification Guide, page 524

**CONTAC®
MAXIMUM STRENGTH
Continuous Action Nasal
Decongestant/Antihistamine
12 Hour Caplets**

Composition: [See table on next page.]
Product Information: Each CONTAC Maximum Strength timed release caplet provides up to 12 hours of relief. Part of the caplet goes to work right away for fast relief; the rest is released gradually to provide up to 12 hours of prolonged relief. With just *one* caplet in the morning and *one* at bedtime, you feel better all day, sleep better at night, breathing freely without congestion. CONTAC Maximum Strength provides:
● A NASAL DECONGESTANT which helps clear nasal passages, shrinks swollen membranes and helps decongest sinus openings.
● AN ANTIHISTAMINE at the maximum level to help relieve itchy, watery eyes, sneezing, and runny nose.

Indications: For temporary relief of nasal congestion due to the common cold, hay fever or other upper respiratory allergies, and nasal congestion associated with sinusitis.

Directions: Adults and children 12 years of age and older: One caplet every 12 hours, not to exceed 2 caplets in 24 hours, or as directed by a doctor. Children under 12 years of age: consult a doctor.
NOTE: The nonactive portion of the caplet that supplies the active ingredients may occasionally appear in your stool as a soft mass.
TAMPER-RESISTANT PACKAGING FEATURES FOR YOUR PROTECTION:
Each caplet is encased in a plastic cell with a foil back; do not use if cell or foil is broken. The name CONTAC appears on each caplet; do not use this product if the CONTAC name is missing.
This carton is protected by a clear overwrap printed with "safety-sealed"; do not use if overwrap is missing or broken.

Warnings: Do not exceed recommended dosage. If nervousness, dizziness or sleeplessness occur, discontinue use and consult a doctor. If symptoms do not improve within 7 days or are accompanied by fever, consult a physician before continuing use. Do not take this product unless directed by a doctor, if you have a breathing problem such as emphysema, heart disease, high blood pressure, thyroid disease, diabetes, or chronic bronchitis, or if you have glaucoma or difficulty in urination due to enlargement of the prostate gland. Do not take this product if you are taking another medication containing phenylpropanolamine. May cause drowsiness; alcohol, sedatives and tranquilizers may increase the drowsiness effect. Avoid alcoholic beverages while taking this product. Do not take this product if you are taking sedatives or tranquilizers, without first consulting your doctor. Do not

drive or operate heavy machinery. May cause excitability, especially in children. Keep this and all drugs out of reach of children. In case of accidental overdose, seek professional assistance or contact a poison control center immediately. As with any drug, if you are pregnant or nursing a baby, seek the advice of a health professional before using this product. Store at controlled room temperature (59°–86°F).

Drug Interaction Precaution: Do not use this product if you are now taking a prescription monoamine oxidase inhibitor (MAOI) (certain drugs for depression, psychiatric or emotional conditions or Parkinson's disease), or for 2 weeks after stopping the MAOI drug. If you are uncertain whether your prescription drug contains an MAOI, consult a health professional before taking this product.

Formula: Active Ingredients: Each Maximum Strength caplet contains Phenylpropanolamine Hydrochloride 75 mg.; Chlorpheniramine Maleate 12 mg. (which is a higher dose of antihistamine than CONTAC capsules). **Inactive Ingredients (listed for individuals with specific allergies):** Acetylated Monoglycerides, Carnauba Wax, Colloidal Silicon Dioxide, Ethylcellulose, Hydroxypropyl Methylcellulose, Lactose, Stearic Acid, Titanium Dioxide.

How Supplied: Consumer packages of 10, 20 and 40 caplets.
Note: There are other CONTAC products. Make sure this is the one you are interested in.
Shown in Product Identification Guide, page 524

**CONTAC®
Continuous Action Nasal
Decongestant/Antihistamine
12 Hour Capsules**

Composition: [See table on next page.]
Product Information: Each CONTAC time release capsule contains over 600 "tiny time pills." Some go to work right away. The rest are scientifically timed to dissolve slowly to give up to 12 hours of relief.

Indications: For temporary relief of nasal congestion due to the common cold, hay fever or other upper respiratory allergies, associated with sinusitis. Helps decongest sinus openings, and passages; temporarily relieves sinus congestion and pressure. For the temporary relief of runny nose, sneezing, itching of the nose and throat, and itchy and watery eyes due to hay fever or other upper respiratory allergies.

Directions: Adults and children over 12 years of age: One capsule every 12 hours, not to exceed 2 capsules in 24 hours, or as directed by a doctor. Children under 12 years of age: consult a doctor.

Continued on next page

SmithKline Beecham—Cont.

TAMPER-RESISTANT PACKAGING FEATURES FOR YOUR PROTECTION:
Each capsule is encased in a plastic cell with a foil back; do not use if cell or foil is broken. Each CONTAC capsule is protected by a red Perma-Seal™ band which bonds the two capsule halves together; do not use if capsule or band is broken.
This carton is protected by a clear overwrap printed with "safety-sealed"; do not use if overwrap is missing or broken.

Warnings: Do not exceed the recommended dosage. If nervousness, dizziness, or sleeplessness occur, discontinue use and consult a doctor. If symptoms do not improve within 7 days or are accompanied by high fever, consult a doctor. Do not take this product, unless directed by a doctor, if you have a breathing problem such as emphysema or chronic bronchitis, or if you have heart disease, high blood pressure, thyroid disease, diabetes, glaucoma or difficulty in urination due to enlargement of the prostate gland. Do not take this product if you are taking another medication containing phenylpropanolamine. Use caution when driving a motor vehicle or operating machinery. May cause drowsiness; alcohol, sedatives and tranquilizers may increase the drowsiness effect. Avoid alcoholic beverages while taking this product. Do not take this product if you are taking sedatives or tranquilizers, without first consulting your doctor. May cause excitability especially in children. KEEP THIS AND ALL DRUGS OUT OF REACH OF CHILDREN. IN CASE OF ACCIDENTAL OVERDOSE, SEEK PROFESSIONAL ASSISTANCE OR CONTACT A POISON CONTROL CENTER IMMEDIATELY. As with any drug, if you are pregnant or nursing a baby, seek the advice of a health professional before using this product. Store at controlled room temperature (59°–86°F).

Drug Interaction Precaution: Do not use this product if you are now taking a prescription monoamine oxidase inhibitor (MAOI) (certain drugs for depression, psychiatric or emotional conditions, or Parkinson's disease), or for 2 weeks after stopping the MAOI drug. If you are uncertain whether your prescription drug contains an MAOI, consult a health professional before taking this product.

Each Capsule Contains: Phenylpropanolamine Hydrochloride 75 mg. and Chlorpheniramine Maleate 8 mg. Also Contains: Benzyl Alcohol, Butylparaben, D&C Red No. 33, D&C Yellow No. 10, Edetate Calcium Disodium, FD&C Red No. 3, FD&C Yellow No. 6, Gelatin, Methylparaben, Pharmaceutical Glaze, Propylparaben, Sodium Lauryl Sulfate, Sodium Propionate, Starch, Sucrose and other ingredients, may also contain: Polysorbate 80.

How Supplied: Consumer packages of 10, 20 and 40 capsules.
Note: There are other CONTAC products. Make sure this is the one you are interested in.
Shown in Product Identification Guide, page 524

CONTAC®
Severe Cold and Flu
Caplets
Analgesic • Decongestant
Antihistamine • Cough Suppressant

Composition: [See table below.]

Product Information: Two caplets every 6 hours to help relieve the discomforts of severe colds with flu-like symptoms.

Product Benefits: CONTAC Severe Cold and Flu contains a Non-Aspirin Analgesic, a Decongestant, an Antihistamine and a Cough Suppressant.

Indications: Provides temporary relief from nasal and sinus congestion, runny nose, sneezing, coughing, fever, headache and minor aches associated with the common cold, sore throat and the flu.

Directions: Adults (12 years and over): Two caplets every 6 hours, not to exceed 8 caplets in any 24-hour period, or as directed by a doctor.
TAMPER-RESISTANT PACKAGING FEATURES FOR YOUR PROTECTION:
Caplets are encased in a plastic cell with a foil back; do not use if cell or foil is broken. The letters SCF appear on each caplet; do not use this product if these letters are missing.
This carton is protected by a clean overwrap printed with "safety-sealed"; do not use if overwrap is missing or broken.

Warnings: Do not take this product for more than 10 days. If symptoms do not improve or are accompanied by fever that lasts for more than 3 days, or if new symptoms occur, consult a doctor. If sore throat is severe, persists for more than 2 days, is accompanied or followed by fever, headache, rash, nausea, or vomiting, consult a doctor promptly. A persistent cough may be a sign of a serious condition. If cough persists for more than 7 days, tends to recur, or is accompanied by rash, persistent headache, fever that lasts for more than 3 days, or if new symptoms occur, consult a doctor. Do not take this product for persistent or chronic cough such as occurs with smoking, asthma, emphysema, or if cough is accompanied by excessive phlegm (mucus) unless directed by a doctor. May cause excitability especially in children. Do not take this product, unless directed by a doctor, if you have a breathing problem such as emphysema or chronic bronchitis, or if you have heart disease, high blood pressure, thyroid disease, diabetes, glaucoma or difficulty in urination due to enlargement of the prostate gland. May cause marked drowsiness: alcohol, sedatives, and tranquilizers may increase the drowsiness effect. Avoid taking alcoholic beverages while taking this product. Do not take this product if you are taking sedatives or tranquilizers, without first consulting your doctor. Use caution when driving a motor vehicle or operating machinery. **Do not exceed recommended dosage.** If nervousness,

---

PDR For Nonprescription Drugs

CONTAC

	CONTACT 12 Hour Cold Caplets	CONTACT 12 Hour Cold Capsules	CONTAC Severe Cold and Flu Caplets (each 2 caplet dose)	CONTAC Severe Cold and Flu Hot Medicine Drink (each Packet dose)	CONTAC Severe Cold and Flu Non-Drowsy Caplet (each 2 caplet dose)	CONTAC Day & Night Cold & Flu Day Caplets	CONTAC Day & Night Cold & Flu Night Caplets
Phenylpropanolamine HCl	75.0 mg	75.0 mg	25.0 mg	—	—	—	—
Chlorpheniramine Maleate	12.0 mg	8.0 mg	4.0 mg	4.0 mg	—	—	—
Pseudoephedrine HCl	—	—	—	60.0 mg	60.0 mg	60.0 mg	60.0 mg
Acetaminophen	—	—	1000.0 mg	650.0 mg	650.0 mg	650.0 mg	650.0 mg
Dextropmethorphan Hydrobromide	—	—	30.0 mg	20.0 mg	30.0 mg	30.0 mg	—
Diphenhydramine HCl	—	—	—	—	—	—	50.0 mg

dizziness, or sleeplessness occur, discontinue use and consult a doctor. **KEEP THIS AND ALL DRUGS OUT OF THE REACH OF CHILDREN.** Prompt medical attention is critical for adults as well as for children even if you do not notice any signs or symptoms. In case of accidental overdose, seek professional assistance or contact a Poison Control Center immediately. As with any drug, if you are pregnant or nursing a baby, seek the advice of a health professional before using this product.

Drug Interaction Precaution: Do not use this product if you are now taking a prescription monoamine oxidase inhibitor (MAOI) (certain drugs for depression, psychiatric or emotional conditions, or Parkinson's disease), or for 2 weeks after stopping the MAOI drug. If you are uncertain whether your prescription drug contains an MAOI, consult a health professional before taking this product.

Formula: Active Ingredients: Each caplet contains Acetaminophen, 500 mg., Dextromethorphan Hydrobromide, 15 mg.; Phenylpropanolamine Hydrochloride, 12.5 mg.; Chlorpheniramine Maleate, 2 mg. **Inactive Ingredients (listed for individuals with specific allergies):** Cellulose, FD&C Blue 1, Hydroxypropyl Methylcellulose, Polyethylene Glycol, Polysorbate 80, Povidone, Sodium Starch Glycolate, Starch, Stearic Acid, Titanium Dioxide.
Avoid storing at high temperature (greater than 100°F).

How Supplied: Consumer packages of 16 and 30 caplets.

Note: There are other CONTAC products. Make sure this is the one you are interested in.
Shown in Product Identification Guide, page 524

CONTAC
Severe Cold and Flu
Non-Drowsy
Caplets
Decongestant * Analgesic
Cough Suppressant

Product Information: Two caplets every 6 hours to help relieve, without drowsiness, the discomfort of severe colds with flu-like symptoms.
Product Benefits: Contac Severe Cold and Flu Non-Drowsy contains a NON-ASPIRIN ANALGESIC, a DECONGESTANT, and a COUGH SUPPRESSANT.

Indications: Provides temporary relief from nasal and sinus congestion, coughing, fever, headache and minor aches associated with the common cold, sore throat and the flu.

Directions: Adults (12 years and older): Two caplets every 6 hours, not to exceed 8 caplets in any 24-hour period, or as directed by a doctor.
TAMPER-RESISTANT PACKAGING FEATURES FOR YOUR PROTECTION: Caplets are encased in a plastic cell with a foil back; do not use if cell or foil is bro-

ken. The letters ND SCF appear on each caplet, do not use this product if these letters are missing.
This carton is protected by a clean overwrap with "safety sealed"; do not use if overwrap is missing or broken.

Warnings: Do not take this product for more than 10 days. If symptoms do not improve or are accompanied by fever that lasts for more than 3 days, or if new symptoms occur, consult a doctor. If sore throat is severe, persists for more than 2 days, is accompanied or followed by fever, headache, rash, nausea, or vomiting, consult a doctor promptly. A persistent cough may be a sign of a serious condition. If cough persists for more than 7 days, tends to recur, or is accompanied by rash, persistent headache, fever that lasts for more than 3 days, or if new symptoms occur, consult a doctor. Do not take this product for persistent or chronic cough such as occurs with smoking, asthma, emphysema, or if cough is accompanied by excessive phlegm (mucus) unless directed by a doctor. May cause excitability especially in children. Do not take this product, unless directed by a doctor, if you have a breathing problem such as emphysema or chronic bronchitis, or if you have heart disease, high blood pressure, thyroid disease, diabetes, glaucoma or difficulty in urination due to enlargement of the prostrate gland. May cause marked drowsiness: alcohol, sedatives, and tranquilizers may increase the drowsiness effect. Avoid taking alcoholic beverages while taking this product. Do not take this product if you are taking sedatives or tranquilizers, without first consulting your doctor. Use caution when driving a motor vehicle or operating machinery. **Do not exceed recommended dosage.** If nervousness, dizziness, or sleeplessness occur, discontinue use and consult a doctor. **KEEP THIS AND ALL DRUGS OUT OF THE REACH OF CHILDREN.** Prompt medical attention is critical for adults as well as for children even if you do not notice any signs or symptoms. In case of accidental overdose, seek professional assistance or contact a Poison Control Center immediately. As with any drug, if you are pregnant or nursing a baby, seek the advice of a health professional before using this product.

Drug Interaction Precaution: Do not use this product if you are now taking a prescription monoamine oxidase inhibitor (MAOI) (certain drugs for depression, psychiatric or emotional conditions, or Parkinson's disease), or for 2 weeks after stopping the MAOI drug. If you are uncertain whether your prescription drug contains an MAOI, consult a health professional before taking this product.

Active Ingredients: Acetaminophen 500 mg, Dextromethorphan Hydrobromide 15 mg, Phenylpropanolamine Hydrochloride 12.5 mg and Chlorpheniramine maleate 2 mg.

Inactive Ingredients: FD&C Blue 1, Cellulose, Hydroxypropyl Methylcellu-

lose, Polyethylene Glycol, Polysorbate 80, Povidone, Sodium Starch Glycolate, Starch, Stearic Acid, and Titanium Dioxide.
Avoid storing at high temperature (greater than 100°F).

How Supplied: Consumer package of 16 and 30 caplets.
Note: There are other Contact products. Make sure this is the one you are interested in.
Shown in Product Identification Guide, page 524

DEBROX® Drops
Ear Wax Removal Aid

Description: Carbamide peroxide 6.5%. Also contains citric acid, glycerin, propylene glycol, sodium stannate, water, and other ingredients.

Actions: DEBROX®, used as directed, cleanses the ear with sustained microfoam. DEBROX Drops foam on contact with earwax due to the release of oxygen. DEBROX Drops provide a safe, nonirritating method of softening and removing ear wax.

Indications: For occasional use as an aid to soften, loosen, and remove excessive earwax.

Directions: FOR USE IN THE EAR ONLY. Adults and children over 12 years of age: tilt head sideways and place 5 to 10 drops into ear. Tip of applicator should not enter ear canal. Keep drops in ear for several minutes by keeping head tilted or placing cotton in the ear. Use twice daily for up to four days if needed, or as directed by a doctor. Any wax remaining after treatment may be removed by gently flushing the ear with warm water, using a soft rubber bulb ear syringe. Children under 12 years of age: consult a doctor.

Warnings: Do not use if you have ear drainage or discharge, ear pain, irritation or rash in the ear, or are dizzy; consult a doctor. Do not use if you have an injury or perforation (hole) of the eardrum or after ear surgery unless directed by a doctor. Do not use for more than four days. If excessive earwax remains after use of this product, consult a doctor. Avoid contact with the eyes.

Cautions: Avoid exposing bottle to excessive heat and direct sunlight. Keep tip on bottle when not in use. Keep this and all drugs out of the reach of children. In case of accidental ingestion, seek professional assistance or contact a poison control center immediately.

How Supplied: DEBROX Drops are available in ½- or 1-fl-oz plastic squeeze bottles with applicator spouts.
Shown in Product Identification Guide, page 524

Continued on next page

SmithKline Beecham—Cont.

ECOTRIN®
Enteric-Coated Aspirin
Antiarthritic, Antiplatelet

Description: 'Ecotrin' is enteric-coated aspirin (acetylsalicylic acid, ASA) available in tablet and caplet forms in 81 mg, 325 mg and 500 mg dosage units. The enteric coating covers a core of aspirin and is designed to resist disintegration in the stomach, dissolving in the more neutral-to-alkaline environment of the duodenum. Such action helps to protect the stomach from injury that may result from ingestion of plain, buffered or highly buffered aspirin (see SAFETY).

Indications: 'Ecotrin' is indicated for:
- conditions requiring chronic or long-term aspirin therapy for pain and/or inflammation, e.g., rheumatoid arthritis, juvenile rheumatoid arthritis, systemic lupus erythematosus, osteoarthritis (degenerative joint disease), ankylosing spondylitis, psoriatic arthritis, Reiter's syndrome and fibrositis,
- antiplatelet indications of aspirin (see the ANTIPLATELET-EFFECT section) and
- situations in which compliance with aspirin therapy may be affected because of the gastrointestinal side effects of plain, i.e., non-enteric-coated, or buffered aspirin.

Dosage: For analgesic indications, the OTC maximum dosage for aspirin is 4000 mg per day in divided doses, i.e., up to 650 mg every 4 hours or 1000 mg every 6 hours.
For antiplatelet effect dosage: see the ANTIPLATELET EFFECT section.
Under a physician's direction, the dosage can be increased or otherwise modified as appropriate to the clinical situation. When 'Ecotrin' is used for anti-inflammatory effect, the physician should be attentive to plasma salicylate levels, and may also caution the patient to be alert to the development of tinnitus as an indicator of elevated salicylate levels. It should be noted that patients with a high frequency hearing loss (such as may occur in older individuals) may have difficulty perceiving the tinnitus. Tinnitus would then not be a reliable indicator in such individuals.

Inactive Ingredients:
ECOTRIN 81 mg—Carnauba Wax, D&C Yellow #10, FD&C Blue #2, FD&C Red #40, FD&C Yellow #6, Hydroxypropyl Methylcellulose, Iron Oxide, Methacrylic Acid Copolymer, Microcrystalline Cellulose, Polyethylene Glycol, Polysorbate 80, Propylene Glycol, Silicon Dioxide, Starch, Stearic Acid, Talc, Titanium Dioxide, Triethyl Citrate.
ECOTRIN 325 mg and 500 mg—Carnauba Wax, Cellulose Acetate Phthalate, Diethyl Phthalate, D&C Yellow #10, FD&C Blue #2, FD&C Red #40, FD&C Yellow #6, Iron Oxide, Microcrystalline Cellulose, Silicon Dioxide, Sodium Starch Glycolate, Starch, Stearic Acid, Titanium Dioxide.

Bioavailability: The bioavailability of aspirin from 'Ecotrin' has been demonstrated in a number of salicylate excretion studies. The studies show levels of salicylate (and metabolites) in urine excreted over 48 hours for 'Ecotrin' do not differ statistically from plain, i.e., non-enteric-coated, aspirin.
Plasma studies, in which 'Ecotrin' has been compared with plain aspirin in steady-state studies over eight days, also demonstrate that 'Ecotrin' provides plasma salicylate levels not statistically different from plain aspirin.
Information regarding salicylate levels over a range of doses was generated in a study in which 24 healthy volunteers (12 male and 12 female) took daily (divided) doses of either 2600 mg, 3900 mg, or 5200 mg of 'Ecotrin'. Plasma salicylate levels generally acknowledged to be anti-inflammatory (15 mg/dL.) were attained at daily doses of 5200 mg, on Day 2 by females and Day 3 by males. At 3900 mg, anti-inflammatory levels were attained at Day 3 by females and Day 4 by males. Dissolution of the enteric coating occurs at a neutral-to-basic pH and is therefore dependent on gastric emptying into the duodenum. With continued dosing, appropriate plasma levels are maintained.

Safety: The safety of 'Ecotrin' has been demonstrated in a number of endoscopic studies comparing 'Ecotrin', plain aspirin, buffered aspirin and highly buffered aspirin preparations. In these studies, all forms of aspirin were dosed to the OTC maximum (3900–4000 mg per day) for up to 14 days. The normal healthy volunteers participating in these studies were gastroscoped before and after the courses of treatment and 14-day drug-free periods followed active drug. Compared to all the other preparations, there was less gastric damage at a statistically significant level during the 'Ecotrin' courses. There was also statistically less duodenal damage when compared with the plain, i.e., non-enteric-coated, aspirin.
Details of studies demonstrating the safety and bioavailability of 'Ecotrin' are available to health care professionals. Write: Professional Services Department, SmithKline Beecham Consumer Healthcare, L.P., P.O. Box 1467, Pittsburgh, Pa. 15230.

WARNINGS: Children and teenagers should not use this product for chicken pox or flu symptoms before a doctor is consulted about Reye Syndrome, a rare but serious illness reported to be associated with aspirin. Do not take this product for pain for more than 10 days or for fever for more than 3 days unless directed by a doctor. If pain or fever persists or gets worse, if new symptoms occur, or if redness or swelling is present, consult a doctor because these could be signs of a serious condition. Do not take this product if you are allergic to aspirin, have asthma, or if you have stomach problems that persist or recur, or if you have ulcers or bleeding problems unless directed by a doctor. If ringing in the ears or a loss of hearing occurs, consult a doctor before taking any more of this product. **Keep this and all drugs out of the reach of children.** In case of accidental overdose, seek professional assistance or contact a poison control center immediately. As with any medicine, if you are pregnant or nursing a baby, seek the advice of a health professional before using this product. **IT IS ESPECIALLY IMPORTANT NOT TO USE ASPIRIN DURING THE LAST 3 MONTHS OF PREGNANCY UNLESS SPECIFICALLY DIRECTED TO DO SO BY A DOCTOR BECAUSE IT MAY CAUSE PROBLEMS IN THE UNBORN CHILD OR COMPLICATIONS DURING DELIVERY.**

Drug Interaction Precaution: Do not take this product if you are taking a prescription drug for anticoagulation (thinning of the blood), diabetes, gout, or arthritis unless directed by a doctor.

Professional Warning: There have been occasional reports in the literature concerning individuals with impaired gastric emptying in whom there may be retention of one or more 'Ecotrin' tablets over time. This unusual phenomenon may occur as a result of outlet obstruction from ulcer disease alone or combined with hypotonic gastric peristalsis. Because of the integrity of the enteric coating in an acidic environment, these tablets may accumulate and form a bezoar in the stomach. Individuals with this condition may present with complaints of early satiety or of vague upper abdominal distress. Diagnosis may be made by endoscopy or by abdominal films which show opacities suggestive of a mass of small tablets *(Ref.: Bogacz, K. and Caldron, P.: Enteric-coated Aspirin Bezoar: Elevation of Serum Salicylate Level by Barium Study. Amer. J. Med. 1987:83, 783–6.).* Management may vary according to the condition of the patient. Options include: gastrotomy and alternating slightly basic and neutral lavage *(Ref.: Baum, J.: Enteric-Coated Aspirin and the Problem of Gastric Retention. J. Rheum., 1984:11, 250–1.).* While there have been no clinical reports, it has been suggested that such individuals may also be treated with parenteral cimetidine (to reduce acid secretion) and then given sips of slightly basic liquids to effect gradual dissolution of the enteric coating. Progress may be followed with plasma salicylate levels or via recognition of tinnitus by the patient.
It should be kept in mind that individuals with a history of partial or complete gastrectomy may produce reduced amounts of acid and therefore have less acidic gastric pH. Under these circumstances, the benefits offered by the acid-resistant enteric coating may not exist.

Antiplatelet Effect Aspirin may be recommended to reduce the risk of death and/or nonfatal myocardial infarction (MI) in patients with a previous infarction or unstable angina pectoris and its use in reducing the risk of transient ischemic attacks in men.

Labeling for both indications follows:

ASPIRIN FOR MYOCARDIAL INFARCTION

Indication: Aspirin is indicated to reduce the risk of death and/or nonfatal myocardial infarction in patients with a previous infarction or unstable angina pectoris.

Clinical Trials: The indication is supported by the results of six, large, randomized multicenter, placebo-controlled studies involving 10,816 predominantly male, post-myocardial infarction (MI) patients and one randomized placebo-controlled study of 1,266 men with unstable angina.[1-7] Therapy with aspirin was begun at intervals after the onset of acute MI varying from less than three days to more than five years and continued for periods of from less than one year to four years. In the unstable angina study, treatment was started within one month after the onset of unstable angina and continued for 12 weeks, and patients with complicating conditions such as congestive heart failure were not included in the study.

Aspirin therapy in MI patients was associated with about a 20 percent reduction in the risk of subsequent death and/or nonfatal reinfarction, a median absolute decrease of 3 percent from the 12 to 22 percent event rates in the placebo groups. In aspirin-treated unstable angina patients, the reduction in risk was about 50 percent, a reduction in event rate to 5% from the 10% in the placebo group over the 12 weeks of the study.

Daily dosage of aspirin in the post-myocardial infarction studies was 300 mg in one study and 900 to 1500 mg in five studies. A dose of 325 mg was used in the study of unstable angina.

Adverse Reactions

Gastrointestinal Reactions: Doses of 1000 mg per day of plain aspirin caused gastrointestinal symptoms and bleeding that in some cases were clinically significant. In the largest postinfarction study (the Aspirin Myocardial Infarction Study [AMIS] with 4,500 people), the percentage incidences of gastrointestinal symptoms of a standard, solid-tablet formulation and placebo-treated subjects, respectively, were: stomach pain (14.5%; 4.4%); heartburn (11.9%; 4.8%); nausea and/or vomiting (7.6%; 2.1%); hospitalization for gastrointestinal disorder (4.9%; 3.5%). In the AMIS and other trials, plain aspirin-treated patients had increased rates of gross gastrointestinal bleeding. Symptoms and signs of gastrointestinal irritation were not significantly increased in subjects treated for unstable angina with buffered aspirin in solution.

Cardiovascular and Biochemical: In the AMIS trial, the dosage of 1000 mg per day of plain aspirin was associated with small increases in systolic blood pressure (BP) (average 1.5 to 2.1 mmHg) and diastolic BP (0.5 to 0.6 mmHg), depending upon whether maximal or last available readings were used. Blood urea nitrogen and uric acid levels were also increased, but by less than 1.0 mg%. Subjects with marked hypertension or renal insufficiency had been excluded from the trial so that the clinical importance of these observations for such subjects or for any subjects treated over more prolonged periods is not known. It is recommended that patients placed on long-term aspirin treatment, even at doses of 300 mg per day, be seen at regular intervals to assess changes in these measurements.

Sodium in Buffered Aspirin for Solution Formulations: One tablet daily of buffered aspirin in solution adds 553 mg of sodium to that in the diet and may not be tolerated by patients with active sodium-retaining states such as congestive heart or renal failure. This amount of sodium adds about 30 percent to the 70 to 90 meq intake suggested as appropriate for dietary hypertension in the 1984 Report of the Joint National Committee on Detection, Evaluation, and Treatment of High Blood Pressure.[8]

Dosage and Administration: Although most of the studies used dosages exceeding 300 mg daily, two trials used only 300 mg and pharmacologic data indicate that this dose inhibits platelet function fully. Therefore, 300 mg or a conventional 325 mg aspirin dose daily is a reasonable, routine dose that would minimize gastrointestinal adverse reactions for both solid oral dosage forms (buffered and plain aspirin) and buffered aspirin in solution.

References:
1. Elwood, P.C., et al.: A Randomized Controlled Trial of Acetylsalicylic Acid in the Secondary Prevention of Mortality from Myocardial Infarction, *Br. Med. J.* 1:436–440, 1974.
2. The Coronary Drug Project Research Group: Aspirin in Coronary Heart Disease, *J. Chronic Dis.* 29:625–642, 1976.
3. Breddin, K., et al.: Secondary Prevention of Myocardial Infarction: A Comparison of Acetylsalicylic Acid, Phenprocoumon or Placebo, *Homeostasis* 470:263–268, 1979.
4. Aspirin Myocardial Infarction Study Research Group: A Randomized Controlled Trial of Aspirin in Persons Recovered from Myocardial Infarction, *J.A.M.A.* 243:661–669, 1980.
5. Elwood, P.C., and Sweetnam, P.M.: Aspirin and Secondary Mortality After Myocardial Infarction, *Lancet* pp. 1313–1315, Dec. 22–29, 1979.
6. The Persantine-Aspirin Reinfarction Study Research Group, Persantine and Aspirin in Coronary Heart Disease, *Circulation* 62: 449–469, 1980.
7. Lewis, H.D., et al.: Protective Effects of Aspirin Against Acute Myocardial Infarction and Death in Men with Unstable Angina, Results of a Veterans Administration Cooperative Study, *N. Engl. J. Med.* 309:396–403, 1983.
8. 1984 Report of the Joint National Committee on Detection, Evaluation, and Treatment of High Blood Pressure, U.S. Department of Health and Human Services and U.S. Public Health Service, National Institutes of Health. NIH Pub. No. 84–1088.

Aspirin for Transient Ischemic Attacks

Indication For reducing the risk of recurrent transient ischemic attacks (TIAs) or stroke in men who have had transient ischemia of the brain due to fibrin platelet emboli. There is inadequate evidence that aspirin or buffered aspirin is effective in reducing TIAs in women at the recommended dosage. There is no evidence that aspirin or buffered aspirin is of benefit in the treatment of completed strokes in men or women.

Clinical Trials The indication is supported by the results of a Canadian study[1] in which 585 patients with threatened stroke were followed in a randomized clinical trial for an average of 26 months to determine whether aspirin or sulfinpyrazone, singly or in combination, was superior to placebo in preventing transient ischemic attacks, stroke or death. The study showed that, although sulfinpyrazone had no statistically significant effect, aspirin reduced the risk of continuing transient ischemic attacks, stroke or death by 19 percent and reduced the risk of stroke or death by 31 percent. Another aspirin study carried out in the United States with 178 patients showed a statistically significant number of "favorable outcomes," including reduced transient ischemic attacks, stroke and death.[2]

Precautions Patients presenting with signs and/or symptoms of TIAs should have a complete medical and neurologic evaluation. Consideration should be given to other disorders that resemble TIAs. Attention should be given to risk factors: it is important to evaluate and treat, if appropriate, other diseases associated with TIAs and stroke, such as hypertension and diabetes.

Concurrent administration of absorbable antacids at therapeutic doses may increase the clearance of salicylates in some individuals. The concurrent administration of nonabsorbable antacids may alter the rate of absorption of aspirin, thereby resulting in a decreased acetylsalicylic acid/salicylate ratio in plasma. The clinical significance of these decreases in available aspirin is unknown. Aspirin at dosages of 1,000 mg per day has been associated with small increases in blood pressure, blood urea nitrogen, and serum uric acid levels. It is recommended that patients placed on long-term aspirin treatment be seen at regular intervals to assess changes in these measurements.

Adverse Reactions: At dosages of 1,000 mg or higher of aspirin per day, gastrointestinal side effects include stomach pain, heartburn, nausea and/or vomiting, as well as increased rates of gross gastrointestinal bleeding.

Dosage and Administration Adult dosage for men is 1,300 mg a day, in

Continued on next page

SmithKline Beecham—Cont.

divided doses of 650 mg twice a day or 325 mg four times a day.

References:
1. The Canadian Cooperative Study Group: Randomized Trial of Aspirin and Sulfinpyrazone in Threatened Stroke, *N. Engl. J. Med.* 299:53, 1978.
2. Fields, W. S., et al.: Controlled Trial of Aspirin in Cerebral Ischemia, *Stroke* 8:301–316, 1980.

How Supplied:
'Ecotrin' Tablets
  81 mg in bottle of 36
  325 mg in bottles of 100*, 250
  500 mg in bottles of 60*, 150
'Ecotrin' Caplets
  500 mg in bottles of 60.
* Without child-resistant caps.

TAMPER-RESISTANT PACKAGE FEATURES FOR YOUR PROTECTION:
- Bottle has imprinted seal under cap.
- The words ECOTRIN LOW or ECOTRIN REG or ECOTRIN MAX appear on each tablet or caplet (see product illustration printed on carton).
- DO NOT USE THIS PRODUCT IF ANY OF THESE TAMPER-RESISTANT FEATURES ARE MISSING OR BROKEN.

Comments or Questions? Call Toll-Free 800-245-1040 weekdays.
Shown in Product Identification Guide, page 524

FEOSOL® CAPSULES   OTC
Hemantinic

Description: 'Feosol' Capsules provide the body with ferrous sulfate—iron in its most efficient form—for simple iron deficiency and iron-deficiency anemia when the need for such therapy has been determined by a physician. The special targeted-release capsule formulation—ferrous sulfate in pellets—reduces stomach upset, a common problem with iron.

Formula: Active ingredients: Each capsule contains 159 mg. of dried ferrous sulfate USP (50 mg. of elemental iron), equivalent to 250 mg. of ferrous sulfate USP. **Inactive Ingredients** (listed for individuals with specific allergies): Benzyl Alcohol, Cetylpyridinium Chloride, D&C Red 33, Yellow 10, FD&C Blue 1, D&C Red 7, Red 40, Gelatin, Glyceryl Stearates, Iron Oxide, Polyethylene Glycol, Povidone, Sodium Lauryl Sulfate, Starch, Sucrose, White Wax and trace amounts of other inactive ingredients.

Dosage: Adults: 1 or 2 capsules daily or as directed by a physician.
Children: As directed by a physician.

TAMPER-RESISTANT PACKAGING FEATURES:
- The carton is protected by a clear overwrap printed with "safety sealed", do not use if overwrap is missing or broken.

- Each capsule is encased in a plastic cell with a foil back; do not use if cell or foil is broken.
- Each FEOSOL capsule is protected by a red Perma-Seal™ band which bonds the two capsule halves together; do not use if capsule is broken or band is missing or broken.

WARNINGS: Do not exceed recommended dosage. The treatment of any anemic condition should be under the advice and supervision of a physician. Since oral iron products interfere with absorption of oral tectracycline antibiotics, these products should not be taken within two hours of each other. Iron-containing medication may occasionally cause constipation or diarrhea. **Keep this and all drugs out of reach of children. Contains iron, which can be harmful or fatal to children in large doses. In case of accidental overdose, seek professional assistance or contact a Poison Control Center immediately.** As with any drug, if you are pregnant or nursing a baby, seek the advice of a health professional before using this product.
Manufactured with methylchloroform, a substance which harms public health and environment by destroying ozone in the upper atmosphere.
Store at controlled room temperature (59°–86°F.).

How Supplied: Packages of 30 and 60 capsules; in Single Unit Packages of 100 capsules (intended for institutional use only).
Also available in Tablets and Elixir.
Shown in Product Identification Guide, page 525

FEOSOL® ELIXIR   OTC
Iron Supplement

Description: 'Feosol' Elixir, an unusually palatable iron elixir, provides the body with ferrous sulfate—iron in its most efficient form. The standard elixir for simple iron deficiency and iron-deficiency anemia when the need for such therapy has been determined by a physician.

Formula: Each 5 ml. (1 teaspoonful) contains ferrous sulfate USP, 220 mg. (44 mg. of elemental iron); alcohol, 5%.
Also contains (listed for individuals with specific allergies): Citric Acid, FD&C Yellow 6 (Sunset Yellow) as a color additive, Flavors, Glucose, Saccharin Sodium, Sucrose, Purified Water.

Dosage: Adults—1 to 2 teaspoonsful three times daily preferably between meals. Children and Infants: As directed by physician. Mix with water or fruit juice to avoid temporary staining of teeth; do not mix with milk or wine-based vehicles.
TAMPER-RESISTANT PACKAGE FEATURE:
IMPRINTED SEAL AROUND BOTTLE CAP: DO NOT USE IF BROKEN.

Warnings: Do not exceed recommended dosage. The treatment of any anemic condition should be under the advice and supervision of a physician. Since oral iron products interfere with absorption of oral tetracycline antibiotics, these products should not be taken within two hours of each other. Occasional gastrointestinal discomfort (such as nausea) may be minimized by taking with meals and by beginning with one teaspoonful the first day, two the second, etc., until the recommended dosage is reached. Iron-containing medication may occasionally cause constipation or diarrhea and liquids may cause temporary staining of the teeth (this is less likely when diluted). **Keep this and all drugs out of reach of children. Contains iron, which can be harmful or fatal to children in large doses. In case of accidental overdose, seek professional assistance or contact a Poison Control Center immediately.** As with any drug, if you are pregnant or nursing a baby, seek the advice of a health professional before using this product.
Store at controlled room temperature. Protect from freezing.

How Supplied: A clear orange liquid in 16 fl. oz. bottle.

Also available: 'Feosol' Tablets, 'Feosol' Capsules
NOTE: There are other Feosol products. Make sure this is the one you are interested in.
Shown in Product Identification Guide, page 525

FEOSOL® TABLETS   OTC
Iron Supplement

Description: 'Feosol' Tablets provide the body with ferrous sulfate, iron in its most efficient form, for iron deficiency and iron-deficiency anemia when the need for such therapy has been determined by a physician. The distinctive triangular-shaped tablet has a coating to prevent oxidation and improve palatability.

Formula: Each tablet contains 200 mg. of dried ferrous sulfate USP (65 mg. of elemental iron), equivalent to 325 mg. (5 grains) of ferrous sulfate USP. Also contains (listed for individuals with specific allergies): Calcium Sulfate, D&C Yellow 10, FD&C Blue 2, Glucose, Hydroxypropyl Methylcellulose, Mineral Oil, Polyethylene Glycol, Sodium Lauryl Sulfate, Starch, Stearic Acid, Talc, Titanium Dioxide, and trace amounts of other inactive ingredients.

Dosage: Adults—one tablet 3 to 4 times daily, after meals and upon retiring or as directed by a physician. Children: As directed by a physician.
TAMPER-RESISTANT PACKAGE FEATURES:
- Bottle has imprinted seal under cap. Do not use if missing or broken.
- FEOSOL Tablets are triangular shaped (see product illustration printed on carton).

CAUTION: DO NOT USE THIS PROD-
UCT IF ANY OF THESE TAMPER-RE-
SISTANT FEATURES ARE MISSING
OR BROKEN.
Comments or Questions?
**Call toll-free 800-245-1040 week-
days.**

Warnings: Do not exceed recommended dosage. The treatment of any
anemic condition should be under the
advice and supervision of a physician.
Since oral iron products interfere with
absorption of oral tetracycline antibiotics, these products should not be taken
within two hours of each other. Occasional gastrointestinal discomfort (such
as nausea) may be minimized by taking
with meals and by beginning with one
tablet the first day, two the second, etc.,
until the recommended dosage is
reached. Iron-containing medication
may occasionally cause constipation or
diarrhea. **Keep this and all drugs out
of reach of children. Contains iron,
which can be harmful or fatal to children in large doses. In case of accidental overdose, seek professional assistance or contact a Poison Control
Center immediately.** As with any drug,
if you are pregnant or nursing a baby,
seek the advice of a health professional
before using this product.
Avoid storing at high temperature
(greater than 100°F.).

How Supplied: Bottles of 100 tablets.
Also available in Capsules and Elixir.
*Shown in Product Identification
Guide, page 525*

GAVISCON® Antacid Tablets
[găv 'ĭs-kŏn]

Composition: Each chewable tablet contains the following active ingredients:
Aluminum hydroxide dried gel... 80 mg
Magnesium trisilicate .... 20 mg
and the following inactive ingredients:
alginic acid, calcium stearate, flavor, sodium bicarbonate, starch (may contain
cornstarch), and sucrose.

Actions: Unique formulation produces
soothing foam which floats on stomach
contents. Foam containing antacid pre-
cedes stomach contents into the esophagus when reflux occurs to help protect
the sensitive mucosa from further irritation. GAVISCON® acts locally without
neutralizing entire stomach contents to
help maintain integrity of the digestive
process. Endoscopic studies indicate that
GAVISCON Antacid Tablets are equally
as effective in the erect or supine patient.

Indications: GAVISCON is specifically formulated for the temporary relief
of heartburn (acid indigestion) due to
acid reflux. GAVISCON is not indicated
for the treatment of peptic ulcers.

Directions: Chew two to four tablets
four times a day or as directed by a physician. Tablets should be taken after meals
and at bedtime or as needed. For best
results follow by a half glass of water or

other liquid. DO NOT SWALLOW
WHOLE.

Warnings: Do not take more than 16
tablets in a 24-hour period or 16 tablets
daily for more than 2 weeks, except under the advice and supervision of a physician. Do not use this product except under the advice and supervision of a physician if you are on a sodium-restricted
diet. Each GAVISCON Tablet contains
approximately 0.8 mEq sodium.

Drug Interaction Precaution: Antacids may interact with certain prescription drugs. If you are presently taking
a prescription drug, do not take this
product without checking with your
physician or other health professional.
Store at a controlled room temperature
in a dry place.
Keep this and all drugs out of the reach
of children. In case of accidental overdose, seek professional assistance or contact a poison control center immediately.

How Supplied: Available in bottles of
100 tablets and in foil-wrapped 2s in
boxes of 30 tablets.
Issued 2/87
*Shown in Product Identification
Guide, page 525*

**GAVISCON® EXTRA STRENGTH
RELIEF FORMULA Antacid Tablets**
[găv 'ĭs-kŏn]

Composition: Each chewable tablet
contains the following active ingredients:
Aluminum hydroxide .... 160 mg
Magnesium carbonate .... 105 mg
and the following inactive ingredients:
alginic acid, calcium stearate, flavor,
mannitol, sodium bicarbonate, stearic
acid, and sucrose.

Directions: Chew 2 to 4 tablets four
times a day or as directed by a physician.
Tablets should be taken after meals and
at bedtime or as needed. For best results
follow by a half glass of water or other
liquid. DO NOT SWALLOW WHOLE.

┌─────────────────────────────┐
FDA Approved Uses: For the relief
of heartburn, sour stomach, and/or
acid indigestion, and upset stomach
associated with heartburn, sour
stomach, and/or acid indigestion.
└─────────────────────────────┘

Warnings: Do not take more than 16
tablets in a 24-hour period or 16 tablets
daily for more than 2 weeks, except under the advice and supervision of a physician. Do not use this product except under the advice and supervision of a physician if you are on a sodium-restricted
diet. Each tablet contains approximately
1.3 mEq sodium.

Drug Interaction Precaution: Antacids may interact with certain prescription drugs. If you are presently taking a
prescription drug, do not take this product without checking with you physician
or other health professional.
Store at a controlled room temperature
in a dry place.

Keep this and all drugs out of the reach
of children.
In case of accidental overdose, seek professional assistance or contact a poison
control center immediately.

How Supplied: Available in bottles of
100 tablets and in foil-wrapped 2s in
boxes of 30.
*Shown in Product Identification
Guide, page 525*

**GAVISCON® EXTRA STRENGTH
RELIEF FORMULA**
Liquid Antacid
[găv 'ĭs-kŏn]

Composition: Each 2 teaspoonfuls
(10 mL) contains the following active
ingredients:
Aluminum hydroxide.................. 508 mg
Magnesium carbonate................. 475 mg
And the following inactive ingredients:
butylparaben, edetate disodium, flavor,
glycerin, propylparaben, saccharin sodium, simethicone emulsion, sodium alginate, sorbitol solution, water, and xanthan gum.

┌─────────────────────────────┐
FDA Approved Uses: For the relief
of heartburn, sour stomach and/or
acid indigestion, and upset stomach
associated with heartburn, sour
stomach and/or acid indigestion.
└─────────────────────────────┘

**Directions: SHAKE WELL BEFORE
USING.** Take 2 to 4 teaspoonfuls four
times a day or as directed by a physician.
GAVISCON Extra Strength Relief Formula Liquid should be taken after meals
and at bedtime, followed by half a glass of
water. Dispense product only by spoon or
other measuring device.

Warnings: Except under the advice
and supervision of a physician, do not
take more than 16 teaspoonfuls in a 24-
hour period or 16 teaspoonfuls daily for
more than 2 weeks. May have laxative
effect. Do not use this product if you have
a kidney disease; do not use this product
if you are on a sodium-restricted diet.
Each teaspoonful contains approximately 0.9 mEq sodium.

Drug Interaction Precaution: Antacids may interact with certain prescription drugs. If you are presently taking a
prescription drug, do not take this product without checking with your physician or other health professional.
Keep tightly closed. Avoid freezing. Store
at a controlled room temperature.
Keep this and all drugs out of the reach
of children.
In case of accidental overdose, seek professional assistance or contact a poison
control center immediately.

How Supplied: Available in 12 fl oz
(355 mL) bottles.
*Shown in Product Identification
Guide, page 525*

Continued on next page

SmithKline Beecham—Cont.

GAVISCON® Liquid Antacid
[găv 'ĭs-kŏn]

Composition: Each tablespoonful (15 ml) contains the following active ingredients:
Aluminum hydroxide .... 95 mg
Magnesium carbonate ....; 358 mg
And the following inactive ingredients: D&C Yellow #10, edetate disodium, FD&C Blue #1, flavor, glycerin, paraben preservatives, saccharin sodium, sodium alginate, sorbitol solution, water, and xanthan gum.

> **FDA Approved Uses:** For the relief of heartburn, sour stomach and/or acid indigestion, and upset stomach associated with heartburn, sour stomach and/or acid indigestion.

Directions: SHAKE WELL BEFORE USING. Take 1 or 2 tablespoonfuls four times a day or as directed by a physician. GAVISCON Liquid should be taken after meals and at bedtime, followed by half a glass of water. Dispense product only by spoon or other measuring device.

Warnings: Except under the advice and supervision of a physician, do not take more than 8 tablespoonfuls in a 24-hour period or 8 tablespoonfuls daily for more than 2 weeks. May have laxative effect. Do not use this product if you have a kidney disease; do not use this product if you are on a sodium-restricted diet. Each tablespoonful of GAVISCON Liquid contains approximately 1.7 mEq sodium.

Drug Interaction Precaution: Antacids may interact with certain prescription drugs. If you are presently taking a prescription drug, do not take this product without checking with your physician or other health professional.
Keep tightly closed. Avoid freezing. Store at a controlled room temperature.
Keep this and all drugs out of the reach of children.
In case of accidental overdose, seek professional assistance or contact a poison control center immediately.

How Supplied: Bottles of 12 fluid ounce (355 ml) and 6 fluid ounce (177 ml).
Shown in Product Identification Guide, page 525

GAVISCON®-2 Antacid Tablets
[găv 'ĭs-kŏn]

Composition: Each chewable tablet contains the following active ingredients: Aluminum hydroxide dried gel...160 mg
Magnesium trisilicate .... 40 mg
and the following inactive ingredients: alginic acid, calcium stearate, flavor, sodium bicarbonate, starch (may contain cornstarch), and sucrose.

Indications: GAVISCON® is specifically formulated for the temporary relief of heartburn (acid indigestion) due to acid reflux. GAVISCON is not indicated for the treatment of peptic ulcers.

Directions: Chew one to two tablets four times a day or as directed by a physician. Tablets should be taken after meals and at bedtime or as needed. For best results follow by a half glass of water or other liquid. DO NOT SWALLOW WHOLE.

Warnings: Do not take more than eight tablets in a 24-hour period or eight tablets daily for more than 2 weeks, except under the advice and supervision of a physician. Do not use this product except under the advice and supervision of a physician if you are on a sodium-restricted diet. Each GAVISCON-2 Tablet contains approximately 1.6 mEq sodium.

Drug Interaction Precaution: Antacids may interact with certain prescription drugs. If you are presently taking a prescription drug, do not take this product without checking with your physician or other health professional.
Store at a controlled room temperature in a dry place.
Keep this and all drugs out of the reach of children. In case of accidental overdose, seek professional assistance or contact a poison control center immediately.

How Supplied: Boxes of 48 foil-wrapped tablets.

Issued 2/87
Shown in Product Identification Guide, page 525

GLY-OXIDE® Liquid

Description: GLY-OXIDE® Liquid contains carbamide peroxide 10%.

Actions: GLY-OXIDE® Liquid has an oxygen-rich formula that works to relieve the pain of canker sores by cleaning and debriding damaged tissue so natural healing can occur. GLY-OXIDE Liquid's dense oxygenating microfoam helps destroy odor-forming germs and flushes out food particles that ordinary brushing can miss.

Administration: Do not dilute. Apply directly from bottle. Replace tip on bottle when not in use.

Indications and Usage: For local treatment and hygienic prevention of minor oral inflammation such as canker sores, denture irritation, and postdental procedure irritation. Place several drops on affected area four times daily, after meals and at bedtime, or as directed by a dentist or physician; expectorate after two or three minutes. Or place 10 drops onto tongue, mix with saliva, swish for several minutes, and expectorate.
As an adjunct to oral hygiene (orthodontics, dental appliances) after regular brushing, swish 10 or more drops vigorously. Continue for two to three minutes; expectorate.
When normal oral hygiene is inadequate or impossible (total care geriatrics, etc), swish 10 or more drops vigorously after meals and expectorate.

Precautions: Severe or persistent oral inflammation, denture irritation, or gingivitis may be serious. If these conditions or unexpected side effects occur, consult a dentist or physician immediately.
Avoid contact with eyes. Protect from heat and direct light. Keep this and all drugs out of the reach of children. In case of accidental overdose, seek professional assistance or contact a poison control center immediately.

How Supplied: GLY-OXIDE® Liquid is available in ½-fl-oz and 2-fl-oz non-spill, plastic squeeze bottles with applicator spouts.
Shown in Product Identification Guide, page 525

MASSENGILL® Douches,　　　OTC
Towelettes and Cleansing Wash
[mas 'sen-gil]

PRODUCT OVERVIEW

Key Facts: Massengill is the brand name for a line of douches which are recommended for routine cleansing and for temporary relief of vaginal itching and irritation. Massengill disposable douches are available in two Vinegar & Water formulas (Extra Mild and Extra Cleansing), a Baking Soda formula, four Cosmetic solutions (Country Flowers, Fresh Baby Powder Scent Mountain Breeze, and Spring Rain Freshness), and a Medicated formula (with povidone-iodine). Massengill also is available in a Non-Medicated liquid concentrate and powder form. Massengill also has products specially designed to safely and gently cleanse the external vaginal area: Massengill Soft Cloth Towelettes (Unscented and Baby Powder), Massengill Medicated Soft Cloth Towelettes and Massingill Feminine Cleansing Wash.

Major Uses: Massengill's Vinegar & Water, Baking Soda & Water, and Cosmetic douches are recommended for routine douching, or for cleansing following menstruation, prescribed use of vaginal medication or use of contraceptives. Massengill Medicated is recommended in a seven day regimen for the symptomatic relief of minor itching and irritation associated with vaginitis due to Candida albicans, Trichomonas vaginalis, and Gardnerella vaginalis. Massengill Feminine Cleansing Wash is a gentle soapfree way to clean the external vaginal area. Massengill Non-medicated Soft Cloth Towelettes are a convenient and portable way to cleanse the external vaginal area and wash odor away. Massengill Medicated Soft Cloth Towelettes provide temporary relief of minor external itching associated with irritation or skin rashes.

Safety Information: Do not douche during pregnancy unless directed by a physician. Douching does not prevent pregnancy. Do not use this product and consult your physician if you are experiencing any of the following symptoms: unusual vaginal discharge, vaginal bleeding, painful and/or frequent urination, lower abdominal/pelvis pain, or you or your sex partner has genital sores or ulcers.

Massengill Vinegar & Water, Baking Soda & Water, and Cosmetic Douches—If vaginal dryness or irritation occurs, discontinue use.

Massengill Medicated — Women with iodine-sensitivity should not use this product. If symptoms persist after seven days, or if redness, swelling or pain develop, consult a physician. Do not use while nursing unless directed by a physician.

PRODUCT INFORMATION
MASSENGILL®
[mas 'sen-gil]
Disposable Douches
MASSENGILL®
Liquid Concentrate
MASSENGILL® Powder

Ingredients: DISPOSABLES: Extra Mild Vinegar and Water—Water and Vinegar.

Extra Cleansing Vinegar and Water —Water, Vinegar, Puraclean™ (Cetylpyridinium Chloride), Diazolidinyl Urea, Disodium EDTA.

*Puraclean is a trademark for cetylpyridinium chloride, a safe, special cleansing ingredient not found in any other vinegar & water douche.

Baking Soda and Water—Sanitized Water, Sodium Bicarbonate (Baking Soda).

Fresh Baby Powder Scent—Water, SD Alcohol 40, Lactic Acid, Sodium Lactate, Octoxynol-9, Cetylpyridinium Chloride, Propylene Glycol (and) Diazolidinyl Urea (and) Methylparaben (and) Propylparaben, Disodium EDTA, Fragrance, FD&C Blue #1.

Country Flowers—Water, SD Alcohol 40, Lactic Acid, Sodium Lactate, Octoxynol-9, Cetylpyridinium Chloride, Propylene Glycol (and) Diazolidinyl Urea (and), Methylparaben (and) Propylparaben, Disodium EDTA, Fragrance, D&C Red #28, FD&C Blue #1.

Mountain Breeze—Water, SD Alcohol 40, Lactic Acid, Sodium Lactate, Octoxynol-9, Cetylpyridinium Chloride, Propylene Glycol (and) Diazolidinyl Urea (and) Methylparaben (and) Propylparaben, Disodium EDTA, Fragrance, D&C Yellow #10, FD&C Blue #1.

Spring Rain Freshness—Water, SD Alcohol 40, Lactic Acid, Sodium Lactate, Octoxynol-9, Cetylpyridinium Chloride, Propylene Glycol (and) Diazolidinyl Urea (and Methylparaben (and) Propylparaben, Disodium EDTA, Fragrance.

LIQUID CONCENTRATE: Water, SD Alcohol 40, Lactic Acid, Sodium Bicarbonate, Octoxynol-9, Methyl Salicylate, Eucalyptol, Menthol, Thymol, D&C Yellow #10, FD&C Yellow #6 (Sunset Yellow).

POWDER: Sodium Chloride, Ammonium alum, PEG-8, Phenol, Methyl Salicylate, Eucalyptus Oil, Menthol, Thymol, D&C Yellow #10, FD&C Yellow #6 (Sunset Yellow).

Indications: Recommended for routine cleansing at the end of menstruation, after use of contraceptive creams or jellies (check the contraceptive package instructions first) or to rinse out the residue of prescribed vaginal medication (as directed by physician).

Actions: The buffered acid solutions of Massengill Douches are valuable adjuncts to specific vaginal therapy following the prescribed use of vaginal medication or contraceptives and in feminine hygiene.

Directions: DISPOSABLES: Twist off flat, wing-shaped tab from bottle containing premixed solution, attach nozzle supplied and use. The unit is completely disposable.

LIQUID CONCENTRATE: Fill cap ¾ full, to measuring line, and pour contents into douche bag containing 1 quart of warm water. Mix thoroughly.

POWDER Packettes: Dissolve the contents of 1 packet in a quart of warm water. Mix thoroughly in a separate container or douche bag.

Container: Dissolve two rounded teaspoonfuls in a douche bag containing 1 quart of warm water. Mix thoroughly.

Warning: Douching does not prevent pregnancy. Do not use during pregnancy except under the advice and supervision of your physician. If vaginal dryness or irritation occurs, discontinue use. Use this product only as directed for routine cleansing. You should douche no more than twice a week except on the advice of your doctor.

An association has been reported between douching and pelvic inflammatory disease (PID), a serious infection of your reproductive system which can lead to sterility and/or ectopic (tubal) pregnancy. PID requires immediate medical attention.

PID's most common symptoms are pain and/or tenderness in the lower part of the abdomen and pelvis. You may also experience a vaginal discharge, vaginal bleeding, nausea or fever. Other sexually transmitted diseases (STDs) have similar symptoms and/or frequent urination, genital sores, or ulcers. Douches should not be used for the self treatment of any STDs or PID. If you suspect you have one of these infections or PID, stop using this product and see your doctor immediately.

See the enclosed insert for important health information concerning sexually transmitted diseases and PID.

How Supplied: Disposable—6 oz. disposable plastic bottle.
Liquid Concentrate—4 oz. plastic bottles.
Powder—4 oz., Packettes—12's.

MASSENGILL Feminine   OTC
Cleansing Wash
[mas 'sen-gil]

Ingredients: Water, sodium laureth sulfate, magnesium laureth sulfate, sodium laureth-8 sulfate, magnesium laureth-8 sulfate, sodium oleth sulfate, magnesium oleth sulfate, lauramidopropyl betaine, myristamine oxide, lactic acid, PEG-120 methyl glucose dioleate, fragrance, sodium methylparaben, sodium ethylparaben, sodium propylparaben, methylchloroisothiazolinone, methylisothiazolinone, D&C Red #33.

Indications: For cleansing and refreshing of external vaginal area.

Actions: Massengill feminine cleansing wash safely and gently cleanses the external vaginal area.

Directions: Pour small amount into palm of hand or wash cloth and lather into wet skin. Rinse clean. Safe to use daily.

How Supplied: 8 fl. oz plastic flip-top bottle.

MASSENGILL®   OTC
[mas 'sen-gil]
Fragrance-Free Soft Cloth Towelette and Baby Powder Scent

Ingredients: Unscented
Water, Octoxynol-9, Lactic Acid, Sodium Lactate, Potassium Sorbate, Disodium EDTA, and Cetylpyridinium Chloride.
Baby Powder Scent
Water, Lactic Acid, Sodium Lactate, Potassium Sorbate, Octoxynol-9, Disodium EDTA, Cetylpyridinium Chloride, and Fragrance.

Indications: For cleansing and refreshing the external vaginal area.

Actions: Massengill Baby Powder Scent and Fragrance-Free Soft Cloth Towelettes safely cleanse the external vaginal area. The towelette delivery system makes the application soft and gentle.

Directions: Remove towelette from foil packet, unfold, and gently wipe. Throw away towelette after it has been used once.

How Supplied: Sixteen individually wrapped, disposable towelettes per carton.

MASSENGILL® Medicated
[mas 'sen-gil]
Disposable Douche

Active Ingredient: Cepticin™ (povidone-iodine)

Indications: For symptomatic relief of minor vaginal irritation or itching associated with vaginitis due to Candida albicans, Trichomonas vaginalis, and Gardnerella vaginalis.

Continued on next page

SmithKline Beecham—Cont.

Action: Povidone-iodine is widely recognized as an effective broad spectrum microbicide against both gram negative and gram positive bacteria, fungi, yeasts and protozoa. While remaining active in the presence of blood, serum or bodily secretions, it possesses virtually none of the irritating properties of iodine.

Warning: Douching does not prevent pregnancy. Do not use during pregnancy or while nursing except under the advice and supervision of your physician. If vaginal dryness or irritation occurs discontinue use. Use this product only as directed. Do not use this product for routine cleansing.

An association has been reported between douching and pelvic inflammatory disease (PID), a serious infection of your reproductive system, which can lead to sterility and/or ectopic (tubal) pregnancy. PID requires immediate medical attention.

PID's most common symptoms are pain and/or tenderness in the lower part of the abdomen and pelvis. You may also experience vaginal discharge, vaginal bleeding, nausea or fever. Other sexually transmitted diseases (STDs) have similar symptoms and/or frequent urination, genital sores, or ulcers. Douches should not be used for self-treatment of any STDs or PID. If you suspect you have one of these infections or PID, stop using this product and see your doctor immediately.

See the enclosed insert for important health information concerning sexually transmitted diseases and PID. Women with iodine sensitivity should not use this product.

Keep out of the reach of children.

Avoid storing at high temperature (greater than 100°F).

Protect from freezing.

Dosage and Administration: Dosage is provided as a single unit concentrate to be added to 6 oz. of sanitized water supplied in a disposable bottle. A specially designed nozzle is provided. After use, the unit is discarded. Use one bottle a day for seven days. Although symptoms may be relieved earlier, treatment should be continued for the full seven days.

How Supplied: 6 oz. bottle of sanitized water with 0.17 oz. vial of povidone-iodine and nozzle.

Shown in Product Identification Guide, page 525

MASSENGILL® Medicated   OTC
[mas'sen-gil]
Soft Cloth Towelette

Active   Ingredient: Hydrocortisone (0.5%).

Inactive Ingredients: Diazolidinyl Urea, DMDM Hydantoin, Isopropyl Myristate, Methylparaben, Polysorbate 60, Propylene Glycol, Propylparaben, Sorbitan Stearate, Steareth-2, Steareth-21, Water.

Also available in non-medicated Baby Powder Scent and Unscented formulas to freshen and cleanse the external vaginal area.

Indications: For soothing relief of minor external feminine itching or other itching associated with minor skin irritations, and rashes. Other uses of this product should be only under the advice and supervision of a physician.

Action: Massengill Medicated Soft Cloth Towelettes contain hydrocortisone, a proven anti-inflammatory, anti-pruritic ingredient. The towelette delivery system makes the application soothing, soft, and gentle.

Warnings: For external use only. Avoid contact with eyes. If condition worsens, symptoms persist for more than seven days, or symptoms recur within a few days, do not use this or any other hydrocortisone product unless you have consulted a physician. If experiencing a vaginal discharge, see a physician. Do not use this product for the treatment of diaper rash.

Keep this and all drugs out of the reach of children. As with any drug, if pregnant or nursing a baby, seek the advice of a health professional before using this product. In case of accidental ingestion, seek professional assistance or contact a Poison Control Center immediately.

Directions: Adults and Children two years of age and older—apply to the affected area not more than three to four times daily. Remove towelette from foil packet, gently wipe, and discard. Throw away towelette after it has been used once. Children under 2 years of age: DO NOT USE.

How   Supplied: Ten   individually wrapped, disposable towelettes per carton.

N'ICE® Medicated Sugarless Sore Throat and Cough Lozenges
[nis]

Active Ingredient: Cherry—Each lozenge contains 5.0 mg. menthol in a sorbitol base. Citrus—Each lozenge contains 5.0 mg. menthol in a sorbitol base. Menthol Eucalyptus—Each lozenge contains 5.0 mg. menthol in a sorbitol base. Cool Peppermint—Each lozenge contains 5.0 mg. menthol in a sorbitol base. N'ICE 'N CLEAR Cherry Eucalyptus—Each lozenge contains 7.0 mg. menthol in a sorbitol base. N'ICE 'N CLEAR. Menthol Eucalyptus—Each lozenge contains 5.0 mg. menthol in a sorbitol base.

Inactive Ingredients: Cherry—Flavors, D&C Red 33, Sorbitol, Tartaric Acid, FD&C Yellow 6. Citrus—Citric Acid, Flavors, Saccharin Sodium, Sodium Citrate, Sorbitol, Yellow 10. Menthol Eucalyptus—Citric Acid, Flavors, Sorbitol. Cool Peppermint—Blue 1, Flavor, Maltitol Solution, Sorbitol, Yellow 10. N'ICE 'N CLEAR Cherry Eucalyptus—Flavors, D&C Red 33, Sorbitol, Tartaric Acid, FD&C Yellow 6. N'ICE 'N CLEAR Menthol Eucalyptus—Citric Acid, Flavors, Sorbitol.

Indications: Temporarily suppresses cough due to minor throat and bronchial irritation associated with a cold or inhaled irritants. Temporarily relieves minor sore throat pain.

Warnings: Do not administer to children under six years of age unless directed by a doctor. A persistent cough may be a sign of a serious condition. If cough or sore throat is severe, persists for more than 2 days, or is accompanied or followed by difficulty in breathing, fever, headache, rash, swelling, nausea, or vomiting, do not use and consult a doctor promptly. Do not take this product for persistent or chronic cough such as occurs with smoking, asthma, emphysema, or if cough is accompanied by excessive phlegm (mucus) unless directed by a doctor. In case of accidental overdose, seek professional assistance. **Keep this and all medications out of the reach of children.** Do not exceed recommended dosage. Avoid storing at high temperature (greater than 100°F).

Drug Interaction: No know drug interaction.

Dosage and Administration: Cherry, Citrus, Menthol Eucalyptus, Cool Peppermint, N'ICE 'N CLEAR Cherry Eucalyptus, N'ICE 'N CLEAR Menthol Eucalyptus—Adults and children six and older: Let lozenge dissolve slowly in the mouth. Repeat every hour as needed, or as directed by a doctor, up to 10 lozenges per day.

Professional Labeling: For the temporary relief of pain associated with tonsillitis, pharyngitis, throat infections or stomatitis.

How Supplied: Available in packages of 16 lozenges. N'ICE Cherry available in packages of 8 and 16 lozenges.

NOVAHISTINE® DMX
[nō"vă-his'tēn]
Cough/Cold Formula & Decongestant

Active Ingredients: Each 5 ml teaspoonful contains Dextromethorphan Hydrobromide 10 mg., Guaifenesin 100 mg., Pseudoephedrine Hydrochloride 30 mg.

Inactive Ingredients: Alcohol 10%, FD & C Red No. 40, FD & C Yellow No. 6, Flavors, Glycerin, Hydrochloric Acid, Invert Sugar, Saccharin Sodium, Sodium Chloride, Sorbitol and Water.

Indications: For temporary relief from cough and nasal congestion due to the common cold. Helps loosen phlegm (sputum) and thin bronchial secretions to rid the bronchial passageways of bothersome mucus. Helps decongest sinus openings and passages; temporarily relieves sinus congestion and pressure.

Warnings: If symptoms do not improve within 7 days or are accompanied by fever, consult a doctor. A persistent cough may be a sign of a serious condition. If cough persists for more than 7 days, tends to recur, or is accompanied by fever, rash, or persistent headache, consult a doctor. Do not take this product for persistent or chronic cough such as occurs with smoking, asthma, chronic bronchitis or emphysema, or where cough is accompanied by excessive phlegm (mucus) unless directed by a doctor. Do not take this product if you have heart disease, high blood pressure, thyroid disease, diabetes, or difficulty in urination due to enlargement of the prostate gland, unless directed by a doctor. **Do not exceed recommended dosage.** If nervousness, dizziness, or sleeplessness occur, discontinue use and consult a doctor. **KEEP THIS AND ALL DRUGS OUT OF THE REACH OF CHILDREN.** In case of accidental overdose, seek professional assistance or contact a Poison Control Center immediately. As with any drug, if you are pregnant or nursing a baby, seek the advice of a health professional before using this product.

Drug Interaction Precaution: Do not use this product if you are now taking a prescription monoamine oxidase inhibitor (MAOI) (certain drugs for depression, psychiatric or emotional conditions, or Parkinson's Disease), or for 2 weeks after stopping the MAOI drug. If you are uncertain whether your prescription drug contains an MAOI, consult a health professional before taking this product.

Contraindications: NOVAHISTINE DMX is contraindicated in patients with severe hypertension, severe coronary artery disease, and in patients on MAOI therapy. Patient idiosyncrasy to adrenergic agents may be manifested by insomnia, dizziness, weakness, tremor, or arrhythmias.
Nursing mothers: Pseudoephedrine is contraindicated in nursing mothers because of the higher than usual risk for infants from sympathomimetic amines.
Hypersensitivity: NOVAHISTINE DMX is contraindicated in patients with hypersensitivity or idiosyncrasy to sympathomimetic amines, dextromethorphan, or to other formula ingredients.

Adverse Reactions: Adverse reactions occur infrequently with usual oral doses of NOVAHISTINE DMX. When they occur, adverse reactions may include gastrointestinal upset and nausea. Because of the pseudoephedrine in NOVAHISTINE DMX, hyperreactive individuals may display ephedrine-like reactions such as tachycardia, palpitations, headache, dizziness or nausea. Sympathomimetic drugs have been associated with certain untoward reactions including fear, anxiety, tenseness, restlessness, tremor, weakness, pallor, respiratory difficulty, dysuria, insomnia, hallucinations, convulsions, CNS depres-

sion, arrhythmias, and cardiovascular collapse with hypotension.
Note: Guaifenesin interferes with the colorimetric determination of 5-hydroxyindoleacetic acid (5-HIAA) and vanillylmandelic acid (VMA).

Directions For Use: Adults and children 12 years and older: 2 teaspoonfuls every 4 hours, not to exceed 8 teaspoonfuls in 24 hours, or as directed by a doctor. Children 6 to under 12 years: 1 teaspoonful every 4 hours, not to exceed 4 teaspoonfuls in 24 hours, or as directed by a doctor. Consult a doctor for the use in children under 6 years of age.

How Supplied: NOVAHISTINE DMX, in 4 fluid ounce bottles. Keep tightly closed. Protect from excessive heat and light. Avoid freezing.
Shown in Product Identification Guide, page 525

NOVAHISTINE® Elixir
[nō″vă-hĭs′tēn]
Cold & Hay Fever Formula

Active Ingredients: Each 5 ml teaspoonful of NOVAHISTINE Elixir contains: Chlorpheniramine Maleate 2 mg. and Phenylephrine Hydrochloride 5 mg.

Inactive Ingredients: Alcohol 5%, D & C Yellow No. 10, FD & C Blue No. 1, Flavors, Glycerin, Sodium Chloride, Sorbitol and Water. Although considered sugar-free, each 5 ml contributes approximately 7 calories from sorbitol.

Indications: For the temporary relief of nasal congestion, runny nose, sneezing, itching of the nose or throat, and itchy watery eyes due to the common cold, hay fever, or other upper respiratory allergies.

Warnings: If symptoms do not improve within 7 days or are accompanied by a fever, consult a doctor. May cause excitability especially in children. Do not take this product, unless directed by a doctor, if you have a breathing problem such as emphysema or chronic bronchitis, or if you have heart disease, high blood pressure, thyroid disease, diabetes, glaucoma, or difficulty in urination due to enlargement of the prostate gland. May cause drowsiness; alcohol, sedatives, and tranquilizers may increase the drowsiness effect. Avoid alcoholic beverages while taking this product. Do not take this product if you are taking sedatives or tranquilizers, without first consulting your doctor. Use caution when driving a motor vehicle or operating machinery. **Do not exceed recommended dosage.** If nervousness, dizziness, or sleeplessness occur, discontinue use and consult a doctor. **KEEP THIS AND ALL DRUGS OUT OF THE REACH OF CHILDREN.** In case of accidental overdose, seek professional assistance or contact a Poison Control Center immediately. As with any drug, if you are pregnant or nursing a baby, seek the advice of a health professional before using this product.

Drug Interaction Precaution: Do not use this product if you are now taking a prescription monoamine oxidase inhibitor (MAOI) (certain drugs for depression, psychiatric or emotional conditions, or Parkinson's Disease), or for 2 weeks after stopping the MAOI drug. If you are uncertain whether your prescription drug contains an MAOI, consult a health professional before taking this product.

Contraindications: NOVAHISTINE Elixir is contraindicated in patients with severe hypertension, severe coronary artery disease, and in patients on MAOI therapy. Patient idiosyncrasy to adrenergic agents may be manifested by insomnia, dizziness, weakness, tremor, or arrhythmias.
NOVAHISTINE Elixir is also contraindicated in patients with narrow-angle glaucoma, urinary retention, peptic ulcer, asthma, emphysema, chronic pulmonary disease, shortness of breath, or difficulty in breathing.
Nursing Mothers: Phenylephrine is contraindicated in nursing mothers.
Hypersensitivity: NOVAHISTINE Elixir is also contraindicated in patients with hypersensitivity or idiosyncrasy to sympathomimetic amines, antihistamines, or to other formula ingredients.

Adverse Reactions: Drugs containing sympathomimetic amines have been associated with certain untoward reactions, including fear, anxiety, tenseness, restlessness, tremor, weakness, pallor, respiratory difficulty, dysuria, insomnia, hallucinations, convulsions, CNS depression, arrhythmias, and cardiovascular collapse with hypotension. Individuals hyperreactive to phenylephrine may display ephedrine-like reactions such as tachycardia, palpitations, headache, dizziness, or nausea.
Phenylephrine is considered safe and relatively free of unpleasant side effects when taken at recommended dosage. Patients sensitive to antihistamine drugs may experience mild sedation. Other side effects from antihistamines may include dry mouth, dizziness, weakness, anorexia, nausea, vomiting, headache, nervousness, polyuria, heartburn, diplopia, dysuria, and very rarely dermatitis.

Directions For Use: Adults (12 years and older): 2 teaspoonfuls every 4 hours, not to exceed 12 teaspoonfuls in 24 hours, or as directed by a doctor. Children 6 to under 12 years: 1 teaspoonful ever 4 hours, not to exceed 6 teaspoonfuls in 24 hours, or as directed by a doctor. Consult a doctor for use in chldren under 6 years of age.

How Supplied: NOVAHISTINE Elixir, in 4 fluid ounce bottles. Keep tightly closed. Protect from excessive heat and light. Avoid freezing.
Shown in Product Identification Guide, page 525

Continued on next page

SmithKline Beecham—Cont.

PANADOL®
Acetaminophen
Tablets and Caplets

Description: Each Maximum Strength PANADOL Caplet or Tablet contains acetaminophen 500 mg.

Indications: For the fast, temporary relief of minor aches, and pains associated with headaches, backaches, muscle aches, toothache, menstrual pain and colds and flu. Also to reduce fever and for temporary relief of minor arthritis pain.

Directions: Adults and children 12 years and over: 2 tablets or caplets every 4 hours as needed, not to exceed 8 tablets or caplets in 24 hours or as directed by a doctor. **Children under 12 years:** Consult a doctor.

Warnings: Do not take this product for pain for more than 10 days or for fever for more than 3 days unless directed by a doctor. If pain or fever persists or gets worse, if new symptoms occur, or if redness or swelling is present, consult a doctor because these could be signs of a serious condition. Keep this and all drugs out of the reach of children. In case of accidental overdose, seek professional assistance or contact a poison control center immediately. Prompt medical attention is critical for adults as well as for children even if you do not notice any signs or symptoms. As with any drug, if you are pregnant or nursing a baby, seek the advice of a health professional before using this product.

Active Ingredient: Acetaminophen 500 mg per tablet or caplet.

Inactive Ingredients: Hydroxypropyl Methylcellulose, Potassium Sorbate, Povidone, Pregelatinized Starch, Starch, Stearic Acid, Talc, and Triacetin.

How Supplied: Tablets (white with "P" and "500" imprint) in bottles of 30 and 60. Caplets (white with "P" and "500" imprint) in bottle of 24.
Shown in Product Identification Guide, page 525

Children's PANADOL®
Acetaminophen Chewable Tablets, Liquid, Drops

Description: Each Children's PANADOL Chewable Tablet contains 80 mg acetaminophen in a fruit-flavored sugar-free tablet. Children's PANADOL Acetaminophen Liquid is fruit-flavored, red in color, and is alcohol-free, sugar-free and aspirin-free. Each ½ teaspoonful contains 80 mg of acetaminophen. Infant's PANADOL Drops are fruit-flavored, red in color, and are alcohol-free, sugar-free and aspirin-free. Each 0.8 mL (one calibrated dropperful) contains 80 mg acetaminophen.

Indications: Acetaminophen, the active ingredient in Children's PANADOL, is the analgesic/antipyretic most widely recommended by pediatricians for fast, effective relief of children's fevers. It also relieves the aches and pains of colds and flu, earaches, headaches, teething, immunizations, tonsillectomy, and childhood illnesses.
Children's PANADOL Tablets, Liquid, and Drops are aspirin-free and contain no alcohol or sugar. The pleasant-tasting formulations are not likely to upset or irritate children's stomachs.

Usual Dosage: Dosing is based on single doses in the range of 10–15 mg/kg body weight. Doses may be repeated every four hours up to 4 or 5 times daily, but not to exceed 5 doses in 24 hours. To be administered to children under 2 years only on advice of a physician.
Children's PANADOL Chewable Tablets: 2–3 yr, 24–35 lb, 2 tablets; 4–5 yr, 36–47 lb, 3 tablets; 6–8 yr, 48–59 lb, 4 tablets; 9–10 yr, 60–71 lb, 5 tablets; 11 yr, 72–95 lb, 6 tablets. May be repeated every 4 hours, up to 5 times in a 24-hour period.
Children's PANADOL Liquid: 4–11 mo, 12–17 lb, ½ teaspoonful; 12–23 mo, 18–23 lb, ¾ teaspoonful; 2–3 yr, 24–35 lb, 1 teaspoonful; 4–5 yr, 36–47 lb, 1½ teaspoonfuls; 6–8 yr, 48–59 lb, 2 teaspoonfuls; 9–10 yr, 60–71 lb, 2½ teaspoonfuls; 11 yr, 72–95 lb, 3 teaspoonfuls. May be repeated every 4 hours up to 5 times in a 24-hour period. May be administered alone or mixed with formula, milk, juice, cereal, etc.
Infant's PANADOL Drops: 0–3 mo, 6–11 lb, ½ dropperful (0.4 mL); 4–11 mo, 12–17 lb, 1 dropperful (0.8 mL); 12–23 mo, 18–23 lb, 1½ dropperfuls (1.2 mL); 2–3 yr, 24–35 lb, 2 dropperfuls (1.6 mL); 4–5 yr, 36–47 lb, 3 dropperfuls (2.4 mL); 6–8 yr, 48–59 lb, 4 dropperfuls (3.2 mL). May be repeated every 4 hours, up to 5 times in a 24-hour period. May be administered alone or mixed with formula, milk, juice, cereal, etc.

Warnings: Do not give this product for pain for more than 5 days or for fever for more than 3 days unless directed by a doctor. If pain or fever persists or gets worse, if new symptoms occur, or if redness or swelling is present, consult a doctor because these could be signs of a serious condition. Keep this and all drugs out of the reach of children. In case of accidental overdose, seek professional assistance or contact a poison control center immediately. Prompt medical attention is critical for adults as well as for children even if you do not notice any signs or symptoms. As with any drug, if you are pregnant or nursing a baby, seek the advice of a health professional before using this product.

Composition:
Chewable Tablets: Active Ingredient: Acetaminophen, 80 mg per tablet. Inactive Ingredients: FD&C Red No. 28, FD&C Red No. 40, flavor, Mannitol, Saccharin Sodium, Starch, Stearic Acid and other ingredients.
Liquid: Active Ingredient: Acetaminophen, 80 mg per ½ teaspoon. Inactive Ingredients: Benzoic acid, FD&C Red No. 40, Flavor, Glycerin, Polyethylene Glycol, Potassium Sorbate, Propylene Glycol, Purified Water, Saccharin Sodium, Sorbitol solution. May also contain Sodium Chloride or Sodium Hydroxide.
Drops: Active Ingredient: Acetaminophen, 80 mg per 0.8mL dropper. Inactive Ingredients: Citric Acid, FD&C Red No. 40, Flavors, Glycerin, Parabens, Polyethylene Glycol, Propylene Glycol, Purified Water, Saccharin Sodium, Sodium Chloride, Sodium Citrate.

How Supplied: Chewable Tablets (colored pink and scored)—bottles of 30. Liquid (colored red)—bottles of 2 fl. oz. and 4 fl. oz. Drops (colored red)—bottles of ½ oz. (15 mL).
All packages listed above have child-resistant safety caps and tamper-resistant features.
Shown in Product Identification Guide, page 525

SINE-OFF®
No Drowsiness Formula
Caplets

Active Ingredients: Each caplet contains: Pseudoephedrine Hydrochloride 30 mg., Acetaminophen 500 mg.

Inactive Ingredients: Crospovidone, FD & C Red 40, Hydroxypropyl Methylcellulose, Magnesium Stearate, Microcrystalline Cellulose, Polyethylene Glycol, Polysorbate 80, Povidone, Starch, and Titanium Dioxide.

Indications: Temporarily relieves headache pain and nasal congestion due to hay fever or other upper respiratory allergies or associated with sinusitis. Promotes nasal and/or sinus drainage; temporarily relieves sinus congestion and pressure.

Directions For Use: Adults (12 years and older): 2 caplets every 6 hours, not to exceed 8 caplets in any 24-hour period, or as directed by a doctor. Children under 12 years of age: Consult a doctor.

Warnings: Do not take this product for more than 10 days. If symptoms do not improve or are accompanied by fever that lasts more than 3 days, or if new symptoms occur, consult a doctor. Do not take this product if you have heart disease, high blood pressure, diabetes, thyroid disease, or difficulty in urination due to enlargement of the prostate gland unless directed by a doctor. **Do not exceed recommended dosage.** If nervousness, dizziness, or sleeplessness occur, discontinue use and consult a doctor. **KEEP THIS AND ALL MEDICATION OUT OF REACH OF CHILDREN.** Prompt medical attention is critical for adults as well as for children even if you do not notice signs or symptoms. In case of accidental overdose, seek professional assistance or contact a Poison Control Center immediately. As with any drug, if you are pregnant or nursing a baby, seek the advice of a health profession before taking this product.

Drug Interaction Precaution: Do not use this product if you are now taking a prescription monoamine oxidase inhibitor (MAOI) (certain drugs for depression, psychiatric or emotional conditions, or Parkinson's disease), or for 2 weeks after stopping the MAOI drug. If you are uncertain whether your prescription drug contains an MAOI, consult a health profesional before taking this product. Note: There are other SINE-OFF products. Make sure this is the one you are interested in.
Also Available: SINE-OFF Sinus Medicine Caplets, 24 and 100 count.

Tamper-Evident Package Features
- Each caplet is encased in a clear plastic cell with a foil back.
- The name SINE-OFF appears on each caplet.
- DO NOT USE THIS PRODUCT IF ANY OF THESE TAMPER-EVIDENT FEATURES ARE MISSING OR BROKEN.

Comments or Questions? Call Toll-Free 1-800-245-1040 Weekdays.
Avoid storing at high temperature (greater than 100°F).

Shown in Product Identification Guide, page 525

SINE–OFF® Sinus Medicine Caplets
Relieves sinus headache, pain, pressure, congestion, runny nose, sneezing & itchy, watery eyes.

Active Ingredients: Each caplet contains: Chlorpheniramine 2 mg, Pseudoephedrine Hydrochloride 30 mg., Acetaminophen 500 mg.

Inactive Ingredients: Carnauba Wax, Hydroxypropyl Methylcellulose, Magnesium Stearate, Microcrystalline Cellulose, Polydextrose, Polyethylene Glycol, Povidone, Sodium Starch Glycolate, Starch, Stearic Acid, Titanium Dioxide, Triacetin, FD & C Yellow #6, D & C Yellow 10.

Indications: Temporarily relieves headache pain and nasal congestion, runny nose, sneezing and itchy, watery eyes due to hay fever or other upper respiratory allergies, associated with sinusitis, or the common cold. Promotes nasal and/or sinus drainage; temporarily relieves sinus congestion and pressure.

Directions: Adults (12 years and older): 2 caplets every 6 hours, not to exceed 8 caplets in any 24-hour period, or as directed by a doctor. Children under 12 of age: Consult a doctor.

Warnings: Do not take this product for more than 10 days. If symptoms do not improve or are accompanied by fever that lasts for more than 3 days, or if new symptoms occur, consult a doctor. Do not take this product, unless directed by a doctor, if you have a breathing problem such as emphysema or chronic bronchitis, or if you have heart disease, high blood pressure, thyroid disease, diabetes, glaucoma or difficulty in urination due to enlargement of the prostate gland. May cause excitability, especially in children. May cause drowsiness; alcohol, sedatives, and tranquilizers may increase the drowsiness effect. Avoid alcoholic beverages while taking this product. Do not take this product if you are taking sedatives or tranquilizers, without first consulting your doctor. Use caution when driving a motor vehicle or operating machinery. **Do not exceed recommended dosage.** If nervousness, dizziness, or sleeplessness occur, discontinue use and consult a doctor. **KEEP THIS AND ALL DRUGS OUT OF THE REACH OF CHILDREN.** Prompt medical attention is critical for adults as well as for children even if you do not notice any signs or symptoms. In case of accidental overdose, seek professional assistance or contact a Poison Control Center immediately. As with any drug, if you are pregnant or nursing a baby, seek the advice of a health professional before using this product.

Drug Interaction Precaution: Do not use this product if you are now taking a prescription monoamine oxidase inhibitor (MAOI) (certain drugs for depression, psychiatric or emotional conditions, or Parkinson's disease), or for 2 weeks after stopping the MAOI drug. If you are uncertain whether your prescription drug contains an MAOI, consult a health professional before taking this product.

How Supplied: Consumer packages of 24 and 100 caplets.
Note: There are other SINE-OFF products. Make sure this is the one you are interested in.
Also Available: SINE-OFF® Maximum Strength No Drowsiness Formula Caplets 24's .

Tamper-Resistant Package Features For Your Protection:
- Outer carton is sealed.
- Each blister unit is sealed in printed foil.
- DO NOT USE THIS PRODUCT IF ANY OF THESE TAMPER-EVIDENT FEATURES ARE MISSING OR BROKEN.

Comments or Questions? Call Toll-Free 1-800-245-1040 Weekdays.
Store at controlled room temperature (59–86°F).

Shown in Product Identification Guide, page 525

SINGLET® For Adults
Decongestant/Antihistamine/ Analgesic (pain reliever)/Antipyretic (fever reducer)

Description: Each pink Singlet tablet contains Pseudoephedrine Hydrochloride 60 mg, Chlorpheniramine Maleate 4 mg, and Acetaminophen 650 mg. Also contains: D&C Red No. 27, D&C Yellow No. 10, FD&C Blue No. 1, Hydroxypropyl Cellulose, Hydroxypropyl Methylcellulose 2910, Magnesium Stearate, Microcrystalline Cellulose, Polyethylene Glycol 8000, Pregelatinized Corn Starch, Sodium Starch Glycolate, Sucrose, and Titanium Dioxide.

Indications: For the temporary relief of nasal congestion, runny nose, occasional sinus headache, fever, sneezing, watery eyes or itching of the nose, throat, and eyes due to colds, hay fever, or other upper respiratory allergies.

Warnings: Do not take this product for more than 7 days. Unless directed by a physician, do not take this product if you have asthma, glaucoma, emphysema, chronic pulmonary disease, heart disease, high blood pressure, thyroid disease, diabetes, shortness of breath, difficulty in breathing, difficulty in urination due to enlargement of the prostate gland, or if you are presently taking a prescription drug for high blood pressure or depression. Do not exceed recommended dosage because severe liver damage, nervousness, dizziness, or sleeplessness may occur. May cause excitability. Consult your physician if symptoms persist, if new symptoms occur, or if redness or swelling is present, because these could be signs of a serious condition. Consult your physician if fever persists for more than 3 days (72 hours) or recurs. May cause drowsiness; alcohol, sedatives, and tranquilizers may increase the drowsiness effect. Avoid alcoholic beverages while taking this product. Do not take this product if you are taking sedatives or tranquilizers without first consulting your physician. Use caution when driving a motor vehicle or operating machinery. If sensitive to any of the ingredients, do not use.
As with any drug, if you are pregnant or nursing a baby, seek the advice of a health professional before using this product. KEEP THIS AND ALL DRUGS OUT OF THE REACH OF CHILDREN. In case of accidental overdose, seek professional assistance or contact a Poison Control Center immediately. Prompt medical attention is critical for adults as well as for children even if you do not notice any signs or symptoms.

Dosage and Administration: Adults and children 12 years and older: one tablet 3 to 4 times a day, taken with water, while symptoms persist. Do not take more than 1 tablet within a 4-hour period. Do not exceed 4 tablets in 24 hours. Children under 12 years of age: consult a physician.

Storage: Protect from excessive heat and moisture.

How Supplied: Bottles of 100.

Continued on next page

SmithKline Beecham—Cont.

SUCRETS® Maximum Strength Wintergreen
SUCRETS® Wild Cherry Regular Strength
SUCRETS® Children's Cherry Flavored
Sore Throat Lozenges
[su 'krets]
SUCRETS® Regular Strength Original Mint
SUCRETS® Regular Strength Vapor Lemon
SUCRETS® Maximum Strength Vapor Black Cherry

Active Ingredient: Maximum Strength Wintergreen: Dyclonine Hydrochloride 3.0 mg. per lozenge. Wild Cherry, Regular Strength: Dyclonine Hydrochloride 2.0 mg. per lozenge. Children's Cherry: Dyclonine Hydrochloride 1.2 mg. per lozenge. Regular Strength–Original Mint: Hexylresorcinol 2.4 mg. per lozenge. Regular Strength–Vapor Lemon: Dyclonine Hydrochloride 2.0 mg. per lozenge. Maximum Strength–Vapor Black Cherry: Dyclonine Hydrochloride 3.0 mg. per lozenge.

Inactive Ingredients: Maximum StrengthWintergreen: Citric Acid, Corn Syrup, Silicon Dioxide, Sucrose, Mineral Oil, Yellow 10. Wild Cherry Regular Strength: Blue 1, Corn Syrup, Flavor, Red 40, Silicon Dioxide, Sucrose, Tartaric Acid. Children's Cherry: Blue 1, Citric Acid, Corn Syrup, Red 40, Silicon Dioxide, Sucrose. Regular Strength–Original Mint: Blue 1, Corn Syrup, Flavors, Silicon Dioxide, Sucrose, Mineral Oil, Yellow 10. Regular Strength–Vapor Lemon: Citric Acid, Corn Syrup, Flavors, Silicon Dioxide, Sucrose, Mineral Oil, Yellow 10. Maximum Strength–Vapor Black Cherry: Blue 1, Corn Syrup, Flavor, Menthol, Red 40, Silicon Dioxide, Sucrose, Tartaric Acid.

Indications: For temporary relief of occasional minor sore throat pain and mouth irritations.

Actions: Dyclonine Hydrochloride's soothing anesthetic action relieves minor throat irritations.

Warnings: If sore throat is severe, persists more than 2 days, is accompanied or followed by fever, headache, rash, nausea, or vomiting, consult a doctor promptly. If sore mouth symptoms do not improve in 7 days, see your dentist or doctor promptly. DO NOT EXCEED RECOMMENDED DOSAGE. KEEP THIS AND ALL MEDICINES OUT OF THE REACH OF CHILDREN. IN CASE OF ACCIDENTAL OVERDOSE, SEEK PROFESSIONAL ASSISTANCE OR CONTACT POISON CONTROL CENTER IMMEDIATELY.

Drug Interaction: No known drug interaction.

Symptoms and Treatment of Oral Overdosage: Reactions due to large overdosage are systemic and involve the central nervous system and cardiovascular system. Central nervous system reactions are characterized by excitation and/or depression. Nervousness, dizziness, blurred vision or tremors may occur. Reactions involving the cardiovascular system include depression of the myocardium, hypotension or bradycardia. Should a large overdose be suspected seek professional assistance. Call your physician, local poison control center or the Rocky Mountain Poison Control Center at 303-592-1710 (Collect), 24 hours a day.

Dosage and Administration: Adults and children 2 years of age or older: Allow one lozenge to dissolve slowly in the mouth. May be repeated every two hours as needed. Children under 2 years of age: Consult a dentist or doctor.

Professional Labeling: For the temporary relief of pain associated with tonsillitis, pharyngitis, throat infections or stomatitis.

How Supplied: Available in plastic packages of 18 lozenges.
Shown in Product Identification Guide, page 526

SUCRETS® 4 HOUR COUGH SUPPRESSANT
[su 'krets]
dextromethorphan hydrobromide

Active Ingredient:
Each cough lozenge contains Dextromethorphan Hydrobromide 15 mg.
Inactive Ingredients:
Menthol Eucalyptus—Corn Syrup, D&C Yellow #10. FD&C Blue #1 Flavor, Magnesium Trisilicate, Menthol, Mineral Oil, Sucrose.
Wild Cherry—Corn Syrup, FD&C Blue #1, FD&C Red #40, Flavor, Magnesium Trisilicate, Menthol, Mineral Oil, Sucrose.

Indications For Use: For effective temporary relief of coughs due to minor sore throat and bronchial irritation associated with colds or inhaled irritants.

Directions: Adults and children twelve years of age and over: Take one (1) cough lozenge every 4 hours as needed. Do not exceed maximum dosage of 6 lozenges in any 24-hour period unless directed by a physician.
Children over six years of age: Take one (1) cough lozenge every 6 hours as needed. Do not exceed maximum dosage of 4 lozenges in any 24-hour period unless directed by a physician.
This product not intended for children under 6 years of age.
Avoid storing at high temperature (greater than 100°F).

Drug Interaction Precaution: Do not use this product (or give this product to your child) if you (or your child) are now taking a prescription monoamine oxidase inhibitor (MAOI) (certain drugs for depression, psychiatric or emotional conditions, or Parkinson's disease), or for 2 weeks after stopping MAOI drug. If you are uncertain whether you or your child's prescription drug contains a MAOI, consult a health professional before taking this product.

Warnings: A persistent cough may be a sign of a serious condition. If cough persists for more than 1 week, tends to recur, or is accompanied by fever, rash or persistent headache, consult a physician. Do not take this product for persistent or chronic cough such as occurs with smoking, asthma, emphysema, or if cough is accompanied by excessive phlegm (mucus) unless directed by a physician. Do not administer to children under 6 years of age unless directed by a physician.
As with any drug, if you are pregnant or nursing a baby, seek the advice of a health professional before using this product.
In case of accidental overdose, seek professional assistance or contact a poison control center immediately.
Keep this and all medication out of the reach of children.
Shown in Product Identification Guide, page 525

TELDRIN®
Chlorpheniramine Maleate/ Phenylpropanolamine Hydrochloride Timed-Release 12 hour Allergy Relief Capsules
IMPROVED!
Now relieves congestion too!
PLEASE NOTE: This description replaces the previous formulation of TELDRIN—Timed Release Allergy Capsules which contained Chlorpheniramine 12 mg. per capsule.

Active Ingredients: Each capsule contains Chlorpheniramine Maleate 8 mg. and Phenylpropanolamine Hydrochloride 75 mg.

Inactive Ingredients: Benzyl Alcohol, Butylparaben, D & C Red No. 33, Edetate Calcium Disodium, FD & C Red No. 3, FD & C Yellow No. 6, Gelatin, Methylparaben, Pharmaceutical Glaze, Propylparaben, Sodium Lauryl Sulfate, Sodium Propionate, Starch, Sucrose, and other ingredients. May also contain Polysorbate 80.

Indications: Temporarily relieves runny nose and reduces sneezing, itching of the nose or throat, and itchy, watery eyes due to hay fever or other upper respiratory allergies. Temporarily relieves nasal congestion due to the common cold, hay fever, or associated with sinusitis.

Direction For Use: Adults and children over 12 years of age: One capsule every 12 hours, not to exceed 2 capsules in 24 hours, or as directed by a doctor. Children under 12 years of age, consult a doctor.

Warnings: Do not exceed recommended dosage. If nervousness, dizziness, or sleeplessness occur, discontinue use and consult a doctor. If symptoms do not improve within 7 days or are accompanied by fever, consult a doctor. Do not take this product unless directed by a doctor, if you have a breathing problem such as emphysema or chronic bronchitis, or if you have heart disease, high blood pressure, thyroid disease, diabetes, glaucoma, or difficulty in urination due to enlargement of the prostate gland. Do not take this product if you are taking another medication containing phenylpropanolamine. May cause excitability, especially in children. May cause drowsiness; alcohol, sedatives, and tranquilizers may increase the drowsiness effect. Avoid alcoholic beverages while taking this product. Do not take this product if you are taking sedatives or tranquilizers without first consulting your doctor. Use caution when driving a motor vehicle or operating machinery. **KEEP THIS AND ALL DRUGS OUT OF THE REACH OF CHILDREN.** In case of accidental overdose, seek professional assistance or contact a Poison Control Center immediately. As with any drug, if you are pregnant or nursing a baby, seek the advice of a health professional before using this product.

Drug Interaction Precaution: Do not use this product if you are now taking a prescription monoamine oxidase inhibitor (MAOI) (certain drugs for depression, psychiatric or emotional conditions, or Parkinson's Disease), or for 2 weeks after stopping the MAOI drug. If you are uncertain whether your prescription drug contains an MAOI, consult a health professional before taking this product.

Tamper-Evident Package Features
- Each capsule is encased in a plastic cell with a foil back.
- Each capsule is protected by a red Perma Seal™ band which bonds the two capsule halves together.
- DO NOT USE THIS PRODUCT IF ANY OF THESE TAMPER-EVIDENT FEATURES ARE MISSING OR BROKEN.

Comments or Questions? Call Toll-Free 1-800-245-1040 Weekdays.
Store in a dry place, at controlled room temperature (59–86°F).

Shown in Product Identification Guide, page 526

TUMS® Antacid Tablets
TUMS E–X® Antacid Tablets
TUMS ULTRA® Antacid Tablets

Indications: For fast relief of acid indigestion, heartburn, sour stomach, and upset stomach associated with these symptoms.

Active Ingredient:
Tums, Calcium Carbonate 500 mg
Tums E-X, Calcium Carbonate 750 mg
Tums ULTRA, Calcium Carbonate 1000 mg

Inactive Ingredients: Flavor(s), Mineral Oil, Sodium Polyphosphate, Starch, Sucrose, Talc. May also contain Adipic Acid, FD&C Blue 1, FD&C Yellow 6, D&C Yellow 10, D&C Red 27, D&C Red 30.

Actions: Tums provides rapid neutralization of stomach acid. Each Tums tablet has an acid-neutralizing capacity (ANC) of 10 mEq. Each Tums E-X tablet has an ANC of 15 mEq and each Tums ULTRA tablet, an ANC of 20 mEq. This high neutralization capacity makes Tums tablets an ideal antacid for management of conditions associated with hyperacidity. It effectively neutralizes free acid yet does not cause systemic alkalosis in the presence of normal renal function. A double-blind placebo-controlled clinical study demonstrated that calcium carbonate taken at a dosage of 16 Tums tablets daily for a two-week period was non-constipating/non-laxative.

Warnings: Tums: Do not take more than 16 tablets in a 24-hour period or use the maximum dosage of this product for more than 2 weeks, except under the advice and supervision of a physician. If symptoms persist for 2 weeks, stop using this product and see a physician. Keep this and all drugs out of the reach of children.
Tums E-X: Do not take more than 10 tablets in a 24-hour period or use the maximum dosage of this product for more than two weeks, except under the advice and supervision of a physician. If symptoms persist for two weeks, stop using this product and see a physician. Keep this and all drugs out of the reach of children.
Tums ULTRA: Do not take more than 8 tablets in 24-hour period or use the maximum dosage of this product for more than two weeks, except under the advice and supervision of a physician. If symptoms persist for two weeks, stop using and see a physician. Keep this and all drugs out of the reach of children.

Drug Interaction Precaution: Antacids may interact with certain prescription drugs. If you are presently taking a prescription drug, do not take this product without checking with your physician or other health professional.

Dosage and Administration:
Tums: Chew 2-4 tablets as symptoms occur. Repeat hourly if symptoms return, or as directed by physician.
Tums E-X: Chew 2-4 tablets as symptoms occur. Repeat hourly if symptoms return, or as directed by a physician.
Tums ULTRA: Chew 2-3 tablets as symptoms occur. Repeat hourly if symptoms return, or as directed by a physician.
Important Dietary Information- As a source of Extra Calcium-
Tums: Chew 2 or 3 tablets after meals or as directed by a physician. Each tablet provides 200mg calcium which is 20% of the U.S. RDA (or Daily Value) for calcium for adults. Five tablets provide 100% of the daily calcium needs for adults. When used as a calcium supplement do not exceed 16 tablets per day. Each tablet contains not more than 2mg sodium.
Tums E-X: Chew 2 or 3 tablets after meals or as directed by a physician. Each

tablet provides 300mg calcium which is 30% of the U.S. RDA (or Daily Value) for calcium for adults. Four tablets provide 120% of the daily calcium needs for adults. When used as a calcium supplement do not exceed 10 tablets per day. Each tablet contains not more than 3mg sodium.
Tums ULTRA: Chew 1 or 2 tablets after meals or as directed by a physician. Each tablet provides 400mg calcium which is 40% of the U.S. RDA (or Daily Value) for calcium for adults. Three tablets provide 120% of the daily calcium needs for adults. When used as a calcium supplement do not exceed 8 tablets per day. Each tablet contains not more than 4mg sodium.

Professional Labeling: Indicated for the symptomatic relief of hyperacidity associated with the diagnosis of peptic ulcer, gastritis, peptic esophagitis, gastric hyperacidity, and hiatal hernia.

How Supplied:
Tums: Peppermint flavor is available in 12-tablet rolls, 3-roll wraps, and bottles of 75 and 150. **Assorted Flavors** (Cherry, Lemon, Orange, and Lime), are available in 12-tablet rolls, 3-roll wraps, and bottles of 75, 150, and 400.
Tums E-X: Wintergreen, Cherry, Assorted Fruit and **Assorted Tropical Fruit Flavors;** 8-tablet rolls, 3-roll wraps and bottles of 48 and 96 tablets. Tropical fruit is also available in bottles of 250 tablets.
Tums ULTRA: Assorted Fruit and **Assorted Mint Flavors;** bottles of 36 and 72 tablets.
This labeling information is current as of January 1, 1995.

Shown in Product Identification Guide, page 526

TUMS Anti-gas /Antacid Formula

Active Ingredients: 500 mg of calcium carbonate and 20 mg of simethicone per tablet.
Tums Anti-gas/Antacid formula Assorted Fruit Flavor Inactive Ingredients: Adipic Acid, Corn Syrup, D&C Red 27, D&C Red 30, D&C Yellow 10, FD&C Blue 1, FD&C Yellow 6, Flavors, Microcrystalline Cellulose, Mineral Oil, Sodium Polyphosphate, Starch, Sucrose, Talc, Triglycerol Monooleate.
Each tablet contains not more than 2 mg of sodium and is considered dietetically sodium free.
The 500 mg of calcium carbonate in each tablet provide 200 mg of elemental calcium.
Non-laxative/non-constipating.

Indications: For fast relief of acid indigestion, heartburn, and sour stomach accompanied by gas and upset stomach associated with these symptoms.

Actions: Calcium carbonate, when tested in vitro neutralizes 10 mEq of 0.1N HCl. This neutralization capacity com-

Continued on next page

SmithKline Beecham—Cont.

bined with a rapid rate of reaction makes calcium carbonate an ideal antacid for management of conditions associated with hyperacidity. It effectively neutralizes free acid yet does not cause systemic alkalosis in the presence of normal renal function.

Warnings: Do not take more than 16 tablets in a 24-hour period or use the maximum dosage of this product for more than 2 weeks, except under the advice and supervision of a doctor. Keep this and all drugs out of the reach of children.

Drug Interaction Precaution: Antacids may interact with certain prescription drugs. If you are presently taking a prescription drug, do not take this product without checking with your physician or other health professional.

Dosage and Administration: Chew 1 or 2 tablets as symptoms occur. Repeat hourly if symptoms return, or as directed by a doctor. No water is required.

Professional Labeling: Indicated for the symptomatic relief of hyperacidity associated with the diagnosis of peptic ulcer, gastritis, peptic esophagitis, gastric hyperacidity, and hiatal hernia.

How Supplied: 60 tablet bottles 4770D

TUMS 500™
Calcium Supplement

Each Tablet Contains: 1,250 mg calcium carbonate, which provides 500 mg elemental calcium (50% of the U.S. RDA, or Daily Value). Each tablet contains less than 4 mg sodium.

Ingredients: Sucrose, Calcium Carbonate, Starch, Talc, Mineral Oil and Sodium Polyphosphate. May also contain Adipic Acid, FD&C Blue 1, FD&C Yellow 6, D&C Yellow 10, D&C Red 27, D&C Red 30.

Directions: Chew one tablet with meals, two to three times a day or as recommended by a physician.

IMPORTANT INFORMATION ON OSTEOPOROSIS

Osteoporosis affects older persons, especially middle-aged, white and Asian women and those whose families tend to have fragile bones in later years. A lifetime of regular exercise and eating a healthful diet that includes enough calcium, especially during teen and early adult years, builds and maintains good bone health and may reduce the risk of osteoporosis later in life. Adequate calcium intake is important, but intakes above 2,000 mg elemental calcium are not likely to provide any additional benefit.

How Supplied: Tums 500™ is available in **Assorted Fruit, Peppermint, Cherry, and Wintergreen** Flavors, in bottles of 60 tablets.

Standard Homeopathic Company
210 WEST 131st STREET
BOX 61067
LOS ANGELES, CA 90061

HYLAND'S ARNICAID™ TABLETS
100% natural temporary relief of symptoms of pain and soreness from muscle overexertion or injury.

Indications: Hyland's Arnicaid Tablets are a homeopathic product indicated for the control and symptomatic relief of acute bruising and soreness due to falls, blows, and muscle strain. Arnicaid provides a 100% natural relief for children and adults. Use after minor accidents or after sports workouts. Arnicaid contains no sucrose, dextrose or fillers. Like all homeopathic products, Arnicaid has no known contraindications or side effects.

Directions: Adults—1–2 tablets every 4 hours, or as needed.
Children over 3 years of age—½ adult dose.

Active Ingredients: Arnica Montana 30X HPUS in a base of lactose USP.

Warnings: Do not use if cap band is broken or missing. If symptoms persist for more than seven days or worsen, contact a licensed health care professional. Do not use in children under three years of age without consulting a licensed health care professional. As with any drug, if you are pregnant or nursing a baby, seek the advice of a licensed health care professional before using this product. Keep this and all medications out of reach of children. In case of accidental overdose, contact a poison control center or the manufacturer at the number provided below.
P&S Laboratories
Los Angeles, CA 90061
Questions? Call us: 800/624-9659
MADE IN USA
Arnicaid and Hyland's are trademarks of Standard Homeopathic Co.

HYLAND'S BED WETTING TABLETS

Active Ingredients: *Equisetum hyemale* (Scouring Rush) 2X HPUS, *Rhus aromatica* (Fragrant Sumac) 3X HPUS, *Belladonna* 3X HPUS (0.0003% Alkaloids).

Inactive Ingredients: Lactose USP.

Indications: A homeopathic combination for the temporary relief of involuntary urination (common bed wetting) in children.

Directions: Children 3 to 12 years: 2 to 3 tablets before meals and at bedtime, or as directed by a licensed health care practitioner. Children over 12 years: double the above recommended dose.

Warnings: If symptoms persist for more than seven days or worsen, consult a Health Care Professional. As with any drug, if you are pregnant or nursing a baby, seek the advice of a health professional before using this product. Keep this and all medication out of the reach of children.

How Supplied: Bottles of 125—one grain sublingual tablets (NDC 54973-7501-01). Store at room temperature.

HYLAND'S CALMS FORTÉ TABLETS

Active Ingredients: *Passiflora* (Passion Flower) 1X triple strength HPUS, *Avena sativa* (Oat) 1X triple strength HPUS, *Humulus lupulus* (Hops) 1X double strength HPUS, *Chamomilla* (Chamomile) 2X HPUS, *Calcarea Phosphorica* (Calcium Phosphate) 3X HPUS, *Ferrum Phosphorica* (Iron Phosphate) 3X HPUS, *Kali Phosphoricum* (Potassium Phosphate) 3X HPUS, *Natrum Phosphoricum* (Sodium Phosphate) 3X HPUS, *Magnesia Phosphoricum* (Magnesium Phosphate) 3X HPUS.

Inactive Ingredients: Lactose USP.

Indications: Temporary symptomatic relief of simple nervous tension and insomnia.

Directions: Adults, As a relaxant: 1 to 2 tablets as needed or 3 times daily between meals. In insomnia: 1 to 3 tablets ½ to 1 hour before retiring. Repeat as needed without danger of side effects. Children, As a relaxant: 1 tablet as needed or 3 times daily before meals. In insomnia: 1 to 2 tablets 1 hour before retiring. Non-habit-forming.

Warnings: If symptoms persist for more than seven days or worsen, consult a Health Care Professional. As with any drug, if you are pregnant or nursing a baby, seek the advice of a health professional before using this product. Keep this and all medication out of the reach of children.

How Supplied: Bottles of 100 four grain tablets (NDC 54973-1121-02). Store at room temperature. Bottles of 50 four grain tablets (NDC 54973-1121-01). Store at room temperature.

HYLAND'S CLEARAC™ TABLETS
All natural ClearAc helps clear up acne, pimples, and acne blemishes.

Indications: Hyland's ClearAc Tablets are a homeopathic combination indicated for the management and symptomatic relief of symptoms of pimples, blackheads, and blemishes associated with common acne (acne vulgaris). ClearAc

Tablets provide a 100% natural approach. Like all homeopathic products, ClearAc Tablets have no known contraindications or side effects. Use in conjunction with a high-quality skin cleanser, such as 100% Natural Hyland's ClearAc Cleanser with Calendula.

Directions: Adults—2–3 tablets every 4 hours, or as needed.

Active Ingredients: Echinacea Ang. 6X HPUS, Berberis Vulg. 6X HPUS, Sulphur Iod. 6X HPUS, Hepar Sulph. 6X HPUS in a base of lactose USP.

Warnings: Do not use if cap band is broken or missing. If symptoms persist or worsen, contact a licensed health care professional. As with any drug, if you are pregnant or nursing a baby, seek the advice of a licensed health care professional before using this product. Keep this and all medications out of reach of children. In case of accidental overdose, contact a poison control center or the manufacturer at the number provided below.
P&S Laboratories
Los Angeles, CA 90061
Questions? Call us: 800/624-9659
MADE IN USA
ClearAc and Hyland's are trademarks of Standard Homeopathic Co.

HYLAND'S COLIC TABLETS

Active Ingredients: *Disocorea* (Wild Yam) 2X HPUS, *Chamomilla* (Chamomile) 3X HPUS, *Colocynth* (Bitter Apple) 3X HPUS.

Inactive Ingredients: Lactose USP.

Indications: A homeopathic combination for the temporary relief of colic and gas pains caused by irritating food, feeding too quickly, swallowing air and similar conditions during teething, colds and other minor upset periods in children.

Directions: For children to 2 years of age: administer 2 tablets dissolved in a teaspoon of water or on the tongue every 15 minutes until relieved; then every 2 hours as required. Children over 2 years: 3 tablets dissolved on the tongue as above; or as recommended by a licensed health care practitioner.

Warnings: If symptoms persist for more than seven days or worsen, consult a Health Care Professional. Keep this and all medication out of the reach of children.

How Supplied: Bottles of 125—one grain sublingual tablets (NDC 54973-7502-01). Store at room temperature.

HYLAND'S COUGH SYRUP WITH HONEY™

Active Ingredients: Each fluid ounce contains: *Ipecacuanha* (Ipecac) 3X HPUS, *Aconitum napellus* (Aconite) 3X HPUS, *Spongia Tosta* (Sponge) 3X HPUS, *Antimonium Tartaricum* (Potassium Antimony Tartrate) 6X HPUS.

Inactive Ingredients: Simple syrup and honey.

Indications: A homeopathic combination for the temporary relief of symptoms of simple, dry, tight or tickling coughs due to colds in children.

Directions: Children 1 to 12 years: 1 to 3 teaspoonfuls as required. Children over 12 years and adults: 3 to 4 teaspoonfuls as required. May be taken with or without water. Repeat as often as necessary to relieve symptoms. For children under 1 year of age, consult a licensed health care practitioner.

Warnings: Do not use this product for persistent or chronic cough such as occurs with asthma, smoking or emphysema; or if cough is accompanied with excessive mucus, unless directed by a licensed health care practitioner. If symptoms persist for more than seven days, tend to recur, or are accompanied by a high fever, rash, or persistent headache, consult a Health Care Professional. As with any drug, if you are pregnant or nursing a baby, seek the advice of a health professional before using this product. Keep this and all medication out of the reach of children.

How Supplied: Bottles of 4 fluid ounces (120 ml) (NDC 54973-7503-02). Store at room temperature.

HYLAND'S C–PLUS™ COLD TABLETS

Active Ingredients: *Eupatorium perfoliatum* (Boneset) 2X HPUS, *Euphrasia officinalis* (Eyebright) 2X HPUS, *Gelsemium sempervirens* (Yellow Jasmine) 3X HPUS, *Kali Iodatum* (Potassium Iodide) 3X HPUS.

Inactive Ingredients: Lactose USP, Natural Raspberry Flavor.

Indications: A homeopathic combination for the temporary relief of symptoms of runny nose and sneezing due to common head colds in children.

Directions: Children 1 to 3 years: 2 tablets every 15 minutes for 4 doses, then hourly until relieved. For children 3 to 6 years: 3 tablets as above; for children 6 and older: 6 tablets as above or as directed by a licensed health care practitioner.

Warnings: If symptoms persist for more than seven days or worsen, consult a Health Care Professional. As with any drug, if you are pregnant or nursing a baby, seek the advice of a health professional before using this product. Keep this and all medication out of the reach of children.

How Supplied: Bottles of 125—one grain sublingual tablets (NDC 54973-7505-01). Store at room temperature.

HYLAND'S DIARREX™ TABLETS
100% natural temporary relief of symptoms of acute gastrointestinal distress associated with nonspecific diarrhea.

Indications: Hyland's Diarrex Tablets are a homeopathic combination indicated for the temporary control and symptomatic relief of acute nonspecific diarrhea. Diarrex provides a 100% natural approach which aids in relief of symptoms of loose stools and associated gastric symptoms. Like all homeopathic products, Diarrex has no known contraindications or side effects.

Directions: Adults—2–3 tablets every 4 hours, or as needed. Children over 3 years of age—½ adult dose.

Active Ingredients: Arsenicum Alb. 6X HPUS, Podophyllum Pelt. 6X HPUS, Chamomilla 6X HPUS, Phosphorus 6X HPUS, Mercurius Viv. 6X HPUS in a base of lactose USP.

Warnings: Do not use if cap band is broken or missing. If symptoms persist for more than two days or worsen, contact a licensed health care professional. Do not use in children under three years of age without consulting a licensed health care professional. Discontinue use if diarrhea is accompanied by a high fever (greater than 101°F), or if blood is present in the stool and contact a licensed health care professional. As with any drug, if you are pregnant or nursing a baby, seek the advice of a licensed health care professional before using this product. Keep this and all medication out of reach of children. In case of accidental overdose, contact a poison control center or the manufacturer at the number provided below.
P&S Laboratories
Los Angeles, CA 90061
Questions? Call us: 800/624-9659
MADE IN USA
Diarrex and Hyland's are trademarks of Standard Homeopathic Co.

HYLAND'S ENURAID™ TABLETS
100% natural temporary relief of symptoms of common incontinence in adults.

Indications: Hyland's EnurAid Tablets are a homeopathic combination indicated for the control and symptomatic relief of involuntary urination (common incontinence) in adults. EnurAid provides a 100% natural approach which aids in relief of symptoms of bladder control and related symptoms. Like all homeopathic products, EnurAid has no known contraindications or side effects.

Directions: Adults—2–3 tablets every 4 hours, or as needed.

Active Ingredients: Belladonna 6X HPUS, Cantharis 6X HPUS, Apis Mell. 6X HPUS, Arnica Mont. 6X HPUS, Allium Cepa 6X HPUS, Rhus Arom. 6X

Continued on next page

Standard Homeopathic—Cont.

HPUS, Equisetum Hyem. 6X HPUS in a base of lactose USP.

Warnings: Do not use if cap band is broken or missing. If symptoms persist for more than seven days or worsen, contact a licensed health care professional. Discontinue use if symptoms are accompanied by a high fever (greater than 101°F), or if blood is present in urine and contact a licensed health care professional. As with any drug, if you are pregnant or nursing a baby, seek the advice of a licensed health care professional before using this product. Keep this and all medications out of reach of children. In case of accidental overdose, contact a poison control center or the manufacturer at the number provided below.
P&S Laboratories
Los Angeles, CA 90061
Questions? Call us: 800/624-9659
MADE IN USA
EnurAid and Hyland's are trademarks of Standard Homeopathic Co.

HYLAND'S TEETHING TABLETS

Active Ingredients: *Calcarea Phosphorica* (Calcium Phosphate) 3X HPUS, *Chamomilla* (Chamomile) 3X HPUS, *Coffea Cruda* (Coffee) 3X HPUS, *Belladonna* 3X HPUS (Alkaloids 0.0003%).

Inactive Ingredients: Lactose USP.

Indications: A homeopathic combination for the temporary relief of symptoms of simple restlessness and wakeful irritability due to cutting of teeth.

Directions: 2 to 3 tablets in a teaspoon of water or on the tongue, 4 times per day. If the child is restless or wakeful, 2 tablets every hour for 6 doses or as directed by a licensed health care practitioner.

Warnings: If symptoms persist for more than seven days or worsen, consult a Health Care Professional. As with any drug, if you are pregnant or nursing a baby, seek the advice of a health professional before using this product. Keep this and all medication out of the reach of children.

How Supplied: Bottles of 125—one grain sublingual tablets (NDC 54973-7504-01). Store at room temperature.

HYLAND'S VITAMIN C FOR CHILDREN™

Active Ingredients: 25 mg Vitamin C as Sodium Ascorbate (30 mg).

Inactive Ingredients: Lactose USP, Natural Lemon Flavor.

Indications: Each tablet provides children with 55% of the daily recommended requirement of Vitamin C. Sodium Ascorbate is preferred to Ascorbic Acid

when gastric irritation may result from free acid.

Directions: Children 2 years and older: 1 to 2 tablets on the tongue or as directed by a licensed health care practitioner.

Warning: Keep this and all medication out of the reach of children.

How Supplied: Bottles of 125—one grain sublingual tablets (NDC 54973-7506-01). Store at room temperature. Tablets may turn brown in color with exposure to light. Color change does not affect potency.

Stellar Pharmacal Corp.
Div./Star Pharmaceuticals, Inc.
1990 N.W. 44TH STREET
POMPANO BEACH, FL
33064-8712

STAR–OTIC® EAR SOLUTION
Antibacterial, Antifungal, Nonaqueous Ear Solution

Active Ingredients: Acetic acid nonaqueous, Burow's solution, Boric acid, in a propylene glycol vehicle, with an acid pH and a low surface tension.

Indications: For the prevention of otitis externa, commonly called "Swimmer's Ear". To inhibit bacterial and fungal growth and maintain the external ear canal's normal acid mantle following swimming or showering.

Actions: Star-Otic Ear Solution is antibacterial, antifungal, hydrophilic, has an acid pH and a low surface tension. Acetic acid and boric acid inhibit the rapid multiplication of microorganisms and help maintain the lining mantle of the ear canal in its normal acid state. Burow's solution (aluminum acetate) is a mild astringent. Propylene glycol reduces moisture in the ear canal.

Warning: Do not use in ear if tympanic membrane (ear drum) is perforated or punctured.

Symptoms and Treatment of Overdosage: Discontinue use if undue irritation or sensitivity occurs.

Dosage and Administration: Adults and Children: To help restore normal pH to the outer ear canal. In susceptible persons, instill 3–5 drops of Star-Otic Ear Solution in each ear before and after swimming or bathing, or as directed by physician.

Professional Labeling: Same as those outlined under Indications.

How Supplied: Available in ½ oz measured drop, safety tip, plastic bottle.

Sterling Health
See Miles Inc.

Thompson Medical Company, Inc.
222 LAKEVIEW AVENUE
WEST PALM BEACH
FLORIDA 33401

ASPERCREME®
[*ăs-per-crēme*]
External Analgesic Rub With Aloe

Description: ASPERCREME® is available as an odor-free creme and lotion for use as a topical massage rub that temporarily relieves minor muscle aches and pains.
Aspercreme does not contain aspirin.

Active Ingredient: Salycin® 10% (Thompson Medical's brand of Trolamine Salicylate).

Other Ingredients: Creme: Aloe Vera Gel, Cetyl Alcohol, Glycerin, Methylparaben, Mineral Oil, Potassium Phosphate, Propylparaben, Stearic Acid, Triethanolamine, Water. Lotion: Aloe Vera Gel, Cetyl Alcohol, Glyceryl Stearate, Isopropyl Palmitate, Lanolin, Methylparaben, Potassium Phosphate, Propylene Glycol, Propylparaben, Sodium Lauryl Sulfate, Stearic Acid, Water.

Actions: External analgesic rub.

Indications: Analgesic rub for temporary relief of minor aches and pains of muscles associated with simple strains and sprains.

Warnings: Use only as directed. If prone to allergic reaction from aspirin or salicylate, consult a physician before using. If redness is present or condition worsens, or if pain persists for more than 7 days or clears up and occurs again within a few days, discontinue use and consult a physician. Do not use on children under 10 years of age. Do not apply if skin is irritated or if irritation develops. As with any drug, if you are pregnant or nursing a baby, seek the advice of a health professional before using this product. For external use only. Avoid contact with eyes. **KEEP THIS AND ALL MEDICINES OUT OF THE REACH OF CHILDREN.** In case of accidental ingestion seek professional assistance or contact a poison control center immediately.

Dosage and Administration: Apply generously to affected area. Massage into painful area until thoroughly absorbed into skin, repeat as necessary, but not more than 4 times daily.

How to Store: Store at controlled room temperature 59°–86°F (15°–30°C).

How Supplied: Creme: 1¼ oz., 3 oz. and 5 oz. tubes. Lotion: 6 oz. bottle.

Shown in Product Identification Guide, page 526

CAPZASIN-P
[Căp-zā-sĭn-P]
Topical Analgesic Creme

Description: Capzasin-P contains purified capsaicin, a natural ingredient that penetrates deep to temporarily relieve minor aches and pains of muscles and joints associated with arthritis, simple backache, strains and sprains. Capzasin-P is so effective that doctors recommend it more than all other topical analgesics combined.

Active Ingredient: Capsaicin 0.025% w/w.

Other Ingredients: Benzyl Alcohol, Cetyl Alcohol, Glyceryl Monostearate, Isopropyl Myristate, Polyoxyl 40 Stearate, Purified Water, Sorbitol Solution, White Petrolatum.

Actions: External analgesic rub.

Indications: For the temporary relief of minor aches and pains of muscles and joints associated with arthritis, simple backache, strains and sprains.

Warnings: For external use only. Avoid contact with the eyes and mucous membranes. If condition worsens, or if symptoms persist for more than 7 days or clear up and occur again within a few days, discontinue use of this product and consult a physician. Do not apply to wounds, damaged or broken (open), irritated skin or if excessive irritation develops. Do not bandage tightly. Do not use with a heating pad. As with any drug, if you are pregnant or nursing a baby, seek the advice of a health professional before using this product. **KEEP THIS AND ALL MEDICINES OUT OF THE REACH OF CHILDREN.** In case of accidental ingestion, seek professional assistance or contact a poison control center immediately.

Dosage and Administration: Adults and children 2 years of age and older: Apply to affected area not more than 3 to 4 times daily. Children under 2 years of age: Consult a physician. Transient burning may occur upon application, but generally disappears in several days. For optimum relief, apply 3 to 4 times daily. **WASH HANDS WITH SOAP AND**

WATER AFTER APPLYING. Read package insert before using.

How to Store: Store at controlled room temperature 15°–30°C (59°–86°F).

How Supplied: 1.5 oz. creme tube.

Shown in Product Identification Guide, page 526

CORTIZONE-5®
Creme and Ointment
CORTIZONE FOR KIDS™ Creme
Anti-itch
(0.5% hydrocortisone)

Description: CORTIZONE-5® creme and ointment are topical anti-itch preparations containing aloe.

Active Ingredient: Hydrocortisone 0.5%.

Other Ingredients: Creme: Aloe Vera Gel, Aluminum Sulfate, Calcium Acetate, Cetearyl Alcohol, Glycerin, Light Mineral Oil, Methylparaben, Potato Dextrin, Propylparaben, Sodium C12–15 Alcohols Sulfate, Sodium Lauryl Sulfate, Water, White Petrolatum, White Wax. Ointment: Aloe Extract, White Petrolatum.

Indications: CORTIZONE-5® is recommended for the temporary relief of itching associated with minor skin irritations, inflammations and rashes due to: eczema, insect bites, poison ivy, oak, sumac, soaps, detergents, cosmetics, jewelry, seborrheic dermatitis, psoriasis, external anal and genital itching. Other uses of this product should be only under the advice and supervision of a physician.

Warnings: For external use only. Avoid contact with the eyes. If condition worsens, or if symptoms persist for more than 7 days or clear up and occur again within a few days, do not use this or any other hydrocortisone product unless you have consulted a physician. Do not use in genital area if you have a vaginal discharge, consult a physician. Do not use for the treatment of diaper rash, or for the treatment of chicken pox, consult a physician.
Warnings For External Anal Itching Users: Do not exceed the recommended daily dosage unless directed by a physician. In case of bleeding, consult a physician promptly. Do not put this product into the rectum by using fingers or any mechanical device or applicator.
KEEP THIS AND ALL MEDICINES OUT OF THE REACH OF CHILDREN. In case of accidental ingestion, seek professional assistance or contact a Poison Control Center immediately.

Dosage and Administration: Adults and children 2 years of age and older: Apply to affected area not more than 3 to 4 times daily. Children under 2 years of age: Do not use, consult a physician.
Directions For External Anal Itching Users: Adults: When practical, cleanse the affected area with mild soap and warm water and rinse thoroughly.

Gently dry by patting or blotting with toilet tissue or a soft cloth before application of this product. Children under 12 years of age: Consult a physician.

How to Store: Store at controlled room temperature 15°–30°C (59°–86°F).

How Supplied: CORTIZONE-5 creme: 1 oz. and 2 oz. tubes. CORTIZONE for KIDS™ creme: ½ oz. and 1 oz. tubes. CORTIZONE-5 ointment: 1 oz. tube.

Shown in Product Identification Guide, page 526

CORTIZONE-10™
Creme and Ointment
CORTIZONE-10™ EXTERNAL ANAL ITCH RELIEF Creme
CORTIZONE-10™ SCALP ITCH FORMULA™ Liquid
Anti-itch
(1.0% hydrocortisone)

Description: CORTIZONE-10™ creme with aloe, ointment and liquid are topical anti-itch preparations. Maximum Strength available without a prescription.

Active Ingredient: Hydrocortisone 1.0%.

Other Ingredients: Creme: Aloe Vera Gel, Aluminum Sulfate, Calcium Acetate, Cetearyl Alcohol, Glycerin, Light Mineral Oil, Methylparaben, Potato Dextrin, Propylparaben, Sodium C12-15 Alcohols Sulfate, Sodium Lauryl Sulfate, Water, White Petrolatum, White Wax. Ointment: White Petrolatum. Liquid: Benzyl Alcohol, Propylene Glycol, Purified Water, SD Alcohol 40-2 (60% v/v).

Indications: Cortizone-10™ is recommended for the temporary relief of itching associated with minor skin irritations, inflammation and rashes due to: eczema, insect bites, poison ivy, oak, sumac, soaps, detergents, cosmetics, jewelry, seborrheic dermatitis, psoriasis, external anal and genital itching. Other uses of this product should be only under the advice and supervision of a physician.

Warnings: For external use only. Avoid contact with the eyes. If condition worsens, or if symptoms persist for more than 7 days or clear up and occur again within a few days, do not use this or any other hydrocortisone product unless you have consulted a physician. Do not use in genital area if you have a vaginal discharge, consult a physician. Do not use for the treatment of diaper rash, consult a physician. **Warnings For External Anal Itching Users:** Do not exceed the recommended daily dosage unless directed by a physician. In case of bleeding, consult a physician promptly. Do not put this product into the rectum by using fingers or any mechanical device or applicator.

Continued on next page

Thompson Medical—Cont.

KEEP THIS AND ALL MEDICINES OUT OF THE REACH OF CHILDREN. In case of accidental ingestion, seek professional assistance or contact a Poison Control Center immediately.

Dosage and Administration: Adults and children 2 years of age and older: Apply to affected area not more than 3 to 4 times daily. Children under 2 years of age: Do not use, consult a physician.

Directions For External Anal Itching Users: Adults: When practical, cleanse the affected area with mild soap and warm water. Rinse thoroughly. Gently dry by patting or blotting with tissue or a soft cloth before application of this product. Children under 12 years of age: Consult a physician.

How to Store: Store at controlled room temperature 15°–30°C (59°–86°F).

How Supplied: CORTIZONE-10™ creme: 1 oz. and 2 oz. tubes. CORTIZONE-10™ ointment: 1 oz. and 2 oz. tubes. CORTIZONE-10™ External Anal Itch Relief creme: 1 oz. tube. CORTIZONE-10™ Scalp Itch Formula™ liquid: 1.5 fl. oz.

Shown in Product Identification Guide, page 526

DEXATRIM® Caplets and Tablets
[*dĕx-a-trĭm*]
Prolonged action anorectic for weight control

DEXATRIM® Maximum Strength Plus Vitamin C/Caplets and Caffeine-Free Caplets
phenylpropanolamine HCl   75mg (time release)
(180 mg Vitamin C, immediate release, added for nutritional supplementation)

DEXATRIM® Maximum Strength Extended Duration Time Tablets
phenylpropanolamine HCl   75mg (time release)

Indication: DEXATRIM® is an aid for effective appetite control to assist weight reduction. It is available in a time release dosage form.

Directions: Adult oral dosage is **one caplet** at mid-morning with a full glass of water. **Exceeding the recommended dose has not been shown to result in greater weight loss.** (This product's effectiveness is directly related to the degree to which you reduce your usual daily food intake.) The use of this product should be limited to periods not exceeding 3 months, because this should be enough time to establish new eating habits. Read and follow the important Diet Plan enclosed.

Warnings: DO NOT TAKE MORE THAN 1 DEXATRIM CAPLET PER DAY (24 HOURS). Exceeding the recommended dose may cause serious health problems. FOR ADULT USE ONLY. Do not give this product to children under 12 years of age. Persons between 12 and 18 or over 60 are advised to consult their physician before using this product.

There have been reports that stroke, seizure, heart attack, arrhythmia, psychosis, and death might be associated with the ingestion of phenylpropanolamine. If you are being treated for depression, an eating disorder or have heart disease, diabetes, thyroid or any other disease, do not take this product except under the supervision of a physician. If nervousness, dizziness, sleeplessness, palpitations or headache occurs, stop taking this medication and consult your physician. Check your blood pressure regularly. If you have high blood pressure, do not use this product and consult your physician. As with any drug, if you are pregnant or nursing a baby, seek the advice of a health professional before using this product. Do not take this product if you are hypersensitive to any of its ingredients.

Drug Interaction Precaution: If you are taking a cough/cold or allergy medication containing any form of phenylpropanolamine, or any oral nasal decongestant, do not take this product. Do not use this product if you are taking any prescription drug, except under the advice and supervision of a physician. Do not use this product if you are presently taking a prescription monoamine oxidase inhibitor (MAOI) for depression or for two weeks after stopping use of an MAOI without first consulting a physician. KEEP THIS AND ALL MEDICATIONS OUT OF THE REACH OF CHILDREN. In case of accidental overdose, seek professional assistance or contact a poison control center immediately.

Dosage and Administration:
Caplet Dosage Forms: DEXATRIM® Maximum Strength Plus Vitamin C, DEXATRIM® Maximum Strength/Caffeine-Free.
Tablet Dosage Form: DEXATRIM® Maximum Strength Extended Duration Time Tablets.
Administration: One caplet or tablet at midmorning with a full glass of water.

How Supplied: All Dexatrim products are supplied in tamper-evident blister packages. Do not use if individual seals are broken.
DEXATRIM® Maximum Strength Plus Vitamin C/Caffeine-Free Caplets: Packages of 20 and 40 with 1250 calorie DEXATRIM Diet Plan.
DEXATRIM® Maximum Strength Extended Duration Time Tablets: Packages of 20 and 40 with 1250 calorie DEXATRIM Diet Plan.

References: Altschuler, S., et. al., *Int J Obesity,* 1982;6:549–556.
Atkinson, RL, Dannels SA, Marlin RL; AM J Clin Nutr, 56 (4); 755; Oct. 1992.
Blackburn, G.L., et. al., *JAMA,* 1989; 261:3267–3272.
Morgan, J.P., et. al., *J Clin Psychopharm,* 1989:9(1):33–38.
Lasagna, L., *Phenylpropanolamine—A Review,* New York, John Wiley and Sons, 1988.
All referenced materials available on request.

Shown in Product Identification Guide, page 526

DEXATRIM® PLUS VITAMINS
[*Dĕx-ă-trĭm Plus Vitamins*]
Prolonged action anorectic for weight control plus a multi-vitamin. Phenylpropanolamine HCl 75 mg (time release) plus a Multi-Vitamin tablet

Indication: DEXATRIM® is an aid for effective appetite control to assist weight reduction. It is available in a time release dosage form. The multi-vitamin, in caplet form, is for dietary supplementation.

Ingredients: Each Maximum Strength Dexatrim Caplet Contains: Active Ingredient: Phenylpropanolamine HCl 75 mg. (appetite suppressant time release). Inactive Ingredients: Vitamin C (Ascorbic Acid) 180 mg., Calcium Sulfate Dihydrate, Croscarmellose Sodium, Ethylcellulose, FD&C Blue No. 1 Aluminum Lake, FD&C Red No. 40 Aluminum Lake, FD&C Yellow No. 6 Aluminum Lake, Hydroxypropyl Methylcellulose, Lactose, Magnesium Stearate, Polyethylene Glycol, Polysorbate 80, Stearic Acid, Titanium Dioxide.

Each Vitamin/Mineral Caplet Contains:		%U.S.RDA[1]
Vitamin A (as Acetate & Beta Carotene)	5,000 IU	100%
Vitamin E (di-Alpha Tocopheryl Acetate)	30 IU	100%
Vitamin C (as Ascorbic Acid)	60 mg.	100%
Folic Acid	0.4 mg.	100%
Vitamin B1 (as Thiamine Mononitrate)	1.5 mg.	100%
Vitamin B2 (as Riboflavin)	1.7 mg.	100%
Niacinamide	20 mg.	100%
Vitamin B6 (as Pyridoxine Hydrochloride)	2 mg.	100%
Vitamin B12 (as Cyanocobalamin)	6 mcg.	100%
Vitamin D	400 IU	100%
Biotin	30 mcg.	10%
Pantothenic Acid (as Calcium Pantothenate)	10 mg.	100%
Calcium (as Dibasic Calcium Phosphate)	162 mg.	16%
Phosphorus (as Dibasic Calcium Phosphate)	125 mg.	13%
Iodine (as Potassium Iodide)	150 mcg.	100%
Iron (as Ferrous Fumarate)	18 mg.	100%
Magnesium (as Magnesium Oxide)	100 mg.	25%
Copper (as Cupric Oxide)	2 mg.	100%
Zinc (as Zinc Oxide)	15 mg.	100%
Manganese (as Manganese Sulfate)	2.5 mg.	*
Potassium (as Potassium Chloride)	40 mg.	*
Chloride (as Potassium Chloride)	36.3 mg.	*

Chromium (as Chromium
Chloride) .... 25 mcg. *
Molybdenum (as Sodium
Molybdate) .... 25 mcg. *
Selenium (as Sodium
Selenate) .... 25 mcg. *
Vitamin K1 (as
Phytonadione) .... 25 mcg. *
Nickel (as Nickel Sulfate) .... 5 mcg. *
Tin (as Stannous Chloride) .... 10 mcg. *
Silicon (as Sodium
Metasilicate & Oxides) .... 2 mg. *
Vanadium (as Sodium
Metavanadate) .... 10 mcg. *
Boron (as Borates) .... 150 mcg. *

[1]U.S.RECOMMENDED DAILY AL-
LOWANCE (U.S. RDA) FOR ADULTS
AND CHILDREN 4 OR MORE YEARS
OF AGE
*NO U.S. RDA HAS BEEN ESTAB-
LISHED.

Other Ingredients: Cellulose, FD&C
Blue No. 1, FD&C Yellow No. 6, Hydroxypropyl Methylcellulose, Magnesium
Stearate, Methylcellulose, Polyethylene
Glycol, Polysorbate 80, Povidone, Propylene Glycol, Titanium Dioxide, Silica, Silicon Dioxide, Starch, Water.

Directions: Adult oral dosage is **one
red caplet marked "dexatrim"** and **one
vitamin/mineral caplet marked
"Complete Vitamin"** at mid-morning
with a full glass of water. Exceeding the
recommended dose has not been shown
to result in greater weight loss. (This
product's effectiveness is directly related
to the degree to which you reduce your
usual daily food intake.) The use of this
product should be limited to periods not
exceeding 3 months, because this should
be enough time to establish new eating
habits. Read and follow important Diet
Plan enclosed.

**WARNINGS: FOR ADULT USE
ONLY. DO NOT TAKE MORE THAN
1 DEXATRIM CAPLET PER DAY (24
HOURS). Exceeding the recommended dose may cause serious
health problems. FOR ADULT USE
ONLY.** Do not give this product to children under 12 years of age. Persons between 12 and 18 or over 60 are advised to
consult their physician before using this
product.
There have been reports that stroke, seizure, heart attack, arrhythmia, psychosis, and death might be associated with
the ingestion of phenylpropanolamine. If
you are being treated for depression, an
eating disorder or have heart disease,
diabetes, thyroid or any other disease, do
not take this product except under the
supervision of a physician. If nervousness, dizziness, sleeplessness, palpitations or headache occurs, stop taking this
medication and consult your physician.
Check your blood pressure regularly. If
you have high blood pressure, do not use
this product and consult your physician.
As with any drug, if you are pregnant or
nursing a baby, seek the advice of a
health professional before using this
product. Do not take this product if you

are hypersensitive to any of its ingredients.
Drug Interaction Precaution: If you
are taking a cough/cold or allergy
medication containing any form of phenylpropanolamine, or any oral nasal decongestant, do not take this product. Do
not use this product if you are taking any
prescription drug, except under the advice and supervision of a physician. Do
not use this product if you are presently
taking a prescription monoamine oxidase inhibitor (MAOI) for depression or
for two weeks after stopping use of
an MAOI without first consulting a
physician.
KEEP THIS AND ALL MEDICATIONS
OUT OF THE REACH OF CHILDREN.
In case of accidental overdose, seek professional assistance or contact a poison
control center immediately.
How Supplied: Dexatrim Plus Vitamins is supplied in tamper-evident blister packaging containing 14 Dexatrim
caplets and 14 multi-vitamin/mineral
caplets or containing 28 Dexatrim
caplets and 28 multi-vitamin/mineral
caplets.
*Shown in Product Identification
Guide, page 526*

ENCARE®
[en'kar]
Vaginal Contraceptive Suppositories

Description: Encare is a safe and effective contraceptive in a convenient
vaginal suppository form available without a prescription. Encare is reliable
because it offers two-way protection:
(1) Encare kills sperm on contact by releasing a precise dose of nonoxynol 9, the
spermicide most recommended by doctors. (2) Encare gently disperses a physical barrier of protection against the cervix to help prevent pregnancy.
Encare is colorless and odorless; it is as
pleasant to use as it is effective.
Encare is an effective contraceptive in
vaginal suppository form.

Active Ingredient: Each Suppository
contains 100 mg Nonoxynol 9.
Other Ingredients: Polyethylene Glycols, Sodium Bicarbonate, Sodium
Citrate, Tartaric Acid.
Indications: Encare is effective in the
prevention of pregnancy.
Action: Encare is 100% free of hormones and free of the serious side effects
associated with oral contraceptives.
Encare is convenient and easy to use.
Women like Encare because each insert
is individually wrapped and can be easily
carried in a pocket or purse. Encare is
approximately as effective as vaginal
foam contraceptives in actual use, yet
there is no applicator, so there is nothing
to fill, remove, or clean. For added protection, Encare may be used in conjunction with other contraceptive methods,
such as a condom or as a second application with a diaphragm.
Because Encare can be inserted as much
as an hour before intercourse, it does not

interfere with spontaneity or ruin the
mood. Many men are not even aware a
woman is using Encare. Encare has been
used successfully by millions of women
throughout Europe and America.

Special Warning: Spermicidal contraceptives should not be used during
pregnancy. Some experts believe that
there may be an increased risk of birth
defects occurring in children whose
mothers used a spermicidal contraceptive at the time of conception or during
pregnancy. If you believe you may be
pregnant, have a pregnancy test before
using a spermicidal contraceptive. If you
have used a spermicidal contraceptive
after becoming pregnant, or used a spermicidal contraceptive when you became
pregnant, discuss this issue with your
doctor.

Cautions: If your doctor has told you
that you should not become pregnant,
consult your doctor as to which method,
(including Encare), is best for you.
If you or your partner experience irritation, discontinue use. If irritation persists, consult your doctor. This product
has not been shown to protect against
HIV (AIDS) and other sexually transmitted diseases.
Do not take orally. **KEEP THIS AND
ALL DRUGS OUT OF THE REACH OF
CHILDREN.** In case of accidental ingestion, call a poison control center,
emergency medical facility or a doctor
immediately.
Keep away from excessive heat and moisture. Store at controlled room temperature: 15°C–30°C (59°–86°F).

Dosage and Administration: For best
protection against pregnancy, it is essential to follow package instructions. At
least 10 minutes before intercourse,
place one Encare insert with your fingertip as far as possible into the vagina, to-
wards the small of your back. Best protection will occur when Encare is placed
deep into the vagina. You may feel a
pleasant sensation of warmth as Encare
effervesces and distributes the spermicide, nonoxynol 9, within the vagina.
This is a natural attribute of the active
ingredient.
IMPORTANT: It is essential to insert
Encare at least 10 minutes before intercourse. If one chooses, Encare can be inserted up to one hour before intercourse.
If intercourse has not taken place within
one hour after insertion, use a new Encare insert. Use a new Encare insert each
time intercourse is repeated. Encare can
be used safely as frequently as needed.
Douching after use of Encare is not required; however, should you desire to do
so, wait at least six hours after intercourse.
**Instructions enclosed in package are
in both English and Spanish.**

How Supplied: Boxes of 12.

References: Barwin, B., *Contraceptive
Delivery System*, 4, 331–334, 1983. Mas-

Continued on next page

Thompson Medical—Cont.

ters, W., et. al. *Fertility and Sterility*, 32, 161–165, 1979.
Dimpfl J., et. al. sexualmedizin 1984; 2: 95-8. Schill WB, Wolff HH. Andrologia 1981; 13(1): 42-9. Stone SC, Cardinale F. AM J Obstet Gynecol 1979; 133: 635-8.

HEMORID™ For Women
Hemorrhoidal Creme, Suppositories, and Cleanser

Description: HEMORID™ For Women is available in Creme, Suppositories and Cleanser.

Ingredients:
Creme: Active Ingredients: White Petrolatum 30.0%, Mineral Oil 20.0%, Pramoxine Hydrochloride 1.0%, Phenylephrine Hydrochloride 0.25%. Other Ingredients: Aloe Vera Gel, Cetyl Alcohol, Methylparaben, Polysorbate 80, PPG-15 Stearyl Ether, Propylparaben, Purified Water, Sorbitan Monooleate, Stearyl Alcohol.
Suppositories: Active Ingredients: Zinc Oxide USP 11.0%, Phenylephrine Hydrochloride USP 0.25%, and Hard Fat 88.25%.
Other Ingredients: Aloe Vera
Cleanser: Contains: Water, Mineral Oil, Petrolatum, Glyceryl Stearate, PEG-100 Stearate, Glycerin, Stearic Acid, Triethanolamine, Squalane, Methylparaben, Cetyl Alcohol, Diazolidinyl Urea, Propylparaben, Orange Blossom Extract.

Indications:
Creme: Temporarily shrinks swollen hemorrhoidal tissue and helps relieve the local pain, burning, itching and discomfort associated with hemorrhoids or anorectal inflammation.
Suppositories: Temporarily shrinks swollen hemorrhoidal tissue and helps relieve the local itching, discomfort, and burning associated with hemorrhoids or anorectal inflammation.
Cleanser: Specifically formulated to cleanse, refresh, and soothe the perianal area. Also may be used for the external vaginal area.
Warnings:
Creme: Do not use in the eyes or nose. If condition worsens or does not improve within 7 days, consult a physician. Do not exceed the recommended daily dosage, unless directed by a physician. Do not apply to large areas of the body. In case of bleeding, consult a physician promptly. Do not put this product into the rectum by using fingers or any mechanical device or applicator. Certain persons can develop allergic reactions to ingredients in this product. If the symptom being treated does not subside or if redness, irritation, swelling, pain or other symptoms develop or increase, discontinue use and consult a physician. Do not use this product if you have heart disease, high blood pressure, thyroid disease, diabetes or difficulty in urination due to enlarge-

ment of the prostate gland, unless directed by a physician. As with any drug, if you are pregnant or nursing a baby, seek the advice of a health professional before using this product.
Suppositories: If condition worsens or does not improve within 7 days, consult a physician. Do not exceed the recommended daily dosage, unless directed by a physician. In case of bleeding, consult a physician promptly. Do not use this product if you have heart disease, high blood pressure, thyroid disease, diabetes or difficulty in urination due to enlargement of the prostate gland, unless directed by a physician. As with any drug, if you are pregnant or nursing a baby, seek the advice of a health professional before using this product.
Cleanser: If irritation persists or worsens, discontinue use and consult a physician. In case of bleeding, consult a physician promptly.

Dosage and Administration:
Creme: **Adults:** When practical, cleanse the affected area with mild soap and warm water and rinse thoroughly. Gently dry by patting or blotting with toilet tissue or a soft cloth before application of this product. Apply externally to the affected area up to 4 times daily. **Children under 12 years of age:** Consult a physician.
Suppositories: Adults: When practical, cleanse the affected area with mild soap and warm water and rinse thoroughly. Gently dry by patting or blotting with toilet tissue or a soft cloth before application of this product. Detach one suppository from strip of suppositories. Holding one suppository upright, carefully remove the wrapper by peeling down both sides starting from the pointed end. Insert into the rectum pointed end first. Avoid excessive handling of the suppository. May be used up to 4 times daily. **Children under 12 years of age:** Consult a physician.
Cleanser: Apply a small amount of the cleanser onto bathroom tissue and wipe skin around the perianal area after bowel movements or when discomfort occurs. To soothe and refresh the external vaginal area, apply a small amount of cleanser onto bathroom tissue and cleanse as needed.
How to Store: Store at controlled room temperature 15°-30°C (59°-86°F).

How Supplied: HEMORID For Women Creme: 1 oz. tube. HEMORID For Women Suppositories: 12's. HEMORID For Women Cleanser: 4 oz. bottle.
Shown in Product Identification Guide, page 526

SLEEPINAL®
Night-time Sleep Aid Capsules and Softgels
(Diphenhydramine HCl)

Description: SLEEPINAL is a nighttime sleep aid. When taken prior to bedtime, it helps to relieve sleeplessness and aids in falling asleep.

Active Ingredient: Diphenhydramine HCl 50 mg.

Other Ingredients: Capsules: FD&C Blue No. 1, Gelatin, Lactose, Magnesium Stearate, Povidone, Talc.
Softgels: D&C Yellow No. 10, FD&C Blue No. 1, Gelatin, Glycerin, Polyethylene Glycol 400, Povidone 30, Propylene Glycol, Sorbitol, Water.

Indications: For relief of occasional sleeplessness.

Action: SLEEPINAL is an antihistamine with anticholinergic and sedative action.

Warnings: **Read before using.** Do not exceed recommended dosage. Do not give to children under 12 years of age. If sleeplessness persists continuously for more than 2 weeks, consult your physician. Insomnia may be a symptom of serious underlying medical illness. Do not take this product, unless directed by a physician, if you have a breathing problem such as emphysema or chronic bronchitis, or if you have glaucoma or difficulty in urination due to the enlargement of the prostate gland. Avoid alcoholic beverages while taking this product. Do not take this product if you are taking sedatives or tranquilizers, without first consulting your physician. As with any drug, if you are pregnant or nursing a baby, seek the advice of a health professional before using this product.
KEEP THIS AND ALL MEDICATIONS OUT OF THE REACH OF CHILDREN. In case of accidental overdose, seek professional assistance or contact a Poison Control Center immediately.

Dosage and Administration: Capsules and Softgels: Adults and children 12 years of age and over: Oral dosage, one at bedtime if needed, or as directed by a physician.

How to Store: Store in a dry place at controlled room temperature 15° C–30° C (59° F–86° F). Protect softgels from light, retain product in box until administered.

How Supplied: Capsules and Softgels: Sleepinal is supplied in tamper-evident blister packages. Do not use if individual seals are broken. Packages of 16 and 32 capsules and 8 and 16 softgels.
Shown in Product Identification Guide, page 526

SPORTSCREME®
[spŏrts-crēme]
External Analgesic Rub

Description: SPORTSCREME® is available as a creme and lotion for use as a topical massage rub that temporarily relieves minor muscle aches and pains. Sportscreme has a clean, fresh scent.

Active Ingredient: Salycin® 10% (Thompson Medical's brand of Trolamine Salicylate).

Other Ingredients: Cetyl Alcohol, FD&C Blue No. 1, FD&C Yellow No. 5,

Fragrance, Glycerin, Methylparaben, Mineral Oil, Potassium Phosphate Monobasic, Propylparaben, Stearic Acid, Triethanolamine, Water.

Actions: External analgesic rub.

Indications: Analgesic rub for temporary relief of minor aches and pains of muscles associated with simple strains and sprains.

Warnings: Use only as directed. If prone to allergic reaction from aspirin or salicylate, consult a physician before using. If redness is present or if condition worsens, or if pain persists for more than 7 days, discontinue use and consult a physician. Do not use on children under ten years of age. Do not apply if skin is irritated or if irritation develops. As with any drug, if you are pregnant or nursing a baby, seek the advice of a health professional before using this product. For external use only. Avoid contact with eyes. KEEP THIS AND ALL MEDICINES OUT OF THE REACH OF CHILDREN. In case of accidental ingestion, seek professional assistance or contact a poison control center immediately.

Dosage and Administration: Apply generously to affected area. Massage into painful area until thoroughly absorbed into skin. Repeat as needed, especially before retiring and in the morning, but not more than 4 times daily.

How to Store: Store at controlled room temperature 15°–30°C (59°–86°F).

How Supplied: Cream: 1.25 oz. and 3 oz. tubes: Lotion: 6 oz. bottle.

TEMPO
[tem-pō]
Soft Antacid

Description: Tempo is a unique, chewable soft antacid that provides fast, effective relief from acid indigestion, heartburn, and gas. Tempo is pleasant tasting, not chalky or gritty.

Active Ingredients: Each drop contains Calcium Carbonate 414 mg., Aluminum Hydroxide 133 mg., Magnesium Hydroxide 81 mg., Simethicone 20 mg.

Other Ingredients: Corn Syrup, Deionized Water, FD&C Blue No. 1, Flavor, Sorbitol, Soy Protein, Starch, Titanium Dioxide, 3.0 mg. Sodium per drop (dietetically sodium free).

Indication: For the relief of heartburn, sour stomach, acid indigestion, gas, and upset stomach associated with these symptoms.

Warnings: Do not take more than 12 drops in a 24-hour period or use the maximum dosage for more than two weeks except under the advice and supervision of a doctor. **KEEP THIS AND ALL DRUGS OUT OF THE REACH OF CHILDREN.**

Drug Interaction Precaution: Antacids may interact with certain prescription drugs. If you are presently taking a prescription drug, do not take this product without checking with your physician or other health professional.

Dosage and Administration: One tablet dosage. Not to exceed more than 12 tablets in a 24-hour period.

How to Store: Store at controlled room temperature 15°–30°C (59°–86°F).

How Supplied: 10, 30, and 60 Pieces
Shown in Product Identification Guide, page 526

Transdermal Technologies, Inc.
P.O. BOX 14804
NORTH PALM BEACH, FL
33408-0804

NDC 58433-100-00
TOPICAL ANALGESIC OINTMENT

Indications: For temporary relief of minor aches and pains of muscles and joints associated with bruises, backache, strains resulting from athletic or other strenuous activity of arthritis.

Directions: Adults and children, 5 years of age and older. Smooth a small amount onto affected area until it disappears. May be applied repeatedly if pain persists until an easing of pain is experienced. Apply not more than 3 or 4 times daily. Children under 5: Consult a physician. Non-staining.

Active Ingredient: Strong ammonia solution.

Warnings: For External Use Only. Avoid contact with eyes. Do not apply to broken or irritated skin. Do not bandage tightly. Do not use if skin irritation develops. If condition worsens, or if symptoms persist for more than 7 days, discontinue use of this product and consult a physician. Do not use in the presence of Poison Oak, Ivy, or Sumac. Persons with known skin sensitivities should consult a physician before using this product. KEEP THIS AND ALL MEDICINES OUT OF THE REACH OF CHILDREN.
Store at room temperature. Made in U.S.A.

Triton Consumer Products, Inc.
561 W. GOLF ROAD
ARLINGTON HEIGHTS, IL 60005

MG 217® PSORIASIS/DANDRUFF MEDICATION
Skin Care: Ointment and Lotion
Scalp: Shampoo

Active Ingredients: Ointment— Coal Tar Solution USP 10%. **Lotion—** Coal Tar Solution USP 5%. **Tar Shampoo—** Coal Tar Solution USP 15%. **Tar-Free Shampoo—** Sulfur 5% and salicylic acid 3%.

Action/Uses: Relief for itching, scaling and flaking of psoriasis, seborrheic dermatitis and/or dandruff.

Warnings: For external use only. Keep out of the reach of children. Avoid contact with eyes. If undue skin irritation occurs, discontinue use.

Administration: Ointment or Lotion —Apply to affected area one to four times daily. **Shampoo**—Shake well before using. Wet hair, then massage liberal amount of MG 217 into scalp and leave on for several minutes. Rinse thoroughly. For best results, use at least twice a week or as directed by a physician.

How Supplied: Ointment—3.8 oz. jars. **Lotion**—4 oz. bottles. **Shampoo**—4 oz. and 8 oz. bottles.

UAS Laboratories
5610 ROWLAND RD #110
MINNETONKA, MN 55343

DDS-ACIDOPHILUS
Capsule, Tablet & Powder free of dairy products, corn, soy, and preservatives

Description: DDS-Acidophilus is the source of a special strain of Lactobacillus acidophilus free of dairy products, corn, soy and preservatives. Each capsule or tablet contains one billion viable DDS-1 L.acidophilus at the time of manufacturing. One gram of powder contains two billion viable DDS-1 L.acidophilus.

Indications and Usages: An aid in implanting the gut with beneficial Lactobacillus acidophilus under conditions of digestive disorders, acne, yeast infections, and following antibiotic therapy.

Administration: One to two capsules or tablets twice daily before meals. One-fourth teaspoon powder can be substituted for two capsules or tablets.

How Supplied: Bottles of 100 capsules or tablets. 12 bottles per case. Powder is available in 2 oz. bottle; 12 bottles per case.

Storage: Keep refrigerated under 40°F.

Continued on next page

UAS—Cont.

DDS-Acidophilus
Booklet describing superior-strain Acidophilus without dairy products, corn, soy, or preservatives. Two billion viable DDS-L. acidopohilus per gram.

The Upjohn Company
KALAMAZOO, MI 49001

CORTAID®
Maximum Strength and Regular Strength
Cream, Ointment and Spray
(hydrocortisone 1% and ½%)
Anti-itch products

Indications: Use CORTAID for the temporary relief of itching associated with minor skin irritations, inflammation, and rashes due to eczema, psoriasis, seborrheic dermatitis, poison ivy, poison oak, or poison sumac, insect bites, soaps, detergents, cosmetics, jewelry, and for external feminine and anal itching. Other uses of this product should be only under the advice and supervision of a physician.

Description: Maximum Strength and Regular Strength CORTAID provide safe, effective relief of many different types of itches and rashes and is the brand recommended most by physicians and pharmacists. Maximum Strength CORTAID is the same strength and form of hydrocortisone relief formerly available only with a prescription. CORTAID is available in 1) a greaseless, odorless vanishing cream that leaves no residue; 2) a soothing, lubricating ointment; 3) a quick-drying non-staining, non-aerosol spray (Maximum Strength only).

Active Ingredients: CORTAID Cream and CORTAID Ointment: hydrocortisone acetate (equivalent to 1% or ½% hydrocortisone).
CORTAID Spray: hydrocortisone 1%.

Other Ingredients:
Maximum Strength Products:
Maximum Strength Cream: butylparaben, cetyl alcohol, glycerin, methylparaben, sodium lauryl sulfate, stearic acid, stearyl alcohol, purified water, and white petrolatum.
Maximum Strength Ointment: butylparaben, cholesterol, methylparaben, microcrystalline wax, mineral oil, and white petrolatum.
Maximum Strength Spray: alcohol, glycerin, methylparaben, and purified water.
Regular Strength Products:
Regular Strength Cream: aloe vera, butylparaben, cetyl palmitate, glyceryl stearate, methylparaben, polyethylene glycol, stearamidoethyl diethylamine, and purified water.

Regular Strength Ointment: aloe vera, butylparaben, cholesterol, methylparaben, mineral oil, white petrolatum, and microcrystalline wax.

Uses: The vanishing action of CORTAID Cream makes it cosmetically acceptable when the skin itch or rash treated is on exposed parts of the body such as the hands or arms. CORTAID Ointment is best used where protection lubrication and soothing of dry and scaly lesions is required. The ointment is also recommended for treating itchy genital and anal areas. CORTAID Spray is a quick-drying, non-staining formulation suitable for covering large areas of the skin.

Warnings: For external use only. Avoid contact with the eyes. If condition worsens, or if symptoms persist for more than 7 days or clear up and occur again within a few days, stop use of this product and do not begin use of any other hydrocortisone product unless you have consulted a physician. Do not use for the treatment of diaper rash. Consult a physician. For external feminine itching, do not use if you have a vaginal discharge. Consult a physician. For external anal itching, do not exceed the recommended daily dosage unless directed by a physician. In case of bleeding, consult a physician promptly. Do not put this product into the rectum by using fingers or any mechanical device or applicator.
Keep this and all drugs out of the reach of children. In case of accidental ingestion, seek professional assistance or contact a poison control center immediately.

Dosage and Administration: *Adults and children 2 years of age and older:* Apply to affected area not more than 3 to 4 times daily. *Children under 2 years of age:* Do not use, consult a physician. *Adults:* For external anal itching, when practical, cleanse the affected area with mild soap and warm water and rinse thoroughly by patting or blotting with an appropriate cleansing pad. Gently dry by patting or blotting with toilet tissue or a soft cloth before application of this product. *Children under 12 years of age:* For external anal itching, consult a physician.

How Supplied:
Cream: ½ oz. and 1 oz. tubes
Ointment: ½ oz. and 1 oz. tubes
Non-Aerosol Spray: 1.5 fluid oz.
Shown in Product Identification Guide, page 526

DOXIDAN® LIQUI-GELS®
Stimulant/Stool Softener Laxative

Indications: DOXIDAN is a safe, reliable laxative for the relief of occasional constipation. The combination of a stimulant/stool softener laxative allows positive laxative action on a softened stool for gentle evacuation without straining. DOXIDAN generally produces a bowel movement in 6 to 12 hours.

Active Ingredients: Each soft gelatin capsule contains 65 mg yellow phenolphthalein and 60 mg docusate calcium.

Inactive Ingredients: May contain Alcohol up to 1.5% (w/w). Also contains corn oil, FD&C Blue #1 and Red #40, gelatin, glycerin, hydrogenated vegetable oil, lecithin, parabens, sorbitol, titanium dioxide, vegetable shortening, yellow wax, and other ingredients.

Dosage and Administration: Adults and children 12 years of age and over: one or two capsules by mouth daily. For use in children under 12, consult a physician.

Warnings: Do not use laxative products when abdominal pain, nausea, or vomiting are present unless directed by a doctor. If you have noticed a sudden change in bowel habits that persists over a period of 2 weeks, consult a doctor before using a laxative. Laxative products should not be used for a period longer than 1 week unless directed by a doctor. Rectal bleeding or failure to have a bowel movement after use of a laxative may indicate a serious condition. Discontinue use and consult your doctor. If skin rash appears, do not use this product or any other preparation containing phenolphthalein. Keep this and all drugs out of the reach of children. In case of accidental overdose, seek professional assistance or contact a poison control center immediately. As with any drug, if you are pregnant or nursing a baby, seek the advice of a health professional before using this product.

How Supplied: Packages of 10, 30, 100 and 1,000 maroon soft gelatin capsules, and Unit Dose 100s (10 × 10 strips). LIQUI-GELS® Reg TM R P Scherer Corp
Shown in Product Identification Guide, page 527

DRAMAMINE® Tablets
(dimenhydrinate USP)
DRAMAMINE® Chewable Tablets
(dimenhydrinate USP)
DRAMAMINE® Children's Liquid
(dimenhydrinate syrup USP)

Indications: For the prevention and treatment of the nausea, vomiting, or dizziness associated with motion sickness.

Description: Dimenhydrinate is the chlorotheophylline salt of the antihistaminic agent diphenhydramine. Dimenhydrinate contains not less than 53% and not more than 56% of diphenhydramine, and not less than 44% and not more than 47% of 8-chlorotheophylline, calculated on the dried basis.

Active Ingredients:
DRAMAMINE Tablets and Chewable Tablets: Dimenhydrinate 50 mg.
DRAMAMINE Children's: Dimenhydrinate 12.5 mg. per 5 ml.

Inactive Ingredients:
DRAMAMINE Tablets: Acacia, Carboxymethylcellulose Sodium, Corn Starch, Magnesium Stearate, and Sodium Sulfate.
DRAMAMINE Children's: FD&C Red No. 40, Flavor, Glycerin, Methylparaben, Sucrose, and Water.
DRAMAMINE Chewable Tablets: Aspartame, Citric Acid, FD&C Yellow No. 6, Flavor, Magnesium Stearate, Methacrylic Acid Copolymer, Sorbitol. Phenylketonurics: Contains Phenylalanine 1.5 mg per tablet.
Contains FD&C Yellow No. 5 (tartrazine) as a color additive.

Actions: While the precise mode of action of dimenhydrinate is not known, it is thought to have a depressant action on hyperstimulated labyrinthine function.

Directions:
DRAMAMINE Tablets and Chewable Tablets: To prevent motion sickness, the first dose should be taken one half to one hour before starting activity.
ADULTS: 1 to 2 tablets every 4 to 6 hours, not to exceed 8 tablets in 24 hours or as directed by a doctor.
CHILDREN 6 TO UNDER 12: ½ to 1 tablet every 6 to 8 hours, not to exceed 3 tablets in 24 hours or as directed by a doctor.
CHILDREN 2 to UNDER 6: ¼ to ½ tablet every 6 to 8 hours not to exceed 1½ tablets in 24 hours or as directed by a doctor.
Children may also be given DRAMAMINE Cherry Flavored Liquid in accordance with directions for use.
DRAMAMINE Children's: To prevent motion sickness, the first dose should be taken one half to one hour before starting activity. CHILDREN 2 TO UNDER 6: 1 to 2 teaspoonfuls every 6 to 8 hours not to exceed 6 teaspoonfuls in 24 hours or as directed by a doctor. Use of a measuring device is recommended for all liquid medication. CHILDREN 6 TO UNDER 12: 2 to 4 teaspoonfuls every 6 to 8 hours, not to exceed 12 teaspoonfuls in 24 hours or as directed by a doctor. CHILDREN 12 YEARS OR OLDER: 4 to 8 teaspoons (5 ml per teaspoonful) every 4 to 6 hours, not to exceed 32 teaspoonfuls in 24 hours or as directed by a doctor.

Warnings: Do not take this product if you have asthma, glaucoma, emphysema, chronic pulmonary disease, shortness of breath, difficulty in breathing, or difficulty in urination due to enlargement of the prostate gland unless directed by a doctor. Do not give to children under 2 years of age unless directed by a doctor. May cause marked drowsiness; alcohol, sedatives, and tranquilizers may increase the drowsiness effect. Avoid alcoholic beverages while taking this product. Do not take this product if you are taking sedatives or tranquilizers, without first consulting your doctor. Use caution when driving a motor vehicle or operating machinery. Not for frequent or prolonged use except on advice of a doctor. Do not exceed recommended dosage.

Keep this and all drugs out of the reach of children. In case of accidental overdose, seek professional assistance or contact a poison control center immediately. As with any drug, if you are pregnant or nursing a baby, seek the advice of a health professional before using this product.

How Supplied: *Tablets* —scored, white tablets available in packets of 12 and 36 and bottles of 100; *Chewables* —scored, orange tablets available in packets of 8 and 24; *Liquid* —Available in bottles of 4 fl oz).

Shown in Product Identification Guide, page 527

DRAMAMINE II™
(Meclizine hydrochloride)

Indications: For the prevention and treatment of the nausea, vomiting, or dizziness associated with motion sickness.

Description: Meclizine hydrochloride is an antihistamine of the piperazine class with antiemetic action.

Actions: While the precise mode of action of meclizine hydrochloride is not known, it is thought to have a depressant action on hyperstimulated labyrinthine function.

Active Ingredients: Each tablet contains 25 mg. meclizine hydrochloride.

Inactive Ingredients: Colloidal silicon dioxide, croscarmellose sodium, dibasic calcium phosphate, D&C yellow no. 10 aluminum lake, microcrystalline cellulose, magnesium stearate.

Directions: To prevent motion sickness, the first dose should be taken one hour before starting your activity.
Adults: Take 1 to 2 tablets daily or as directed by a doctor. Do not exceed 2 tablets in 24 hours.

Warnings: Do not take this product if you have asthma, glaucoma, emphysema, chronic pulmonary disease, shortness of breath, difficulty in breathing, or difficulty in urination due to enlargement of the prostate gland unless directed by a doctor. Do not give to children under 12 years of age unless directed by a doctor. May cause drowsiness; alcohol, sedatives, and tranquilizers may increase the drowsiness effect. Avoid alcoholic beverages while taking this product. Do not take this product if you are taking sedatives or tranquilizers without first consulting your doctor. Use caution when driving a motor vehicle or operating machinery. Do not exceed recommended dosage. Keep this and all drugs out of reach of children. In case of accidental overdose, seek professional assistance or contact a poison control center immediately. As with any drug, if you are pregnant or nursing a baby, seek the advice of a health professional before using this product.

How Supplied: Dramamine II is supplied as a yellow tablet in packages of 8.
Shown in Product Identification Guide, page 527

KAOPECTATE®
Anti-Diarrheal,
Regular Flavor, Peppermint Flavor and Children's Cherry Flavored Liquids. Maximum Strength Caplets.

Indications: For the fast relief of diarrhea and cramping.

Active Ingredients: Each tablespoon or caplet contains 750 mg attapulgite.

Inactive Ingredients: Liquids: flavors, gluconodelta-lactone, magnesium, aluminum silicate, methylparaben, sorbic acid, sucrose, titanium dioxide, xanthan gum and purified water; Peppermint flavor and Children's Cherry flavor contain FD&C Red #40. Maximum Strength Caplets: Carnauba Wax, Croscarmellose Sodium, Hydroxypropyl Cellulose, Hydroxypropyl Methylcellulose, Methylparaben, Pectin, Propylene Glycol, Propylparaben, Sucrose, Titanium Dioxide, Zinc Stearate. May also contain Talc.

Dosage and Administration: Liquids: For best results, take full recommended dose at first sign of diarrhea and after each subsequent bowel movement. (Maximum 7 times in 24 hours.) Adults and children 12 years of age and over: 2 tablespoons. Children 6 to under 12 years of age: 1 tablespoon. Children 3 to 6 years of age: ½ tablespoon. Maximum Strength Tablets: Swallow whole caplets with water; do not chew. For best results, take full recommended dose. Adults: Take 2 caplets after the initial bowel movement and 2 caplets after each subsequent bowel movement, not to exceed 12 caplets in 24 hours. Children 6 to 12 years of age: Take 1 caplet after the initial bowel movement and 1 caplet after each subsequent movement, not to exceed 6 caplets in 24 hours. Children 3 to under 6 years of age: Use Children's Cherry Flavored Liquid or Advanced Formula KAOPECTATE Liquid.

Warnings: Unless directed by a physician, do not use Kaopectate Liquids in infants and children under 3 years of age or Kaopectate Caplets in infants or children under 6 years of age or for more than two days in the presence of high fever. Keep this and all drugs out of the reach of children. In case of accidental overdose, seek professional assistance or contact a poison control center immediately.

How Supplied: Regular flavor available in 8 oz., 12 oz. and 16 oz. bottles. Peppermint flavor available in 8 oz. and 12 oz. bottles. Children's Cherry flavor available in 6 oz. bottle. Maximum Strength Caplets available in blister packs of 12 and 20 caplets.

Shown in Product Identification Guide, page 527

Continued on next page

Upjohn—Cont.

KAOPECTATE 1-D™
Caplets
Anti-Diarrheal

Indications: Controls the symptoms of diarrhea.

Active Ingredient: Each caplet contains 2 mg Loperamide HCl.

Inactive Ingredients: Corn starch, lactose, magnesium stearate, microcrystalline celluose.

Dosage and Administration: Swallow whole caplets with water; do not chew. For best results, take full recommended dose.
Adults and Children 12 years of age and older: Take 2 caplets after the first loose bowel movement and 1 caplet after each subsequent loose bowel movement but no more than 4 caplets a day for no more than 2 days.
Children 9–11 years (60–95 lbs): Take 1 caplet after the first bowel movement and ½ caplet after each subsequent loose bowel movement but no more than 3 caplets a day for no more than 2 days.
Children 6–8 years (48–59 lbs): Take 1 caplet after the first loose bowel movement and ½ caplet after each subsequent loose bowel movement but no more than 2 caplets a day for no more than 2 days. Under 6 years old (up to 47 lbs): Consult a physician. Not intended for use in children under 6 years old.

Warnings: Do not use for more than two days unless directed by a physician. Do not use if diarrhea is accompanied by high fever (greater than 101°F), or if blood or mucus is present in the stool, or if you have had a rash or other allergic reaction to loperamide HCl. If you are taking antibiotics or have a history of liver disease, consult a physician before using this product. As with any drug, if you are pregnant or nursing a baby, seek the advice of a health professional before using this product. Keep this and all drugs out of the reach of children. In case of accidental overdose, seek professional assistance or contact a poison control center immediately.

How Supplied: Available in blister packs of 6 and 12 caplets.

MOTRIN® IB
Caplets, Tablets and Gelcaps
(ibuprofen, USP)
Pain Reliever/Fever Reducer

WARNING: ASPIRIN-SENSITIVE PATIENTS. Do not take this product if you have had a severe allergic reaction to aspirin, eg—asthma, swelling, shock or hives because even though this product contains no aspirin or salicylates, cross-reactions may occur in patients allergic to aspirin.

Indications: For the temporary relief of headache, muscular aches, minor pain of arthritis, toothache, backache, minor aches and pains associated with the common cold, pain of menstrual cramps, and for reduction of fever.

Directions: Adults: Take 1 caplet, tablet or gelcap every 4 to 6 hours while symptoms persist. If pain or fever does not respond to 1 caplet, tablet or gelcap, 2 caplets, tablets or gelcaps may be used, but do not exceed 6 caplets, tablets or gelcaps in 24 hours, unless directed by a doctor. The smallest effective dose should be used. Take with food or milk, if stomach or stomach pain occurs with use.
Consult a doctor if these symptoms are more than mild or if they persist. Children: Do not give this product to children under 12 except under the advice and supervision of a doctor.

Warnings: Do not take for pain for more than 10 days or for fever for more than 3 days unless directed by a doctor. If pain or fever persists or gets worse, if new symptoms occur, or if the painful area is red or swollen, consult a doctor. These could be signs of serious illness. If you are under a doctor's care for any serious condition, consult a doctor before taking this product. As with aspirin and acetaminophen, if you have any condition which requires you to take prescription drugs or if you have had any problems or serious side effects from taking any nonprescription pain reliever, do not take MOTRIN® IB without first discussing it with your doctor. If you experience any symptoms which are unusual or seem unrelated to the condition for which you took ibuprofen, consult a doctor before taking any more of it.
Although ibuprofen is indicated for the same conditions as aspirin and acetaminophen, it should not be taken with them except under a doctor's direction. Do not combine this product with any other ibuprofen-containing product.
As with any drug, if you are pregnant or nursing a baby, seek the advice of a health professional before using this product. IT IS ESPECIALLY IMPORTANT NOT TO USE IBUPROFEN DURING THE LAST 3 MONTHS OF PREGNANCY UNLESS SPECIFICALLY DIRECTED TO DO SO BY A DOCTOR BECAUSE IT MAY CAUSE PROBLEMS IN THE UNBORN CHILD OR COMPLICATIONS DURING DELIVERY.
Keep this and all drugs out of the reach of children. In case of accidental overdose, seek professional assistance or contact a poison control center immediately. **Store at room temperature. Avoid excessive heat 40°C (104°F).**

Active Ingredient: Each caplet, tablet or gelcap contains ibuprofen 200 mg.

Other Ingredients: Carnauba wax, cornstarch, hydroxypropyl methylcellulose, propylene glycol, silicon dioxide, pregelatinized starch, stearic acid, titanium dioxide. Gelcaps also contain benzyl alcohol, butylparaben, butyl alcohol, castor oil, colloidal silicon dioxide, edetate calcium disodium, FDC Yellow No. 6, gelatin, iron oxide black, magnesium stearate, methylparaben, microcrystalline cellulose, povidone, propylparaben, SDA 3A starch, propylparaben, SDA 3A alcohol, sodium lauryl sulfate, sodium propionate, and sodium starch glycolate.

How Supplied: Bottles of 24, 50, 100, 130 and 165 Caplets or Tablets. Bottles of 24 and 50 Gelcaps. Vial of 8 caplets.
Shown in Product Identification Guide, page 527

MOTRIN® IB Sinus
Caplets and Tablets
(Ibuprofen/Pseudoephedrine)
Pain Reliever/Fever Reducer/
Nasal Decongestant

WARNING: ASPIRIN-SENSITIVE PATIENTS. Do not take this product if you have had a severe allergic reaction to aspirin, eg—asthma, swelling, shock or hives because even though this product contains no aspirin or salicylates, cross-reactions may occur in patients allergic to aspirin.

Indications: For the temporary relief of symptoms associated with sinusitis, the common cold or flu including nasal congestion, headache, body aches, pains, and fever.

Directions: *Adults and children 12 years of age and older:* Take 1 caplet or tablet every 4 to 6 hours while symptoms persist. If symptoms do not respond to 1 caplet or tablet, 2 caplets or tablets may be used but do not exceed 6 caplets or tablets in 24 hours. Take with food or milk if occasional and mild heartburn, upset stomach, or stomach pain occurs with use. Consult a doctor if these symptoms are more than mild or if they persist. *Children:* Do not give this product to children under 12 years of age except under the advice and supervision of a doctor.

Warnings: Do not take for colds for more than 7 days or for fever for more than 3 days unless directed by a doctor. If the cold or fever persists or gets worse or if new symptoms occur, consult a doctor. These could be signs of serious illness. As with aspirin and acetaminophen, if you have any condition which requires you to take prescription drugs or if you have had any problems or serious side effects from taking any non-prescription pain reliever, do not take this product without first discussing it with your doctor. IF YOU EXPERIENCE ANY SYMPTOMS WHICH ARE UNUSUAL OR SEEM UNRELATED TO THE CONDITION FOR WHICH YOU TOOK THIS PRODUCT, CONSULT A DOCTOR BEFORE TAKING ANY MORE OF IT. If you are under a doctor's care for any serious condition, consult a doctor before taking this product. Do not exceed recommended dosage because at higher doses nervousness, dizziness or sleeplessness may occur. Do not take this product if you have high blood pressure, heart disease, diabetes, thyroid disease or difficulty in urination due to enlargement of the prostate gland, except under the advice and supervision of a doctor.

Drug Interaction Precaution: Do not take this product if you are presently taking a prescription drug for high blood pressure or depression without first consulting your doctor. Do not combine this product with other non-prescription pain relievers. Do not combine this product with any other ibuprofen-containing product.

As with any drug, if you are pregnant or nursing a baby, seek the advice of a health professional before using this product. IT IS ESPECIALLY IMPORTANT NOT TO USE THIS PRODUCT DURING THE LAST 3 MONTHS OF PREGNANCY UNLESS SPECIFICALLY DIRECTED TO DO SO BY A DOCTOR BECAUSE IT MAY CAUSE PROBLEMS IN THE UNBORN CHILD OR COMPLICATIONS DURING DELIVERY.

Keep this and all drugs out of the reach of children. In case of accidental overdose, seek professional assistance or contact a poison control center immediately. **Store at room temperature. Avoid excessive heat above 40°C (104°F).**

Active Ingredient: Each caplet or tablet contains ibuprofen 200 mg and pseudoephedrine HCL 30 mg.

Other Ingredients: Cellulose, Corn Starch, Glyceryl Triacetate, Hydroxypropyl Methylcellulose, Silicon Dioxide, Sodium Lauryl Sulfate, Sodium Starch Glycolate, Stearic Acid, Titanium Dioxide, Red #40 Aluminum Lake.

How Supplied: Available in blister packages of 20 and 40 caplets or 20 tablets.

Shown in Product Identification Guide, page 527

**Maximum Strength
MYCITRACIN®
Triple Antibiotic First Aid Ointment
MYCITRACIN® Plus Pain Reliever**

Indications: Maximum Strength MYCITRACIN and MYCITRACIN Plus Pain Reliever are first aid ointments to help prevent infection in minor burns, cuts, nicks, scrapes, scratches and abrasions.

Description: MYCITRACIN combines three topical antibiotics in a soothing, non-irritating petrolatum base that does not sting, aids healing, and helps prevent infection. MYCITRACIN Plus Pain Reliever also temporarily relieves pain.

Directions: *For adults and children (all ages):* Clean the affected area. Apply a small amount of MYCITRACIN (an amount equal to the surface area of the tip of a finger) on the affected area 1 to 3 times daily. If desired, cover the affected area with a sterile bandage.

Warnings: For external use only. Do not use in the eyes or apply over large areas of the body. In case of deep or puncture wounds, animal bites, or serious burns, consult a physician. Stop use and consult a physician if the condition persists or gets worse. Do not use longer

than 1 week unless directed by a physician. Keep this and all medications out of the reach of children. In case of accidental ingestion, seek professional assistance or contact a poison control center immediately.

Active Ingredients:
Maximum Strength MYCITRACIN: Each gram contains bacitracin, 500 units; neomycin sulfate equiv. to 3.5 mg neomycin; polymyxin B sulfate, 5,000 units.
MYCITRACIN Plus Pain Reliever: Each gram contains bacitracin, 500 units; neomycin sulfate equiv. to 3.5 mg neomycin; polymyxin B sulfate, 5000 units; lidocaine, 40 mg.

Other Ingredients:
Maximum Strength MYCITRACIN: butylparaben, cholesterol, methylparaben, microcrystalline wax, mineral oil, and white petrolatum.
MYCITRACIN Plus Pain Reliever: butylparaben, cholesterol, methylparaben, microcrystalline wax, mineral oil, and white petrolatum.

How Supplied:
½ oz. tubes, 1 oz. tubes and $\frac{1}{32}$ oz. foil packets (144 per carton)
Shown in Product Identification Guide, page 527

**SURFAK® LIQUI-GELS®
Stool Softener Laxative**

Indications: SURFAK is indicated for the relief of occasional constipation. SURFAK generally produces a bowel movement in 12 to 72 hours. SURFAK is useful when only stool softening (without propulsive action) is required to relieve constipation.

Active Ingredients: Each soft gelatin capsule contains 240 mg docusate calcium.

Inactive Ingredients: May contain Alcohol up to 3% (w/w). Also contains corn oil, FD&C Blue #1 and Red #40, gelatin, glycerin, parabens, sorbitol, and other ingredients.

Dosage and Administration: Adults and children 12 years of age and over: one capsule by mouth daily for several days or until bowel movements are normal. For use in children under 12, consult a physician.

Warnings: Do not use laxative products when abdominal pain, nausea, or vomiting are present unless directed by a doctor. If you have noticed a sudden change in bowel habits that persists over a period of 2 weeks, consult a doctor before using a laxative. Laxative products should not be used for a period longer than 1 week unless directed by a doctor. Rectal bleeding or failure to have a bowel movement after use of a laxative may indicate a serious condition. Discontinue use and consult your doctor. Keep this and all drugs out of the reach of children. In case of accidental overdose, seek professional assistance or contact a poison

control center immediately. As with any drug, if you are pregnant or nursing a baby, seek the advice of a health professional before using this product.

How Supplied: Packages of 10, 30, 100 and 500 red soft gelatin capsules and Unit Dose 100s (10 × 10 strips). LIQUI-GELS® Reg TM R P Scherer Corp
Shown in Product Identification Guide, page 527

Wakunaga of America Co., Ltd.

**Subsidiary of Wakunaga
Pharmaceutical Co., Ltd.
23501 MADERO
MISSION VIEJO, CA 92691**

**BeSure™
Prevents flatulence**

Indications: Take 1–2 capsules with offending foods.

Ingredients: Contains GRAS food enzymes from *Saccharomyces* and *Aspergillus*.

**KYOLIC®
Odor Modified Garlic**

Active Ingredient: Aged Garlic Extract.™

Indications: Dietary Supplement.

Suggested Use: Average serving, four capsules or tablets a day during or after meals.

How Supplied: LIQUID FORMULAS —Kyolic-Aged Garlic Extract Flavor and Odor Modified: *Plain or* Enriched with Vitamin B_1 and B_{12} *2 or 4 fl. oz; with or without gelatin capsules.*
TABLET/CAPSULE FORMULAS (Ingredients per Tablet/Capsule)
KYOLIC—Super Formula 100 *Tablets & Capsules:* Aged Garlic Extract Powder (300 mg), Whey; Bottles of 100 and 200.
KYOLIC—Super Formula 101 *Tablets & Capsules:* Garlic Plus® Aged Garlic Extract (270 mg), *Whey,* Brewer's Yeast (27 mg), Kelp (9 mg); Bottles of 100 and 200.
KYOLIC—Super Formula 102 *Tablets & Capsules:* Aged Garlic Extract Powder (350 mg), "Kyolic Enzyme Complex™" [Amylase, Protease, Cellulase and Lipase] (30 mg), Bottles of 100 and 200.
KYOLIC—Super Formula 103 *Capsules:* Aged Garlic Extract Powder (220 mg), Ester C® [Calcium Ascorbate] (150 mg), Astragulus membranaceous (100 mg), calcium citrate (50 mg), bottles of 100 and 200.
KYOLIC—Super Formula 104 *Capsules:* Aged Garlic Extract Powder (300 mg), Lecithin (200 mg), Bottles of 100 and 200.
KYOLIC—Super Formula 105 *Capsules:* Aged Garlic Extract Powder *(200 mg), Vitamin C as Calcium Asorbate (145 mg), 10,000 I.U. of Vitamin A as Beta Carotene*

Continued on next page

Wakunaga—Cont.

60 IU Vitamin E as d-α-Tocopheryl Succinate, 50 µg L-Selenomethionine, Green Tea; Bottles of 100 and 200.
KYOLIC®—Super Formula 106 Capsules: Aged Garlic Extract Powder (300 mg), Hawthorne Berry 50 mg, 100 IU Vitamin E as d-α-Tocopheryl Succinate, Cayenne Pepper (10 mg), Bottles of 100 and 200.
KYOLIC® RESERVE™ Capsules: Aged Garlic Extract Powder (600 mg); Bottles of 60 and 120.
KYOLIC® Aged Garlic Extract Caplets: Aged Garlic Extract Powder (600 mg) Boxes of 30.
KYO-CHROME™ Caplets: Aged Garlic Extract Powder (500 mg); Niacin (20 mg); Chromium as picolinate (200 µg); Boxes of 30.
KYO-CHROME™ Capsules: Aged Garlic Extract Powder (200 mg); Niacin (10 mg); Chromium as picolinate (100 µg); Bottles of 90.
PREMIUM KYOLIC® ®-EPA Gel Caps: Aged Garlic Extract (120 mg) with 1000 mg of fish oil; Bottles of 90.
GINGKO BILOBA PLUS™ Capsules: Ginkgo Biloba Extract, Aged Garlic Extract (200 mg) & Siberian Ginseng Extract; Bottles of 45 and 90.
Professional label "SGP" is available in Aged Garlic Extract powder forms.
Shown in Product Identification Guide, page 527

Kyo-Dophilus®
Probiotic Dietary Supplements

Suggested Use: 1 capsule/tablet, twice daily with meals to replace beneficial bacteria.

How Supplied: Kyo-Dophilus® Capsules: 1.5 billion cells of *L. acidophilus, B. bifidum, & B. longum*
Kyo-Dophilus® Tablets: 1 billion live cells of *L. acidophilus*
Acidophilasé Capsules: 1 billion live cells of *L. acidophilus, B. bifidum,* Amylase, Protease, & Lipase.

Kyo-Green®

Powdered formula: Barley & Wheat Grass, Chlorella, Kelp, & Brown Rice As a dietary supplement, 2 tsp. provide nutrients of a serving of vegetables.

EDUCATIONAL MATERIAL

From Soil to Shelf
Brochure describing our company, garlic fields, aging tanks and factory, plus our product line.

Wallace Laboratories
P.O. BOX 1001
HALF ACRE ROAD
CRANBURY, NJ 08512

MALTSUPEX®
(malt soup extract)
Powder, Liquid, Tablets

Composition: MALTSUPEX is a nondiastatic extract from barley malt, which is available in powder, liquid, and tablet form. Each MALTSUPEX product has a gentle laxative action and promotes soft, easily passed stools. Each Tablet contains 750 mg of Malt Soup Extract and approximately 0.15 to 0.25 mEq of potassium. Tablet Ingredients: D&C Yellow No. 10, FD&C Red No. 40, flavor (artificial), hydroxypropyl methylcellulose, methylparaben, polyethylene glycol, propylparaben, povidone, simethicone emulsion, stearic acid, talc, titanium dioxide.
Powder: Each level scoop provides approximately 8 g of Malt Soup Extract.
Liquid: Each tablespoonful (½ fl. oz.) contains approximately the equivalent of 16 g Malt Soup Extract Powder. Other ingredients: Sodium propionate and potassium sorbate.

EFFECTIVE, NON-HABIT-FORMING

Indications: For relief of occasional constipation. This product generally produces a bowel movement in 12 to 72 hours.

Warnings: Do not use laxative products when abdominal pain, nausea or vomiting are present unless directed by a physician. If constipation persists, consult a physician.
If you have noticed a sudden change in bowel habits that persists over a period of 2 weeks, consult a physician before using a laxative.
Keep this and all medications out of the reach of children.

Laxative products should not be used for a period longer than one week unless directed by a physician. Rectal bleeding or failure to have a bowel movement after use of a laxative may indicate a serious condition. Discontinue use and consult a physician.
As with any drug, if you are pregnant or nursing a baby, seek the advice of a health professional before using this product.
MALTSUPEX Powder and Liquid only—Do not use these products except under the advice and supervision of a physician if you have kidney disease.

Precautions: Allow for carbohydrate content in diabetic diets and infant formulas.
Liquid: (67%, 14 g/tablespoon, or 56 calories/tablespoon)
Powder: (83%, 6 g or 24 calories per scoop)
Tablets: 0.6 g per tablet or 3 calories.
MALTSUPEX **Liquid** contains approximately 23 mg of sodium per tablespoonful. Each scoop of **Powder** contains the equivalent of 8 g of Malt Soup Extract Powder and 1.5 to 2.75 mEq of potassium.

Directions: General—Drink a full glass (8 ounces) of liquid with each dose. The recommended daily dosage of MALTSUPEX may vary. Use the smallest dose that is effective and lower dosage as improvement occurs.
MALTSUPEX **Powder**—Each bottle contains a scoop. Each scoopful (which is the equivalent to a standard measuring tablespoon) should be levelled with a knife.

Usual Dosage—Powder:
[See table below.]
Usual Dosage—Liquid:
[See table at top of next page.]
MALTSUPEX **Tablets:** Adult Dosage: The recommended daily dosage of MALTSUPEX may vary from 12 to 64 g.

AGE	CORRECTIVE*	MAINTENANCE
12 years to ADULTS	Up to 4 scoops twice a day (Take a full glass [8 oz.] of liquid with each dose.)	2 to 4 scoops at bedtime
CHILDREN 6–12 years of age	Up to 2 scoops twice a day (Take a full glass [8 oz.] of liquid with each dose.)	
CHILDREN 2–6 years of age	1 scoop twice a day (Take a full glass [8 oz.] of liquid with each dose.)	
BOTTLE FED INFANTS (Over 1 month)	1 to 2 scoops per day in formula	½ to 1 scoop per day in formula
BREAST FED INFANTS (Over 1 month)	½ scoop in 2–4 oz. of water or fruit juice twice a day	

* Full corrective dosage should be used for 3 or 4 days or until relief is noted. Then continue on maintenance dosage as needed. Use a clean, dry scoop to remove powder. Replace cover tightly to keep out moisture.

AGE	CORRECTIVE*	MAINTENANCE
12 years to ADULTS	2 tablespoonfuls twice a day (Take a full glass [8 oz.] of liquid with each dose.)	1 to 2 tablespoonfuls at bedtime
CHILDREN 6–12 years of age	1 to 2 tablespoonfuls once or twice a day (Take a full glass [8 oz.] of liquid with each dose.)	
CHILDREN 2–6 years of age	½ tablespoonful twice a day (Take a full glass [8 oz.] of liquid with each dose.)	
BOTTLE FED INFANTS (Over 1 month)	½ to 2 tablespoonfuls per day in formula	1 to 2 teaspoonfuls per day in formula
BREAST FED INFANTS (Over 1 month)	1 to 2 teaspoonfuls in 2 to 4 oz. water or fruit juice once or twice a day	

* Full corrective dosage should be used for 3 or 4 days or until relief is noted. Then continue on maintenance dosage as needed. Use a clean, dry scoop to remove the liquid. Replace cover tightly after use.

Start with four tablets (3 g) four times daily (with meals and at bedtime) and adjust dosage according to response. Drink a full glass of (8 oz.) of liquid with each dose.

Preparation Tips: Powder—Add dosage to milk, water, or fruit juice and stir until dissolved. Mixing is easier if added to warm milk or warm water. May be flavored with vanilla or cocoa to make "malteds."

Excellent with warm milk at bedtime. Also available in tablet and liquid forms.

Note: Although shade, texture, taste, and height of contents may vary between bottles, action remains the same.

Liquid: Mixing is easier if MALT-SUPEX Liquid is added to an ounce or two of warm water and stirred. Then add milk, water, or fruit juice and stir until dissolved. May be flavored with vanilla or cocoa to make "malteds." Excellent with warm milk at bedtime. Also available in tablet and powder forms.

How Supplied: MALTSUPEX is supplied in 8 ounce (NDC 0037-9101-12) and 16 ounce (NDC 0037-9101-08) jars of MALTSUPEX Powder; 8 fluid ounce (NDC 0037-9051-12) and 1 pint (NDC 0037-9051-08) bottles of MALTSUPEX Liquid; and in bottles of 100 MALT-SUPEX Tablets (NDC 0037-9201-01).

MALTSUPEX **Powder** and **Liquid** are Distributed by

WALLACE LABORATORIES
Division of
CARTER-WALLACE, INC.
Cranbury, New Jersey 08512

MALTSUPEX **Tablets** are Manufactured by

WALLACE LABORATORIES
Division of
CARTER-WALLACE, INC.
Cranbury, New Jersey 08512
Rev. 9/92

Shown in Product Identification Guide, page 527

RYNA®
(Liquid)
RYNA–C® ℂ
(Liquid)
RYNA–CX® ℂ
(Liquid)

Description:
RYNA Liquid—Each 5 mL (one teaspoonful) contains:
Chlorpheniramine maleate .... 2 mg
Pseudoephedrine hydrochloride....30 mg
Other ingredients: flavor (artificial), glycerin, malic acid, purified water, sodium benzoate, sorbitol in a clear, colorless to slightly yellow-colored, lemon-vanilla flavored demulcent base containing no sugar, dyes, or alcohol.
RYNA-C Liquid—Each 5 mL (one teaspoonful) contains, in addition:
Codeine phosphate ....10 mg
(WARNING: May be habit-forming)
Other ingredients: flavor (artificial), glycerin, malic acid, purified water, saccharin sodium, sodium benzoate, sorbitol in a clear, colorless to slightly yellow, cinnamon flavored demulcent base containing no sugar, dyes, or alcohol.
RYNA-CX Liquid—Each 5 mL (one teaspoonful) contains:
Codeine phosphate ....10 mg
(WARNING: May be habit-forming)
Pseudoephedrine hydrochloride....30 mg
Guaifenesin ....100 mg
Other ingredients: flavors (artificial), glycerin, glycine, malic acid, povidone, propylene glycol, purified water, saccharin sodium, sorbitol in a clear, colorless to slightly yellow or straw-colored, cherry-vanilla-menthol flavored demulcent base containing no sugar, dyes, or alcohol.

Actions:
Chlorpheniramine maleate in RYNA and RYNA-C is an antihistamine that antagonizes the effects of histamine.

Codeine phosphate in RYNA-C and RYNA-CX is a centrally-acting antitussive that relieves cough.

Pseudoephedrine hydrochloride in RYNA, RYNA-C and RYNA-CX is a sympathomimetic nasal decongestant that acts to shrink swollen mucosa of the respiratory tract.

Guaifenesin in RYNA-CX is an expectorant, the action of which promotes or facilitates the removal of secretions from the respiratory tract. By increasing sputum volume and making sputum less viscous, guaifesesin facilitates expectoration of retained secretions.

Indications:
RYNA: For the temporary relief of nasal congestion due to the common cold, hay fever or other upper respiratory allergies. Temporarily relieves runny nose, sneezing, itching of the nose or throat, and itchy, watery eyes due to hay fever or other respiratory allergies such as allergic rhinitis.

RYNA-C: Temporarily relieves cough, nasal congestion, runny nose and sneezing as may occur with the common cold.

RYNA-CX: Temporarily relieves cough due to minor throat and bronchial irritation and nasal congestion as may occur with the common cold or inhaled irritants. Calms the cough control center and relieves coughing. Helps loosen phlegm (mucus) and thin bronchial secretions to rid the bronchial passageways of bothersome mucus, drain bronchial tubes, and make coughs more productive.

Warnings:
For RYNA:
Do not give this product to children taking other medication or to children under 6 years except under the advice and supervision of a doctor. Do not exceed recommended dosage because nervousness, dizziness or sleeplessness may occur. Do not take this product for more than 7 days. If symptoms do not improve or are accompanied by fever, consult a doctor. Do not take this product except under the advice and supervision of a doctor if you have any of the following symptoms or conditions: high blood pressure; heart disease; thyroid disease; diabetes; asthma; glaucoma; emphysema; chronic pulmonary disease; shortness of breath; difficulty in breathing; or difficulty in urination due to enlargement of the prostate.

For RYNA-C and RYNA-CX:
Adults and children who have a chronic pulmonary disease or shortness of breath, or children who are taking other drugs, should not take these products unless directed by a doctor. Do not give these products to children under 6 years of age except under the advice and supervision of a doctor. A persistent cough may be a sign of a serious condi-

Continued on next page

Wallace—Cont.

tion. If cough persists for more than one week, tends to recur, or is accompanied by fever, rash or persistent headache, consult a doctor. Do not take these products for persistent or chronic cough such as occurs with smoking, asthma, emphysema, or if cough is accompanied by excessive phlegm (mucus) unless directed by a doctor. Do not take these products if you have glaucoma, asthma, emphysema, difficulty in breathing, difficulty in urination due to enlargement of the prostate gland, heart disease, high blood pressure, thyroid disease, or diabetes unless directed by a doctor. May cause or aggravate constipation.

Do not take these products or give to children for more than 7 days. If symptoms do not improve or are accompanied by fever, consult a doctor. Unless directed by a doctor, do not exceed recommended dosage because nervousness, dizziness or sleeplessness may occur at higher doses.

For RYNA and RYNA-C:
These products contain an antihistamine which may cause excitability, especially in children, or may cause drowsiness. Alcohol may increase the drowsiness effect. Do not drive motor vehicles, operate machinery, or drink alcoholic beverages while taking these products.

As with any drug, if you are pregnant or nursing a baby, seek the advice of a health professional before using these products.

Drug Interaction Precaution: Do not use these products without first consulting your doctor if you are presently taking a prescription drug for high blood pressure or depression. [Do not use this product if you are now taking a prescription monoamine oxidase inhibitor (MAOI) (certain drugs for depression, psychiatric or emotional conditions, or Parkinson's disease), or for 2 weeks after stopping the MAOI drug. If you are uncertain whether your prescription drug contains an MAOI, consult a health professional before taking this product.]

Dosage and Administration:
Adults: 2 teaspoonfuls every 6 hours
Children 6 to under 12 years: 1 teaspoonful every 6 hours.
Children under 6 years: Do not take except under the advice and supervision of a doctor.
DO NOT EXCEED 4 DOSES IN 24 HOURS.
Ryna-C and Ryna-CX:
A special measuring device should be used to give an accurate dose of these products to children under 6 years of age. Giving a higher dose than recommended by a doctor could result in serious side effects for the child.

How Supplied:
RYNA: bottles of 4 fl oz (NDC 0037-0638-66) and one pint (NDC 0037-0638-68).
RYNA-C: bottles of 4 fl oz (NDC 0037-0522-66) and one pint (NDC 0037-0522-68).

RYNA-CX: bottles of 4 fl oz (NDC 0037-0801-66) and one pint (NDC 0037-0801-68).
TAMPER-RESISTANT BAND ON CAP PRINTED "WALLACE LABORATORIES." DO NOT USE IF BAND IS MISSING OR BROKEN.

Storage:
RYNA: Store at controlled room temperature 15°–30°C (59°–86°F).
RYNA-C and RYNA-CX: Store at controlled room temperature 15°–30°C (59°–86°F). Dispense in a tight, light-resistant container.
KEEP THESE AND ALL DRUGS OUT OF THE REACH OF CHILDREN. IN CASE OF ACCIDENTAL OVERDOSE, SEEK PROFESSIONAL ASSISTANCE OR CONTACT A POISON CONTROL CENTER IMMEDIATELY.
WALLACE LABORATORIES
Division of
CARTER-WALLACE, Inc.
Cranbury, New Jersey 08512
Rev. 8/92
Shown in Product Identification Guide, pages 527 and 528

Warner-Lambert Company
Consumer Health Products Group
201 TABOR ROAD
MORRIS PLAINS, NJ 07950

CELESTIAL SEASONINGS® SOOTHERS™ Herbal Throat Drops

Active Ingredients: Menthol and pectin.

Inactive Ingredients: HONEY-LEMON CHAMOMILE–Chamomile Flower Extract; Citric Acid; Corn Syrup; Honey; Lemon Juice; Natural Flavoring; Oils of Angelica Root, Anise Star, Ginger, Lemon grass, Sage and White Thyme; Sucrose; Tea Extract. HARVEST CHERRY–Cherry, Elderberry and Pineapple Juices; Citric Acid; Corn Syrup; Natural Flavoring; Oils of Angelica Root, Anise Star, Ginger, Lemon Grass, Sage and White Thyme; Sucrose. HERBAL ORANGE SPICE–Beta Carotene; Citric Acid; Corn Syrup; Natural Flavoring; Oils of Angelica Root, Anise Star, Cassia Bark, Ginger, Lemon Grass, Sage and White Thyme; Orange Juice; Sucrose.

Indications: For temporary relief of occasional minor irritation, pain, sore mouth and sore throat. Provides temporary protection of irritated areas in sore mouth and sore throat.

Warnings: If sore throat is severe, persists for more than 2 days, is accompanied or followed by fever, headache, rash, nausea, or vomiting, consult a doctor promptly. If sore mouth symptoms do not improve in 7 days, see your dentist or doctor promptly. Keep this and all drugs out of the reach of children.

Dosage and Administration: Adults and children 5 years and over: Dissolve 2 drops (one at a time) slowly in the mouth.

May be repeated every 2 hours as needed or as directed by a dentist or doctor. Children under 5 years: Consult a dentist or doctor.

How Supplied: Celestial Seasonings Soothers Throat Drops are available in bags of 24 drops. They are available in three flavors: Honey-Lemon Chamomile, Harvest Cherry and Herbal Orange Spice.
Shown in Product Identification Guide, page 528

HALLS® MENTHO–LYPTUS® Cough Suppressant Tablets

Active Ingredients: Each tablet contains eucalyptus oil and menthol.

Inactive Ingredients: Glucose Syrup, Flavoring, Sugar and Artificial Colors.

Indications: For temporary relief of minor throat irritation and coughs due to colds or inhaled irritants. Makes nasal passages feel clearer.

Warning: A persistent cough or sore throat may be a sign of a serious condition. If cough persists for more than 1 week, tends to recur, or is accompanied by fever, rash or persistent headache, or if sore throat is severe, persistent or accompanied by high fever, headache, nausea, and vomiting, consult a doctor. Do not take this product for sore throat lasting more than 2 days or persistent or chronic cough such as occurs with smoking, asthma, emphysema, or if cough is accompanied by excessive phlegm (mucus) unless directed by a doctor. Keep this and all drugs out of the reach of children.

Dosage and Administration: Adults and children 5 years and over: dissolve one tablet slowly in mouth. Repeat every hour as needed or as directed by a doctor. Children under 5 years: consult a doctor.

How Supplied: Halls Mentho-Lyptus Cough Suppressant Tablets are available in single sticks of 9 tablets each, and in bags of 30 and 60 tablets. They are available in five flavors: Regular Mentho-Lyptus, Cherry, Honey-Lemon, Ice Blue–Peppermint, and Spearmint.
Shown in Product Identification Guide, page 528

HALLS® SUGAR FREE MENTHO-LYPTUS® Cough Suppressant Tablets

Active Ingredients: BLACK CHERRY and CITRUS BLEND–Menthol 5 mg and Eucalyptus Oil 2.8 mg per tablet. MOUNTAIN MENTHOL–Menthol 6 mg and Eucalyptus Oil 2.8 mg per tablet.

Inactive Ingredients: BLACK CHERRY–Acesulfame Potassium, Blue 1, Flavoring, Isomalt and Red 40. CITRUS BLEND–Acesulfame Potassium, Flavoring, Isomalt and Yellow 5 (Tartrazine). MOUNTAIN MENTHOL–Acesulfame Potassium, Flavoring and Isomalt.

Indications: For temporary relief of minor throat irritation and coughs due to colds, or inhaled irritants. Makes nasal passages feel clearer.

Warnings: A persistent cough or sore throat may be a sign of a serious condition. If cough persists for more than 1 week, tends to recur, or is accompanied by fever, rash or persistent headache, or if sore throat is severe, persistent or accompanied by high fever, headache, nausea, and vomiting, consult a doctor. Do not take this product for sore throat lasting more than 2 days or persistent or chronic cough such as occurs with smoking, asthma, emphysema, or if cough is accompanied by excessive phlegm (mucus) unless directed by a doctor. Keep this and all drugs out of the reach of children. Excess consumption may have a laxative effect.

Dosage and Administration: Adults and children 5 years and over: dissolve one tablet slowly in mouth. Repeat every hour as needed or as directed by a doctor. Children under 5 years: consult a doctor.

Additional Information: Diabetics: This product may be useful in your diet on the advice of a physician.

> **Exchange Information*:**
> 1 Tablet = Free Exchange.
> 10 Tablets = 1 Fruit.

* The dietary exchanges are based on the *Exchange Lists for Meal Planning*, Copyright ©1989 by the American Diabetes Association, Inc. and the American Dietetic Association.

How Supplied: Halls Sugar Free Mentho-Lyptus Cough Suppressant Tablets are available in bags of 25 tablets. They are available in three flavors: Black Cherry, Citrus Blend and Mountain Menthol.
Shown in Product Identification Guide, page 528

MAXIMUM STRENGTH HALLS® PLUS
Cough Suppressant Tablets

Active Ingredients: Menthol 10 mg. per centerfilled tablet.

Inactive Ingredients: Mentho-Lyptus: Corn Syrup, Flavoring, Glycerin, High Fructose Corn Syrup and Sucrose. Cherry: Corn Syrup, FD&C Blue No. 2, FD&C Red No. 40, Flavoring, Glycerin, High Fructose Corn Syrup and Sucrose. Honey-Lemon: Acesulfame Potassium, Corn Syrup, D&C Yellow No. 10, FD&C Yellow No. 6, Flavoring, Glycerin, High Fructose Corn Syrup, Honey and Sucrose.

Indications: For temporary relief of minor throat irritation and coughs due to colds or inhaled irritants. Makes nasal passages feel clearer.

Warnings: A persistent cough or sore throat may be a sign of a serious condition. If cough persists for more than 1 week, tends to recur, or is accompanied

by fever, rash or persistent headache or if sore throat is severe, persistent or accompanied by high fever, headache, nausea, and vomiting, consult a doctor. Do not take this product for sore throat lasting more than 2 days or persistent or chronic cough such as occurs with smoking, asthma, emphysema, or if cough is accompanied by excessive phlegm (mucus) unless directed by a doctor. Keep this and all drugs out of the reach of children.

Dosage and Administration: Adults and children 5 years and over: for cough dissolve 1 tablet slowly in mouth-repeat every hour as needed or as directed by a doctor; for sore throat dissolve either 1 tablet or 2 tablets (one at a time) slowly in mouth-repeat every 2 hours as needed or as directed by a doctor. Children under 5 years; consult a doctor.

How Supplied: Maximum Strength Halls Plus Cough Suppressant Tablets are available in single sticks of 10 tablets each and in bags of 25 tablets. They are available in three flavors: Regular Mentho-Lyptus, Cherry and Honey-Lemon.
Shown in Product Identification Guide, page 528

HALLS® Vitamin C Drops

Description: Halls Vitamin C Drops are a delicious way to get 100% of the U.S. Recommended Daily Allowance of Vitamin C. Each drop provides 60 mg. of Vitamin C (100% U.S. RDA).

Ingredients: Sugar, Glucose Syrup, Sodium Ascorbate, Citric Acid, Ascorbic Acid, Natural Flavoring and Artificial Color (Including Yellow 5 and Yellow 6).

Indication: Dietary Supplementation.

How Supplied: Halls Vitamin C Drops are available in single sticks of 9 drops each and in bags of 30 drops. They are available in an all-natural citrus flavor assortment: (lemon, sweet grapefruit and orange).
Shown in Product Identification Guide, page 528

ROLAIDS® Antacid Tablets
Original Flavor and Spearmint

Active Ingredient: Calcium Carbonate 412 mg. and Magnesium Hydroxide 80 mg.

Inactive Ingredients: Flavoring, Light Mineral Oil, Magnesium Stearate, Mannitol, Microcrystalline Cellulose, Polyethylene Glycol, Pregelatinized Starch, Silicon Dioxide and Sucrose.

Indications: For the relief of heartburn, sour stomach or acid indigestion and upset stomach associated with these symptoms.

Actions: Rolaids® provides rapid neutralization of stomach acid. Each tablet has acid-neutralizing capacity of 11 mEq and the ability to maintain the pH of stomach contents to 3.5 or greater for a

significant period of time. Each tablet provides 16% of the nutritional Daily Value for calcium and 8% of the nutritional Daily Value for magnesium and contains less than 0.4 mg. of sodium.

Warnings: Do not take more than 14 tablets in a 24-hour period or use the maximum dosage of this product for more than 2 weeks except under the advice and supervision of a physician. Keep this and all drugs out of the reach of children.

Drug Interaction Precaution: Antacids may interact with certain prescription drugs. If you are presently taking a prescription drug, do not take this product without checking with your physician or other health professional.

Dosage and Administration: Chew 1 or 2 tablets as symptoms occur. Repeat hourly if symptoms return or as directed by a physician.

How Supplied: One roll contains 12 tablets; 3-pack contains three 12-tablet rolls; one bottle contains 75 tablets; one bottle contains 150 tablets.
Shown in Product Identification Guide, page 528

CALCIUM RICH/SODIUM FREE ROLAIDS® Antacid Tablets
Cherry and Assorted Fruit Flavors

Active Ingredient: Calcium Carbonate 550 mg. per tablet.

Inactive Ingredients:
Cherry Flavor: Colors (Red 27 and Titanium Dioxide), Corn Starch, Flavoring, Light Mineral Oil, Magnesium Stearate, Mannitol, Pregelatinized Starch, Silicon Dioxide and Sucrose.
Assorted Fruit Flavors: Colors (Blue 1, Red 27, Red 40, Titanium Dioxide, Yellow 5 [Tartrazine] and Yellow 6), Corn Starch, Flavoring, Light Mineral Oil, Magnesium Stearate, Mannitol, Pregelatinized Starch, Silicon Dioxide and Sucrose.

Indications: For the relief of heartburn, sour stomach or acid indigestion and upset stomach associated with these symptoms.

Actions: Calcium Rich/Sodium Free Rolaids provides rapid neutralization of stomach acid. Each tablet has an acid-neutralizing capacity of 11 mEq and the ability to maintain the pH of stomach contents at 3.5 or greater for a significant period of time. Each tablet provides 22% of the nutritional Daily Value for calcium and contains less than 0.4 mg. of sodium.

Warnings: Do not take more than 14 tablets in a 24-hour period or use the maximum dosage of this product for more than 2 weeks except under the advice and supervision of a physician. Keep this and all drugs out of the reach of children.

Continued on next page

Warner-Lambert—Cont.

Drug Interaction Precaution: Antacids may interact with certain prescription drugs. If you are presently taking a prescription drug, do not take this product without checking with your physician or other health professional.

Dosage and Administration: Chew 1 or 2 tablets as symptoms occur. Repeat hourly if symptoms return or as directed by a physician.

How Supplied: One roll contains 12 tablets; 3-pack contains three 12-tablet rolls; one bottle contains 75 tablets; one bottle contains 150 tablets.
Shown in Product Identification Guide, page 528

Warner Wellcome
Consumer HealthCare Products
Warner-Lambert Company
201 TABOR ROAD
MORRIS PLAINS, NJ 07950
(See also Warner-Lambert)

ACTIFED® Tablets
[ăk 'tuh-fĕd]

Product Benefits: Each ACTIFED® Tablet contains two maximum strength ingredients for temporary relief from symptoms of the common cold, seasonal allergies (hay fever) and sinus congestion.
The **ANTIHISTAMINE** (triprolidine) temporarily dries runny nose and relieves sneezing associated with the common cold, hay fever or other upper respiratory allergies. Also relieves itching of the nose or throat, and itchy, watery eyes due to hay fever.
The **DECONGESTANT** (pseudoephedrine) temporarily relieves nasal congestion due to the common cold, hay fever or other upper respiratory allergies, or associated with sinusitis. Temporarily relieves nasal stuffiness. Reduces the swelling of nasal passages; shrinks swollen membranes; and temporarily restores freer breathing through the nose. Also, helps to decongest sinus openings and passages; relieves sinus pressure.

Each Actifed Tablet Contains: pseudoephedrine hydrochloride 60 mg and triprolidine hydrochloride 2.5 mg. Also contains: flavor, hydroxypropyl methylcellulose, lactose, magnesium stearate, polyethylene glycol, potato starch, povidone, sucrose, and titanium dioxide.

Directions: Adults and children 12 years of age and over, 1 tablet every 4 to 6 hours. Children 6 to under 12 years of age, ½ tablet every 4 to 6 hours. Do not exceed 4 doses in 24 hours. Children under 6 years of age, consult a doctor.

Warnings: May cause drowsiness; alcohol, sedatives, and tranquilizers may increase the drowsiness effect. Avoid alcoholic beverages while taking this product. Do not take this product if you are

taking sedatives or tranquilizers, without first consulting your doctor. Use caution when driving a motor vehicle or operating machinery. May cause excitability, especially in children. Do not exceed recommended dosage because at higher doses nervousness, dizziness or sleeplessness may occur. If symptoms do not improve within 7 days or are accompanied by high fever, consult a doctor before continuing use. Do not take this product, unless directed by a doctor, if you have high blood pressure, heart disease, diabetes, thyroid disease, glaucoma, a breathing problem such as emphysema or chronic bronchitis, or difficulty in urination due to enlargement of the prostate gland. As with any drug, if you are pregnant or nursing a baby, seek the advice of a health professional before using this product.
Drug Interaction Precaution: Do not take this product if you are presently taking a prescription antihypertensive or antidepressant drug containing a monoamine oxidase inhibitor except under the advice and supervision of a doctor.
KEEP THIS AND ALL DRUGS OUT OF THE REACH OF CHILDREN. In case of accidental overdose, seek professional assistance or contact a Poison Control Center immediately.
Store at 15° to 25°C (59° to 77°F) in a dry place and protect from light.

How Supplied: Boxes of 12, 24, 48 and bottles of 100; unit dose pack box of 100.
Shown in Product Identification Guide, page 528

ACTIFED® ALLERGY DAYTIME/ NIGHTTIME CAPLETS
[ăk 'tuh-fĕd]

> This package contains 2 separate products: Actifed® Allergy DAYTIME (white caplets) is a no-drowsiness product. Actifed® Allergy NIGHTTIME (blue caplets) may cause marked drowsiness. Read directions carefully for both products.

ACTIFED® ALLERGY DAYTIME (white caplets)
ANTIHISTAMINE-FREE. CONTAINS NO INGREDIENTS THAT MAY CAUSE DROWSINESS.

Product Benefits: The **DAYTIME** no-drowsiness product (white caplets) contains a nasal decongestant (pseudoephedrine) that provides temporary relief of nasal congestion due to hay fever or other upper respiratory allergies. Helps decongest sinus openings and passages; relieves sinus pressure; reduces swollen nasal passages.

Directions: Adults and children 12 years and over, **2 caplets every 4 to 6 hours** during waking hours. Do not exceed a total of 8 caplets (Daytime or Nighttime) in 24 hours. **Do not take Actifed Allergy Daytime within 4 hours**

of Actifed Allergy Nighttime. Not recommended for children under 12.

Each Actifed Allergy Daytime Caplet Contains: pseudoephedrine hydrochloride 30 mg. Also contains: carnauba wax, crospovidone, hydroxypropyl methylcellulose, lactose, magnesium stearate, microcrystalline cellulose, polyethylene glycol, and titanium dioxide.

ACTIFED® ALLERGY NIGHTTIME (blue caplets) **MAY CAUSE MARKED DROWSINESS.**

Product Benefits: The **NIGHTTIME** product (blue caplets) contains a nasal decongestant (pseudoephedrine) and an antihistamine (diphenhydramine) that provide temporary relief of nasal congestion, sinus pressure, swollen nasal passages, runny nose, and sneezing due to hay fever or other upper respiratory allergies. Also relieves itching of the nose or throat and itchy, watery eyes due to hay fever.

Directions: Adults and children 12 years and over, **2 caplets at bedtime.** Due to potential marked drowsiness, do not take during waking hours unless confined to bed or resting at home; 2 caplets then may be taken every 4 to 6 hours. Do not exceed a total of 8 caplets (Daytime and/or Nighttime) in 24 hours. **Do not take Actifed Allergy Nighttime within 4 hours of Actifed Daytime.** Not recommended for children under 12.

Warning: May cause marked drowsiness; alcohol, sedatives and tranquilizers may increase the drowsiness effect. Avoid alcoholic beverages while taking Actifed Allergy Nighttime. Do not take this product if you are taking sedatives or tranquilizers, without first consulting your doctor. Use caution when driving a motor vehicle or operating machinery.

Each Actifed Allergy Nighttime Caplet Contains: diphenhydramine hydrochloride 25 mg and pseudoephedrine hydrochloride 30 mg. Also contains: carnauba wax, crospovidone, FD&C Blue No. 1 Lake, hydroxypropyl methylcellulose, lactose, magnesium stearate, microcrystalline cellulose, polyethylene glycol, polysorbate 80, and titanium dioxide.

ACTIFED DAYTIME/NIGHTTIME products do not contain triprolidine hydrochloride, the antihistamine found in other ACTIFED products.

Warnings: Do not exceed a combined total of 8 caplets (Actifed Allergy Daytime *plus* Actifed Allergy Nighttime) in 24 hours. These products may cause excitability, especially in children. Do not exceed recommended dosage for these products because at higher doses nervousness, dizziness, or sleeplessness may occur. If symptoms do not improve within 7 days or are accompanied by high fever, consult a doctor before continuing use. Do not take these products, unless directed by a doctor, if you have high blood pressure, heart disease, thyroid disease, glaucoma, a breathing problem such as emphysema or chronic bronchitis, or difficulty in urination due to enlargement of the prostate gland. As with any drug, if you are pregnant or nursing a baby, seek the advice of a health professional before using these products.

Drug Interaction Precaution: Do not take these products if you are presently taking a prescription antihypertensive or antidepressant drug containing a monoamine oxidase inhibitor except under the advice and supervision of a doctor.
KEEP THESE AND ALL DRUGS OUT OF THE REACH OF CHILDREN. In case of accidental overdose, seek professional assistance or contact a Poison Control Center immediately.
Store at 15° to 25°C (59° to 77°F) in a dry place and protect from light.

How Supplied: Package contains 24 Daytime caplets and 8 Nighttime Caplets.
Shown in Product Identification Guide, page 528

ACTIFED® PLUS Caplets
[ăk ′tuh-fĕd]

Product Benefits: Each dose of ACTIFED® PLUS contains three maximum strength ingredients for temporary relief from symptoms of the common cold, seasonal allergies (hay fever) and sinus congestion.
The **ANTIHISTAMINE** (triprolidine) temporarily dries runny nose and relieves sneezing associated with the common cold, hay fever or other upper respiratory allergies. Also relieves itching of the nose or throat, and itchy, watery eyes due to hay fever.
The **DECONGESTANT** (pseudoephedrine) temporarily relieves nasal congestion due to the common cold, hay fever or other upper respiratory allergies, or associated with sinusitis. Temporarily relieves nasal stuffiness. Reduces the swelling of nasal passages; shrinks swollen membranes; and temporarily restores freer breathing through the nose. Also, helps to decongest sinus openings and passages; relieves sinus pressure.
The non-aspirin **ANALGESIC** (acetaminophen) temporarily relieves occasional minor aches, pains and headache, and reduces fever due to the common cold.

Each ACTIFED® PLUS Coated Caplet Contains: acetaminophen 500 mg, pseudoephedrine hydrochloride 30 mg and triprolidine hydrochloride 1.25 mg. Also contains: carnauba wax, crospovidone, FD&C Blue No. 1 Lake, D&C Yellow No. 10 Lake, hydroxypropyl methylcellulose, magnesium stearate, microcrystalline cellulose, polyethylene glycol, polysorbate 80, povidone, pregelatinized corn starch, stearic acid, and titanium dioxide.

Directions: Adults and children 12 years of age and over, 2 caplets every 6 hours. Do not exceed 8 caplets in 24 hours. Not recommended for children under 12 years of age.

Warnings: May cause drowsiness; alcohol, sedatives, and tranquilizers may increase the drowsiness effect. Avoid alcoholic beverages while taking this product. Do not take this product if you are taking sedatives or tranquilizers, without first consulting your doctor. Use caution when driving a motor vehicle or operating machinery. May cause excitability, especially in children. Do not exceed recommended dosage because at higher doses nervousness, dizziness, or sleeplessness may occur. Do not take this product for more than 7 days. If symptoms do not improve or are accompanied by fever that lasts for more than 3 days, or if new symptoms occur, consult a doctor. Do not take this product, unless directed by a doctor, if you have high blood pressure, heart disease, diabetes, thyroid disease, glaucoma, a breathing problem such as emphysema or chronic bronchitis, or difficulty in urination due to enlargement of the prostate gland. As with any drug, if you are pregnant or nursing a baby, seek the advice of a health professional before using this product.

Drug Interaction Precaution: Do not take this product if you are presently taking a prescription antihypertensive or antidepressant drug containing a monoamine oxidase inhibitor except under the advice and supervision of a doctor.
KEEP THIS AND ALL DRUGS OUT OF THE REACH OF CHILDREN. In case of accidental overdose, seek professional assistance or contact a Poison Control Center immediately. Prompt medical attention is critical for adults as well as for children even if you do not notice any signs or symptoms.

Store at 15° to 25°C (59° to 77°F) in a dry place and protect from light.

How Supplied: Boxes of 20, 40.
Shown in Product Identification Guide, page 528

ACTIFED® PLUS Tablets
[ăk ′tuh-fĕd]

Product Benefits: Each dose of ACTIFED® PLUS contains three maximum strength ingredients for temporary relief from symptoms of the common cold, seasonal allergies (hay fever) and sinus congestion.
The **ANTIHISTAMINE** (triprolidine) temporarily dries runny nose and relieves sneezing associated with the common cold, hay fever or other upper respiratory allergies. Also relieves itching of the nose or throat, and itchy, watery eyes due to hay fever.
The **DECONGESTANT** (pseudoephedrine) temporarily relieves nasal congestion due to the common cold, hay fever or other upper respiratory allergies, or associated with sinusitis. Temporarily relieves nasal stuffiness. Reduces the swelling of nasal passages; shrinks swollen membranes; and temporarily restores freer breathing through the nose. Also,

helps to decongest sinus openings and passages; relieves sinus pressure.
The non-aspirin **ANALGESIC** (acetaminophen) temporarily relieves occasional minor aches, pains and headache, and reduces fever due to the common cold.

Each ACTIFED® PLUS Coated Tablet Contains: acetaminophen 500 mg, pseudoephedrine hydrochloride 30 mg and triprolidine hydrochloride 1.25 mg. Also contains: carnauba wax, crospovidone, FD&C Blue No. 1 Lake, D&C Yellow No. 10 Lake, hydroxypropyl methylcellulose, magnesium stearate, microcrystalline cellulose, polyethylene glycol, polysorbate 80, povidone, pregelatinized corn starch, stearic acid, and titanium dioxide.

Directions: Adults and children 12 years of age and over, 2 tablets every 6 hours. Do not exceed 8 tablets in 24 hours. Not recommended for children under 12 years of age.

Warnings: May cause drowsiness: alcohol, sedatives, and tranquilizers may increase the drowsiness effect. Avoid alcoholic beverages while taking this product. Do not take this product if you are taking sedatives or tranquilizers, without first consulting your doctor. Use caution when driving a motor vehicle or operating machinery. May cause excitability, especially in children. Do not exceed recommended dosage because at higher doses nervousness, dizziness, or sleeplessness may occur. Do not take this product for more than 7 days. If symptoms do not improve, or are accompanied by fever that lasts for more than 3 days, or if new symptoms occur, consult a doctor. Do not take this product, unless directed by a doctor, if you have high blood pressure, heart disease, diabetes, thyroid disease, glaucoma, a breathing problem such as emphysema or chronic bronchitis, or difficulty in urination due to enlargement of the prostate gland. As with any drug, if you are pregnant or nursing a baby, seek the advice of a health professional before using this product.

Drug Interaction Precaution: Do not take this product if you are presently taking a prescription antihypertensive or antidepressant drug containing a monoamine oxidase inhibitor except under the advice and supervision of a doctor.
KEEP THIS AND ALL DRUGS OUT OF THE REACH OF CHILDREN. In case of accidental overdose, seek professional assistance or contact a Poison Con-

Continued on next page

This product information was prepared in November 1994. On these and other Warner Wellcome Consumer HealthCare Products, detailed information may be obtained by addressing Warner Wellcome Consumer HealthCare Products, Warner-Lambert, Morris Plains, NJ 07950

Warner Wellcome—Cont.

trol Center immediately. Prompt medical attention is critical for adults as well as for children even if you do not notice any signs or symptoms.

Store at 15° to 25°C (59° to 77°F) in a dry place and protect from light.

How Supplied: Boxes of 20, 40.
Shown in Product Identification Guide, page 528

ACTIFED® SINUS DAYTIME/ NIGHTTIME Tablets and Caplets
[ak'tuh-fĕd]

> This package contains 2 separate products: Actifed® Sinus DAYTIME (white tablets or caplets) is a no-drowsiness product; Actifed® Sinus NIGHTTIME (blue tablets or caplets) may cause marked drowsiness. Read directions carefully for both products.

ACTIFED® SINUS DAYTIME (white tablets and caplets)
CONTAINS NO INGREDIENTS THAT MAY CAUSE DROWSINESS.

Product Benefits: The **DAYTIME** no-drowsiness product (white tablets or caplets) contains a non-aspirin pain reliever (acetaminophen) and nasal decongestant (pseudoephedrine) that provide temporary relief of sinus headache pain, sinus pressure and nasal congestion due to the common cold, hay fever, or other allergies.

Directions: Adults and children 12 years and over, **2 tablets or caplets** every 6 hours during waking hours. Do not exceed a total of 8 tablets (Daytime and/ or Nighttime) in 24 hours. **Do not take Actifed Sinus Daytime within 6 hours of Actifed Sinus Nighttime.** Not recommended for children under 12.

Each Actifed Sinus Daytime Tablet or Caplets Contains: acetaminophen 500 mg and pseudoephedrine hydrochloride 30 mg. Also contains: carnauba wax, crospovidone, hydroxypropyl methylcellulose, magnesium stearate, microcrystalline cellulose, polyethylene glycol, povidone, pregelatinized corn starch, stearic acid, and titanium dioxide.

ACTIFED® SINUS NIGHTTIME (blue tablets and caplets)
MAY CAUSE MARKED DROWSINESS.

Product Benefits: The **NIGHTTIME** product (blue tablets or caplets) contains a non-aspirin pain reliever (acetaminophen), a nasal decongestant (pseudoephedrine), and an antihistamine (diphenhydramine) that provide temporary relief of sinus headache pain, sinus pressure, nasal congestion, runny nose, and sneezing due to the common cold, hay fever, or other allergies. Also relieves itching of the nose or throat and itchy, watery eyes due to hay fever.

Directions: Adults and children 12 years and over, **2 tablets or caplets at bedtime.** Due to potential marked drowsiness, do not take during waking hours unless confined to bed or resting at home; 2 tablets or caplets then may be taken every 6 hours. Do not exceed a total of 8 tablets or caplets (Daytime and/or Nighttime) in 24 hours. **Do not take Actifed Sinus Nighttime within 6 hours of Actifed Sinus Daytime.** Not recommended for children under 12.

Warning: May cause marked drowsiness; alcohol, sedatives, and tranquilizers may increase the drowsiness effect. Avoid alcoholic beverages while taking Actifed Sinus Nighttime. Do not take this product if you are taking sedatives or tranquilizers, without first consulting your doctor. Use caution when driving a motor vehicle or operating machinery.

Each Actifed Sinus Nighttime Tablet or Caplet Contains: acetaminophen 500 mg, diphenhydramine hydrochloride 25 mg and pseudoephedrine hydrochloride 30 mg. Also contains: carnauba wax, crospovidone, FD&C Blue No. 1 Lake, hydroxypropyl methylcellulose, magnesium stearate, microcrystalline cellulose, polyethylene glycol, polysorbate 80, povidone, pregelatinized corn starch, sodium starch glycolate, stearic acid, and titanium dioxide.
ACTIFED DAYTIME/NIGHTTIME products do not contain triprolidine hydrochloride, the antihistamine found in other ACTIFED products.

Warnings: Do not exceed a combined total of 8 tablets or caplets (Actifed Sinus Daytime *plus* Actifed Sinus Nighttime) in 24 hours. These products may cause excitability, especially in children. Do not exceed recommended dosage for these products because at higher doses nervousness, dizziness, or sleeplessness may occur. Do not take these products for more than 7 days. If symptoms do not improve or are accompanied by fever that lasts for more than 3 days, or if new symptoms occur, consult a doctor. Do not take these products, unless directed by a doctor, if you have high blood pressure, heart disease, diabetes, thyroid disease, glaucoma, a breathing problem such as emphysema or chronic bronchitis, or difficulty in urination due to enlargement of the prostate gland. As with any drug, if you are pregnant or nursing a baby, seek the advice of a health professional before using these products.

Drug Interaction: Do not take these products if you are presently taking a prescription antihypertensive or antidepressant drug containing a monoamine oxidase inhibitor except under the advice and supervision of a doctor.
KEEP THESE AND ALL DRUGS OUT OF THE REACH OF CHILDREN. In case of accidental overdose, seek professional assistance or contact a Poison Control Center immediately. Prompt medical attention is critical for adults as well as for children even if you do not notice any signs or symptoms.
Store at 15° to 25°C (59° to 77°F) in a dry place and protect from light.

How Supplied: Package contains 18 Daytime Tablets or Caplets and 6 Nighttime Tablets or Caplets.
Shown in Product Identification Guide, page 528

ACTIFED® Syrup
[ăk'tuh-fĕd]

Product Benefits: ACTIFED® Syrup contains two maximum strength ingredients for temporary relief from symptoms of the common cold, seasonal allergies (hay fever) and sinus congestion.
The **ANTIHISTAMINE** (triprolidine) temporarily dries runny nose and relieves sneezing associated with the common cold, hay fever, or other upper respiratory allergies. Also relieves itching of the nose or throat, and itchy, watery eyes due to hay fever.
The **DECONGESTANT** (pseudoephedrine) temporarily relieves nasal congestion due to the common cold, hay fever or other upper respiratory allergies, or associated with sinusitis. Temporarily relieves nasal stuffiness. Reduces the swelling of nasal passages; shrinks swollen membranes; and temporarily restores freer breathing through the nose. Also, helps to decongest sinus openings and passages; relieves sinus pressure.

Each 5 mL (1 teaspoonful) Actifed® Syrup Contains: pseudoephedrine hydrochloride 30 mg and triprolidine hydrochloride 1.25 mg. Also contains: methylparaben 0.1% and sodium benzoate 0.1% (added as preservatives), D&C Yellow No. 10, glycerin, purified water, and sorbitol.

Directions: Adults and children 12 years and over, 2 teaspoonfuls every 4 to 6 hours. Children 6 to under 12 years, 1 teaspoonful every 4 to 6 hours. Do not exceed 4 doses in 24 hours. Children under 6, consult a doctor.

Warnings: May cause drowsiness; alcohol, sedatives, and tranquilizers may increase the drowsiness effect. Avoid alcoholic beverages while taking this product. Do not take this product if you are taking sedatives or tranquilizers, without first consulting your doctor. Use caution when driving a motor vehicle or operating machinery. May cause excitability, especially in children. Do not exceed recommended dosage because at higher doses nervousness, dizziness or sleeplessness may occur. If symptoms do not improve within 7 days or are accompanied by high fever, consult a doctor before continuing use. Do not take this product, unless directed by a doctor, if you have high blood pressure, heart disease, diabetes, thyroid disease, glaucoma, a breathing problem such as emphysema or chronic bronchitis, or difficulty in urination due to enlargement of the prostate gland. As with any drug, if you are pregnant or nursing a baby, seek the advice of a health professional before using this product.

Drug Interaction Precaution: Do not take this product if you are presently taking a prescription antihypertensive or antidepressant drug containing a monoamine oxidase inhibitor except under the advice and supervision of a doctor.

KEEP THIS AND ALL DRUGS OUT OF THE REACH OF CHILDREN. In case of accidental overdose, seek professional assistance or contact a Poison Control Center immediately.
Store at 15° to 25°C (59° to 77°F) and protect from light.

How Supplied: Bottles of 4 fl oz (118 mL) and 1 pint. (473 mL)

ANUSOL®
[ă′nŭ-sōl″]
Hemorrhoidal Suppositories/ Ointment

Description:
Anusol Suppositories: Active Ingredient: Topical Starch 51%. Also contains: Benzyl Alcohol, Partially Hydrogenated Soy Bean Oil with Sorbitan Tristearate, Tocopheryl Acetate.
Anusol Ointment: Active ingredients: Pramoxine HCl 1%, Mineral Oil 46.7% and Zinc Oxide 12.5%. Also contains: Benzyl Benzoate, Calcium Phosphate Dibasic, Cocoa Butter, Glyceryl Monooleate, Glyceryl Monostearate, Kaolin, Peruvian Balsam and Polyethylene Wax.

Actions: Anusol Suppositories and Anusol Ointment help to relieve burning, itching and discomfort arising from irritated anorectal tissues. They have a soothing, lubricant action on mucous membranes. Pramoxine Hydrochloride in Anusol Ointment is a rapidly acting local anesthetic for the skin and mucous membranes of the anus and rectum. Pramoxine HCl is also chemically distinct from procaine, cocaine, and dibucaine and can often be used in the patient previously sensitized to other surface anesthetics. Surface analgesia lasts for several hours.

Indications: Anusol Ointment: Temporarily relieves the pain, soreness, and burning of hemorrhoids and other anorectal disorders while it forms a temporary protective coating over inflamed tissues. Anusol Ointment is to be applied externally or in the lower portion of the anal canal (The enclosed dispensing cap is designed to control dispersion of the ointment to the affected area in the lower portion of the anal canal only.) Anusol Suppositories: Gives temporary relief from the itching, burning and discomfort of hemorrhoids and other anorectal disorders, and temporarily provides a coating for relief of anorectal discomforts and protects the irritated areas.

Contraindications: Anusol Suppositories and Anusol Ointment are contraindicated in those patients with a history of hypersensitivity to any of the components of the preparations. Upon application of Anusol Ointment, which contains Pramoxine HCl, a patient may occasionally experience burning, especially if the anoderm is not intact. Sensitivity reactions have been rare; discontinue medication if suspected. Certain persons can develop allergic reactions to ingredients in this product.

Warnings: Anusol Ointment: Certain persons can develop allergic reactions to ingredients in this product. If the symptom being treated does not subside, if condition worsens or does not improve within 7 days, if redness, irritation, swelling, pain, or other symptoms develop or increase, discontinue use and consult a physician. In case of bleeding, consult a physician promptly. Do not exceed the recommended daily dosage unless directed by a physician. Do not put this product into the rectum by using fingers or any mechanical device or applicator. Keep this and all drugs out of the reach of children. In case of accidental ingestion seek professional advice or contact a Poison Control Center immediately. Anusol Suppositories: Do not exceed recommended daily dosage unless directed by a physician. If condition worsens or does not improve within 7 days, consult a physician. In case of bleeding, consult a physician promptly. Keep this and all drugs out of the reach of children. In case of accidental ingestion seek professional assistance or contact a Poison Control Center immediately. As with any drug, if you are pregnant or nursing a baby, seek the advice of a health professional before using this product.

Directions: Anusol Suppositories: Adults: When practical, cleanse the affected area with Tucks® Hemorrhoidal Pads or mild soap and warm water. Rinse thoroughly. Gently dry by patting or blotting with toilet tissue or soft cloth before application of this product.
1. Detach one suppository from the strip of suppositories.
2. Remove wrapper before inserting into the rectum. Hold suppository upright (with words "pull apart" at top) and carefully separate foil by inserting tip of fingernail at foil split.
3. Peel foil slowly and evenly down both sides, exposing suppository.
4. Avoid excessive handling of suppository which is designed to melt at body temperature.
5. Insert one (1) suppository rectally up to 6 times daily or after each bowel movement.
6. If suppository seems soft, hold in foil wrapper under cold water for 2 or 3 minutes.
Children under 12 years of age: consult a physician.
Anusol Ointment: Adults: When practical, cleanse the affected area with

Tucks® Hemorrhoidal Pads or mild soap and warm water and rinse thoroughly. Gently dry by patting or blotting with toilet tissue or soft cloth before application of this product. Apply ointment externally to the affected area up to five (5) times daily. To use dispensing cap, attach it to tube, lubricate well, then gently insert part way into the anus. Squeeze tube to deliver medication. Thoroughly cleanse dispensing cap after use. Children under 12 years of age: Consult a physician.

How Supplied: Anusol Suppositories— boxes of 12 or 24 in silver foil strips.
Anusol Ointment—1-oz tubes and 2-oz tubes with plastic applicator.
Ointment: Store between 15° and 30°C (59° and 86°F).
Suppositories: Do not store above 86°F or suppositories may melt.
Shown in Product Identification Guide, page 528

ANUSOL HC-1
Anti-Itch Hydrocortisone Ointment

Active Ingredient: Hydrocortisone Acetate (equivalent to 1% Hydrocortisone).

Inactive Ingredients: Diazolidinyl Urea, Methylparaben, Microcrystalline Wax, Mineral Oil, Propylene Glycol, Propylparaben, Sorbitan Sesquioleate and White Petrolatum.

Indications: For temporary relief of external anal itching associated with minor skin irritations, inflammation and rashes. Other uses of this product should be only under the advice and supervision of a physician.

Warnings: For external use only. Avoid contact with the eyes. If condition worsens, or if symptoms persist for more than 7 days or clear up and occur again within a few days, stop use of this product and do not begin use of any other hydrocortisone product unless you have consulted a physician. Do not exceed the recommended daily dosage unless directed by a physician. In case of bleeding, consult a physician promptly. Do not put this product into the rectum by using fingers or any mechanical device or applicator. Do not use for treatment of diaper rash. Consult a physician. Keep this and all drugs out of the reach of children. In case of accidental ingestion seek professional assistance or contact a Poison Control Center immediately.

Continued on next page

This product information was prepared in November 1994. On these and other Warner Wellcome Consumer HealthCare Products, detailed information may be obtained by addressing Warner Wellcome Consumer HealthCare Products, Warner-Lambert, Morris Plains, NJ 07950

Warner Wellcome—Cont.

Directions: Adults: when practical cleanse affected area with mild soap and warm water. Rinse thoroughly. Gently dry by patting or blotting with tissue or soft cloth before application of this product. Apply to affected area not more than 3 to 4 times daily. Children under 12 years: do not use, consult a physician.

How Supplied: Anusol HC-1 Ointment in 0.7 oz tube. Store at Room Temperature 59°–86°F.

Shown in Product Identification Guide, page 528

BENADRYL® Allergy
[bĕ'nă-drĭl]
Tablets and Kapseals®

Active Ingredients: Each Tablet/Kapseal contains: Diphenhydramine Hydrochloride 25 mg.

Inactive Ingredients: Each Tablet contains: Candelilla Wax, Croscarmellose Sodium, Dibasic Calcium Phosphate Dihydrate, D&C Red No. 27 Aluminum Lake, Hydroxypropyl Methylcellulose, Microcrystalline Cellulose, Polyethylene Glycol, Polysorbate 80, Pregelantinized Starch, Stearic Acid, Titanium Dioxide, and Zinc Stearate.
Each Kapseal contains: Lactose and Magnesium Stearate. The Kapseals capsule shell contains: D&C Red No. 28, FD&C Red No. 3, FD&C Red No. 40, FD&C Blue No. 1, Gelatin, Glyceryl Monooleate, and Titanium Dioxide.

Indications: Temporarily relieves runny nose and sneezing, itching of the nose or throat, and itchy, watery eyes due to hay fever or other upper respiratory allergies, and runny nose and sneezing associated with the common cold.

Warnings: May cause excitability especially in children. Do not take this product, unless directed by a doctor, if you have a breathing problem such as emphysema or chronic bronchitis, or if you have glaucoma or difficulty in urination due to enlargement of the prostate gland. May cause marked drowsiness; alcohol, sedatives, and tranquilizers may increase the drowsiness effect. Avoid alcoholic beverages while taking this product. Do not take this product if you are taking sedatives or tranquilizers, without first consulting your doctor. Use caution when driving a motor vehicle or operating machinery. Do not use any other products containing diphenhydramine while using this product. As with any drug, if you are pregnant or nursing a baby, seek the advice of a health professional before using this product. KEEP THIS AND ALL DRUGS OUT OF REACH OF CHILDREN. In case of accidental overdose, seek professional assistance or contact a Poison Control Center immediately.

Directions: Adult and children 12 years of age and over is 25 to 50 mg (1 to 2 tablets/kapseals) every 4 to 6 hours. Not to exceed 12 tablets/kapseals in 24 hours. Children 6 to under 12 years of age: oral dosage is 12.5 mg* to 25 mg (1 tablet/kapseal) every 4 to 6 hours, not to exceed 6 tablets/kapseals in 24 hours. For children under 6 years of age consult your doctor.

How Supplied: Benadryl tablets are supplied in boxes of 24, kapseals are supplied in boxes of 24 and 48.
Store at room temperature 15°–30° C (59°–86° F). Protect from moisture.

___

* This dosage is not available in this package. Do not attempt to break tablet/kapseal. This dosage is available in a pleasant tasting Benadryl Allergy Liquid Medication.

Shown in Product Identification Guide, page 528

BENADRYL®
[bĕ'nă-drĭl]
Allergy Decongestant Tablets

Active Ingredients: Each tablet contains: Benadryl® (Diphenhydramine Hydrochloride USP) 25 mg. and Pseudoephedrine Hydrochloride 60 mg.

Inactive Ingredients: Each tablet contains: Corn Starch, Croscarmellose Sodium, Dibasic Calcium Phosphate Dihydrate, FD&C Blue No. 1 Aluminum Lake, Hydroxypropyl Methylcellulose, Microcrystalline Cellulose, Polyethylene Glycol, Polysorbate 80, Pregelatinized Starch, Stearic Acid, Titanium Dioxide and Zinc Stearate.

Indications: Temporarily relieves nasal congestion; runny nose and sneezing, itching of the nose or throat, and itchy, watery eyes due to hay fever or other upper respiratory allergies, and runny nose, sneezing, and nasal congestion associated with the common cold.

Warning: Do not exceed recommended dosage. If nervousness, dizziness, or sleeplessness occur, discontinue use and consult a doctor. If symptoms do not improve within 7 days or are accompanied by fever, consult a doctor. Do not take this product, unless directed by a doctor, if you have a breathing problem such as emphysema or chronic bronchitis, heart disease, high blood pressure, thyroid disease, diabetes, or if you have glaucoma or difficulty in urination due to enlargement of the prostate gland. May cause excitability especially in children. May cause marked drowsiness; alcohol, sedatives, and tranquilizers may increase the drowsiness effect. Avoid alcoholic beverages while taking this product. Do not take this product if you are taking sedatives or tranquilizers, without first consulting your doctor. Use caution when driving a motor vehicle or operating machinery. Do not use any other products containing diphenhydramine while using this product. As with any drug, if you are pregnant or nursing a baby, seek the advice of a health professional before using this product. KEEP THIS AND ALL DRUGS OUT OF THE REACH OF CHILDREN. In case of accidental overdose, seek professional assistance or contact a Poison Control Center immediately.

Drug Interaction Precaution: Do not use this product if you are now taking a prescription monoamine oxidase inhibitor (MAOI) (certain drugs for depression, psychiatric or emotional conditions, or Parkinson's disease), or for 2 weeks after stopping the MAOI drug. If you are uncertain whether your prescription drug contains an MAOI, consult a health professional before taking this product.

Directions: Adults and children over 12 years of age: 1 tablet every 4 to 6 hours not to exceed 4 tablets in 24 hours. For children under 12 consult your doctor.

How Supplied: Benadryl Allergy Decongestant Tablets are supplied in boxes sp. of 24.
Store at room temperature 15°–30° C (59°–86° F).
Protect from moisture.

Shown in Product Identification Guide, page 529

BENADRYL®
**Allergy Decongestant
Liquid Medication**

Active Ingredients: Each teaspoonful (5 mL) contains: Diphenhydramine Hydrochloride) 12.5 mg. and Pseudoephedrine Hydrochloride 30 mg. Also contains: Citric Acid, FD&C Blue No. 1, FD&C Red No. 40, Flavors, Glycerin, Poloxamer 407, Polysorbate 20, Purified Water, Saccharin Sodium, Sodium Benzoate, Sodium Chloride, Sodium Citrate and Sorbitol Solution.

Indications: Temporarily relieves nasal congestion, runny nose, and sneezing, itching of the nose or throat, and itchy, watery eyes due to hay fever or other upper respiratory allergies, and runny nose, sneezing and nasal congestion associated with the common cold.

Directions: Follow dosage recommendations below, or use as directed by your doctor.

Benadryl® Allergy Decongestant
Liquid Medication

AGE	DOSAGE
Children Under 6 years of age	Consult a Doctor
Children 6 to under 12 years of age	One (1) teaspoonful every 4 to 6 hours. Not to exceed 4 teaspoonfuls in 24 hours.

| Adults and Children 12 years of age and over | Two (2) teaspoonfuls every 4 to 6 hours. Not to exceed 8 teaspoonfuls in 24 hours. |

Warnings: Do not exceed recommended dosage. If nervousness, dizziness, or sleeplessness occur, discontinue use and consult a doctor. If symptoms do not improve within 7 days or are accompanied by fever, consult a doctor. Do not take this product, unless directed by a doctor, if you have a breathing problem such as emphysema or chronic bronchitis, heart disease, high blood pressure, thyroid disease, diabetes, or if you have glaucoma or difficulty in urination due to enlargement of the prostate gland. May cause excitability, especially in children. May cause marked drowsiness; alcohol, sedatives, and tranquilizers may increase the drowsiness effect. Avoid alcoholic beverages while taking this product. Do not take this product if you are taking sedatives or tranquilizers, without first consulting your doctor. Use caution when driving a motor vehicle or operating machinery. Do not use any other products containing diphenhydramine while using this product. As with any drug, if you are pregnant or nursing a baby, seek the advice of a health professional before using this product. KEEP THIS AND ALL DRUGS OUT OF THE REACH OF CHILDREN. In case of accidental overdose, seek professional assistance or contact a Poison Control Center immediately.

Drug Interaction Precaution: Do not use this product if you are now taking a prescription monoamine oxidase inhibitor (MAOI) (certain drugs for depression, psychiatric or emotional conditions, or Parkinson's disease), or for 2 weeks after stopping the MAOI drug. If you are uncertain whether your prescription drug contains an MAOI, consult a health professional before taking this product.

How Supplied: Benadryl Allergy Decongestant Liquid Medication is supplied sp. in 4 fl. oz. bottles.
Store at room temperature (59°–86°F). Protect from freezing.
Shown in Product Identification Guide, page 529

BENADRYL® Allergy Liquid Medication

Active Ingredient: Each teaspoonful (5 mL) contains Diphenhydramine Hydrochloride 12.5 mg.

Inactive Ingredients: Each teaspoonful (5 mL) contains: Citric Acid, D&C Red No. 33, FD&C No. 40, Flavors, Glycerin, Poloxamer 407, Polysorbate 20, Saccharin Sodium, Sodium Benzoate, Sodium Citrate, Sugar, and Water.

Indications: Benadryl temporarily relieves runny nose and sneezing, itching of the nose or throat and itchy, watery eyes due to hay fever or other upper respiratory allergies and runny nose and sneezing associated with the common cold.

Directions: Follow dosage recommendations below or use as directed by your doctor.

Benadryl® Allergy
Liquid Medication

AGE	DOSAGE
Children Under 6 years of age	Consult a Doctor
Children 6 to under 12 years of age	1 to 2 teaspoonfuls (12.5 to 25 mg.) every 4 to 6 hours. Not to exceed 12 teaspoonfuls in 24 hours.
Adults and Children 12 years of age and over	2 to 4 teaspoonfuls (25 to 50 mg.) every 4 to 6 hours. Not to exceed 24 teaspoonfuls in 24 hours.

Warnings: May cause excitability, especially in children. Do not take this product, unless directed by a doctor, if you have a breathing problem such as emphysema, or chronic bronchitis, or if you have glaucoma or difficulty in urination due to enlargment of the prostate gland. May cause marked drowsiness; alcohol, sedatives, and tranquilizers may increase the drowsiness effect. Avoid alcoholic beverages while taking this product. Do not take this product if you are taking sedatives or tranquilizers, without first consulting your doctor. Use caution when driving a motor vehicle or operating machinery. Do not use any other products containing diphenhydramine while using this product. As with any drug, if you are pregnant or nursing a baby seek the advice of a health professional before using this product. KEEP THIS AND ALL DRUGS OUT OF THE REACH OF CHILDREN. In case of accidental overdose, seek professional assistance or contact a Poison Control Center immediately.

How Supplied: Benadryl Allergy Liquid Medication is supplied in 4 and 8 fluid ounce bottles.

Store at room temperature (59°–86°F). Protect from freezing.

Shown in Product Identification Guide, page 528

BENADRYL® Allergy Sinus Headache

Active Ingredients: Each caplet contains Diphenhydramine Hydrochloride 12.5 mg, Pseudoephedrine Hydrochloride 30 mg and Acetaminophen 500 mg.

Inactive Ingredients: Candelilla Wax, Croscarmellose Sodium, D&C Yellow No. 10 Aluminum Lake, FD&C Blue No. 1 Aluminum Lake, FD&C Yellow No. 6 Aluminum Lake, Hydroxypropyl Cellulose, Hydroxypropyl Methylcellulose, Microcrystalline Cellulose, Polyethylene Glycol, Polysorbate 80, Pregelatinized Starch, Sodium Starch Glycolate, Starch, Stearic Acid, Titanium Dioxide, and Zinc Stearate.

Indications: For the temporary relief of minor aches, pains, and headache, runny nose and sneezing, itching of the nose or throat, and itchy, watery eyes due to hay fever, and nasal congestion due to the common cold, hay fever, or other upper respiratory allergies. Helps decongest sinus openings and passages; temporarily relieves sinus congestion and pressure.

Action: BENADRYL ALLERGY/SINUS/HEADACHE is specially formulated to provide effective relief of your upper respiratory allergy symptoms complicated by sinus and headache problems. It combines the strength of BENADRYL to relieve your runny nose: sneezing; itchy water eyes; itchy nose or throat with a maximum strength NASAL DECONGESTANT to relieve nasal and sinus congestion and a maximum strength non-aspirin PAIN RELIEVER to relieve sinus pain and headache.

Warnings: Do not exceed recommended dosage. If nervousness, dizziness, or sleeplessness occur, discontinue use and consult a doctor. Do not take this product for more than 10 days. If symptoms do not improve or are accompanied by fever that lasts for more than 3 days, or if new symptoms occur, consult a doctor. Do not take this product, unless directed by a doctor, if you have a breathing problem such as emphysema or chronic bronchitis, heart disease, high blood pressure, thyroid disease, diabetes, or if you have glaucoma or difficulty in urination due to enlargement of the prostate gland. May cause excitability especially in children. May cause marked drowsiness; alcohol, sedatives, and tranquilizers may increase the drowsiness effect. Avoid alcoholic beverages while taking this product. Do not take this product if you are taking sedatives or tranquilizers, without first consulting your doctor. Use caution when driving a motor vehicle or operating machinery. Do not use any other products containing diphenhydramine while using this product. As with any drug, if you are pregnant or nursing a baby, seek the advice of a health professional before using this

Continued on next page

This product information was prepared in November 1994. On these and other Warner Wellcome Consumer HealthCare Products, detailed information may be obtained by addressing Warner Wellcome Consumer HealthCare Products, Warner-Lambert, Morris Plains, NJ 07950

Warner Wellcome—Cont.

product. KEEP THIS AND ALL DRUGS OUT OF THE REACH OF CHILDREN. In case of accidental overdose seek professional assistance or contact a Poison Control Center immediately. Prompt medical attention is critical for adults as well as for children even if you do not notice any signs or symptoms.

Drug Interaction Precaution: Do not use this product if you are now taking a prescription monoamine oxidase inhibitor (MAOI) (certain drugs for depression, psychiatric or emotional conditions, or Parkinson's disease), or for 2 weeks after stopping the MAOI drug. If you are uncertain whether your prescription drug contains an MAOI, consult a health professional before taking this product.

Directions: Adults and children 12 years of age and over.—two (2) caplets every 6 hours, not to exceed 8 caplets in 24 hours. For children under 12 years of age consult a doctor for recommended dosage.

How Supplied: Benadryl Allergy Sinus Headache is available in boxes of 24 caplets. Store at room temperature, 15°–30°C (59°–86°F).

*Shown in Product Identification
Guide, page 529*

BENADRYL® Dye-Free Allergy Liqui-gel® Softgels

Active Ingredients: Each softgel contains: Diphenhydramine Hydrochloride 25 mg.

Inactive Ingredients: Gelatin, Glycerin, Polyethylene Glycol and Sorbitol.

Indications: Temporarily relieves runny nose and sneezing, itching of the nose or throat, and itchy, watery eyes due to hay fever or other upper respiratory allergies, and runny nose and sneezing associated with the common cold.

Directions: Follow dosage recommendations below, or use as directed by your doctor.

Benadryl® Dye-Free Allergy
Liqui-Gels® Softgel

AGE	DOSAGE
Adults and Children 12 years of age and over	25 to 50 mg. (1 to 2 softgels) every 4 to 6 hours. Not to exceed 12 softgels in 24 hours.
Children 6 to under 12 years of age See ** symbol below	12.5 to 25 mg. (1 softgel) every 4 to 6 hours. Not to exceed 6 softgels in 24 hours.
Children Under 6 years of age	Consult a Doctor

**12.5 mg. dosage strength is not available in this package. Do not attempt to break softgels. This dosage is available in a fruit flavored Benadryl® Dye-Free Allergy Liquid Medication.

Warnings: May cause excitability, especially in children. Do not take this product, unless directed by a doctor, if you have a breathing problem such as emphysema or chronic bronchitis, or if you have glaucoma or difficulty in urination due to enlargement of the prostate gland. May cause marked drowsiness; alcohol, sedatives, and tranquilizers may increase the drowsiness effect. Avoid alcoholic beverages while taking this product. Do not take this product if you are taking sedatives or tranquilizers, without first consulting your doctor. Use caution when driving a motor vehicle or operating machinery. Do not use any other products containing diphenhydramine while using this product. As with any drug, if you are pregnant or nursing a baby, seek the advice of a health professional before using this product. KEEP THIS AND ALL DRUGS OUT OF THE REACH OF CHILDREN. In case of accidental overdose, seek professional assistance or contact a Poison Control Center immediately.

How Supplied: Benadryl® Dye-Free Allergy Liqui-Gels® Softgels are supplied in boxes of 24.
Store at 59°–77°F.
Protect from heat and humidity.

*Shown in Product Identification
Guide, page 529*

BENADRYL® Dye-Free Allergy Liquid Medication

Active Ingredients: Each teaspoonful (5 mL.) contains Diphenhydramine HCL 6.25 mg.

Inactive Ingredients: Each teaspoonful (5 mL.) contains: Carboxymethylcellulose sodium, Citric Acid, Flavor, Glycerin, Saccharin Sodium, Sodium Benzoate, Sodium Citrate, Sorbitol Solution and Water.

Indications: Temporarily relieves runny nose and sneezing, itching of the nose or throat, and itchy, watery eyes due to hay fever or other upper respiratory allergies, and runny nose and sneezing associated with the common cold.

Directions: Follow dosage recommendations below, or use as directed by your doctor.

Benadryl® Dye-Free Allergy
Liquid Medication

AGE	DOSAGE
Children Under 6 years of age	Consult a Doctor
Children 6 to under 12 years of age	2–4 Teaspoonfuls (12.5 to 25 mg) every 4 to 6 hours. Not to exceed 24 teaspoonfuls in 24 hours.
Adults and Children 12 years of age and over	4–8 teaspoonfuls (25 to 50 mg) every 4 to 6 hours. Not to exceed 48 teaspoonfuls in 24 hours.

Warnings: May cause excitability especially in children. Do not take this product, unless directed by a doctor, if you have a breathing problem such as emphysema or chronic bronchitis, or if you have glaucoma or difficulty in urination due to enlargement of the prostate gland. May cause marked drowsiness; alcohol, sedatives, and tranquilizers may increase the drowsiness effect. Avoid alcoholic beverages while taking this product. Do not take this product if you are taking sedatives or tranquilizers, without first consulting your doctor. Use caution when driving a motor vehicle or operating machinery. Do not use any other products containing diphenhydramine while using this product. As with any drug, if you are pregnant or nursing a baby, seek the advice of a health professional before using this product. KEEP THIS AND ALL DRUGS OUT OF THE REACH OF CHILDREN. In case of accidental overdose, seek professional assistance or contact a Poison Control Center immediately.

How Supplied: Benadryl Dye-Free Allergy Liquid Medication is supplied in 8 fl. oz. bottles.

Store at room temperature (59°–86°F). Protect from freezing.

*Shown in Product Identification
Guide, page 529*

BENADRYL® Itch Relief Stick
[bĕ'nă-drĭl]
Maximum Strength 2%
Topical Analgesic/Skin Protectant

Active Ingredients: Benadryl® (Diphenhydramine Hydrochloride) 2%, Zinc Acetate 0.1%.

Inactive Ingredients: Also contains: Alcohol 73.5%, Aloe Vera, Glycerin, Povidone, Purified Water, and Tromethamine.

Indications: For the temporary relief of itching and pain associated with insect bites or minor skin irritations.

Warnings: FOR EXTERNAL USE ONLY. Do not use on chicken pox, measles, blisters, or on extensive areas of skin, except as directed by a physician. Avoid contact with the eyes. If condition worsens, or if symptoms persist for more than 7 days or clear up and occur again within a few days, discontinue use of this product and consult a physician. Do not use on children under 6 years of age without consulting a physician. Do not use any other drugs containing diphenhydramine while using this product. KEEP THIS AND ALL DRUGS OUT OF THE REACH OF CHILDREN. In case of accidental ingestion, seek professional assistance or contact a Poison Control Center immediately. Flammable. Keep away from fire or flame.

Directions: For adults and children 6 years of age and older; apply to the affected area not more than three to four times daily. For children under 6 years of age: consult a physician.
Store at room temperature (59°–86°F).

How Supplied: Benadryl® Itch Relief Stick is available in a .47 oz (14 mL) dauber.
Shown in Product Identification Guide, page 529

BENADRYL
Itch Relief Cream Children's Formula
BENADRYL Itch Relief Cream
Maximum Strength, 2%

Active Ingredients: Children's Formula contains Benadryl® (diphenhydramine hydrochloride) 1% and Zinc Acetate 0.1%; Maximum Strength contains Benadryl® (diphenhydramine hydrochloride) 2%, and Zinc Acetate 0.1%.

Inactive Ingredients: Aloe Vera, Cetyl Alcohol, Diazolidinyl Urea, Methylparaben, Polyethylene Glycol Monostearate 1000, Propylene Glycol, Propylparaben, and Purified Water.

Indications: For the temporary relief of itching and pain associated with insect bites, minor skin irritations and rashes due to poison ivy, poison oak or poison sumac. Dries the oozing and weeping of poison ivy, poison oak and poison sumac.

Actions: Benadryl is the most prescribed topical antihistamine available. It contains the histamine blocker Benaryl® to block the itch, and provides topical anesthetic action to stop the pain. Benadryl gives you the kind of itch and pain relief you can't get from hydrocortisone. Benadryl cream is a soothing, greaseless, vanishing cream.

Warnings: For external use only. Do not use on chicken pox, measles, blisters, or on extensive areas of skin except as directed by a physician. Avoid contact with the eyes. If condition worsens, or if symptoms persist for more than 7 days, or clear up and occur again within a few days, discontinue use of this product and consult a physician. Do not use any other drugs containing diphenhydramine while using this product. KEEP THIS AND ALL DRUGS OUT OF THE REACH OF CHILDREN. In case of accidental ingestion, seek professional assistance or contact a Poison Control Center immediately.

Directions: Children's Formula: For children 2 years of age and older: Apply to affected area not more than three to four times daily, or as directed by a phy-

sician. **For children under 2 years of age: consult a physician.**
Maximum Strength 2%—For adults and children 12 years of age and older: Apply to affected area not more than three to four times daily, or as directed by a physician. **For children under 12 years of age: consult a physician.**
Store at room temperature (59°–86°F).

How Supplied: Benadryl Itch Relief Cream is available in ½ oz. (14.2g) Children's Formula and ½ oz. (14.2g) Maximum Strength tubes.
Shown in Product Identification Guide, page 529

BENADRYL® Itch Relief Spray
Children's Formula
BENADRYL® Itch Relief Spray
Maximum Strength 2%

Active Ingredients: Children's Formula contains Benadryl® (diphenhydramine hydrochloride) 1%, Zinc Acetate 0.1%; Maximum Strength contains Benadryl® (diphenhydramine hydrochloride) 2%, Zinc Acetate 0.1%.

Inactive Ingredients: Alcohol, Aloe Vera, Glycerin, Povidone, Tromethamine and Purified Water.

Indications: For the temporary relief of itching and pain associated with insect bites, allergic itches, minor skin irritations and rashes due to poison ivy, poison oak, or poison sumac. Dries the oozing and weeping of poison ivy, poison oak, and poison sumac.

Actions: Benadryl is the most prescribed topical antihistamine available. It contains the histamine blocker Benadryl® to block the itch, and provides topical anesthetic action to stop the pain. Benadryl gives you the kind of itch and pain relief you can't get from hydrocortisone. The spray feature allows soothing relief without touching or rubbing the affected area.

Warnings: FOR EXTERNAL USE ONLY. Do not use on chicken pox, measles, blisters, or extensive areas of skin except as directed by a physician. Avoid contact with the eyes. If condition worsens, or if symptoms persist for more than 7 days or clear up and occur again within a few days, discontinue use of this product and consult a physician. Do not use any other drugs containing diphenhydramine while using this product. KEEP THIS AND ALL DRUGS OUT OF THE REACH OF CHILDREN. In case of accidental ingestion, seek professional assistance or contact a Poison Control Center immediately. Flammable. Keep away from fire or flame.

Directions: Children's Formula—For children 2 years of age and older: Apply to the affected area not more than three to four times daily, or as directed by a physician. **For children under 2 years of age: consult a physician. Maximum Strength 2%**—For adults and children 12 years of age or older: Apply

to the affected area not more than three to four times daily, or as directed by a physician. **For children under 12 years of age: consult a physician.**
Store at room temperature (59°–86°F).

How Supplied: Benadryl® Spray is available in a 2 oz. (59 mL) pump spray bottle.
Shown in Product Identification Guide, page 529

BENADRYL® Itch Stopping Gel
[bĕ′nă-drĭl]
Children's Formula and
Maximum Strength 2%

Active Ingredients: Children's Formula contains: Benadryl® (Diphenhydramine Hydrochloride) 1%, Zinc Acetate 1%. **Maximum Strength contains:** Benadryl® (Diphenhydramine Hydrochloride) 2%, Zinc Acetate 1%.

Inactive Ingredients: Also contains: SD Alcohol 38B 2.5% v/v, Camphor, Citric Acid, Diazolidinyl Urea, Glycerin, Hydroxypropyl Methylcellulose, Methylparaben, Propylene Glycol, Propylparaben, Purified Water, Sodium Citrate.

Indications: For the temporary relief of itching and pain associated with insect bites, minor skin irritations, and rashes due to poison ivy, poison oak or poison sumac. Dries the oozing and weeping of poison ivy, poison oak and poison sumac.

Actions: Benadryl Itch Stopping Gel contains the Histamine Blocker Benadryl® to block the itch. And, it has added drying action for the oozing and weeping associated with some rashes. The nonrunny, clear gel is packaged in a pump dispenser for easy application. Benadryl, the kind of itch and pain relief that you can't get from hydrocortisone or calamine.

Warnings: FOR EXTERNAL USE ONLY. Do not use on chicken pox, measles, blisters, or on extensive areas of skin except as directed by a physician. Avoid contact with the eyes. If condition worsens, or if symptoms persist for more than 7 days or clear up and occur again within a few days, discontinue use of this product and consult a physician. Do not use any other drugs containing diphenhydramine while using this product. Keep this and all drugs out of the reach of children. In case of accidental ingestion, seek professional assistance or contact a Poison Control Center immediately.

Continued on next page

This product information was prepared in November 1994. On these and other Warner Wellcome Consumer HealthCare Products, detailed information may be obtained by addressing Warner Wellcome Consumer HealthCare Products, Warner-Lambert, Morris Plains, NJ 07950

Warner Wellcome—Cont.

Directions: Children's Formula: Shake well. For children 6 years of age or older: apply to affected area sparingly not more than 3 to 4 times daily, or as directed by a physician. **For children under 6 years of age: consult a physician.**

Maximum Strength: Shake well. Adults and children 12 years of age or older: Apply to affected area sparingly not more than 3 to 4 times daily, or as directed by a physician. **For children under 12 years of age: consult a physician.**

Store at room temperature (59°–86°F).

How Supplied: Benadryl Itch Stopping Gel is supplied in 4 fl oz tubes.
Shown in Product Identification Guide, page 529

BENYLIN® Multisymptom

Active Ingredients: Each teaspoonful (5 mL) contains Dextromethorphan HBr 5 mg, Pseudoephedrine HCl 15 mg and Guaifenesin 100 mg. Also contains Caramel, Citric Acid, D&C Red No. 33, Disodium Edetate, FD&C Red No. 40, Flavors, Poloxamer 407, Polyethylene Glycol, Propyl Gallate, Propylene Glycol, Sodium Benzoate, Sodium Chloride, Sodium Citrate, Sodium Saccharin, Sorbitol Solution and Water.

Indications: For temporary relief of cough due to minor throat and bronchial irritation and nasal congestion as may occur with the common cold. Helps loosen phlegm (mucus) and thin bronchial secretions to drain bronchial tubes and make coughs more productive.

Warnings: A persistent cough may be a sign of a serious condition. If cough persists for more than one week, tends to recur, or is accompanied by fever, rash, or persistent headache, consult a physician. Do not take this product if the following symptoms are present unless directed by a physician: (1) persistent or chronic cough such as occurs with smoking, asthma, chronic bronchitis or emphysema or where cough is accompanied by excessive phlegm (mucus); (2) if you have heart disease, high blood pressure, thyroid disease, diabetes or difficulty in urination due to enlargement of the prostate gland. Do not exceed recommended dosage because at higher doses nervousness, dizziness, or sleeplessness may occur. As with any drug, if you are pregnant or nursing a baby seek the advice of a health care professional before using this product. KEEP THIS AND ALL DRUGS OUT OF THE REACH OF CHILDREN. In case of accidental overdose, seek professional assistance or contact a Poison Control Center immediately.

Drug Interaction Precaution: Do not use this product if you are now taking a prescription monoamine oxidase inhibitor (MAOI) (certain drugs for depression, psychiatric or emotional conditions, or Parkinson's disease), or for 2 weeks after stopping the MAOI drug. If you are uncertain whether your prescription drug contains an MAOI, consult a health professional before taking this product.

Directions for Use: Follow dosage recommendations below or use as directed by your physician. Repeat every 4 hours not to exceed 4 doses in 24 hours.

Benylin® Multisymptom

AGE	DOSAGE
12 years & older	4 teaspoonfuls
6 to under 12 years	2 teaspoonfuls
2 to under 6 years	1 teaspoonful
Under 2 years	Consult Physician

How Supplied: Benylin Multisymptom is available in 4 oz bottles. Store at 59–86 F.
Shown in Product Identification Guide, page 529

BENYLIN® Expectorant

Active Ingredients: Each teaspoonful (5mL) contains Dextromethorphan HBr 5 mg and Guaifenesin 100 mg. Also contains: Caramel, Citric Acid, D&C Red No. 33, Disodium Edetate, FD&C Red No. 40, Flavors, Poloxamer 407, Polyethylene Glycol, Propyl Gallate, Propylene Glycol, Sodium Benzoate, Sodium Chloride, Sodium Citrate, Sodium Saccharin, Sorbitol Solution and Water.

Indications: Maximum strength, nonnarcotic cough suppressant for temporary relief of cough due to minor throat and bronchial irritation as may occur with the common cold or inhaled irritants. Helps loosen phlegm (mucus) and thin bronchial secretions to drain bronchial tubes and make coughs more productive.

Warning: A persistent cough may be a sign of a serious condition. If cough persists for more than one week, tends to recur, or is accompanied by fever, rash, or persistent headache, consult a physician. Do not take this product for persistent or chronic cough such as occurs with smoking, asthma, emphysema, or if cough is accompanied by excessive phlegm (mucus), unless directed by a physician. As with any drug, if you are pregnant or nursing a baby, seek the advice of a health professional before using this product. KEEP THIS AND ALL DRUGS OUT OF THE REACH OF CHILDREN. In case of accidental overdose seek professional assistance or contact a Poison Control Center immediately.

Drug Interaction Precaution: Do not use this product if you are now taking a prescription monoamine oxidase inhibitor (MAOI) (certain drugs for depression, psychiatric or emotional conditions, or Parkinson's disease), or for 2 weeks after stopping the MAOI drug. If you are uncertain whether your prescription drug contains an MAOI, consult a health professional before taking this product.

Directions For Use: Follow dosage recommendations below, or use as directed by your physician. Repeat every 4 hours. Do not exceed the following doses in a 24 hour period: 12 years and older-24 teaspoonfuls, 6 to under 12 years-12 teaspoonfuls, 2 to 6 years-6 teaspoonfuls.

Benylin® Expectorant

AGE	DOSAGE
12 years & older	2 to 4 teaspoonfuls
6 to under 12 years	1 to 2 teaspoonfuls
2 to under 6 years	½ to 1 teaspoonful
Under 2 years	Consult Physician

How Supplied: Benylin Expectorant is available in 4 oz. bottles.
Store at room temperature (59°–86°F)
Shown in Product Identification Guide, page 529

BENYLIN® Adult Formula Cough Suppressant

Active Ingredient: Each teaspoonful (5 mL) contains: Dextromethorphan HBr 15 mg. Also contains: Caramel, Citric Acid, D&C Red No. 33, FD&C Red No. 40, Flavors, Glycerin, Poloxamer 407, Polysorbate 20, Sodium Benzoate, Sodium Carboxymethyl Cellulose, Sodium Citrate, Sodium Saccharin, Sorbitol Solution, and Water.

Warnings: A persistent cough may be a sign of a serious condition. If cough persists for more than one week, tends to recur, or is accompanied by fever, rash or persistent headache, consult a physician. Do not take this product for persistent or chronic cough such as occurs with smoking, asthma, emphysema, or if cough is accompanied by excessive phlegm (mucus), unless directed by a physician. As with any drug, if you are pregnant or nursing a baby, seek the advice of a health professional before using this product. KEEP THIS AND ALL DRUGS OUT OF THE REACH OF CHILDREN. In case of accidental overdose, seek professional assistance or contact a Poison Control Center immediately.

Drug Interaction Precaution: Do not use this product if you are taking a prescription monoamine oxidase inhibitor

(MAOI) (certain drugs for depression, psychiatric or emotional conditions, or Parkinson's disease), or for 2 weeks after stopping the MAOI drug. If you are uncertain whether your prescription drug contains an MAOI, consult a health professional before taking this product.

Indication: Maximum strength, non-narcotic cough suppressant for temporary relief of cough due to minor throat and bronchial irritation as may occur with the common cold or inhaled irritants.

Directions For Use: Follow dosage recommendations below, or use as directed by your physician. Repeat every 6 to 8 hours, not to exceed 4 doses in a 24 hour period.

Benylin® Adult Formula

AGE	DOSAGE
12 years & older	2 teaspoonfuls
6 to under 12 years	1 teaspoonful
2 to under 6 years	½ teaspoonful
under 2 years	Consult Physician

How Supplied: Benylin Adult Formula is supplied in 4 oz. bottles. Store at room temperature (59–86°F) See bottom flap for lot number and expiration date.
Shown in Product Identification Guide, page 529

BENYLIN® Pediatric Cough Suppressant

Active Ingredient: Each teaspoonful (5 mL) contains: Dextromethorphan HBr 7.5 mg. Also contains: Citric Acid, FD&C Blue No. 1, FD&C Red No. 40, Flavors, Glycerin, Poloxamer 407, Polysorbate 20, Sodium Benzoate, Sodium Carboxymethyl Cellulose, Sodium Citrate, Sodium Saccharin, Sorbitol Solution, and Water.

Indications: Non-narcotic cough suppressant for temporary relief of cough due to minor throat and bronchial irritation as may occur with the common cold or inhaled irritants.

Warnings: A persistent cough may be a sign of a serious condition. If cough persists for more than one week, tends to recur, or is accompanied by fever, rash, or persistent headache, consult a physician. Do not take this product for persistent or chronic cough such as occurs with smoking, asthma, emphysema, or if cough is accompanied by excessive phlegm (mucus), unless directed by a physician. As with any drug, if you are pregnant or nursing a baby, seek the advice of a health professional before using

this product. KEEP THIS AND ALL DRUGS OUT OF THE REACH OF CHILDREN. In case of accidental overdose, seek professional assistance or contact a Poison Control Center immediately.

Drug Interaction Precaution: Do not use this product if you are now taking a prescription monoamine oxidase inhibitor (MAOI) (certain drugs for depression, psychiatric or emotional conditions, or Parkinson's disease), or for 2 weeks after stopping the MAOI drug. If you are uncertain whether your prescription drug contains an MAOI, consult a health professional before taking this product.

Directions for Use: Follow dosage recommendations below or use as directed by your physician. Repeat every 6 to 8 hours not to exceed 4 doses in a 24 hour period.

Benylin® Pediatric

AGE	DOSAGE
Under 2 years	Consult Physician
2 to under 6 years	1 teaspoonful
6 to under 12 years	2 teaspoonfuls
12 years & older	4 teaspoonfuls

How Supplied: 4 oz bottles
Shown in Product Identification Guide, page 529

BOROFAX® Skin Protectant
[bôr 'uh-făks]

Indications: Helps treat and prevent diaper rash. Protects chafed skin due to diaper rash and helps seal out wetness.

Directions: Change wet and soiled diapers promptly, cleanse the diaper area, and allow to dry. Apply ointment liberally as often as necessary, with each diaper change, especially at bedtime or anytime when exposure to wet diapers may be prolonged.

Warnings: For external use only. Avoid contact with the eyes. If condition worsens or does not improve within 7 days, consult a doctor. Keep this and all drugs out of the reach of children. In case of accidental ingestion, seek professional assistance or contact a Poison Control Center immediately.

Active Ingredients: Zinc oxide 15% and white petrolatum 68.6%.
Also contains: Lanolin, mineral oil, and fragrance.
Store at 15° to 25°C (59° to 77°F).

How Supplied: Tube, 1.8 oz (50 g)
Shown in Product Identification Guide, page 529

CALADRYL® Lotion
[că 'lă drĭl "]
CALADRYL Cream For Kids
CALADRYL Clear Lotion

Active Ingredients: Caladryl Lotion and Caladryl Cream For Kids; Calamine 8%, and Pramoxine HCl 1%.
Caladryl Clear Lotion; Pramoxine HCl 1% and Zinc Acetate 0.1%.

Inactive Ingredients: Caladryl Lotion —SD Alcohol 38B% v/v, Camphor, Diazolidinyl Urea, Fragrance, Hydroxypropyl Methylcellulose, Methylparaben, Polysorbate 80, Propylene Glycol, Propylparaben, Water and Xanthan Gum.
Caladryl Cream for Kids—Camphor, Cetyl Alcohol, Cyclomethicone, Diazolidinyl Urea, Fragrance, Methylparaben, Polysorbate 60, Propylene Glycol, Propylparaben, Sorbitan Stearate, Soya Sterol and Water.
Caladryl Clear Lotion—SD Alcohol 38B 2.5% v/v, Camphor, Citric Acid, Diazolidinyl Urea, Fragrance, Glycerin, Hydroxypropyl Methylcellulose, Methylparaben, Polysorbate 40, Propylene Glycol, Propylparaben, Purified Water and Sodium Citrate.

Indications: For the temporary relief of itching and pain associated with rashes due to poison ivy, poison oak or poison sumac, insect bites and minor irritations. Dries the oozing and weeping of poison ivy, poison oak and poison sumac.

Warnings: For external use only. Avoid contact with the eyes. If condition worsens, or symptoms persist for more than 7 days or clear up and occur again within a few days, discontinue use of this product and consult a physician. KEEP THIS AND ALL DRUGS OUT OF THE REACH OF CHILDREN. In case of accidental ingestion seek professional assistance or contact a Poison Control Center immediately.

Directions: For adults and children 2 years of age and older: Apply to the affected area no more than three to four times daily. Before each application, cleanse skin with soap and water and dry affected area. **Children under 2 years of age: Consult a physician.**
Additional instructions for only Lotion and Clear Lotion: Shake Well.

How Supplied: Caladryl Cream for Kids—1½ oz tubes
Caladryl Clear Lotion—6 fl. oz. bottles
Caladryl Lotion—6 fl. oz. bottles
Shown in Product Identification Guide, page 529

Continued on next page

This product information was prepared in November 1994. On these and other Warner Wellcome Consumer HealthCare Products, detailed information may be obtained by addressing Warner Wellcome Consumer HealthCare Products, Warner-Lambert, Morris Plains, NJ 07950

Warner Wellcome—Cont.

EMPIRIN® ASPIRIN Tablets
[ĕm 'puh-rŭn]

For relief of headache, minor muscular aches and pains, toothache, discomfort and fever of colds and flu, pain of the premenstrual and menstrual periods, and temporary relief of minor arthritis pain (see CAUTION below).

Directions: Adults: 1 or 2 tablets with a full glass of water. Repeat every 4 hours as needed, up to 12 tablets a day.
Children: Consult a physician (see WARNINGS).

Caution: In arthritic conditions, if pain persists for more than 10 days or redness is present, consult a physician immediately.

Warnings: Children and teenagers should not use this medicine for chicken pox or flu symptoms before a doctor is consulted about Reye syndrome, a rare but serious illness reported to be associated with aspirin. Keep this and all medicines out of children's reach. In case of accidental overdose, contact a physician immediately.

High or continued fever, severe or persistent sore throat especially when accompanied by high fever, headache, nausea or vomiting, may be serious. Consult your physician. Do not exceed dose unless directed by a physician. Do not take this product if you are allergic to aspirin, have asthma, a gastric ulcer or its symptoms, or are taking a medication that affects the clotting of blood, except under the advice of a physician. As with any drug, if you are pregnant or nursing a baby, seek the advice of a health professional before using this product.
IT IS ESPECIALLY IMPORTANT NOT TO USE ASPIRIN DURING THE LAST 3 MONTHS OF PREGNANCY UNLESS SPECIFICALLY DIRECTED TO DO SO BY A DOCTOR BECAUSE IT MAY CAUSE PROBLEMS IN THE UNBORN CHILD OR COMPLICATIONS DURING DELIVERY.

Active Ingredients: Each tablet contains aspirin 325 mg (5 gr).

Inactive Ingredients: microcrystalline cellulose and potato starch.

Store at 15° to 25°C (59° to 77°F) in a dry place.

How Supplied: Bottles of 50, 100.

---

e·p·t® PREGNANCY TEST
You can find out whether or not you're pregnant by testing any time of day and as early as the first day of your missed period.
With just one easy step **e·p·t** gives you clear results in just 3 minutes. **e·p·t Pregnancy Test.** The name more women trust™

Before You Begin The Test. Please read the instructions carefully. Registered nurses are available to confidentially answer your calls regarding **e·p·t.** If you have any questions about **e·p·t.** call toll-free 1-800-562-0266 (8:30 am to 8:00 pm EST) or 1-800-223-0182 (8:30 am to 5:00 pm EST) weekdays.

To Use e·p·t.
Only for external use (not for internal use). Remove the test stick from the foil pouch and throw away the freshness packet.

Slide back the clear splashguard to expose the absorbent tip and protect the results and control windows.
[See table below.]
Hold the test stick by the thumb grip with the exposed **absorbent tip pointing downward and directly into your urine stream** for at least 5 seconds until it is thoroughly wet.

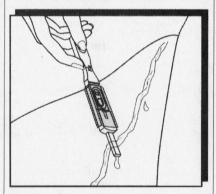

Do not urinate on the windows. (If you prefer, you can urinate into a clean dry cup or container. **Dip only the absorbent tip of the stick** in the urine for at least 5 seconds.)
Lay the test stick down on a flat surface with the windows facing upward while you wait for the test result. (If you wish, you can slide forward the clear splashguard to cover the saturated area.)
As the test begins to work, you may notice a light pink color moving across the windows.

To Read The Results.
Wait at least 3 minutes to read the result. After 3 minutes, a line will appear in the square Control Window to tell you that the test is finished. Once the line appears in the square Control Window, you may read the result.
Do not read the results after 20 minutes have passed. The round Results Window shows you test results.

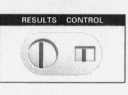

2 LINES— PREGNANT
If you see one line in each window as illustrated, the test has indicated that you are pregnant.
(One line can be darker than the other. The two lines can be any shade of pink and can be lighter or darker than the color picture. However, you should see two clear parallel lines as indicated.)

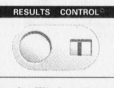

1 LINE–NOT PREGNANT
If you see a line in the square Control Window but no line in the round Results Window, the test has indicated that you are not Pregnant.

Frequently Asked Questions
How Does e·p·t Work?
e·p·t detects a hormone in your urine that the body produces only during pregnancy (hCG human Chorionic Gonadotropin).
Do I Have To Test in the Morning?
No. You can use **e·p·t** any time of day. You do not have to use first morning urine.
How Soon Can I use e·p·t?
e·p·t can detect hCG hormone levels in your urine as early as the first day your period is late. **e·p·t** can be used on the day of your missed period as well as any day thereafter.
What If I Don't Think The Results of the Test are Correct?
If it is hard to tell whether there is a line or not in the round Results Window, repeat the test after 2–3 days with a new stick—if the result is positive, the line should be darker. If you follow the instructions carefully, you should not get a false result. Certain drugs which contain hCG or that are used in combination with hCG (such as Pegnyl, Profasi, Pergonal) and rare medical conditions may give a false result. Alcohol, analgesics, antibiotics, birth control pills, hormone

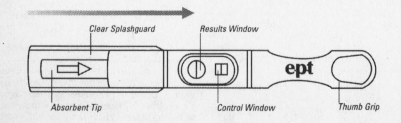

Clear Splashguard   *Results Window*

ept

Absorbent Tip   *Control Window*   *Thumb Grip*

therapies containing clomiphene citrate (such as Clomid, Serophen) or painkillers **should not** affect the test result. If you repeat the test and continue to get an unexpected result, contact your doctor.

The test may give a false positive result if you have recently had a miscarriage, or if you have recently given birth. This is because the test may detect hCG still in your system from a previous pregnancy. You should ask your doctor for help in interpreting the results of your **e·p·t** test if you have recently been pregnant.

What if the Line in the Round Results Window is Dark but the Line in the Square Control Window is Very Faint?

The result is positive (2 lines).

What Should I Do If the Result is Positive (Pregnant)?

If the result is positive, you should see your doctor to discuss your pregnancy and next steps. Early prenatal care is important to ensure the health of you and your baby.

What Should I do if the Result is Negative (Not Pregnant)?

If the result is negative, no pregnancy hormone (hCG) has been detected and you are probably not pregnant. However, you may have miscalculated when your period was due, especially if you have irregular periods. If your period does not start within a week, repeat the test. If you still get a negative result and your period has not started, you should see your doctor.

What If I Don't Wait the Full 3 Minutes Before Reading the Test Result?

If you read the test result before 3 minutes, you may not give the test enough time to work, and the results may be inaccurate. The appearance of a line in the square control window will tell you that the test is finished and you may read the results.

Shown in Product Identification Guide, page 529

GELUSIL®

[jěl 'ū-sĭl "]

Antacid–Anti-gas
Liquid/Tablets
Sodium Free

Each teaspoonful (5 mL) of Gelusil Liquid contains: Aluminum Hydroxide Gel (equivalent to 200 mg of Aluminum Hydroxide Dried Gel), Magnesium Hydroxide 200 mg and Simethicone 25 mg (an antiflatulent).

Each Gelusil Tablet contains: Aluminum Hydroxide Dried Gel 200 mg, Magnesium Hydroxide 200 mg and Simethicone 25 mg (an antiflatulent).

Also contains: Liquid: Ammonia Solution Strong; Calcium Hypochlorite; Citric Acid; Flavors; Hydroxypropyl Methylcellulose; Menthol; Sodium Saccharin; Sorbitol Solution; Water; Xanthan Gum. Tablets: Flavors; Magnesium Stearate; Mannitol; Sorbitol; Sugar.

Advantages:
- High acid-neutralizing capacity
- Sodium free

- Simethicone for antiflatulent activity
- Good taste for better patient compliance
- Fast dissolution of chewed tablets for prompt relief

Indications: For the relief of heartburn, sour stomach, acid indigestion and to alleviate or relieve symptoms of gas.

Directions for Use: Two or more teaspoonfuls or tablets one hour after meals and at bedtime, or as directed by a physician.

Tablets should be chewed.
Liquid: Shake well before use.

Warnings: Do not take more than 12 tablets or teaspoonfuls in a 24-hour period, or use this maximum dosage for more than two weeks, or use this product if you have kidney disease, except under the advice and supervision of a physician.

Keep this and all drugs out of the reach of children.

Professional Warnings: Prolonged use of aluminum-containing antacids in patients with renal failure may result in or worsen dialysis osteomalacia. Elevated tissue aluminum levels contribute to the development of the dialysis encephalopathy and osteomalacia syndromes. Small amounts of aluminum are absorbed from the gastrointestinal tract and renal excretion of aluminum is impaired in renal failure. Aluminum is not well removed by dialysis because it is bound to albumin and transferrin, which do not cross dialysis membranes. As a result, aluminum is deposited in bone, and dialysis osteomalacia may develop when large amounts of aluminum are ingested orally by patients with impaired renal function. Aluminum forms insoluble complexes with phosphate in the gastrointestinal tract, thus decreasing phosphate absorption. Prolonged use of aluminum-containing antacids by normophosphatemic patients may result in hypophosphatemia if phosphate intake is not adequate. In its more severe forms, hypophosphatemia can lead to anorexia, malaise, muscle weakness, and osteomalacia.

Drug Interaction Precaution: Antacids may interact with certain prescription drugs. If you are presently taking a prescription drug, do not take this product without checking with your physician or other health professional.

How Supplied:
Liquid—In plastic bottles of 12 fl oz. (355 mL)
Tablets—White, embossed Gelusil P-D 034—individual strips of 10 in boxes of 100.
Store at Room Temperature 59°–86°F (15°–30°C).

Shown in Product Identification Guide, page 530

LISTERMINT®
Alcohol-Free Mouthrinse

Ingredient: Water, Glycerin, Poloxamer 335, PEG 600, Flavors, Sodium Lauryl Sulfate, Sodium Benzoate, Sodium Saccharin, Benzoic Acid, Zinc Chloride, D&C Yellow #10, FD&C Green #3.

Indications: Freshens breath; contains no fluoride.

Directions: Rinse with 30 ml (1 fl. oz.) for 30 seconds to freshen breath in the morning and after meals as needed.

Warnings: Do not swallow. Keep out of reach of children.

How Supplied: Listermint® is supplied to consumers in 18 and 32 fl. oz. bottles and available to professionals in 3 fl. oz. bottles and in gallons.

Shown in Product Identification Guide, page 530

LISTERINE® Antiseptic

Active Ingredients: Thymol 0.064%, Eucalyptol 0.092%, Methyl Salicylate 0.060% and Menthol 0.042%. Also contains: Water, Alcohol 26.9%, Benzoic Acid, Poloxamer 407 and Caramel.

Indications: To help prevent and reduce plaque and gingivitis/For bad breath.

Actions: Listerine® Antiseptic has been shown to help prevent and reduce supragingival plaque accumulation and gingivitis when used in a conscientiously applied program of oral hygiene and regular professional care. Its effect on periodontitis has not been determined. Listerine is the only leading nonprescription mouthrinse that has received the American Dental Association's Council on Dental Therapeutics Seal of Acceptance for helping to prevent and reduce plaque above the gumline and gingivitis.

Directions: Rinse full strength for 30 seconds with 20 ml (⅔ fl. ounce or 4 teaspoonfuls) morning and night. If bad breath persists, see your dentist.

Warnings: Do not administer to children under twelve years of age. Keep this and all drugs out of the reach of children. Do not swallow. In case of accidental overdose, seek professional assistance or contact a Poison Control Center immediately.

How Supplied: Listerine® Antiseptic is supplied in 250 ml, 500 ml, 1.0 liter and

Continued on next page

This product information was prepared in November 1994. On these and other Warner Wellcome Consumer HealthCare Products, detailed information may be obtained by addressing Warner Wellcome Consumer HealthCare Products, Warner-Lambert, Morris Plains, NJ 07950

Warner Wellcome—Cont.

1.5 liter bottles, as well as 3 and 58 fl. oz. bottles. It is also available to professionals in 3 and 48 fl. oz. bottles and in gallons.

Shown in Product Identification Guide, page 530

COOL MINT LISTERINE®

Active Ingredients: Thymol 0.064%, Eucalyptol 0.092%, Methyl Salicylate 0.060% and Menthol 0.042%.

Inactive Ingredients: Water, Sorbitol Solution, Alcohol 21.6%, Poloxamer 407, Benzoic Acid, Flavoring, Sodium Saccharin, Sodium Citrate, Citric Acid and FD&C Green #3.

Indications: To help prevent and reduce plaque and gingivitis/For bad breath.

Actions: Cool Mint Listerine® Antiseptic has been shown to help prevent and reduce supragingival plaque accumulation and gingivitis when used in a conscientiously applied program of oral hygiene and regular professional care. Its effect on periodontitis has not been determined. Listerine is the only leading nonprescription mouthrinse that has received the American Dental Association's Council on Dental Therapeutics Seal of Acceptance for helping to prevent and reduce plaque above the gumline and gingivitis.

Directions: Rinse full strength for 30 seconds with 20 ml (⅔ fl. ounce or 4 teaspoonfuls) morning and night. If bad breath persists, see your dentist.

Warnings: Do not administer to children under twelve years of age. Keep this and all drugs out of the reach of children. Do not swallow. In case of accidental overdose, seek professional assistance or contact a Poison Control Center immediately.

How Supplied: Cool Mint Listerine® Antiseptic is supplied in 250 ml, 500 ml, 1.0 liter and 1.5 liter bottles, as well as 3 and 58 fl. oz. bottles. It is also available to professionals in 3 and 48 fl. oz. bottles and in gallons.

Shown in Product Identification Guide, page 530

FRESHBURST LISTERINE®

Active Ingredients: Thymol 0.064%, Eucalyptol 0.092%, Methyl Salicylate 0.060% and Menthol 0.042%.

Inactive Ingredients: Water, Sorbitol Solution, Alcohol 21.6%, Poloxamer 407, Benzoic Acid, Flavoring, Sodium Saccharin, Sodium Citrate, Citric Acid, D&C Yellow #10 and FD&C Green #3.

Indications: To help prevent and reduce plaque and gingivitis/For bad breath.

Actions: FreshBurst Listerine® Antispetic has been shown to help prevent and reduce supragingival plaque accumulation and gingivitis when used in a conscientiously applied program of oral hygiene and regular professional care. Its effect on periodontitis has not been determined. Listerine is the only leading nonprescription mouthrinse that has received the American Dental Association's Council on Dental Therapeutics Seal of Acceptance for helping to prevent and reduce plaque above the gumline and gingivitis.

Directions: Rinse full strength for 30 seconds with 20 ml (⅔ fl. ounce or 4 teaspoonfuls) morning and night. If bad breath persists, see your dentist.

Warnings: Do not administer to children under twelve years of age. Keep this and all drugs out of the reach of children. Do not swallow. In case of accidental overdose, seek professional assistance or contact a Poison Control Center immediately.

How Supplied: FreshBurst Listerine® Antiseptic is supplied in 250 ml, 500 ml, 1.0 liter and 1.5 liter bottles, as well as 3 and 58 fl. oz. bottles. It is also available to professionals in 3 and 48 fl. oz. bottles and in gallons.

Shown in Product Identification Guide, page 530

LUBRIDERM® LOTION
Dry Skin Care Lotion

Composition:
Scented—Contains Water, Mineral Oil, Petrolatum, Sorbitol, Lanolin, Stearic Acid, Lanolin Alcohol, Cetyl Alcohol, Tri (PPG-3 Myristyl Ether) Citrate, Triethanolamine, Methylparaben, Methyldibromo Glutaronitrile/Phenoxyethanol, Fregrance, Ethylparaben, Propylparaben, Butylparaben, Sodium Chloride.
Fragrance Free—Contains Water, Mineral Oil, Petrolatum, Sorbitol, Lanolin, Stearic Acid, Lanolin Alcohol, Cetyl Alcohol, Tri (PPG-3 Myristyl Ether) Citrate, Triethanolamine, Methylparaben, Methyldibromo Glutaronitrile/Phenoxyethanol, Ethylparaben, Propylparaben, Butylparaben, Sodium Chloride.

Actions and Uses: Lubriderm Lotion is an oil-in-water emulsion indicated for use in softening, soothing and moisturizing dry chapped skin. Lubriderm relieves the roughness, tightness and discomfort associated with dry or chapped skin and helps protect the skin from further drying.
Lubriderm's formula smoothes easily into skin without leaving a greasy feeling.

Administration and Dosage: Apply as often as needed to hands and body to restore and maintain the skin's natural suppleness.

Precautions: For external use only.

How Supplied:
Scented: Available in 1, 6, 10 and 16 fl. oz. plastic bottles, and a 2.5 ounce tube.
Fragrance Free: Available in 1, 6, 10 and 16 fl. oz. plastic bottles, and a 2.5 ounce tube.

Shown in Product Identification Guide, page 530

LUBRIDERM® BATH AND SHOWER OIL

Composition: Contains Mineral Oil, PPG-15 Stearyl Ether, Oleth-2, Nonoxynol-5, Fragrance, D&C Green No. 6.

Actions and Uses: Lubriderm Bath and Shower Oil is a lanolin-free, mineral oil–based, bath oil designed for softening and soothing dry skin during the bath. The formula disperses into countless droplets of oil that coat the skin and help lubricate and soften. It is equally effective in hard or soft water and provides an excellent way to moisturize the skin and help counterbalance the drying effects of harsh soaps and hot water.

Administration and Dosage: One to two capfuls in bath, or apply with hand or moistened cloth in shower and rinse. For use as a skin cleanser, rub into wet skin and rinse.

Precautions: Avoid getting in eyes; if this occurs, flush with clear water. When using any bath and shower oil, take precautions against slipping. For external use only.

How Supplied: Available in 8 fl. oz. plastic bottles.

Shown in Product Identification Guide, page 530

LUBRIDERM® Moisture Recovery
Alpha Hydroxy Formula
Creme/Lotion

Composition: Creme—Contains Water, Isostearic Acid, Stearic Acid, Sodium Lactate, PPG-12/SMDI Copolymer, Lactic Acid, Steareth-21, Steareth-2, Mineral Oil, Cetyl Alcohol, Magnesium Aluminum Silicate, Imidurea, Potassium Sorbate, Xanthan Gum, Fragrance. Lotion—Contains Water, Isostearic Acid, Stearic Acid, Steareth-21, Sodium Lactate, PPG-12/SMDI Copolymer, Lactic Acid, Steareth-2, Magnesium Aluminum Silicate, Cetyl Alcohol, Imidurea, Potassium Sorbate, Xanthan Gum, Fragrance.

Actions and Uses: Lubriderm Moisture Recovery Alpha Hydroxy Formula is ideal for patients with severely dry skin. It accelerates the process of exfoliation, allowing newer, healthier looking skin to emerge. The patented alpha hydroxy delivery system provides long lasting, concentrated healing of severely dry skin.

Administration and Dosage: Apply creme to rough, dry skin areas like feet, knees, and elbows. The lotion is ideal for overall body moisturization.

Precautions: For external use only. Avoid contact with the eyes.

How Supplied:
Creme—Available in 4 oz. plastic tubes.
Lotion—Available in 8 oz. plastic tubes.

Shown in Product Identification Guide, page 530

LUBRIDERM® Moisture Recovery GelCreme

Composition: Contains Water, Cetyl Alcohol, Glycerin, Mineral Oil, Cyclomethicone Fluid, Propylene Glycol Dicaprylate/Dicaprate, PEG-40 Stearate, Isopropyl Isostearate, Emulsifying Wax, Lecithin, Carbomer 940, Diazolidinyl Urea, Titanium Dioxide, Sodium Benzoate, BHT, Tri(PPG-3 Myristyl Ether) Citrate, Disodium Edetate, Retinyl Palmitate, Tocopheryl Acetate, Sodium Pyruvate, Iodopropynyl Butylcarbamate, Sodium Hydroxide, Xanthan Gum.

Actions and Uses: Lubriderm Moisture Recovery GelCreme is recommended for patients with severely dry skin. It's patented emollient system contains vitamins, nutrients, and antioxidants to heal and protect dry skin. The unique formulation combines the richness of a creme with the light feel of a gel.

Administration and Dosage: Apply to hands and body.

Precautions: For external use only.

How Supplied: Available in 4 and 7.5 oz. plastic bottles.

Shown in Product Identification Guide, page 530

LUBRIDERM® Seriously Sensitive Lotion

Composition: Contains Water, Butylene Glycol, Glycerin, Mineral Oil, Petrolatum, Cetyl Alcohol, Propylene Glycol Dicaprylate/Dicaprate, Peg-40 Stearate, C11-C13 Isoparaffin, Glyceryl Stearate, Tri (PPG-3 Myristyl Ether) Citrate, Emulsifying Wax, Dimethicone, DMDM Hydantoin, Methylparaben, Carbomer 940, Ethylparaben, Propylparaben, Titanium Dioxide, Disodium EDTA, Sodium Hydroxide, Butylparaben, Xanthan Gum.

Action and Uses: Lubriderm Seriously Sensitive Lotion is recommended for patients with sensitive skin. Its unique combination of emollients provides sensitive dry skin with the moisture it needs while helping to create a protective layer. Seriously Sensitive Lotion is hypoallergenic, noncomedogenic, and 100% lanolin free, fragrance free, and dye free. It is lightweight, nongreasy, and absorbs quickly.

Administration and Dosage: Apply to hands and body to help protect and heal sensitive dry skin.

Precautions: For external use only.

How Supplied: Available in 6 and 10 oz. plastic bottles.

Shown in Product Identification Guide, page 530

MYADEC® Tablets
High Potency Multivitamin
Multimineral Formula

Each Tablet Represents:		% of US Recommended Daily Allowances (US RDA)
VITAMINS		
Vitamin A**	5,000 IU*	100%
Vitamin D	400 IU	100%
Vitamin E	30 IU	100%
Vitamin C	60 mg	100%
Folic Acid	400 mcg	100%
Vitamin B₁	1.7 mg	113%
Vitamin B₂	2.0 mg	118%
Niacin	20 mg	100%
Vitamin B₆	3 mg	150%
Vitamin B₁₂	6 mcg	100%
Biotin	30 mcg	10%
Pantothenic Acid	10 mg	100%
Vitamin K	25 mcg	***
MINERALS		
Calcium	162 mg	16%
Phosphorus	125 mg	13%
Iodine	150 mcg	100%
Iron	18 mg	100%
Magnesium	100 mg	25%
Copper	2 mg	100%
Zinc	15 mg	100%
Manganese	2.5 mg	***
Potassium	40 mg	***
Chloride	36.3 mg	***
Chromium	25 mcg	***
Molybdenum	25 mcg	***
Selenium	25 mcg	***
Nickel	5 mcg	***
Tin	10 mcg	***
Silicon	10 mcg	***
Vanadium	10 mcg	***
Boron	150 mcg	***

* International Units
** as Acetate and Beta Carotene
*** No US Recommended Daily Allowance (US RDA) has been established for this nutrient.

Ingredients: Dicalcium phosphate, magnesium oxide, potassium chloride, ascorbic acid, dl-alpha tocopheryl acetate, ferrous fumarate, modified starch glycolate, starch, cellulose, modified cellulose gum, niacinamide, silica, zinc oxide, polyethylene glycol, d-calcium pantothenate, beta carotene, vitamin A acetate, manganese sulfate, magnesium stearate, pyridoxine hydrochloride, phytonadione, biotin, cupric oxide, riboflavin, thiamine mononitrate, cyanocobalamin, vitamin D, folic acid, potassium iodide, sodium potassium borates, chromium chloride, sodium selenate, sodium molybdate, stannous chloride, sodium metasilicate, sodium metavanadate, nickelous sulfate, pharmaceutical glaze, methylcellulose, polysorbate, titanium dioxide (color), Yellow #6, Red #40, Blue #2, povidone, propylene glycol, hydroxypropylcellulose.

Warning: Close tightly and keep out of the reach of children. Contains iron, which can be harmful or fatal to children in large doses. In case of accidental overdose, seek professional assistance or contact a Poison Control Center immediately.

Actions and Uses: High potency vitamin supplement with minerals for adults.

Dosage: One tablet daily with a full meal.

How Supplied: In bottles of 130. Store below 30°C (86°F). Protect from moisture.

NEOSPORIN® Ointment
[nē 'uh-spō 'rŭn]

Indications: First aid to help prevent infection in minor cuts, scrapes, and burns.

Directions: Clean the affected area. Apply a small amount of this product (an amount equal to the surface area of the tip of a finger) on the area 1 to 3 times daily. May be covered with a sterile bandage.

Warnings: For external use only. Stop use and consult a physician if the condition persists or gets worse, or if a rash or other allergic reaction develops. Do not use this product if you are allergic to any of the listed ingredients. Do not use in the eyes or apply over large areas of the body. In case of deep or puncture wounds, animal bites, or serious burns, consult a physician. Do not use longer than 1 week unless directed by a physician. Keep this and all drugs out of the reach of children. In case of accidental ingestion, seek professional assistance or contact a Poison Control Center immediately.

Each Gram Contains: polymyxin B sulfate 5,000 units, bacitracin zinc 400 units and neomycin 3.5 mg in a special white petrolatum base.

Store at 15° to 25°C (59° to 77°F).

How Supplied: Tubes, ½ oz (14.2 g) (with applicator tip), 1 oz (28.4 g); 1/32 oz (0.9 g) (approx.) foil packets packed 10 per box (Neo To Go™) or 144 per box.

Professional Labeling: Consult *1995 Physicians' Desk Reference®*.

Shown in Product Identification Guide, page 530

Continued on next page

This product information was prepared in November 1994. On these and other Warner Wellcome Consumer HealthCare Products, detailed information may be obtained by addressing Warner Wellcome Consumer HealthCare Products, Warner-Lambert, Morris Plains, NJ 07950

Warner Wellcome—Cont.

NEOSPORIN® PLUS MAXIMUM STRENGTH Cream
[nē ''uh-spō 'rŭn]

Indications: First aid to help prevent infection and provide temporary relief of pain or discomfort in minor cuts, scrapes, and burns.

Directions: Adults and children 2 years of age and older: Clean the affected area. Apply a small amount of this product (an amount equal to the surface area of the tip of a finger) on the area 1 to 3 times daily. May be covered with a sterile bandage. **Children under 2 years of age: Consult a physician.**

Warnings: For external use only. If condition worsens, or if symptoms persist for more than 1 week or clear up and occur again within a few days, or if a rash or other allergic reaction develops, discontinue use of this product and consult a physician. Do not use this product if you are allergic to any of the listed ingredients. Do not use in the eyes or apply over large areas of the body. Do not use in large quantities, particularly over raw surfaces or blistered areas. In case of deep or puncture wounds, animal bites, or serious burns, consult a physician. Do not use longer than 1 week unless directed by a physician. Keep this and all drugs out of the reach of children. In case of accidental ingestion, seek professional assistance or contact a Poison Control Center immediately.

Each Gram Contains: polymyxin B sulfate 10,000 units, neomycin 3.5 mg, and lidocaine 40 mg. Also contains: methylparaben 0.25% (added as a preservative), emulsifying wax, mineral oil, poloxamer 188, propylene glycol, purified water, and white petrolatum. Store at 15° to 25°C (59° to 77°F).

How Supplied: ½ oz (14.2 g) tubes.
Shown in Product Identification Guide, page 530

NEOSPORIN® PLUS MAXIMUM STRENGTH Ointment
[nē ''uh-spō 'rŭn]

Indications: First aid to help prevent infection and provide temporary relief of pain or discomfort in minor cuts, scrapes, and burns.

Directions: Adults and children 2 years of age and older: Clean the affected area. Apply a small amount of this product (an amount equal to the surface area of the tip of a finger) on the area 1 to 3 times daily. May be covered with a sterile bandage. **Children under 2 years of age: Consult a physician.**

Warnings: For external use only. If condition worsens, or if symptoms persist for more than 1 week or clear up and occur again within a few days, or if a rash or other allergic reaction develops, dis-

continue use of this product and consult a physician. Do not use this product if you are allergic to any of the listed ingredients. Do not use in the eyes or apply over large areas of the body. Do not use in large quantities, particularly over raw surfaces or blistered areas. In case of deep or puncture wounds, animal bites, or serious burns, consult a physician. Do not use longer than 1 week unless directed by a physician. Keep this and all drugs out of the reach of children. In case of accidental ingestion, seek professional assistance or contact a Poison Control Center immediately.

Each Gram Contains: polymyxin B sulfate 10,000 units, bacitracin zinc 500 units, neomycin 3.5 mg, and lidocaine 40 mg in a special white petrolatum base. Store at 15° to 25°C (59° to 77°F).

How Supplied: ½ oz (14.2 g) and 1 oz (28.4 g) tubes.
Shown in Product Identification Guide, page 530

NIX®
Permethrin
Lice Treatment

Product Benefits: Nix Creme Rinse kills lice and their unhatched eggs with only one application. Nix protects against head lice reinfestation for a full 14 days. The unique creme rinse formula leaves hair manageable and easy to comb.

Indications: For the treatment of head lice.
Shake well before using.

Directions for Use: Nix Creme Rinse should be used after hair has been washed with your regular shampoo, rinsed with water and towel dried. A sufficient amount should be applied to saturate hair and scalp (especially behind the ears and on nape of the neck). Leave on hair for 10 minutes but no longer. Rinse with water. A single application is sufficient. Retreatment is required in less than 1% of patients. If live lice are observed seven days or more after the first application of this product, a second treatment should be given. For proper head lice management, remove nits with the nit comb provided.
Head lice live on the scalp and lay small white eggs (nits) on the hair shaft close to the scalp. The nits are most easily found on the nape of the neck or behind the ears. All personal headgear, scarfs, coats, and bed linen should be disinfected by machine washing in hot water and drying, using the hot cycle of a dryer for at least 20 minutes. Personal articles of clothing or bedding that cannot be washed may be dry-cleaned, sealed in a plastic bag for a period of about 2 weeks, or sprayed with a product specifically designed for this purpose. Personal combs and brushes may be disinfected by soaking in hot water (above 130°F) for 5 to 10 minutes. Thorough vacuuming of

rooms inhabited by infected patients is recommended.

Warnings: For external use only. Itching, redness, or swelling of the scalp may occur. If skin irritation persists or infection is present or develops, discontinue use and consult a doctor. Do not use near the eyes or permit contact with mucous membranes. If product gets into the eyes, immediately flush with water. Consult a doctor if infestation of eyebrows or eyelashes occurs. This product may cause breathing difficulty or an asthmatic episode in susceptible persons. This product should not be used on children less than 2 months of age. As with any drug, if you are pregnant or nursing a baby, seek the advice of a health professional before using this product. Keep this and all drugs out of the reach of children. In case of accidental ingestion, seek professional assistance or contact a Poison Control Center immediately.

Each Fluid Ounce Contains: permethrin 280 mg (1%). Inactive ingredients are: balsam canada, cetyl alcohol, citric acid, FD&C Yellow No. 6, fragrance, hydrolyzed animal protein, hydroxyethylcellulose, polyoxyethylene 10 cetyl ether, propylene glycol, and stearalkonium chloride. Also contains: isopropyl alcohol 5.6 g (20%) and added as preservatives, methylparaben 56 mg (0.2%) and propylparaben 22 mg (0.08%). Store at 15° to 25°C (59° to 77°F).

How Supplied: Bottles of 2 fl oz (50 mL) with special comb and Family Pack of 2 bottles, 2 fl oz (50 mL) each, with special comb.
Shown in Product Identification Guide, page 530

POLYSPORIN® Ointment
[pŏl 'ē-spō 'rŭn]

Indications: First aid to help prevent infection in minor cuts, scrapes, and burns.

Directions: Clean the affected area. Apply a small amount of this product (an amount equal to the surface area of the tip of a finger) on the area 1 to 3 times daily. May be covered with a sterile bandage.

Warnings: For external use only. Stop use and consult a physician if the condition persists or gets worse, or if a rash or other allergic reaction develops. Do not use this product if you are allergic to any of the listed ingredients. Do not use in the eyes or apply over large areas of the body. In case of deep or puncture wounds, animal bites, or serious burns, consult a physician. Do not use longer than 1 week unless directed by a physician. Keep this and all drugs out of the reach of children. In case of accidental ingestion, seek professional assistance or contact a Poison Control Center immediately.

Each Gram Contains: polymyxin B sulfate 10,000 units and bacitracin zinc 500 units in a special white petrolatum base.

Store at 15° to 25°C (59° to 77°F).

How Supplied: Tubes, ½ oz (14.2 g) with applicator tip, 1 oz (28.4 g); ¹⁄₃₂ oz (0.9 g) (approx.) foil packets packed in cartons of 144.
Shown in Product Identification Guide, page 530

POLYSPORIN® Powder
[pŏl ´ē-spō ´rŭn]

Indications: First aid to help prevent infection in minor cuts, scrapes, and burns.

Directions: Clean the affected area. Apply a light dusting of the powder on the area 1 to 3 times daily. May be covered with a sterile bandage.

Warnings: For external use only. Stop use and consult a physician if the condition persists or gets worse, or if a rash or other allergic reaction develops. Do not use this product if you are allergic to any of the listed ingredients. Do not use in the eyes or apply over large areas of the body. In case of deep or puncture wounds, animal bites, or serious burns, consult a physician. Do not use longer than 1 week unless directed by a physician. Keep this and all drugs out of the reach of children. In case of accidental ingestion, seek professional assistance or contact a Poison Control Center immediately.

Each Gram Contains: polymyxin B sulfate 10,000 units and bacitracin zinc 500 units in a lactose base.

Store at 15° to 25°C (59° to 77°F). Do not store under refrigeration.

How Supplied: 0.35 oz (10 g) shaker-vial.
Shown in Product Identification Guide, page 530

REPLENS® Vaginal Moisturizer
[ree ´plenz]

Description: Replens relieves the discomfort of vaginal dryness for days with a single application. Replens non-hormonal vaginal moisturizer provides natural feeling moisture to continuously hydrate vaginal tissue. Replens is non-staining, fragrance free, non-greasy and non-irritating Estrogen-Free.

Actions: When used as directed, Replens provides long-lasting relief from the discomfort of vaginal dryness by providing continuous hydration to the vaginal tissue.

Ingredients: Purified water, glycerin, mineral oil, polycarbophil, Carbomer 934P, hydrogenated palm oil glyceride, and sorbic acid.

Warnings: Keep out of the reach of children. Replens is not a contraceptive. Does not contain spermicide.

Usage: Use as needed. One application approximately once every 2 to 3 days is recommended.

How Supplied: Replens is available in boxes containing 3 or 8 pre-filled disposable applicators. Each applicator delivers 2.5 grams.
Shown in Product Identification Guide, page 530

SINUTAB® Non-Drying Liquid Caps

Indications: Temporarily relieves nasal congestion associated with sinusitis. Helps loosen phlegm (mucus) and thin bronchial secretions to drain bronchial tubes.

Active Ingredients: Each liquid cap contains: Pseudoephedrine Hydrochloride 30 mg., Guaifenesin 200 mg.

Inactive Ingredients: FD&C Blue No. 1, Gelatin, Glycerin, Polyethylene Glycol, Povidone, Propylene Glycol, and Sorbitol.

Warnings: Do not exceed recommended dosage. If nervousness, dizziness, or sleeplessness occur, discontinue use and consult a doctor. If symptoms do not improve within 7 days or are accompanied by fever, consult a doctor. Do not take this product if you have heart disease, high blood pressure, thyroid disease, diabetes, or difficulty in urination due to enlargement of the prostate gland unless directed by a doctor. Do not take this product for persistent or chronic cough such as occurs with smoking, asthma, chronic bronchitis, or emphysema, or where cough is accompanied by excessive phlegm (mucus) unless directed by a doctor. A persistent cough may be a sign of a serious condition. If cough persists for more than 1 week, tends to recur, or is accompanied by a fever, rash, or persistent headache, consult a doctor. As with any drug, if you are pregnant or nursing a baby, seek the advice of a health professional before using this product.

Drug Interaction Precaution: Do not use this product if you are now taking a prescription monoamine oxidase inhibitor (MAOI) (certain drugs for depression, psychiatric or emotional conditions, or Parkinson's disease), or for 2 weeks after stopping the MAOI drug. If you are uncertain whether your prescription drug contains an MAOI, consult a health professional before taking this product.

Precaution: KEEP THIS AND ALL DRUGS OUT OF THE REACH OF CHILDREN.

Symptoms and Treatment of Oral Overdosage: In case of accidental overdose, seek professional assistance or contact a Poison Control Center immediately.

Dosage and Administration: Adults and children 12 years of age and over: swallow 2 liquid caps every 4 hours, not to exceed 8 liquid caps in 24 hours, or as directed by a doctor. Children under 12 years of age, consult a doctor.

How Supplied: Sinutab® Non-Drying supplied in a box of 24 liquid caps.
Shown in Product Identification Guide, page 531

SINUTAB® Sinus Medication, Regular Strength Without Drowsiness Formula, Tablets

Indications: Specially formulated to provide fast, temporary relief of sinus pain and congestion due to colds, flu, allergy and hay fever without drowsiness.

Active Ingredients: Each tablet contains: Acetaminophen 325 mg., pseudoephedrine hydrochloride 30 mg.

Inactive Ingredients: Croscarmellose sodium, D&C Red No. 33, FD&C Red No. 40, hydroxypropyl cellulose, hydroxypropyl methylcellulose, magnesium stearate, microcrystalline cellulose, propylene glycol, simethicone, starch pregelatinized, titanium dioxide, zinc stearate.

Actions: Sinutab® Sinus Medication, Regular Strength Without Drowsiness Formula, Tablets contain an analgesic (acetaminophen) to relieve pain and a decongestant (pseudoephedrine hydrochloride) to reduce congestion of the nasopharyngeal mucosa.
Acetaminophen is both analgesic and antipyretic. Because acetaminophen is not a salicylate, Sinutab® Sinus Medication, Regular Strength Without Drowsiness Formula, Tablets can be used by patients who are allergic to aspirin.
Pseudoephedrine hydrochloride, a sympathomimetic drug, provides vasoconstriction of the nasopharyngeal mucosa resulting in a nasal decongestant effect. The absence of antihistamine in the formula provides the added benefit of reduced likelihood of drowsiness side effects.

Warnings: Do not exceed recommended dosage. If symptoms persist, do not improve within 7 days, or are accompanied by high fever, or if new symptoms occur, see your doctor before continuing use. Do not take this product if you have high blood pressure, heart disease, diabetes, thyroid disease, or difficulty in urination due to an enlarged prostate gland, except under doctor's supervision. Do not take this product for more than 10 days. As with any drug, if you are pregnant or nursing a baby, seek the advice of a health professional before using this product. Keep this and all drugs out of the reach of children. In case of accidental overdose, seek professional

Continued on next page

This product information was prepared in November 1994. On these and other Warner Wellcome Consumer HealthCare Products, detailed information may be obtained by addressing Warner Wellcome Consumer HealthCare Products, Warner-Lambert, Morris Plains, NJ 07950

Warner Wellcome—Cont.

help or contact a Poison Control Center immediately.

Drug Interaction: Do not take this product if you are presently taking a prescription drug for high blood pressure or depression without first consulting your doctor.

Dosage and Administration: Adults 2 tablets every 4 hours, not to exceed 8 tablets in 24 hours, or as directed by physician. Children under 12 should use only as directed by a physician.

How Supplied: Sinutab® Sinus Medication, Regular Strength Without Drowsiness Tablets are supplied in child-resistant blister packs of 24 tablets.

Store at room temperature (59°–86°F).

SINUTAB® Sinus Allergy Medication, Maximum Strength Formula, Tablets and Caplets

Indications: Specially formulated to provide fast, maximum strength relief of sinus pain and congestion due to allergies. Sinutab Sinus Allergy Medication is a complete allergy and hay fever medication relieving runny nose, itchy watery eyes and sneezing.

Active Ingredients: Each tablet/caplet contains: Acetaminophen 500 mg., chlorpheniramine maleate 2 mg., pseudoephedrine hydrochloride 30 mg.

Inactive Ingredients:
Tablets contain: Croscarmellose Sodium, Crospovidone, D&C Yellow No. 10 Aluminum Lake, FD&C Yellow No. 6 Alluminum Lake, Microcrystalline Cellulose, Povidone, Pregelatinized Starch, Stearic Acid, and Zinc Stearate.
Caplets contain: Carnauba Wax, Croscarmellose Sodium, Crospovidone, D&C Yellow No. 10 Aluminum Lake, FD&C Yellow No. 6 Aluminum Lake, Hydroxypropyl Cellulose, Hydroxypropyl Methylcellulose, Microcrystalline Cellulose, Polyethylene Glycol, Povidone, Pregelatinized Starch, Stearic Acid, Titanium Dioxide, and Zinc Stearate.

Actions: Sinutab® Sinus Allergy Medication, Maximum Strength Formula, Tablets and Caplets contain an analgesic (acetaminophen) to relieve pain, a decongestant (pseudoephedrine hydrochloride) to reduce congestion of the nasopharyngeal mucosa, and an antihistamine (chlorpheniramine maleate) to help control allergic symptoms.
Acetaminophen is both analgesic and antipyretic. Because acetaminophen is not a salicylate, Sinutab® Sinus Allergy Medication, Maximum Strength Formula, Tablets and Caplets can be used by patients who are allergic to aspirin.
Pseudoephedrine hydrochloride, a sympathomimetic drug, provides vasoconstriction of the nasopharyngeal mucosa resulting in a nasal decongestant effect. Chlorpheniramine maleate is an antihistamine incorporated to provide relief of running nose, sneezing, itching of the nose or throat, and itchy and watery eyes as may occur in allergic rhinitis.

Warnings: Do not exceed recommended dosage. If symptoms persist, do not improve within 7 days, or are accompanied by high fever, or if new symptoms occur, see your doctor before continuing use. Do not take this product if you have high blood pressure, heart disease, diabetes, thyroid disease, glaucoma, or difficulty in urination due to an enlarged prostate gland, except under doctor's supervision. Do not take this product for more than 10 days. May cause drowsiness; alcohol, sedatives and tranquilizers may increase the drowsiness effect. Avoid alcoholic beverages, driving a motor vehicle or operating machinery while taking this product. Do not take this product if you are taking sedatives or tranquilizers, without first consulting your doctor. As with any drug, if you are pregnant or nursing a baby, seek the advice of a health professional before using this product. Keep this and all drugs out of the reach of children. In case of accidental overdose, seek professional help or contact a Poison Control Center immediately.

Drug Interaction: Do not take this product if you are presently taking a prescription drug for high blood pressure or depression without first consulting your doctor.

Dosage and Administration: Adults 2 tablets or caplets every 6 hours, not to exceed 8 tablets or caplets in 24 hours, or as directed by physician. Children under 12 should use only as directed by physician.

How Supplied: Sinutab® Sinus Allergy Medication, Maximum Strength Formula, Caplets and Tablets are supplied in child-resistant blister packs in boxes of 24 tablets or caplets.

Store at room temperature (59°–86°F).
Shown in Product Identification Guide, page 531

SINUTAB® Sinus Medication, Maximum Strength Without Drowsiness Formula, Tablets and Caplets

Indications: Specially formulated to provide fast, maximum strength relief of sinus pain and congestion due to colds, flu and allergies. Sinutab relieves sinus headache and pressure without drowsiness.

Active Ingredients: Each tablet/caplet contains: Acetaminophen 500 mg., pseudoephedrine hydrochloride 30 mg.

Inactive Ingredients:
Tablets contain: Croscarmellose Sodium, Crospovidone, D&C Yellow No. 10 Aluminum Lake, FD&C Yellow No. 6 Aluminum Lake, Microcrystalline Cellulose, Povidone, Pregelatinized Starch, Stearic Acid, and Zinc Stearate.
Caplets contain: Carnauba Wax, Croscarmellose Sodium, Crospovidone, D&C Yellow No. 10 Aluminum Lake, FD&C Yellow No. 6 Aluminum Lake, Hydroxypropyl Cellulose, Hydroxypropyl Methylcellulose, Microcrystalline Cellulose, Polyethylene Glycol, Povidone, Pregelatinized Starch, Stearic Acid, Titanium Dioxide, and Zinc Stearate.

Actions: Sinutab® Sinus Medication, Maximum Strength Without Drowsiness Formula, Tablets and Caplets contain an analgesic (acetaminophen) to relieve pain, and a decongestant (pseudoephedrine hydrochloride) to reduce congestion of the nasopharyngeal mucosa.
Acetaminophen is both analgesic and antipyretic. Because acetaminophen is not a salicylate, Sinutab® Sinus Medication, Maximum Strength Without Drowsiness Formula, can be used by patients who are allergic to aspirin.
Pseudoephedrine hydrochloride, a sympathomimetic drug, provides vasoconstriction of the nasopharyngeal mucosa resulting in a nasal decongestant effect. The absence of antihistamine in the formula provides the added benefit of reduced likelihood of drowsiness side effects.

Warnings: Do not exceed recommended dosage. If symptoms persist, do not improve within seven days, or are accompanied by high fever, or if new symptoms occur, see your doctor before continuing use. Do not take this product if you have high blood pressure, heart disease, diabetes, thyroid disease, or difficulty in urination due to an enlarged prostate gland except under doctor's supervision. Do not take this product for more than 10 days. As with any drug, if you are pregnant or nursing a baby, seek the advice of a health professional before using this product. Keep this and all drugs out of the reach of children. In case of accidental overdose, seek professional help or contact a Poison Control Center immediately.

Drug Interaction: Do not take this product if you are presently taking a prescription drug for high blood pressure or depression without first consulting your doctor.

Dosage and Administration: Adults, 2 tablets or caplets every 6 hours, not to exceed 8 tablets or caplets in 24 hours or as directed by physician. Children under 12 should use only as directed by physician.

How Supplied: Sinutab® Sinus Medication, Maximum Strength Without Drowsiness Formula, Caplets and Tablets are supplied in child-resistant blister packs in boxes of 24 tablets or caplets or in boxes of 48 caplets.
Shown in Product Identification Guide, page 531

SUDAFED® 12 Hour Caplets
[sū 'duh-fĕd]

Each coated extended-release caplet contains pseudoephedrine hydrochloride 120 mg in a capsule-shaped tablet. Also contains: hydroxypropyl methylcellulose, magnesium stearate, microcrystalline cellulose, polyethylene glycol, povidone, and titanium dioxide. Printed with edible blue ink.

Indications: For temporary relief of nasal congestion due to the common cold, hay fever, or other upper respiratory allergies, and nasal congestion associated with sinusitis; promotes nasal and/or sinus drainage.

Directions: Adults and children 12 years and over—One caplet every 12 hours, not to exceed two caplets in 24 hours. Sudafed 12 Hour is not recommended for children under 12 years of age.

Warnings: Do not exceed recommended dosage because at higher doses, nervousness, dizziness, or sleeplessness may occur. Do not take this product if you have heart disease, high blood pressure, thyroid disease, diabetes, or difficulty in urination due to enlargement of the prostate gland unless directed by a doctor. If symptoms do not improve within 7 days or are accompanied by fever, consult your doctor before continuing use. As with any drug, if you are pregnant or nursing a baby, seek the advice of a health professional before using this product.

Drug Interaction Precaution: Do not take this product if you are presently taking a prescription drug for high blood pressure or depression, without first consulting your doctor.
KEEP THIS AND ALL DRUGS OUT OF THE REACH OF CHILDREN. In case of accidental overdose, seek professional assistance or contact a Poison Control Center immediately.

Store at 15° to 25°C (59° to 77°F) in a dry place and protect from light.

How Supplied: Boxes of 10 and 20.
Shown in Product Identification Guide, page 531

SUDAFED® Tablets 30 mg
[sū 'duh-fĕd]

Each tablet contains pseudoephedrine hydrochloride 30 mg. Also contains: acacia, carnauba wax, dibasic calcium phosphate, FD&C Red No. 40 Lake and Yellow No. 6 Lake, magnesium stearate, pharmaceutical glaze, polysorbate 60, potato starch, povidone, sodium benzoate, stearic acid, talc, and titanium dioxide. Printed with edible black ink.

Indications: For temporary relief of nasal congestion due to the common cold, hay fever or other upper respiratory allergies, and nasal congestion associated with sinusitis; promotes nasal and/or sinus drainage.

Directions: To be given every 4 to 6 hours. Do not exceed 4 doses in 24 hours. Adults and children 12 years of age and over, 2 tablets. Children 6 to under 12 years of age, 1 tablet. Children 2 to under 6 years of age, use Children's Sudafed Liquid. For children under 2 years of age, consult a physician.

Warnings: Do not exceed recommended dosage because at higher doses nervousness, dizziness or sleeplessness may occur. If symptoms do not improve within 7 days, or are accompanied by a high fever, consult a physician before continuing use. Do not take this preparation if you have high blood pressure, heart disease, diabetes, thyroid disease, or difficulty in urination due to enlargement of the prostate gland, except under the advice and supervision of a physician. As with any drug, if you are pregnant or nursing a baby, seek the advice of a health professional before using this product.

Drug Interaction Precaution: Do not take this product if you are presently taking a prescription antihypertensive or antidepressant drug containing a monoamine oxidase inhibitor, except under the advice and supervision of a physician.
KEEP THIS AND ALL MEDICINES OUT OF CHILDREN'S REACH. In case of accidental overdose, seek professional assistance or contact a Poison Control Center immediately.

Store at 15° to 25°C (59° to 77°F) in a dry place and protect from light.

How Supplied: Boxes of 24, 48. Bottles of 100. Institutional Pack, Carton of 500 x 2.
Shown in Product Identification Guide, page 531

SUDAFED® Tablets 60 mg (Adult Strength)
[sū 'duh-fĕd]

Each tablet contains pseudoephedrine hydrochloride 60 mg. Also contains: acacia, carnauba wax, corn starch, dibasic calcium phosphate, hydroxypropyl methylcellulose, magnesium stearate, pharmaceutical glaze, polysorbate 60, sodium starch glycolate, stearic acid, sucrose, talc, and titanium dioxide. Printed with edible red ink.

Indications: For temporary relief of nasal congestion due to the common cold, hay fever or other upper respiratory allergies, and nasal congestion associated with sinusitis; promotes nasal and/or sinus drainage.

Directions: To be given every 4 to 6 hours. Do not exceed 4 doses in 24 hours. Adults and children 12 years of age and over, 1 tablet. Children 6 to under 12 years of age, use Sudafed 30 mg Tablets. Children 2 to under 6 years of age, use Children's Sudafed Liquid. For children under 2 years of age, consult a physician.

Warnings: Do not exceed recommended dosage because at higher doses nervousness, dizziness or sleeplessness may occur. If symptoms do not improve within 7 days, or are accompanied by a high fever, consult a physician before continuing use. Do not take this preparation if you have high blood pressure, heart disease, diabetes, thyroid disease, or difficulty in urination due to enlargement of the prostate gland, except under the advice and supervision of a physician. As with any drug, if you are pregnant or nursing a baby, seek the advice of a health professional before using this product.

Drug Interaction Precaution: Do not take this product if you are presently taking a prescription antihypertensive or antidepressant drug containing a monoamine oxidase inhibitor, except under the advice and supervision of a physician.
KEEP THIS AND ALL MEDICINES OUT OF CHILDREN'S REACH. In case of accidental overdose, seek professional assistance or contact a Poison Control Center immediately.

Store at 15° to 25°C (59° to 77°F) in a dry place and protect from light.

How Supplied: Bottles of 100.
Shown in Product Identification Guide, page 531

Children's SUDAFED® Liquid
[sū 'duh-fĕd]

Each 5 mL (1 teaspoonful) contains pseudoephedrine hydrochloride 30 mg. Also contains: methylparaben 0.1% and sodium benzoate 0.1% (added as preservatives), citric acid, FD&C Red No. 40, flavor, glycerin, purified water, sorbitol and sucrose.

Indications: For temporary relief of nasal congestion due to the common cold, hay fever or other upper respiratory allergies and nasal congestion associated with sinusitis; promotes nasal and/or sinus drainage.

Directions: To be given every 4 to 6 hours. Do not exceed 4 doses in 24 hours. Children 6 to under 12 years of age, 1 teaspoonful. Children 2 to under 6 years of age, ½ teaspoonful. For children under 2 years of age, consult a physician.

Warnings: Do not exceed recommended dosage because at higher doses

Continued on next page

This product information was prepared in November 1994. On these and other Warner Wellcome Consumer HealthCare Products, detailed information may be obtained by addressing Warner Wellcome Consumer HealthCare Products, Warner-Lambert, Morris Plains, NJ 07950

Warner Wellcome—Cont.

nervousness, dizziness or sleeplessness may occur. Do not give this product to children for more than 7 days. If symptoms do not improve or are accompanied by high fever, consult a physician. Do not give this product to children who have heart disease, high blood pressure, thyroid disease, or diabetes unless directed by a physician.

Drug Interaction Precaution: Do not give this product to a child who is taking a prescription drug for high blood pressure or depression, without first consulting the child's physician.

KEEP THIS AND ALL MEDICINES OUT OF CHILDREN'S REACH. In case of accidental overdose, seek professional assistance or contact a Poison Control Center immediately.

Store at 15° to 25°C (59° to 77°F) and protect from light.

How Supplied: Bottles of 4 fl oz. (118 mL)

Shown in Product Identification Guide, page 531

SUDAFED® COLD AND COUGH LIQUIDCAPS
[*sū duh 'fĕd*]

Indications: The COUGH SUPPRESSANT (dextromethorphan) temporarily relieves cough due to the common cold. The DECONGESTANT (pseudoephedrine) temporarily relieves stuffy nose and sinus congestion due to the common cold. The non-aspirin PAIN RELIEVER/FEVER REDUCER (acetaminophen) temporarily relieves minor sore throat pain, headache, fever, and body aches due to the common cold or flu. The EXPECTORANT (guaifenesin) helps loosen phlegm (mucus) to drain bronchial tubes and make coughs more productive.

Directions: Adults and children 12 years of age and over, 2 liquid caps every 4 hours, not to exceed 8 liquid caps in 24 hours. Not recommended for children under 12 years of age.

Each Liquid Cap Contains: acetaminophen 250 mg, dextromethorphan hydrobromide 10 mg, guaifenesin 100 mg, and pseudoephedrine hydrochloride 30 mg. Also contains D&C Yellow No. 10, FD&C Red No. 40, gelatin, glycerin, polyethylene glycol, povidone, propylene glycol, purified water, and sorbitol. Printed with edible white ink.

Warnings: Do not exceed recommended dosage because at higher doses nervousness, dizziness, or sleeplessness may occur. Do not take this product for more than 7 days. A persistent cough may be a sign of a serious condition. If cough or other symptoms persist for more than 7 days, tend to recur, or are accompanied by rash, persistent headache, fever that lasts for more than 3 days, or if new symptoms occur, consult a

physician. Do not take this product for persistent or chronic cough such as occurs with smoking, asthma, chronic bronchitis, emphysema, or where cough is accompanied by excessive phlegm (mucus) unless directed by a physician. If sore throat is severe, persists for more than 2 days, is accompanied or followed by fever, headache, rash, nausea, or vomiting, consult a physician promptly. Do not take this product if you have high blood pressure, heart disease, diabetes, thyroid disease, or difficulty in urination due to enlargement of the prostate gland except under the advice and supervision of a physician. As with any drug, if you are pregnant or nursing a baby, seek the advice of a health professional before using this product.

Drug Interaction Precaution: Do not use this product if you are now taking a prescription monoamine oxidase inhibitor (MAOI) (certain drugs for depression, psychiatric or emotional conditions, or Parkinson's disease), or for 2 weeks after stopping the MAOI drug. If you are uncertain whether your prescription drug contains an MAOI, consult a health professional before taking this product.

KEEP THIS AND ALL DRUGS OUT OF THE REACH OF CHILDREN. In case of accidental overdose, seek professional assistance or contact a Poison Control Center immediately. Prompt medical attention is critical for adults as well as children even if you do not notice any signs or symptoms.

Store at 15° to 25°C (59° to 77°F) in a dry place and protect from light.

How Supplied: Box of 10 and 20.
Shown in Product Identification Guide, page 531

SUDAFED® Cough Syrup
[*sū 'duh-fĕd*]

Each 5 mL (1 teaspoonful) contains pseudoephedrine hydrochloride 15 mg, dextromethorphan hydrobromide 5 mg and guaifenesin 100 mg. Also contains: alcohol 2.4%, methylparaben 0.1% and sodium benzoate 0.1% (added as preservatives), citric acid, D&C Yellow No. 10, FD&C Blue No. 1, flavor, glycerin, purified water, sodium chloride and sucrose.

Indications: For temporary relief of cough due to minor throat and bronchial irritation as may occur with the common cold or inhaled irritants. For temporary relief of nasal congestion due to the common cold. Helps loosen phlegm (mucus) and thin bronchial secretions to rid the bronchial passageways of bothersome mucus.

Directions: To be given every 4 hours. Do not exceed 4 doses in 24 hours. Adults and children 12 years of age and over, 4 teaspoonfuls. Children 6 to under 12 years of age, 2 teaspoonfuls. Children 2 to under 6 years of age, 1 teaspoonful. For children under 2 years of age, consult a physician.

Warnings: Do not give this product to children under 2 years of age unless directed by a physician. Do not exceed recommended dosage because at higher doses nervousness, dizziness or sleeplessness may occur. Do not take this product for persistent or chronic cough such as occurs with smoking, asthma, chronic bronchitis, or emphysema, or where cough is accompanied by excessive phlegm (mucus) unless directed by a physician. A persistent cough may be a sign of a serious condition. If cough persists for more than 1 week, tends to recur, or is accompanied by fever, rash, or persistent headache, consult a physician. Do not take this preparation if you have high blood pressure, heart disease, diabetes, thyroid disease, or difficulty in urination due to enlargement of the prostate gland, except under the advice and supervision of a physician. As with any drug, if you are pregnant or nursing a baby, seek the advice of a health professional before using this product.

Drug Interaction Precaution: Do not take this product if you are presently taking a prescription antihypertensive or antidepressant drug containing a monoamine oxidase inhibitor except under the advice and supervision of a physician.

KEEP THIS AND ALL DRUGS OUT OF THE REACH OF CHILDREN. In case of accidental overdose, seek professional assistance or contact a Poison Control Center immediately.

Store at 15° to 25°C (59° to 77°F).
DO NOT REFRIGERATE.

How Supplied: Bottles of 4 fl oz (118 mL).

Shown in Product Identification Guide, page 531

SUDAFED PLUS® Liquid
[*sū 'duh-fĕd*]

Product Benefits: For the temporary relief of nasal or sinus congestion, sneezing, runny nose, and itchy, watery eyes associated with the common cold, hay fever, or other upper respiratory allergies.

EACH 5 mL (1 TEASPOONFUL) SUDAFED PLUS® LIQUID CONTAINS: pseudoephedrine hydrochloride 30 mg and chlorpheniramine maleate 2 mg. Also contains: methylparaben 0.1% and sodium benzoate 0.1% (added as preservatives), citric acid, D&C Yellow No. 10, FD&C Yellow No. 6, flavor, glycerin, purified water and sucrose.

Directions: Adults and children 12 years and over, 2 teaspoonfuls every 4 to 6 hours. Children 6 to under 12 years, 1 teaspoonful every 4 to 6 hours. Do not exceed 4 doses in 24 hours. Children under 6, consult a doctor.

Warnings: May cause drowsiness; alcohol, sedatives, and tranquilizers may increase the drowsiness effect. Avoid alcoholic beverages while taking this product. Do not take this product if you are taking sedatives or tranquilizers, without first consulting your doctor. Use caution when driving a motor vehicle or operating machinery. May cause excitability, especially in children. Do not exceed recommended dosage because at higher doses nervousness, dizziness or sleeplessness may occur. If symptoms do not improve within 7 days, or are accompanied by a high fever, consult a doctor before continuing use. Do not take this product, unless directed by a doctor, if you have high blood pressure, heart disease, diabetes, thyroid disease, glaucoma, a breathing problem such as emphysema or chronic bronchitis, or difficulty in urination due to enlargement of the prostate gland. As with any drug, if you are pregnant or nursing a baby, seek the advice of a health professional before using this product.

Drug Interaction Precaution: Do not take this product if you are presently taking a prescription antihypertensive or antidepressant drug containing a monoamine oxidase inhibitor except under the advice and supervision of a doctor.

KEEP THIS AND ALL DRUGS OUT OF THE REACH OF CHILDREN. In case of accidental overdose, seek professional assistance or contact a Poison Control Center immediately.

Store at 15° to 25°C (59° to 77°F) and protect from light.

How Supplied: Bottles of 4 fl oz (118 mL).

Shown in Product Identification Guide, page 531

SUDAFED PLUS® Tablets
[sū'duh-fĕd]

Product Benefits: For the temporary relief of nasal or sinus congestion, sneezing, runny nose, and itchy, watery eyes associated with the common cold, hay fever, or other upper respiratory allergies.
EACH SUDAFED PLUS® TABLET CONTAINS: pseudoephedrine hydrochloride 60 mg and chlorpheniramine maleate 4 mg. Also contains: lactose, magnesium stearate, potato starch and povidone.

Directions: Adults and children 12 years and over, 1 tablet every 4 to 6 hours. Children 6 to under 12 years, ½ tablet every 4 to 6 hours. Do not exceed 4 doses in 24 hours. Children under 6, consult a doctor.

Warnings: May cause drowsiness; alcohol, sedatives, and tranquilizers may increase the drowsiness effect. Avoid alcoholic beverages while taking this product. Do not take this product if you are taking sedatives or tranquilizers, without first consulting your doctor. Use caution when driving a motor vehicle or operating machinery. May cause excitability, especially in children. Do not exceed

recommended dosage because at higher doses nervousness, dizziness or sleeplessness may occur. If symptoms do not improve within 7 days, or are accompanied by a high fever, consult a doctor before continuing use. Do not take this product, unless directed by a doctor, if you have high blood pressure, heart disease, diabetes, thyroid disease, glaucoma, a breathing problem such as emphysema or chronic bronchitis, or difficulty in urination due to enlargement of the prostate gland. As with any drug, if you are pregnant or nursing a baby, seek the advice of a health professional before using this product.

Drug Interaction Precaution: Do not take this product if you are presently taking a prescription antihypertensive or antidepressant drug containing a monoamine oxidase inhibitor except under the advice and supervision of a physician.

KEEP THIS AND ALL DRUGS OUT OF THE REACH OF CHILDREN. In case of accidental overdose, seek professional assistance or contact a Poison Control Center immediately.

Store at 15° to 25°C (59° to 77°F) in a dry place and protect from light.

How Supplied: Boxes of 24, 48.
Shown in Product Identification Guide, page 531

SUDAFED® Severe Cold Formula Caplets
[sū'duh-fĕd]

Product Benefits: Maximum allowable levels of nasal decongestant, cough suppressant, and non-aspirin pain reliever/fever reducer provide temporary relief from symptoms of the common cold and flu. This product contains no ingredients that may cause drowsiness. The **DECONGESTANT** (pseudoephedrine) temporarily relieves nasal and sinus congestion due to the common cold. It temporarily relieves nasal stuffiness; reduces the swelling of nasal passages; shrinks swollen membranes; and temporarily restores freer breathing through the nose. The **COUGH SUPPRESSANT** (dextromethorphan) temporarily relieves cough due to the common cold. The non-aspirin **PAIN RELIEVER/FEVER REDUCER** (acetaminophen) temporarily relieves headache, body aches and pains, minor sore throat pain, and reduces fever due to the common cold.

Directions: Adults and children 12 years of age and over, 2 caplets every 6 hours, not to exceed 8 caplets in 24 hours. Not recommended for children under 12 years of age.

Each Coated Caplet Contains: acetaminophen 500 mg, dextromethorphan hydrobromide 15 mg, and pseudoephedrine hydrochloride 30 mg. Also contains: carnauba wax, crospovidone, hydroxypropyl methylcellulose, magnesium stearate, microcrystalline cellulose, polyeth-

ylene glycol, povidone, pregelatinized corn starch, stearic acid, and titanium dioxide.

Warnings: Do not exceed recommended dosage because at higher doses nervousness, dizziness or sleeplessness may occur. Do not take this product for more than 10 days. A persistent cough may be a sign of a serious condition. If cough persists for more than 7 days, tends to recur, or is accompanied by rash, persistent headache, fever that lasts for more than 3 days, or if new symptoms occur, consult a physician. Do not take this product for persistent or chronic cough such as occurs with smoking, asthma, emphysema, or if cough is accompanied by excessive phlegm (mucus) unless directed by a physician. If sore throat is severe, persists for more than 2 days, is accompanied or followed by fever, headache, rash, nausea, or vomiting, consult a physician promptly. Do not take this product if you have high blood pressure, heart disease, diabetes, thyroid disease, or difficulty in urination due to enlargement of the prostate gland except under the advice and supervision of a physician. As with any drug, if you are pregnant or nursing a baby, seek the advice of a health professional before using this product.

Drug Interaction Precaution: Do not use this product if you are now taking a prescription monoamine oxidase inhibitor (MAOI) (certain drugs for depression, psychiatric or emotional conditions, or Parkinson's disease), or for 2 weeks after stopping the MAOI drug. If you are uncertain whether your prescription drug contains an MAOI, consult a health professional before taking this product.

KEEP THIS AND ALL DRUGS OUT OF THE REACH OF CHILDREN. In case of accidental overdose, seek professional assistance or contact a Poison Control Center immediately. Prompt medical attention is critical for adults as well as for children even if you do not notice any signs or symptoms.

Store at 15° to 25°C (59° to 77°F) in a dry place.

How Supplied: Boxes of 10, 20.
Shown in Product Identification Guide, page 531

Continued on next page

This product information was prepared in November 1994. On these and other Warner Wellcome Consumer HealthCare Products, detailed information may be obtained by addressing Warner Wellcome Consumer HealthCare Products, Warner-Lambert, Morris Plains, NJ 07950

Warner Wellcome—Cont.

SUDAFED® Severe Cold Formula Tablets
[sū' duh-fĕd]

Product Benefits: Maximum allowable levels of nasal decongestant, cough suppressant, and non-aspirin pain reliever/fever reducer provide temporary relief from symptoms of the common cold and flu. This product contains no ingredients that may cause drowsiness. The **DECONGESTANT** (pseudoephedrine) temporarily relieves nasal and sinus congestion due to the common cold. It temporarily relieves nasal stuffiness; reduces the swelling of nasal passages; shrinks swollen membranes; and temporarily restores freer breathing through the nose. The **COUGH SUPPRESSANT** (dextromethorphan) temporarily relieves cough due to the common cold. The non-aspirin **PAIN RELIEVER/FEVER REDUCER** (acetaminophen) temporarily relieves headache, body aches and pains, minor sore throat pain, and reduces fever due to the common cold.

Directions: Adults and children 12 years of age and over, 2 tablets every 6 hours, not to exceed 8 tablets in 24 hours. Not recommended for children under 12 years of age.

Each Coated Tablet Contains: acetaminophen 500 mg, dextromethorphan hydrobromide 15 mg, and pseudoephedrine hydrochloride 30 mg. Also contains: carnauba wax, crospovidone, hydroxypropyl methylcellulose, magnesium stearate, microcrystalline cellulose, polyethylene glycol, povidone, pregelatinized corn starch, stearic acid, and titanium dioxide.

Warnings: Do not exceed recommended dosage because at higher doses nervousness, dizziness or sleeplessness may occur. Do not take this product for more than 10 days. A persistent cough may be a sign of a serious condition. If cough persists for more than 7 days, tends to recur, or is accompanied by rash, persistent headache, fever that lasts for more than 3 days, or if new symptoms occur, consult a physician. Do not take this product for persistent or chronic cough such as occurs with smoking, asthma, emphysema, or if cough is accompanied by excessive phlegm (mucus) unless directed by a physician. If sore throat is severe, persists for more than 2 days, is accompanied or followed by fever, headache, rash, nausea, or vomiting, consult a physician promptly. Do not take this product if you have high blood pressure, heart disease, diabetes, thyroid disease, or difficulty in urination due to enlargement of the prostate gland except under the advice and supervision of a physician. As with any drug, if you are pregnant or nursing a baby, seek the advice of a health professional before using this product.

Drug Interaction Precaution: Do not use this product if you are now taking a prescription monoamine oxidase inhibitor (MAOI) (certain drugs for depression, psychiatric or emotional conditions, or Parkinson's disease), or for 2 weeks after stopping the MAOI drug. If you are uncertain whether your prescription drug contains an MAOI, consult a health professional before taking this product.
KEEP THIS AND ALL DRUGS OUT OF THE REACH OF CHILDREN. In case of accidental overdose, seek professional assistance or contact a Poison Control Center immediately. Prompt medical attention is critical for adults as well as for children even if you do not notice any signs or symptoms.

Store at 15° to 25°C (59° to 77°F) in a dry place.

How Supplied: Boxes of 10, 20.
Shown in Product Identification Guide, page 531

SUDAFED® SINUS Caplets
[sū' duh-fĕd]

Product Benefits:
● Maximum allowable levels of non-aspirin pain reliever and nasal decongestant provide temporary relief of sinus headache pain, pressure and nasal congestion due to colds and flu or hay fever and other allergies.
● Contains no ingredients which may cause drowsiness.

Directions: Adults and children 12 years and over, 2 caplets every 6 hours, not to exceed 8 caplets in a 24-hour period. Not recommended for children under 12 years of age.

Each Coated Caplet Contains: acetaminophen 500 mg and pseudoephedrine hydrochloride 30 mg. Also contains: carnauba wax, crospovidone, FD&C Yellow No. 6 Lake, hydroxypropyl methylcellulose, magnesium stearate, microcrystalline cellulose, polyethylene glycol, polysorbate 80, povidone, pregelatinized corn starch, stearic acid, and titanium dioxide.

Warnings: Do not exceed recommended dosage because at higher doses nervousness, dizziness, or sleeplessness may occur. Do not take this product for more than 10 days. If symptoms do not improve or are accompanied by fever that lasts for more than 3 days, or if new symptoms occur, consult a physician. Do not take this product if you have high blood pressure, heart disease, diabetes, thyroid disease, or difficulty in urination due to enlargement of the prostate gland except under the advice and supervision of a physician. As with any drug, if you are pregnant or nursing a baby, seek the advice of a health professional before using this product.

Drug Interaction Precaution: Do not take this product if you are presently taking a prescription antihypertensive or antidepressant drug containing a monoamine oxidase inhibitor except un-

der the advice and supervision of a physician.
KEEP THIS AND ALL DRUGS OUT OF THE REACH OF CHILDREN. In case of accidental overdose, seek professional assistance or contact a Poison Control Center immediately. Prompt medical attention is critical for adults as well as children even if you do not notice any signs or symptoms.

Store at 15° to 25°C (59° to 77°F) in a dry place and protect from light.

How Supplied: Boxes of 24 and 48.
Shown in Product Identification Guide, page 531

SUDAFED® SINUS Tablets
[sū' duh-fĕd]

Product Benefits:
● Maximum allowable levels of non-aspirin pain reliever and nasal decongestant provide temporary relief of sinus headache pain, pressure and nasal congestion due to colds and flu or hay fever and other allergies.
● Contains no ingredients which may cause drowsiness.

Directions: Adults and children 12 years and over, 2 tablets every 6 hours, not to exceed 8 tablets in a 24-hour period. Not recommended for children under 12 years of age.

Each Coated Tablet Contains: Acetaminophen 500 mg and pseudoephedrine hydrochloride 30 mg. Also contains: carnauba wax, crospovidone, FD&C Yellow No. 6 Lake, hydroxypropyl methylcellulose, magnesium stearate, microcrystalline cellulose, polyethylene glycol, polysorbate 80, povidone, pregelatinized corn starch, stearic acid, and titanium dioxide.

Warnings: Do not exceed recommended dosage because at higher doses nervousness, dizziness, or sleeplessness may occur. Do not take this product for more than 10 days. If symptoms do not improve or are accompanied by fever that lasts for more than 3 days, or if new symptoms occur, consult a physician. Do not take this product if you have high blood pressure, heart disease, diabetes, thyroid disease, or difficulty in urination due to enlargement of the prostate gland except under the advice and supervision of a physician. As with any drug, if you are pregnant or nursing a baby, seek the advice of a health professional before using this product.

Drug Interaction Precaution: Do not take this product if you are presently taking a prescription antihypertensive or antidepressant drug containing a monoamine oxidase inhibitor except under the advice and supervision of a physician.
KEEP THIS AND ALL DRUGS OUT OF THE REACH OF CHILDREN. In case of accidental overdose, seek professional assistance or contact a Poison Control Center immediately. Prompt medi-

cal attention is critical for adults as well as children even if you do not notice any signs or symptoms.

Store at 15° to 25°C (59° to 77°F) in a dry place and protect from light.

How Supplied: Boxes of 24 and 48.
Shown in Product Identification Guide, page 531

TUCKS® Clear Hemorrhoidal Gel

Indications: For prompt temporary relief of itching, burning and discomfort associated with inflamed hemorrhoidal tissues.

Directions: For External Use Only. Adult: When practical, cleanse the affected area with Tucks® Medicated Pads or with mild soap and warm water and rinse thoroughly. Gently dry by patting or blotting with toilet tissue or soft cloth before application of this product. Apply gel externally to the affected area up to 6 times daily or after each bowel movement. Children under 12 years of age: consult a physician.

Warnings: If condition worsens or does not improve within 7 days, consult a physician. Do not exceed recommended daily dosage unless directed by a physician. In case of bleeding, consult a physician promptly. Do not put this product into the rectum by using fingers or any mechanical device or applicator. Keep this and all drugs out of the reach of children. In case of accidental ingestion, seek professional assistance or contact a Poison Control Center immediately.

Active Ingredients: Witch Hazel 50% and Glycerin 10%. Also contains: Benzyl Alcohol, Carbomer 974 P, Disodium Edetate, Propylene Glycol, Sodium Hydroxide and Water.
Store at room temperature 15°–30°C (59°–86°F).

How Supplied: Tucks Clear Gel is supplied in 0.7 oz (19.8g) tubes.
Shown in Product Identification Guide, page 531

TUCKS®
Pre-moistened Hemorrhoidal/Vaginal Pads

Indications: For prompt, temporary relief of minor external itching, burning and irritation associated with hemorrhoids.

Uses:
Hemorrhoids: Tucks extra-soft cloth pads allow for the gentlest possible care of tender inflamed hemorrhoidal tissue.
Hygienic Wipe: Tucks Pads are effective for everyday personal hygienic use on outer rectal and vaginal areas. Used in place of toilet tissue, Tucks Pads gently and thoroughly remove irritation-causing matter. They are especially handy during menstrual periods.
Moist Compress: For additional relief, Tucks Pads can be folded and used as a compress on inflamed tissue. Tucks Pads are particularly helpful in relieving dis-

comfort following childbirth, rectal or vaginal surgery.

Directions: For external use only. *As a hemorrhoidal treatment* —Adults: When practical, cleanse the affected area with mild soap and warm water, and rinse thoroughly. Gently dry by patting or blotting with toilet tissue or soft cloth before each application of this product. Gently apply to affected area by patting and then discard. Can be used up to six times daily. Children under 12 years of age: consult a physician.
As a hygienic wipe —Use as a wipe instead of toilet tissue.
As a moist compress —For soothing relief, fold pad and place in contact with irritated tissue. Leave in place for 5 to 15 minutes. Repeat as needed.

Warnings: If condition worsens or does not improve within 7 days, consult a physician. Do not exceed recommended daily dosage unless directed by a physician. In case of bleeding, consult a physician promptly. Do not put this product in the rectum by using fingers or any mechanical device or applicator. Keep this and all drugs out of the reach of children. In case of accidental ingestion, seek professional assistance or contact a Poison Control Center immediately.

Active Ingredients: Soft pads premoistened with a solution containing 50% Witch Hazel. Also contains: Water, Glycerin, Alcohol 7%, Propylene Glycol, Sodium Citrate, Diazolidinyl Urea, Citric Acid, Methylparaben, Aloe Vera Gel, Propylparaben.

How Supplied: Jars of 50 and 125. Also available as Tucks Take-Alongs®, individual, foil-wrapped, nonwoven 6 Two-Packs) pads..
Shown in Product Identification Guide, page 531

Wellness International Network, Ltd.
**1501 LUNA ROAD, BLDG. 102
CARROLLTON, TX 75006**

BIO-COMPLEX 5000™
Gentle Foaming Cleanser

Uses: BIO-COMPLEX 5000™ Gentle Foaming Cleanser, with alpha-hydroxy acids, aloe vera, and botanical infusions, is an advanced cleansing gel designed for all skin types. BIO-COMPLEX 5000 Gentle Foaming Cleanser protects the skin while gently removing surface impurities, make-up, and pollution.

Inactive Ingredients: Aloe Vera Gel, Infusion of Sage, Infusion of Chamomile, Ammonium Lauryl Sulfate, Lauramidopropyl Betaine, Glycerin, Lauramide DEA, Cetyl Betaine, Tocopherol, Citric Acid, Lactic Acid, Malic Acid, Ascorbic Acid, Methylchloroisothiazolinone, Methylisothiazolinone, Propylparaben, Methylparaben.

Directions: Splash warm water onto face. Place a small amount of gel on fingertips. Apply evenly to face and neck in circular motions, massaging skin gently but thoroughly. Rinse completely and pat dry with a soft towel.

How Supplied: 8 fluid ounce/236 ml. bottle.

BIO-COMPLEX 5000™
Revitalizing Conditioner

Uses: BIO-COMPLEX 5000™ Revitalizing Conditioner, with vitamins, antioxidants, and sunscreen, helps restore moisture to dried-out, heat-styled hair. Its nourishing formula contains the essence of awapuhi, a Hawaiian ginger plant extract known for its healing qualities. This advanced conditioner enhances hair with silkening agents and detangles hair after shampooing. Hair is left clean, soft, manageable, and protected against styling aids and environmental elements. BIO-COMPLEX 5000 Revitalizing Conditioner is excellent for all hair types, especially damaged or over-processed hair.

Inactive Ingredients: Water, Stearyl Alcohol, Propylene Glycol, Stearamidopropyl Dimethalymine, Cyclomethicone, Polyquaternium - 11, Stearalkonium Chloride, Cetearyl Alcohol, PEG - 40 Hydrogenated Castor Oil, Citric Acid, Tocopherol, Ascorbic Acid, Retinyl Palmitate, Octyl Methoxycinnamate, Awapuhi Fragrance, Ceteth - 20, Soluble Animal Keratin, Imidazolidinyl Urea, Propylparaben, Methylparaben.

Directions: After shampooing with BIO-COMPLEX 5000™ Revitalizing Shampoo, apply to wet hair. Massage through hair, paying special attention to the ends. Leave on 2–3 minutes. Rinse thoroughly. Towel dry and style as usual.

How Supplied: 12 fluid ounce bottle.

BIO-COMPLEX 5000™
Revitalizing Shampoo

Uses: BIO-COMPLEX 5000™ Revitalizing Shampoo, with vitamins, anti-oxidants, and sunscreen, cleanses and moisturizes hair for excellent manageability. Specially formulated with the essence of awapuhi, a Hawaiian ginger plant extract known for its healing qualities, this formula contains the mildest blend of surfactants and a wealth of natural conditioning ingredients to provide body, luster, and healthier-looking hair.

Inactive Ingredients: Water, Ammonium Lauryl Sulfate, Tea Lauryl Sulfate, Cetyl Betaine, Lauramide DEA, Cocamidopropyl Betaine, Glycerin, Ascorbic Acid, Tocopherol, Retinyl Palmitate, Citric Acid, Hydrolyzed Wheat Protein, Awapuhi Fragrance, Octyl Methoxycinnamate, PEG - 7 Glyceryl Cocoate,

Continued on next page

Wellness International—Cont.

Methylchloroisothiazolinone, Methylisothiazolinone, Caramel.

Directions: Apply a small amount to wet hair and massage gently into scalp, creating a generous lather. Rinse and repeat if necessary. For best results, follow with BIO-COMPLEX 5000™ Revitalizing Conditioner.

How Supplied: 12 fluid ounce bottle.

BIOLEAN®
Herbal & Amino Acid Food Supplement

Uses: BIOLEAN® is a unique combination of Chinese herbal extracts and pharmaceutical grade amino acids specifically designed to help raise overall health, participate in individual life extension programs, and enhance athletic performance. It has been shown to be extremely effective in promoting the healthy loss of excess body fat while helping to maintain lean body mass and potent energy levels. BIOLEAN, when used as a daily nutritional supplement, has been shown to stimulate immune function in individuals with blunted sympathetic nervous systems, especially overweight and obese persons. It also acts as a positive stimulator to immune functions involved in protection from environmental and dietary carcinogens. Components in BIOLEAN are known to cause fat loss through thermogenic activity and altered fuel metabolism resulting from sympathomimetic response to stimulation of beta receptors in adipose and muscle cells. The positive immune response, though not completely understood, is at least partially attributable to beta stimulation in adipocytes and the adaptogenic and tonifying activity of certain of the herbal extracts. This has been demonstrated in their long history of use in tradional Chinese herbal medicine as well as current scientific research which points to, among other possibilities, the extremely potent antioxidant properties found in some of the component plants, most notably in the Green Tea and Schizandrae extracts. BIOLEAN may increase athletic performance and endurance through three pathways: 1) increased oxygen uptake in the lungs as a result of expanding bronchial passages; 2) enhanced mental acuity and response resulting from sympathetic nervous system stimulus; and 3) increasing the employment of fatty acids as fuel in muscle mitochondria while simultaneously sparing muscle glycogen and nitrogen.
The herbal extracts in BIOLEAN are produced in a unique and exclusive process which is proprietary to this product. Instead of creating extracts based on a set quantity of one particular active within many which may be present in any particular plant, BIOLEAN components are concentrated to maintain the natural and complete spectrum of biolog-ically active factors, in the same ratio presented by the unprocessed plant.

Directions: Adults take one white capsule and one to three tablets with low-calorie food mid to late morning. If using BIOLEAN for the first time, take one capsule and one tablet on days 1 and 2, one capsule and two tablets on days 3 and 4, and one capsule and three tablets beginning day 5. Needs vary with the individual. Some persons may require less than three tablets daily or wish to spread the taking of the tablets throughout morning and early afternoon to achieve optimum results. Do not exceed recommended daily amounts. It is recommended that you drink at least eight glasses of water daily.

Warnings: Phenylketonurics: Contains Phenylalanine. Not for use by children. Consult your physician before using this product if you are taking asthma medications, appetitie suppressing drugs, antidepressants, or cardiovascular medication. Do not consume if you are pregnant or lactating, or have high blood pressure, cardiovascular disease, diabetes, prostatic hypertrophy, glaucoma, hyperthyroidism, psychosis, or thyroid disease. If symptoms of allergy develop, discontinue use.

Ingredients: *Capsules:* 400 mg. of the following mix: L-Phenylalanine, L-Tyrosine, L-Carnitine. *Tablets:* 650 mg. of the following herbal mix: Ma Huang, Green Tea, Schizandrae Berry, Rehmannia Root, Hawthorne Berry, Jujube Seed, Alisma Root, Angelicae Dahuricae Root, Epemidium, Poria Cocos, Rhizoma Rhei, Stephania Root, Angelicae Sinensis Root, Codonopsis Root, Eucommium Bark, and Notoginseng Root.

How Supplied: One box contains 14 packets. One capsule and three tablets per packet.

BIOLEAN ACCELERATOR™
Herbal & Amino Acid Formulation

Uses: BIOLEAN ACCELERATOR™ is a unique combination of Chinese herbal extracts and pharmaceutical grade amino acids specifically designed to complement BIOLEAN® by extending and accelerating its actions. BIOLEAN is, in the traditional view of Chinese herbal medicine, a strong Yang blend. This means that it is energy or heat-producing at its core, though the addition of the amino acids and certain of the herbal components lends a very definite restorative, or Yin element, as well. BIOLEAN ACCELERATOR is a strong Yin herbal formula, intended to augment the lesser replenishing Yin elements of BIOLEAN. Though the physiological actions of many herbs are complex and not totally understood, the formula in BIOLEAN ACCELERATOR extends the adaptogenic, thermogenic, restorative, and detoxifying results experienced with BIOLEAN, with an emphasis on the restorative and adaptogenic effects. The herbal formula is a combination of tonifiers traditionally used in China for the lungs, liver, and kidneys.

Directions: For maximum effectiveness, use in conjunction with original BIOLEAN. Take one tablet in the morning with original BIOLEAN. BIOLEAN ACCELERATOR™ may also be taken in the afternoon with or without additional BIOLEAN if desired. As with original BIOLEAN, maximum absorption will be attained if taken with low-calorie food.

Warnings: Phenylketonurics: Contains Phenylalanine. Not for use by children. Consult your physician before using this product if you are taking appetite suppressing drugs or antidepressants. If symptoms of allergy develop, discontinue use.

Ingredients: Each tablet contains 250 mg. herbal mix (Black Sesame Seed, Raw Chinese Foxglove Root, Chinese Wolfberry Fruit, Achyranthes Root, Cornelian Cherry Fruit, Chinese Yam, Eclipta Herb, Rose Hips, Privet Fruit, Mulberry Fruit-Spike, Polygonati Rhizome, Cooked Chinese Foxglove Root, Poria Cocos, Cuscuta Seed, Foxnut Seed, Alisma Rhizome, Moutan Bark, Phellodendron Bark, Anemarrhena Rhizome, Schisandra Berry, Royal Jelly), L-Tyrosine, L-Phenylalanine.

How Supplied: One bottle contains 28 tablets.

BIOLEAN LIPOTRIM™
All-Natural Dietary Supplement

Uses: LipoTrim™ is a highly active, synergistic combination of garcinia cambogia extract and chromium polynicotinate. The method of action is by inhibition of lipolysis and regulation of blood glucose levels. Serum glucose derived from dietary carbohydrates and not immediately converted to energy or glycogen tends to be converted into fat stores and cholesterol. In individuals with excess body fat stores or slow basal metabolism, this tendency is thought to be higher. The garcinia cambogia extract present in LipoTrim is verified by HPLC analysis to be no less that 50%(-) hydroxycitrate (HCA). HCA inhibits ATP-citrate lyase which retards Acetyl CoA synthesis, severely restricting conversion of excess glucose into fatty acids and cholesterol. Animal studies have shown post-meal fatty acid synthesis reduction of 40–80% on an 8–12 hour period. When glucose to fat/cholesterol conversion is retarded, glycogen conversion continues, increasing liver stores and causing satiety signals to be sent to the brain resulting in appetite suppression. In situations of intense physical exercise, increased glycogen stores have been shown to result in enhanced endurance and recovery. By restricting the activity of insulin, chromium has been shown to exhibit a regulating effect on blood glucose levels thus extending the benefits of HCA.

Directions: As a dietary supplement, take one capsule three times daily, 30 minutes before each meal. LipoTrim should be used in conjunction with a healthy diet and exercise plan.

Ingredients: CitriMax™* (garcinia cambogia), ChromeMate®* (chromium polynicotinate).

How Supplied: One bottle contains 42 easy-to-swallow capsules.

*CitriMax™ is a trademark of Inter-Health.
ChromeMate® is a registered trademark of InterHealth.

INCHES AWAY™
BIOLEAN® Body Shaping Lotion

Uses: Inches Away™ is a non-exercise option for men and women wishing to maintain a toned appearance.

Directions: Apply a thin layer of lotion to the skin surface and massage deeply into skin. Allow for complete epidermal absorption. For best results, submerge bottle in hot tap water for five minutes and apply immediately after a hot shower or bath. Use twice a day, morning and night. For maximum effectiveness, use as a part of the total BIOLEAN weight management system.

Warnings: Use only as directed. Do not microwave. Keep out of the reach of children. Do not take internally. Avoid direct contact with facial and genital areas. If you currently have a rash or any skin problems, do not use. If skin irritation develops, discontinue use.

Inactive Ingredients: Deionized Water, Glyceryl Stearate, Hexyl Laurate, Dimethicone, C12-20 Acid PEG-8 Ester, PEG-100 Stearate, Aminophylline, Methylsilanetriol Theophylline Acetate, Propylene Glycol, Cetearyl Octanoate, Octyl Palmitate, Sorbitol, Glycerin, Sorbitan Stearate, Tocopherol Acetate, Octyl Methoxycinnamate, Aloe Vera Gel, Sodium Cetearyl Sulfate, Methylsilanol Mannuronate, Sodium Dehydroacetate, Methylparaben, Disodium EDTA, Propylparaben, Imidazolidinyl Urea.

How Supplied: Net Wt. 4.0 oz.

BIOLEAN MEAL™
Nutritional Meal Replacement Drink

Uses: BIOLEAN MEAL™ is formulated specifically for use with the other products in the BIOLEAN®System. It has a natural chocolate flavor which mixes instantly, without need for blending, to form a creamy drink which is equally delicious in water, milk, or milk substitutes, including rice and soy base. BIOLEAN MEAL is a low-calorie, nonfat, low-lactose powder designed to provide an optimum, alternative blend of protein, carbohydrates, and dietary fiber to individuals who have unhealthy or insufficient dietary habits, are on a fat loss program, or desire to enhance their athletic ability.

BIOLEAN MEAL has been biologically engineered to contain a 1:1 ratio of casein proteins to whey proteins. This represents a significant improvement in taste, solubility, nutritional content, and BV (biological value) compared to caseinates, soy defatted whole egg, and egg white protein, the latter historically being the standard of comparison for all protein sources. There are several factors contributing to this higher BV. Bovine milk has a ratio of casein to whey of 4:1, whereas human milk is 2:3. The amino acid composition, absorption, and utilization of whey protein is superior to other sources of supplemental dietary protein. This is especially true for individuals with limited or compromised GI function which often accompanies situations involving physical and emotional stress, illness, disease, and trauma. Athletes with increased protein requirements will also benefit from a higher BV protein source. Whey protein has the highest ratio of essential to nonessential amino acids and contains the highest quantity of Branched Chain Amino Acids (BCAA), especially Leucine, which is double that of egg protein. Leucine is consumed in large amounts during periods of exercise, trauma, infection, and caloric restriction. Muscle recovery, fuel production, and immune function are dependent upon adequate supply and replacement of Leucine. Research has also shown that tissues stores of glutathione are increased by the regular intake of whey protein.

The immune enhancing effects of whey protein, combined with the high nutritive value of milk protein isolate, promotes the loss of body fat and the retention and growth of lean body mass (muscle, bone, and internal organs) as well as supporting all other normal physiological processes such as immune function and cellular replacement, especially during periods of added stress brought on by dieting, illness, and athletic activity.

Directions: Add contents to 8 ounces of water or nonfat milk and stir or shake until completely mixed. For a thicker drink, blend for 10 seconds and drink immediately. For pudding, blend for 30 seconds and refrigerate. BIOLEAN MEAL has been formulated specifically for use with the other products in the BIOLEAN System.

Warnings: Phenylketonurics: Contains Phenylalanine.

Ingredients: Myotein (Proprietary bio-engineered protein blend of specially isolated fat and lactose free milk proteins and whey protein concentrate), Fructose, Maltodextrin, Nonfat Milk Solids, Naturally Processed Cocoa, Natural Flavor Complex (Chocolate, Vanilla, and Vanilla Cream), Cellulose Gel, Guar Gum, Corn Starch, Aspartame.

How Supplied: One box contains 14 packets. Serving size equals one packet.

FOOD FOR THOUGHT™
Choline-Enriched Nutritional Drink

Uses: A great-tasting citrus cooler, this choline-enriched nutritional beverage provides nutrients important for mental fitness. Food For Thought™ is ideal for work, school or any time performance is needed. For vigor of body, mind and spirit, this tangy citrus beverage delivers essential minerals and vitamins to the body.

Directions: Add 6 ounces of chilled water or fruit juice to one packet of mix. Stir briskly. Consume 1–2 times per day. Keep in a cool, dry place.

Warnings: Not for use by children, pregnant or lactating women. Persons taking medications should seek medical advice before taking this product. Persons with ulcers or a history of ulcers should consult their physician before using a choline supplement. Do not consume more than four servings per day. Avoid the use of antacids containing aluminum with this product.

Ingredients: Fructose, Choline Bitartrate, Calcium Pantothenate, Natural Flavor, Glycine, Ascorbic Acid, Vitamin E Acetate, Niacinamide, Lysine, Silicon Dioxide, Zinc Gluconate, Chromium Aspartate, Niacin, Magnesium Gluconate, Pyridoxine Hydrochloride, Thiamin Mononitrate, Riboflavin, Copper Gluconate, Vitamin B12.

How Supplied: One box contains 14 packets of drink mix. Serving size equals one packet.

STEPHAN™ BIO-NUTRITIONAL
Daytime Hydrating Creme

Uses: Hypo-allergenic STEPHAN™ BIO-NUTRITIONAL Daytime Hydrating Creme hydrates the skin and maintains the moisture level of the upper layers of the epidermis. It is an excellent day cream for both men and women who wish to combat the visible signs of aging skin, the appearance of wrinkles or lines, and the loss of that firm look of facial features and contours. These light emulsions are absorbed rapidly by the skin and leave an invisible protective film which hydrates the epidermis, regulates the moisture level, and leaves skin feeling supple and soft.

Inactive Ingredients: Water, Stearic Acid, Isodecyl Neopentanoate, Isostearyl Stearoyl Stearate, DEA Cetyl Phosphate, C12-15 Alkyl Benzoate, Squalane, Dimethicone, Aloe Vera Gel, Tocopherol, Cetyl Esters, Carbomer, Fragrance, Benzophenone-3, Triethanolamine, Imidazolidinyl Urea, Propylparaben, Methylparaben, Annatto.

Directions: Apply evenly on a completely cleansed face and neck. May be used around the eye area, avoiding direct

Continued on next page

Wellness International—Cont.

contact with the eyes. Suitable for all skin types.

Warnings: For external use only. Avoid contact with eyes.

How Supplied: Net Wt. 1.75 oz.

STEPHAN™ BIO-NUTRITIONAL
Eye-Firming Concentrate

Uses: Hypo-allergenic STEPHAN™ BIO-NUTRITIONAL Eye-Firming Concentrate is specially formulated to revitalize the delicate area around the eyes. This non-oily fluid pampers sensitive eyes, reduces the look of puffiness and dark circles around eyes, and smoothes and softens the appearance of fine lines in the eye area.

Inactive Ingredients: Infusion of Chamomile, Cornflower Extract, Horsetail Extract, Sugar Cane Extract, Citrus Extract, Apple Extract, Green Tea Extract, Methyl Gluceth-20, Panthenol, Cyanocobalamin, Propylene Glycol, Laureth-4, Hydrolyzed Wheat Protein, Tissue Respiratory Factors, Plant Pseudocollagen, Aloe Vera Gel, Triethanolamine, Dimethicone Copolyol, PEG-30 Glyceryl Laurate, Phenethyl Alcohol, Carbomer, Xanthan Gum, Benzophenone-4, Disodium EDTA, Methylchloroisothiazolinone, Methylisothiazolinone, Methylparaben, Propylparaben.

Directions: Apply in the morning, or any time of the day, in small quantities to the skin around the eyes with light, tapping motions, avoiding direct contact with the eyes. In the evening, apply gently to the entire eye contour area.

Warnings: For external use only. Avoid direct contact with eyes.

How Supplied: 1 fl. oz.

STEPHAN™ BIO-NUTRITIONAL
Nightime Moisture Creme

Uses: Hypo-allergenic STEPHAN™ BIO-NUTRITIONAL Nightime Moisture Creme is a heavier, richer cream for mature, dry, or sun-damaged skin. This advanced formula is excellent for dehydrated skin, promoting suppleness and moisture, and improving the appearance of fine lines and wrinkles.

Inactive Ingredients: Water, Caprylic/Capric Triglyceride, Propylene Glycol, Stearic Acid, Polysorbate 60, Cetyl Alcohol, Octyl Palmitate, Beeswax, Sorbitan Stearate, Canola Oil, Avocado Oil, Safflower Oil, Squalane, Liposomes, Soluble Collagen, Dimethicone, Bisabolol, Aloe Vera Gel, Fragrance, C12-15 Alkyl Benzoate, Hydroxyethylcellulose, Octyl Methoxycinnamate, Disodium EDTA, Sodium Borate, Benzophenone-3, Allantoin, Phenoxyethanol, Methylparaben, Propylparaben, Butylparaben, Ethyl-

paraben, FD&C Yellow No. 10, Caramel.

Directions: In the evening, apply by lightly massaging onto a thoroughly cleansed face and neck. Avoid direct contact with eyes. For drier skin, it may be used during the day as a moisturizer, under make-up, or after sun bathing.

Warning: For external use only. Avoid contact with eyes.

How Supplied: Net Wt. 1.75 oz.

STEPHAN™ BIO-NUTRITIONAL
Refreshing Moisture Gel

Uses: Hypo-allergenic STEPHAN™ BIO-NUTRITIONAL Refreshing Moisture Gel is specially formulated to refine pores and promote a clear, clean, and smooth-looking complexion. It is designed to deeply cleanse and super-stimulate the skin. This gel is suitable for all skin types, especially problem areas. A quick "pick-me-up," STEPHAN BIO-NUTRITIONAL Refreshing Moisture Gel immediately restores the radiant, firm, and youthful appearance of the face while acting as a cumulative, revitalizing beauty treatment.

Inactive Ingredients: Water, Propylene Glycol, Glycerin, Hydroxyethylcellulose, Sugar Cane Extract, Citrus Extract, Apple Extract, Green Tea Extract, Hydrolyzed Wheat Protein, Tissue Respiratory Factors, Panthenol, Aloe Vera Gel, Laureth-4, Magnesium Aluminum Silicate, Tetrasodium EDTA, Benzophenone-3, Imidazolidinyl Urea, Methylchloroisothiazolinone, Methylisothiazolinone, Methylparaben, Propylparaben, Phenethyl Alcohol, FD&C Yellow No. 10, FD&C Red No. 40, FD&C Yellow No. 5.

Directions: After thoroughly cleansing in the morning or evening, apply a liberal layer to the face, neck and eye area, avoiding eye contact. Remove after 20–30 minutes with warm water. Suitable for all skin types.

Warnings: For external use only. Avoid contact with eyes.

How Supplied: Net Wt. 1.75 oz.

STEPHAN™ BIO-NUTRITIONAL
Ultra Hydrating Fluid

Uses: Hypo-allergenic STEPHAN™ BIO-NUTRITIONAL Ultra Hydrating Fluid is a complete treatment to help firm the skin, soften fine lines, and preserve youthful-looking, radiant skin. STEPHAN BIO-NUTRITIONAL Ultra Hydrating Fluid helps combat the aged look of the skin.

Inactive Ingredients: Water, Glycerin, Panthenol, Sodium Hyaluronate, Phenethyl Alcohol, Aloe Vera Gel, Methyl Gluceth-20, PEG-30 Glyceryl Laurate, Methylsilanol Hydroxyproline Aspartate, Xanthan Gum, Methyl-

chloroisothiazolinone, Methylisothiazolinone.

Directions: Gently apply all over the face, neck, and eye contour area, preferably in the morning. Use as a part of a regular daily skin care routine or as an occasional preventive treatment.

Warnings: For external use only. Avoid direct contact with eyes.

How Supplied: 1 fl. oz.

STEPHAN™ CLARITY
Nutritional Supplement

Uses: Designed for both men and women, STEPHAN™ Clarity contains selected tissue proteins supported by vitamins, minerals, amino acids, and herbs regarded as important to memory and concentration.

Directions: Take one to two capsules per day.

Warnings: Phenylketonurics: Contains Phenylalanine.

Ingredients: Lecithin, Bee Pollen, Glutamic Acid, Vitamin C, Ribonucleic Acid, Ginkgo Biloba (as 8:1 extract), Aspartic Acid, Vitamin E, Vitamin B-3, Leucine, Arginine, Lysine, Phenylalanine, Serine, Valine, Proline, Isoleucine, Alanine, Glycine, Threonine, Tyrosine, Vitamin B-5, Vitamin B-1, Histidine, Methionine, Cysteine, Adenosine Triphosphate, Vitamin B-6, Vitamin B-2, Vitamin A, Folic Acid, Biotin, Vitamin D-3, Vitamin B-12.

How Supplied: One bottle contains 30 easy-to-swallow capsules.

STEPHAN™ ELASTICITY
Nutritional Supplement

Uses: A nutritional food supplement for men and women, STEPHAN™ Elasticity contains a scientifically balanced mixture of specific tissue proteins (in the form of nutrients) supported by vitamins, minerals, amino acids, and herbs which are established as important for skin tone, texture, and appearance.

Directions: Take one capsule per day.

Warning: Phenylketonurics: Contains Phenylalanine.

Ingredients: Equisetum Arvense, Protein Isolates (Alanine, Arginine, Aspartic Acid, Cysteine, Glutamic Acid, Glycine, Histidine, Isoleucine, Leucine, Lysine, Methionine, Phenylalanine, Proline, Serine, Threonine, Tyrosine, Valine), Fucus, Vitamine E (Dl-Alpha), Zinc (Amino Acid Chelate), Vitamin C, Ribonucleic Acid, Calcium (Amino Acid Chelate), Magnesium (Amino Acid Chelate), Iron (Amino Acid Chelate), Manganese (Amino Acid Chelate), Selenium (Amino Acid Chelate), Chromium (Amino Acid Chelate), Adenosine Triphosphate, Vitamin A (Acetate).

How Supplied: One bottle contains 30 easy-to-swallow capsules.

STEPHAN™ ELIXIR
Nutritional Supplement

Uses: Formulated with an exclusive blend of specific proteins, STEPHAN™ Elixir is ideal for both men and women. These tissue proteins are supported by vitamins, minerals, amino acids, and herbs recognized as important for general health and well being.

Directions: Take one capsule per day.

Warnings: Phenylketonurics: Contains Phenylalanine.

Ingredient: Soya Isolate (Alanine, Arginine, Aspartic Acid, Cysteine, Glutamic Acid, Glycine, Histidine, Isoleucine, Leucine, Lysine, Methionine, Phenylalanine, Proline, Serine, Threonine, Tyrosine, Valine), Bee Pollen, Vitamin C, Malic Acid, Ginkgo Biloba (8:1 extract), Citric Acid, Ribonucleic Acid, Vitamin E, Vitamin B-3, Zinc (Amino Acid Chelate), Iron (Amino Acid Chelate), Calcium Pantothenate, Vitamin B-1, Vitamin B-5, Adenosine Triphosphate, Vitamin B-6, Vitamin B-2, Vitamin A, Folic Acid, Selenium (Amino Acid Chelate), Biotin, Vitamin D-3, Vitamin B-12.

How Supplied: One bottle contains 30 easy-to-swallow capsules.

STEPHAN™ ESSENTIAL
Nutritional Supplement

Uses: Designed for both men and women, STEPHAN™ Essential is a nutritional food supplement which contains specific tissue proteins supported by vitamins, minerals, herbs, and amino acids which have long been established as being important for the health of the heart and circulatory system.

Directions: Take one to two capsules per day.

Warnings: Phenylketonurics: Contains Phenylalanine.

Ingredients: Bee Pollen, L-Carnitine, Omega 3 Oil, Glutamic Acid, Ribonucleic Acid, Aspartic Acid, Vitamin E, Leucine, Arginine, Lysine, Magnesium (Amino Acid Chelate), Phenylalanine, Serine, Valine, Proline, Isoleucine, Alanine, Glycine, Threonine, Tyrosine, Histidine, Methionine, Cysteine, Adenosine Triphosphate, Selenium (Amino Acid Chelate).

How Supplied: One bottle contains 30 easy-to-swallow capsules.

STEPHAN™ FEMININE
Nutritional Supplement

Uses: Specifically designed for women, STEPHAN™ Feminine contains selected tissue proteins supported by vitamins, minerals, and amino acids regarded as important to the ever-changing female body.

Directions: Take one to two capsules per day.

Warnings: Phenylketonurics: Contains Phenylalanine.

Ingredients: Magnesium Oxide, Glutamic Acid, Ribonucleic Acid, Aspartic Acid, Vitamin E, Leucine, Arginine, Lysine, Phenylalanine, Serine, Valine, Proline, Isoleucine, Alanine, Glycine, Threonine, Tyrosine, Histidine, Methionine, Cysteine, Boron (Amino Acid Chelate), Adenosine Triphosphate, Selenium.

How Supplied: One bottle contains 30 easy-to-swallow capsules.

STEPHAN™ FLEXIBILITY
Nutritional Supplement

Uses: A nutritional supplement for both men and women, STEPHAN™ Flexibility is rich with exclusive proteins which are supported by vitamins, minerals, and amino acids recognized as beneficial to the health of joint and soft tissues.

Directions: Take one to two capsules per day.

Warnings: Phenylketonurics: Contains Phenylalanine.

Ingredients: Vitamin C, Ribonucleic Acid, Vitamin E, Vitamin B-3, Glutamic Acid, Zinc (Amino Acid Chelate), Calcium (Amino Acid Chelate), Aspartic Acid, Bee Pollen, Leucine, Arginine, Lysine, Vitamin B-5, Vitamin B-1, Phenylalanine, Serine, Valine, Proline, Isoleucine, Alanine, Glycine, Threonine, Tyrosine, Histidine, Cysteine, Adenosine Triphosphate, Vitamin B-6, Boron (Amino Acid Chelate), Vitamin B-2, Methionine, Vitamin A, Folic Acid, Selenium (Amino Acid Chelate), Biotin, Vitamin D-3, Vitamin B-12.

How Supplied: One bottle contains 30 easy-to-swallow capsules.

STEPHAN™ LOVPIL
Nutritional Supplement

Uses: STEPHAN™ Lovpil is a nutritional food supplement for men and women of all ages. STEPHAN Lovpil is formulated with vitamins, minerals, herbs, amino acids, and selected proteins recognized as important for general health and vitality.

Directions: Take one capsule per day.

Warnings: Phenylketonurics: Contains Phenylalanine.

Ingredients: Calcium Carbonate, Vitamin C, Damiana Powder, Zinc (Amino Acid Chelate), Ribonucleic Acid, Soya Isolate (Isoleucine, Phenylalanine, Leucine, Threonine, Lysine, Methionine, Valine, Alanine, Glycine, Histidine, Arginine, Proline, Aspartic Acid, Serine, Cys-

---

teine, Tyrosine, Glutamic Acid), Manganese (Amino Acid Chelate), Adenosine Triphosphate, Vitamin A (Acetate), Folic Acid, Vitamin D (Cholecalciferol), Selenium (Methionine), Vitamin B12.

How Supplied: One bottle contains 30 easy-to-swallow capsules.

STEPHAN™ MASCULINE
Nutritional Supplement

Uses: A nutritional food supplement formulated for the adult male, STEPHAN™ Masculine contains a special blend of nutrients with vitamins, minerals, herbs, and amino acids.

Directions: Take one to two capsules per day.

Ingredients: L-Histidine, Calcium (Carbonate), Bee Pollen, Parsley, Ribonucleic Acid, Zinc (Amino Acid Chelate), Magnesium (Amino Acid Chelate), Adenosine Triphosphate.

How Supplied: One bottle contains 30 easy-to-swallow capsules.

STEPHAN™ PROTECTOR
Nutritional Supplement

Uses: STEPHAN™ Protector is a nutritional food supplement that combines specific proteins, vitamins, minerals, and amino acids recognized as important for the health of areas associated with the human immune system. STEPHAN Protector may be used by men and women of all ages.

Directions: Take one capsule per day.

Warnings: Phenylketonurics: Contains Phenylalanine.

Ingredients: Bee Pollen, Astragalus, Kelp, Glutamic Acid, Ribonucleic Acid, Aspartic Acid, Leucine, Arginine, Lysine, Phenylalanine, Serine, Proline, Valine, Isoleucine, Alanine, Glycine, Threonine, Tyrosine, Histidine, Methionine, Cysteine, Adenosine Triphosphate.

How Supplied: One bottle contains 30 easy-to-swallow capsules.

STEPHAN™ RELIEF
Nutritional Supplement

Uses: Designed for both men and women, STEPHAN™ Relief has been formulated with a special combination of nutrients, vitamins, minerals, amino acids, and herbs which are recognized as important to the digestive and excretory systems.

Directions: Take one to two capsules per day.

Ingredients: Fucus, Parsley (extract 4:1), Psyllium, Leucine, Isoleucine, Valine, Bee Pollen, Ribonucleic Acid,

Continued on next page

Wellness International—Cont.

Calcium Pantothenate, Adenosine Triphosphate.

How Supplied: One bottle contains 30 easy-to-swallow capsules.

STEPHAN™ TRANQUILITY
Nutritional Supplement

Uses: Designed for both men and women, STEPHAN™ Tranquility is a nutritional food supplement which contains a blend of vitamins, minerals, and amino acids recognized as important to areas involved in stress management.

Directions: Take one to two capsules per day.

Warnings: Phenylketonurics: Contains Phenylalanine.

Ingredients: Lecithin, Choline Bitartrate, Myo-Inositol, Vitamin C, Valerian (As 4:1 extract), Ribonucleic Acid, Vitamin E, Vitamin B-3, Glutamic Acid, Aspartic Acid, Calcium (Amino Acid Chelate), Leucine, Arginine, Lysine, Phenylalanine, Serine, Valine, Proline, Isoleucine, Alanine, Glycine, Threonine, Tyrosine, Vitamin B-5, Vitamin B-1, Histidine, Magnesium, Methionine, Cysteine, Adenosine Triphosphate, Vitamin B-6, Vitamin B-2, Vitamin A, Folic Acid, Biotin (Amino Acid Chelate), Vitamin D-3, Vitamin B-12.

How Supplied: One bottle contains 30 easy-to-swallow capsules.

WINRGY™
Nutritional Drink with Vitamin C

Uses: A delicious, Vitamin C-enriched beverage, WINRGY™ was formulated with a special blend of nutrients designed to offer a nutritional alternative to coffees and colas.

Directions: Add 6 ounces of chilled water or fruit juice to one packet of mix. Stir briskly. Consume 1–2 times per day. Keep in a cool, dry place.

Warnings: Phenylketonurics: Contains Phenylalanine. Not for use by children, pregnant or lactating women. Persons taking medications should seek medical advice before taking this product. Do not consume more than four servings per day. Avoid the use of antacids containing aluminum with this product.

Ingredients: Fructose, L-Phenylalanine, Natural Flavors, Citric Acid, Taurine, Glycine, Ascorbic Acid, Caffeine, Niacinamide, Vitamin E Acetate, Calcium Pantothenate, Silicon Dioxide, Potassium Aspartate, Manganese Aspartate, Chromium Aspartate, Pyridoxine Hydrochloride, Zinc Gluconate, Riboflavin, Thiamin Mononitrate, Copper Gluconate, Folic Acid, Vitamin B12.

How Supplied: One box contains 14 packets. Serving size equals one packet.

Whitehall Laboratories
**American Home
Products Corporation
FIVE GIRALDA FARMS
MADISON, NJ 07940-0871**

ADVIL®
[ad 'vil]
**Ibuprofen Tablets, USP
Ibuprofen Caplets***
**Pain Reliever/Fever Reducer
*Oval-Shaped Tablets**

WARNING: **ASPIRIN-SENSITIVE PATIENTS. Do not take this product if you have had a severe allergic reaction to aspirin, e.g.—asthma, swelling, shock or hives, because even though this product contains no aspirin or salicylates, cross-reactions may occur in patients allergic to aspirin.**

Active Ingredient: Each tablet or caplet contains Ibuprofen 200 mg.

Inactive Ingredients: Acetylated Monoglyceride, Beeswax and/or Carnauba Wax, Croscarmellose Sodium, Iron Oxides, Lecithin, Methylparaben, Microcrystalline Cellulose, Pharmaceutical Glaze, Povidone, Propylparaben, Silicon Dioxide, Simethicone, Sodium Benzoate, Sodium Lauryl Sulfate, Starch, Stearic Acid, Sucrose, Titanium Dioxide.

Indications: For the temporary relief of minor aches and pains associated with the common cold, headache, toothache, muscular aches, backache, for the minor pain of arthritis, for the pain of menstrual cramps and for reduction of fever.

Dosage and Administration: Adults: Take one tablet or caplet every 4 to 6 hours while symptoms persist. If pain or fever does not respond to one tablet or caplet, two tablets or caplets may be used but do not exceed six tablets or caplets in 24 hours unless directed by a doctor. The smallest effective dose should be used. Take with food or milk if occasional and mild heartburn, upset stomach, or stomach pain occurs with use. Consult a doctor if these symptoms are more than mild or if they persist. Children: Do not give this product to children under 12 years of age except under the advice and supervision of a doctor.

Warnings: Do not take for pain for more than 10 days or for fever for more than 3 days unless directed by a doctor. If pain or fever persists or gets worse, if new symptoms occur, or if the painful area is red or swollen, consult a doctor. These could be signs of serious illness. If you are under a doctor's care for any serious condition, consult a doctor before taking this product. As with aspirin and acetaminophen, if you have any condition which requires you to take prescription drugs or if you have had any problems or serious side effects from taking any nonprescription pain reliever, do not take this product without first discussing it with your doctor. **IF YOU EXPERIENCE ANY SYMPTOMS WHICH ARE UNUSUAL OR SEEM UNRELATED TO THE CONDITION FOR WHICH YOU TOOK IBUPROFEN, CONSULT A DOCTOR BEFORE TAKING ANY MORE OF IT.** Although ibuprofen is indicated for the same conditions as aspirin and acetaminophen, it should not be taken with them except under a doctor's direction. Do not combine this product with any other ibuprofen-containing product. As with any drug, if you are pregnant or nursing a baby, seek the advice of a health professional before using this product. **IT IS ESPECIALLY IMPORTANT NOT TO USE IBUPROFEN DURING THE LAST 3 MONTHS OF PREGNANCY UNLESS SPECIFICALLY DIRECTED TO DO SO BY A DOCTOR BECAUSE IT MAY CAUSE PROBLEMS IN THE UNBORN CHILD OR COMPLICATIONS DURING DELIVERY.** Keep this and all drugs out of the reach of children. In case of accidental overdose, seek professional assistance or contact a poison control center immediately.

How Supplied: Coated tablets in bottles of 4, 8, 24, 50 (non-child resistant size), 72 (E-Z Cap) 100, 165 and 250. Coated caplets in bottles of 24, 50 (non-child resistant size), 72 (E-Z Cap) 100, 165, and 250. Coated tablets in thermoform packaging of 8.

Storage: Store at room temperature; avoid excessive heat (40°C, 104°F).

Shown in Product Identification Guide, page 531

ADVIL® Cold and Sinus
**Ibuprofen/Pseudoephedrine HCl
Caplets* and Tablets
Pain Reliever/Fever Reducer/Nasal Decongestant**

***Oval-Shaped tablets**

WARNING: ASPIRIN-SENSITIVE PATIENTS. Do not take this product if you have had a severe allergic reaction to aspirin, eg, asthma, swelling, shock or hives, because even though this product contains no aspirin or salicylates, cross-reactions may occur in patients allergic to aspirin.

Indications: For temporary relief of symptoms associated with the common cold, sinusitis or flu, including nasal congestion, headache, fever, body aches, and pains.

Directions: *Adults:* Take 1 caplet or tablet every 4 to 6 hours while symptoms persist. If symptoms do not respond to 1 caplet or tablet, 2 caplets or tablets may be used, but do not exceed 6 caplets or tablets in 24 hours unless directed by a doctor. The smallest effective dose should be used. Take with food or milk if occasional and mild heartburn, upset stomach, or stomach pain occurs with use. Consult a doctor if these symptoms are more than mild or if they persist. *Children:* Do not give this product to children under 12 years of age except under the advice and supervision of a doctor.

Warnings: Do not take for colds for more than 7 days or for fever for more than 3 days unless directed by a doctor. If the cold or fever persists or gets worse, or if new symptoms occur, consult a doctor. These could be signs of serious illness. As with aspirin and acetaminophen, if you have any condition which requires you to take prescription drugs or if you have had any problems or serious side effects from taking any nonprescription pain reliever, do not take this product without first discussing it with your doctor. IF YOU EXPERIENCE ANY SYMPTOMS WHICH ARE UNUSUAL OR SEEM UNRELATED TO THE CONDITION FOR WHICH YOU TOOK THIS PRODUCT, CONSULT A DOCTOR BEFORE TAKING ANY MORE OF IT. If you are under a doctor's care for any serious condition, consult a doctor before taking this product.
Do not exceed recommended dosage because at higher doses nervousness, dizziness, or sleeplessness may occur. Do not take this product if you have high blood pressure, heart disease, diabetes, thyroid disease or difficulty in urination due to enlargement of the prostate gland, except under the advice and supervision of a doctor.

Drug Interaction Precaution: Do not take this product if you are presently taking a prescription drug for high blood pressure or depression without first consulting your doctor. Do not combine this product with other non-prescription pain relievers. Do not combine this product with any other ibuprofen-containing product. As with any drug, if you are pregnant or nursing a baby, seek the advice of a health professional before using this product.
IT IS ESPECIALLY IMPORTANT NOT TO USE THIS PRODUCT DURING THE LAST 3 MONTHS OF PREGNANCY UNLESS SPECIFICALLY DIRECTED TO DO SO BY A DOCTOR BECAUSE IT MAY CAUSE PROBLEMS IN THE UNBORN CHILD OR COMPLICATIONS DURING DELIVERY. Keep this and all drugs out of the reach of children. In case of accidental overdose, seek professional assistance or contact a poison control center immediately.

Active Ingredients: Each caplet or tablet contains Ibuprofen 200 mg and Pseudoephedrine HCl 30 mg.

Inactive Ingredients: Carnauba or Equivalent Wax, Croscarmellose Sodium, Iron Oxides, Methylparaben, Microcrystalline Cellulose, Propylparaben, Silicon Dioxide, Sodium Benzoate, Sodium Lauryl Sulfate, Starch, Stearic Acid, Sucrose, Titanium Dioxide.

How Supplied: Advil® Cold and Sinus is an oval-shaped tan-colored caplet or tan-colored tablet supplied in consumer bottles of 40 and blister packs of 20. Medical samples are available in a 2's pouch dispenser.

Storage: Store at room temperature; avoid excessive heat (40°C, 104°F).
Shown in Product Identification Guide, page 531

CLEARBLUE EASY®
Pregnancy Test Kit

Clearblue Easy is one of the easiest and fastest pregnancy tests available because all a woman has to do is hold the absorbent tip in her urine stream and in 3 minutes she can read the result. A blue line appears in the small window to show that the test is complete and the large window shows the test result. If there is a blue line in the large window, the woman is pregnant. If there is no line, she is not pregnant.

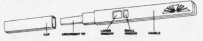

Clearblue Easy is a rapid, one-step pregnancy test for home use, which detects the pregnancy hormone HCG (human chorionic gonadotropin) in the urine. This hormone is produced in increasing amounts during the first part of pregnancy. Clearblue Easy uses sensitive monoclonal antibodies to detect the presence of this hormone from the first day of a missed period.
A negative result means that no pregnancy hormone was detected and the woman is probably not pregnant. If the menstrual period does not start within a week, she may have miscalculated the day her period was due. She should repeat the test using another Clearblue Easy test. If the second test still gives a negative result and she still has not menstruated, she should see her doctor.
Clearblue Easy is specially designed for easy use at home. However, if there are any questions about the test or results, give the Clearblue Easy TalkLine a call at 1-800-883-EASY. A specially trained staff of advisors is available to answer your questions.
Manufactured by Unipath Ltd., Bedford, U.K. Unipath, Clearblue Easy and the fan device are trademarks.
Distributed by Whitehall Laboratories, Madison, NJ 07940-0871.
Shown in Product Identification Guide, page 532

CLEARPLAN EASY™
One-Step Ovulation Predictor

CLEARPLAN EASY is one of the easiest home ovulation predictor tests to use because of its unique technological design. It consists of just one piece and involves only one step to get results. To use CLEARPLAN EASY, a woman simply holds the absorbent tip in her urine stream (a woman can test any time of day) for 5 seconds, and after 5 minutes, she can read the results. A blue line will appear in the small window to show her that the test has worked correctly. The large window indicates the presence of

luteinizing hormone (LH) in her urine. If there is a line in the large window which is similar to or darker than the line in the small window, she has detected her LH surge.

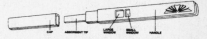

Laboratory tests confirm that CLEARPLAN EASY is over 98% accurate in detecting the LH surge as shown by radioimmunoassay (RIA).
CLEARPLAN EASY employs highly sensitive monoclonal antibody technology to accurately predict the onset of ovulation, and, consequently, the best time each month for a woman to try to become pregnant. The test monitors the amount of LH in a woman's urine. Small amounts of LH are present during most of the menstrual cycle, but the level normally rises sharply about 24 to 36 hours before ovulation (which is when an egg is released from the ovary). CLEARPLAN EASY detects this LH surge preceding ovulation so that a woman knows 24–36 hours beforehand the time she is most able to become pregnant.
A woman will be most fertile during the 1 to 3 days after an LH surge is detected. Sperm can fertilize an egg for many hours after sexual intercourse. So, if sexual intercourse occurs during the 1–3 days after a similar or darker line appears in the large window, the chances of getting pregnant are maximized.

CLEARPLAN EASY contains 5 days of tests. If, because a woman's cycles are irregular or if for any other reason a woman does not detect her LH surge after 5 days of testing, she should continue testing with a second CLEARPLAN EASY kit. CLEARPLAN EASY offers users the support of a TalkLine (1-800-883-EASY). This service is operated by trained advisors who are available to answer any questions about using the test or reading the results.

Produced by Unipath Ltd., Bedford, U.K.
Unipath, CLEARPLAN EASY and the fan device are trademarks.
Distributed by Whitehall Laboratories, Madison, NJ 07940-0871.
Shown in Product Identification Guide, page 532

PREPARATION H®
[prep-e'rā-shen-āch]
Hemorrhoidal Ointment and Cream
PREPARATION H®
Hemorrhoidal Suppositories

Description: Preparation H is available in ointment, cream and suppository product forms. The <u>Ointment</u> contains Petrolatum 71.9%, Mineral Oil 14%, Shark Liver Oil 3% and Phenylephrine HCl 0.25%.
The **Cream** contains Petrolatum 18%, Glycerin 12%, Shark Liver Oil 3% and Phenylephrine HCl 0.25%.

Continued on next page

Whitehall—Cont.

The **Suppositories** contain Cocoa Butter 79% and Shark Liver Oil 3%.

Indications: Preparation H Ointment and Cream temporarily shrink hemorrhoidal tissue and give temporary relief of the itching, burning and discomfort associated with hemorrhoids. Preparation H Suppositories provide temporary relief of the itching, burning, and discomfort associated with hemorrhoids.

Warnings: In case of bleeding, or if condition worsens or does not improve within 7 days, consult a doctor promptly. Do not exceed the recommended daily dosage unless directed by a doctor. Keep this and all drugs out of the reach of children. In case of accidental ingestion, seek professional assistance or contact a poison control center immediately. As with any drug, if you are pregnant or nursing a baby, seek the advice of a health professional before using this product.
Ointment/Cream: Do not use this product if you have heart disease, high blood pressure, thyroid disease, diabetes, or difficulty in urination due to enlargement of the prostate gland unless directed by a doctor.
Ointment: Do not use this product with an applicator if the introduction of the applicator into the rectum causes additional pain. Consult a doctor promptly.
Cream: Do not put this product into the rectum by using fingers or any mechanical device or applicator.

Drug Interaction Precaution: Ointment/Cream—Do not use this product if you are presently taking a prescription drug for high blood pressure or depression, without first consulting your doctor.

Dosage and Administration:
Ointment/Cream/Suppositories—
ADULTS—When practical, cleanse the affected area by patting or blotting with an appropriate cleansing tissue. Gently dry by patting or blotting with toilet tissue or a soft cloth before application of this product.
Children under 12 years of age: consult a doctor.
Ointment—Apply to the affected area up to 4 times daily, especially at night, in the morning or after each bowel movement. Regular application and lubrication with Preparation H Ointment provide continual therapy for relief of hemorrhoidal symptoms. FOR INTRARECTAL USE: Before applying, remove protective cover from applicator. Attach applicator to tube. Lubricate applicator well, then gently insert applicator into the rectum. Thoroughly cleanse applicator after each use and replace protective cover. Also apply ointment to external area.
Cream—Apply externally to the affected area up to 4 times daily, especially at night, in the morning, or after each bowel movement. Preparation H Cream is to be applied externally or in the lower portion of the anal canal only. The enclosed dispensing cap is designed to control dispersion of the cream to the affected area in the lower portion of the anal canal. Before applying, remove protective cover from dispensing cap. Attach cap to tube. Lubricate dispensing cap well, then gently insert dispensing cap part way into the anus. Thoroughly cleanse dispensing cap after each use and replace protective cover. Regular application and lubrication with Preparation H Cream provide continual therapy for relief of hemorrhoidal symptoms.
Suppositories—Remove wrapper before inserting into the rectum. Insert one suppository into the rectum up to 6 times daily, especially at night, in the morning or after each bowel movement. Regular application and lubrication with Preparation H Suppositories provide continual therapy for relief of hemorrhoidal symptoms.

Inactive Ingredients: Ointment—Beeswax, Benzoic Acid, BHA, Corn Oil, Glycerin, Lanolin, Lanolin Alcohol, Methylparaben, Paraffin, Propylparaben, Thyme Oil, Tocopherol, Water.
Cream—BHA, Carboxymethylcellulose Sodium, Cetyl Alcohol, Citric Acid, Edetate Disodium, Glyceryl Oleate, Glyceryl Stearate, Lanolin, Methylparaben, Propyl Gallate, Propylene Glycol, Propylparaben, Simethicone, Sodium Benzoate, Sodium Lauryl Sulfate, Stearyl Alcohol, Tocopherol, Xanthan Gum, Water.
Suppositories—Ascorbyl Palmitate, Benzoic Acid, BHA, Corn Oil, Edetate Disodium, Glycerin, Methylparaben, PEG-12 Dilaurate, Propylparaben, Tocopherol, Water, White Wax.

How Supplied: Ointment: Net Wt. 1 oz. and 2 oz. **Cream:** Net wt. 0.9 oz. and 1.8 oz. **Suppositories:** 12's, 24's and 48's.
Store at room temperature in cool place but not over 80° F.
Shown in Product Identification Guide, page 532

PREPARATION H®
HYDROCORTISONE 1%
[prep-e 'ra-shen-ach]
Anti-Itch Cream

Description: Preparation H® Hydrocortisone 1% is an antipruritic cream containing 1% Hydrocortisone.

Indications: For the temporary relief of external anal itch and itching associated with minor skin irritations and rashes. Other uses of this product should be only under the advice and supervision of a doctor.

Warnings: For external use only. Avoid contact with the eyes. If condition worsens, or if symptoms persist for more than 7 days or clear up and occur again within a few days, stop use of this product and do not begin use of any other hydrocortisone product unless you have consulted a doctor. Do not exceed the recommended daily dosage unless directed by a doctor. In case of bleeding, consult a doctor promptly. Do not put this product into the rectum by using fingers or any mechanical device or applicator. Do not use for the treatment of diaper rash; consult a doctor. Keep this and all drugs out of the reach of children. In case of accidental ingestion, seek professional assistance or contact a Poison Control Center immediately.

Directions: Adults: When practical, cleanse the affected area by patting or blotting with an appropriate cleansing tissue. Gently dry by patting or blotting with toilet tissue or soft cloth before application of this product. Apply to affected area not more than 3 to 4 times daily.
Children under 12 years of age: consult a doctor.

Inactive Ingredients: BHA, Cellulose Gum, Cetyl Alcohol, Citric Acid, Disodium EDTA, Glycerin, Glyceryl Oleate, Glyceryl Stearate, Lanolin, Methylparaben, Petrolatum, Propyl Gallate, Propylene Glycol, Propylparaben, Simethicone, Sodium Benzoate, Sodium Lauryl Sulfate, Stearyl Alcohol, Water, Xanthan Gum.

How Supplied: Available in Net Wt. 0.9 oz. tube. Store at room temperature or in cool place but not over 80°F. If cellophane tear strip is missing or if cellophane wrap is broken or missing when purchased, do not use.
Shown in Product Identification Guide, page 532

PRIMATENE® Dual Action Formula
[prīm 'a-tēn]
Tablets

Description: Primatene Dual Action Tablets contain Theophylline Anhydrous 60 mg, Ephedrine Hydrochloride 12.5 mg, and Guaifenesin 100 mg.

Indications: For temporary relief of shortness of breath, tightness of chest, and wheezing due to bronchial asthma. Eases breathing for asthma patients by reducing spasms of bronchial muscles and helps loosen phlegm and thin bronchial secretions to rid bronchial passageways of mucus and make coughs more productive.

Warnings: Do not use this product unless a diagnosis of asthma has been made by a doctor. Do not use this product if you have heart disease, high blood pressure, thyroid disease, diabetes, or difficulty in urination due to enlargement of the prostate gland unless directed by a doctor. Do not use this product if you have ever been hospitalized for asthma or if you are taking any prescription drug for asthma unless directed by a doctor. Do not continue to use this product, but seek medical assistance immediately if symptoms are not relieved within 1 hour or become worse. Some users of this product may experience nervousness, tremor, sleeplessness, nausea, and loss of appetite. If these symptoms persist or become worse, consult your doctor. Do not take this product for persistent chronic cough such as occurs with smoking, asthma, chronic bronchitis, or emphysema or where cough is accompanied by excessive phlegm (mucus) unless directed by a doctor. A persistent cough may be a sign of a serious condition. If cough persists for more than one week, tends to recur, or is accompanied by a fever, rash, or persistent headache, consult a doctor. As with any drug, if you are pregnant or nursing a baby, seek the advice of a health professional before using this product. Keep this and all drugs out of the reach of children. In case of accidental overdose, seek professional assistance or contact a Poison Control Center immediately.

Drug Interaction Precaution: Do not use this product if you are now taking a prescription monoamine oxidase inhibitor (MAOI) (certain drugs for depression, psychiatric or emotional conditions, or Parkinson's disease), or for 2 weeks after stopping the MAOI drug. If you are uncertain whether your prescription drug contains an MAOI, consult a health professional before taking this product.

Directions: Adults and children 12 years of age and over, 2 tablets initially, then two every 4 hours, as needed, not to exceed 12 tablets in 24 hours. Do not exceed recommended dosage unless directed by a doctor. Children (under 12 years of age)—consult a doctor.

Inactive Ingredients: Calcium Stearate, Hydrogenated Vegetable Oil, Microcrystalline Cellulose

How Supplied: Available in 24 and 60 tablet thermoform blister cartons. Store at room temperature between 20°C and 25°C (68°F to 77°F).
Shown in Product Identification Guide, page 532

PRIMATENE®
[prĭm'a-tēn]
Mist
(Epinephrine Inhalation Aerosol Bronchodilator)

Description: Primatene Mist contains Epinephrine 5.5 mg/mL.

FDA approved uses.

Indications: For temporary relief of shortness of breath, tightness of chest, and wheezing due to bronchial asthma. Eases breathing for asthma patients by reducing spasms of bronchial muscles.

Directions: Inhalation dosage for adults and children 12 years of age and over, and children 4 to under 12 years of age: Start with one inhalation, then wait at least 1 minute. If not relieved, use once more. Do not use again for at least 3 hours. The use of this product by children should be supervised by an adult. Children under 4 years of age: Consult a physician. Each inhalation delivers 0.22 mg of epinephrine.

Warnings: Do not use this product unless a diagnosis of asthma has been made by a physician. Do not use this product if you have heart disease, high blood pressure, thyroid disease, diabetes, or difficulty in urination due to enlargement of the prostate gland unless directed by a physician. As with any drug, if you are pregnant or nursing a baby, seek the advice of a health professional before using this product. Do not use this product if you have ever been hospitalized for asthma or if you are taking any prescription drug for asthma unless directed by a physician. Keep this and all drugs out of the reach of children. In case of accidental overdose, seek professional assistance or contact a poison control center immediately. **DO NOT CONTINUE TO USE THIS PRODUCT BUT SEEK MEDICAL ASSISTANCE IMMEDIATELY IF SYMPTOMS ARE NOT RELIEVED WITHIN 20 MINUTES OR BECOME WORSE. DO NOT USE THIS PRODUCT MORE FREQUENTLY OR AT HIGHER DOSES THAN RECOMMENDED UNLESS DIRECTED BY A PHYSICIAN.** EXCESSIVE USE MAY CAUSE NERVOUSNESS AND RAPID HEART BEAT AND POSSIBLY, ADVERSE EFFECTS ON THE HEART.

Drug Interaction Precaution: Do not use this product if you are now taking a prescription monoamine oxidase inhibitor (MAOI) (certain drugs for depression, psychiatric or emotional conditions, or Parkinson's disease), or for 2 weeks after stopping the MAOI drug. If you are uncertain whether your prescription drug contains an MAOI, consult a health professional before taking this product.

Caution: Contents under pressure. Do not puncture or throw container into incinerator. Using or storing near open flame or heating above 120° F (49° C) may cause bursting. Store at room temperature 59° F to 86° F (15° C to 30° C).

Directions For Use of Mouthpiece: The Primatene Mist mouthpiece, which is enclosed in the Primatene Mist 15 mL size (not the refill size), should be used for inhalation only with Primatene Mist.

1. Take plastic cap off mouthpiece. (For refills, use mouthpiece from previous purchase.)
2. Take plastic mouthpiece off bottle.
3. Place other end of mouthpiece on bottle.
4. Turn bottle upside down. Place thumb on bottom of mouthpiece over circular button and forefinger on top of vial. Empty the lungs as completely as possible by exhaling.
5. Place mouthpiece in mouth with lips closed around opening. Inhale deeply while squeezing mouthpiece and bottle together. Release immediately and remove unit from mouth. Complete taking the deep breath, drawing the medication into your lungs and holding breath as long as comfortable.
6. Exhale slowly keeping lips nearly closed. This helps distribute the medication in the lungs.
7. Replace plastic cap on mouthpiece.

Care of the Mouthpiece:
The Primatene Mist mouthpiece should be washed once daily with soap and hot water, and rinsed thoroughly. Then it should be dried with a clean, lint-free cloth.
If the unit becomes clogged and fails to spray, please send the clogged unit to:
Whitehall Laboratories
5 Giralda Farms
Madison, N.J. 07940

Inactive Ingredients: Alcohol 34%, Ascorbic Acid, Fluorocarbons (Propellant), Water. Contains No Sulfites.

Warning: Contains CFC 12, 114, substances which harm public health and environment by destroying ozone in the upper atmosphere.

How Supplied:
1/3 Fl. oz. (10 mL) With Mouthpiece.
1/2 Fl. oz. (15 mL) With Mouthpiece.
1/2 Fl. oz. (15 mL) Refill
3/4 Fl. oz. (22.5 mL) Refill
Shown in Product Identification Guide, page 532

PRIMATENE®
[prĭm'a-tēn]
Tablets

Description: Primatene Tablets contain Theophylline Anhydrous 130 mg and Ephedrine Hydrochloride 24 mg.

Indications: For temporary relief of shortness of breath, tightness of chest, and wheezing due to bronchial asthma. Eases breathing for asthma patients by reducing spasms of bronchial muscles.

Warnings: Do not use this product unless a diagnosis of asthma has been made by a doctor. Do not use this product if you have heart disease, high blood pressure, thyroid disease, diabetes or difficulty in urination due to enlargement of the prostate gland unless directed by a doctor. Do not use this product if you have ever been hospitalized for asthma or if you are taking any prescription drug for asthma unless directed by a doctor. **DRUG INTERACTION PRECAUTION:** Do not use this product if you are now taking a prescription monoamine oxidase inhibitor (MAOI) (certain drugs for depression, psychiatric or emotional conditions or Parkinson's disease), or for 2 weeks after stopping the MAOI drug. If you are uncertain whether your prescription drug contains an MAOI, consult a health professional before taking this product. Do not continue to use this product but seek medical assistance immediately if symptoms are not relieved within 1 hour or become worse. Some users of this product may experience nervousness, tremor, sleeplessness, nausea, and loss of appetite. If these symptoms persist or become worse, consult your doctor. As with any drug, if you are pregnant or nursing a baby, seek the advice of a health profes-

Continued on next page

Whitehall—Cont.

sional before using this product. Keep this and all drugs out of the reach of children. In case of accidental overdose, seek professional assistance or contact a poison control center immediately.

Directions: Adults and children 12 years of age and over: 1 tablet initially and then one every 4 hours, as needed, not to exceed 6 tablets in 24 hours. For children under 12 years of age, consult a doctor.

Inactive Ingredients:
Croscarmellose Sodium, D&C Yellow No. 10 Lake, FD&C Yellow No. 6 Lake, Magnesium Stearate, Microcrystalline Cellulose, Silica, Starch, Stearic Acid.

How Supplied: Available in 24 and 60 tablet thermoform blister cartons.
Store at room temperature, between 20°C and 25°C (68°F to 77°F).

Shown in Product Identification Guide, page 532

SEMICID®
[sĕm ′ē-sĭd]
Vaginal Contraceptive Inserts

Indication: For the prevention of pregnancy.

Warnings: DO NOT INSERT SEMICID IN URINARY OPENING (urethra). If you accidentally insert Semicid into the urinary opening, you may have increased burning when urinating, difficulty in starting to urinate, you may also notice a pink color of your urine or have abdominal pain. If these symptoms occur, drink large amounts of water in order to urinate as frequently as possible (even if urinating causes discomfort), and consult your doctor or clinic immediately. If you accidentally insert Semicid into the urinary opening and become aware of this before intercourse, do not proceed with sexual activity. If your doctor has told you that you should not become pregnant, ask your doctor if you can use this product for contraception. Any delay in your menstrual period may be an early sign of pregnancy. If this happens, consult your doctor or clinic as soon as possible. If you or your partner think you have had an allergic reaction to the spermicide (nonoxynol-9) in this product, do not use Semicid. A small number of men and women may be sensitive to nonoxynol-9. Therefore, if you or your partner experience irritation, burning or itching in the genital area, discontinue use. If these symptoms persist, consult your doctor or clinic. If douching is desired, always wait at least 6 hours after intercourse before douching. Keep this and all drugs out of the reach of children. In case of accidental ingestion, seek professional assistance or contact a poison control center immediately.

Directions for Use: BEFORE using Semicid, it is important that you read the package insert carefully for complete instructions and warnings.

FOR USE ALONE OR WITH A CONDOM.
EACH INSERT IS INDIVIDUALLY SEALED FOR YOUR PROTECTION. IF SEAL ON IMPRINTED STRIP IS OPENED WHEN PURCHASED, DO NOT USE.
For best protection against pregnancy, follow these instructions exactly:
1. Separate one insert packet along the perforation from the strip of inserts. To open a single insert packet, hold the packet with the arrows pointed upward, grasp the tab at the top of the packet and tear apart.
2. Use the forefinger and thumb to position the unwrapped insert as deeply as possible into the VAGINAL OPENING, the same opening from which the menstrual flow leaves the body (and where a tampon is placed). EXTREME CARE SHOULD BE TAKEN NOT TO INSERT SEMICID INTO THE URINARY OPENING (URETHRA), the opening from which urine passes out of the body.
3. It is ESSENTIAL that Semicid be inserted at least 15 minutes before intercourse so it can dissolve in the vagina. If intercourse is delayed for more than one (1) hour after insertion or if intercourse is repeated at any time, another insert must be used. It is safe to use Semicid as frequently as needed, however, "Directions for Use" should be carefully followed each time.

Active Ingredients: Each insert contains Nonoxynol-9, 100 mg.

Inactive Ingredients: Benzethonium Chloride, Citric Acid, D&C Red 21 Lake, D&C Red 33 Lake, Methylparaben, Polyethylene Glycol, Water.
How Supplied: Strip Packaging of 9 or 18 inserts.
Keep Semicid at room temperature (not over 86°F or 30°C).

Shown in Product Identification Guide, page 532

TODAY®
[tü-dā]
Vaginal Contraceptive Sponge

Description: Today Vaginal Contraceptive Sponge is a soft polyurethane foam sponge containing nonoxynol-9, a spermicide used by millions of women for over 25 years.
Today Sponge is effective, safe, and convenient. Today Sponge provides 24-hour contraceptive protection without hormones, allowing spontaneity. Today Sponge is easy to use, nonmessy and disposable.

Active Ingredient: Each Today Sponge contains nonoxynol-9, one gram.

Inactive Ingredients: Benzoic acid, citric acid, sodium dihydrogen citrate, sodium metabisulfite, sorbic acid, water in a polyurethane foam sponge.

Indication: For the prevention of pregnancy.

Actions: Used as directed, Today Vaginal Contraceptive Sponge prevents pregnancy in three ways: 1) the spermicide nonoxynol-9 kills sperm before they can reach the egg; 2) Today Sponge traps and absorbs sperm; 3) Today Sponge blocks the cervix so that sperm cannot enter.
Today Sponge is designed for easy insertion into the vagina. It is positioned against the cervix, and while in place provides protection against pregnancy for 24 hours. The soft polyurethane foam sponge is formulated to feel like normal vaginal tissue and has a specially designed ribbon loop attached to an interior web for maximum strength.
In clinical trials of Today Sponge since 1979, in over 1,800 women worldwide who completed over 12,000 cycles of use, the method-effectiveness, i.e., the level of effectiveness seen in women who followed the printed instructions exactly and who used Today Sponge every time that they had intercourse, was 89 to 91%. In women who did not use Today Sponge consistently and properly, the effectiveness was 84 to 87%.

Instructions: For best protection against pregnancy, follow instructions exactly. Remove one Today Sponge from airtight inner pack, wet thoroughly with clean tap water, and squeeze gently several times until it becomes very sudsy. The water activates the spermicide. Fold the sides of Today Sponge upward until it looks long and narrow and then insert it deeply into the vagina with the string loop dangling below. Protection begins immediately and continues for 24 hours. Today Vaginal Contraceptive Sponge must be inserted *before* intercourse begins. Once the penis enters the vagina, there may be leakage of sperm without ejaculation. Once ejaculation occurs, sperm reach the fallopian tubes quickly. It is not necessary to add creams, jellies, foams, or any other additional spermicide as long as Today Sponge is in place, no matter how many acts of intercourse may occur during a 24-hour period. Always wait 6 hours after your last act of intercourse before removing Today Sponge. If you have intercourse when Today Sponge has been in place for 24 hours, it must be left in place an additional 6 hours after intercourse before removing it. It is unlikely that Today Sponge will fall out. During a bowel movement or other form of internal straining, it may be pushed down to the opening of the vagina and perhaps fall out. If you suspect this is happening, simply insert a finger into your vagina and push the sponge back. If it should fall into the toilet, moisten a new sponge and insert it immediately.
To remove Today Sponge, place a finger in the vagina and reach up and back to find the string loop. Hook a finger around the loop. Slowly and gently pull the Sponge out. Difficulty in removing Today Sponge has been reported by a small number of women. If the vaginal muscles seem to be holding it tightly, wait a few minutes and try again. If re-

moval is still difficult, use the following exercise to relax your vaginal muscles: Tighten vaginal muscles as hard as you can and hold for 10 seconds, then relax and let go. Repeat. As you relax, breathe out slowly while bearing down. Now remove the sponge as you continue to relax. If you still have difficulty after reading the instructions for removing the sponge from your vagina or if you remove only a portion of the sponge, contact the Today Talkline (1-800-223-2329) or consult your physician or clinic immediately.

If there is a noticeable odor when you remove the Sponge this is not usually cause for concern. However, discoloration or a foul smell may be an indication of a vaginal infection. If you notice these signs of infection, see your clinic or physician immediately.

Warnings: Some cases of Toxic Shock Syndrome (TSS) have been reported in women using barrier contraceptives including the diaphragm, cervical cap and Today Sponge. Although the occurrence of TSS is uncommon, some studies indicate that there is an increased risk of non-menstrual TSS with the use of barrier contraceptives, including Today Sponge. Today Sponge should not be left in place for more than 30 hours after insertion. If you experience two or more of the warning signs of TSS including fever, vomiting, diarrhea, muscular pain, dizziness, and rash similar to sunburn, consult your physician or clinic immediately. If you have difficulty removing the sponge from your vagina or you remove only a portion of the sponge, contact the Today TalkLine or consult your physician or clinic immediately. Today Sponge should not be used during the menstrual period. After childbirth, miscarriage or other termination of pregnancy, it is important to consult your physician or clinic before using this product. If you have ever had Toxic Shock Syndrome do not use Today Sponge.

A small number of men and women may be sensitive to the spermicide in this product (nonoxynol-9) and should not use this product if irritation occurs and persists. Of the women in the clinical trials, between 2–3% discontinued use of the sponge because of itching, irritation, or rash, and 1–3% discontinued because of allergic reactions. If you or your partner have ever experienced an allergic reaction to the spermicide used in this product, it is best to consult a physician before using Today Vaginal Contraceptive Sponge. If either you or your partner develops burning or itching in the genital area, stop using this product and contact your physician.

A higher degree of protection against pregnancy will be afforded by using another method of contraception in addition to a spermicidal contraceptive. This is especially true during the first few months, until you become familiar with the method. In our clinical studies, approximately one-half of all accidental pregnancies occurred during the first

three months of use. Where avoidance of pregnancy is essential, the choice of contraceptive should be made in consultation with a doctor or a family planning clinic. Any delay in your menstrual period may be an early sign of pregnancy. If this happens, consult your physician or clinic as soon as possible. Keep this and all drugs out of reach of children. In case of accidental ingestion of Today Sponge, call a poison control center, emergency medical facility or doctor. (For most people ingestion of small amounts of the spermicide alone should not be harmful.) As with any drug, if you are pregnant or nursing a baby, seek professional advice before using this product.

How To Store: Store at normal room temperature.

How Supplied: Packages of 3s, 6s, and 12s.

J.B. Williams Company, Inc.
65 HARRISTOWN ROAD
GLEN ROCK, NJ 07452

CĒPACOL®/CĒPACOL MINT
[sē'pǝ-cŏl]
Mouthwash/Gargle

Ingredients: Cēpacol Mouthwash contains: Ceepryn® (cetylpyridinium chloride) 0.05%. Also contains: Alcohol 14%, Edetate Disodium, FD&C Yellow No. 5 (tartrazine) as a color additive, Flavors, Glycerin, Polysorbate 80, Saccharin, Sodium Biphosphate, Sodium Phosphate, and Water.
Cēpacol Mint Mouthwash contains: Ceepryn® (cetylpyridinium chloride) 0.05%. Also contains: Alcohol 14.5%, D&C Yellow No. 10, FD&C Green No. 3, Flavor, Glucono Delta-Lactone, Glycerin, Poloxamer 407, Saccharin Sodium, Sodium Gluconate, and Water.

Actions: Cēpacol/Cēpacol Mint is a soothing, pleasant-tasting mouthwash/gargle. It kills germs that cause bad breath for a fresher, cleaner mouth.
Cēpacol/Cēpacol Mint has a low surface tension, approximately ½ that of water. This property is the basis of the spreading action in the oral cavity as well as its foaming action. Cēpacol/Cēpacol Mint leaves the mouth feeling fresh and clean and helps provide soothing, temporary relief of dryness and minor mouth irritations.

Uses: Recommended as a mouthwash and gargle for daily oral care; as an aromatic mouth freshener to provide a clean feeling in the mouth; as a soothing, foaming rinse to freshen the mouth.
Used routinely before dental procedures, helps give patient confidence of not offending with mouth odor. Often employed as a foaming and refreshing rinse before, during, and after instrumentation and dental prophylaxis. Convenient as a mouth-freshening agent after taking dental impressions. Helpful in reducing

the unpleasant taste and odor in the mouth following gingivectomy.
Used in hospitals as a mouthwash and gargle for daily oral care. Also used to refresh and soothe the mouth following emesis, inhalation therapy, and intubations, and for swabbing the mouths of patients incapable of personal care.

Warning: Keep out of the reach of children. Do not use in children under 6 years of age. If more than a small amount has been accidentally swallowed, seek professional assistance or contact a Poison Control Center.

Directions for Use: Rinse vigorously before or after brushing or any time to freshen the mouth. Particularly useful after meals or before social engagements. Cēpacol/Cēpacol Mint leaves the mouth feeling refreshingly clean.
Use full strength every two or three hours as a soothing, foaming gargle, or as directed by a physician or dentist. May also be mixed with warm water.
Product label directions are as follows: Use full strength. Rinse mouth thoroughly before or after brushing or whenever desired or use as directed by a physician or dentist.

How Supplied:
Cēpacol Mouthwash: 12 oz, 18 oz, 24 oz, and 32 oz. 4 oz trial size.
Shown in Product Identification Guide, page 532

CĒPACOL®
[sē'pǝ-cŏl]
Throat Lozenges
Original, Cherry, Honey-Lemon, Menthol-Eucalyptus Flavors
Anesthetic Lozenges

Ingredients: (per lozenge)

Original: Ceepryn® (cetylpyridinium chloride) 1.4 mg, D&C Yellow No. 10, FD&C Yellow No. 6, Flavor, Glucose, and Sucrose.

Cherry: Active Ingredient: Menthol 3.6 mg. Also contains: Cetylpyridinium Chloride, D&C Red No. 33, FD&C Red No. 40, Flavor, Glucose, and Sucrose.

Honey-Lemon: Active Ingredient: Menthol 3.6 mg. Also contains: Caramel, Cetylpyridinium Chloride, D&C Yellow No. 10, FD&C Yellow No 6. Flavors, Glucose, and Sucrose.

Menthol-Eucalyptus: Active Ingredient: Menthol 5.0 mg. Also contains: Cetylpyridinium Chloride, Eucalyptol, Glucose, and Sucrose.

Anesthetic: Active Ingredient: Benzocaine 10 mg. Also contains Cetylpyridinium Chloride, D&C Yellow No. 10, FD&C Blue No. 2, Flavors, Glucose, and Sucrose.

Actions: Cherry, Honey-Lemon, Menthol-Eucalyptus: Menthol provides a mild anesthetic effect and cooling sensation for symptomatic relief of occasional

Continued on next page

J.B. Williams—Cont.

minor sore throat pain and minor throat irritations. **Anesthetic:** Stimulates salivation to relieve dryness of the mouth and provide a mild anesthetic effect for sore throat pain relief.

Indications: Original: For soothing, temporary relief of dryness of the mouth and throat. **Cherry, Honey-Lemon, Menthol-Eucalyptus and Anesthetic:** For fast, temporary relief of occasional minor sore throat pain and dry, scratchy throat.

Warnings: If sore throat is severe, persists for more than 2 days, is accompanied or followed by fever, headache, rash, nausea, or vomiting, consult a physician promptly. If sore mouth symptoms do not improve in 7 days, see your dentist or physician promptly. Do not administer to children under 6 years of age unless directed by physician or dentist. Keep this and all drugs out of the reach of children. In case of accidental overdose, seek professional assistance or contact a Poison Control Center immediately. As with any drug, if you are pregnant or nursing a baby, seek the advice of a health professional before using this product.

Dosage and Administration: Adults and children 6 years of age and older: Allow product to dissolve slowly in the mouth. May be repeated every 2 hours as needed or as directed by a dentist or physician.

How Supplied:

Trade package:
18 lozenges in 2 pocket packs of 9 each.

Professional package: Original: 648 lozenges in 72 blisters of 9 each. Anesthetic: shelf pack of 324 lozenges in 36 blisters of 9 each.
Store at room temperature, below 86°F (30°C). Protect contents from humidity.
Shown in Product Identification Guide, page 532

Wyeth-Ayerst Laboratories
Division of American Home Products Corporation
P.O. BOX 8299
PHILADELPHIA, PA 19101

Wyeth-Ayerst Tamper-Resistant/Evident Packaging

Statements alerting consumers to the specific type of Tamper-Resistant/Evident Packaging appear on the bottle labels and cartons of all Wyeth-Ayerst over-the-counter products. This includes plastic cap seals on bottles, individually wrapped tablets or suppositories, and sealed cartons. This packaging has been developed to better protect the consumer.

ALUDROX®
[al'ū-drox]
Antacid
(alumina and magnesia)
ORAL SUSPENSION

Composition: *Suspension*—each 5 ml teaspoonful contains 307 mg aluminum hydroxide [Al(OH)$_3$] as a gel and 103 mg of magnesium hydroxide. The inactive ingredients present are artificial and natural flavors, benzoic acid, butylparaben, glycerin, hydroxypropyl methylcellulose, methylparaben, propylparaben, saccharin, simethicone, sorbitol solution, and water. Sodium content is 0.10 mEq per 5 ml suspension.

Indications: For temporary relief of heartburn, upset stomach, sour stomach, and/or acid indigestion.

Directions: *Suspension*—Two teaspoonfuls (10 ml) every 4 hours or as directed by a physician. Medication may be followed by a sip of water if desired.

Warnings: Do not take more than 12 teaspoonfuls (60 ml) of suspension in a 24-hour period or use maximum dosage for more than two weeks except under the advice and supervision of a physician. Prolonged use of aluminum-containing antacids in patients with renal failure may result in or worsen dialysis osteomalacia. Elevated tissue aluminum levels contribute to the development of dialysis encephalopathy and osteomalacia syndromes. Also, a number of cases of dialysis encephalopathy have been associated with elevated aluminum levels in the dialysate water. Small amounts of aluminum are absorbed from the gastrointestinal tract and renal excretion of aluminum is impaired in renal failure. Prolonged use of aluminum-containing antacids in such patients may contribute to increased plasma levels of aluminum. Aluminum is not well removed by dialysis because it is bound to albumin and transferrin, which do not cross dialysis membranes. As a result, aluminum is deposited in bone, and dialysis osteomalacia may develop when large amounts of aluminum are ingested orally by patients with impaired renal function. As with any drug, if you are pregnant or nursing a baby, seek the advice of a health professional before using this product.

Drug Interaction Precautions: Do not take this product if you are presently taking a prescription antibiotic drug containing any form of tetracycline.
Keep at Room Temperature, Approx. 77°F (25°C).
Suspension should be kept tightly closed and shaken well before use. Avoid freezing.
Keep this and all drugs out of the reach of children.

How Supplied: *Oral Suspension*—bottles of 12 fluidounces.
Shown in Product Identification Guide, page 532

Professional Labeling: Consult *1995 Physicians' Desk Reference.*

AMPHOJEL®
[am'fo-jel]
Antacid
(aluminum hydroxide gel)
ORAL SUSPENSION • TABLETS

Composition: *Suspension—Peppermint flavored*—Each teaspoonful (5 mL) contains 320 mg aluminum hydroxide [Al(OH)$_3$] as a gel, and not more than 0.10 mEq of sodium. The inactive ingredients present are calcium benzoate, glycerin, hydroxypropyl methylcellulose, menthol, peppermint oil, potassium butylparaben, potassium propylparaben, saccharin, simethicone, sorbitol solution, and water. *Suspension—Without flavor*—Each teaspoonful (5 mL) contains 320 mg of aluminum hydroxide [Al (OH)$_3$] as a gel. The inactive ingredients present are butylparaben, calcium benzoate, glycerin, hydroxypropyl methylcellulose, methylparaben, propylparaben, saccharin, simethicone, sorbitol solution, and water. *Tablets* are available in 0.3 and 0.6 g strengths. Each contains, respectively, the equivalent of 300 mg and 600 mg aluminum hydroxide as a dried gel. The inactive ingredients present are artificial and natural flavors, cellulose, hydrogenated vegetable oil, magnesium stearate, polacrilin potassium, saccharin, starch, and talc. The 0.3 g (5 grain) strength is equivalent to about 1 teaspoonful of the suspension and the 0.6 g (10 grain) strength is equivalent to about 2 teaspoonfuls. Each 0.3 g tablet contains 0.08 mEq of sodium and each 0.6 g tablet contains 0.13 mEq of sodium.

Indications: For temporary relief of heartburn, upset stomach, sour stomach, and/or acid indigestion.

Directions: *Suspension*—Two teaspoonfuls (10 ml) to be taken five or six times daily, between meals and on retiring or as directed by a physician. Medication may be followed by a sip of water if desired. *Tablets*—Two tablets of the 0.3 g strength, or one tablet of the 0.6 g strength, five or six times daily, between meals and on retiring or as directed by a physician. It is unnecessary to chew the 0.3 g tablet before swallowing with water. After chewing the 0.6 g tablet, sip about one-half glass of water.

Warnings: Do not take more than 12 teaspoonfuls (60 ml) of suspension, or more than twelve (12) 0.3 g tablets, or more than six (6) 0.6 g tablets in a 24-hour period or use this maximum dosage for more than two weeks except under the advice and supervision of a physician. May cause constipation. Prolonged use of aluminum-containing antacids in patients with renal failure may result in or worsen dialysis osteomalacia. Elevated tissue aluminum levels contribute to the development of dialysis encephalopathy and osteomalacia syndromes. Also, a number of cases of dialysis encephalopathy have been associated with elevated aluminum levels in the dialysate water. Small amounts of aluminum are absorbed from the gastrointestinal tract and renal excretion of aluminum is impaired in renal failure. Prolonged use of aluminum-containing antacids in such patients may contribute to increased plasma levels of aluminum. Aluminum is not well removed by dialysis because it is bound to albumin and transferrin, which do not cross dialysis membranes. As a result, aluminum is deposited in bone, and dialysis osteomalacia may develop when large amounts of aluminum are ingested orally by patients with impaired renal function. As with any drug, if you are pregnant or nursing a baby, seek the advice of a health professional before using this product.

Drug Interaction Precaution: Antacids may interact with certain prescription drugs. Do not use this product if you are presently taking a prescription antibiotic containing any form of tetracycline. If you are presently taking a prescription drug, do not take this product without checking with your physician. Keep tightly closed and store at room temperature, Approx. 77°F (25°C). Suspension should be shaken well before use. Avoid freezing. Keep this and all drugs out of the reach of children.

How Supplied: *Suspension*—Peppermint flavored; without flavor—bottles of 12 fluidounces. *Tablets*—a convenient auxiliary dosage form—0.3 g (5 grain) bottles of 100; 0.6 g (10 grain), boxes of 100.

Shown in Product Identification Guide, page 532

Professional Labeling: Consult *1995 Physicians' Desk Reference.*

BASALJEL®
[bā 'sel-jel]
(basic aluminum carbonate gel)
ORAL SUSPENSION • CAPSULES • TABLETS

Composition: *Suspension*—each 5 mL teaspoonful contains basic aluminum carbonate gel equivalent to 400 mg aluminum hydroxide [Al(OH)₃]. The inactive ingredients present are artificial and natural flavors, butylparaben, calcium benzoate, glycerin, hydroxypropyl methylcellulose, methylparaben, mineral oil, propylparaben, saccharin, simethicone, sorbitol solution, and water. *Capsule* contains dried basic aluminum carbonate gel equivalent to 608 mg of dried aluminum hydroxide gel or 500 mg aluminum hydroxide [Al(OH)₃]. The inactive ingredients present are D&C Yellow 10, FD&C Blue 1, FD&C Red 40, FD&C Yellow 6, gelatin, polacrilin potassium, polyethylene glycol, talc, and titanium dioxide. *Tablet* contains dried basic aluminum carbonate gel equivalent to

608 mg of dried aluminum hydroxide gel or 500 mg aluminum hydroxide. The inactive ingredients present are cellulose, hydrogenated vegetable oil, magnesium stearate, polacrilin potassium, starch, and talc.

Indications: For the symptomatic relief of hyperacidity, associated with the diagnosis of peptic ulcer, gastritis, peptic esophagitis, gastric hyperacidity, and hiatal hernia.

Warnings: Do not take more than 24 tablets/capsules/teaspoonsful of BASALJEL in a 24-hour period, or use this maximum dosage for more than two weeks except under the advice and supervision of a physician. Dosage should be carefully supervised since continued overdosage, in conjunction with restriction of dietary phosphorus and calcium, may produce a persistently lowered serum phosphate and a mildly elevated alkaline phosphatase. A usually transient hypercalciuria of mild degree may be associated with the early weeks of therapy. Prolonged use of aluminum-containing antacids in patients with renal failure may result in or worsen dialysis osteomalacia. Elevated tissue aluminum levels contribute to the development of dialysis encephalopathy and osteomalacia syndromes. Also, a number of cases of dialysis encephalopathy have been associated with elevated aluminum levels in the dialysate water. Small amounts of aluminum are absorbed from the gastrointestinal tract and renal excretion of aluminum is impaired in renal failure. Prolonged use of aluminum-containing antacids in such patients may contribute to increased plasma levels of aluminum. Aluminum is not well removed by dialysis because it is bound to albumin and transferrin, which do not cross dialysis membranes. As a result, aluminum is deposited in bone, and dialysis osteomalacia may develop when large amounts of aluminum are ingested orally by patients with impaired renal function. As with any drug, if you are pregnant or nursing a baby, seek the advice of a health professional before using this product.

Dosage and Administration: *Suspension*—two teaspoonsful (10 mL) in water or fruit juice taken as often as every two hours up to twelve times daily. Two teaspoonsful have the capacity to neutralize 23 mEq of acid. *Capsules*—two capsules as often as every two hours up to twelve times daily. Two capsules have the capacity to neutralize 24 mEq of acid. *Tablets*—two tablets as often as every two hours up to twelve times daily. Two tablets have the capacity to neutralize 25 mEq of acid. The sodium content of each dosage form is as follows: 0.13 mEq/5 mL for the suspension, 0.12 mEq per capsule, and 0.12 mEq per tablet.

Precautions: May cause constipation. Adequate fluid intake should be maintained in addition to the specific medical or surgical management indicated by the patient's condition.

Drug Interaction Precaution: Alumina-containing antacids should not be used concomitantly with any form of tetracycline therapy.

How Supplied: Suspension—bottles of 12 fluidounces.
Capsules—bottles of 100 and 500.
Tablets (scored)—bottles of 100.
Shown in Product Identification Guide, page 532

Professional Labeling: Consult *1995 Physicians' Desk Reference.*

BONAMIL®
[bŏn 'ă-mil]
Infant Formula with Iron
• Powder

Bonamil is a casein predominant infant formula intended to meet the nutritional needs of infants and children who are not breastfed and who are not allergic to cow's milk protein and/or intolerant to lactose.
IMPORTANT NOTICE: BREAST MILK IS BEST FOR BABIES. Infant formula is intended to replace or supplement breast milk when breast-feeding is not possible or is insufficient, or when mothers elect not to breast-feed. PROFESSIONAL ADVICE SHOULD BE FOLLOWED ON THE NEED FOR AND PROPER METHOD OF USE OF INFANT FORMULA AND ON ALL MATTERS OF INFANT FEEDING.

Ingredients: NONFAT MILK, LACTOSE, SOYBEAN OIL AND COCONUT OIL, SOY LECITHIN, POTASSIUM BICARBONATE, ASCORBIC ACID, CHOLINE CHLORIDE, FERROUS SULFATE, TAURINE, ALPHA TOCOPHERYL ACETATE, ZINC SULFATE, NIACINAMIDE, CUPRIC SULFATE, VITAMIN A PALMITATE, CALCIUM PANTOTHENATE, THIAMINE HYDROCHLORIDE, RIBOFLAVIN, PYRIDOXINE HYDROCHLORIDE, MANGANESE SULFATE, BETA CAROTENE, FOLIC ACID, PHYTONADIONE, BIOTIN, CHOLECALCIFEROL, CYANOCOBALAMIN.
WHEN DILUTED ACCORDING TO DIRECTIONS, EACH 5 FL. OZ. (150 mL) CONTAINS 100 CALORIES.

NUTRIENTS:	PER 100 Cal	
PROTEIN	2.3	g
FAT	5.4	g
CARBOHYDRATE	10.7	g
WATER	135	g
LINOLEIC ACID	1300	mg
VITAMINS:		
VITAMIN A	300	IU
VITAMIN D	60	IU
VITAMIN E	2.85	IU
VITAMIN K	8	mcg
THIAMINE (VIT. B₁)	100	mcg
RIBOFLAVIN (VIT. B₂)	150	mcg
VITAMIN B₆	63	mcg
VITAMIN B₁₂	0.2	mcg
NIACIN	750	mcg
FOLIC ACID (FOLACIN)	7.5	mcg

Continued on next page

Wyeth-Ayerst—Cont.

PANTOTHENIC ACID	315	mcg
BIOTIN	2.2	mcg
VITAMIN C (ASCORBIC ACID)	8.3	mg
CHOLINE	15	mg

MINERALS:

CALCIUM	69	mg
PHOSPHORUS	54	mg
MAGNESIUM	6	mg
IRON	1.8	mg
ZINC	0.75	mg
MANGANESE	15	mcg
COPPER	70	mcg
IODINE	5	mcg
SODIUM	27	mg
POTASSIUM	93	mg
CHLORIDE	63	mg

Directions For Preparation And Use: Carefully measure and mix formula to avoid health hazards.
Always wash hands before mixing. **Wash and rinse can top before opening.** Clean bottles, nipples, caps, and utensils and boil in water for 5 minutes. Boil additional water for formula for 5 minutes, then let cool to lukewarm temperature. For normal dilution (20 calories per fl. oz.), pour required amount of previously boiled water into nursing bottle(s). Using the measuring scoop enclosed in the can, add one level unpacked scoop (8.3 g) of powder for each 2 fl. oz. (60 mL) of water. Always add the powder to the water. Cap bottle and shake well. **Refrigerate prepared formula and use within 24 hours, warming to body temperature and shaking well before use.** After feeding, discard any remaining formula. To ensure freshness, cover opened can with plastic lid and store in a cool, dry place. DO NOT REFRIGERATE OR FREEZE. Use contents within one month after opening.
Warning: Do not use microwave to prepare or warm formula. Serious burns may occur.
Using standard mixing instructions, 1 lb. (453 g) of powder yields approximately 120 fl. oz. of infant formula (20 calories/fl. oz.).
Questions or Comments:
1-800-999-9384
W-YETH

Shown in Product Identification Guide, page 532

CEROSE®DM
[se-ros 'DM]
Antihistamine/Nasal Decongestant/ Cough Suppressant

Description: Each teaspoonful (5 mL) contains 15 mg dextromethorphan hydrobromide, 4 mg chlorpheniramine maleate, and 10 mg phenylephrine hydrochloride. Alcohol 2.4%. The inactive ingredients present are artificial flavors, citric acid, edetate disodium, FD&C Yellow 6, glycerin, saccharin sodium, sodium benzoate, sodium citrate, sodium propionate, and water.

Indications: For the temporary relief of cough due to minor throat and bronchial irritation as may occur with the common cold or with inhaled irritants. Temporarily relieves nasal congestion, runny nose, and sneezing due to the common cold, hay fever, or other upper respiratory allergies.

Directions: Adults and children 12 years of age and over: One teaspoonful every four hours as needed. Children 6 to under 12 years of age: One-half teaspoonful every four hours as needed. Do not exceed six doses in a 24-hour period. For children under 6 years, consult a doctor.

Drug Interaction Precaution: Do not use this product if you are now taking a prescription monoamine oxidase inhibitor (MAOI) (certain drugs for depression, psychiatric or emotional conditions, or Parkinson's disease), or for 2 weeks after stopping the MAOI drug. If you are uncertain whether your prescription drug contains an MAOI, consult a health professional before taking this product. Do not take this product if you are presently taking a prescription drug for high blood pressure or depression without first consulting your doctor.

Warnings: May cause marked drowsiness; alcohol may increase the drowsiness effect. Avoid alcoholic beverages while taking this product. Use caution when driving a motor vehicle or operating machinery. Do not take this product if you have heart disease, high blood pressure, thyroid disease, diabetes, asthma, glaucoma, emphysema, chronic pulmonary disease, shortness of breath, difficulty in breathing, or difficulty in urination due to enlargement of the prostate gland unless directed by a doctor. This product may cause excitability, especially in children. Do not exceed recommended dosage because at higher doses nervousness, dizziness, or sleeplessness may occur. Do not take this product for more than 7 days. A persistent cough may be a sign of a serious condition. If symptoms persist for more than one week, tend to recur, or are accompanied by fever, rash, or persistent headache, consult a doctor. Do not take this product for persistent or chronic cough such as occurs with smoking, or if cough is accompanied by excessive phlegm (mucus) unless directed by a doctor. As with any drug, if you are pregnant or nursing a baby, seek the advice of a health professional before using this product.

Keep this and all drugs out of the reach of children. In case of accidental overdose, seek professional assistance or contact a Poison Control Center immediately.

How Supplied: Cases of 12 bottles of 4 fl. oz.; bottles of 1 pint.
Keep tightly closed—Store below 77° F (25° C).

Shown in Product Identification Guide, page 532

COLLYRIUM for FRESH EYES
[ko-lir 'e-um]
a neutral borate solution
EYE WASH

Description: Soothing Collyrium Eye Wash for Fresh Eyes is specially formulated to soothe, refresh, and cleanse irritated eyes. Collyrium Eye Wash is a neutral borate solution that contains boric acid, sodium borate, benzalkonium chloride (as a preservative), and water.

Indications: To cleanse the eye, loosen foreign material, air pollutants or chlorinated water.

Recommended Uses:
Home—For emergency flushing of foreign bodies or whenever a soothing eye rinse is necessary.
Hospitals, dispensaries and clinics— For emergency flushing of chemicals or foreign bodies from the eye.

Directions: Remove the eyecup from blister. Puncture bottle by twisting threaded eyecup down onto bottle; then remove it from the bottle. Rinse eyecup with clean water immediately before and after each use. Avoid contamination of rim and interior surface of eyecup. Fill eyecup one-half full with Collyrium Eye Wash. Apply cup tightly to the affected eye to prevent the escape of the liquid and tilt head backward. Open eyelid wide and rotate eyeball to thoroughly wash eye. Rinse cup with clean water after use and recap by twisting threaded eyecup on the bottle for storage.

Warnings: Do not use if solution changes color or becomes cloudy, or with a wetting solution for contact lenses or other eye care products containing polyvinyl alcohol.
This product contains benzalkonium chloride as a preservative. Do not use this product if you are sensitive to benzalkonium chloride.
To avoid contamination do not touch tip of container to any surface. Replace cap after using. If you experience eye pain, changes in vision, continued redness, irritation of the eye, or if the condition worsens or persists, consult a doctor. Obtain immediate medical treatment for all open wounds in or near the eye.
The Collyrium for Fresh Eyes bottle is sealed for your protection. Prior to first use, remove cap and squeeze bottle. If bottle leaks, do not use.
Keep this and all medication out of the reach of children.
Keep bottle tightly closed at Room Temperature, Approx. 77°F (25°C).

How Supplied: Bottles of 4 fl. oz. (118 ml) with eyecup.

Shown in Product Identification Guide, page 533

COLLYRIUM FRESH™
[ko-lir 'e-um]
Sterile Eye Drops
Lubricant
Redness Reliever

Description: Collyrium Fresh is a specially formulated sterile eye drop which can be used, up to 4 times daily, to relieve redness and discomfort due to minor eye irritations caused by dust, smoke, smog, swimming, or sun glare.
The active ingredients are tetrahydrozoline HCl (0.05%) and glycerin (1.0%). Other ingredients include benzalkonium chloride (0.01%) and edetate disodium (0.1%) as preservatives, boric acid, hydrochloric acid and sodium borate.

Indications: For the temporary relief of redness due to minor eye irritations or discomfort due to burning or exposure to wind or sun.

Directions: Tilt head back and squeeze 1 to 2 drops into each eye up to 4 times daily, or as directed by a physician.

Warnings: Do not use if solution changes color or becomes cloudy. Remove contact lenses before using. If you have glaucoma, do not use this product except under the advice and supervision of a physician. Overuse of this product may produce increased redness of the eye. To avoid contamination, do not touch tip of container to any surface. Replace cap after using. If you experience eye pain, changes in vision, continued redness or irritation of the eye, or if the condition worsens or persists for more than 72 hours, discontinue use and consult a physician.
Keep this and all medication out of the reach of children.
Retain carton for complete product information.
Keep bottle tightly closed at Room Temperature, Approx. 77°F (25°C).

How Supplied: Bottles of ½ fl. oz. (15 ml) with built-in eye dropper.
Shown in Product Identification Guide, page 533

DONNAGEL®
[don 'nă-jel]
Liquid and Chewable Tablets

Each tablespoon (15 mL) of **Donnagel Liquid** contains: 600 mg Attapulgite, USP.

Inactive Ingredients: Alcohol 1.4%, Benzyl Alcohol, Carboxymethylcellulose Sodium, Citric Acid, FD&C Blue 1, Flavors, Magnesium Aluminum Silicate, Methylparaben, Phosphoric Acid, Propylene Glycol, Propylparaben, Saccharin Sodium, Sorbitol, Titanium Dioxide, Water, Xanthan Gum.

	Liquid	Chewable Tablets
Adults	2 Tablespoons	2 Tablets
Children		
12 years and over	2 Tablespoons	2 Tablets
6 through 11 years	1 Tablespoon	1 Tablet
3 through 5 years	½ Tablespoon	½ Tablet
Under 3 years	Consult Physician	

Liquid should be shaken well. Tablets should be chewed thoroughly and swallowed.

Each **Donnagel Chewable** Tablet contains: 600 mg Attapulgite, USP.

Inactive Ingredients: D&C Yellow 10 Aluminum Lake, FD&C Blue 1 Aluminum Lake, Flavors, Magnesium Stearate, Mannitol, Saccharin Sodium, Sorbitol, Water.

Indications: Donnagel is indicated for the symptomatic relief of diarrhea. It reduces the number of bowel movements, improves consistency of loose, watery bowel movements and relieves cramping.

Warnings: Patients are told that diarrhea may be serious. They are warned not to use this product for more than 2 days, or in the presence of fever, or in children under 3 years of age unless directed by a physician.
This product should not be taken by patients who are hypersensitive to any of the ingredients. As with any drug, women who are pregnant or nursing a baby should seek the advice of a health professional before using this product.

Dosage and Administration: Full recommended dose should be administered at the first sign of diarrhea and after each subsequent bowel movement, NOT TO EXCEED 7 DOSES IN A 24-HOUR PERIOD.
[See table above.]

How Supplied: Donnagel Liquid (green suspension) in 4 fl. oz. (NDC 0008-0888-02), 8 fl. oz. (NDC 0008-0888-04), and 16 fl. oz. (NDC 0008-0888-05).
Donnagel Chewable Tablets (light-green, flat-faced, beveled-edged, round tablets with darker green flecks; one side engraved "W", obverse engraved Donnagel) in consumer blister packages of 18 (NDC 0008-0889-02.)
Store at Controlled Room Temperature, between 15°C and 30°C (59°F and 86°F).
Shown in Product Identification Guide, page 533

NURSOY®
[nur-soy]
Soy protein isolate formula
READY-TO-FEED
CONCENTRATED LIQUID
POWDER

Breast milk is best for babies. NURSOY® milk-free, lactose-free formula is intended to meet the nutritional needs of infants and children who are not breast-fed and are allergic to cow's milk protein and/or intolerant to lactose. It should not be used in infants and children allergic to soybean protein.

NURSOY Ready-to-Feed and Concentrated Liquid are corn free and contain only sucrose as their carbohydrate.

NURSOY Powder contains corn syrup solids and sucrose as its carbohydrate. Professional advice should be followed.

NURSOY's fat blend closely resembles the fatty acid composition of human milk and has physiologic levels of linoleic and linolenic acid.

NURSOY contains beta-carotene, a component of human milk. The estimated renal solute load of NURSOY is relatively low.

Ingredients (in normal dilution supplying 20 calories per fluidounce): 87% water; 6.7% sucrose; 3.4% oleo, coconut, oleic (safflower) and soybean oils; 2.0% soy protein isolate; and less than 1% of each of the following: potassium citrate; monobasic sodium phosphate; calcium carbonate; dibasic calcium phosphate; magnesium chloride; calcium chloride; soy lecithin; calcium carrageenan; calcium hydroxide; L-methionine; sodium chloride; potassium bicarbonate; taurine; ferrous, zinc, and cupric sulfates; L-carnitine; potassium iodide; ascorbic acid; choline chloride; alpha-tocopheryl acetate; niacinamide; calcium pantothenate; riboflavin; vitamin A palmitate; thiamine hydrochloride; pyridoxine hydrochloride; beta-carotene; phytonadione; folic acid; biotin; cholecalciferol; cyanocobalamin.

PROXIMATE ANALYSIS
at 20 calories per fluidounce
READY-TO-FEED, CONCENTRATED LIQUID, and POWDER

	(W/V)
Protein	1.8 %
Fat	3.6 %
Carbohydrate	6.9 %
Water	87.0 %
Crude fiber ... not more than	0.01 %
Calories/fl. oz.	20

Continued on next page

Wyeth-Ayerst—Cont.

Vitamins, Minerals: In normal dilution, each liter contains:

A	2,000	IU
D$_3$	400	IU
E	9.5	IU
K$_1$	100	mcg
C (ascorbic acid)	55	mg
B$_1$ (thiamine)	670	mcg
B$_2$ (riboflavin)	1000	mcg
B$_6$	420	mcg
B$_{12}$	2	mcg
Niacin	5000	mcg
Pantothenic acid	3000	mcg
Folic acid (folacin)	50	mcg
Choline	85	mg
Inositol	27	mg
Biotin	35	mcg
Calcium	600	mg
Phosphorus	420	mg
Sodium	200	mg
Potassium	700	mg
Chloride	375	mg
Magnesium	67	mg
Manganese	200	mcg
Iron	12.0	mg
Copper	470	mcg
Zinc	5	mg
Iodine	60	mcg

Preparation: *Ready-to-Feed* (32 fl. oz. cans of 20 calories per fluidounce formula)—shake can, open and pour into previously sterilized nursing bottle; attach nipple and feed. Cover opened can and immediately store in refrigerator. Use contents of can within 48 hours of opening.
Prolonged storage of can at excessive temperatures should be avoided.
Expiration date is on top of can.
WARNING: DO NOT USE A MICROWAVE TO PREPARE OR WARM FORMULA. SERIOUS BURNS MAY OCCUR.
Concentrated Liquid —For normal dilution supplying 20 calories per fluidounce, use equal amounts of NURSOY® liquid and cooled, previously boiled water.
Note: Prepared formula should be used within 24 hours.
Prolonged storage of can at excessive temperatures should be avoided.
Expiration date is on top of can.
WARNING: DO NOT USE A MICROWAVE TO PREPARE OR WARM FORMULA. SERIOUS BURNS MAY OCCUR.
Powder —For normal dilution supplying 20 calories per fluidounce, add 1 level measuring scoop to 2 fluidounces of water.
Note: Prepared formula should be used within 24 hours.
Prolonged storage of can at excessive temperatures should be avoided.
Expiration date is on bottom of can.
WARNING: DO NOT USE A MICROWAVE TO PREPARE OR WARM FORMULA. SERIOUS BURNS MAY OCCUR.

How Supplied: *Ready-to-Feed* —presterilized and premixed, 32 fluidounce (1 quart) cans, cases of 6 cans;
Concentrated Liquid —13 fluidounce cans, cases of 12 cans;

Powder —1 pound cans, cases of 6 cans.
Questions or Comments regarding NURSOY: 1-800-99-WYETH.
Shown in Product Identification Guide, page 533

SMA®
Iron fortified
Infant formula
READY–TO–FEED
CONCENTRATED LIQUID
POWDER

Breast milk is best for babies. Infant formula is intended to replace or supplement breast milk when breast feeding is not possible or is insufficient, or when mothers elect not to breast feed.
Good maternal nutrition is important for the preparation and maintenance of breast feeding. Extensive or prolonged use of partial bottle feeding, before breast feeding has been well established, could make breast feeding difficult to maintain. A decision not to breast feed could be difficult to reverse.
Professional advice should be followed on all matters of infant feeding. Infant formula should always be prepared and used as directed. Unnecessary or improper use of infant formula could present a health hazard. Social and financial implications should be considered when selecting the method of infant feeding.
SMA® is close in nutrient composition to human milk with its physiologic fat blend, whey-dominated protein composition, and inclusion of beta-carotene and nucleotides.
SMA, utilizing a hybridized safflower (oleic) oil, became the first infant formula offering fat and calcium absorption closest to that of human milk, with physiologic levels of linoleic acid and linolenic acid. Thus, the fat blend in SMA provides a ready source of energy, helps protect infants against neonatal tetany and produces a ratio of vitamin E to polyunsaturated fatty acids (linoleic acid) more than adequate to prevent hemolytic anemia and yields a serum lipid profile close to that of the breast-fed infant.
By combining reduced minerals whey with skimmed cow's milk, SMA reduces the protein content to fall within the range of human milk, adjusts the whey-protein to casein ratio to that of human milk, and subsequently reduces the mineral content to a physiologic level.
The resultant 60:40 whey-protein to casein ratio provides protein nutrition superior to a casein-dominated formula. In addition, the essential amino acids, including cystine, are present in amounts close to those of human milk. So the protein in SMA is of high biologic value.
Five nucleotides found in higher amounts in human milk compared to infant formula have been added to SMA at the levels found in breast milk.
The physiologic mineral content makes possible a low renal solute load which helps protect the functionally immature

infant kidney, increases expendable water reserves and helps protect against dehydration.
Use of lactose as the carbohydrate results in a physiologic stool flora and a low stool pH, decreasing the incidence of perianal dermatitis.

Ingredients: SMA Concentrated Liquid or Ready-to-Feed. Water; nonfat milk; reduced minerals whey; oleo, coconut, oleic (safflower or sunflower), and soybean oils; lactose; soy lecithin; taurine; cytidine-5'-monophosphate; calcium carrageenan; adenosine-5'-monophosphate; disodium uridine-5'-monophosphate; disodium inosine-5'-monophosphate; disodium guanosine-5'-monophosphate; *Minerals:* Potassium bicarbonate and chloride; calcium chloride and citrate; sodium bicarbonate and citrate; ferrous, zinc, cupric, and manganese sulfates. *Vitamins:* ascorbic acid, alpha tocopheryl acetate, niacinamide, vitamin A palmitate, calcium pantothenate, thiamine hydrochloride, riboflavin, pyridoxine hydrochloride, beta-carotene, folic acid, phytonadione, biotin, cholecalciferol, cyanocobalamin.

SMA Powder. Lactose; oleo, coconut, oleic (safflower or sunflower), and soybean oils; nonfat milk; whey protein concentrate; soy lecithin; taurine; cytidine-5'-monophosphate; adenosine-5'-monophosphate; disodium uridine-5'-monophosphate; disodium inosine-5'-monophosphate; disodium guanosine-5'-monophosphate. *Minerals:* Potassium phosphate; calcium hydroxide; magnesium chloride; calcium chloride; sodium bicarbonate; ferrous sulfate; potassium hydroxide; potassium bicarbonate; zinc, cupric, and manganese sulfates; potassium iodide. *Vitamins:* Ascorbic acid, choline chloride, inositol, alpha tocopheryl acetate, niacinamide, calcium pantothenate, vitamin A palmitate, riboflavin, thiamine hydrochloride, pyridoxine hydrochloride, beta-carotene, folic acid, phytonadione, biotin, cholecalciferol, cyanocobalamin.

PROXIMATE ANALYSIS
at 20 calories per fluidounce
READY-TO-FEED, POWDER, and
CONCENTRATED LIQUID:

	(W/V)
Fat	3.6 %
Carbohydrate	7.2 %
Protein	1.5 %
60% Lactalbumin (whey protein)	0.9 %
40% Casein	0.6 %
Crude Fiber	None
Total Solids	12.6 %
Calories/fl. oz.	20

Vitamins, Minerals: In normal dilution, each liter contains:

A	2000	IU
D$_3$	400	IU
E	9.5	IU
K$_1$	55	mcg
C (ascorbic acid)	55	mg
B$_1$ (thiamine)	670	mcg
B$_2$ (riboflavin)	1000	mcg
B$_6$	420	mcg
(pyridoxine hydrochloride)		

B₁₂	1.3	mcg
Niacin	5000	mcg
Pantothenic Acid	2100	mcg
Folic Acid (folacin)	50	mcg
Choline	100	mg
Biotin	15	mcg
Calcium	420	mg
Phosphorus	280	mg
Sodium	150	mg
Potassium	560	mg
Chloride	375	mg
Magnesium	45	mg
Manganese	100	mcg
Iron	12	mg
Copper	470	mcg
Zinc	5	mg
Iodine	60	mcg

Preparation: *Ready-to-Feed* (8 and 32 fl. oz. cans of 20 calories per fluid-ounce formula)—shake can, open and pour into previously sterilized nursing bottle; attach nipple and feed immediately. Cover opened can and immediately store in refrigerator. Use contents of can within 48 hours of opening.
Prolonged storage of can at excessive temperatures should be avoided.
Expiration date is on top of can.
WARNING: DO NOT USE A MICRO-WAVE TO PREPARE OR WARM FORMULA. SERIOUS BURNS MAY OCCUR.
Powder—(1 pound and 2 pound 3 ounce cans)—For normal dilution supplying 20 calories per fluidounce, use 1 level measuring scoop to 2 fluidounces of cooled, previously boiled water.
Prolonged storage of can of powder at excessive temperatures should be avoided.
Expiration date is on bottom of can.
WARNING: DO NOT USE A MICRO-WAVE TO PREPARE OR WARM FORMULA. SERIOUS BURNS MAY OCCUR.
Concentrated Liquid—For normal dilution supplying 20 calories per fluidounce, use equal amounts of SMA® liquid and cooled, previously boiled water.
Prolonged storage of can at excessive temperatures should be avoided.
Expiration date is on top of can.
WARNING: DO NOT USE A MICRO-WAVE TO PREPARE OR WARM FORMULA. SERIOUS BURNS MAY OCCUR.
Note: Prepared formula should be used within 24 hours.

How Supplied: *Ready-to-Feed*—pre-sterilized and premixed, 32 fluidounce (1 quart) cans, cases of 6 cans; 8 fluidounce cans, cases of 24 (4 carriers of 6 cans). *Powder*—1 pound and 2 pound 3 ounce cans with measuring scoop, cases of 6 cans. *Concentrated Liquid*—13 fluidounce cans, cases of 24 cans.
Also Available: SMA® lo-iron. Those who appreciate the particular advantages of SMA® infant formula, close in nutrient composition to mother's milk, sometimes need or wish to recommend a formula that does not contain a high level of iron. SMA® lo-iron has all the benefits of regular SMA® but with a reduced level of iron of 1.4 mg per quart.

Infants should receive supplemental dietary iron from an outside source to meet daily requirements.
Concentrated Liquid—13 fl. oz. cans, cases of 12 cans. *Powder*—1 pound cans with measuring scoop, cases of 6 cans. *Ready-to-Feed*—32 fl. oz. cans, cases of 6 cans.
Preparation of the standard 20 calories per fluidounce formula of SMA® lo-iron is the same as SMA® iron fortified given above.
Questions or Comments regarding SMA: 1-800-99-WYETH.
Shown in Product Identification Guide, page 533

STUART PRENATAL® Tablets
Multivitamin/Multimineral
Supplement

One Tablet Daily Provides
VITAMINS

A*	4,000 IU
D	400 IU
E	11 mg
C	100 mg
Folic Acid	0.8 mg
B₁	1.84 mg
(thiamin mononitrate)	
B₂	1.7 mg
(riboflavin)	
Niacinamide	18 mg
B₆	2.6 mg
(pyridoxine hydrochloride)	
B₁₂	4 mcg
(cyanocobalamin)	

MINERALS

Calcium	200 mg
Iron	60 mg
Zinc	25 mg
(zinc oxide)	

---

*Input as vitamin A acetate and beta carotene. STUART PRENATAL contains no added dyes, flavors or sweeteners.

Ingredients
Each tablet contains:
Active: calcium sulfate, ferrous fumarate, ascorbic acid, dl-alpha tocopheryl acetate, zinc oxide, niacinamide, vitamin A acetate, beta carotene, pyridoxine hydrochloride, riboflavin, thiamin mononitrate, folic acid, cholecalciferol, cyanocobalamin. Inactive: croscarmellose sodium, hydroxypropyl methylcellulose, microcrystalline cellulose, pregelatinized starch, red iron oxide, titanium dioxide.

Indications: STUART PRENATAL is a nonprescription multivitamin/multimineral supplement for use before, during, and after pregnancy. It provides essential vitamins and minerals, including 60 mg of elemental iron as well-tolerated ferrous fumarate, and 200 mg of elemental calcium (nonalkalizing and phosphorus-free), and 25 mg zinc. STUART PRENATAL also contains 0.8 mg folic acid.

Directions: Before, during and after pregnancy, one tablet daily, or as directed by a physician.

Warning: As with all medications keep out of the reach of children. In case of accidental overdose, seek professional assistance or contact a Poison Control Center immediately.

How Supplied: Bottles of 100 light pink tablets imprinted "Wyeth 794". A child-resistant safety cap is standard on 100 tablet bottles as a safeguard against accidental ingestion by children.
NDC 0008-0794-01.
Shown in Product Identification Guide, page 533

WYANOIDS® Relief Factor
[*wi′a-noids*]
Hemorrhoidal Suppositories

Description: Active Ingredients: Cocoa Butter 79% and Shark Liver Oil 3%. **Inactive Ingredients:** Ascorbyl Palmitate, Benzoic Acid, BHA, Corn Oil, Edetate Disodium, Glycerin, Methylparaben, PEG-12 Dilaurate, Propylparaben, Tocopherol, Water, White Wax.

Indications: Gives temporary relief of the itching, discomfort and burning associated with hemorrhoids and protects irritated areas.

Directions: *Adults*—When practical, cleanse the affected area by patting or blotting with an appropriate cleansing pad. Gently dry by patting or blotting with toilet tissue or a soft cloth before application of this product. Remove wrapper before inserting into the rectum. Insert one suppository into the rectum up to 6 times daily or after each bowel movement. *Children under 12 years of age*—Consult a doctor.

Warnings: In case of bleeding or if the condition worsens or does not improve within 7 days, the patient should consult a physician promptly. Keep this and all medicines out of the reach of children. In case of accidental ingestion, seek professional assistance or contact a Poison Control Center immediately. As with any drug, if you are pregnant or nursing a baby, seek the advice of a health professional before using this product.
Do not store above 80°F.
Do Not Use if Cellophane Safety Tear Strip is Missing or Cellophane Safety Wrap is Broken or Missing When Purchased.

How Supplied: Boxes of 12.
Shown in Product Identification Guide, page 533

EDUCATIONAL MATERIAL

Audiovisual Programs
The **Wyeth-Ayerst Audiovisual Catalog,** listing audiovisual programs available through the Wyeth-Ayerst Audiovisual Library or on loan through the

Continued on next page

Wyeth-Ayerst—Cont.

local Wyeth-Ayerst representative, can be obtained by writing Professional Service, Wyeth-Ayerst Laboratories, P.O. Box 8299, Philadelphia, PA 19101.

Zila Pharmaceuticals, Inc.
5227 NORTH 7th STREET PHOENIX, AZ 85014-2817

ZILACTIN® Medicated Gel
ZILACTIN®-L Liquid
ZILACTIN®-B Medicated Gel
with Benzocaine
DERMAFLEX® Topical Anesthetic Gel Coating

Description: **Zilactin** Medicated Gel stops pain and speeds healing of canker sores, fever blisters and cold sores. Zilactin forms a tenacious, occlusive film which holds the medication in place while controlling pain. Intra-orally, the film can last up to 8 hours, usually allowing pain-free eating and drinking. Extra-orally, the film will last much longer.

Zilactin-L is a non film-forming liquid that treats and relieves the pain, itching and burning of developing and existing cold sores and fever blisters. Zilactin-L is specially formulated to treat the initial signs of tingling, itching or burning that signal an oncoming cold sore or fever blister. Zilactin-L can often prevent developing cold sores or fever blisters from breaking out. If a lesion does occur, Zilactin-L will significantly reduce the size and the duration of the outbreak.

Zilactin-B is a medicated gel containing benzocaine that forms a smooth, flexible and occlusive film on the oral mucosa. It's specially formulated to control pain and shield the mouth sores, canker sores, cheek bites and gum sores that occur from dental appliances from the environment of the mouth. The film can last up to 8 hours.

DermaFlex is a topical anesthetic gel "bandage" that provides temporary relief from and protects minor skin irritations including the pain and itching associated with scrapes, minor cuts, insect bites and minor rashes. DermaFlex forms a flexible, invisible, waterproof bandage which holds the active ingredient (pain relieving lidocaine) in place for hours while protecting the affected skin.
Clinical studies on the effectiveness of Zila's products are available on request.

Active Ingredients: **Zilactin**—Benzyl Alcohol (10%); **Zilactin-L**—Lidocaine (2.5%); **Zilactin-B**—Benzocaine (10%); **DermaFlex**—Lidocaine (2.5%)

Application: **Zilactin:** FOR USE IN THE MOUTH AND ON LIPS. Apply every four hours for the first three days and then as needed. Dry the affected area. Apply a thin coat of Zilactin and allow 60 seconds for the gel to dry into a film. Outside the mouth, Zilactin forms a transparent film. Inside the mouth, the film is white.

Zilactin-L: FOR USE ON THE LIPS AND AROUND THE MOUTH. Apply every 1-2 hours for the first three days and then as needed. For maximum effectiveness use at first signs of tingling or itching. Moisten a cotton swab with several drops of Zilactin-L. Apply on lip area where symptoms are noted or directly on existing cold sore or fever blister and allow to dry for 15 seconds.

Zilactin-B: FOR USE IN THE MOUTH. Apply every four hours for the first three days and then as needed. Dry the affected area. Apply a thin coat of Zilactin-B and allow 60 seconds for the gel to dry into a film.

DermaFlex: FOR EXTERNAL USE. Apply as needed (not more than 3-4 times daily). Dry the affected area. Apply a thin coat of DermaFlex and allow 60 sec-

onds for the gel to dry into a transparent film. Apply a thin second coat and allow it to dry. Additional coats are applied directly over existing film bandage.

Warning: A mild, temporary stinging sensation may be experienced when applying Zilactin, Zilactin-L, Zilactin-B or DermaFlex to an open cut, sore or blister. This may be minimized by first applying ice for a minute before application of the medication. DO NOT USE IN OR NEAR EYES. In the event of accidental contact with the eye, flush with water immediately and continuously for ten minutes. Seek immediate medical attention if pain or irritation persists. For temporary relief only. As with all medications, keep out of the reach of children. Do not use Zilactin-L, Zilactin-B, or DermaFlex if you have a history of allergy to local anesthetics such as benzocaine, lidocaine or other "caine" anesthetics.

How Supplied: Zila products are non-prescription and carried by most drug wholesalers, retail chains and independent pharmacies. Each product is available to physicians and dentists directly from Zila in single use packages.

For further information call or write:
Zila Pharmaceuticals, Inc.
5227 N. 7th Street, Phoenix, AZ 85014-2817, (602) 266-6700

U.S. patent numbers 4,285,934; 4,381,296; 5,081,157 and 5,081,158
Shown in Product Identification Guide, page 533

EDUCATIONAL MATERIAL

Samples and literature are available to medical professionals on request.

DRUG INFORMATION CENTERS

For additional information on overdosage, adverse reactions, drug interactions, and any other medication problem, specialized drug information centers are strategically located throughout the nation. Use the directory that follows to find the center nearest you. Listings are alphabetical by state and city.

ALABAMA

BIRMINGHAM
Drug Information Service University of Alabama Hospital
619 S. 19th St.
Birmingham, AL 35233
Mon.-Fri. 8 AM-5 PM
Tel.: 205-934-2162
Fax: 205-934-3501

Global Drug Information Center Samford University School of Pharmacy
800 Lakeshore Dr.
Birmingham, AL 35229
Mon.-Fri. 8 AM-4:30 PM
Tel.: 205-870-2891
Fax: 205-870-2016

HUNTSVILLE
Huntsville Hospital Drug Information Center
101 Sivley Rd.
Huntsville, AL 35801
Mon.-Fri. 8 AM-5 PM
Tel.: 205-517-8288
Fax: 205-517-6558

ARIZONA

TUCSON
Arizona Poison and Drug Information Center Arizona Health Sciences Center University Medical Center
1501 N. Campbell Ave.
Room 1156
Tucson, AZ 85724
7 days/week, 24 hours
Tel.: 602-626-6016
       800-362-0101 (AZ)
Fax: 602-626-2720

ARKANSAS

LITTLE ROCK
Arkansas Poison and Drug Information Center College of Pharmacy-UAMS
4301 W. Markham St.
Little Rock, AR 72205
7 days/week, 24 hours
Tel.: 800-376-4766 (AR)
Fax: 501-686-7357

CALIFORNIA

LOS ANGELES
Los Angeles Regional Drug & Poison Information Center LAC & USC Medical Center
1200 N. State St.
RM 1107 A & B
Los Angeles, CA 90033
7 days/week, 24 hours
Tel: 213-226-2622
       800-777-6476 (CA)
Fax: 213-226-4194

SAN DIEGO
Drug Information Analysis Service Veterans Administration Medical Center
3350 La Jolla Village Dr.
San Diego, CA 92161
Mon.-Fri. 8 AM-4:30 PM
Tel.: 619-552-8585
Fax: 619-552-7452

Drug Information Center U.S. Naval Hospital
34800 Bob Wilson Dr.
San Diego, CA 92134
Mon.-Fri. 8 AM-4 PM
Tel.: 619-532-8414

Drug Information Service University of California San Diego Medical Center
200 West Arbor Dr.
San Diego, CA 92103
Mon.-Fri. 9 AM-5 PM
Tel.: 1-900-288-8273
Fax: 619-692-1867

SAN FRANCISCO
Drug Information Analysis Service University of California
P.O. Box 0622
San Francisco, CA 94143
Mon.-Fri. 8 AM-5 PM
Tel.: 415-476-4346

SANTA MONICA
Drug Information Services St. Johns Hospital and Health Center
1328 22nd St.
Santa Monica, CA 90404
Mon.-Fri. 24 hours
Tel.: 310-829-8243
       310-829-8250
       (after hours)

STANFORD
Drug Information Center Stanford University Hospital Dept. of Pharmacy H0301
300 Pasteur Dr.
Stanford, CA 94305
Mon.-Fri. 9 AM-5 PM
Tel.: 415-723-6422
Fax: 415-725-5028

COLORADO

DENVER
Rocky Mountain Drug Consultation Center
645 Bannock St.
Denver, CO 80204
Mon.-Fri. 8:30 AM-4 PM
Tel.: 303-893-3784
Fax: 303-623-1119
Outside Denver County
900-285-3784
$2.95 first minute
$1.95 each additional minute

Drug Information Center University of Colorado Health Science Center
4200 E. 9th Ave.
Campus Box C239
Denver, CO 80262
Mon.-Fri. 8:30 AM-4:30 PM
Tel.: 303-270-8489
Fax: 303-270-3353

CONNECTICUT

FARMINGTON
Drug Information Service University of Connecticut Health Center
263 Farmington Ave.
Farmington, CT 06030
Mon.-Fri. 8 AM-4:30 PM
Tel.: 203-679-2783

HARTFORD
Drug Information Center Hartford Hospital
P.O. Box 5037
80 Seymour St.
Hartford, CT 06102
Mon.-Fri. 8:30 AM-5 PM
Tel.: 203-545-2221
       203-545-2961 (after hours)
Fax: 203-545-2415

NEW HAVEN

Drug Information Center
Yale-New Haven Hospital
20 York St.
New Haven, CT 06504
Mon.-Fri. 8:15 AM-4:45 PM
Tel.: 203-785-2248
Fax: 203-737-4229

DISTRICT OF COLUMBIA

Drug Information Center
Washington Hospital
Center
110 Irving St., NW
Washington, DC 20010
Mon.-Fri. 7:30 AM-4 PM
Tel.: 202-877-6646
Fax: 202-877-5428

Drug Information Service
Howard University
Hospital
2041 Georgia Ave. NW
Washington, DC 20060
Mon.-Fri. 9 AM-5 PM
Tel.: 202-865-1325
Fax: 202-745-3731

FLORIDA

GAINESVILLE

Drug Information &
Pharmacy Resource
Center
Shands Hospital at
University of Florida
P.O.Box 100316
Gainesville, FL 32610
Mon.-Fri. 9 AM-5 PM
Tel.: 904-395-0408
Fax: 904-338-9860
For healthcare
professionals only.

JACKSONVILLE

Drug Information Service
University Medical Center
655 W. 8th St.
Jacksonville, FL 32209
Mon.-Fri. 8 AM-5 PM
Tel.: 904-549-4095
Fax: 904-549-4272

MIAMI

Drug Information
Center (119)
Miami VA Medical Center
1201 NW 16th St.
Miami, FL 33125
Mon.-Fri. 7:30 AM-4:00 PM
Tel.: 305-324-3237
Fax: 305-324-3386

NORTH MIAMI BEACH

Drug Information Service
NOVA/Southeastern
University of the Health
Sciences
1750 NE 168th St.
N. Miami Beach, FL 33162
Mon.-Fri. 9 AM-5 PM
Tel.: 305-948-8255

GEORGIA

ATLANTA

Emory University Hospital
Dept. of Pharmaceutical
Services
1364 Clifton Rd. NE
Atlanta, GA 30322
Mon.-Fri. 8:30 AM-5 PM
Tel.: 404-727-4644
Fax: 404-727-3302

Drug Information Service
Northside Hospital
1000 Johnson Ferry Rd.
Atlanta, GA 30342
Mon.-Fri. 9 AM-4 PM
Tel.: 404-851-8676
Fax: 404-851-8682

Drug Information Center
Grady Memorial Hospital
and Mercer University
80 Butler St., SE
P.O. Box 26041
Atlanta, GA 30335-3801
Mon.-Fri. 8 AM-4 PM
Tel.: 404-616-7725
Fax: 404-616-7727

AUGUSTA

Drug Information Center
University of Georgia
Medical College of GA
Rm. BIW201
1120 15th St.
Augusta, GA 30912-5600
Mon.-Fri. 8:30 AM-5 PM
Tel.: 706-721-2887
Fax: 706-721-3827

IDAHO

POCATELLO

Idaho Drug Information
Service
Box 8092
Pocatello, ID 83209
Mon.-Fri. 8 AM-5 PM
Tel.: 208-236-4689
Fax: 208-236-4687

ILLINOIS

BLOOMINGTON

Drug Information Center
BroMenn Life Care Center
807 N. Main St.
Bloomington, IL 61701
7 days/week, 24 hours
Tel.: 309-829-0755
Fax: 309-829-0760

CHICAGO

Drug Information Center
Northwestern
Memorial Hospital
250 E. Superior St.
Wesley 153
Chicago, IL 60611
Mon.-Fri. 8:30 AM-5 PM
Tel.: 312-908-7573
Fax: 312-908-7956

Flo Manzano
Director of Pharmacy
Services
Saint Joseph Hospital
2900 N. Lake Shore Dr.
Chicago, IL 60657
Tel.: 312-665-3140

Drug Information Services
University of Chicago
5841 S. Maryland Ave.
MC 0010
Chicago, IL 60637
Mon.-Fri. 8 AM-5 PM
Tel.: 312-702-1388
Fax: 312-702-6631

Drug Information Center
University of Illinois
at Chicago
Room C300, MC 883
1740 W. Taylor St.
Chicago, IL 60612
Mon.-Fri. 8 AM-4 PM
Tel.: 312-996-0209
Fax: 312-996-0906

HARVEY

Drug Information Center
Ingalls Memorial Hospital
1 Ingalls Dr.
Harvey, IL 60426
Mon.-Fri. 8 AM-4:30 PM
Tel.: 708-333-2300
x 4430
Fax: 708-210-3108

HINES

Drug Information Service
Hines Veterans
Administration Hospital
Inpatient Pharmacy
(119B)
Hines, IL 60141
Mon.-Fri. 8 AM-4 PM
Tel.: 708-343-7200

PARK RIDGE

Drug Information Center
Lutheran General Hospital
1775 Dempster St.
Park Ridge, IL 60068
Mon.-Fri. 7:30 AM-4 PM
Tel.: 708-696-8128

ROCKFORD

Drug Information Center
Swedish-American
Hospital
1400 Charles St.
Rockford, IL 61104
7 days/week, 24 hours
Tel.: 815-968-4400
x 4577, 4800

INDIANA

INDIANAPOLIS

Drug Information Center
St. Vincent Hospital and
Health Services
2001 W. 86th St.
P.O. Box 40970
Indianapolis, IN 46240
Mon.-Fri. 8 AM-4 PM
Tel: 317-338-3200

Indiana University Medical
Center/Pharmacy
Dept. UH1410
550 N. University Blvd.
Indianapolis, IN 46202
Mon.-Fri. 8 AM-4:30 PM
Tel.: 317-274-3581
Fax: 317-274-2327

IOWA

DES MOINES

Drug Information Center
Mercy Hospital Medical
Center
400 University Ave.
Des Moines, IA 50314
Mon.-Fri. 8 AM-4:30 PM
Tel.: 515-247-3286
Fax: 515-247-3966

Mid-Iowa Poison and Drug
Information Center
Iowa Methodist Medical
Center
1200 Pleasant St.
Des Moines, IA 50309
7 days/week, 24 hours
Tel.: 515-241-6254
800-362-2327 (IA)
Fax: 515-241-5085

IOWA CITY

Drug Information Center
University of Iowa
Hospital and Clinics
200 Hawkins Dr.
Iowa City, IA 52242
Mon.-Fri. 8 AM-5 PM
Tel.: 319-356-2600

KANSAS

KANSAS CITY

Drug Information Center
University of Kansas
Medical Center
3901 Rainbow Blvd.
Kansas City, KS 66160
Mon.-Fri. 8:30 AM-4:30 PM
Tel.: 913-588-2328

KENTUCKY

LEXINGTON

Drug Information Center
Chandler Medical Center
College of Pharmacy
University of Kentucky
800 Rose St., C-117
Lexington, KY 40536
Mon.-Fri. 8 AM-5 PM
Tel.: 606-323-5320
Fax: 606-323-2049

LOUISIANA

MONROE

Drug Information Center
St. Francis Medical
Center
309 Jackson St.
Monroe, LA 71201
7 days/week, 24 hours
Tel.: 318-327-4250
Fax: 318-327-4125

NEW ORLEANS

Xavier University Drug
Information Center
Tulane Medical Center
Hospital and Clinic
Box #C12
1415 Tulane Ave.
New Orleans, LA 70112
Mon.-Fri. 9 AM-5 PM
Tel.: 504-588-5670
Fax: 504-588-5862

MARYLAND

ANDREWS AFB

Drug Information Services
89th Med Gp/SGSAP
1050 W. Perimeter Rd.
Suite B1-39
Andrews AFB, MD 20331
Mon.-Fri. 7:30 AM-6 PM
Tel.: 301-981-4209
Fax: 301-981-4544

ANNAPOLIS

Drug Information Services
The Anne Arundel
Medical Center
Franklin & Cathedral
Streets
Annapolis, MD 21401
7 days/week, 24 hours
Tel.: 410-267-1130
          410-267-1000
Fax: 410-267-1628

BALTIMORE

Drug Information Center
Franklin Square
Hospital Center
9000 Franklin Square Dr.
Baltimore, MD 21237
Mon.-Fri. 8 AM-4:30 PM
Tel.: 410-682-7700
          410-682-7374
          (after hours)

Drug Information Service
Johns Hopkins
Medical Center
600 N. Wolfe St.
Halstead 503
Baltimore, MD 21287
Mon.-Fri. 8:30 AM-5 PM
Tel.: 410-955-6348
Fax: 410-955-8283

Drug Information Center
University of Maryland
at Baltimore
School of Pharmacy
Baltimore, MD 21201
Mon.-Fri. 8:30 AM-5 PM
Tel.: 410-706-7568
Fax: 410-706-7184

BETHESDA

Drug Information Service
Pharmacy Department
Warren G. Magnuson
Clinical Center National
Institutes of Health
9000 Rockville Pike
(Bldg.10)
Bethesda, MD 20892
Mon.-Fri. 8:30 AM-5 PM
Tel.: 301-496-2407
Fax: 301-496-0210

EASTON

Drug Information Center
Memorial Hospital
219 S. Washington St.
Easton, MD 21601
7 days/week, 24 hours
Tel.: 410-822-1000
          x 5645
Fax: 410-822-4958

MASSACHUSETTS

BOSTON

Drug Information Service
Brigham and Women's
Hospital
75 Frances St.
Boston, MA 02115
Mon.-Fri. 7 AM-3:30 PM
Tel.: 617-732-7166
Fax: 617-566-2396

Drug Information Service
New England Medical
Center Pharmacy
750 Washington St.
Box 420
Boston, MA 02111
Mon.-Fri. 8 AM-4:30 PM
Tel.: 617-956-5380
Fax: 617-956-5638

WORCESTER

Drug Information Center
U.M.M.C. Hospital
55 Lake Ave. North
Worcester, MA 01605
Mon.-Fri. 8:30 AM-5 PM
Tel.: 508-856-3456
          508-856-2775
Fax: 508-856-1850

MICHIGAN

ANN ARBOR

Drug Information Service
University of Michigan
Medical Center
1500 East Medical Center
Dr.
UHB2 D301 Box 0008
Ann Arbor, MI 48109
Mon.-Fri. 8 AM-5 PM
Tel.: 313-936-8200
          313-936-8251
          (after hours)
Fax: 313-936-7027

DETROIT

Drug Information Center
Henry Ford Hospital
2799 W. Grand Blvd.
Detroit, MI 48202
Mon.-Fri. 8 AM-5 PM
Tel.: 313-876-1229
Fax: 313-876-1302

Drug Information Services
Harper Hospital
3990 John R. St.
Detroit, MI 48201
Mon.-Fri. 8 AM-5 PM
Tel.: 313-745-2006
          313-745-8638
          (after hours)

LANSING

Drug Information Center
Sparrow Hospital
1215 E. Michigan Ave.
Lansing, MI 48912
Mon.-Fri. 8 AM-4:30 PM
Tel.: 517-483-2444
Fax: 517-483-2088

PONTIAC

Drug Information Center
St. Joseph Mercy Hospital
900 Woodward
Pontiac, MI 48341
Mon.-Fri. 8 AM-4:30 PM
Tel.: 810-858-3055
Fax: 810-858-6036

ROYAL OAK

Drug Information Services
William Beaumont
Hospital
3601 West 13 Mile Rd.
Royal Oak, MI 48073
Mon.-Fri. 8 AM-4:30 PM
Tel.: 810-551-4077
Fax: 810-551-2426

SOUTHFIELD

Drug Information Service
Providence Hospital
16001 West 9 Mile Rd.
P.O. Box 2043
Southfield, MI 48075
Mon.-Fri. 8 AM-4:30 PM
Tel.: 810-424-3125
Fax: 810-424-5364

MINNESOTA

ROCHESTER

Drug Information Center
St. Mary's Hospital
1216 2nd St., SW
Rochester, MN 55902
Mon.-Fri. 8 AM-5 PM
Tel.: 507-255-5062
          507-255-5732
          (after hours)
Fax: 507-255-7556

ST. PAUL

Drug Information Service
United Hospital and
Children's Hospital of
St. Paul
333 N. Smith Ave.
St. Paul, MN 55102
Mon.-Fri. 9 AM-5 PM
Tel.: 612-220-8566
Fax: 612-220-5323

MISSISSIPPI

JACKSON

Drug Information Center
University of Mississippi
Medical Center
2500 N. State St.
Jackson, MS 39216
Mon.-Fri. 8 AM-5 PM
(on call 24 hours)
Tel.: 601-984-2060
Fax: 601-984-2063

MISSOURI

SPRINGFIELD

Drug Information &
Clinical Research Services
1235 E. Cherokee
Springfield, MO 65804
Mon.-Fri. 7:30 AM-4:30 PM
Tel.: 417-885-3488
Fax: 417-888-7788

ST. JOSEPH

Drug Information Service
Heartland Hospital West
801 Faraon St.
St. Joseph, MO 64501
7 days/week, 7 AM-10 PM
Tel.: 816-271-7582
Fax: 816-271-7590

NEBRASKA

OMAHA

Drug Information Service
School of Pharmacy
Creighton University
2500 California Plaza
Omaha, NE 68178
Mon.-Fri. 8:30 AM-4:30 PM
Tel.: 402-280-5101
Fax: 402-280-5147

Drug Information and
Education Services
University of Nebraska
Medical Center
600 S. 42nd St.
Omaha, NE 68198-1090
Mon.-Fri. 8 AM-4:30 PM
Tel.: 402-559-4114
Fax: 402-559-4907

NEW HAMPSHIRE

LEBANON

Drug Information Center
Dartmouth-Hitchcock
Medical Center
1 Medical Center Dr.
Lebanon, NH 03756
Mon.-Fri. 7:30 AM-4 PM
Tel.: 603-650-5590

NEW MEXICO

ALBUQUERQUE

New Mexico Poison &
Drug Information Center
University of New Mexico
Albuquerque, NM 87131
7 days/week, 24 hours
Tel.: 505-843-2551
    800-432-6866 (NM)
Fax: 505-277-5892

NEW YORK

BRONX

Drug Information Center
Dept. of Pharmacy
RM BN32
Bronx Municipal
Hospital Center
Pelham Pkwy. South and
Eastchester Rd.
Bronx, NY 10461
Mon.-Fri. 9 AM-5 PM
Tel.: 718-918-4556
Fax: 718-918-7848

BROOKLYN

International Drug
Information Center
Long Island University
Arnold & Marie Schwartz
College of Pharmacy
1 University Plaza
Brooklyn, NY 11201
Mon.-Fri. 9 AM-5 PM
Tel.: 718-488-1064

BUFFALO

Drug Information Center
Erie County Medical
Center
462 Grider St.
Buffalo, NY 14215
Mon.-Fri. 8 AM-5 PM
Tel.: 716-898-3000
For healthcare
professionals only.

COOPERSTOWN

Drug Information Center
The Mary Imogene
Bassett Hospital
1 Atwell Rd.
Cooperstown, NY 13326
Mon.-Fri. 8:30 AM-5 PM
Tel.: 607-547-3686
Fax: 607-547-3629

NEW HYDE PARK

Drug Information Center
St. John's University at
Long Island Jewish
Medical Center
270-05 76th Ave.
New Hyde Park, NY
11042 Mon.-Fri. 9 AM-3 PM
Tel.: 718-470-DRUG
Fax: 718-470-1742

NEW YORK

Drug Information Center
Lenox Hill Hospital
100 E. 77th St.
New York, NY 10021
Mon.-Fri. 9 AM-5 PM
Tel.: 212-434-3190
Fax: 212-434-3176

Drug Information Center
Memorial Sloan-Kettering
Cancer Center
1275 York Ave.
New York, NY 10021
Mon-Fri. 9 AM-5 PM
Tel.: 212-639-7552
Fax: 212-639-2171

Drug Information Center
Mount Sinai Medical
Center
1 Gustave Levy Place
New York, NY 10029
Mon.-Fri. 9 AM-5 PM
Tel.: 212-241-6619
Fax: 212-348-7927

Drug Information Service
Bellevue Hospital Center
462 1st Ave.
New York, NY 10016
Mon.-Fri. 9 AM-5 PM
Tel.: 212-561-6504
Fax: 212-561-6503

Drug Information Service
The New York Hospital
525 E. 68th St.
New York, NY 10021
Mon.-Fri. 9 AM-5 PM
Tel.: 212-746-0741
Fax: 212-746-8506

ROCHESTER

Drug Information Service
Dept. of Pharmacy
University of Rochester at
Strong Memorial Hospital
601 Elmwood Ave.
Rochester, NY 14642
Mon.-Fri. 8 AM-5 PM
Tel.: 716-275-3718
    716-275-2681
    (after hours)
Fax: 716-473-9842

STONY BROOK

Suffolk Drug
Information Center
University Hospital
S.U.N.Y.-Stony Brook
Room 3 - 561, Z7310
Stony Brook, NY 11794
Mon.-Fri. 8 AM-4:30 PM
Tel.: 516-444-2672
    516-444-2680
    (after hours)
Fax: 516-444-7669

NORTH CAROLINA

BUIES CREEK

Drug Information Center
School of Pharmacy
Campbell University
P.O. Box 1090
Buies Creek, NC 27506
Mon.-Fri. 8:30 AM-4:30 PM
Tel: 800-327-5467 (NC)
    910-893-1200 x 2701
Fax: 910-893-1476

CHAPEL HILL

Drug Information Center
University of North
Carolina Hospitals
101 Manning Dr.
Chapel Hill, NC 27514
Mon.-Fri. 8 AM-5 PM
Tel.: 919-966-2373
Fax: 919-966-3069

GREENSBORO

Triad Poison Center
Moses H. Cone
Memorial Hospital
1200 N. Elm St.
Greensboro, NC 27401
7 days/week, 24 hours
Tel.: 910-574-8105
Fax: 910-574-7910

GREENVILLE

Eastern Carolina Drug
Information Center
Pitt County Memorial
Hospital/Department of
Pharmacy Services
2100 Stantonsburg Rd.
Greenville, NC 27835
Mon.-Fri. 8 AM-4:30 PM
Tel.: 919-816-4257
Fax: 919-816-7425

WINSTON-SALEM

**Drug Information
Service Center
NC Baptist Hospital
Bowman-Gray
Medical Center**
Medical Center Blvd.
Winston-Salem, NC 27157
Mon.-Fri. 8 AM-5 PM
Tel.: 910-716-2037
Fax: 910-716-2186

OHIO

ADA

**Drug Information Center
Raabe College of
Pharmacy, Ohio Northern
University**
Ada, OH 45810
Mon.-Fri. 9 AM-5 PM
Tel.: 419-772-2289
Fax: 419-772-1917

CLEVELAND

**Cleveland Clinic
Foundation Drug
Information Center**
9500 Euclid Ave.
Cleveland, OH 44195
Mon.-Fri. 8 AM-4:30 PM
Tel.: 216-444-6456
Fax: 216-444-0158

COLUMBUS

**Central Ohio Poison
Center
Columbus Children's
Hospital**
700 Children's Drive
Columbus, OH 43205
Tel.: 513-222-2227
Fax: 614-221-2672

**Drug Information Center
Dept. of Pharmacy
Doan Hall 368
Ohio State University
Hospital**
410 W. 10th Ave.
Columbus, OH 43210
Mon.-Fri. 8 AM-4 PM
Tel.: 614-293-8679
Fax: 614-293-3165

**Drug Information Center
Riverside Methodist
Hospitals**
3535 Olantangy River
Road Columbus, OH 43214
Mon.-Fri. 8 AM-5 PM
Tel.: 614-566-5425
Fax: 614-566-5447

PARMA

**Clinical Pharmacy
Services
Kaiser Permanente Drug
Information Center**
12301 Snow Rd.
Parma, OH 44130
Tel: 216-265-4400
       216-362-2727
       pager 3133

TOLEDO

**Drug Information Service
The Toledo Hospital**
2142 N. Cove Blvd.
Toledo, OH 43606
Mon.-Fri. 8 AM-4:30 PM
Tel.: 419-471-2171
       419-471-5637
       (after hours)
Fax: 419-479-6926

ZANESVILLE

**Drug Information/
Poison Center
Bethesda Hospital**
2951 Maple Ave.
Zanesville, OH 43701
7 days/week, 24 hours
Tel.: 614-454-4221
       800-686-4221 (OH)
Fax: 614-454-4059

OKLAHOMA

OKLAHOMA CITY

**Drug Information Center
Baptist Medical Center**
3300 Northwest
Expressway
Oklahoma City, OK 73112
Mon. -Fri. 8 am to 4:30 pm
Tel: 405-949-3660
Fax: 405-945-5858

**Drug Information Center
Presbyterian Hospital**
700 NE 13th St.
Oklahoma City, OK 73104
Mon.-Fri. 7 AM-3:30 PM
Tel.: 405-271-6226
Fax: 405-271-3460

**Drug Information Service
University of Oklahoma
Health Sciences Center**
Rm LIB-380 A
1000 S.L. Young Blvd.
Oklahoma City, OK 73117
Mon.-Fri. 8 AM-5 PM
Tel.: 405-271-8080
Fax: 405-271-3297

TULSA

**Drug Information Service
St. Francis Hospital**
6161 S. Yale Ave.
Tulsa, OK 74136
Mon.-Fri. 9 AM-5:30 PM
Tel.: 918-494-6339
Fax: 918-494-1893

OREGON

PORTLAND

**University Drug
Consultation Service
Oregon Health
Sciences University**
3181 SW Sam Jackson
   Park Rd.
Portland, OR 97201
Mon.-Fri. 8:30 AM-5 PM
Tel.: 503-494-7530
Fax: 503-494-0011

PENNSYLVANIA

ERIE

**Pharmacy and Drug
Information Services
Hamot Medical Center**
201 State St.
Erie, PA 16550
7 days/week, 24 hours
Tel.: 814-877-6022
Fax: 814-877-6108

PHILADELPHIA

**Drug Information Center
Temple University
Hospital Dept. of
Pharmacy**
Broad and Ontario St.
Philadelphia, PA 19140
Mon.-Fri. 8 AM-4:30 PM
Tel.: 215-701-4644
Fax: 215-701-3463

**Drug Information Center
Thomas Jefferson
University Hospital**
111 S. 11th and Walnut
St. Philadelphia, PA 19107
Mon.-Fri. 8 AM-5 PM
Tel.: 215-955-8877

PITTSBURGH

**The Center for Drug
Information
The Mercy Hospital
of Pittsburgh**
1400 Locust St.
Pittsburgh, PA 15219
Mon.-Fri. 8 AM-4:30 PM
Tel.: 412-232-7903
       412-232-7907
Fax: 412-232-8422

**Drug Information and
Pharmacoepidemiology
Center
University of Pittsburgh
Medical Center**
137 Victoria Bldg.
Pittsburgh, PA 15261
Mon.-Fri. 8 AM-6 PM
Tel.: 412-624-3784
Fax: 412-642-6350

**Drug Information Center
Allegheny General
Hospital**
320 E. North Ave.
Pittsburgh, PA 15212
Mon.-Fri. 8 AM-4:30 PM
Tel.: 412-359-3192
Fax: 412-359-4806

UPLAND

**Drug Information Center
Crozer-Chester
Medical Center**
1 Medical Ctr. Blvd.
Upland, PA 19013
Mon.-Fri. 8 AM-4:30 PM
Tel.: 610-447-2851
       610-447-2862
       (after hours)
Fax: 215-447-2820

WILLIAMSPORT

**Drug Information Center
Williamsport Hospital and
Medical Center**
777 Rural Ave.
Williamsport, PA 17701
Mon.-Fri. 8 AM-4 PM
Tel.: 717-321-3289
Fax: 717-321-3230

PUERTO RICO

SAN JUAN

**Centro Informacion
Medicamentos
Escuela de Farmacia RCM**
P.O. Box 365067
San Juan, PR 00936
Mon.-Fri. 8 AM-4 PM
Tel.: 809-758-2525 x 1516
Tel. & Fax: 809-763-0196

RHODE ISLAND

PROVIDENCE

**Drug Information Service
Dept. of Pharmacy
Rhode Island Hospital**
593 Eddy St.
Providence, RI 02903
Mon.-Fri. 8:30 AM-5 PM
Tel.: 401-444-5547
Fax: 401-444-8062

Drug Information Center
University of Rhode Island
Roger Williams
Medical Center
825 Chalkstone Ave.
Providence, RI 02908
Mon.-Fri. 8 AM-4 PM
Tel.: 401-456-2260
Fax: 401-456-2510

SOUTH CAROLINA

CHARLESTON

Drug Information Service
Medical University of
South Carolina
154 Ashley Ave.
Charleston, SC 29403
Mon.-Fri. 8 AM-5:30 PM
Tel.: 803-792-3896
      800-922-5250
Fax: 803-792-5532

SPARTANBURG

Drug Information Center
Spartanburg Regional
Medical Center
101 E. Wood St.
Spartanburg, SC 29303
Mon.-Fri. 8 AM-5 PM
Tel.: 803-560-6910
      803-560-6779
      (after hours)
Fax: 803-560-6017

SOUTH DAKOTA

BROOKINGS

South Dakota Drug
Information Center
300 22nd Ave.
Brookings, SD 57006
7 days/week, 8 AM-4:30 PM
Tel.: 800-456-1004

SIOUX FALLS

Drug Information Center
McKennan Hospital
800 E. 21st St.
Sioux Falls, SD 57117
7 days/week, 24 hours
Tel.: 605-336-3894
      800-952-0123 (SD)
      800-843-0505
      (MN, IA, NE)
Fax: 605-333-8206

TENNESSEE

KNOXVILLE

Drug Information Center
University of Tennessee
Medical Center
1924 Alcoa Hwy.
Knoxville, TN 37920
Mon.-Fri. 8 AM-4:30 PM
Tel.: 615-544-9125

MEMPHIS

Drug Information Center
University of Tennessee
800 Madison Ave.
Memphis, TN 38163
Mon.-Fri. 8 AM-5 PM
Tel.: 901-448-5555
Fax: 901-448-5419

South East Regional Drug
Information Center
VA Medical Center
1030 Jefferson Ave.
Memphis, TN. 38104
Mon.-Fri. 7:30 AM-4 PM
Tel.: 901-523-8990, x 5191

TEXAS

GALVESTON

Drug Information Center
University of Texas
Medical Branch
301 University Blvd. -
G01 Galveston, TX 77555
Mon.-Fri. 8 AM-5 PM
Tel.: 409-772-2734
Fax: 409-772-8408

HOUSTON

Drug Information Center
Ben Taub General Hospital
Texas Southern University
College of Pharmacy and
Health Sciences
1504 Taub Loop
Houston, TX 77030
Mon.-Fri. 8 AM-10 PM
Tel.: 713-793-2915
      713-793-2937

Drug Information Center
Methodist Hospital
6565 Fannin (DB1-09)
Houston, TX 77030
Mon.-Fri. 8 AM-5 PM
Tel.: 713-790-4190
Fax: 713-793-1224

LACKLAND A.F.B.

Drug Information Center
Dept. of Pharmacy
Wilford Hall Medical
Center
2200 Berquist Dr., Suite
1 Lackland A.F.B., TX 78236
Mon.-Fri. 7:30 AM-5 PM
Tel.: 210-670-6291

LUBBOCK

Methodist Hospital
Drug Information &
Consultation Service
3615 19th St.
Lubbock, TX 79410
Mon.-Fri. 8 AM-5 PM
Tel.: 806-793-4012
Fax: 806-784-5322
      (Attn: Pharmacy)

TEMPLE

Drug Information Center
Scott and White
Memorial Hospital
2401 S. 31st. St.
Temple, TX 76508
Mon.-Fri. 8 AM-6 PM
Tel.: 817-724-4636

UTAH

SALT LAKE CITY

Drug Information Center
Dept. of Pharmacy
Services Room A-050
University of Utah
Hospital
50 N. Medical Dr.
Salt Lake City, UT 84132
Mon.-Fri. 8:30 AM-4:30 PM
Tel.: 801-581-2073
Fax: 801-585-6688

VIRGINIA

HAMPTON

Drug Information Center
Sentara Hampton
General Hospital
3120 Victoria Blvd.
Hampton, VA 23669
7 days/week,
7 AM-Midnight
Tel.: 804-727-7185

RICHMOND

Drug Information Center
St. Mary's Hospital
5801 Bremo Rd.
Richmond, VA 23226
Mon.-Fri. 24 hrs.
Tel.: 804-281-8058
Fax: 804-285-4411

WASHINGTON

SPOKANE

Drug Information Center
Washington State
University College
of Pharmacy
601 W. 1st Ave.
Spokane, WA 92204
Mon.-Fri. 8 AM-4 PM
Tel.: 509-456-4409

WEST VIRGINIA

MORGANTOWN

West Virginia Drug
Information Center
West Virginia University-
Robert C. Byrd
Health Sciences Center
1124 HSN
P.O.Box 9520
Morgantown, WV 26506
Mon.-Fri. 9 AM-5 PM
Tel.: 304-293-5101
      800-352-2501 (WV)
Fax: 304-293-5483

WISCONSIN

MADISON

Drug Information Center
Univ. of Wisconsin
Hospital & Clinics
600 Highland Ave.
Madison, WI 53792
7 days/week,
7:30 AM-10:30 PM
Tel.: 608-262-1315
Fax: 608-263-9424

WYOMING

LARAMIE

Drug Information Center
University of Wyoming
P.O.Box 3375
Laramie, WY 82071
Mon.-Fri. 8 AM-5 PM
Tel.: 307-766-6128
Fax: 307-766-2953